Sex- and Gender-Based Women's Health

Sarah A. Tilstra • Deborah Kwolek
Julie L. Mitchell • Brigid M. Dolan
Michael P. Carson
Editors

Sex- and Gender-Based Women's Health

A Practical Guide for Primary Care

Springer

Editors
Sarah A. Tilstra
University of Pittsburgh School of Medicine
Division of General Internal Medicine
Department of Medicine
Pittsburgh, PA
USA

Julie L. Mitchell
Medical College of Wisconsin
Milwaukee, WI
USA

Michael P. Carson
Hackensack Meridian School of Medicine
at Seton Hall, Jersey Shore University
Medical Center
Department of Medicine
Neptune, NJ
USA

Deborah Kwolek
Harvard Medical School, Massachusetts General
Hospital
Department of Medicine
Boston, MA
USA

Brigid M. Dolan
Northwestern University Feinberg School
of Medicine, Division of General Internal
Medicine and Geriatrics
Department of Medicine
Chicago, IL
USA

ISBN 978-3-030-50694-0 ISBN 978-3-030-50695-7 (eBook)
https://doi.org/10.1007/978-3-030-50695-7

This Springer imprint is published by the registered company Springer Nature Switzerland AG
The registered company address is: Gewerbestrasse 11, 6330 Cham, Switzerland

Continuing Medical Education Information

Earn up to 41.0 Continuing Medical Education (CME) AMA PRA Category 1 Credits and 41.0 MOC Points

These activities have been planned and implemented in accordance with the Essential Areas and Policies of the Accreditation Council for Continuing Medical Education (ACCME) through the joint providership of the Society of General Internal Medicine (SGIM) and the University of Alabama School of Medicine (UASOM).

Accreditation

The University of Alabama School of Medicine is accredited by the Accreditation Council for Continuing Medical Education to provide continuing medical education for physicians.

The University of Alabama School of Medicine designates this enduring material for a maximum of 41.0 *AMA PRA Category 1 Credit*™. Physicians should claim only the credit commensurate with the extent of their participation in the activity.

The boards of nursing in many states, including Alabama, recognize Category 1 continuing medical education courses as acceptable activities for the renewal of license to practice nursing.

Disclaimer

Dosages, indications, and methods of use of any drug referred to in this publication may reflect the clinical experience of the authors, clinical literature, or other clinical resources. Therefore, please see the full prescribing information before using any product mentioned. UAB is an equal opportunity/affirmative action institution.

ABIM MOC Credit

Successful completion of this CME activity, which includes participation in the evaluation component, enables the participant to earn up to 41 MOC points in the American Board of Internal Medicine's (ABIM) Maintenance of Certification (MOC) program. Participants will earn MOC points equivalent to the amount of CME credits claimed for the activity. It is the CME activity provider's responsibility to submit participant completion information to ACCME for the purpose of granting ABIM MOC credit.

Method of Participation and Fees

Each chapter in this book is eligible for CME/MOC credits. Additional information, including how to purchase and earn CME/MOC credits, is available at www.sgim.org/Womens_Health_CME.

Upon purchase and completion of reflective statements for each chapter, you will be able to obtain CME/MOC credit. These enduring material products, in accordance with ACCME guidelines, are required to provide an assessment of the learner that measures achievement of the educational purpose and/or objectives of the activity. CME/MOC credit will be provided upon completion of the evaluation and reflective statements for each respective chapter individually.

Those who request MOC will be required to provide their ABIM# and Month and Day of Birth; this information will used for ACCME reporting purposes only.

CME/MOC Fee Per Chapter = $7.50 for SGIM Members; $15.00 for non-members.

In order to purchase and obtain CME/MOC credits, please go to www.sgim.org/Womens_Health_CME.

Preface

Women's health had traditionally been envisioned as breast, reproductive, and gynecologic care historically addressed by our obstetrics and gynecology partners, but beginning in the 1990s, primary care physicians began to take an active role in providing women's healthcare, developing teaching curricula and performing research specific to women's health issues. We, as physicians providing primary care, appreciate that women and gender diverse patients are much more complex. The optimal care of our patients requires knowledge and skills which integrate primary medical care, mental health care, breast care, and gynecologic care into each evaluation with attention to adept communication, trust building, and an understanding of social factors. In one afternoon, we see patients with concerns ranging from osteoporosis, depression, intimate partner violence, vaginal bleeding, irritable bowel syndrome, headaches, and urinary incontinence—sometimes in a single encounter. As primary providers, we must also have expertise in family planning, cancer screening, and well-woman examinations. Our patients expect comprehensive care, yet studies of residency training reveal that few residency programs in internal medicine offer dedicated training in women's health, and upon graduation many residents feel unprepared and are unable to demonstrate competency to care for female patients [1, 2].

In response to this need, it is with great pride that we present this sex- and gender-based women's health curriculum written by a host of women's health physician educators, researchers, and clinicians. This work fulfills our long-term goal to produce a resource written explicitly for primary care providers to both guide the care of women and gender diverse patients and to educate learners in this discipline. This book does not serve as a comprehensive review of all available literature, but instead is tailored to the essential components necessary to care for the sex- and gender-specific preventive, medical, psychological, and social needs of our patients. This text is based upon the principles of evidenced-based medicine and includes review of clinical guidelines. Expert opinion and pearls from senior women's health experts have been added to provide nuance in patient care and to fill knowledge gaps on subjects not well studied as of this writing.

There is no right or wrong way to use this book. It can be used as a quick point-of-care clinical reference for a specific topic (i.e., contraception) or as a longitudinal curriculum for learners. While this text is organized into eight parts of related content, the reading of this text is not intended to be strictly linear. To assist non-linear readers, chapters are extensively cross-referenced.

We focus on practical issues in the outpatient setting and we do not intend to limit our audience to a single specialty or credential. This text is for generalist physicians, nurse practitioners, and other practitioners in primary care. In the same way that we have chosen to be inclusive in the definition of the female patient (women and gender diverse people), we encourage interprofessional discussion and learning of this content.

We are passionate about promoting sex- and gender-based women's health (SGBWH) education for learners at all levels; thus, we have designed this book to aid educators. Each chapter has clear, measurable learning objectives and multiple-choice questions to check understanding. Clinician-educators preparing a discussion or lecture on a selected topic could assign a chapter to residents, fellows, or students as a pre- or post-read. We encourage providers who have a large population of women patients to consider reading the book in its entirety. Academic leaders seeking to raise awareness of SGBWH could use this book as part of a developmental effort.

We are extremely honored and grateful to have been trained, mentored, and inspired by a cadre of fierce women's health advocates, expert clinicians, research pioneers, and gifted educators. It would be a disservice to them to write this book and ignore the history and evolution of the work that preceded us. This book is the result of the intersection of female academic leadership; the advancement of women's health policy, research, and education; the understanding of the health impact of social and gender disparities; and the integration of women's health with sex-and gender-based medicine. With great esteem, we dedicate Chaps. 1 and 2 to Drs. Melissa McNeil, Carol Bates, Paula Johnson, Ann Nattinger, Molly Carnes, Sandra Levison, Ana Nunez. Lucia Beck Weiss, Karen Carlson, Karen Freund, Saralyn Mark, Janet Henrich, Wendy Klein, Jan Werbinski, Abby Spencer, Marjorie Jenkins, Vivian Pinn, Pam Charney, Peter Garner, Richard V. Lee, Karen Rosene-Montella, Bill Baron, and many, many others. We also acknowledge and thank the original leaders in the women's health centers of excellence program and the women's health movement in general, and those who now continue to carry on the important work of promoting women's health and sex- and gender-based medicine regionally, nationally, and internationally.

We must express our deepest gratitude to all of the phenomenal contributing authors of this book: for their energy, patience, time, and willingness to contribute to this text on their days off, during their scarce free time, and after their kids and partners were asleep. We are deeply appreciative of our chairs, chiefs, and clinical colleagues who supported us, covered for us, and in many other ways supported our work over the past 2 years. Thank you to Springer and especially Ms. Stephanie Frost, our Deputy Editor, for her constant support, admirable laugh, organizational skills, and persistent emails. We dedicate this book to our patients, who are the reason we practice medicine. Your wisdom has inspired us to keep learning, researching, teaching, and finding ways to improve the way we provide care and has kept us grounded as advocates and role models. To our mentees and learners, this book is for you. Thank you for pushing us to be the best versions of ourselves, to reflect on our faults, and for motivating us to do everything better the next day.

Finally, and most importantly, we are forever indebted to our families and friends: our parents, partners, and children who have literally sacrificed so that this volume could be completed. Without your love and support, none of this would have been possible.

We conclude with the hope of improving the healthcare of our patients through interdisciplinary collaboration and education, and inspiring a new generation of women's health providers.

Sarah A. Tilstra Pittsburgh, PA, USA
Deborah Kwolek Boston, MA, USA
Julie L. Mitchell Milwaukee, WI, USA
Brigid M. Dolan Chicago, IL, USA
Michael P. Carson Neptune, NJ, USA

References

1. Spencer AL, Kern LM. Primary care program directors' perceptions of women's health education: a gap in graduate medical education persists. J Women's Health. 2008;17:549–56.
2. Hsieh E, Nunez-Smith M, Henrich JB. Needs and priorities in women's health training: perspectives from an internal medicine residency program. J Women's Health. 2013;22:667–72.

In Gratitude

Most importantly to my wife Miriam who pulled, and still pulls, double duty creating and maintaining our Home, and the boy and the girl, Evan and Leah. They are why I walk so quickly on rounds: to complete all the work that needs to be done for our patients, but then get home for dinner ASAP. Albie and Karen who got me here, passed on the ability to do it, and taught me how to get through the toughest of times. My high school (yes high school) lacrosse coach and teammates for lessons on focus, support, and striving for excellence.

The Obstetric Medicine pioneers and mentors who created this awesome career path with clinical challenges and research opportunities for a guy who is apparently blissfully naïve enough not to be afraid, and who trained me to be a true diagnostician and internist. To the people I've met through NASOM and SGIM, my academic homes that provide the deepest sense of family and professional satisfaction. The residents and students who by their growth let me know directly and indirectly that my passion for what I do is appreciated and does achieve my goal of at least playing some role in helping them develop as professionals. The people who offer the highest compliment by trusting me to be their doctor, and Dr. Elliot Frank who trusted me with the resources to pursue research and academic projects. Finally, to my co-editor-siblings who taught me, and allowed me to join them to be the favorite brother on this project.

- *Michael P. Carson*

Thank you to our fearless leader, Dr. Sarah Tilstra, and to the community of women's health educators and researchers who have collaborated on this book; I appreciate having had the opportunity to learn from the knowledge and wisdom of the group. I am eternally grateful for the village of mentors who led me to a career in women's health and education—particularly Dr. Raquel Buranosky, Dr. Melissa McNeill, Dr. Jane Sillman, Dr. Paula Johnson, and Dr. Lori Tishler—and the students, residents, and patients who provide continual inspiration. My efforts on this book and otherwise in life are steadfastly supported by Curtis and Connor D, whose laughter and kindness bring joy into every day.

- *Brigid M. Dolan*

Lovingly dedicated to my mother Rena Thorstensen-Gomez, who lives with the Lord, and to my father Robert Gomez, who is a devoted scholar and teacher. To my extraordinary husband, Dr. Christopher Kwolek, my true love and best friend since our first day of medical school at UCSF. To our daughters and sons—Sarah, Rachel, Bekah, Maddy, Josh, Danny, Robert, Jonathan, and Joel. Thank you for your loving support, sacrifice, and encouragement. To my sisters Terri, Jeanne, Rebekah, and Jessica and their daughters. To Cecilia, Lucie, the extended family, and the life group. To my patients, thank you for the privilege of allowing me to serve as your physician. A special thanks to my MGMG practice family, and to the leadership at MGH. To the inspirational leaders, mentors, teachers, colleagues, trainees, and students who together have worked towards the advancement of women's health especially at the University of Kentucky, the VA Women's Health Program, Harvard Medical School, SGIM, and beyond. Chapter 1 was written in your honor. To Sarah, Julie, Michael, and Brigid, thank you for the joyful opportunity of working with you on this project, for your collegiality, and for your incredible tenacious commitment to scholarship in women's health.

- *Deborah Kwolek*

My contribution to this text would not be possible without the love and support of my husband Rob Thielke and our children Jim, John, and Charlotte Thielke. I must also thank Dr. Sarah Tilstra for her vision for the book and her confidence in me, Dr. Ann Nattinger for her longstanding, wise mentorship, and my co-editors who I can now call my BFFs. I have found inspiration from my teachers, my learners, and of course my patients. This work has truly been my privilege.

- *Julie L. Mitchell*

This work would not have been possible without the support and mentorship of the Pitt Women's Health Program under the guidance of Dr. Melissa McNeil, where I am honored to have been trained, sponsored, influenced, and inspired. To my mentors and work wives, Drs. Raquel Buranosky, Carla Spagnoletti, Rachel Bonnema, Meg McNamara, Deborah DiNardo, Jen Corbelli, and Anna Donovan, from whom I have learned to work smarter, and am forever grateful for your encouragement, friendship, and laughs. To Jeremy, my boys Brandon and Zachary, and Nana, for your love, sacrifice, and sanity. To Julie Mitchell, Deborah Kwolek, Brigid Dolan, and Michael Carson—my new forever family, thank you for your trust in this project, comic relief, perseverance, attention to detail, and dedication to excellence. Finally, to my patients and learners who make this work so special, foster humility, challenge my curiosity, and facilitate joy—even on the hardest days—thank you.

- *Sarah A. Tilstra*

Contents

Contributors

Benjamin D. Beran, MD Froedtert & Medical College of Wisconsin, Department of Obstetrics and Gynecology, Wauwatosa, WI, USA

Lisa B. Bernstein, MD Emory University School of Medicine, Department of Medicine, Atlanta, GA, USA

Eliana Bonifacino, MD, MS University of Pittsburgh Medical Center, Division of General Internal Medicine, Pittsburgh, PA, USA

Rachel A. Bonnema, MD, MS, FACP University of Texas Southwestern Medical Center, Dallas, TX, USA

Sonya Borrero, MD, MS Center for Women's Health Research and Innovation (CWHRI), University of Pittsburgh School of Medicine, Pittsburgh, PA, USA

Center for Health Equity Research and Promotion (CHERP), VA Pittsburgh Healthcare System, Department of Medicine, Pittsburgh, PA, USA

Rachel Brook, MD David Geffen School of Medicine, UCLA, Department of Internal Medicine, Los Angeles, CA, USA

Raquel A. Buranosky, MD, MPH University of Pittsburgh Medical Center, Department of Medicine, Pittsburgh, PA, USA

Michael P. Carson, MD Hackensack Meridian School of Medicine at Seton Hall, Jersey Shore University Medical Center, Department of Medicine, Neptune, NJ, USA

Andrea E. Carter, MD, MS University of Pittsburgh School of Medicine, Division of General Internal Medicine, Pittsburgh, PA, USA

Rachel S. Casas, MD, EdM Division of General Internal Medicine, Penn State Milton S. Hershey Medical Center, Hershey, PA, USA

Cynthia H. Chuang, MD, MSc Division of General Internal Medicine, Penn State Milton S. Hershey Medical Center, Hershey, PA, USA

Jennifer Corbelli, MD, MS University of Pittsburgh Medical Center, Division of General Internal Medicine, Pittsburgh, PA, USA

Jill C. Costello, MD Department of Medicine/Division of Rheumatology, Medical College of Wisconsin, Milwaukee, WI, USA

Meredith O. Cruz, MD, MPH/MBA Froedtert and the Medical College of Wisconsin, Department of Obstetrics and Gynecology, Milwaukee, WI, USA

Aarati Didwania, MD, MSCI Northwestern University, Feinberg School of Medicine, Division of General Medicine & Geriatrics, Chicago, IL, USA

Deborah DiNardo, MD, MS VA Pittsburgh Healthcare System, Department of Medicine, Pittsburgh, PA, USA

University of Pittsburgh School of Medicine, Pittsburgh, PA, USA

Brigid M. Dolan, MD, MEd Northwestern University Feinberg School of Medicine, Division of General Internal Medicine and Geriatrics, Department of Medicine, Chicago, IL, USA

Nicole M. Donnellan, MD Magee-Womens Hospital of University of Pittsburgh Medical Center, Department of Obstetrics, Gynecology, and Reproductive Sciences, Pittsburgh, PA, USA

Anna K. Donovan, MD, MS IM Residency Training Program, University of Pittsburgh Medical Center-Presbyterian, Department of Medicine, Division of General Internal Medicine, Pittsburgh, PA, USA

Amy H. Farkas, MD, MS Department of Internal Medicine, Medical College of Wisconsin, Clement Zablocki VA, Milwaukee, WI, USA

Aletia Farmer, MD University of Kentucky, Department of Internal Medicine/Women's Health, Lexington, KY, USA

Molly Ainsman Fisher, MD Allegheny Health Network, Pittsburgh, PA, USA

Jacqueline Carey Fister, MD University of Kentucky, Department of Internal Medicine/ Women's Health, Lexington, KY, USA

Amy Fitzpatrick, MD, MS Boston Medical Center/Boston University School of Medicine, Department of Internal Medicine, Boston, MA, USA

Jordana Friedman, MD, FACP Northwestern University, Feinberg School of Medicine, Department of Internal Medicine, Chicago, IL, USA

Rebecca Gitlin, PhD Los Angeles County Department of Mental Health, Los Angeles, CA, USA

Mita Sanghavi Goel, MD, MPH Northwestern University, Feinberg School of Medicine, Division of General Medicine & Geriatrics, Chicago, IL, USA

Anna Golob, MD Department of Medicine, University of Washington and VA Puget Sound Healthcare System, Seattle, WA, USA

Alda Maria R. Gonzaga, MD, MS University of Pittsburgh School of Medicine, Departments of Medicine and Pediatrics, Pittsburgh, PA, USA

Alexandra M. Goodwin, MD New York University, Bellevue Hospital Center, Department of General Internal Medicine and Clinical Innovation, New York, NY, USA

Whitfield Board Growdon, MD Massachusetts General Hospital, Department of Obstetrics, Gynecology and Reproductive Medicine, Division of Gynecologic Oncology, Boston, MA, USA

Rachel K. Harrison, MD Medical College of Wisconsin, Department of Obstetrics and Gynecology, Milwaukee, WI, USA

Jana G. Hashash, MD, MSc Department of Internal Medicine, Division of Gastroenterology, Hepatology, and Nutrition, University of Pittsburgh, Pittsburgh, PA, USA

American University of Beirut, Beirut, Lebanon

Marjorie R. Jenkins, MD, MEdHP, FACP University of South Carolina School of Medicine Greenville, Greenville, SC, USA

Kay M. Johnson, MD, MPH Department of Medicine, University of Washington and VA Puget Sound Healthcare System, Seattle, WA, USA

Amanda Johnson, MD University of Colorado School of Medicine, Department of Obstetrics and Gynecology, Aurora, CO, USA

Akeira L. Johnson, MD Clement Zablocki VA, Department of General Internal Medicine, Milwaukee, WI, USA

Sarah A. Jones, MD, MS University of Pittsburgh Medical Center, Department of Internal Medicine, Pittsburgh, PA, USA

Anna Kho, MD Emory University School of Medicine, Department of Medicine, Atlanta, GA, USA

Juliana M. Kling, MD, MPH, NCMP Mayo Clinic, Department of Women's Health Internal Medicine, Rochester, NY, USA

Agnes Koczo, MD University of Pittsburgh Medical Center, Department of Internal Medicine, Pittsburgh, PA, USA

Sumana Koduri, MD Medical College of Wisconsin, Froedtert Memorial Lutheran Hospital, Department of Obstetrics and Gynecology, Milwaukee, WI, USA

Deborah Kwolek, MD Harvard Medical School, Massachusetts General Hospital, Department of Medicine, Boston, MA, USA

Anita Leon-Jhong, MD University of Pittsburgh Medical Center, Division of General Internal Medicine, Pittsburgh, PA, USA

Beth Lewis, MD, MPH Jacobi Medical Center, Department of Obstetrics and Gynecology, Bronx, NY, USA

Amy D. Lu, MD San Francisco VA Medical Center, University of San Francisco Medical Center, San Francisco, CA, USA

Michael Lund, MD Department of Obstetrics and Gynecology, Medical College of Wisconsin, Milwaukee, WI, USA

Jennifer S. McCall-Hosenfeld, MD, MSc The Pennsylvania State University College of Medicine, Department of Medicine, Hershey, PA, USA

Kerri Palamara, MD Center for Physician Well-Being, Massachusetts General Hospital, Department of Medicine, Boston, MA, USA

Megan McNamara, MD, MS Case Western Reserve University School of Medicine, Louis Stokes Cleveland VA Medical Center, Department of Medicine, Cleveland, OH, USA

Melissa A. McNeil, MD, MPH University of Pittsburgh Medical Center, Department of Internal Medicine, Pittsburgh, PA, USA

University of Pittsburgh School of Medicine, Division of General Internal Medicine, Pittsburgh, PA, USA

Sarah Merriam, MD, MS VA Pittsburgh Healthcare System, Department of Medicine, Pittsburgh, PA, USA

Alexandra E. Mieczkowski, MD, MS UPMC Presbyterian Shadyside and Children's Hospital of Pittsburgh of UPMC, Division of General Internal Medicine, General Academic Pediatrics, Pittsburgh, PA, USA

Julie L. Mitchell, MD, MS, FACP Medical College of Wisconsin, Milwaukee, WI, USA

Raj Narayan, MD, FRCOG, FACOG Froedtert & Medical College of Wisconsin, Department of Obstetrics and Gynecology, Wauwatosa, WI, USA

Azadeh Nasseh, MD, MSc Boston Medical Center, Boston University School of Medicine, Department of Internal Medicine, Section of GIM, Boston, MA, USA

Nicolette A. Oleng', MD Boston University School of Medicine, Department of General Internal Medicine, Boston Medical Center, Boston, MA, USA

Christine A. Prifti, MD Boston University Medical Center, Department of Medicine, Women's Health Unit, Boston, MA, USA

Christina I. Ramirez, MD Magee-Womens Hospital of University of Pittsburgh Medical Center, Department of Obstetrics, Gynecology, and Reproductive Sciences, Pittsburgh, PA, USA

Sophia M. Reljanovic, MD Case Western Reserve University School of Medicine, Louis Stokes Cleveland VA Medical Center, Department of Women's Health, Cleveland, OH, USA

Brianna Rossiter, MD VA Pittsburgh Healthcare System, Pittsburgh, PA, USA

University of Pittsburgh School of Medicine, Department of Medicine, Division of General Internal Medicine, Pittsburgh, PA, USA

Jennifer Rusiecki, MD, MS University of Chicago, Department of General Internal Medicine, Chicago, IL, USA

Janice Ryden, MD, FACP Johns Hopkins University School of Medicine, Johns Hopkins Community Physicians, Department of Internal Medicine (*retired*), Baltimore, MD, USA

Jenna Sarvaideo, BA, DO Medical College of Wisconsin, Department of Medicine, Division of Endocrinology, Milwaukee, WI, USA

Alfred Shoukry, MD UPMC, Department of Internal Medicine, Pittsburgh, PA, USA

Swati Shroff, MD, MS Sidney Kimmel Medical College, Thomas Jefferson University, Department of Medicine, Philadelphia, PA, USA

Jane S. Sillman, MD Brigham and Women's Hospital, Department of Medicine, Boston, MA, USA

Halle G. Sobel, MD, FACP Robert Larner MD, College of Medicine at The University of Vermont, Department of General Internal Medicine, Burlington, VT, USA

Carla Spagnoletti, MD, MS University of Pittsburgh, Department of Medicine, Pittsburgh, PA, USA

Brielle M. Spataro, MD, MS University of Pittsburgh Medical Center, Department of Internal Medicine, Pittsburgh, PA, USA

Traci A. Takahashi, MD, MPH Department of Medicine, University of Washington and VA Puget Sound Healthcare System, Seattle, WA, USA

Holly N. Thomas, MD, MS University of Pittsburgh, Department of Medicine, Pittsburgh, PA, USA

Sarah A. Tilstra, MD, MS, FACP University of Pittsburgh School of Medicine, Division of General Internal Medicine, Department of Medicine, Pittsburgh, PA, USA

Katherine E. Twist, MD University of Kentucky, Department of Internal Medicine, Lexington, KY, USA

Eloho Ufomata, MD, MS University of Pittsburgh School of Medicine, Department of Internal Medicine, Pittsburgh, PA, USA

Rachel Vanderberg, MD, MS Division of General Internal Medicine, University of Pittsburgh, Pittsburgh, PA, USA

Emmanuelle Yecies, MD Advanced Fellow in Women's Health, Department of Medicine, VA Pittsburgh Healthcare System, Pittsburgh, PA, USA

Department of General Internal Medicine, University of Pittsburgh School of Medicine, Pittsburgh, PA, USA

Glossary of Commonly Used Abbreviations and Acronyms

ACOG	American College of Obstetricians and Gynecologists
ACS	American Cancer Society
AI	Aromatase inhibitor
ASCO	American Society of Clinical Oncology
BMD	Bone mineral density
BMI	Body mass index
BMP	Basic metabolic panel (includes sodium, potassium, chloride, bicarbonate, blood urea nitrogen, creatinine, glucose, calcium)
BPS	Bladder pain syndrome
BRCA	BReast CAncer gene
BSO	Bilateral salpingo-oophorectomy
BV	Bacterial vaginitis
CA-125	Cancer antigen 125
CAD	Coronary artery disease
CBC	Complete blood count
CBE	Clinical breast exam
CBT	Cognitive behavioral therapy
CDC	Center for Disease Control and Prevention
CMP	Comprehensive metabolic panel (includes a BMP + total protein, albumin, bilirubin, alkaline phosphatase, aspartate amino transferase, alanine amino transferase)
COC	Combined oral contraceptive
COPD	Chronic obstructive pulmonary disease
CT	Computed tomography
CVD	Cardiovascular disease
DCIS	Ductal carcinoma in situ
DEXA or DXA	Dual energy x-ray absorptiometry
DHEA-S	Dehydroepiandrosterone sulfate
DM	Diabetes mellitus
DSM V	Diagnostic and Statistical Manual of Mental Disorders, Fifth Edition
ED	Emergency department
EMG	Electromyography
FDA	US Food and Drug Administration
FRAX	Fracture Risk Assessment Tool
FSH	Follicular stimulating hormone
GAD-7	Generalized Anxiety Disorder-7
GDM	Gestational diabetes mellitus
GERD	Gastroesophageal reflux disease
GSM	Genitourinary syndrome of menopause
HCV	Hepatitis C virus
HIV	Human immunodeficiency virus
HMO	Health Maintenance Organization

HPA	Hypothalamic-pituitary-adrenal axis
HPV	Human papillomavirus
HR	Hazard ratio
HT	Hormone therapy
HTN	Hypertension
IC	Interstitial cystitis
ICS	Inhaled corticosteroid
ICU	intensive care unit
IOM	Institute of Medicine (now known as NAM)
IUD	Intrauterine device
LABA(s)	Long acting beta$_2$ agonist(s)
LCIS	Lobular carcinoma in situ
LEEP	Loop Electrosurgical Excision Procedure
LGBTQ	Lesbian, gay, bisexual, transgender, queer/questioning
LH	Luteinizing hormone
LV	Left ventricle or left ventricular
IHD	Ischemic heart disease
INR	International normalized ratio
IPV	Interpersonal violence
MAOI	Monoamine oxidase inhibitors
MDI	Metered-dose inhaler
MHT	Menopausal hormone therapy
MRI	Magnetic resonance imaging
MSM	Men who have sex with men
NAM	National Academy of Medicine (formerly IOM)
NAMS	North American Menopause Society
NIH	National Institutes of Health
NCCN	National Comprehensive Cancer Network
NNT	Number needed to treat
NSAID	Nonsteroidal anti-inflammatory drug
OC	Oral contraceptive
OCP	Oral contraceptive pill
OR	Odds ratio
PCOS	Polycystic ovary syndrome
PCP	Primary care provider
PET	Positron emission tomography
PHQ-9	Patient Health Questionnaire-9
PID	Pelvic inflammatory disease
POP	Progestin only pill
RCT	Randomized controlled trial
RR	Relative risk
SBE	Self-breast exam
SERM	Selective estrogen receptor modulators
SNRI	Serotonin-norepinephrine reuptake inhibitors
SSRI	Selective serotonin reuptake inhibitors
STI	Sexually transmitted infection
TAH	Total abdominal hysterectomy
TAHBSO	Total abdominal hysterectomy with bilateral salpingo-oophorectomy
TCA	Tricyclic antidepressant
TSH	Thyroid stimulating hormone
WHO	World Health Organization
US	Ultrasound
USPSTF	United States Preventive Services Task Force

Part I

Foundations of Women's Health and Gender Based Medicine

Women's Health and Sex- and Gender-Based Medicine: Past, Present, and Future

1

Deborah Kwolek and Marjorie R. Jenkins

Learning Objectives

1. Describe the evolution of the women's health movement from reproductive health to the comprehensive sex- and gender-informed care of women.
2. Discuss major research advances in women's health that affect clinical care.
3. Give examples of nonreproductive sex-based differences that are clinically relevant in primary care.
4. Describe how the knowledge and skills needed for breast care, gynecologic care, mental health care, and health-care delivery are integrated in the primary care of women.
5. Discuss women's health and sex- and gender-based medicine curricula for medical student, interprofessional, resident, and continuing education.
6. List educational interventions to advance education in sex- and gender-based care for all learners.
7. Explain urgent needs, persistent gaps, and future directions in the field of sex- and gender-based women's health.

Lidia, a 42-year-old cisgender woman (pronouns she/her/hers), presents to her primary care provider for an annual exam. She has no new complaints except for occasional insomnia and hot flashes. She has a history of a breast biopsy and two pregnancies complicated by preeclampsia and gestational diabetes, but the provider did not ask about breast or reproductive history and therefore this data is not revealed. She is given a physical without breast or gynecologic examination.

Introduction

> Every cell has a sex, and all bodies are influenced by gender. Integrating results from research investigating sex and gender differences into medical education, training, and clinical practice will improve care for all [1].

Women's health is much more than reproductive health. The field of women's health has evolved over the years from a focus on reproductive organs to an understanding that sex-based differences exist throughout the body, and that gynecologic care, medical care, breast care, and mental health care must be integrated to take care of the whole woman. Sex- and gender-based medicine (SGBM) is a newer field which emerged from the women's health movement. SGBM studies sex as a biological variable (SABV) and applies findings individually to all persons in the context of gender influences [2–5]. Sex- and gender-based women's health (SGBWH) is the integration of SGBM and women's health.

To advance the field of SGBWH, researchers and educators in women's health join forces with the proponents of sex- and gender-based medicine and use an interprofessional approach to promote sex-based research, education, and clinical care. Persistent deficits, including the lack of SGBWH knowledge and skills among health professionals, and the lack of research studies that report findings according to sex and gender variables, must be remediated [5].

D. Kwolek (✉)
Harvard Medical School, Massachusetts General Hospital, Department of Medicine, Boston, MA, USA
e-mail: dkwolek@mgh.harvard.edu

M. R. Jenkins
University of South Carolina School of Medicine Greenville, Greenville, SC, USA

S. A. Tilstra et al. (eds.), *Sex- and Gender-Based Women's Health*, https://doi.org/10.1007/978-3-030-50695-7_1

This volume is part of the solution, providing a core curriculum for primary health-care providers that covers common women's health issues as seen through the lens of SGBM. The mastery of the material in this book will provide a solid foundation to provide sex- and gender-informed care to all women within the broader goal of excellent primary care for all persons.

Foundations of Women's Health and Sex- and Gender-Based Medicine

Defining Sex- and Gender-Based Women's Health

What is sex- and gender-based women's health (SGBWH), and what distinguishes a SGBWH provider or curriculum? SGBWH is a mindset, a paradigm shift, and a set of core competencies. It takes on a number of public health issues, employs a way of doing research which includes women as participants, asks whether and why sex and gender differences exist, and, most importantly, poses the question, "Are these differences clinically meaningful?" SGBWH is a body of knowledge, a set of skills, and a model of comprehensive, integrated, and informed clinical services. SGBWH is concerned with community outreach and addressing disparities through advocacy, so as to care for the underserved, members of minority populations, low-income individuals, and immigrants, with equity. SGBWH values promoting women and underrepresented minorities into leadership positions, and accommodating providers in their roles as family caregivers while pursuing their professional career.

SGBWH is patient-centered and considers the whole person in the context of their social environment and cultural context. It affirms that sex is a biological variable (SABV) and that gender is a social construct; both factors influence the health of every person. In order to personalize health care, sex and gender must be factored into the care of each and every patient [6–8]. A suggested definition of SGBWH is displayed in Table 1.1 and is adapted from an original definition of women's health from 1997. The terminology used to describe the concept of women's health has changed over the years, but the basic principles and core values have persisted and progressed.

The ideal women's health provider takes women's concerns seriously and acknowledges biopsychosocial factors that impact health. The provider is knowledgeable of hormonal and reproductive conditions unique to women and of relevant differences between men and women in nonreproductive conditions. Providers should be skilled at painless exams, respectful interactions, effective communication, and shared decision-making methods. For specialists, knowledge of sex and gender differences in their specialty is required.

Table 1.1 Definition of sex- and gender-based women's health (SGBWH)

Sex- and gender-based women's health (SGBWH) is devoted to facilitating the: Preservation of wellness. Prevention of illness. Patient-centered approach to conditions.
SGBWH includes conditions which: Are unique to women. Have epidemiology, manifestations, management strategies, and/or prognoses which are affected by sex and gender.
A SGBWH approach: Cultivates the study of sex and gender differences. Recognizes the contribution of multidisciplinary and interprofessional teams. Incorporates the individual's personal experience of health and illness. Recognizes the diversity of health needs over the life cycle and how these needs reflect differences in race, class, ethnicity, culture, sexual orientation, gender, levels of education, and access to medical care. Includes the empowerment of women, as for all patients, to be informed participants in their own health care with shared decision-making. Seeks to help resolve gaps, inequities and disparities within health care.

Adapted from the National Academy for Women's Health Medical Education (NAWHME) Women's Health in the Curriculum [9]

Lidia self-refers for mammography, and afterwards she is notified that she has calcifications seen on her mammogram that should be biopsied. She is anxious about her referral to the breast center, stating that she had a bad experience in the past with doctors "who did not explain anything to her" and did not listen to her concerns.

Core Values: What Do Patients Want?

A guiding principle in SGBWH is to provide excellent health care which aligns with the priorities and values of patients. An interdisciplinary, inclusive approach to health care based on sex- and gender-specific data is sought by consumers of health care, especially women [10]. To answer the question of what patients want, the authors propose the following core values based on decades of literature on deficiencies in women's health, focus groups, and studies of consumer demands in women's health and primary care [9–12]:

1. *The respect for the value of an informed patient's choice.* Patients have the right to self-determination based on adequate and accurate information and a presentation of options which is understandable to the patient. Individuals want the opportunity to ask questions and for providers to respect their autonomy in making medical decisions. Informed consent is an example of this component and, more recently, shared decision-making.

- Clinical example: A 40-year-old's primary care provider has explained the increased risk of false-positive mammogram results, which might require additional diagnostic interventions, but supports the patient's ultimate decision to begin mammography at 40.

2. *The respect for a patient's values and the patient's perspective.* The values and beliefs that are important to patients should be honored by the provider and taken seriously.
   - Clinical example: A woman with ductal carcinoma in situ (DCIS) chooses bilateral mastectomy for treatment and prophylaxis. This patient should subsequently be supported in her decision, even if some providers might view the chosen treatment as "overkill."
3. *The right to comprehensive, integrated care.* Fragmentation is a problem within medical care and especially for women patients who have breast and gynecologic issues.
   - Clinical example: Models of integrated care include one-stop shopping women's health centers, collaborative care, and primary care with seamless referral networks to specialists.
4. *The right to sensitive, private, painless care including permission-seeking, proper draping, gentle positioning, skilled providers and care teams, and trauma-informed care.* Clinical settings and patient encounters should feel safe to patients.
   - Clinical example: Extra care should be taken to drape patients, pull curtains, and prevent interruptions and intrusions at all times and especially when a patient is undergoing a breast, genital, or rectal examination.
5. *The right to be cared for by providers who are knowledgeable and skilled in women's health and sex- and gender-based medicine.* Women assume that their healthcare providers are knowledgable about common breast issues, gynecologic issues, mental health issues, menopause, and sex- and gender-informed aspects of care.
   - Clinical example: Perimenopausal and menopausal symptoms with hot flashes, night sweats, poor sleep, and irritability are common. Providers should recognize this constellation of symptoms and be familiar with treatment options and understand their own limits and scope of practice.
6. *The right to evidence-based health care that is supported by data from scientific studies which included women and reported outcomes by sex.*
   - Clinical example: Aspects of cardiovascular disease (CVD) have significant similarities and differences between men and women which impact risk, evaluation, treatment, and prognosis. Primary care providers should take an obstetric history from all women and recognize that the obstetrical complications of gestational diabetes and hypertensive disorders of pregnancy increase a woman's future risk of CVD [9, 13].

Paradigm for the Scope of Practice in the Primary Care of Women

Early in the women's health movement, a paradigm for primary women's health care was put forth as the integration of primary care gynecology, primary care psychiatry, and primary care medicine [9]. We suggest that the paradigm be modified: (1) adding breast health and medical care of the pregnant patient as essential components of the primary care of women, (2) including sex and gender aspects, (3) expanding psychiatry to include the psychosocial aspects of sex and gender, and (4) emphasizing the influence of the reproductive hormonal influences and sex- and gender-based differences in all domains (see Fig. 1.1 below).

Sex- and gender-based primary care for women integrates breast health, ob-gyn, primary care, and behavioral health. Each patient is also understood within the context of gender identity, gender expression, natal sex, sexual orientation, sexual behavior, family composition and dynamics, educational level, employment, cultural background, religious background, ethnic heritage, racial identity, genetic heritage, lifestyle habits, and life phase.

Lidia returns to clinic with multiple issues. Her biopsy revealed atypical hyperplasia, and she is debating whether to take tamoxifen for chemoprevention. She is also having hot flashes and bloating and is feeling depressed and anxious. She is pleased to hear that these issues can all be addressed by her primary care provider, who explains that hot flashes affect sleep, and sleep affects mood. Further, tamoxifen can make hot flashes worse. After a lengthy discussion of risks and benefits, she decides to start tamoxifen and venlafaxine.

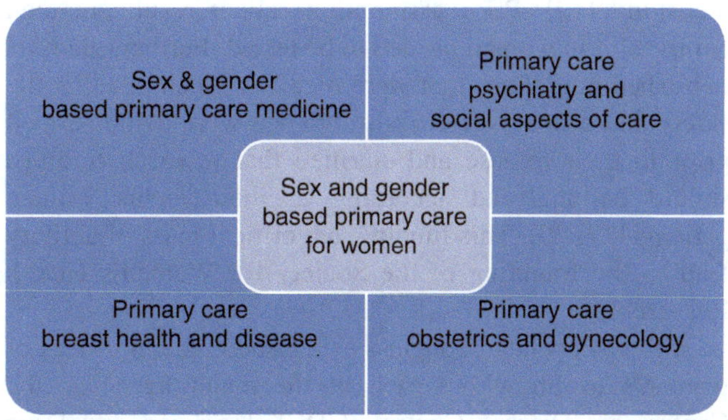

Fig. 1.1 The integration of multiple domains in the primary care of women

The History of Women's Health and Sex- and Gender-Based Medicine

The women's health movement of the 1960s began as women became dissatisfied with the lack of information available to them and the lack of choices regarding their medical care [14]. Medicine was taught without reference to sex and gender except for in the reproductive system. The 70 kg man was presented as the normal human body, and women's bodies were thus considered as "other" [4]. Pressure mounted for women's rights, and in 1985, the National Institutes of Health (NIH) commissioned a task force to study the need for increased research with women as subjects. The report documented the dearth of research on women and the lack of inclusion of women in clinical trials. Medical research at that time did not include women subjects as they were a "protected population," which meant that there was little data on the risks and benefits of medications and treatments in women [15, 16].

Women's Health 1990–1999: An Explosion of Research and New Initiatives

Federal Action and Funding The Women's Health Equity Act of 1990 created the Office for Research in Women's Health (ORWH) at the NIH, with an initial $14 million budget. The ORWH provided the blueprint for decades of medical research and support for the women's health movement to the present. The mandate for women's health research included every organ system, the effects of sex hormones throughout the body, and the psychosocial aspects of health [17, 18].

In the largest trial of its time, the Women's Health Initiative was funded with $625 million in 1991 to longitudinally study the influence of hormone replacement therapy (as it was called then) and diet on cardiovascular disease and colon cancer. Osteoporosis was another major focus of the study [19]. Prior assumptions about results in men being valid in women needed to be tested. Further, the NIH published guidelines that were modified to ensure that the safety and efficacy of drugs in women were demonstrated prior to their release and clarified that research findings should be analyzed according to men versus women patients [17, 20]. This funding and critical mass of activity lead to the founding of the Society for Women's Health Research.

A few years later, congress established federal offices of women's health within each of the major agencies: the Centers for Disease Control (CDC), the Food and Drug Administration (FDA), the Health Research and Services Administration (HRSA), the Veteran's Administration (VA), and the Department of Health and Human Services (DHHS).

Industry and the Private Sector Alongside federal actions, pharmaceutical companies, managed care organizations, private foundations, and nonprofit organizations provided dollars and held educational conferences to fuel an explosion of research and public awareness in women's health. Pharmaceutical companies established women's health divisions to study and market hormone replacement, antidepressants, statins, and osteoporosis treatments. Estrogen replacement therapy (ERT) was viewed as a fountain of youth because early observational studies supported its use for the prevention of cardiovascular disease and osteoporosis. Managed care organizations viewed women, who constitute more than half the American population and almost two-thirds of the population aged 65 and older, as the key consumers to decide where families would spend their healthcare dollars. Women are greater users of healthcare services than men, and women strongly influence health care utilization because they often manage health care for their family. For these reasons, increased attention was paid to the wants and needs of women patients.

In the 1990s, the state of both women's medical care and of education in women's health was described as "a patchwork quilt with gaps" because it was fragmented and had not adequately prepared physicians to deliver comprehensive care to women [6]. In response, models of integrated clinical care for women were created.

Professional Education in Women's Health Whereas women's health had previously been equated with reproductive health, attention was drawn toward the content of medical curricula and residency programs to train providers in the comprehensive care of women. The American Association of Medical Colleges (AAMC) surveyed medical curricula and found that women's health topics were generally not covered in medical curricula outside of obstetrics and gynecology (ob-gyn) [3].

The traditional internal medicine curriculum covered only two-thirds of necessary skills for the care of women [21, 22], with deficiencies primarily in gynecology. Family medicine residencies traditionally included more gynecology than internal medicine programs, but many program directors in family medicine reported that teaching on women's health issues apart from traditional ob-gyn topics was inadequate [23]. Competencies were established at multiple levels to improve women's health education; curricula were analyzed and modified to expand the knowledge and skills of healthcare providers.

During this time, there was an explosion of interest and participation in women's health education at all levels, in research in women's health, and in improving clinical services to women. The first textbooks on women's health for primary care were written, interdisciplinary women's health clinics were founded, and many regional and national conferences focusing on women's health were held [24–26].

Academia and Centers of Excellence in Women's Health Academic centers applied for grant dollars which were earmarked for women's health concerns. Federal funding to establish academic centers of excellence (COEs) in women's health was made available, and academic medical centers competed to receive COE designation and funding. The COE program was funded from 1995 to 2007; necessary components were: research, clinical care, education, community outreach, and leadership. Concurrent action by the Veterans Affairs (VA) Administration offered competitive grant funding for women's health fellowships in partnership with medical schools creating women's health clinics and, in so doing, trained faculty to facilitate future training and research.

Additionally, women's health and SGBM research had new outlets to disseminate their findings. The Journal of Women's Health and Gender-Based Medicine launched in 1992; the publication continued as the Journal of Women's Health in 2002 and became the official journal of the American Medical Women's Association (AMWA) in 2008.

Women's Health 2000–2009: Establishing Sex- and Gender-Based Medicine

Growth in Women's Health Throughout the next decade, women's health continued to grow and expand. The NIH published a six-volume Agenda for Research in Women's Health for the twenty-first Century [27] which revealed a blueprint of continued needs in research across all aspects of health. Research programs enrolled women subjects, and the effects of female hormones throughout the body were topics of intense research. The NIH started the Building Interdisciplinary Research Careers in Women's Health (BIRCWH) program, which is a mentored career-development program to promote careers in women's health and sex differences research. Since the program was created in 2000, at least 77 grants to 41 institutions supporting more than 613 junior faculty members have been awarded by ORWH and BIRCWH program cosponsors [28].

The curricula at schools of dentistry, nursing, pharmacy, and allied health professions were analyzed for content in women's health. Interprofessional education expanded. Education in women's health increased and improved at all levels. (See section on Education below.)

Establishing Sex- and Gender-Based Medicine Marianne Legato, MD, who subsequently wrote the textbook *Principles of Gender-Specific Medicine* observed, "When we make the unwarranted assumptions that results in men will apply equally to women, we miss the opportunities that studying women would give us: to define new questions, to understand more clearly the nature of human biology and how it is compromised by disease, and to develop more effective treatments for disease in both sexes" [29, 30].

Proponents of women's health in the 1990s included sex- and gender-based differences as part of the definition and scope of women's health. The NIH revised its guidelines on the inclusion of women and minorities in clinical research in 1994, stating that all studies were expected to analyze results and conclusions for women and men [20].

It was in 2001, however, when the Institute of Medicine (IOM) published the report "Does Sex Matter?", that the sex- and gender-based medicine movement became more universally recognized and moved into the mainstream [5].

Scientific discovery has elucidated sex differences throughout the human body and gender influences on diagnosis and care delivery (Table 1.2). It is now accepted that sex is a biological variable based on chromosomal complement (XX, XY, and other sex chromosome combinations), having an impact on anatomy and physiology, and must be addressed in scientific research. Gender is a social construct which, among other concepts, includes self-representation to society and the environment's response based on that representation. The textbook *Principles of Gender-Specific Medicine* (Legato et al) had international contributors and was published in 2004 [29].

Table 1.2 Examples of sex and gender factors relevant to research and clinical care

Genetic and cellular	Anatomic and physiological
Individual gene expression and mutations. Chromosomal variations. Cellular level differences. Cellular receptors for hormones.	Size of organs and blood vessels. Body size. Body composition. Pharmacodynamics and pharmacokinetics. Liver metabolism of drugs. Breast tissue in women versus men. Reproductive organs. Sex differences in organ function. Surgical alterations of anatomy.
Hormonal	**Psychosocial**
In utero hormonal milieu. Hormonal effects on cells, tissues, and organs. Hormonal fluctuations across the life span: Puberty, menstruation, pregnancy, lactation, and menopause. Reproductive potential. Exogenous hormones.	In utero influences/ stressors. Psychosocial stressors. Caregiving demands. Gendered societal expectations. Adverse childhood events. Trauma and intimate partner violence.

Lidia calls asking for a refill of zolpidem 10 mg nightly which was started by another provider several years ago. She admits that she is often sleepy the next day after she takes the medication. Lidia's provider tells her that the approved maximum dose of zolpidem is 5 mg for women, as opposed to 10 mg for men. Lidia learns that there are differences in drug metabolism between the sexes and that women, more than men, have high zolpidem levels the day following drug ingestion.

Sex and Gender Differences That Make a Difference Many sex and gender differences are clinically meaningful. Examples include:

1. After consuming the same amount of alcohol, women have higher blood alcohol levels than men, even allowing for size differences, which is partly because women have lower levels of alcohol dehydrogenase in their stomachs than men [31].
2. Multiple studies have demonstrated that, compared to men, women generally have a lesser extent of both overt and subclinical coronary atherosclerosis [32], but traditionally feminine gender traits, such as being a care-giver versus a primary income producer for a family, negatively affects the prognosis in recovery from acute coronary syndromes more than sex of the patient [33].
3. Women are more likely to develop Heart Failure with preserved Ejection Fraction (HFpEF) than men [34].
4. Women are more susceptible to fatal torsades de pointes than men when taking the anti-arrhythmic medications sotalol, disopyramide, or amiodarone [35].
5. Women are more likely than men to suffer a second heart attack within one year of their first heart attack [36].
6. Autoimmune diseases are more common in women than men, and the XX sex chromosome complement has been shown to be disease promoting in some autoimmune diseases as compared to XY. Pregnancy reduces relapse in cell-mediated but not antibody-mediated diseases, suggesting a protective role for high levels of estrogen [37].
7. After menopause, women lose more bone mass than men, which is why 80% of people with osteoporosis are women. However, men are more likely than women to die after an osteoporotic hip fracture. The majority of research on osteoporosis is conducted in women, and less is known about treatment efficacy in men [38].
8. Cluster headaches are more common in men but are more common in women than previously believed. Aura with cluster headache is equally common in both sexes, but women are much more likely to experience sensory, language, and brainstem auras than men [39].
9. Chronic obstructive pulmonary disease (COPD) is more severe despite lower smoking exposure in female patients as compared to male patients [40].
10. Zolpidem has different dosage recommendations for men and women. Zolpidem is metabolized more slowly in women leading to dangerously high doses persisting until the next day, with an increased incidence of subsequent car accidents [41].

Some Signs of Stalled Women's Health Efforts Sex- and gender-based knowledge increased over the decades because of research in women's health and sex and gender differences. With the increased emphasis on sex and gender, however, there was concern that the original mandate to integrate women's health throughout health professional education might become sidelined [42].

The COE program was defunded in 2007, and the survival of women's health centers was dependent upon each home institution's willingness to continue the previously established programs. Enthusiasm and dollars to explore hormonal therapies decreased when preliminary reports from the women's health initiative found that postmenopausal hormone therapy use was not universally beneficial, with concern for breast cancer risk and increased cardiovascular events [19].

Many of the original leaders who pushed the women's health movement forward subsequently retired, focused on other areas of academia, or otherwise lost steam due to reduced resources and institutional support. Increased interest and funding for primary care centers of excellence (not specific to women), the study and correction of disparities, the rise of interprofessional education (formerly called multidisciplinary education in older literature), and the emphasis on sex and gender as unique variables in the care of patients replaced much of the prior focus on women's health.

Although in the late 2000s the emphasis on women's health education began to wane, in 2008, the American Medical Women's Association (AMWA) renewed their commitment to defining and disseminating a shared curriculum in women's health. The goal of complete curricular reform with the inclusion of women's health and sex- and gender-based medicine gained momentum in the following decade and continues into the present [43, 44].

Lasting impact from the COE program was achieved at a large number of centers in the form of continued research in women's health, expansion beyond traditional women's health through sex- and gender-based medicine, persistence of many women's health clinics, and continued influence in many medical, dental, nursing, pharmacy, allied health, and public health educational curricula. Women were promoted in academic medicine, endowed chairs in women's health were funded, and many graduates of women's health fellowships were productive in academic careers.

The Collaboration of Women's Health and Sex and Gender Medicine 2010 to 2020: Addressing Gaps in Research

Women's health, as a movement, was at a nadir in the early 2010's. The general consensus appeared to be that focused women's health educational efforts were no longer needed, having been adequately addressed and remediated. At the same time, the Institute of Medicine (IOM) published a report which showed that large gaps remained in research on women's health concerns [45]. A closer look at research efforts found that, although women were included in research studies and clinical trials at increasing rates, the analysis of data by sex or gender was often not completed or reported. There are many barriers to changing the status quo of sex- and gender-blind reporting within the scientific literature (discussed in more detail below; see section on future directions).

On the basic science level, there was an increased awareness that cellular research must be conducted with knowledge of the sex of the cell, whether XX, XY, or other. Animal research should be conducted on female and male animals, as appropriate, with the results indicating the sex of the animals.

A subsequent national IOM workshop summary on sex-specific reporting of scientific research disputed the notion that gaps in SGBM and WH had been adequately remediated and urged that further efforts were needed [46]. Governmental and funding agencies started taking note of gender and sex disparities. In 2010, the Canadian Institutes of Health Research established policies requiring researchers to include both sex and gender as critical variables in all studies or clinical trials, as did the European Commission in 2013. In 2016, the NIH began requiring that US grant proposals include information as to how sex, but not necessarily gender, would be incorporated as a biological variable in research studies. The World Health Organization urges that sex and gender be incorporated into health-care policy worldwide [47].

The field of SGBM has grown over the last two decades, but as a grassroots effort, not with an influx of monetary resources. Collaboration was forged between prior leaders in WH and the proponents of SGBM, and the two fields were merged into a new focus. The Sex and Gender Women's Health Collaborative (SGWHC) was formed in 2012 and spurred renewed efforts at research, educational, and clinical reform. Founding organizations included the American Medical Women's Association, the American College of Women's Health Physicians, and the Society for Women's Health Research. Collaborating institutions include the Laura W. Bush Institute for Women's Health and multiple national and international academic institutions. The Sex and Gender Women's Health Collaborative website lists resources for practitioners and patients interested in SGBWH, including a sex and gender bibliography, a national sex- and gender-based physician registry, and links to educational materials [1]. The Collaborative has taken a leading role in curricular reform in sex and gender-based health education, including several summits in sex- and gender-based education [1, 44, 48–50].

Lidia, now age 53, took tamoxifen for 5 years without complication and is now postmenopausal. She presents with substernal chest pain on exertion. She is screened by her PCP for diabetes, tobacco use, cholesterol, and family history for cardiovascular risk factors. On further questioning, her provider discovers that Lidia has a history of gestational diabetes and preeclampsia. Lidia undergoes an exercise stress test which is negative, but because of her prenatal risk factors, she is referred to a cardiologist who has a special interest in heart disease in women.

Models of Clinical Care for Women

In response to women's demands and market forces, many integrated clinics providing women's health have been established.

Obstetrics and gynecology practices and maternity care centers hired more female doctors and widwives, provided private birthing rooms for deliveries, upgraded facilities, and became more comprehensive in scope. Fertility centers and abortion services have also been called women's health centers, despite the narrow foci. Research of women's preferences in the past found that patients of reproductive age were often more satisfied with their care from ob-gyns than from internal medicine primary care providers, suggesting that young women highly value providers with expertice in reproductive health [51].

Diagnostic women's health centers arose, providing mammography, DXA scans, and other radiological services. Some centers provided needle biopsies when needed.

Comprehensive breast centers were formed to improve the quality of breast services. These centers were multidisciplinary and offered mammography often with same-day interpretation. Consultation with a multidisciplinary team of dedicated breast surgeons, oncologists, plastic surgeons, and radiation oncologists became the norm for patients diagnosed with cancer in some areas. Volunteer groups and national organizations, including the Susan Komen Foundation [52], assisted women with patient education and comprehensive care including spiritual care, help with wigs and fashion, lymphedema treatment, support groups, and other services.

Primary care-based women's health clinics, staffed by primarily women providers and often interprofessional in nature, employed physicians, NPs, social workers, and/or mental health providers working together. A key example was the Women's Health Associates at Massachusetts General Hospital, founded in 1985 by Dr. Karen Carlson. The US Department of Health and Human Services used this clinic as a model to subsequently aid in the development of numerous National Centers of Excellence in Women's Health [53].

Many women's health clinics added elements across disciplines and increased care integration. Centers might have included primary care, gynecologic care, osteoporosis screening, prevention and treatment, menopausal care, breast screening, diabetic education, urinary incontinence screening and treatment, and the primary treatment of depression, anxiety, and premenstrual syndrome (PMS) in one clinical space. Referral networks identified providers in various specialties with a special interest in women's health including women's cardiology, women's health gastroenterology specializing in functional bowel problems, rheumatologists who treated women with fibromyalgia, and mental health providers who were sensitive to women with a history of trauma, and skilled in the gender-specific needs of women. These clinics enjoyed strong relationships with ob-gyn and breast centers. In some cases, all of these elements were brought together in the same physical space to make a truly comprehensive women's health center. In other cases, a "Center Without Walls" was founded which did not exist in a single physical space but consisted of a network of providers, clinics, and services for the comprehensive care of women.

Veterans Affairs In 1990, the Veterans Administration (VA) recognized and acknowledged that it was not providing adequate care to its growing number of women veterans who had the same rights to health care as male veterans. Many women veterans had experienced sexual abuse or harassment in the military or had a history of trauma prior to enlisting in service. The VA assigned Women Veterans Coordinators at each medical center who acted as case managers to address the needs of women veterans. The VA funded women's health centers throughout the VA system and mandated that women veterans' clinical care be sensitive to the privacy and safety concerns of its patients [54]. The VA held continuing education conferences on women's issues and veteran-specific issues to train its providers. The conferences addressed post-traumatic stress disorder (PTSD), sexual traumas, mental health, and other subjects in interprofessional care. The VA clinics serve as training sites for medical students, residents, and fellows [55]. The VA further provided funding for women's health clinical fellowships which have trained many leaders in women's health [56]. (See Chap. 38 on Care of the Female Veteran.)

Three months later, Lidia's symptoms have progressed, and she is evaluated by a cardiologist. Given her symptoms and risk factors of gestational diabetes and preeclampsia, she is sent for a nuclear stress test. The stress test is positive, and cardiac catheterization reveals significant coronary artery disease. Lidia would like to know if her sex and ethnic background as an Indian American affect her prognosis.

Community Outreach, Disparities, and Health Equity

Sex- and gender-based women's health (SGBWH) is concerned with public health and barriers to care for patients: literacy issues, minority issues, socioeconomic issues, cultural competency, care of underserved populations, and the interaction between medicine and social, societal, and legal factors. The original COEs were each required to focus attention on a specific underserved population. Campaigns to raise awareness of women's health issues and to empower and educate women have been a priority among women's health advocates. In the 1980s, the AIDS epidemic cast attention on the needs and health issues of the gay community, but less was known about lesbian health and the needs of transgender individuals. From the beginning, the women's health movement partnered with women's studies experts to address the needs of lesbian women. (See Chap. 36 on Care of Sexual Minority Women and Chap. 37 on Transgender Care.) Today, women's, minority, and LGBT issues are often housed together in offices on disparities and/or equity at individual academic institutions.

Disparities result in disproportionate morbidity and mortality, and providers should be aware of the lower screening rates, suboptimal diagnostic testing, loss of patients to follow-up, less comprehensive treatment, and overall worse prognosis in certain demographic groups, including immigrants and sexual minorities (See section on disparities in Chap. 14 on Cervical Cancer and Human Papillomavirus). Women are overrepresented in the United States within the poor and underserved populations. There is a need for culturally sensitive patient education and strategies to overcome barriers to care for populations at risk. For instance, in the United States, HPV vaccination is widely available and free for children. Culturally sensitive reframing of the vaccine debate allowed parents who were initially concerned that HPV vaccination would lead to teenage promiscuity to instead understand HPV vaccination as routine care. Gaps still remain for those who have poor access to health care (e.g., rural and low-income populations) in the United States and worldwide. (See Chap. 2 on High-Value Health Care.)

The women's health construct recognizes race as a complex factor in health care which is affected by country of birth, country of residence, income, educational level, diet, and activity. While ignoring race as a factor is not advised, defining race can be problematic. In the United States and elsewhere, populations are becoming more racially mixed. Many shared decision-making tools and risk calculators include race as a variable, but validation for various races may be limited. An example is the Gail model that: was developed in White women, underestimates risk in Black women, is not well validated in Hispanic or Asian women, and has no data on women from India [57]. Another example is genetic screening; the BRCA 1 and 2 genes are known to be very common (1 in 40) in the Ashkenazi Jewish population. What is less well known is that BRCA genes have been found to be relatively common in Hispanic women in the Southwest United States; 25% tested positive for BRCA in a high-risk breast cancer clinic population [58].

There is further concern that bucketing women into racial categories may lead to unintended differences in health-care delivery processes—that is, when the intention is to call out important disparities in order to address them, sometimes, the action of labeling itself may lead to disparate treatments. One must proceed with caution when collecting sociodemographic history to assess risk and design an approach to management. Standard processes and treatments for all people, regardless of race or other kinds of minority status, are both the goal and a core strategy to address disparities and counteract unconscious bias. Women's health education teaches that variation is expected, and an emphasis is placed upon competence for culturally sensitive care of every person [59].

Lidia is very grateful for the excellent sex- and gender-based care she has received and wants to know why more health-care providers do not seem to know about women's health and sex and gender differences relevant to clinical care.

Education in Women's Health and Sex- and Gender-Based Medicine

> Women will never receive optimal care until all health-care providers are fully trained to meet their needs. The goal is to improve training in the care of women in the full range of women's health issues and thus end the fragmentation of women's health care [60].

The road to educational changes in women's health and sex- and gender-based medicine began in the 1990s and has been filled with challenges. In 1995, the Council on Graduate Medical Education's (COGME) *Fifth Report on Women and Medicine* found that many women receive incomplete and poorly coordinated care for their routine and comprehensive health concerns, in part due to deficiencies in the education of physicians. The Council stated that changes in undergraduate and graduate medical education, in addition to continuing medical education, were needed to adequately address the comprehensive health needs of women [3]. In 1998, systematic surveys of american medical school curricula by the Association of American Medical Colleges (AAMC) found significant gaps in medical education concerning women's health, and changes were recommended [42, 61]. Studies of curricula in dental, pharmacy, nursing, public health, and allied health professional schools had similar findings, and an expert panel convened to make recommendations for interprofessional collaboration in women's health curricula in 2012 [62].

Importantly, studies found that most medical schools did not routinely offer material on women's health and gender-based physiology as a focused course of study, except as preclinical and clinical electives with limited influence on the overall curriculum [60, 61]. Traditional clerkship rotations fragmented the care of women: internal medicine and surgery presented nonreproductive aspects of care, and ob-gyn focused on reproductive- and gender-specific issues. As a result, relevant menstrual, obstetrical, gynecologic, and sexual histories were often omitted in the history and physical notes written by students and residents during non-ob-gyn rotations [9, 60, 63].

Women's health was a catalyst for reform in medical education in which sex- and gender-based content and women's health beyond reproductive health are weaved into undergraduate curricula. Concepts in complexity science and physiological variation, together with advances in medical educational methods, facilitated the curricular change [59].

Throughout the next decade, there were continued efforts to advance women's health education at all levels, and interdisciplinary curricula were developed (see section on resources at the end of the chapter) [9, 64, 65]. Despite national attention to women's health education, however, the women's health content in medical education at most institutions continued to be suboptimal [42, 66, 67]. Innovative instructional methods used to introduce women's health knowledge and skills into medical curricula included problem-based learning cases [68–70], web-based modules [71], standardized patient workshops, and structured clinical instructional modules (SCIM), which are a form of modified objective structured clinical examinations (OSCE) [72, 73]. Substantial curricular changes required support from the highest levels of academic institutions, faculty development, awareness campaigns, and the designation of a center or program to spearhead efforts [74–76].

An early model for integrating women's health issues into the entire medical school curriculum and the barriers and solutions to implementing the new curriculum were detailed in publications from educational innovators at Drexel's (formerly MCP Hahnemann) Center of Excellence in Women's Health [70, 76]. Other institutions, especially the Centers of Excellence in Women's Health, were also successful in integrating women's health into their curricula, leveraging grant money, institutional support, and buy-in from leaders in the academic medical centers. Federal mandates and commitment from organizations such as the AAMC provided incentive for the efforts. At that time, women's health curricula were disseminated to partnering institutions and adapted to an interprofessional audience of learners [77–80].

As the emphasis on sex- and gender-based medicine has increased, the Sex and Gender Women's Health Collaborative (SGWHC) and seasoned educators have worked toward the inclusion of sex- and gender-based medicine into medical and interprofessional curricula [44, 48–50]. In 2011, in collaboration with the National Board of Medical Examiners (NBME), the SGWHC audited the National Board of Medical Examiners (NBME) exams for women's health and sex and gender content [1, 48]. In 2012, the first sex and gender educational summit was held, and a plan was outlined to introduce sex and gender content into medical curricula [49]. In 2015, 2018, and 2020, additional summits were held with increased participation and expanding scope to include interprofessional education and international partners [44, 50].

In order to influence lasting and meaningful change, education must occur at all levels: undergraduate education in all health professional schools, graduate medical education, faculty development, and continuing education. Faculty development and resident education are critical for the improvement of direct patient care and equally important for teaching students in the classrooms and inpatient care settings. It is essential that basic knowledge, attitudes, and skills in women's health and sex- and gender-based medicine are disseminated throughout all aspects, and to all members, of the medical enterprise [42, 59, 76, 81, 82].

Despite the many activities, reports, and roundtable discussions focusing on SGBWH, curricular integration of sex- and gender-based medicine in US medical schools is not widespread [83–86]. Changes at a small school or program or in individual courses are easier than changing the whole curriculum at a large school or program [59]. Barriers to integration include the saturation of curricula and competition for instructional time, a lack of buy-in from leadership, limitations on finances, and the shortage of champions and experts in sex- and gender-based medicine and women's health within the faculty. A major challenge is the lack of tangible resources, such as a curricular roadmaps or tool kits, to readily guide faculty, staff, and learners through the organizational navigation, institutional negotiation, and resource allocation needed to sustain curricular change [76, 86].

Another challenge is that SGBWH often lacks an academic home within health professional schools, and therefore, resources and opportunities for promotion and influence among SGBWH faculty can be limited. Furthermore, SGBWH adherents are diverse in terms of field of study and specialty, which makes concerted efforts to cohesively advance the field difficult. Academic meetings tend to cater to one field or specialty, and faculty members often have limited funds for travel. Lastly, most faculty who focus on women's health are women taking care of women, and there is concern that the field is marginalized within professional education and academics partly for this reason [42, 76, 86].

Potential solutions to the continued challenge of integrating women's health and sex- and gender-based medicine into curricula include defining interprofessional competencies and learning objectives, developing shared curricula, raising awareness, obtaining external and internal funding, auditing and inclusion of SGBWH content on licensure and board examinations, enhancing faculty development programs, establishing dedicated offices or programs within academic centers, encouraging participation of key faculty on curriculum committees, developing faculty rewards for scholarship in SGBWH, and enforcing faculty accountability for including relevant sex- and gender-based information in their teaching, research, and clinical endeavors. Curricular change teams which include curriculum influencers, student or resident champions, institutional leaders, and content experts can be particularly effective as change agents [49]. Ob-gyn, as the only medical specialty wholly devoted to women, has provided leadership nationally and locally in the women's health arena and continues to be a key ally in this intrinsically multidisciplinary and interprofessional effort [1, 76, 85, 86]. Key steps in the planning and integration of SGBWH content into existing curricula are detailed in Table 1.3.

Graduate Medical Education: Resident Curricula and Fellowship Training

The American Board of Internal Medicine (ABIM) and the American Academy of Family Physicians (AAFP) have stated that the knowledge and clinical skills required for the care of women must be addressed within the context of the general skills acquired by residents. Traditionally, internal medicine (IM) residencies have had limited training in gynecology, and no training in obstetrics, and for this reason, focused attention in women's health-care training is needed in IM [21–23]. Competency in women's health among primary care providers is important for both patient safety and patient satisfaction. There is concern that IM residents are not adequately prepared to care for women of reproductive age, women aged 18–34 years, which may lead to decreased patient satisfaction and quality of care [51, 87–89].

Table 1.3 Integrating sex- and gender-based women's health (SGBWH) into curricula [9, 70, 76, 85, 86]

1. Identify and recognize barriers.
(a) Saturation of curriculum and competition for instructional time.
(b) Lack of an academic home for women's health and sex- and gender-based medicine.
(c) Lack of faculty and residents familiar with sex- and gender-based medicine.
(d) Lack of clinical opportunities for students and trainees.
(e) Lack of funding to support programming, administration, and faculty time.
(f) Lack of women or key supporters in leadership to promote the importance and inclusion of SGBWH subject matter.
2. Develop an implementation plan.
(a) Obtain internal or external funding if possible.
(b) Develop and perform a needs assessment to (1) identify targeted learners, (2) audit and review the existing curricula to determine gaps in SGBWH content, and (3) identify the information that is most needed by the learners.
(c) Assess institutional readiness and available resources: Buy-in from the leadership within a professional school, department, or residency program director is essential. Meet with the dean, chairs, program directors, course directors, and clerkship directors.
(d) Determine scope of what is to be taught: List of competencies and learning objectives.
(e) Teach: Identify opportunities to integrate SGBWH content into existing curricula, and highlight relevant sex and gender differences wherever possible. Develop new courses, lectures, small group sessions, cases, and clinical opportunities.
(f) Identify key faculty, residents, and students for collaboration and influence
(i) Form a task force to meet regularly and to build and sustain momentum for change
(ii) Designate representatives to represent SGBWH education on curricular committees and case discussion meetings
(g) Provide faculty development and faculty rewards to increase participation
(h) Build a searchable repository of information references, cases, lectures, and resources
3. Execute the plan.
(a) Thread awareness of SGBWH throughout the curriculum by asking all speakers to address issues of sex and gender differences in lectures and tutorials. The expectation can be specified in the letter of invitation to speakers.
(b) Ask "what if?" ask all teachers and learners to reflect on the incorporation of diversity and gender issues into their lectures and case discussions. Ask, "what if this was a woman, a transgender individual, an uninsured patient? How would this change the teaching points discussed?"
(c) Augment curricula and faculty development with SGBWH additions such as special speakers, SGBWH grand rounds, and clinical elective experiences.
(d) Add innovative online modules, podcasts, and health informational technology (IT) education.
(e) Implement SGBWH clinical skills workshops utilizing models or standardized patients.
4. Review: Assess, evaluate, and respond to feedback.
(a) Develop evaluation tools.
(b) Regularly evaluate and assess using continuous improvement cycles to check and adjust.
(c) Involve learners and perhaps patients in the reflective critique.

Interdisciplinary educational and patient care partnerships between ob-gyns and primary care providers, which help bridge this gap, have been well received by trainees and promote a comprehensive view in the care of women patients [1, 64, 90–96].

When developing a curriculum in women's health for IM residents, there are numerous resources which may be of use. The ABIM expectations for women's health competencies and the published blueprint of topics for the ABIM exam define the scope of training required for all internal medicine residents [97–99]. The ABIM exam blueprint lists primary medical content categories and the percentage assigned to each for a typical exam: obstetrics-gynecology and psychiatry make up 3% and 4%, respectively, of the total examination questions. Moreover, women's health and preventive health care are listed as "cross-content areas" and are relevant to all of the content categories. Together, women's health and prevention comprise 12% of the examination questions [99]. Other sources which inform the development of women's health curricula include lists of competencies; surveys of residents, residency directors, and graduated residents; preventive services guidelines; and recommendations from experts and educators in women's health [21, 100–104].

To prepare residents in the comprehensive care of women patients, topics specific to women and reproductive health issues, menopause, breast care, preconception care, and care of the pregnant patient must be included in the curriculum. Sex- and gender-based concepts, that acknowledge sex as a biological variable, should be woven throughout all aspects of the broader curriculum [21, 100–104].

A summary of current curricular recommendations for all internal medicine residents is outlined in Table 1.4. The list aligns closely with the content of this book. The ABIM blueprint of what internists should know and the Federated Council for Internal Medicine (FCIM) recommendations are comprehensive in the list of topics required. The Women's Preventive Services Initiative (WPSI) lists the knowledge needed for screening and prevention, and these topics should be addressed as an integral part of primary care and wellness visits. Surveys of residents, program directors, and women's health experts identify areas of greatest continued need, specifically topics which may not be covered sufficiently in existing internal medicine curricula.

In addition to specific topics for inclusion in internal medicine curricula, interrelationships between reproductive and nonreproductive aspects of care are critical to patient care. Specifically, breast and ob-gyn histories belong in complete history and physical examinations performed on each patient; for example, complications of pregnancy, gestational diabetes, and preeclampsia influence the risk of diabetes and cardiovascular disease in later life, and a history of atypical hyperplasia of the breast increases the future risk of breast

Table 1.4 Summary of women's health curricular content needs for internal medicine residencies [21, 22, 90, 99–104]

Domains	Knowledge and skills topics	ABIM Blueprint/ABIM recs[a]/FICM[b]	WPSI: Well-woman care[c]	Greatest need per PD, resident[d], and women's health expert[e] surveys
Health maintenance	Lifestyle: Diet, activity, and obesity	X	X	N/A
	Habits: Alcohol, tobacco, and substance use	X	X	N/A
	Immunizations	X	X	N/A
	Health screening	X	X	N/A
Breast health	General breast care	X	X	X = E
	Risk assessment and BRCA testing	X	X	X = S, C
	Prevention: Chemoprevention	X	X	x
	Benign breast conditions: Lumps, pain, and discharge	X	–	X = E, D,M
	Cancer principles of management	X	–	X = M
	Survivor care	X	–	X
Family planning	Assess reproductive plans	X	X	X = C
	Preconception counseling	X	X	X = C
	Contraception: OC, IUD, and LARC	X	X	X = C, P
	EC, medical abortion, abortion, and infertility	X	–	N/A
Pregnancy and postpartum care	Medical problems in pregnancy	X	X	X
	Ectopic pregnancy	X	–	X
	Mastitis and breastfeeding	X	X	x
Gynecology	Sexually transmitted infections	X	X	X = D,M
	Vaginitis/vulvovaginal disorder	X	X	X = D, M
	Abnormal bleeding/menstrual disorders	X	–	X = D
	Dysmenorrhea	X	–	X = M
	Pelvic pain: Fibroids, endometriosis, and ovarian cysts	X	–	X = D
	Sexual function/dysfunction	X	–	X = D
Menopause	Symptoms	X	–	X = M
	Hormonal therapy	X	–	X = C, P
	Genitourinary atrophy	X	–	X
Mental health/ social aspects of health	Depression/mental health disorders	X	X	X = D,M
	Intimate partner violence	X	X	X = S
	Sexual trauma/rape	X	–	X = S
	Eating disorders	X	–	X = D
	Chronic pain	X	–	x
	Lesbian/bisexual health care	X	–	X = M
Urogynecology	Urinary incontinence	X	X	X = D,M
	Urinary tract infections	X	X	N/A
Cancer screening and principles of management	Breast	X	X	X = E, S
	Cervical	X	X	X = E, S, D, R
	Colon and lung	X	X	N/A
	Uterine, ovarian, and vulvar/vaginal	X	–	N/A
Medical topics relevant to SGBWH	Cardiovascular disease in women	X	X	X
	Osteoporosis and fall prevention	X	X	X = S, M
	PCOS/endocrine disorders	X	–	X = D
	Irritable bowel syndrome	X	–	X = M
	Migraine headache	X	–	N/A
	Sex- and gender-related differences	X	–	N/A

Abbreviations: *X* included in competency recommendations, guidelines, or high priorities as identified by surveys, *x* lower priority topics as identified by surveys, (–) outside scope of recommendations, *BRCA* breast cancer gene, *CVD* cardiovascular disease, *DM* diabetes mellitus, *EC* emergency contraception, *HTN* hypertension, *IUD* intrauterine device, *LARC* long-acting reversible contraceptive, *N/A* not applicable, content not included in surveys, *OC* oral contraceptives, *PCOS* polycystic ovary syndrome, *PD* program director, *recs* recommendations

[a]Recommended from the American Board of Internal Medicine (ABIM) and certifying exam blueprint [21, 99]

[b]FCIM = the Federated Council for Internal Medicine [22]

[c]WPSI = the women's preventive services initiative: evidence-based prevention and screening [90]

[d]Surveys of residents and program directors [100–103]

[e]Most important women's health educational topics for inclusion in residency training per internal medicine women's health experts. Recommendations are further classified as C = counsel, E = exam, S = screen, D = diagnose, R = refer, and M = prescribe or manage [104]

Table 1.5 Resident surveys: the value of clinical experiences in women's health and relevance for practice after residency [100, 102]

Clinical experiences listed in descending order of priority by current residents[a]	• Women's cardiology[b] • STI and HIV • Menopausal health • Bone metabolism/ osteoporosis • Intimate partner violence/ women's shelter[b] • Breast health • Mental health • Gynecology • Sports injuries in women[b] • Urogynecology • Maternal medicine • Reproductive endocrinology
Women's health topics needing increased emphasis in residency[a,c]	• STI and HIV • Menopausal health • Bone metabolism/ osteoporosis • Breast health • Mental health • Gynecology • Urogynecology

HIV human immunodeficiency virus, *STI* sexually transmitted infection
[a]Residents in a single IM program [102]
[b]Topics not included in survey
[c]Women's health subjects that graduated physicians from a single IM program felt least prepared for but were most needed in practice after residency [100]

Table 1.6 Curriculum implementation opportunities [76, 86]

	Opportunities	Tips
Teaching forums and formats	• Clinical skills workshops • Standardized patients • Noon conferences • Resident reports • Preclinical conferences • Ground rounds • Directed readings • Problem-based learning modules • Journal clubs • Women's health seminars • Continuity clinic experiences • Specialty clinic experiences • Online modules, webinars, materials	• Audit content of current curriculum • Letter to presenters asking all faculty to address sex and gender biology and clinical differences in teaching and lectures as appropriate • Sex and gender distinctions taught across all subjects • Identify faculty with special expertise or interest and form women's health education working group
Faculty development and Continuing Medical Education (CME)	• Annual faculty development workshops • Grand rounds presentations • Women's health conferences • Online modules, webinars, materials	• It is essential that all faculty are on board with respect to sex as a biological variable and essential women's health content

cancer. Essential residency training in medical procedures relevant to women's health includes the Pap test and obtaining endocervical cultures [9, 91].

Clinical experiences, especially time spent in specialty clinics, are effective for developing competency and are highly valued by residents. Surveys of current and graduated residents, however, suggest that the current level of training in women's health during residency is not adequately preparing trainees for practice after residency [100, 102, 105]. (See Table 1.5).

Ideally, residency programs should use a written curriculum in women's health. Opportunities to include women's health in curricula include didactics, reading lists, case-based learning, workshops, and clinical experiences in continuity and specialty clinics [9]. Many methods of instruction in women's health are described in literature, but few have been vigorously evaluated [106]. Direct clinical experiences are superior, when available for provider education. Faculty development, especially for continuity clinic preceptors, is essential to reinforce learning introduced in didactic sessions or through assigned readings [70, 76, 82, 107]. Interdisciplinary clinical training between IM and ob-gyn residents has been shown to be effective in women's health education and is valued by trainees [1, 65, 74, 89, 91, 94, 95]. (See Table 1.6).

Primary Care Residents in Internal Medicine The knowledge and skills in women's health recommended for primary care residents are more advanced than those required of categorical residents. Primary care residents, in addition to general awareness of sex and gender issues within the subspecialties, should have increased training in gynecology and breast care, STI evaluation, menopausal treatment, osteoporosis screening, and primary mental health care. Supplemental clinical experiences in gynecology, bone health, women's cardiology, endocrinology, psychiatry, and breast health should be offered if available. Additional training in gynecologic procedures, such as IUD insertion, is of interest to some residents [21]. A survey of program directors in primary care revealed that areas of relative weakness in existing curricula include preconception counseling, contraception, abnormal bleeding, mental health, intimate partner violence (IPV), menopause, sexual trauma, rape, urinary incontinence, osteoporosis, and polycystic ovary syndrome (PCOS). In contrast, relative strengths include depression, pelvic examinations, cancer screening, hypertension, diabetes mellitus, and cholesterol treatment [105].

Women's Health Tracks in Internal Medicine Tracks in women's health typically focus the majority of the continuity care experience for residents on women patients. Additional seminars, journal clubs, and specialty clinical training bring an advanced level of women's health focus to these trainees. The women's health track (WH track)—the first of its kind—was established in 1994 by Dr. Melissa McNeil for residents with a strong interest in developing expertise in health issues that are unique to women, are more common in women, and present differently in women [108]. There are approximately eight known women's health track residencies available in internal medicine that offer additional experience in gynecology, mental health, endocrine, comprehensive women's health or VA women's clinics, and breast centers [109]. Although there are women's health tracks as well as post-graduate women's health fellowships, there is no additional ACGME distinction accrediting the women's health focus and expertise. Published works provide descriptions of women's health tracks and provide data showing that graduates of women's health tracks tend to become leaders in women's health and to be academically productive [110–112].

Women's Health Fellowships Women's health fellowships train health-care providers in the multidisciplinary and advanced needs of women patients within the paradigm of SGBWH as defined in this chapter. Dr. Saralyn Mark described the first fellowship, which incorporated advanced learning in endocrinology, gynecology, psychiatry, cardiology, breast health, domestic violence, and the medical care of pregnant patients [113]. The VA women's health fellowships were instituted in 1993 and included additional curricula on the health needs of women veterans, post-traumatic stress disorder (PTSD), sexual trauma, assault, and harassment. These multidisciplinary fellowships were supported by academic departments and included training in research and investigation. Other similar fellowships not associated with the VA followed. Graduates of women's health fellowships have been shown to become leaders in women's health in academic medical centers and to have academically productive careers. A review of fellowships and a listing of known fellowships are available in published form [56, 109, 114].

There is debate on whether women's health fellowship training should be a separate certification within internal medicine, like geriatrics, or remain as an uncertified area of concentration. Thoughtful articles have been written detailing the pros and cons of such a proposal, and at present, there is no additional women's health specialty certification or recognition within internal medicine [114, 115].

Faculty Development and Continuing Education for Health Professionals

Faculty Development and Continuing Education There is continued need for programs to possess a cadre of trained educators who are fully equipped to teach trainees and peers about women's health and gender-based medicine [2, 59]. A survey of internal medicine and family medicine teaching faculty at five academic medical centers found that internal medicine faculty perceived a significantly greater need than family medicine attending physicians for faculty development in women's health, especially in breast care, medical problems in pregnancy, and gynecologic topics [82]. Similar results were found in a survey of primary care providers (PCPs) when asked about continuing medical education (CME) in women's health. Breast care, heart disease in women, osteoporosis, intimate partner violence, mental health, and gynecologic topics were in high demand [81]. Grand rounds and other seminars, continuing education conference opportunities, and focused faculty development in women's have been described as effective and as being well received among medical educators [74–78, 82].

Interprofessional Education (IPE) IPE is an international movement relevant to health-care redesign that fits nicely with the SGBWH paradigm: patient-centered and holistic. Women's health care in the past has been fragmented, and IPE promotes a remedy for fragmented care: the collaborative care of patients. Nurse practitioners, nurses, and midwives provide excellent gender-sensitive care to patients and comprise a large proportion of attendees at CME conferences focusing on primary care women's health. Nurse practitioners in women's health have held their own annual women's health conference for over 20 years [116].

Education in SGBWH should be integrated throughout the curriculum of all health professions students, not just medical students. In an early project, women's health was integrated into the curricula of the medical, dental, pharmacy, nursing, and allied health schools as well as the internal medicine residency at one institution. This adapted curriculum was spread further to 15 health-care professional schools throughout the country [77, 78]. Today, more health-care professionals in dentistry, pharmacy, public health, and allied health fields are benefiting from increased women's health curricula in the classroom and have interest and expertise in topics specific to SGBWH. Examples of relevent clinical topics include oral and facial pain, bone loss in the jaw, hormonal impacts on gum disease, pharmacokinetic and medication efficacy differences between the sexes, ligamental laxity in women, sports injuries in women, best practices in health communication, social determinants of health, and public health issues related to SGBWH.

In 2013, the Health Research and Services Administration (HRSA) published "Women's Health Curricula: Final Report on Expert Panel Recommendations for Interprofessional Collaboration Across the Health Professions" [62]. The report defined core competencies, examined existing women's health education efforts and literature, and made recommendations for the dissemination of women's health curricula across the health professions: medicine, nursing, pharmacy, dentistry, public health, and social work. The report also contains a model to assess institutional readiness for integrating sex- and gender-based women's health across disciplines.

In 2018, the American Dental Education Association (ADEA) and the NIH ORWH cosponsored an expert roundtable titled "Women's Health in Interprofessional Education and Collaborative Care." The convening report, logic model, and strategies for medicine, dentistry, nursing, pharmacy, and public health are available electronically to health and allied professions schools and organizations to use in curriculum development, collaborative care, and experiential treatment and learning [117]. The growth of interprofessional education provides a plethora of opportunities for the various disciplines to work together to promote women's health education throughout undergraduate and graduate education. Medical education research engages clinician educators, whose promotion may depend on scholarly activity and research endeavors, to develop platforms outside of the traditional biomedical research environments.

Research in SGBWH

The women's health movement spurred awareness and created a community, which in turn led to funding streams, policies, and new organizations that then allowed an explosion of research in women's health and sex- and gender-based medicine (see section on history above) [18, 85, 118]. Many women's health and SGBM investigations were sorely needed, for example, studies of postmenopausal estrogen and progestins and of breast-conserving surgery for breast cancer. Once conducted, the results of these studies changed practice and further demonstrated the need. The concurrent emphasis on women's health curricula and training as well as leadership development in women's health built a pipeline of interested researchers and topics of study. The research that followed fills the chapters of this textbook.

Lidia is now 62 and feeling well. She is very grateful for the excellent sex- and gender-based women's health care she has received. She would like to invest in the future of health care and agrees to fund a Chair in Women's Health from her business profits.

Leadership and Advancement: Challenges and Solutions

> We conclude with recommendations to promote progress beyond the apparent glass ceiling that is preventing further advancement of women's health and women leaders. We emphasize the need to move beyond 'fixing the women' to a systemic, institutional approach that acknowledges and addresses the impact of unconscious, gender-linked biases that devalue and marginalize women and issues associated with women, such as their health [85].

Although leaders and champions of both sexes are needed to make progress in the fields of sex and gender medicine and women's health, senior women are especially needed in leadership so that changes within academia are not just pieces and happenstance [59]. The issue of leadership development for women came into focus as an area of great need as academic centers acknowledged the very low numbers of women, and especially women with children, in the fields of science and medicine, in academics or the highest ranks of those respective fields, in politics, and in other positions of leadership. The underrepresentation of women and minorities was a problem because those in leadership set the tone and the agenda and made decisions concerning priorities and resources. Additionally, the optics of majority race men dominating these areas limited the self-advocacy of women and vulnerable groups [119, 120].

At academic institutions, tenure clocks made it extremely difficult for women to be promoted on the traditional "7 year up or out" if they parented children or bore children during this time. Part-time and flextime positions are not universally available at academic institutions, and when they were, part-time positions often came with distinct disadvantages: faculty must often be full-time to have tenure or to sit on important committees such as the university senate. Maternity leave was generally not available or was limited, and only full-time faculty were eligible for full benefits. Some women were expected to go back to work full-time at the hospital after a one- to two-week break after giving birth [120].

Although many men take substantial responsibility for the care of children, women traditionally bore a disproportionate load of household responsibilities and were more likely to work part-time than men due to parenting responsibilities [121–123]. Further, the physical and biological challenges of pregnancy, childbirth, and lactation are experienced nearly exclusively by women. The problem this poses for women in academics was eloquently explained by the American Association of University Professors in 2000:

> Raising a child takes 20 years, not one semester. American women, who still do the vast majority of child care, will not achieve equality in academia so long as the ideal academic is defined as someone who takes no time off for child-rearing. With teaching, research, committee assignments, and other responsibilities, pre-tenure academics commonly work many hours of overtime. Defining job requirements in this way tends to eliminate virtually all mothers, so it is not surprising the percentage of tenured women in U.S. colleges and universities has climbed so slowly [120].

Over the past few decades, there have been notable improvements in workplace options and procedures: pregnancy protections, the Family Medical Leave Act (FMLA), maternity leave, modified responsibilities, unpaid leave opportunities, and leave for adoption. Despite these changes, there are persistent areas of need: paid maternity leave, paternity leave, childcare issues, and work schedules that coincide with school schedules. The COVID crisis of 2020 brought these issues into sharp focus as schools and daycares were closed, causing academic and clinical productivity to plummet for many faculty.

Furthermore, there are issues which require careful attention for continued improvement: biases toward women and minorities in hiring and promotions, sexual harassment, and career trajectories which are compatible with child-rearing and work-life balance. Regardless of sex or gender, students, residents, faculty, and community physicians are encouraged to be creative and assertive with their supervisors, deans, program directors, and department heads to explore flextime and part-time job offers, shared positions, "reduced full-time" 9–11 month faculty appointments, modified responsibilities, and reentry programs to allow parents to attend to child-rearing or other personal and family responsibilities while remaining active in the health care community. Telehealth and virtual visits, which became the norm in the setting of the COVID crisis, and the flexiblity afforded by virtual clinics and meetings, may be a positive addition to the options available to physicians trying to manage academic and family demands. Most importantly, parents should be able to advocate for workweek expectations that are compatible with both successful careers and raising the next generation without feeling targeted, marginalized, or inadequate.

In order to advance women in medicine, the COE program included a leadership development component which was not limited to women [124]. National organizations and institutions started leadership trainings, such as the Association of American Medical Colleges (AAMC) women in leadership courses for junior and senior faculty and the Executive Leadership in Academic Medicine (ELAM) program. The NIH, in addition to its career development awards, has grants which help women return to research careers who have taken time off for child-rearing. The Building Interdisciplinary Research Careers in Women's Health (BIRCWH) program continues to fund individuals to prepare them for research careers and advancement in academic medicine.

Women's health as an academic focus in research and education, combined with leadership programs, has enabled many qualified women to advance in academic medicine and other arenas of leadership, as most women's health researchers and educators are, in fact, women. Providers who have completed fellowships in women's health have become leaders within the women's health field and in academia [56]. Endowed chairs in women's health provide top leaders in women's health with the resources and gravitas needed to make a continued impact in academic medicine [125].

Future Directions in SGBWH

To end the perpetual fragmentation of women's health across the health-care delivery environment, educators and clinicians in primary care must be well versed in conditions specific to women such as pregnancy, menopause, and gynecological cancers and also be able to apply clinically meaningful sex and gender differences into clinical practice. Concrete steps toward addressing current gaps include the following:

- Using precise terminology for sex and gender.
- Continuing research into sex and gender differences and the dissemination of significant findings.
- Integrating sustainable sex- and gender-based curricula throughout health professional education.
- Increasing attention to training in ob-gyn topics within internal medicine and other primary care programs.
- Conducting innovative medical education research to determine best practices in SGBWH education.
- Promoting leadership and advancement of faculty committed to SGBWH in the academic environment.
- Advocating for the funding and promotion of SGBWH research and educational programs.
- Supporting clinicians, faculty, and staff so that they can provide an empathic experience for all patients.

It is time to conceptualize women's health in the context of primary care which is personalized to each individual based on sex, gender, and genetics. This conceptual shift will require collaborative and parallel efforts on three fronts: research, education, and clinical care. Researchers need to consider sex and gender as biological variables in study design to provide the evidence on which to base clinical practice. Publishers and editors need to ensure accuracy in the reporting of data by sex and gender, and professional societies need to develop sex- and gender-specific protocols and guidelines. Educators need to incorporate concepts of sex- and gender-based evidence into all levels of health-care education. Primary care providers must incorporate women-specific knowledge and skills and broad concepts of sex and gender into all aspects of health care [48, 50, 85].

Selected Organizations and Resources

The Society of General Internal Medicine (SGIM)

The Women's Health Education Interest Group was formed within the Society of General Internal Medicine (SGIM) in 2001 to foster the ability of women's health educators to network, share resources, lobby, develop uniform curricula, and keep abreast of scientific discoveries. The membership quickly grew to include faculty members from throughout the country. Many of those individuals and their mentees are authors in this book. SGIM has an active commission which sponsors and promotes events in SGBWH and advocates for the promotion of women in academia. The SGIM annual meeting program provides many faculty development opportunities in SGBWH. SGIM, along with other national organizations, are helping to achieve the promise of providing all physicians with a solid foundation for providing the gender-sensitive and specific care that women want and expect (https://www.sgim.org/) [126].

Directory of Residency and Fellowship Programs in Women's Health

Sponsored by the Association of Academic Women's Health Programs (AAWHP), https://womenshealth.vcu.edu/pdf2015/2015DirectoryofResidency.pdf [127], and published in the Journal of Women's Health, the directory describes active programs and provides contact information. "The mission of the AAWHP is to improve the health of women through leadership in research, education clinical models, and community partnerships. This mission is carried out through networking, leadership and mentoring collaborative projects, lobbying and advocacy, political and social commentary, education of policymakers, partnership with national organizations, and creation of interdisciplinary innovative models."

The American Medical Women's Association (AMWA)

AMWA was one of the first organizations concerned with advancing the field of women's health and developed the Advanced Curriculum on Women's Health for faculty development and continuing education (https://www.amwa-doc.org/) [128]. AMWA also sponsors an annual congress on women's health. AMWA is committed to the integration of sex and gender evidence into health professionals' curricula. To this end, AMWA has been a premier sponsor for the 2015, 2018, and 2020 Sex and Gender Health Education Summits (www.sghesummit2018.org) [44].

The Sex and Gender Women's Health Collaborative (SGWHC)

The Sex and Gender Women's Health Collaborative (SGWHC) is now formally a part of AMWA. Founding organizations included the American Medical Women's Association, the College of Women's Health Physicians, and the Society for Women's Health Research. The SGWHC initiated and continues to build a novel digital resource library of sex- and gender-specific materials to be adopted and adapted into medical education and clinical practice, residing at http://www.sgwhc.org [1]. The website also includes a national practitioner database, links to educational materials, and other resources:

- The 2011 collaboration with the National Board of Medical Examiners (NBME) to evaluate the examinations' women's health and sex and gender content [48].
- The 2012 Sex and Gender Medical Education Summit hosted by Mayo Clinic. Online conference report: https://www.liebertpub.com/doi/full/10.1089/jwh.2012.4193 [49].
- The 2015 Sex and Gender Health Education Summit. Online proceedings: https://bsd.biomedcentral.com/articles/supplements/volume-7-supplement-1 [51].
- The 2018 International Sex and Gender Health Education Summit: Advancing Curricula Through a Multidisciplinary Lens. Online proceedings: https://www.sghesummit2018.com/ [44].

Texas Tech Health Sciences Center's Laura W. Bush Institute (TTUHSC LWBI)

TTUHSC LWBI is widely viewed as a global leader for sex and gender health curricular materials. Their website www.sexandgenderhealth.org [129] houses a repository of peer-reviewed sex and gender educational resources. These resources, including slide sets with speaker notes, simulation cases, and interactive modules, have been adapted for use across schools of medicine, pharmacy, nursing, and allied health. LWBI has equally partnered with AMWA and Mayo Clinic on the 2015 and 2018 Sex and Gender Health Education Summits and is committed to future Summit sponsorships.

American College of Obstetricians and Gynecologists: The Women's Preventive Services Initiative (WPSI)

An Advisory Panel comprised of representatives from the American College of Obstetricians and Gynecologists (ACOG) and three other major professional organizations representing the majority of women's health-care providers, including the American Academy of Family Physicians (AAFP), the American College of Physicians (ACP), and the National Association of Nurse Practitioners in Women's Health (NPWH). In addition, three individuals who were members of the Institute of Medicine's 2011 Committee on Preventive Services for Women serve as Advisory Panel members. The Advisory Panel will guide the work of the WPSI and ensure that the initiative delivers a consistent message (https://www.womenspreventivehealth.org/) [130]. ACOG provides numerous resources for the care of women patients, and for patient education through its organization.

National Association of Nurse Practitioners in Women's Health (NPWH)

This organization provides women's health continuing education through a society journal and annual conferences. In addition, there is a mobile app to be used at well-women visits. Members can have joint membership with ACOG (https://npwomenshealthcare.com/about-npwh/) [131].

The National Institutes of Health (NIH) Office for Research on Women's Health (ORWH)

The NIH Sex as a Biological Variable and Inclusion policies help to ensure that women and female biology in general are factored into every stage of research. Sex and gender influence health and disease, and considering these factors in research informs the development of prevention strategies and treatment interventions for both women and men (https://orwh.od.nih.gov/) [132]. A no-cost online course is available to educate clinicians and researchers in the issues related to studying sex and gender differences: https://orwh.od.nih.gov/sex-gender/online-courses-sex-gender-differences [133].

The Society for Women's Health Research

The Society for Women's Health Research (SWHR) is a national nonprofit dedicated to promoting research on biological differences in disease and improving women's health through science, policy, and education (https://swhr.org/) [134].

The Association of American Medical Collges: Group on Women in Medicine and Science

The Association of American Medical Colleges (AAMC) Group on Women in Medicine and Science (GWIMS) "advances the full and successful participation and inclusion of women within academic medicine by addressing gender equity, recruitment and retention, awards and recognition, and career advancement. Advocates for women's advancement and leadership may become members of GWIMS, and those members may be either from the faculty or administration at AAMC member medical schools and teaching hospitals. Their portfolio, formal or informal, may include: gender equity, career advancement, women's recognition, including awards, and women's recruitment and retention throughout the continuum of academic medicine" [from website] (https://www.aamc.org/members/gwims/) [135].

The American College of Physicians (ACP)

The ACP offers learning resources for physicians, with multiple modules applicable to women's health and many offering CME and MOC. Most activities are free to ACP members (https://www.acponline.org/online-learning-center/womens-health) [136].

The American Academy of Famiy Physicians (AAFP)

The AAFP offers its members learning resources and conferences specific to women's health, and is a participant in the multidisicplinary WPSI (https://www.aafp.org) [137].

Summary Points

1. Women's health began as reproductive health but has expanded to include the knowledge that every cell has a sex and that sex and gender aspects of care apply to the whole women.
2. Major research advances include the inclusion of women and minorities in research studies and the realization that sex as a biological variable must be acknowledged in all medical research.
3. Examples of sex-based differences include drug dosages, differences in coronary artery disease between the sexes, and the effect of estrogen in nonreproductive organ systems.
4. The comprehensive primary care of women requires the integration of medical, gynecologic, mental, and breast health domains.
5. Education in SGBWH includes both add-on topics and the integration of sex and gender throughout all topics.
6. The integration of sex- and gender-based women's health into curricula requires needs assessments, champions, learner advocates, content experts, edits of cases through a sex and gender lens, and the support of institutional leaders.
7. Urgent needs and persistent gaps in the sex- and gender-specific care of women include an increased knowledge of genetics, appropriate use of sex and gender terminology, and sex- and gender-based research which breaks out findings by sex and gender.

Review Questions

1. In what year did the National Institutes of Health (NIH) first mandate the inclusion of women in medical research?
   A. 1975
   B. 1980
   C. 1990
   D. 2016
   The correct answer is C. In 1985, the NIH established a task force to study the inclusion of women in medical research. The report led to the mandate that women be included in medical research in 1990. In 1994, the NIH clarified that research results should be reported as men or women, but it was not until 2016 that the NIH required sex as a biological variable be included in all NIH proposals [20, 27, 46].
2. Which of the following is an example of a sex-based difference?
   A. Women like to wear dresses more often than men.
   B. Women are more likely to stay home with children than men.
   C. Women's cells usually have two X chromosomes.
   D. Women tend to be more emotionally expressive than men.
   The correct answer is C. Answers A, B, and D are examples of potential gender differences, which can be studied for their impact on health [46].
3. Which of the following subjects is most neglected in internal medicine training according to surveys of program directors and residents?
   A. Addressing reproductive plans with women.
   B. Mammography screening.
   C. Pelvic exams and Pap tests.
   D. Cardiac risk factors.
   The correct answer is A. Surveys and studies of internal medicine programs reveal that a great need exists for increased training in issues related to reproduction. Addressing reproductive plans, contraception, preconception counseling, and the care of common medical problems during pregnancy are relevant to all primary care but are not sufficiently taught in residency programs. Mammography screening, pelvic exams, and Pap tests and cardiac risk factors are among the women's health subjects which appear to be covered well in many programs. It is important to note that gestational diabetes and hypertensive disorders in pregnancy are sex-specific cardiac risk factors [100–103].
4. Which of the following statements is true about women in academic medicine?
   A. Academic tenure criteria, as a rule, make allowances for the time required for child-raising responsibilities.
   B. Advances in women's health in the 1990s have led to an equal number of women and men ranked as full professors in US medical schools.
   C. Inequities in the pay between men and women faculty vanished in academic medicine due to actions by professional societies.
   D. Promoting leadership for women faculty is considered an important component in the success of women's health programs and curricular change.
   The correct answer is D. The promotion of women to positions of leadership is considered to be a critical step in the sustainability of women's health as a focus in medicine beyond ob-gyn. However, women continue to be underrepresented at the highest ranks of academic medicine despite the increased number of women entering medical school as students. The reasons for inequities in pay and promotion are complex and continue to need remediation within academia. Child-bearing and child-rearing are time-consuming activities over the course of a lifetime, and the impact of this commitment is not fully addressed by tenure and promotion criteria [85, 125].

References

1. Sex and Gender Women's Health Collaborative. http://sgwhc.org/. Accessed April 4, 2019.
2. Kwolek DS. Women's health education: progress and promises. J Gen Intern Med. 2003;18(6):490–1. https://doi.org/10.1046/j.1525-1497.2003.30421.x.
3. Council on Graduate Medical Education. Fifth report on women and medicine. Rockville: U.S. Department of Health and Human Services; 1995.
4. Harrison M. Woman as other: the premise of medicine. JAMWA. 1990;45:225–6.
5. Institute of Medicine. Exploring the biological contributions to human Health: does sex matter? Washington, DC: National Academy Press; 2001.
6. Clancy CM, Massion CT. American women's health care: a patchwork quilt with gaps. JAMA. 1992;268(14):1918–20. https://doi.org/10.1001/jama.268.14.1918.
7. Office of Research on Women's Health. Highlights of NIH Women's Health and Sex Difference Research 1990-2010. https://orwh.od.nih.gov/sites/orwh/files/docs/ORWH-Highlights-2010.pdf. Accessed April 25, 2019.
8. Miller LR, Marks C, Becker JB, et al. Considering sex as a biological variable in preclinical research. FASEB J. 2017;31(1):29–34. https://doi.org/10.1096/fj.201600781R.
9. Donoghue GD. Women's Health in the curriculum: a resource guide for faculty. Philadelphia: National Academy on Women's Health Medical Education; 1996.
10. Pinn VW. Sex and gender factors in medical studies: implications for health and clinical practice. JAMA. 2003;289(4):397–400. https://doi.org/10.1001/jama.289.4.397.
11. James G. Winning in the Women's Health care marketplace: a comprehensive plan for Health care strategists. San Francisco: Jossey-Bass Publishers; 2000.
12. Roter DL, Hall JA, Aoki Y. Physician gender effects in medical communication: a meta-analytic review. JAMA. 2002;288(6):756–64. https://doi.org/10.1001/jama.288.6.756.
13. Carson MP. Society for maternal and fetal medicine workshop on pregnancy as a window to future health: clinical utility of classifying women with metabolic syndrome. Semin Perinatol. 2015;39(4):284–9. https://doi.org/10.1053/j.semperi.2015.05.007.

14. Boston Women's Health Book Collective, Norsigian J. Our Bodies, Ourselves. New York: Simon & Schuster; 2011.
15. Women's health. Report of the public health service task force on women's health issues. Public Health Rep. 1985;100(1):73–106. https://www.ncbi.nlm.nih.gov/pmc/articles/PMC1424718/?page=1 Accessed April 25, 2019
16. McCarthy CR. Historical background of clinical trials involving women and minorities. Acad Med. 1994;69(9):695–8. https://doi.org/10.1097/00001888-199409000-00002.
17. Report of the National Institutes of Health: Opportunities for research on Women's Health (full report) NIH publication no. 92–3457.1993.
18. Pinn VW, Clayton JA, Begg L, Sass SE. Public partnerships for a vision for women's health research in 2020. J Women's Health. 2010;19(9):1603–7. https://doi.org/10.1089/jwh.2010.2386.
19. Women's Health Initiative. The Women's Health Initiative. https://www.whi.org/SitePages/WHI%20Home.aspx. Accessed February 14, 2019.
20. National Institutes of Health. NIH guidelines on the inclusion of women and minorities as subjects in clinical research NIH Guide. 23(11). March 18, 1994. https://grants.nih.gov/grants/guide/notice-files/not94-100.html. Published March 18, 1994. Accessed April 25, 2019.
21. Cassel C, Blank L, Braunstein G, Burke W, Fryhofer SA, Pinn V. What internists need to know: core competencies in women's health. ABIM Subcommittee on Clinical Competence in Women's Health. Am J Med. 1997;102(6):507–12.
22. The Federation Council for Internal Medicine Task Force on Internal Medicine Residency Curriculum. Graduate education in internal medicine: a resource guide to curriculum development. Philadelphia: American College of Physicians; 1997.
23. American Academy of Family Physicians. Recommended core education guidelines for family practice residents: women's health. AAFP Reprint No. 282, April 1994.
24. Carlson KJ, Eisenstat SA. Primary Care of Women. 1st ed: Mosby; 1995.
25. Carr PL, Freund KM. Somani S. The medical care of women. Philadelphia: Saunders; 1995.
26. Wallis LA, Kasper AS. Textbook of Women's Health. Philadelphia: Lippincott-Raven; 1998.
27. U.S. Public Health Service. Agenda for Research on Women's Health for the 21st Century. A Report of the Task Forces on the NIH Women's Health Research Agenda for the 21st Century. National Institutes of Health, pub No 99–4385, Bethesda 1999.
28. Office of Research on Women's Health. Building Interdisciplinary Research in Women's Health (BIRCWH). https://orwh.od.nih.gov/career-development/building-interdisciplinary-research-careers-womens-health-bircwh. Accessed on April 25, 2019.
29. Legato MJ. Principles of gender-specific medicine: Academic Press. Elsevier Academic Press, London, UK; 2004.
30. Legato MJ. Research on the biology of women will improve health care for men, too. Chronicle of Higher Ed May 15, 1998.
31. Frezza M, Padova CD, Pozzato G, Terpin M, Baraona E, Lieber CS. High blood alcohol levels in women. The role of decreased gastric alcohol dehydrogenase activity and first-pass metabolism. N Engl J Med. 1990;322(2):95–9. https://doi.org/10.1056/nejm199001113220205.
32. McClelland RL, Chung H, Detrano R, Post W, Kronmal RA. Distribution of coronary artery calcium by race, gender, and age: results from the Multi-Ethnic Study of Atherosclerosis (MESA). Circulation. 2006;113(1):30–7. https://doi.org/10.1161/circulationaha.105.580696.
33. Pelletier R, Khan NA, Cox J, et al. Sex versus gender-related characteristics. J Am Coll Cardiol. 2016;67(2):27–135. https://doi.org/10.1016/j.jacc.2015.10.067.
34. Scantlebury DC, Borlaug BA. Why are women more likely than men to develop heart failure with preserved ejection fraction? Curr Opin Cardiol. 2011;26(6):562–8. https://doi.org/10.1097/hco.0b013e32834b7faf.
35. Makkar RR, Fromm BS, Steinman RT, Meissner MD, Lehmann MH. Female gender as a risk factor for torsades de pointes associated with cardiovascular drugs. JAMA. 1993;270(21):2590–7. https://doi.org/10.1001/jama.1993.03510210076031.
36. Ubrich R, Barthel P, Haller B, et al. Sex differences in long-term mortality among acute myocardial infarction patients: results from the ISAR-RISK and ART studies. PLoS One. 2017;12(10). https://doi.org/10.1371/journal.pone.0186783.
37. Voskuhl R. Sex differences in autoimmune diseases. Biol Sex Differ. 2011;2(1):1. https://doi.org/10.1186/2042-6410-2-1.
38. Haentjens P, Magaziner J, Colón-Emeric CS, Vanderschueren D, Milisen K, Velkeniers B, et al. Meta-analysis: excess mortality after hip fracture among older women and men. Ann Intern Med. 2010;152(6):380–90. https://doi.org/10.7326/0003-4819-152-6-201003160-00008.
39. Rozen TD, Fishman RS. Female cluster headache in the United States of America: what are the gender differences? J Neurol Sci. 2012;317(1–2):17–28. https://doi.org/10.1016/j.jns.2012.03.006.
40. Sørheim I, Johannessen A, Gulsvik A, Bakke PS, Silverman EK, DeMeo DL. Gender differences in COPD: are women more susceptible to smoking effects than men? Thorax. 2010;65(6):480–5. https://doi.org/10.1136/thx.2009.122002.
41. FDA Drug Safety. FDA requires lower recommended doses for certain drugs containing zolpidem (Ambien, Ambien CR, Edluar, and Zolpimist). January 10, 2013. https://wwwfdagov/drugs/drug-safety/ucm352085htm Accessed April 24, 2019.
42. Henrich JB. Women's health education initiatives: why have they stalled? Acad Med. 2004;79(4):283–8.
43. Werbinski J. AMWA's role in women's health curriculum. J Women's Health. 2008;17(10):1555.
44. Sex and Gender Health Education Summit. Sex and gender Health education summit: advancing curricula through a multidisciplinary Lens https://www.sghesummit2018.com/. Accessed April 24, 2019.
45. Institute of Medicine (IOM). Women's Health Research: progress, pitfalls and promise. Washington, DC: The National Academies Press; 2010.
46. Institute of Medicine (US) Board on Population Health and Public Health Practice. Sex-specific reporting of scientific research: a workshop summary. 2012. https://doi.org/10.17226/13307.
47. Conger K. Of mice, men and women making research more inclusive. Stanford Medicine Magazine. Spring 2017. https://stanmed.stanford.edu/2017spring/how-sex-and-gender-which-are-not-the-same-thing-influence-our-health.html. Accessed April 25, 2019.
48. McGregor AJ, Templeton K, Kleinman MR, Jenkins MR. Advancing sex and gender competency in medicine: sex & gender women's health collaborative. Biol Sex Differ. 2013;4(1):11. https://doi.org/10.1186/2042-6410-4-11.
49. Miller VM, Rice M, Schiebinger L, et al. Embedding concepts of sex and gender health differences into medical curricula. J Women's Health. 2013;22(3):194–202. https://doi.org/10.1089/jwh.2012.4193.
50. Chin EL, Hoggatt M, McGregor AJ, Rojek MK, Templeton K, Casanova R, Klein WS, Miller VM, Jenkins M. Sex and gender in medical education, and proceedings from the 2015 Sex and Gender Education Summit. Biol Sex Differ. 2016;7(Suppl 1) https://bsd.biomedcentral.com/articles/supplements/volume-7-supplement-1. Accessed April 24, 2019
51. Henderson J, Weisman C. Women's patterns of provider use across the lifespan and satisfaction with primary care coordination

and comprehensiveness. Med Care. 2005;43(8):826–33. https://doi.org/10.1097/01.mlr.0000170422.73033.eb.
52. Susan G Komen for the Cure. Breast Cancer Foundation. https://ww5.komen.org/. Updated 2019. Accessed April 24, 2019.
53. Massachusetts General Hospital. About Women's Health Associates. https://www.massgeneral.org/wha/about/ Accessed February 14, 2019.
54. VA Health Care for Women: Despite Progress, improvements needed. HRD-92-23: Published: Jan 23, 1992. Publicly Released: Feb 3, 1992. https://www.gao.gov/products/HRD-92-23 Accessed April 24, 2019.
55. Kwolek DS, Popham J, Caudill TS. VA Women's Health Center as an ambulatory training site. Acad Med. 1998;73(5):606.
56. Tilstra SA, Kraemer KL, Rubio DM, Mcneil MA. Evaluation of VA women's health fellowships: developing leaders in academic women's health. J Gen Intern Med. 2013;28(7):901–7. https://doi.org/10.1007/s11606-012-2306-z.
57. Challa VR, Swamyvelu K, Shetty N. Assessment of the clinical utility of the Gail model in estimating the risk of breast cancer in women from the Indian population. Ecancermedicalscience. 2013;7:363. https://doi.org/10.3332/ecancer.2013.363.
58. Weitzel JN, Clague J, Martir-Negron A, et al. Prevalence and type of BRCA mutations in Hispanics undergoing genetic cancer risk assessment in the southwestern United States: a report from the Clinical Cancer Genetics Community Research Network [published correction appears in J Clin Oncol. 2013 May 1;31(13):1702]. J Clin Oncol. 2012;31(2):210–6. https://doi.org/10.1200/JCO.2011.41.0027.
59. Donoghue GD, Hoffman E, Magrane D. Special theme issue: a new and wider view-women's health as a catalyst for reform of medical education. Acad Med. 2000;75(11):1056–60.
60. Adapted from: Lowey NM. Women's health and medical school curricula. Acad Med. 1994;69(4):280–1.
61. Women's health in the medical school curriculum: Report of a survey and recommendations. Corp author(s): United States; Health Resources and Services Administration; National Institutes of Health (U.S.); Office of Research on Women's Health; United States; Public Health service; office on Women's Health. Publication: [Rockville, Md.]: U.S. Dept. of Health and human services, Health Resources and Services Administration: National Institutes of Health, Year: 1997.
62. Women's Health curricula: final report on expert panel recommendations for Interprofessional collaboration across the Health professions May 2013 U.S. Department of Health and Human Services Health Resources and Services Administration Office of Women's Health. https://www.hrsa.gov/sites/default/files/about/organization/bureaus/owh/report111413.pdf.
63. Bartman BA, Weiss KB. Women's primary care in the United States: a study of practice variations among physician specialties. J Women's Health. 1993;2(3):261–8.
64. Magrane DM. Women's health education for medical students: an interdisciplinary response. Womens Health Issues. 1997;7(4):248–52.
65. Cain JM, Donoghue GD, Magrane DM, Rusch RB. APGO interdisciplinary Women's Health education retreat. Executive summary. Am J Obstet Gynecol. 2002;187(Suppl 3):S4–8.
66. Henrich JB, Viscoli CM. What do medical schools teach about women's health and gender differences? Acad Med. 2006;81(5):476–82. https://doi.org/10.1097/01.ACM.0000222268.60211.fc.
67. Henrich JB, Viscoli CM, Abraham GD. Medical students' assessment of education and training in women's health and in sex and gender differences. J Womens Health (Larchmt). 2008;17(5):815–27. https://doi.org/10.1089/jwh.2007.0589.
68. Kuzma MA, Rutenberg CL, Gracely E, Nieman LZ. The effect of incorporating women's health into a PBL curriculum on students' tendencies to identify learning issues in an ambulatory care setting. Acad Med. 1997;72(10):913–5.
69. Robertson PA, Brown JS, Flanagan TA, et al. The Women's Health curriculum by problem-based learning method from medical students at the University of California, San Francisco. Am J Obstet Gynecol. 1997;176(6):1368–73.
70. Levison SP, Weiss LB, Puglia CD, Nieman LZ, Donoghue GD. A model for integrating women's health issues into a problem-based curriculum. J Women's Health. 1998;7(9):1113–24.
71. Zebrack JR, Mitchell JL, Davids SL, Simpson DE. Web-based curriculum. A practical and effective strategy for teaching women's health. J Gen Intern Med. 2005;20(1):68–74. https://doi.org/10.1111/j.1525-1497.2005.40062.x.
72. Kwolek DS, Blue AV, Griffith CH 3rd. Integrating women's health issues into third-year medical and surgical curricula. Acad Med 1997;72(5):422.
73. Kwolek DS, Blue AV, Griffith CH 3rd, Wilson JF, Haist SA. Gender differences in clinical evaluation: narrowing the gap with women's health clinical skills workshops. Acad Med. 1998;73(Suppl 10):S88–90.
74. Kwolek DS, Grigsby DG, Nora LM. Chancellor's educational retreat for interdisciplinary faculty development in women's health. Acad Med. 2000;75(5):557–8.
75. Kwolek DS, Nora LM, Nash P. A women's health course for education in internal medicine. Acad Med. 1999;74(5):593–4.
76. Weiss LB, Lee S, Levison SP. Barriers and solutions to implementing a new curriculum: lessons from the women's health education program at MCP Hahnemann School of Medicine. J Womens Health Gend Based Med. 2004;9(2):153–60. https://doi.org/10.1089/152460900318641.
77. Nunez A, Kwolek D, McLean A, Taylor A. The consortium for Women's Health education. J Womens Health Gend Based Med. 2000;9(4):458.
78. Kwolek DS, Grigsby D, Norman C, Skelton J, West K. "Multidisciplinary Instructional Models for Women's Health Education". Fund for the Improvement of Post Secondary Education, Current Project Descriptions Office of Post Secondary Education/U.S. Department of Education/November 2000.
79. Jensen LA, Lock SE, Kwolek DS. An interdisciplinary approach to women's health education using the structured clinical instructional module. In: Guberski T, editor. New paradigms in advanced nursing practice: teaching and technological strategies in nurse practitioner education. Washington, DC: National Organization of Nurse Practitioner Faculties; 2003. p. 28–31.
80. Skelton J, West K, Kwolek D. Curriculum assessment of gender/sex issues by student dentists. J Womens Health Gend Based Med. 2000;9(4):457.
81. Kwolek DS, Donnelly MB, Carr E, Sloan DA, Haist SA. Need for comprehensive women's health continuing medical education among primary care physicians. J Contin Educ Heal Prof. 2000;20(1):33–8. https://doi.org/10.1002/chp.1340200107.
82. Kwolek DS, Witzke D, Sloan DA. Assessing the need for faculty development in women's health among internal medicine and family practice teaching faculty. J Wo Health Gend Based Med. 1999;8(9):1195–201. https://doi.org/10.1089/jwh.1.1999.8.1195.
83. Jenkins MR, Herrmann A, Tashjian A, et al. Sex and gender in medical education: a national student survey. Biol Sex Differ. 2016;7(Suppl 1) https://doi.org/10.1186/s13293-016-0094-6.
84. Song MM, Jones BG, Casanova RA. Auditing sex- and gender-based medicine (SGBM) content in medical school curriculum: a student scholar model. Biol Sex Differ. 2016;7(Suppl 1):40. https://doi.org/10.1186/s13293-016-0102-x.
85. Jenkins MR, Miller V. 21st century Women's Health: refining with precision. Mayo Clin Proc. 2016;91(6):695–700. https://doi.org/10.1016/j.mayocp.2016.03.017.
86. Chin EL, Hoggatt M, McGregor AJ, et al. Sex and gender medical education summit: a roadmap for curricular innovation.

Biol Sex Differ. 2016;7(Suppl 1):52. https://doi.org/10.1186/s13293-016-0091-9.
87. Spagnoletti CL, Rubio DM, McNeil MA. Internal medicine residents' preparedness to care for reproductive-age and pregnant women. Teach Learn Med. 2007;19(3):257–63. https://doi.org/10.1080/10401330701366549.
88. Day SC, Cassel CK, Kimball HR. Training internists in women's health: recommendations for educators. Am J Med. 1996;100(4):375–9.
89. https://www.acog.org/About-ACOG/ACOG-Departments/Annual-Womens-Health-Care/Womens-Preventive-Services-InitiativeWomen's Preventive Services Initiative. Recommendations for well-woman care: a well-woman chart. Washington, DC: ACOG Foundation; 2018.
90. American Board of Obstetrics and Gynecology Bulletin for 1997. Dallas, Texas: American board of. Obstet Gynecol. 1996;
91. Parsey KS, Bastian LA, Couchman GM, Slack KD, Simel DL. The development of a primary care curriculum for obstetrics/gynecology residents. JAMWA. 1998;53(Suppl 3):137–9.
92. Lowey NM. Review of APGO women's health curricula proposal. Womens Health Issues. 1996;6(4):192–3.
93. Nelson M, Nicolette J, Johnson K. Integration or evolution: women's health as a model for interdisciplinary change in medical education. Acad Med. 1997;72(9):737–40.
94. Spencer AL, McNeil M. Interdisciplinary curriculum to train internal medicine and obstetrics-gynecology residents in ambulatory women's health: adapting problem-based learning to residency education. J Womens Health (Larchmt). 2009;18(9):1369–75. https://doi.org/10.1089/jwh.2008.1253.
95. Henrich JB, Chambers JT, Steiner JL. Development of an interdisciplinary women's health training model. Acad Med. 2003;78(9):877–84.
96. Carson MP, Ehrenthal D. Medical issues from preconception through delivery: a roadmap for the internist. Med Clin North Am. 2008;92(5):1193–225. https://doi.org/10.1016/j.mcna.2008.04.010.
97. The American College of Physicians. Comprehensive women's health care: the role and commitment of internal medicine. Am J Med. 1997;103:451–7.
98. American Board of Internal Medicine. Policies and Procedures for Certification. June 2019. https://www.abim.org/~/media/ABIM%20Public/Files/pdf/publications/certification-guides/policies-and-procedures.pdf Accessed April 24, 2019.
99. ABIM Exam Content and Blue Print. https://www.abim.org/~/media/ABIM%20Public/Files/pdf/exam-blueprints/certification/internal-medicine.pdf. Accessed 5/30/2019.
100. Wayne DB, DaRosa DA. Evaluating and enhancing a women's health curriculum in an internal medicine residency program. J Gen Intern Med. 2004;19(7):754–9. https://doi.org/10.1111/j.1525-1497.2004.30017.x.
101. Davisson L, Nuss M, Cottrell S. Women's health curriculum for internal medicine residents: development, implementation, and evaluation. J Grad Med Educ. 2010;2(3):398–403. https://doi.org/10.4300/JGME-D-09-00069.1.
102. Hsieh E, Nunez-Smith M, Hendrich JB. Needs and priorities in women's health training: perspectives from an internal medicine residency program. J Women's Health. 2013;22(8):667–72. https://doi.org/10.1089/jwh.2013.4264.
103. Casas RS, Hallett LD, Rich CA, Gerber MR, Battaglia TA. Program directors' perceptions of resident education in women's health: a national survey. J Women's Health. 2017;26(2):133–40. https://doi.org/10.1089/jwh.2016.5860.
104. Farkas AH, Tilstra S, Borrero S, McNeil M. Establishing consensus on residency education in women's health. J Women's Health. 2017;26(1):13–7. https://doi.org/10.1089/jwh.2016.5859.
105. Spencer AL, Kern LM. Primary care program directors' perceptions of women's health education: a gap in graduate medical education persists. J Womens Health (Larchmt). 2008;17(4):549–56. https://doi.org/10.1089/jwh.2007.0473.
106. Zhang CM, Insetta ER, Caufield-Noll C, Levine RB. Women's health curricula in internal medicine residency programs: a scoping review. J Womens Health (Larchmt). 2019; https://doi.org/10.1089/jwh.2018.7317.
107. Dixon JG, Bognar BA, Keyserling TC, et al. Teaching women's health skills: confidence, attitudes and practice patterns of academic generalist physician. J Gen Intern Med. 2003;18(6):411–8. https://doi.org/10.1046/j.1525-1497.2003.10511.x.
108. Internal Medicine Residency Program of UPMC and the University of Pittsburgh. Women's Health Track. https://residency.dom.pitt.edu/program/tracks/womens-health/. Accessed April 25, 2019.
109. Directory of Residency and Fellowship Programs in Women's Health. Directory of residency and fellowship programs in Women's Health, 2016. J Women's Health. 2016;25(5) https://doi.org/10.1089/jwh.2016.dir10.
110. Pursley HG, Kwolek DS. A women's health track for internal medicine residents using evidence-based medicine. Acad Med. 2002;77(7):743–4.
111. Spencer AL, Bost JE, McNeil M. Do women's health internal medicine residency tracks make a difference? J Womens Health (Larchmt). 2007;16(8):1219.
112. Farkas AH, Vanderberg R, McNeil M, et al. The impact of women's health residency tracks on career outcomes. J Womens Health (Larchmt). 2018;27(7):927–32. https://doi.org/10.1089/jwh.2017.6739.
113. Donoghue GD, National Academy on Women's Health Medical Education (NAWHME). In Donoghue GD, editor. Women's Health in the curriculum: a resource guide for the faculty. 1st ed. NAWHME;1996.
114. Foreman H, Weber L, Thacker HL. Update: a review of women's health fellowships, their role in interdisciplinary health care, and the need for accreditation. J Womens Health (Larchmt). 2015;24(5):336–40. https://doi.org/10.1089/jwh.2014.5187.
115. Carnes M, Vogelman B. Women's health fellowships: examining the potential benefits and harms of accreditation. J Womens Health (Larchmt). 2015;24(5):341–8. https://doi.org/10.1089/jwh.2015.5289.
116. Nurse Practitioners in Women's Health (NPWH). 22nd Annual Premier Women's Healthcare Conference (19–03). NPWH. https://www.npwh.org/events/conferences/details/44. Accessed May 31, 2019.
117. 2018 ADEA and ORWH co-sponsor expert roundtable Women's Helath in Interprofessional Education and Collaborative Care ADEA Bulletin of Dental Education> November 2018, Volume 51, Issue 11 > ADEA Co-sponsors Convening on Women's Health in Interprofessional Education and Collaborative Care https://www.adea.org/ADEA/Blogs/Bulletin_of_Dental_Education/ADEA_Co-sponsors_Convening_on_Women_s_Health_in_Interprofessional_Education_and_Collaborative_Care.html.
118. FDA Office of Women's Health research impact and outcomes framework guide to developing an organizational impact and outcomes measurement tool for program assessment and reporting, April 2018. https://www.fda.gov/downloads/ScienceResearch/SpecialTopics/WomensHealthResearch/UCM603175.pdf. Accessed June 15, 2019.
119. Drago R, Williams J. A half-time tenure-track proposal. Change: The Magazine of Higher Learning. 2000;32(6):47–8. https://doi.org/10.1080/00091380009601787.
120. https://www.aaup.org/AAUP/pubsres/policydocs/contents/workfam-stmt.htm#b7. Accessed May 31, 2109.
121. Russell A. The second shift Hochschild 2012.
122. Jacobson CC, Nguyen JC, Kimball AB. Gender and parenting significantly affect work hours of recent dermatology program graduates. Arch Dermatol. 2004;140(2):191–6. https://doi.org/10.1001/archderm.140.2.191.

123. Jolly S, Griffith KA, DeCastro R, Stewart A, Ubel P, Jagsi R. Gender differences in time spent on parenting and domestic responsibilities by high-achieving young physician-researchers. Ann Intern Med. 2014;160(5):344–53. https://doi.org/10.7326/m13-0974.
124. Carnes M, Morrissey C, Geller SE. Women's health and women's leadership in academic medicine: hitting the same glass ceiling? J Womens Health (Larchmt). 2008;17(9):1453–62. https://doi.org/10.1089/jwh.2007.0688.
125. Carnes M, Johnson P, Klein W, Jenkins M, Merz CNB. Advancing women's health and women's leadership with endowed chairs in women's health. Acad Med. 2017;92(2):167–74. https://doi.org/10.1097/ACM.0000000000000142.
126. The Society of General Internal Medicine (SGIM). https://www.sgim.org/. Accessed June 15, 2019.
127. Directory of Residency and Fellowship Programs in Women's Health Sponsored by the Association of Academic Women's Health Programs (AAWHP), https://womenshealth.vcu.edu/pdf2015/2015DirectoryofResidency.pdf. Accessed June 15, 2019.
128. The American Medical Women's Association (AMWA). https://www.amwa-doc.org/. Accessed August 29, 2019.
129. Texas Tech Health Sciences Center's Laura W. Bush Institute (TTUHSC LWBI). http://www.sgwhc.org. Accessed June 15, 2019.
130. The Women's Preventive Services Initiative (WPSI). https://www.womenspreventivehealth.org/. Accessed June 15, 2019.
131. National Association of Nurse Practitioners in Women's Health (NPWH). https://npwomenshealthcare.com/about-npwh/. Accessed June 15, 2019.
132. The NIH Office for Research on Women's Health. https://orwh.od.nih.gov/. Accessed June 15, 2019.
133. https://orwh.od.nih.gov/sex-gender/online-courses-sex-gender-differences. Accessed June 15, 2019.
134. The Society for Women's Health Research. https://swhr.org/. Accessed June 15, 2019.
135. The American Association of Medical Colleges (AAMC) Group on Women in Medicine and Science (GWIMS). https://www.aamc.org/members/gwims/. Accessed June 15, 2019.
136. The American College of Physicians (ACP). https://www.acponline.org/online-learning-center/womens-health. Accessed June 15, 2019.
137. The American Academy of Family Physicians. https://aafp.org/. Accessed August 30, 2020.

High-Value Health Care: Perspectives from the Sex- and Gender-based Care Lens

2

Julie L. Mitchell

Learning Objectives

1. Describe the elements of the quadruple aim and gender differences in access, quality, cost, and care experience.
2. Compare and contrast examples of low-value and high-value care in women.
3. Describe strategies to achieve high-value care for women including systems engineering, shared decision-making, and best use of care teams.
4. Explain how pay-for-value arrangements can improve care in women.
5. Discuss the impact of care disparities and social determinants of health and the importance of gender equity and advocacy.

Barb, a 68-year-old retired administrative assistant, returns to your office for a prevention visit. She explicitly requests this visit be coded as a Medicare annual wellness visit. Barb asks for ovarian cancer screening, specifically an ultrasound and CA-125 test, as has been done the last few years annually. About 10 years ago, her sister had ductal breast cancer in situ, *and she has always been worried about cancer. She also comes to her appointment with a newspaper article on cholesterol medications and has some questions about it.*

Quadruple Aim: Better Care, Healthier People, Smarter Spend, and Joy in Work

Excellence in health care is a balancing act: It is the art of providing the right care at the right time in the right place to the right person in the right way. High-value care means timely access to necessary care and not more. It means care is provided in the emergency department when it is an emergency, in the hospital when the condition is acute, and in the clinic or at home otherwise. Moreover, it means care that is individualized to the needs of the patient and put into the context of the woman's life (medical, social, psychologic, and spiritual). Primary care providers, with comprehensive training, continuity practices, and relationship-centered attitudes, are well suited to provide high-value care and, indeed, they do [1].

The triple aim of quality, affordability, and patient experience was first described as "care, health, and cost" by Don Berwick and others [2]. Recognizing the potential to burn out providers while attempting to meet the triple aim, Bodenheimer and Sinsky added a fourth aim: "improved work life of health-care providers," shortened to "joy in work" [3]. Underscoring the importance of this fourth aim, one set of primary care redesign architects found that achieving health-care excellence was critically dependent on the engagement of the physicians and other team members providing care [4].

Access to Care Including Prevention

One component of high-value care is access to care, which is dependent on insurance status for American women. In a 2016 survey, 59% of women aged 18–64 years were enrolled in employer-sponsored health insurance, a rate that is similar to men [5]. Yet women are more likely than men to be covered by government-sponsored insurance: 21% of non-elderly adult women report Medicaid or other public insurance vs. 17% of men, and 55% of Medicaid beneficiaries

J. L. Mitchell (✉)
Medical College of Wisconsin, Milwaukee, WI, USA
e-mail: jmitchel@mcw.edu

S. A. Tilstra et al. (eds.), *Sex- and Gender-Based Women's Health*, https://doi.org/10.1007/978-3-030-50695-7_2

are female. Medicaid covers low-income women and children, but eligibility varies notably by state statute and policies. For example, the percent of women aged 18–64 years reporting Medicaid insurance ranges from 8 to 31% by state [5]. Women who are older than 65 or who are disabled are eligible for Medicare; 55% of Medicare beneficiaries are women [5].

Prevention is a coverage requirement for all health plans compliant with the Affordable Care Act. United States Preventive Services Task Force (USPSTF) grade A–B recommendations are the standard for preventive benefits [6]. In practice, many women nonetheless end up paying some out-of-pocket costs for prevention: women in private health plans reported some personal expenditures for Pap and related services (23%) and for mammograms (16%) [7].

For women enrolled in Medicare, like in our case, the annual wellness visit (AWV) is an opportunity to review risks, provide preventive care, and choose evidence-based high-value services. Medicare purposefully designed their benefits to include a free annual visit for prevention with its own billing code. Non-Medicare plans also accept an annual prevention visit billed with a prevention code. The use of these prevention codes saves out-of-pocket costs for patients and potentially assists in tracking for continuous process improvement.

Experience of Care: Communication, Relationships, and Teams

Patient experience has become an established, measurable dimension of high-value care [8]. Some have argued that "patient satisfaction" isn't a valid measure of quality either because patients, as laypersons, are unable to assess care or because patients are only satisfied when they are happy, healthy, or receive the services (tests, medications) they think they need. However, several studies have shown correlation between patient experience ratings and more traditional measures of quality, such as adherence to clinical treatment guidelines, and this correlation persists when adjusted for patient mix and when patients are directed to evaluate their experience (not their feelings). Patient-reported experience surveys are best used to evaluate patient-provider interactions, especially when specific to a certain event or service (such as a hospitalization) and closely timed to that event or service. Additionally, there is evidence that when patients are more engaged with their care, patients may choose less resource use rather than more [8].

Women's roles in society and unique needs as patients can lead to expectations and preferences that differ from those of male patients. For all patients, communication is a critical part of high-value care; history taking, shared decision-making, patient education, motivational interviewing, and documenting a care plan all require effective communication skills. While patients from both genders prefer a participatory decision-making style [9], there are gender differences in expectations that affect patients' satisfaction with care. For example, in clinic visits, women base their satisfaction level on "informational content, continuity of care, and multidisciplinarity," while men look to "personal interest shown in them by their providers" [10].

Some women prefer female providers, clinics set up for only women and one-stop shopping for women's health care. To that end, specialized women's health clinics meet a marketing need, although it is not clear if these clinics provide care of higher value [11]. Women of reproductive age can receive primary care either from primary care specialties (like internal medicine or family medicine) or from obstetrics-gynecology; this care may or may not be coordinated. Health-care organizations who wish to be successful in providing high-value care must seek to create comprehensive, coordinated options for women.

In contrast to men, women are more likely to serve as the family caregiver, bringing kids and older adults to their doctor appointments and influencing the motivations and health behaviors of the adult men in their lives. In a 2016 survey, 79% of mothers indicated they usually decide about their children's doctor, compared to only 22% in a similar survey of fathers [7]. Additionally, about 80% of those working in health care, a field that employs about 10% of American workers, are women; yet only 40% of health-care leaders are women [12]. These roles in society may influence women's expectations and agendas when coming to care.

To help provide high-value care, primary care physicians working in advanced medical homes lead care teams consisting of nurses, medical assistants, patient care representatives, and others. These care teams can extend the reach of physicians, improve care quality, and bring improved job satisfaction to all care team members [4, 13, 14]. To achieve these outcomes, all team members must work collaboratively with clear, standard processes and have the tools they need to do their job. Everyone on the team can benefit from working at the top of their license and actively incorporating the expertise each team member brings.

There are many ways care teams can create high value. Some examples include constructing visits for specific time with care team members depending on the visit concern; using pre-visit planning, rooming, and outreach to address clinical care gaps; and training nurses in patient education and shared decision-making. For instance, a clinic appointment may have 10 min budgeted for rooming, with an appointment time for check-in and an appointment time for the physician 10 min later. At rooming, a nurse may provide and review preventive care pamphlets or electronic links, a scribe may document the history and exam, and a nurse may pend the requested diagnostic code/revenue code combination for the physician to sign. Finally, care teams may help patients by extending their reach outside the health system, connecting patients with community organizations (such as support groups or city health departments), and taking advantage of medical management resources (such as a nurse line or social workers) at patients' health insurance companies.

In addition to improved job satisfaction, advanced medical homes with features of accessible coordinated care, patient-centered communication, and team-based care are associated with higher patient experience ratings [15]. Moreover, patient experience ratings suffer when physicians turnover [16]: further evidence to the interdependence of the elements of the quadruple aim.

Your medical assistant enters Barb's concerns (annual wellness visit, requests for ovarian cancer screening, newspaper article on cholesterol medications) in your electronic health record while you review previous testing. For the past 10 years, Barb has had annual pelvic ultrasounds and CA-125 tests that have been negative. On history, she has no symptoms of ovarian or breast cancer and no updates to her family history.

High-Value Care and Strategies to Improve Value

Value is defined as quality divided by cost. High-value care may be care that provides clinical excellence (high quality), is inexpensive (low cost), or, more commonly, is both. Low-value care is care that is ill-advised, expensive, or both. Currently, American health-care practices include substantial waste: About one-fifth of care is likely unnecessary, and about one-fifth of our spend is likely wasted, based on surveys of physicians and published reports [17, 18]. In an analysis of 1.5 million commercially insured patients, Reid found 8% received low-value services in 2013, representing $33 million or $22 per person [19]. In Oregon, Charlesworth found similar rates of low-value services (11–15%) between populations insured by Medicaid and commercial plans, with geographic variations suggesting physician practice patterns are the primary explanation [20]. In Medicare populations, Schwartz found 25% of beneficiaries were affected by low-value services [21].

In general, one can define high-value preventive care as care that is recommended as Grade A or B by the USPSTF (see Table 2.1). High-value care interventions can be found in evidence-based guidelines that weigh cost as well as quality. Increasingly, research studies are reporting not only the

Table 2.1 High-value preventive services in women, defined as USPSTF recommendations with Grades A–B (including only those recommendations that are different than for men) [6]

Population	Recommendation	USPSTF Grade
Age-based recommendations		
Women aged 21–65 years	The USPSTF recommends screening for cervical cancer every 3 years with cervical cytology alone in women aged 21–29 years. For women aged 30 to 65 years, the USPSTF recommends screening every 3 years with cervical cytology alone, every 5 years with high-risk human papillomavirus (hrHPV) testing alone, or every 5 years with hrHPV testing in combination with cytology (cotesting)	A
Women of reproductive age	The USPSTF recommends that clinicians screen for intimate partner violence (IPV) and provide or refer women who screen positive to ongoing support services	B
Women aged 50–74 years	The USPSTF recommends biennial screening mammography	B
Women 65 years and older	The USPSTF recommends screening for osteoporosis with bone measurement testing to prevent osteoporotic fractures	B
In pregnant women		
All pregnant women	The USPSTF recommends that clinicians screen all pregnant women for HIV, including those who present in labor who are untested and whose HIV status is unknown	A
	The USPSTF recommends screening for hepatitis B virus (HBV) infection in pregnant women at their first prenatal visit	A
	The USPSTF recommends early screening for syphilis infection in all pregnant women	A
	The USPSTF recommends screening for preeclampsia in pregnant women with blood pressure measurements throughout pregnancy	B
	The USPSTF recommends that clinicians ask all pregnant women about tobacco use, advise them to stop using tobacco, and provide behavioral interventions for cessation to pregnant women who use tobacco	A
Pregnant women and new mothers	The USPSTF recommends providing interventions during pregnancy and after birth to support breastfeeding	B

(continued)

Table 2.1 (continued)

Population	Recommendation	USPSTF Grade
Pregnant women, during the first pregnancy-related care visit	The USPSTF strongly recommends Rh(D) blood typing and antibody	A
Pregnant women at 12–16 weeks' gestation	The USPSTF recommends screening for asymptomatic bacteriuria with urine culture for pregnant women at 12–16 weeks' gestation or at their first prenatal visit, if later	A
Asymptomatic pregnant women, after 24 weeks of gestation	The USPSTF recommends screening for gestational diabetes mellitus (GDM)	B
Selected pregnant women		
Pregnant women who are at high risk for preeclampsia	The USPSTF recommends the use of low-dose aspirin (81 mg/day) as preventive medication after 12 weeks of gestation	B
Unsensitized Rh(D)-negative pregnant women	The USPSTF recommends repeated Rh(D) antibody testing for all unsensitized Rh(D)-negative women at 24–28 weeks' gestation, unless the biological father is known to be Rh(D) negative	B
Women at increased risk		
Postmenopausal women younger than 65 years at increased risk of osteoporosis	The USPSTF recommends screening for osteoporosis with bone measurement testing to prevent osteoporotic fractures in postmenopausal women younger than 65 years who are at increased risk of osteoporosis, as determined by a formal clinical risk assessment tool	B
Women who have family members with breast, ovarian, tubal, or peritoneal cancer	The USPSTF recommends that primary care providers screen with one of several screening tools designed to identify a family history that may be associated with an increased risk for potentially harmful mutations in breast cancer susceptibility genes (*BRCA1* or *BRCA2*). Women with positive screening results should receive genetic counseling and, if indicated after counseling, BRCA testing	B
Women who are at increased risk for breast cancer	The USPSTF recommends that clinicians engage in shared, informed decision-making with women who are at increased risk for breast cancer about medications to reduce their risk. For women who are at increased risk for breast cancer and at low risk for adverse medication effects, clinicians should offer to prescribe risk-reducing medications, such as tamoxifen or raloxifene	B
Sexually active women		
Sexually active women	The USPSTF recommends screening for chlamydia and gonorrhea in sexually active women age 24 years and younger and in older women who are at increased risk for infection	B
Women who are planning or capable of pregnancy	The USPSTF recommends that all women who are planning or capable of pregnancy take a daily supplement containing 0.4–0.8 mg (400–800 µg) of folic acid	A

health outcomes of interventions but also their cost-effectiveness in terms of dollars per quality-adjusted life-year (QALY) [22]. This measure serves to compare a variety of interventions in a standard way, though it is difficult to pick a single cutoff for "high-value care," given that society's willingness to pay for a given service depends on the context (high-resource or low-resource environment), the case (the age of the individual, the condition, and the alternatives), and individual patient preferences. For these reasons, there is no universally accepted threshold for cost-effective care. Importantly, physicians and provider groups can increase high-value care by improving adherence to evidence-based practices. This is the usual quality work many hospitals and clinics perform and certainly a goal of primary care. A critical complementary strategy is to avoid *low-value* care. Commonly performed low-value care services are starting to be defined, particularly by the Choosing Wisely campaign [23] and researchers studying overuse in Medicare populations [24]. The common low-value services in these lists are manageable in number, and so adjusting practice patterns to address these services may also be manageable. While an important starting point, some argue that these lists focus more on clinical practices that have little value ("no value care") rather than looking critically at the cost-effectiveness [25]. For example, only 2% of the Choosing Wisely recommendations cited cost-effectiveness research [25].

In prioritizing the implementation of interventions that increase value, it is useful for both providers and patients to remember that we all take responsibility for the overall cost of health care, and we all pay for it as well, since the market reacts to high spending by increasing premiums or refusing to pay for certain services. Moreover, "when society spends on low-value healthcare, it's coming at the expense of doing things like hiring more teachers, hiring more police officers, rebuilding our schools, and rebuilding our infrastructure" [26]. While these principles apply to women's as well as men's health care, the overall cost of care for women is higher than for men, primarily because of maternity care, and so improving the rate of high-value care in women may have more impact overall.

In the future, precision medicine may help us better define the circumstances that make services high value. Consider breast cancer screening with mammography, where the current recommendations are largely based simply on age. Yet like all screening tests, the effectiveness of mammography in reducing cancer deaths depends on the risk of the population for breast cancer. While age is the strongest risk factor for breast cancer, other epidemiologic and genetic risk factors change the pretest probability. What if we screened based on risk, omitting routine mammography on low-risk individuals over age 50? In a modeling study, Pashayan and colleagues demonstrated that risk-stratified screening, compared to age-based screening, resulted in 71% fewer overdiagnoses and about $720,000 in savings, with the trade-off of 9.6% fewer breast cancer deaths averted [27]. In terms of absolute risk, this model resulted in 262 breast cancer deaths, 23 more than if using an age-based strategy, but also only 30 cases of overdiagnosis, 75 less than if using an age-based strategy. This risk-stratified scenario, where the threshold for high risk was a 10-year risk of 3.24%, had the highest net monetary benefit, was cost-effective (about $26,000 per QALY), improved the benefit-to-harm ratio, and largely maintained the benefits of screening. Notably, a shift from age-based to precision-based screening requires a shift in thinking; currently, the barriers are numerous, including de-implementation of low-risk screening, a willingness to prioritize preventing the harms of screening, and incorporation of genomic testing into practice [28].

In our case, the patient requested ovarian cancer tests and imaging, which is a preventive service since she has no signs or symptoms. Ovarian cancer screening is not recommended by the USPSTF [6]. Additionally, Choosing Wisely specifically calls this out as a low-value service [29]. A sample of low-value services, including services with Grade D rating by the USPSTF, relevant recommendations from Choosing Wisely, and items specific to women and on researchers' low-value lists, is in Table 2.2.

Table 2.2 A sample of low-value women's health services [6, 21, 29]

Population	Recommendation	Reference
Asymptomatic women who do not have a high-risk hereditary cancer syndrome	The USPSTF, Society for Gynecologic Oncologists, and ACOG recommend against screening for ovarian cancer in asymptomatic women	[6, 29]
Asymptomatic women	American Society of Clinical Pathologists recommends against population-based screening for 25-OH vitamin D deficiency	[29]
Nonpregnant women	American Academy of Family Physicians recommends against performing pelvic exams on asymptomatic women, unless necessary for guideline-appropriate screening for cervical cancer	[29]
Women who have never smoked	The USPSTF recommends against screening for abdominal aortic aneurysms	[6]
Women not at increased risk for breast cancer	The USPSTF recommends against both 1) routine genetic counseling or BRCA testing in women whose family history is not associated with an increased risk for potentially harmful mutations in the BRCA1 or BRCA2 genes and 2) the routine use of medications, such as tamoxifen or raloxifene, for risk reduction of primary breast cancer in women who are not at increased risk for breast cancer	[6]
Women older than 65 years and women younger than 21 years	The USPSTF, ACOG, and the American Academy of Family Physicians recommend against screening for cervical cancer in women older than 65 years who have had adequate prior screening and are not otherwise at high risk for cervical cancer and women younger than 21 years	[6, 21, 29]
Women who have had a hysterectomy	The USPSTF recommends against screening for cervical cancer in women who have had a hysterectomy with removal of the cervix and do not have a history of a high-grade precancerous lesion (i.e., cervical intraepithelial neoplasia [CIN] grade 2 or 3) or cervical cancer	[6, 29]
Postmenopausal women considering hormone therapy for primary prevention of chronic conditions	The USPSTF recommends against the use of combined estrogen and progestin in postmenopausal women and against the use of estrogen alone in postmenopausal women who have had a hysterectomy for primary prevention	[6]
Postmenopausal women	The USPSTF recommends against daily supplementation with 400 IU or less of vitamin D and 1000 mg or less of calcium for the primary prevention of fractures in community-dwelling, postmenopausal women	[6]
Women with a history of bone mineral density testing	American College of Rheumatology recommends against a repeat BMD test within 2 years	[21, 29]
Women with vertebral osteoporotic fractures	Literature recommends against vertebroplasty or kyphoplasty	[21]
Women with overactive bladder	American Urogynecological Society recommends against cystoscopy, urodynamics, or diagnostic renal and bladder ultrasound in the initial workup of an uncomplicated overactive bladder (OAB) patient	[29]

(continued)

Table 2.2 (continued)

Population	Recommendation	Reference
Women with irregular or abnormal bleeding	American Society for Reproductive Medicine recommends against obtaining follicle-stimulating hormone (FSH) levels in women in their 40s to identify the menopausal transition as a cause of irregular or abnormal menstrual bleeding	[29]
Women with suspected thyroid disease	American Society of Clinical Pathology recommends against multiple tests in the initial evaluation of a patient with suspected thyroid disease. Order thyroid-stimulating hormone (TSH), and if abnormal, follow up with additional evaluation or treatment depending on the findings	[29]
Pregnant women	American Academy of Family Physicians and ACOG recommend against scheduled elective, non-medically indicated inductions of labor or Cesarean deliveries before 39 weeks, 0 days gestational age	[29]

While a provider may wish to avoid low-value services, talking with patients about making choices based on value can be challenging. An NEJM perspectives roundtable gives several practical tips on conversing with patients about low-value services [26]. First, providers should be transparent with patients about their reasoning, clearly describing their practice norms and expectations and citing society guidelines or Choosing Wisely to back up their statements. Generally, providers should focus on the clinical harms more than the dollar costs. Second, providers should have a script for common scenarios, such as Paps or pelvics after 65 years, and sum up their script with a recommendation to avoid a low-value service. If the provider questions whether a generally low-value service has value for a certain individual, he or she can begin a discussion with a lead-in such as "On the whole, {this service} is doing all that harm to get very little benefit. Given that, what do you think you want to do?"

You have a frank conversation with the patient about ovarian cancer screening, her concerns, and goals of care. You discuss the downstream effects of over-testing and check for understanding. She agrees that screening ultrasounds and blood tests are not needed. Your visit then turns to other prevention recommendations. According to your records, her last mammogram was three years ago and her last Pap was normal at age 63. Using the atherosclerotic cardiovascular disease pooled cohort calculator, Barb has a 10-year risk of a cardiovascular event of 7.5%.

Test Characteristics

The reason ovarian cancer screening tests are not recommended is that the available tests have unacceptably high false-negative and false-positive rates. In other words, the predictive value of a positive and the predictive value of a negative test are too low.

Table 2.3 Applying test characteristics to a screening test. Example test with 95% sensitivity and 95% specificity in a hypothetical population of 1000 persons with 0.1% point prevalence of the condition. In this example, the positive predictive value is 2% (1/51)

	Disease is present	Disease is absent	
Test is positive	1 True positive[a]	50 False positive	51 All with positive test
Test is negative	0 False negative[a]	949 True negative	949 All with negative test
	1 All with disease	999 All who are well	1000 All population

[a]95% sensitivity would yield 0.95 with a true-positive and 0.05 with a false-negative test; numbers are rounded to whole numbers

In screening, where, by definition, we are testing a low- or average-risk population, most people do not have the problem for which we are screening. Thus, a good screening test needs a very high specificity. For example (see Table 2.3), if the test's specificity (the percent of persons without the problem that test negative, the true negative rate) is 95%, the remainder with a positive test will actually be well, making a 5% false-positive rate. The impact of a 5% false-positive rate is amplified when screening because so many of the population are well. Continuing the example, in a population that has a 0.1% point prevalence (1 out of 1000 have the problem), a 5% false-positive rate means 50 of 1000 people test positive but are well. Since we know 1 of these 1000 has the problem, there would be 51 positive tests, but only 1 of those 51 actually has the problem. The positive test yields meaningful information only 2% of the time, thus a low positive predictive value.

Only half of clinicians have a working knowledge of these concepts [30]. And yet understanding when to order tests and how to interpret the results is critical to high-value care, lest physicians fall prey to ordering unnecessary tests or placing too much importance on a positive result. Providers who lack understanding of critical test characteristics can underestimate the harm caused by an inappropriately ordered test.

Shared Decision-Making

Shared decision-making involves talking with patients to help explain the concepts of value, test characteristics, and best practices to come to a joint decision when selecting appropriate preventive care or other services. Often, there is no one "right answer"; thus, primary care providers frequently face situations where the next best step is shared decision-making. Using the breast cancer screening (Chap. 18) and cervical cancer screening (Chap. 14) recommendations and the information given, most providers would appropriately advise the patient in our case to obtain a mammogram and forego a Pap without much hesitation. However, her borderline cardiac risk (Chap. 21) should direct the clinician to a shared decision-making discussion.

Engaging patients in shared decision-making can be a challenge. First, it can be time-consuming and difficult to fit in a prevention visit, particularly one with multiple prevention items needing a discussion within a limited appointment duration. Of note, women have more prevention recommendations than men (see Table 2.1). Second, situations that require shared decision-making often are the same situations where data is lacking, recommendations are conflicting, or relatively new information changes established practices. Thus, these are situations where providers may not have an internal script for the discussion, may not have materials to help aid the conversation, or may bring their own biases. For example, regarding mammographic screening of women in their forties, Keating and Pace describe several factors preventing a practice change to shared decision-making instead of reflexively ordering a mammogram. These include general biases toward testing, concerns about litigation, more payment for testing and less payment for conversations, disagreement with the guidelines, and inaccurate understanding of the harms, such as overdiagnosis [31]. Third, we must be aware that risk is frequently processed emotionally rather than cognitively [32]. Often, both clinicians and patients anticipate and try to avoid the regret of *not* doing something rather than understand the harms of doing something. In breast cancer screening, this harm is overdiagnosis, which remains largely invisible. It is difficult to disentangle values and beliefs from facts when discussing risk, but the primary care provider is in a very good position to elicit what matters to the patient.

Tips in Providing Shared Decision-Making The best way to address these challenges is a combination of patient-centered materials, appropriate pre-visit preparations and during-visit education conducted by medical home care team members, and managed agendas to match the time available. Decision aids and patient education materials with easy-to-understand graphics on risk improve decision-making discussions [31]. Examples of decision aids can be found on the Internet: The Mayo Clinic website [33] tools include osteoporosis management, and Health Decisions [34] includes cardiovascular prevention and breast cancer screening. Similarly, pamphlets [35] and videos [36] directed at educating patients are available and can be selected to match the patient's learning style and technology savvy. It is important to have diverse materials, picturing individuals of all colors, available in multiple languages to engage all patients. Additionally, sometimes decision aids ask for a race or ethnicity designation but unfortunately don't allow for all realities such as women who are more than one race or who are American Indian; often, this is because calculators are based on research populations that didn't include these designations. For women in this situation, providers can choose between the option with the best fit or not answering. Finally, providers who need training on shared decision-making can use Agency for Healthcare Research and Quality's SHARE materials online [37].

Systems Engineering and Process Improvement

Systems engineering is a way of thinking that allow providers to achieve the quadruple aim by solving problems like finding time for shared decision-making. Health-care organizations that use systems engineering tools like Lean [38] or Six Sigma have a set of reproducible process to discover problems and solve them. This often means improving the process itself but, in other cases, requires adjusting the management system, how processes coordinate, and how people interact with the process.

The use of systems engineering to enhance the care of women is best illustrated with an example. Consider breast cancer screening. The USPSTF recommends mammographic screening at least every 2 years. If an organization has a quality goal of breast cancer screening and patients are not meeting this goal, the organization labels "failure to meet breast cancer screening goal" as the problem and then takes the first step to map out the processes in place that address breast cancer screening. It may be that a standard process is lacking—for example, the only identified process is to expect PCPs to note the gap and order mammograms when due. Other organizations, may have a process or combination of processes, such as (1) outreach between visits by non-physician care team members, (2) pre-visit processes and/or point-of-care reminders for care team members to order mammograms before the visit or on rooming, (3) heightened awareness of the goal and current performance with visual boards and team meetings, or (4) expanding the impact of primary care physicians with

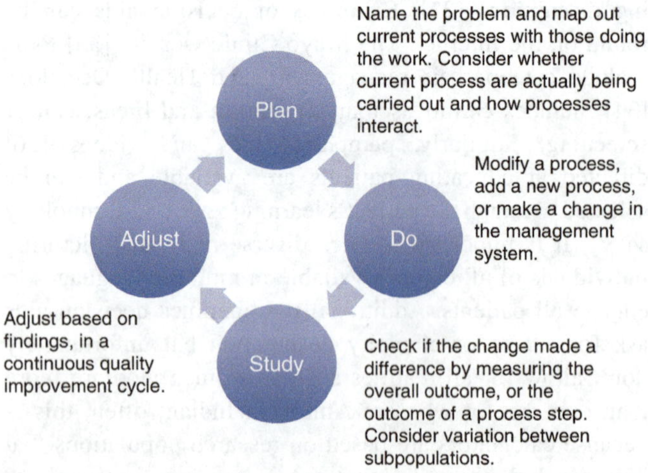

Fig. 2.1 Quality improvement cycle

advance practice providers or in coordination with obstetrics-gynecology clinicians.

Mapping the current process means developing a diagram of who does exactly what when. The care team members who perform the work must be part of the mapping process, both to understand what is truly happening and then to participate in brainstorming for improvement. This mapping process may be done when a problem is identified but ideally happens periodically to continually improve a working process. In a PDSA (Plan/Do/Study/Act or Adjust) improvement cycle model [39], this mapping is the "plan" step. The next step would be to "do," that is, select a modification or an addition to the current process to make the improvement. See Fig. 2.1.

For example, if the current state is a practice where annual mammography was left to PCPs to order at the point of care, a strategy to increase the rate of mammography would be to ensure that patients are coming in at least every 1–2 years for preventive care. For patients insured by Medicare, health-care organizations can take advantage of the annual wellness visit (AWV) benefit and set up systems to remind patients that an appointment is due every 12 months. If physician visits are limited due to demand, practices can develop a process where advanced practice providers (APPs) see the patients for the AWV and partner with physicians to provide any needed complex medical services at another visit.

Once the process is improved, it is incumbent on the team to measure if the change made a difference. The idea is to not only name the problem but to decide on how the problem is measured and tracked. For example, did the breast cancer screening rates improve? If not, did patients at least receive an AWV yearly? This step is called "study" in a PDSA cycle. The final step would be to "adjust" to make the process better.

Often, even a perfect process is not enough to achieve the goal. If the process that the organization's leaders ("management") expect is not the process that is actually happening, barriers must be identified and addressed. In a primary care clinic, "management" may not be simply defined: Is it the physician in a physician-led care team? Is it the medical director or clinic manager? Are all stakeholders on the same page? If the answers to these questions are not clear, it's time to map out the management system.

Alternately, the process may work but only for selected patients (seen by a certain clinician or with a given insurance type or of a certain socioeconomic group) or only for breast cancer screening and not cervical cancer screening. Here, performance or outcome data, preferably with drill-down capability, can help identify the root cause of the problem. The problem may be a matter of training, motivation, or resources. Alternatively, it may be that populations respond differently to interventions. For example, studies have demonstrated that in the case of breast cancer screening, Black women may have a distrust of mammograms, and therefore a phone call alone may be less likely to convince them to schedule the overdue exam [40]. Finally, the problem may be a lack of data. Women, because of fragmented care, often get screenings in multiple systems, and reports may not be appropriately sent or scanned into the primary care providers' system.

Your medical assistant, in a pre-visit planning process, identified that Barb was overdue for a mammogram according to your records and called Barb before the visit about the need for a mammogram. In response to that call, Barb brings in her records of a mammogram done last year that was ordered by an ob-gyn in a health system closer to her home. The mammogram was normal.

Public Reporting and Pay-for-Performance Measures

To highlight high-quality care and assist patients in selecting high-quality providers, facilities, and health insurance plans, organizations such as the Center for Medicare Services [41], National Committee for Quality Assurance [42], and regional health improvement organizations publicly report performance. These publicly available scorecards often include measures of prevention, chronic condition management, patient experience, and cost and utilization, and health systems or providers are compared against an average or benchmark. In general, metrics are selected if they represent services or conditions that are relevant for a large number of people, and consensus exists regarding the best practice for that service or condition that can reliably be measured. While simply the act of public reporting increases transparency and likely quality, more often these measure sets have an impact if they are used in pay-for-performance programs for providers or hospitals or used to hold payers accountable [43].

Pay-for-Value Programs CMS uses pay-for-performance programs to incent high-value care for providers and hospitals [41]. The program for physicians and other eligible clinicians is called the Quality Payment Program, and this program was legislated by the 2015 law called the Medicare Access and CHIP Reauthorization Act (MACRA). Most providers in large groups need to participate in one of two tracks or be subject to a fine. To participate in the Merit-based Incentive Payment System (MIPS), providers select from a list of over 100 metrics (including core measure sets for primary care and for obstetrics-gynecology), report their results to CMS, and then are paid or fined in a zero-sum program. Alternatively, providers and their health systems can participate in the Advanced Alternate Payment Models track, where the model for payment meaningfully shifts from traditional fee-for-service to value-based payment. Quality, cost, and experience measures are publicly shared on either Physician Compare for providers or Hospital Compare for hospitals.

Many services for women are linked to commonly reported measures. For example, breast cancer screening, cervical cancer screening, and chlamydia screening are posted on regional quality improvement organizations' sites [44, 45], at NCQA's rating of health plans [42], and are available for MIPS reporting [41]. Similiarly, Hospital Compare reports the elective delivery and mammogram follow-up rates [41]; the National Healthcare Quality and Disparity Report reports breast cancer mortality, HPV vaccination, and advanced cervical cancer rates [46]; and CMS's Star Ratings Program for Medicare health plans includes breast cancer screening, osteoporosis management after a fracture, and improving bladder control rates [41]. State-run Medicaid plans often have similar measures. As these measures are more strongly linked to payment models, improving high-value care for women becomes not only the right thing to do but also a sound business decision.

Alternative Payment Models and Value-Based Insurance Design

As mentioned, governmental and commercial insurance carriers are increasingly paying providers and facilities based on the value they provide rather than simply based on the services rendered. There are a wide variety of payment arrangements, for instance (1) paying for an outcome like a quality metric (discussed above), (2) sharing in savings or risk determined by the total cost of care, or (3) paying based on the size of the population (number of members) rather than the number of services, called population-based payments. Another arrangement is paying for an "episode of care," such as a joint surgery or a pneumonia hospitalization as a bundle, including all related care in a time window such as 30-days.

Like publicly reported services, quality or cost measures that are linked to a payment often include women's health services. Obstetric care is often paid as an episode; there is a single "global payment" for all services associated with the pregnancy and delivery, up until 6 weeks of delivery, with the fee often dependent on the complexity of the pregnancy. This arrangement encourages coordinated care throughout the pregnancy and the use of the least expensive yet appropriate level of care. For example, episode-based payment encourages hospitals to keep costs of supplies and durable medical equipment low, to only admit when necessary, and to avoid unnecessary days in the hospital. At the same time, episode-based payment encourages providers to manage diabetes, appropriately vaccinate for influenza, and screen for infections to limit complications in pregnant women. The advantages of the bundled payment arrangement end with the end date of the bundle, however. Postpartum care and other health care may become uncoordinated or unavailable (as happens in some state Medicaid plans) at the 6-week postpartum mark [47].

Insurance programs, both commercial and governmental, can also be designed to incentivize patients to be more cost-conscious. Consumer-driven health plans shift first payments and a higher percentage of costs to patients by using high deductibles and co-insurance. These benefit designs do lower overall costs, as patients defer services, some of which are unnecessary or low value [48]. However, some of these deferred services are high value. In a study of Medicare managed health plans before the enactment of the Affordable Care Act, the biennial mammography rate was 8% less among women who had to share in the cost of a mammogram [49]. More rigorous study and innovation are needed to realize the benefits of these plans without putting patients at risk for skipping needed care.

Cost of Care for Women

When considering systems design and insurance payments, it is important to remember that per capita lifetime expenses are generally higher for women (about $360k) than for men (about $270k). About 40% of this difference can be explained by the longer life span of women [50]. Women live about 8% longer than men, and about half of all health-care expenses occur in people over the age of 65 years independent of gender (due to medical conditions, disability, and end-of-life care that occur in older patients). The remainder of the difference in expenditure is likely due to pregnancy and childbirth [51], a necessary burden of health-care services that is carried by only women, despite the fact that both sexes are often required for pregnancy to occur.

Currently, US law does not allow differences in insurance premiums by gender, also known as "gender rating," and most Americans agree with this core principle of the Affordable Care Act [52]. Additionally, the American College of Physicians states in a position paper "health insurers should not be allowed to charge women higher premiums or impose higher cost sharing on women because of their sex or gender" [53].

Thus, care for women is an important target for organizations aiming to improve affordability. In value-based arrangements, providers, payers, and patients all benefit from reducing the cost of care in women. Moreover, when measures like breast cancer screening are part of a population-based payment arrangement, these payments can be earmarked for care teams to assist primary care providers in closing care gaps.

At the conclusion of your clinic session, you huddle with your care team and review your quality measures. Your mammogram rate is 88%, which is better than the average in your clinic. However, your rate for Black women is 77%, while your rate for White women is 95%. Your care team enacts its process for continual quality improvement to address this disparity.

Equity and Disparities

As mentioned, population health refers to the health outcomes of a group of individuals, but it also includes the "distribution of such outcomes within the group" [54]. Thus, equity of care—in terms of both patient characteristics (sex and gender, race, creed, sexuality, or certain conditions) and system processes and outcomes (access, effective communication, costs of care, or care team support)—is also a critical component of the quadruple aim. While pursuing high-value care for women, systems engineering and team-based care programs must address and work to eliminate health disparities.

In the pages that follow, this textbook includes many examples of gender differences in the receipt of care and the outcomes of care. For example, the conditions that affect women veterans are different than in men; heart disease manifests differently in women, with different risk factors, and worse outcomes; and sexually transmitted infections have different and often more severe consequences in women. Just as gender impacts health equity, race affects care and outcomes in women. To illustrate, Black women die of breast cancer at twice the rate of Latinas or Asian women; American Indian women are much less likely to receive prenatal care than Asian or White women; and White women are more likely to receive birth control than Hispanic or Black women. The origins and solutions to sex-based disparities can inform and complement understanding and problem-solving for other disparities.

One foundational step providers can take to address inequity is to look in the mirror. Often, without conscious recognition, we make assessments and decisions based on our backgrounds and experiences; in other words, we harbor implicit bias. To change that bias, we must first be aware of it. Providers can learn of their implicit biases by taking an online survey [55]. Armed with the results, providers might feel empowered to identify biases when they see them, use their names (e.g., call out "racism"), and shift from the majority perspective to the minority perspective [56]. Many institutions and specialty organizations are focused on working with providers to reduce the impact of implicit bias; availing oneself of these opportunities when offered may be the first needed step in providing the equitable care we all aspire to give.

Social Determinants of Health

While most of this text is about "health care," the provision of health care determines only about 10% of health [57]. Far more important are behavior and genetics (together 70%), plus "social circumstances," which contribute about 15% to premature death. Social determinants of health include financial resource strain, education, food and housing security, social support, employment, and insurance status. These factors contribute to one another and to health behaviors, as do the living environment, cultural background.

Since insurance eligibility often depends on employment, income, marriage to a spouse with insurance benefits, and/or minor children, instability in any of these factors can lead to fragmentation in care, limited access, or frequent changes of the enrolled health insurance plan. This is especially the case for women, who are more likely than men to rely on government programs, marriage, and being a parent for care. Women, like men, can experience gaps in insurance coverage, yet rates of uninsured declined markedly with the enactment of the Affordable Care Act. In 2016, 11% of non-elderly adult women were uninsured (down from 18% in 2013); meanwhile, 13% of men (down from 20% in 2013) were uninsured [5].

The presence of insurance doesn't mean unlimited access to health care; some high-deductible health plans have such high out-of-pocket costs that, outside of a catastrophe, beneficiaries are priced out of access beyond preventive care.

About half of uninsured women delayed or went without care because of costs, but 21% of those with private insurance and 25% of those with Medicaid also delayed care or went without [7]. Comparing women overall to men overall, 26% of women delayed care or went without care compared to 19% of men. Women, who on average earn less than men, may be more affected by the rising costs of health care. Finally, 42% of women who have trouble paying for medical bills report difficulty paying for basic necessities such as food and housing because of medical bills.

Getting to the doctor also requires time and transportation. About one-quarter of women delayed or went without care because they couldn't take time off work; that number rises to one-third of low-income women [7]. Similarly, 9% of women delayed or went without care because of transportation barriers, a figure that increases to 19% when considering only low-income women. Further, these transportation problems are significantly worse among Black and Hispanic women.

Covid-19 and Public Health

The Covid-19 pandemic is a stark reminder that the U.S. healthcare system is primarily a system of clinical care delivery to individuals. In contrast, public health functions such as controlling epidemics, contact tracing, and return-to-work or return-to-school strategies are the domain of governments and local health departments. While men and women have similar infection rates when exposed, men tend to have a more severe disease course and worse outcomes. However, Covid-19 has deepened existing disparities based on socioeconomic determinants of health. Women are more likely to work in healthcare (essential work with exposure risk), work part-time or in the informal economy (which does not supply health insurance), and be the primary caregiver of children (forcing a choice between employment/insurance and caregiving for school-aged children at home during the pandemic). Thus, Covid-19 may have a more significant indirect impact on women.

Health Policy and Advocacy

While this textbook largely works to help guide our actions at the bedside in hospitals or in clinics, critical elements of high-value care for women and LGBTQ populations are most impacted when providers influence societal attitudes and/or health policy. This textbook does not suggest providers enter the world of partisan politics. Indeed, providers must remain impartial and care for all persons, as dictated by the 2017 World Medical Association Declaration of Geneva [58]. Yet physicians must be aware of how of our voices and professional societies can and should make a difference [59]. At our core, we are advocates, putting the interests of our patients before our own. Interested readers are directed to relevant society's position papers such as ACP's position on women's health [53], ACOG's position on access [60], and the AAFP's position on violence [61]. Advocacy efforts by health professionals are another important, if often overlooked, avenue toward high-value care for women.

Summary Points

1. The quadruple aim is a four-part goal to achieve high-quality care, a meaningful care experience for patients, job satisfaction for providers, and all at an affordable cost. Access to health care is often dictated by health insurance status; about 60% of non-elderly women have employer-sponsored health insurance and 20% have Medicaid.
2. Examples of high-value care include recommended prevention measures such as breast cancer screening in 50- to 74-year-old women, chlamydia screening in sexually active women 24 years and younger, or supporting breastfeeding interventions in pregnant women and new mothers. In contrast, low-value care may be measures that aren't evidence-based (such as screening for vitamin D deficiency), with limited cost-effectiveness (such as routine BRCA genetic testing) or both (such as elective delivery before 39 weeks).
3. Health care organizations can put systems in place to improve care for women and LGBTQ populations by using teams to promote timely preventive care and chronic disease management, creating a culture of continuous quality improvement, and prioritizing shared decision-making.
4. Measures targeting women such as breast cancer screening are commonly included in pay-for-value arrangements and publicly reported scorecards of performance. Achieving high-value care requires attention to care for women, including maternity care.
5. Population health management means improving the outcomes of the group as well as the outcomes within the group. Gender equity, reducing disparities, addressing social determinants, and professional advocacy are important components of high-value care.

Review Questions

1. One population health tenet is to achieve all four objectives of the "quadruple aim." Which objective is included in the quadruple aim?

A. Reducing health system costs such as clinical informatics and analytics
B. Improving the quality of care such as the rate of breast cancer screening
C. Decreasing the number of for-profit health-care organizations to improve coordination with community organizations
D. Increasing the number of patients seen per day to improve access

The correct answer is B. The quadruple aim is to improve the experience, quality, and vitality of providers while keeping spend in check [3]. Reducing costs are aimed at reducing low-value care or bringing transparent discussions of cost into treatment plans when options are available. Clinical informatics and analytics often develop or inform process improvement which can increase high-value care. Access is an important aspect of patient experience; the ways to improve access are to decrease rate of uninsured and to make clinicians available by ensuring adequate number of primary care physicians and using alternate methods of patient encounters such as advance practice providers.

2. Which of the following is an example of a low-value service?
A. Annual cervical cancer screening in ages 21–64
B. Osteoporosis screening at age 65 years
C. Elective delivery after 40 weeks gestational age
D. Breast MRI for breast cancer screening in BRCA mutation carriers

The answer is A. Low-value services are listed by Choosing Wisely [29]; one example is scheduling an elective delivery before 39 weeks of gestation. High-value preventive care is Grade A–B rating by USPSTF [6]. USPSTF recommends cervical cancer screening every 3–5 years depending on patient factors, osteoporosis screening beginning at age 65 years, and breast cancer screening, including MRI in those at high-risk for breast cancer in women aged 50–74 years.

3. Your health-care organizations' breast cancer screening rate is 55%, using a numerator of at least every 2-year mammogram and a denominator of women ages 50–74 years. The rate for White women is 60%, and the rate for Black women is 45%. Your current efforts to address breast cancer screening include multilingual patient education materials, electronic best-practice alerts at a visit if a mammogram is due, and setting up an annual follow-up appointment for all women in the age range at the end of a visit. Which of the following is the next best step to improve this process?
A. Change the standard follow-up appointment to every 2 years (rather than every 1 year), so as not to schedule unnecessary appointments
B. Hire a medical assistant to call all women in the age range who are due for a mammogram to come in for a mammogram
C. Poll a convenience sample of Black women served by your clinic about why they aren't getting mammograms
D. Map the current process and use performance data informed by observations of the care team to identify less effective and missing steps

The correct answer is D. The core tenet of systems engineering quality improvement is to understand current state before planning a future state [38]. Often, the best ideas for planning the future state come from those doing the work, so the map of the current state and its review should include persons directly involved. After this, it may be that the suggestion is to outreach to those due for mammograms or poll patients.

4. Your health care organization is part of an accountable care organization that has an opportunity for shared savings in a pay-for-value contract. However, to be eligible for shared savings, your organization must meet a quality performance threshold. This threshold includes measures such as breast cancer screening, chlamydia screening, patient experience ratings, and prenatal care visits. Your composite rate is 55%, but the required threshold is 70%. To achieve maximum shared savings, your best next step is to
A. Plan a team meeting to study your composite performance
B. Lower the rate of uninsured at your clinic
C. Reduce the rate of early elective Cesarean sections
D. Reduce your breast cancer spending

The correct answer is A. Pay-for-value contracts encourage health-care organizations and payers to work together as they both benefit from reducing unnecessary spending and low-value care [43]. In this scenario, your group may not share in savings even if it is achieved because the quality composite score is not at threshold, so your best bet is to work on the quality score in a PDSA cycle with your team.

References

1. Koller CF, Khullar D. Primary care spending rate — a lever for encouraging investment in primary care. N Engl J Med. 2017;377:1709–11.
2. Berwick DM, Nolan TW, Whittington J. Triple aim: care, health, and cost. Health Aff. 2008;27(3):759–69.
3. Bodenheimer T, Sinsky C. From triple to quadruple aim: care of the patient requires care of the provider. Ann Fam Med. 2014;12(6):573–6.
4. Reid R, Coleman K, Johnson EA, Fishman PA, Hsu C, et al. The group health medical home at year two: cost savings, higher patient satisfaction, and less burnout for providers. Health Aff. 2010;29(5):835–43.

5. Henry J. Kaiser Family Foundation. Health coverage and uninsured. Based on analysis of March 2017 Current Population Survey, U.S. Census Bureau. https://www.kff.org/state-category/health-coverage-uninsured/health-insurance-status-by-gender/. Accessed 21 Oct 2018.
6. USPSTF. Recommendations for primary care practice, current as of September 2017. https://www.uspreventiveservicestaskforce.org/Page/Name/recommendations. Accessed 27 Oct 2018.
7. Henry J. Kaiser Family Foundation. Women's coverage, access, and affordability: key findings from the 2017 Kaiser Women's Health Survey. March 13, 2018. https://www.kff.org/womens-health-policy/issue-brief/womens-coverage-access-and-affordability-key-findings-from-the-2017-kaiser-womens-health-survey/. Accessed 21 Oct 2018.
8. Manary MP, Boulding W, Staelin S, Glickman SW. The patient experience and health outcomes. N Engl J Med. 2013;368:201–3. https://doi.org/10.1056/NEJMp1211775.
9. Cooper-Patrick L, Gallo JJ, Gonzales JJ, et al. Race, gender, and partnership in the patient-physician relationship. JAMA. 1999;282(6):583–9. https://doi.org/10.1001/jama.282.6.583.
10. Weisman CS, Rich DE, Rogers J, Crawford KG, Grayson CE, Henderson JT. Gender and patient satisfaction with primary care: tuning in to women in quality measurement. J Women's Health Gender-Based Med. 2000;9(6):657–65.
11. Phelan EA, Burke W, Deyo RA, Koepsell TD, LaCroix AZ. Delivery of primary care to women. J Gen Int Med. 2000;15:8–15. https://doi.org/10.1046/j.1525-1497.2000.12178.x.
12. Diamond D. Women make up 80% of healthcare workers but just 40% of executives. August 26, 2014. Advisory Board Daily Briefing Blog. https://www.advisory.com/daily-briefing/blog/2014/08/women-in-leadership. Accessed 21 Oct 2018.
13. O'Malley AS, Gourevitch R, Draper K, Bond A, Tirodkar MA. Overcoming challenges to teamwork in patient-centered medical homes: a qualitative study. J Gen Intern Med. 2015 Feb;30(2):183–92. https://doi.org/10.1007/s11606-014-3065-9.
14. Sinsky CA, Willard-Grace R, Schutzbank AM, Sinsky TA, Margolius D, Bodenheimer T. In search of joy in practice: a report of 23 high-functioning primary care practices. Ann Fam Med. 2013;11:272–8. https://doi.org/10.1370/afm.153.
15. Nelson KM, Helfrich C, Sun H, et al. Implementation of the patient-centered medical home in the veterans health administration associations with patient satisfaction, quality of care, staff burnout, and hospital and emergency department use. JAMA Intern Med. 2014;174(8):1350–8. https://doi.org/10.1001/jamainternmed.2014.2488.
16. Reddy A, Pollack CE, Asch DA, Canamucio A, Werner RM. The effect of primary care provider turnover on patient experience of care and ambulatory quality of care. JAMA Intern Med. 2015;175(7):1157–62. https://doi.org/10.1001/jamainternmed.2015.1853.
17. Carroll AE. The high costs of unnecessary care. JAMA. 2017;318(18):1748–9. https://doi.org/10.1001/jama.2017.16193.
18. Berwick DM, Hackbarth AD. Eliminating waste in US health care. JAMA. 2012;307(14):1513–6. https://doi.org/10.1001/jama.2012.362.
19. Reid RO, Rabideau B, Sood N. Low-value health care services in a commercially insured population. JAMA Intern Med. 2016;176(10):1567–71. https://doi.org/10.1001/jamainternmed.2016.5031.
20. Charlesworth CJ, Meath THA, Schwartz AL, McConnell KJ. Comparison of low-value care in Medicaid vs commercially insured populations. JAMA Intern Med. 2016;176(7):998–1004. https://doi.org/10.1001/jamainternmed.2016.2086.
21. Schwartz AL, Chernew ME, Landon BE, McWilliams JM. Changes in low-value services in year 1 of the Medicare pioneer accountable care organization program. JAMA Intern Med. 2015;175(11):1815–25. https://doi.org/10.1001/jamainternmed.2015.4525.
22. Neumann PJ, Cohen JT, Weinstein MC. Updating cost-effectiveness — the curious resilience of the $50,000-per-QALY threshold. N Engl J Med. 2014;371:796–7.
23. Morden NE, Colla CH, Sequist TD, Rosenthal MB. Choosing wisely — the politics and economics of labeling low-value services. N Engl J Med. 2014;370:589–92.
24. Schwartz AL, Landon BE, Elshaug AG, Chernew ME, McWilliams JM. Measuring low-value care in Medicare. JAMA Intern Med. 2014;174(7):1067–76. https://doi.org/10.1001/jamainternmed.2014.1541.
25. Pandya A. Adding cost-effectiveness to define low-value care. JAMA. 2018;319(19):1977–8. https://doi.org/10.1001/jama.2018.2856.
26. Gawande SS, Colla CH, Halpern SD, Landon BE. Avoiding low-value care. N Engl J Med. 2014;370:e21.
27. Pashayan N, Morris S, Gilbert FJ, Pharoah PDP. Cost-effectiveness and benefit-to-harm ratio of risk-stratified screening for breast cancer a life-table model. JAMA Oncol. 2018;4(11):1504–10. https://doi.org/10.1001/jamaoncol.2018.1901.
28. Roberts MC. Implementation challenges for risk-stratified screening in the era of precision medicine. JAMA Oncol. 2018;4(11):1484–5. https://doi.org/10.1001/jamaoncol.2018.1940.
29. Choosing Wisely Clinician lists. http://www.choosingwisely.org/clinician-lists/. Accessed 21 Oct 2018.
30. Morgan D. What the tests don't show. October 5, 2018, Washington Post.
31. Keating NL, Pace LE. Breast cancer screening in 2018Time for shared decision making. JAMA. 2018;319(17):1814–5. https://doi.org/10.1001/jama.2018.3388.
32. Rosenbaum L. Invisible risks, emotional choices — mammography and medical decision making. N Engl J Med. 2014;371:1549–52.
33. Mayo Clinic Shared Decision Making Resource Center. https://shareddecisions.mayoclinic.org. Accessed 4 Nov 2018.
34. HealthDecision Tools, copywrite 2018. https://www.healthdecision.com/products. Accessed 4 Nov 2018.
35. Breast cancer screening: It's your choice. 2013. http://asksharenow.com.au/wp-content/uploads/2017/07/It's-your-choice-New-information-to-help-women-aged-about-50-to-make-a-decision-includes-overdiagnosis.pdf. Accessed 4 Nov 2018.
36. Jett L. Making decisions about breast cancer screening. Feb 28, 2018. https://www.youtube.com/watch?v=lTnw2CpeGN4&feature=youtu.be
37. ARHQ. SHARE. https://www.ahrq.gov/professionals/education/curriculum-tools/shareddecisionmaking/index.html
38. Womack JP, Jones DT. Lean thinking. London: Simon and Schuster; 2010.
39. Scoville R, Little K. Comparing lean and quality improvement. IHI white paper. Cambridge, MA: Institute for Healthcare Improvement; 2014. Available at ihi.org
40. Peek ME, Sayad JV. Markwardt R. J Gen Intern Med. 2008;23:1847. https://doi.org/10.1007/s11606-008-0756-0.
41. CMS. https://www.cms.gov
42. NCQA Health insurance ratings. http://healthinsuranceratings.ncqa.org/2018/HprPlandetails.aspx?id=57
43. Nyweide DJ, Lee W, Cuerdon TT, et al. Association of Pioneer Accountable Care Organizations vs traditional Medicare fee for service with spending, utilization, and patient experience. JAMA. 2015;313(21):2152–61. https://doi.org/10.1001/jama.2015.4930.
44. Wisconsin Collaborative for Healthcare Quality. http://wchq.org/
45. Minnesota Community Measurement. http://mncm.org/reports-and-websites/reports-and-data/health-care-quality-report/
46. National Healthcare Quality and Disparity Reports. https://nhqrnet.ahrq.gov/inhqrdr/

47. Murray Horwitz ME, Molina RL, Snowden JM. Postpartum care in the United States — new policies for a new paradigm. N Engl J Med. 2018;379:1691–3.
48. Baicker K, Levy H. The insurance value of Medicare. N Engl J Med. 2012;367:1773–5.
49. Trivedi AN, Rakowski W, Ayanian JZ. Effect of cost sharing on screening mammography in Medicare health plans. N Engl J Med. 2008;358:375–83.
50. Alemayehu B, Warner KE. The lifetime distribution of health care costs. Health Serv Res. 2004;39(3):627–42.
51. Mustard CA, Kaufert P, Kozyrskyj A, Mayer T. Sex differences in the use of health care services. N Engl J Med. 1998;338(23):1678–83.
52. KFF Health Reform. https://www.kff.org/health-reform/perspective/public-opinion-on-gender-rating/. Accessed 9 Nov 2018.
53. Daniel H, Erickson SM, Bornstein SS. Women's health policy in the United States: an American College of Physicians position paper. Ann Intern Med. 2018;168:874–5.
54. Kindig D, Stoddart G. What is population health? Am J Public Health. 2003;93(3):380–3.
55. Project Implicit. 2011. https://implicit.harvard.edu/implicit/. Accessed 11 Nov 2018.
56. Hardeman RR, Medina EM, Kozhimannil KB. Structural racism and supporting black lives — the role of health professionals. N Engl J Med. 2016;375:2113–5.
57. Schroeder SA. We can do better—improving the health of the American people. N Engl J Med. 2007;357:1221–8.
58. Parsa-Parsi RW. The revised declaration of Geneva: a modern-day physician's pledge. JAMA. 2017;318(20):1971–2.
59. Berwick DM. Politics and health care. JAMA. 2018;320(14):1437–8.
60. ACOG Statement of Policy: access to women's health care. Reaffirmed July 2016. https://www.acog.org/-/media/Statements-of-Policy/Public/64AccesstoWomenHlthCare2016-1.pdf?dmc=1&ts=20181020T1955330547
61. American Academy of Family Medicine: Violence (position paper). 2014. https://www.aafp.org/about/policies/all/violence.html

The Female Sex- and Gender-Specific History and Examination

3

Eliana Bonifacino and Jennifer Corbelli

Learning Objectives

1. Describe the components of a female gender-specific history and review of systems.
2. List the components of a standard pelvic examination.
3. List key differences among major guidelines on the indications for pelvic examinations.
4. Identify populations that may require adaptations of the pelvic examination.
5. Describe the components of a standard clinical breast examination.

The Female Gender-Specific History

Introduction

A gender-specific history is often performed as part of a comprehensive annual examination or a well-woman visit to elicit information about relevant past medical history, screen for sexual dysfunction, discuss family planning and contraceptive choices, and uncover potential risk factors for future health conditions. Due to the nature of the information discussed in this encounter, some women may feel uncomfortable or anxious discussing their health history. This requires that providers practice sensitive and culturally conscious care.

In general, it is optimal to begin a new patient visit with the patient dressed and sitting on a chair, as opposed to gowned, or on the examination table. When taking a history, language should be sensitive to patient concerns: avoiding implied judgment, colloquial terms, or innuendo [1]. Prior to asking questions that may be uncomfortable in nature, the provider can introduce the topic (e.g., "In the next part of our visit, I will be asking questions regarding your gynecologic health") and "normalize" the interview by explaining that these are common and important health-related questions that are asked of all patients. A female gender-specific history contains the components outlined in Table 3.1.

- *Menstrual History*: Includes the age of menarche, menstrual cycle length, date of last menstrual period, and age of menopause, if indicated. Record bleeding patterns and quantity, and note menses that are absent, irregular, very long and heavy, or if there is intermenstrual bleeding. In appropriate patients, providers should ask about menopausal symptoms including menstrual irregularity, hot flushes, and vaginal dryness. Postmenopausal bleeding should be recorded as it could reflect underlying pathology. (See Chap. 7 on Abnormal Uterine Bleeding and Chap. 8 on Menopause).
- *Contraception*: The patient's current method of contraception, previous methods utilized, and duration of hormonal treatments are noted. If the patient is not using contraception, explore facilitators and barriers to the use of contraceptive methods, and ask the patient their immediate plans should they become pregnant (See Chap. 4 on Patient-Centered Contraceptive Counseling).
- *Obstetrical History and Reproductive Plans*: Future reproductive plans, previous pregnancies, pregnancy complications, and medical comorbidities of pregnancy are recorded. Exploring a patient's future reproductive plans allows providers to discuss preconception counseling or offer appropriate contraceptive counseling. Determine the number of prior pregnancies, and record age of first birth which is applicable to breast cancer risk. Terminations, miscarriages, or ectopic pregnancies, mode of delivery, and gestational age at delivery are recorded (See Chap. 39 on Obstetric Medicine).
  - *Gravidity and Parity*: Two conventional systems exist for documenting a patient's obstetric history. One system for documenting obstetric history includes a descriptive prefix $G_XP_XTab_XSab_XEct_XLC_X$, representing

E. Bonifacino (✉) · J. Corbelli
University of Pittsburgh Medical Center, Division of General Internal Medicine, Pittsburgh, PA, USA
e-mail: bonifacinoe@upmc.edu

S. A. Tilstra et al. (eds.), *Sex- and Gender-Based Women's Health*, https://doi.org/10.1007/978-3-030-50695-7_3

Table 3.1 Essential components of the female sex- and gender-specific history

Chief complaint/HPI/medications/allergies/past medical and surgical history
Gynecologic and reproductive history

Menstrual history:
  Age at menarche.
  Menstrual pattern.
  Age of menopause.
Contraception:
  Current/prior methods.
  Facilitators/barriers.
  Family planning.
Obstetrical history and reproductive plans:
  Gravity/parity/age at first live birth/future plans.
  Complications of pregnancy: DM, HTN, preeclampsia, other.
  Lactation/length of lactation/plans.
Gynecologic history:
  History of STIs/cervical cancer screen/HPV.
  Other gynecologic diagnoses.
Sexual history/activity:
  Sexual orientation/practices/partners.
  Sexual function.

Breast history
History of chest radiation. Family history of breast or ovarian cancer/risk genetic mutation. Mammogram and breast density. History of breast biopsy and result/treatments/breast surgery.
Family and genetic history
Cancers: Breast, ovarian, fallopian tube, endometrial, uterine cancer. GI malignancy, other cancers. Known mutation in patient or family member, genetic testing, and result. CAD/DM/HTN. Osteoporosis.
Social history
Living situation. Job/occupation/education. Intimate partner violence.
Lifestyle habits
Exercise/diet. Smoking/alcohol use/substances.
Review of systems
Breast: Pain/lump/discharge/axillary mass/breast awareness. Gyn: Bleeding/ pain/discharge/prolapse/pruritus/external lesions/ dyspareunia/bloating/menopausal symptoms. Urinary: Incontinence/retention/dysuria/frequency.

Abbreviations: *HPI* history of present illness, *DM* diabetes mellitus, *HTN* hypertension, *HPV* human papillomavirus, *CAD* coronary artery disease, *STI* sexually transmitted infection, *GI* gastrointestinal

the patient's gravidity (G), parity (P), therapeutic abortions (Tab), spontaneous abortions (Sab), ectopic pregnancies (Ect), and living children (LC). Each of these is followed by the number of each event a patient has experienced [2]. $G_2P_2TAB_1LC_2$ would describe a patient who has had two pregnancies, two births, one abortion, and who currently has two live children. This system requires less memorization and communicates essential information to other providers. Another, though similar, system follows the format G_xP_{TPAL}. In this system, the number of pregnancies in a patient's life is designated as gravidity (G), with X representing the total number. The numbers following the patient's parity (P) designate outcomes of the patient's pregnancies: term deliveries (T), preterm deliveries (P), all other pregnancies (A), and living children (L). Using this system, G_3P_{1112} would refer to a patient who has had two pregnancies, one full term, one with a preterm birth, and one abortion, who currently has two live children [2].

- *Complications of Pregnancy*: A history of obstetric complications, even past a woman's childbearing years, may affect risk of cardiovascular disease and diabetes and should be recorded. A history of gestational diabetes, preeclampsia, preterm delivery, placental abruption, and infants who were small for gestational age can increase the patient's risk for premature heart disease and cardiac death [3, 4]. Gestational diabetes greatly increases risk of the development of future maternal diabetes.
- Record maternal complications of pregnancy: peripartum cardiomyopathy, pulmonary edema, or gestational hypertension. Hypertensive or placental insufficiency syndromes include preeclampsia/eclampsia, HELLP (Hemolysis, Elevated Liver enzymes, Low Platelet count) syndrome, AFLP (Acute Fatty Liver of Pregnancy), or HUS/TTP (Hemolytic Uremic Syndrome/Thrombotic Thrombocytopenic Purpura).

- *Lactation*: Providers should discuss breastfeeding history or plans for lactation. Lactation is protective for breast cancer and has protective associations with multiple maternal cardiovascular risk factors [5].
- *Gynecologic History*: Human Papillomavirus (HPV) vaccination doses, date and results of prior Papanicolaou (pap) test and HPV screening, and evaluation of any abnormal pap tests are recorded. Colposcopies and treatments of any cervical intraepithelial neoplastic (CIN) lesions should be noted. (See Chap. 14 on Cervical Cancer and Human Papillomavirus).
- Past or current gynecologic diagnoses: ovarian cysts, uterine fibroids, polycystic ovary syndrome (PCOS), infertility, endometriosis, structural abnormalities, cervical or uterine polyps, procedural, and gynecologic surgical histories should be noted.
- *Sexual History*: The comprehensive wellness visit also presents an ideal time to perform a complete sexual history. Providers should practice sensitivity when asking questions regarding a patient's sexual history as some patients may feel uncomfortable disclosing this information. This history includes questions about sexual practices, sexual dysfunction, sexual orientation, characteristics and number of partners, types of sexual intercourse, history of sexually transmitted infections (STI), use of barrier

contraception, presence of dyspareunia, vaginal bleeding with intercourse, and decreased sexual libido. One should always aim to assess patients for high-risk sexual behavior for contraction of sexually transmitted infections such as human immunodeficiency virus (HIV) and be sure to counsel appropriately. (See Chap. 4 on Patient-Centered Contraceptive Counseling, Chap. 9 on Female Sexual Function and Dysfunction, and Chap. 13 on Sexually Transmitted Infections).

- *Breast Health and Screening History*: Age and frequency of mammograms; history of abnormal mammograms; breast density; prior breast biopsies and results; personal history of breast cancer; history of breast surgery including cosmetic surgery, breast reduction, benign breast conditions; and breast changes including masses, focal pain, discharge, pruritus, or change in the appearance of skin (including erythema and flaking) are recorded [6]. Family history is discussed below, but a cancer history is extremely important to assess for cancer risk. If a woman is at high risk for breast cancer because of a very strong family history, known genetic mutations, a history of atypical hyperplasia, lobular carcinoma in situ (LCIS), or a greater than 20% lifetime risk of breast cancer, then preventive measures such as screening MRIs, chemoprevention, genetic testing, and referrals to or evaluations by breast surgeons should be recorded (See Chap. 17 on the Primary Prevention of Breast Cancer). Lactation history should be recorded, as discussed above.
- *Family and Genetic History*: Asking specifically about a family history of breast, ovarian, fallopian tube, uterine, and colorectal cancer is important as certain genes have been linked to familial cancer syndromes. All cancers in first-, second-, and third-degree relatives may be relevant to breast and ovarian cancer risk. The age that the relative was diagnosed with cancer is important. A family history of known or suspected genetic syndromes which increase breast cancer risk should be recorded. A family history of colonic polyps or colon cancer is very relevant. For example, a patient whose aunt had early-onset colorectal cancer at age 39 may be at higher risk of ovarian, uterine, and gastrointestinal tract cancers if they have the genetic mutation for Lynch syndrome. (For further information see the section on "genetic screening" in Chap. 17, the Primary Prevention of Breast Cancer.) Family history of diabetes, hypertension, hyperlipidemia, and cardiovascular disease with age of onset should be noted (See Chap. 21 on Cardiovascular Disease in Women Part 1: Sex and Gender Differences in Cardiovascular Conditions and Risk Factors.)
- *Social History*: Should contain information on living situation, occupation, and education. Intimate partner violence screening and history of trauma are part of the social history.
  - *Screening for Intimate Partner Violence (IPV)*: The United States Preventive Task Force (USPSTF), American College of Obstetricians and Gynecologists (ACOG), and other professional societies recommend that IPV screening be performed at well-women visits [7, 8]. Language used in charting should be specific and factual such as "Patient states that…." and should clearly document symptoms and physical exam findings. Providers should keep in mind that the medical record may be viewed by the patient or possibly others and should exercise appropriate care. A recent systematic review found that screening for IPV increased the rates of identification of patients/survivors. It has been harder to prove that increased screening decreases IPV; however, identifying victims to offer support is important [9]. For more information, see chapter on IPV and sexual trauma for a complete discussion of interviewing techniques.
- *Lifestyle Habits*: Exercise/diet/smoking/alcohol and other substance use.

Review of Systems (ROS) Note that the following categories may not be included on a standard ROS template and may need to be asked directly:

1. Breast: pain/lump/discharge/galactorrhea/axillary mass/breast awareness.
2. Gynecologic: abnormal or irregular bleeding/pain/discharge/prolapse/pruritus/external lesions/dyspareunia/bloating/menopausal symptoms.
3. Urinary: incontinence/retention/dysuria/frequency.

The Pelvic Examination

Indications

A pelvic examination is indicated in women with a gynecologic symptom or concern including vaginal discharge, abnormal bleeding patterns, pelvic pain, urinary incontinence, dyspareunia, sexual concerns, or abdominal pain. Additionally, a pelvic examination may be needed for cervical cancer screening and evaluation of some sexually transmitted infections. There is controversy regarding the utility of routine screening pelvic examinations beyond what is described above.

Guidelines for Screening Pelvic Examinations

In 2014, the American College of Physicians (ACP) published guidelines for screening pelvic examinations, in asymptomatic, nonpregnant women, based on the results of a systematic review of the literature [10]. No conclusion could be drawn about the effect of screening pelvic examination on the diagnosis of asymptomatic pelvic inflammatory disease (PID), benign gynecologic conditions, or malignancy, excluding cervical and ovarian. Harms associated with screening pelvic examination include patient's pain, fear, and embarrassment, as well as the potential for increased unnecessary surgical procedures. Based on the results of this review, the ACP recommended against performing routine screening pelvic examinations in asymptomatic, nonpregnant women. Several other national and international organizations support this stance [11, 12].

The USPSTF and ACOG, however, do not support or refute this recommendation. The USPSTF published a recommendation statement after review of the literature on screening pelvic examinations, concluding that there is insufficient evidence to support or refute the performance of a routine screening pelvic examination in asymptomatic women [9]. ACOG published an independent review of the literature and, in 2018, concluded that current data is inadequate to support or refute an annual screening pelvic examination. ACOG recommends that obstetrician-gynecologists should discuss the risks and potential benefits of pelvic examination for asymptomatic women with their patients and reach a shared decision about whether or not to perform an exam [13].

Conflicting guidelines may impact patient understanding and adherence to routine gynecologic care. In a recent cross-sectional study examining patient beliefs regarding pelvic examination guidelines, over half of patients believed that they should undergo yearly screening pelvic examination, and over half were unaware of the new guidelines released by ACP [14]. The lack of awareness poses challenges for shared decision-making between provider and patient as knowledge about guidelines can impact decisions. In another study, women who were given the ACP guideline summary to review were much less likely to report wanting to undergo routine pelvic examination when compared to women who had read a previous ACOG guideline recommending continued screening pelvic examinations (OR 0.12) [11].

The editors agree that yearly routine pelvic examinations are unnecessary for asymptomatic women; however, periodic exams to obtain cervical cancer screening samples may be performed according to guidelines. Any complaint of pain, bleeding, or sexual dysfunction should be investigated with a pelvic exam, and the vulva (external exam) should be examined periodically as part of a routine skin check since many dermatologists do not examine this area. Students and residents training for primary care should be adequately trained to perform external and internal pelvic examinations.

Discontinuation of Pelvic Examinations

The choice to discontinue the screening pelvic examination can be considered in patients who have undergone total hysterectomy and bilateral salpingo-oophorectomy for benign causes who are asymptomatic. Care should be taken to ensure that the cervix was removed because patients may not be aware of the details of their surgery. Forgoing this routine internal examination should only be considered in patients who have no history of HIV and immunosuppression, no exposure to diethylstilbestrol (DES) in utero, and no prior cancer or precancerous lesions such as vulvar intraepithelial neoplasia or cervical intraepithelial neoplasia II or III [12]. Periodic external exams and exams for symptoms are still appropriate. For further information, see Chap. 14 on Cervical Cancer and Human Papillomavirus and Chap. 15 on Gynecologic Malignancies.

Chaperones

A chaperone is a trained health-care worker who accompanies the patient and provider in the exam room during an intimate exam. Friends and family members cannot serve as chaperones but can be in the room at the time of the exam at the patient's discretion. No uniform policy exists among US state medical or osteopathic boards regarding the presence of a chaperone in the examination room for intimate examinations [15]. Many studies suggest that patient preferences regarding the presence of chaperones vary, although many patients may prefer not having a chaperone present [16]. An ACOG committee opinion statement specifies that a chaperone should be available upon patient request regardless of the provider's gender and that the patient should have the opportunity to talk with the provider in the absence of the chaperone [17]. Chaperones can provide many benefits including attending to patient's emotions and positioning, assisting with equipment and testing samples, and acting as a third-party witness should there be a disagreement between patient and provider about what occurred during the examination. One should check with institutional policies regarding chaperones as many institutions require chaperones during all sensitive exams.

Positioning

During a typical pelvic examination, the patient assumes the dorsal lithotomy position. Although the patient's feet are commonly placed in footholds, or stirrups, some data suggest that examination without the use of footholds decreases patient discomfort with pelvic examination [18]. The perineum should rest about 2 inches off the end of the exam table as this allows for better access to the pelvic organs. If footholds are not used, the speculum handle will need to face upward to obtain a cervical sample. Alternate positions may be necessary for women with mobility limitations.

Mitigating Patient Anxiety

Some women report feeling fear, anxiety, or embarrassment about pelvic examinations. A 2014 systematic review evaluating the harms of pelvic examination found that between 10% and 80% of women experience these emotions during or before pelvic examination. Many women also experienced pain or discomfort during pelvic examinations, ranging between 10% and 60%. Of concern, this review also points out that many studies indicate an association of pain or discomfort with decreased likelihood of returning for a subsequent examination [10].

In addition to assuring proper privacy, draping, and room temperature, providers can do several things to mitigate patient anxiety. Woman should be asked about history of sexual intercourse. Women who have not previously had penetrative vaginal intercourse, are not currently sexually active, have dyspareunia, or are postmenopausal are at risk of an uncomfortable or painful examination. Women with anxiety, post-traumatic stress disorder, or a history of trauma are also at risk. Interventions to ensure a painless exam and mitigate anxiety include discussing the exam in advance: communicate that the patient is in control of the examination and can request for it to end at any moment, and explain the procedure prior to starting as well as during each step [19]. Throughout the examination, providers should continue to interact with the patient and frequently assess for signs of discomfort. Signs of distress can include breath holding, gripping the table or gown, and squinting the eyes shut. Vocalization by the patient, such as gasping, mumbling, cursing, or yelling, or physical reactions, such as kicking, moving further away from the examiner, or closing one's legs, are obvious signs of severe distress [20]. In order to mitigate mild distress, providers can instruct the patient in deep rhythmic breathing [21] or to Valsalva to relax the pelvic floor. Other potential techniques to mitigate patient's moderate to severe distress include using mental imagery, progressive muscle relaxation, and meditation [20]. Difficult cases should be referred to a gynecologist. In cases of severe physical or emotional distress and in clinical scenarios where pelvic exam is needed, pelvic examination can be performed under anesthesia.

In postmenopausal women, estrogen treatment for 6 weeks prior to the exam can be offered if the patient is not sexually active or has significant dyspareunia. If there is any concern that the exam will be uncomfortable, the initial step can be examination with one gloved finger which is moistened either with water or with a small amount of water-based lubricant (be aware that lubrication may interfere with adequate sampling for a pap test; check with your facility). The exam should be gentle, and gentle downward pressure should be applied to the posterior introitus to induce relaxation of the levator ani. If the examiner cannot perform this procedure without pain, then the exam should not be attempted, and alternative methods of evaluation including possible referral should be considered.

Components of a Pelvic Examination

The pelvic examination traditionally consists of three major components: (1) examination of the external genitalia; (2) internal examination of the vagina and cervix, performed with a speculum; and (3) bimanual examination of the uterus, adnexa, ovaries, and pelvic muscles [12].

1. *Examination of External Genitalia.*

   This component of the pelvic examination involves visual inspection of the perineum, mons pubis, and labia majora and minora. During this inspection, providers may identify any areas suspicious for neoplasia, folliculitis, candida infections, condylomas, other lesions, or ulcers. Providers can also note hair distribution, and in appropriate patients, can help determine Tanner stages. As a component of an external examination, the provider can also examine for Bartholin and Skene glands. Bartholin glands, which are not usually palpable in normal states, are located immediately internal to the hymen and are located bilaterally in the upper third of the vaginal introitus. Skene glands, also not usually palpable in healthy states, are located adjacent to the urethral orifice. Clitoromegaly or virilization should be noted.

2. *The Speculum Examination.*

   The speculum examination involves visualizing the vaginal canal and cervix. A speculum is inserted into the vagina in a downward motion, allowing the provider to examine the vaginal mucosa for lesions or atrophy. The provider can also observe for the presence of discharge and note color, consistency, and odor. Next, the speculum is carefully advanced, and the blades are opened to reveal the patient's cervix. After location of the cervix, the provider notes any discolorations, lesions, or masses on the cervix, as well as locating strings from an intrauterine contraceptive device, if appropriate. Samples for pap and STI testing are taken and then the speculum should be removed. The speculum is removed by gently backing the blades off the cervix and then allowing the blades to fall closed while still in the vaginal vault. This avoids closing the blades on the cervix and allows the speculum to be withdrawn from the vagina completely closed. Providers should take care to avoid pinching vaginal mucosa, skin, or hair between the blades as they close. The walls of the vagina should be visually inspected for lesions, especially if using a clear plastic speculum, while withdrawing the speculum. The speculum is then completely withdrawn, concluding this part of the exam.

Providers are sometimes unable to see the cervix when the speculum blades are opened. In these occasions, providers can first slowly retract the speculum a small amount which can bring the cervix into view. If adjustments to position do not allow providers to visualize the cervix, removing the speculum and performing a bimanual exam may help providers localize the relative position prior to reinsertion of the speculum [20]. Alternatively, a single gloved finger can be inserted prior to the speculum insertion to assess the position of the cervix.

3. *Bimanual Examination.*

The next portion of a comprehensive pelvic examination is a bimanual examination. To perform a bimanual examination, the provider inserts their index and middle finger of one hand into the vagina and places the other hand on the patient's lower abdomen. Using the inserted fingers, providers can locate the cervix and, by moving the cervix, can assess for cervical motion tenderness. Subsequently by lifting the cervix with the internal fingers and performing a downward sweeping motion with the external hand on the abdomen, the provider can assess the uterine position and approximate size. In order to assess the adnexa and ovaries, the inserted fingers can be angled toward each vaginal fornix individually, and the abdominal hand can again sweep downward in an attempt to push the ovary toward the inserted hand for palpation. In this portion of the examination, the ovaries and adnexa would be palpable only by the inserted fingers, not the abdominal hand, for size, tenderness, and irregularities. Note it is uncommon to feel both ovaries in a patient; body habitus and ovary position make it difficult to palpate the entire ovary and adequately characterize its position and size.

Tissue paper should be offered to patients at the conclusion of the exam for cleaning purposes, and a menstrual pad should be offered if any bleeding is noted, which is common if any sample are obtained from the cervix.

Teaching Pelvic Examinations

The intimate nature of a pelvic examination poses challenges in training providers to perform these examinations. Many studies have evaluated the benefits of the use of standardized patients to teach pelvic examinations to a variety of clinical trainees. The use of standardized patients was associated with improved clinical performance when assessed through clinical assessment, objective-structured clinical examinations, self-assessment, and location of abnormalities [22]. Additionally, the use of simulation for teaching pelvic examinations has been shown to lead to improved examination skills when compared to no intervention [23]. Other resources include online video demonstrations [24].

Pelvic Examinations with Accommodations

Examination of the Patient with Disabilities

The examination of a patient with physical or developmental disability poses unique challenges for patients and providers. Despite the challenges, reproductive health care is as imperative in disabled patients as it is in nondisabled patients. Patients with disabilities are as likely as their nondisabled counterparts to engage in sexual activity [25] and more likely to have experienced sexual assault [26, 27]. Given the diversity of types of disability, an individualized approach is often best.

For patients with disabilities, provision of additional time for examination, tables with adjustable heights to facilitate transfer to and from wheelchairs, and wheelchair-accessible clinics should be provided. Depending on the specific physical disability, alternative positions for pelvic examination could be considered including knee-chest positions (laying sideways) and frog or diamond positions [28]. Additionally, providers should be aware of disease-specific considerations for examination, including the avoidance of latex in patients with spina bifida due to the high rates of allergy [29]. The speculum positioning may need to be modified to accommodate various positions.

Examination of Adolescents

The frequency of screening pelvic examination of the adolescent patient is declining due to changes in age recommendations for cervical cancer screening and newer methods to screen for sexually transmitted diseases. However, external pelvic examination is recommended by the American Academy of Pediatrics as part of a routine comprehensive physical exam [30]. A diagnostic speculum and bimanual exam may be indicated when a patient presents with symptoms, menstrual irregularities, or a report of abuse. When performing a pelvic examination on an adolescent patient, there are several key considerations. An examination may be anxiety-provoking and communication regarding steps of the examination is important. Some examination techniques include providing the patient with a mirror to engage the patient in the examination, or examining a child in the mother's lap [31]. A narrower Huffman speculum may be used in younger adolescents. Contrary to guidelines for adults, a chaperone is strongly recommended for pelvic examinations in adolescent patients [30].

Examination of Women Aged 65 and Over

Though the older adult may not need further screening pelvic examinations, diagnostic pelvic examinations may be indicated. When a pelvic examination is needed in an older adult, several considerations are appropriate. Many older women may have difficulty with the traditional dorsal lithotomy position due to arthritis, contractures, or other medical conditions. Providers performing pelvic examination should consider alternative positions, similar to women with physical disabilities [32]. Given the increased incidence of atrophic vaginitis in this population, the liberal use of lubricant can also be considered. Many older women have had a total hysterectomy for either a benign or malignant reason. The remaining vaginal cuff can be very proximal to the introitus or very deep. To prevent discomfort or injury to the cuff, be cautious when inserting a speculum into this area when the depth of the vaginal cuff is unknown. Preexamination with one finger as described above is recommended.

Examination of Patients with Atrophic Vaginitis

Patients that have undergone menopause or that are on testosterone for gender-affirming therapy are at risk of developing atrophic vaginitis. Due to lack of the vaginal lubrication and thinned mucosae that are characteristics of the condition, patients with atrophic vaginitis can experience pain or even traumatic ecchymosis or laceration with pelvic examinations [33]. As in examination of the older woman, generous lubrication may be used. Vaginal estrogen used 2–6 weeks prior to examination, as well as topical lidocaine, may be used with pelvic examination; however, no studies have examined the efficacy of these strategies [1]. Using the smallest speculum to adequately visualize the cervix will be most comfortable for the patient. For cervical cancer screening, vaginal sampling for HPV may be sufficient. (See Chap. 14 on Cervical Cancer and Human Papillomavirus.)

Examination of Patients with Pelvic Organ Prolapse

Pelvic organ prolapse is a common condition, and a specific exam procedure is required to accurately diagnose it and its severity. This specialized examination should occur either when women present with urinary leakage, stool incontinence, pelvic pressure, the feeling of a vaginal or pelvic bulge or something "falling out" or when prolapse is seen grossly during the pelvic exam for other reasons. Pelvic organ prolapse occurs when the bladder, uterus, or rectum descends into the vaginal space due to weakness in the pelvic floor and supporting ligaments and tissues. Risk factors include pregnancy, especially vaginal delivery, age, and less so obesity, pelvic surgery, and occupations requiring heavy lifting [34].

In the dorsal lithotomy position, the patient should be asked to strain or "bear down" to visualize the vaginal walls and any descent of the pelvic organs near the introitus. The speculum can then be split in half so that it makes two "L"-shaped single-blade specula. One single speculum blade is then placed posteriorly to retract the posterior wall of the vagina while the provider observes the anterior wall for prolapse of the bladder (cystocele) while the patient bears down. The procedure is repeated, this time retracting the anterior vaginal wall with the single blade placed anteriorly, paying attention not to press against the urethra or clitoris and observing the posterior vaginal wall for prolapsed rectum (rectocele). During both these exams, the provider should also observe the cervix for prolapse of the uterus. Validated and standardized scoring systems are useful for documentation to compare severity of prolapse over time and avoid subjective ratings that may otherwise differ between providers. The authors recommend either routine use of the simplified Pelvic Organ Prolapse Quantification System [35] or at a minimum, recording the level of descent in terms of the number of centimeters distal or proximal to the introitus and its location (central, anterior, or posterior). See Chap. 23 on Urinary Incontinence to learn more about the treatment of prolapse.

Examination of Patients with Vulvodynia

Patients who have vaginismus or vulvodynia may experience discomfort with pelvic examinations, particularly with palpation of the labia and introitus and speculum insertion. In order to mitigate this discomfort, generous amount of lubricant or topical lidocaine may be utilized. If spasm occurs, the exam may need to be deferred [1]. In patients with vulvodynia, cues to "relax" by the provider feel frustrating and do not lead to relaxation of the pelvic muscles [36]. See Chap. 31 on Chronic Pelvic Pain for more information regarding physical exam techniques in patients with pelvic pain and the evaluation of vulvodynia.

Examination of Sexual or Gender Minority Patients

Significant health-care disparities exist among patients who are from sexual minority groups. Women who identify as lesbian or bisexual are less likely to present for annual physical examinations and less likely to have had cervical cancer screening than heterosexual women [37]. Cultural competence is of utmost importance when performing a pelvic examination for sexual or gender minority patients. It is important to discuss each patient's individual history without making prior assumptions based on external expressions of gender. For further information on sexual and gender minorities, see Chap. 36 on Care of Sexual Minority Women and Chap. 37 on Transgender Care.

Examination of Patients with a History of Sexual Trauma

Patients with a history of sexual trauma are found to be at highest risk for distress associated with pelvic examination [38]. A 2014 systematic review found nine studies that reported on harms of pelvic examination for women with a history of sexual violence. The majority of studies reporting fear, anxiety, distress, or embarrassment found that women who had experienced sexual trauma were at higher risk for experiencing these emotions [10]. Though patients may not always disclose sexual abuse in clinical situations, the majority of patients favor being asked by a provider regarding physical and sexual abuse history [39]. In addition to the strategies referenced in the "Mitigating Patient Anxiety" section above, providers can offer the option of counseling, make a statement to normalize anxiety, offer chaperone or gender concordant care, and at times can be offered anxiolytic therapy [1].

Clinical Breast Examination

The clinical breast examination is frequently performed as part of a comprehensive physical examination. Prior to beginning the examination, the patient should be situated on the exam table with a gown opened in the front. The clinical breast examination includes two primary components: inspection and palpation. The inspection portion begins with the patient sitting with her hands on her hips. Providers should then visually inspect the breasts for symmetry, skin changes, or other abnormalities. Subsequently, the axillary and supraclavicular lymph nodes should be examined. In order to examine the lymph nodes, the patient's arm should be supported at a 45-degree angle with the elbow relaxed. Using finger pads, the axillae should be palpated, taking care to examine the entire anterior, posterior, and media wall. The supraclavicular lymph nodes should be examined subsequently, palpating along the length of the superior aspect of the clavicle.

For the next part of the examination, the provider should assist the patient to lie flat on the examination table. With the patient's arm resting above her head, the provider or patient can expose the breast to be examined. In order to best examine all breast tissue, borders of the examination field should include the clavicle, the sternum, the midaxillary line, and across the ribs inferior to the breast [40]. Overall, a standardized technique is best, with studies indicating that a vertical-strip, or "lawn mower," pattern is most effective [41, 42]. For palpation, the index, middle, and ring fingers should be used together, creating small circles with three different levels of pressure: light, medium, and deep. The nipple should be palpated in the same method as the rest of the breast, without squeezing or attempting to express fluid.

Factors associated with superior accuracy of the breast examination for detection of masses included longer duration of examination, use of correct technique, and greater experience of the examiner [42]. The recommended amount of time for the examination is 3 minutes per breast [43].

Examination does not differ in women who have had breast implants or mastectomy. In women who have had mastectomy, the vertical-strip pattern can be used to palpate the chest wall.

Self-Breast Examination

The self-breast examination (SBE) is no longer routinely recommended as a way to screen for breast cancer as SBE has been shown to increase the rate of breast biopsies for benign findings without any decrease in breast cancer mortality [44]. However, many women practice SBE and often ask questions about SBE. It should be encouraged for women to have "breast awareness" and that any abnormal finding including a mass or lump, breast pain, nipple discharge, or axillary nodularity be brought to the attention of the provider. Women should also alert the provider of any change in family history which might increase the risk of breast- or ovarian-inherited malignancy. See Chap. 18 on Breast Cancer Screening regarding the guidelines and utility of self- and clinical breast examination.

Summary Points

1. In addition to a comprehensive general medical history, a complete female gender-specific history should include a complete sexual history, a pregnancy-specific history including maternal and obstetric complications, a breast history, screening for female cancer risk, a female specific review of systems, and a comprehensive menstrual history from menarche to menopause.
2. A standard complete pelvic examination includes both an external and internal examination, including visual inspection of the external genitalia, speculum examination of the vagina and cervix, and a bimanual examination of the uterus, adnexa, and pelvic floor muscles.

3. There are disparate guidelines that address indications for a screening bimanual examination, with many major medical organizations (ACP, AAFP) recommending against and some stating that there is insufficient evidence to make a definitive conclusion (USPSTF, ACOG).
4. There are many populations of patients in which pelvic examination accommodations may need to be made: those patients with vaginal atrophy, patients with a history of sexual trauma, patients with physical and developmental disabilities, and patients who identify as sexual or gender minority. Health-care providers should be aware of potential challenges and provide empathic and sensitive care.
5. Though there are no official standards, a clinical breast examination should include visual inspection and palpation.

Review Questions

1. A 20-year-old woman presents to her primary care provider's office for an annual wellness examination. She is currently sexually active with one male partner and uses condoms for contraception regularly. Her last menstrual period was 2 weeks ago, and she is concerned about some thin vaginal discharge and mild spotting but denies menorrhagia, itching, abdominal pain, or excessive menstrual cramping. Due to her vaginal discharge, you opt to perform a pelvic examination. Upon insertion of the speculum, the patient has no discomfort, anxiety, or evidence of atrophy of the vaginal mucosae; however, you are unable to visualize the cervix.

   What is the best next step in this physical examination?

   A. Removal of the speculum and localization of cervix through bimanual examination.
   B. Removal of the speculum and use of additional lubricant on reinsertion.
   C. Omitting visualization of the cervix given her primary concern is vaginal discharge.
   D. Omitting visualization of the cervix and assessing for cervical motion tenderness.

   The correct answer is A. The best next step is to remove the speculum and identify the approximate location of the cervix through a bimanual examination. Use of additional lubricant may be indicated when examining a patient who has vulvodynia or atrophic vaginitis; however, these conditions are not present in this patient. Omitting visualization of the cervix based on her primary concern would not be indicated as assessment for cervical lesions is appropriate in this patient who presents with spotting and discharge. While assessing for cervical motion tenderness is appropriate for this patient, this should be in addition to visualization of the cervix and not in lieu of [38].
2. A 40-year-old woman presents to her primary care provider's office for a Pap test. She has no significant past medical history. Her last menstrual period occurred 2 weeks ago, and she reports regular 28-day cycles with no excessive bleeding or cramping. She uses a levonorgestrel intrauterine device (IUD) for contraception and reports one male sexual partner. She expresses anxiety about the pelvic examination.

   Which of the following factors is known to contribute to increased anxiety surrounding pelvic examination?

   A. History of sexual trauma.
   B. History of IUD placement.
   C. History of remote childbirth.
   D. History of sexually transmitted infection.

   The correct answer is A. In a 2014 systematic review, women who had a history of sexual trauma were more likely to experience fear, anxiety, distress, or embarrassment with pelvic examination. History of IUD placement, history of remote childbirth, and history of sexually transmitted infections have not been found to be associated with increased anxiety surrounding pelvic examination [14, 41].

References

1. Bates CK, Carroll N, Potter J. The challenging pelvic examination. J Gen Intern Med. 2011;26(6):651–7.
2. Creinin MD, Simhan HN. Can we communicate gravidity and parity better? Obstet Gynecol. 2009;113(3):709–11.
3. Silverberg O, Park AL, Cohen E, Fell DB, Ray JG. Premature cardiac disease and death in women whose infant was preterm and small for gestational age: a retrospective cohort study. JAMA Cardiol. 2018;3(3):247–51.
4. DeRoo L, Skjaerven R, Wilcox A, Klungsoyr K, Wikstrom AK, Morken NH, et al. Placental abruption and long-term maternal cardiovascular disease mortality: a population-based registry study in Norway and Sweden. Eur J Epidemiol. 2016;31(5):501–11.
5. Perrine CG, Nelson JM, Corbelli J, Scanlon KS. Lactation and maternal cardio-metabolic health. Annu Rev Nutr. 2016;36:627–45.
6. Saslow D, Hannan J, Osuch J, Alciati MH, Baines C, Barton M, et al. Clinical breast examination: practical recommendations for optimizing performance and reporting. CA Cancer J Clin. 2004;54(6):327–44.
7. Force USPST. Final recommendation statement: intimate partner violence and abuse of elderly and vulnerable adults: screening. 2016. Available from: https://www.uspreventiveservicestaskforce.org/Page/Document/RecommendationStatementFinal/intimate-partner-violence-and-abuse-of-elderly-and-vulnerable-adults-screening.
8. ACOG Committee Opinion No. 518: Intimate partner violence. Obstet Gynecol. 2012;119(2 Pt 1):412–7.
9. Force USPST, Bibbins-Domingo K, Grossman DC, Curry SJ, Barry MJ, Davidson KW, et al. Screening for gynecologic conditions with pelvic examination: US Preventive Services Task Force Recommendation Statement. JAMA. 2017;317(9):947–53.

10. Bloomfield HE, Olson A, Greer N, Cantor A, MacDonald R, Rutks I, et al. Screening pelvic examinations in asymptomatic, average-risk adult women: an evidence report for a clinical practice guideline from the American College of Physicians. Ann Intern Med. 2014;161(1):46–53.
11. Sawaya GF, Smith-McCune KK, Gregorich SE, Moghadassi M, Kuppermann M. Effect of professional society recommendations on women's desire for a routine pelvic examination. Am J Obstet Gynecol. 2017;217(3):338 e1–7.
12. Committee on Gynecologic P. Committee opinion No. 534: well-woman visit. Obstet Gynecol. 2012;120(2 Pt 1):421–4.
13. ACOG Committee Opinion No. 754: the utility of and indications for routine pelvic examination. Obstet Gynecol. 2018;132:e174–80.
14. Kling JM, Vegunta S, Al-Badri M, Faubion SS, Fields HE, Shah AA, et al. Routine pelvic examinations: a descriptive cross-sectional survey of women's attitudes and beliefs after new guidelines. Prev Med. 2017;94:60–4.
15. Stagno SJ, Forster H, Belinson J. Medical and osteopathic boards' positions on chaperones during gynecologic examinations. Obstet Gynecol. 1999;94(3):352–4.
16. Fiddes P, Scott A, Fletcher J, Glasier A. Attitudes towards pelvic examination and chaperones: a questionnaire survey of patients and providers. Contraception. 2003;67(4):313–7.
17. Committee on Ethics ACoO, Gynecologists. ACOG Committee Opinion No. 373: sexual misconduct. Obstet Gynecol. 2007;110(2 Pt 1):441–4.
18. Seehusen DA, Johnson DR, Earwood JS, Sethuraman SN, Cornali J, Gillespie K, et al. Improving women's experience during speculum examinations at routine gynaecological visits: randomised clinical trial. BMJ. 2006;333(7560):171.
19. Oscarsson MG, Benzein EG, Wijma BE. The first pelvic examination. J Psychosom Obstet Gynaecol. 2007;28(1):7–12.
20. Williams AA, Williams M. A guide to performing pelvic speculum exams: a patient-centered approach to reducing iatrogenic effects. Teach Learn Med. 2013;25(4):383–91.
21. Hennigen L, Kollar LM, Rosenthal SL. Methods for managing pelvic examination anxiety: individual differences and relaxation techniques. J Pediatr Health Care. 2000;14(1):9–12.
22. Jha V, Setna Z, Al-Hity A, Quinton ND, Roberts TE. Patient involvement in teaching and assessing intimate examination skills: a systematic review. Med Educ. 2010;44(4):347–57.
23. Dilaveri CA, Szostek JH, Wang AT, Cook DA. Simulation training for breast and pelvic physical examination: a systematic review and meta-analysis. BJOG. 2013;120(10):1171–82.
24. Edelman A, Anderson J, Lai S, Braner DAV, Tegtmeyer K. Pelvic examination. N Engl J Med. 2007;356(26):e26.
25. Cheng MM, Udry JR. Sexual behaviors of physically disabled adolescents in the United States. J Adolesc Health. 2002;31(1):48–58.
26. Martin SL, Ray N, Sotres-Alvarez D, Kupper LL, Moracco KE, Dickens PA, et al. Physical and sexual assault of women with disabilities. Violence Against Women. 2006;12(9):823–37.
27. Mitra M, Manning SE, Lu E. Physical abuse around the time of pregnancy among women with disabilities. Matern Child Health J. 2012;16(4):802–6.
28. Abells D, Kirkham YA, Ornstein MP. Review of gynecologic and reproductive care for women with developmental disabilities. Curr Opin Obstet Gynecol. 2016;28(5):350–8.
29. Birmingham PK, Dsida RM. Latex precautions should be used in all spina bifida patients. Pediatr Neurosurg. 1992;18(4):224.
30. Braverman PK, Breech L, Committee on A. American Academy of Pediatrics. Clinical report–gynecologic examination for adolescents in the pediatric office setting. Pediatrics. 2010;126(3):583–90.
31. Simms-Cendan J. Examination of the pediatric adolescent patient. Best Pract Res Clin Obstet Gynaecol. 2018;48:3–13.
32. Richman SM, Drickamer MA. Gynecologic care of elderly women. J Am Med Dir Assoc. 2007;8(4):219–23.
33. Bachmann GA, Nevadunsky NS. Diagnosis and treatment of atrophic vaginitis. Am Fam Physician. 2000;61(10):3090–6.
34. Jelovsek JE, Maher C, Barber MD. Pelvic organ prolapse. Lancet. 2007;369(9566):1027–38.
35. Manonai J, Mouritsen L, Palma P, Contreras-Ortiz O, Korte JE, Swift S. The inter-system association between the simplified pelvic organ prolapse quantification system (S-POP) and the standard pelvic organ prolapse quantification system (POPQ) in describing pelvic organ prolapse. Int Urogynecol J. 2011;22(3):347–52.
36. Albrecht KB. "How-to" guide to pelvic floor muscle dysfunction. Clin Obstet Gynecol. 2015;58(3):546–50.
37. Blosnich JR, Farmer GW, Lee JG, Silenzio VM, Bowen DJ. Health inequalities among sexual minority adults: evidence from ten U.S. states, 2010. Am J Prev Med. 2014;46(4):337–49.
38. Weitlauf JC, Finney JW, Ruzek JI, Lee TT, Thrailkill A, Jones S, et al. Distress and pain during pelvic examinations: effect of sexual violence. Obstet Gynecol. 2008;112(6):1343–50.
39. Friedman LS, Samet JH, Roberts MS, Hudlin M, Hans P. Inquiry about victimization experiences. A survey of patient preferences and physician practices. Arch Intern Med. 1992;152(6):1186–90.
40. Pennypacker HS, Naylor L, Sander AA, Goldstein MK. Why can't we do better breast examinations? Nurse Pract Forum. 1999;10(3):122–8.
41. Saunders KJ, Pilgrim CA, Pennypacker HS. Increased proficiency of search in breast self-examination. Cancer. 1986;58(11):2531–7.
42. Barton MB, Harris R, Fletcher SW. The rational clinical examination. Does this patient have breast cancer? The screening clinical breast examination: should it be done? How? JAMA. 1999;282(13):1270–80.
43. McDonald S, Saslow D, Alciati MH. Performance and reporting of clinical breast examination: a review of the literature. CA Cancer J Clin. 2004;54(6):345–61.
44. Hackshaw AK, Paul EA. Breast self-examination and death from breast cancer: a meta-analysis. Br J Cancer. 2003;88(7):1047–53.

Part II

Gynecologic Health and Disease

Patient-Centered Contraceptive Counseling

4

Emmanuelle Yecies and Sonya Borrero

Learning Objectives

1. Compare different patient-centered approaches for eliciting reproductive goals, preferences, and priorities from patients related to contraception and pregnancy.
2. List currently available contraceptive methods.
3. Compare and contrast the mechanism of action, efficacy, duration of action, and return to fertility of the various contraceptive methods.
4. Discuss side effect profiles, contraindications, and noncontraceptive benefits of each method.
5. Provide counseling regarding emergency contraception and abortion for patients with contraceptive failure or for patients at risk of unwanted pregnancy who are not using prescription contraception.

Jenna is a 22-year-old woman who presents for routine medical care. Her medical history includes hypothyroidism treated with levothyroxine and migraines with aura treated with topiramate. She is a daily smoker but does not drink alcohol or use any illicit substances. She is sexually active with two to three partners per year. Her menses are regular, lasting 5 days every 28 days, with minimal pain and moderate bleeding.

E. Yecies
Section of Women's Health, VA Palo Alto Healthcare System, Palo Alto, CA, USA

S. Borrero (✉)
Center for Women's Health Research and Innovation (CWHRI), University of Pittsburgh School of Medicine, Pittsburgh, PA, USA

Center for Health Equity Research and Promotion (CHERP), VA Pittsburgh Healthcare System, Department of Medicine, Pittsburgh, PA, USA
e-mail: borrsp@upmc.edu

Reproductive Goals Counseling

Despite advances in contraceptive technology and access, 45% of pregnancies in the United States are reported as unintended, with higher rates reported among women of color and low-income women [1]. In recent years, experts and organizations, including the American College of Obstetricians and Gynecologists (ACOG) and the Centers for Disease Control and Prevention (CDC), have recommended that physicians and other care team members discuss reproductive goals with patients [2]. Using patient-centered approaches, providers can gather information about patients' reproductive goals, desires, and/or preferences in order to guide counseling with an end goal of helping patients to achieve healthy pregnancies when desired and prevent unwanted pregnancies [3].

Often implicit in reproductive goals assessments is the assumption that women hold clear and binary pregnancy intentions: that is, at a given time, women either do or do not desire pregnancy. The subsequent counseling strategy (either preconception counseling or contraceptive counseling) is then dependent on which of these opposing goals women express. However, research demonstrates that women often have nuanced feelings and thoughts about pregnancy that can be conflicting, even contradictory, and can fluctuate sometimes rapidly. Thus, open-ended, nonjudgmental questions regarding reproductive goals can elicit richer, more nuanced preferences that can guide meaningful, patient-centered discussions that may include both preconception and contraceptive counseling [4].

S. A. Tilstra et al. (eds.), *Sex- and Gender-Based Women's Health*, https://doi.org/10.1007/978-3-030-50695-7_4

One widely promoted strategy to assess reproductive goals, developed by the Oregon Foundation for Reproductive Health, is called One Key Question™ (OKQ) [5]. This initiative encourages providers to ask all women of childbearing capacity, "Would you like to become pregnant in the next year?" The advantage of this strategy is its simplicity, particularly in short clinical visits, and it is a valuable starting point for providers developing their counseling skills. A potential downside of this method is that it may be perceived by patients as a binary yes/no question and may not elicit or accommodate ambivalent, indifferent, or ambiguous thoughts and feelings about pregnancy.

Another approach to reproductive goals assessment published in the literature is the PATH questions, which can help to elicit long-term goals as well as short-term needs. These questions explicitly leave room for women to express ambivalence about pregnancy desires [4]. The PATH questions include three open-ended questions that assess **p**regnancy **at**titudes, **t**iming, and **h**ow important prevention is to the patient:

1. *Do you think you might like to have (more) children at some point?*
2. If considering future parenthood, *when do you think that might be?*
3. *How important is it to you to prevent pregnancy (until then)?*

As data, including comparative data, on these approaches and others are still lacking, there is no clear optimal approach to eliciting reproductive goals. Providers should consider using either method, or another patient-centered approach altogether, tailored to their comfort and patient population.

Nonpermanent Contraceptive Options

Jenna shares her responses to the PATH questions, revealing that she would like to delay having children for at least a couple of years. Preventing pregnancy is very important to her until then as she is completing a rigorous social work program and wants to graduate before juggling parenthood. She currently uses condoms when needed but is interested in learning more about her contraceptive options.

This section reviews currently available reversible contraceptive methods. For each method, special attention will be placed on mechanism of action, effectiveness, duration of action, and return to fertility. In addition, accessibility and convenience, menstrual changes, and side effects will be covered to guide providers in counseling their patients. Finally, common noncontraceptive benefits and contraindications will be outlined for each method to guide safe and appropriate selection.

There are various frameworks that can be used to organize currently available reversible contraceptive methods. Here, we have chosen to cluster the methods in three general categories related to duration of action and method effectiveness with typical use: long-acting reversible contraceptives (LARCs), short-acting reversible contraceptives (SARCs), and nonhormonal/barrier methods.

In addition to the information presented here, providers may refer to the US Selected Practices Recommendations (US SPR) for further information on initiating and managing different contraceptive methods and the US Medical Eligibility Criteria for Contraceptive Use (US MEC) for guidance on absolute and relative contraindications to specific contraceptive methods [6, 7]. Additional Web-based resources available to both providers and patients include plannedparenthood.org and bedsider.org [8, 9]. Finally, providers should remember to counsel patients that only condoms protect patients against the transmission of sexually transmitted infections (STIs). Condoms may be paired with any other method of contraception if there is any concern about STI exposure.

Long-Acting Reversible Contraceptives

Intrauterine Devices (IUDs)

Intrauterine devices (IUDs) are inserted into the uterus to provide long-acting reversible contraception. Two categories of IUDs have been approved in the United States: copper-containing (nonhormonal) IUDs (ParaGard™) and progestin-releasing IUDs (Mirena™, Kyleena™, Liletta™, Skyla™). Specific considerations about these subtypes are listed below. IUD effectiveness is approximately 99%, with failure rates less than 1% with both perfect and typical use [10]. IUDs may be offered to women of all ages and parities [11–13]; both the American Academy of Family Physicians (AAFP) and ACOG specifically recommend offering these methods to adolescents and nulliparous women [13, 14] as the belief that nulliparous women are not eligible for IUDs remains a barrier to access.

IUDs are placed by trained providers, and requirements for credentialing vary across different institutions. Contraindications to placement include cervical cancer, endometrial cancer, structural pelvic diseases, acute infection, and pregnancy [7]. Providers should determine the patient's last menstrual period and date of last unprotected sexual intercourse, assess the risk of pregnancy, and perform a pregnancy test prior to insertion (Fig. 4.1). If a patient has a high risk of pregnancy but has a negative pregnancy test at

How To Be Reasonably Certain a Woman Is Not Pregnant

A healthcare provider can be reasonably certain that a woman is not pregnant is she has no symptoms or signs of pregnancy and she meets any of the following criteria:

- is ≤ 7 days after the start of normal menses
- has not had sexual intercourse since the start of last normal menses
- has been correctly and consistently using a reliable method of contraception
- is ≤ 7 days after spontaneous or induced abortion
- is within 4 weeks post-partum. In addition
- is fully or nearly fully breastfeeding (exclusively breastfeeding or the vast majority [≥85%] of feeds are breastfeeds), amenorrheic, and < 6 months post-partum

Fig. 4.1 How to determine if a woman is not pregnant [6]. (Adapted from Curtis et al. [6])

insertion, a pregnancy test should be performed 2–3 weeks after insertion.

If STI screening is indicated according to STI screening guidelines, screening may be done at the time of IUD placement and, if positive, antibiotics may be given with the IUD being placed. If, however, there is evidence on exam of active purulent cervicitis, IUD insertion should be delayed until after treatment and documented clearance of the infection [6, 15]. There is no data to support self-IUD string checks, but a follow-up visit with a provider may be scheduled based on provider and patient preference [6]. Return to fertility is prompt after IUD removal, and pregnancy can occur almost immediately after removal, even though return of regular menses typically occurs in 1–2 months for levonorgestrel-IUD users [16, 17].

Copper IUDs

One copper-containing IUD has been approved in the United States, TCu380A (ParaGard™). It is believed to prevent pregnancy in two ways: an inflammatory reaction to the foreign body in the uterus and local changes caused by copper release, including sperm toxicity and impaired implantation [18, 19]. The copper IUD has been FDA approved for contraception for up to 10 years and has been used off-label for up to 12 years [20]. In addition, copper IUDs may be placed for emergency contraception within five days of unprotected intercourse [21, 22]. The most common side effect of copper IUDs is an increase in length, discomfort, and/or heaviness of menstrual bleeding, although this rarely causes significant drops in hemoglobin in previously non-anemic women [23, 24].

Progestin IUDs

Currently, four progestin-containing IUDs have been approved in the United States, which release varying amounts of levonorgestrel (LNg). Progestin IUDs are believed to prevent pregnancy by causing the same foreign body reaction as copper IUDs in addition to providing local progestin effects: thickened cervical mucus and changes in the endometrial lining [18, 25]. These IUDs have various FDA-approved duration of use from 3 to 5 years, though the Mirena™ IUD has been used off-label for up to 7 years [26]. These devices are not currently approved for emergency contraception, though studies are underway. The most common side effect is irregular bleeding, particularly in the first year [23]. By 2 years of use, amenorrhea is reported by 12% (13.5 mg IUDs) up to 30–50% (52 mg IUDs) of women [27, 28]. Other reported side effects include acne, vaginal discharge, and abdominal pain [29]. In addition to broad IUD contraindications, levonorgestrel-releasing IUDs are also contraindicated in breast cancer [7]. Noncontraceptive benefits of the 52 mg LNg IUDs include decrease in menorrhagia and dysmenorrhea (FDA approved for this indication), reduction in endometriosis-related pain and endometrial hyperplasia, and lower rates of endometrial, ovarian, and cervical cancer [30–33].

Subdermal Implant

The subdermal implant (Nexplanon) is a single-rod implant containing etonogestrel, a progestin metabolite. The progestins present in the implant provide contraceptive effects via two mechanisms [34]. First, etonogestrel decreases sperm migration by causing changes in cervical mucus and tubal motility. Second, the high doses of etonogestrel present in the implant inhibit gonadotropin hormone secretion, leading to the inhibition of follicle maturation and ovulation. The implant is greater than 99% effective, with typical and perfect use failure rates less than 1% [35]. The implant has been approved for contraception for up to 3 years, although evidence suggests that it may be effective for longer durations [36]. Studies of prior subdermal implants have demonstrated that circulating levels of hormones are undetectable 1 week after removal [37]. As a result, return of ovulation occurs within 3 months of removal in 91% of women [38].

The implant can be inserted and removed in the office by providers who have been trained in the procedure. This 3-h training is offered by Merck and covers counseling, insertion, and removal, allowing providers to quickly expand their ability to initiate this method in their own practice [39]. No physical examination or testing is necessary prior to insertion. The implant is placed in the inner upper arm. It should be easily palpable, but the device is radio-opaque and can be seen on plain films if its location is in question.

The safety and side effect profile of etonogestrel implants are well studied [35]. Irregular, unscheduled bleeding is the most common side effect and also the most common reason for discontinuation [35]. The number of bleeding days and spotting is highest in the first 3 months of use and stabilizes during the second and third years of use. After the initial bleeding patterns plateau, approximately 20% of women report amenorrhea. However, a study of 90-day reference periods demonstrated that 17% of women had bleeding episodes lasting longer than 14 days, and 6% had more than five bleeding episodes. Headaches are reported in up to 16% of users. Weight gain averaged around 2.8 pounds after 1 year and 3.7 pounds after 2 years of use and was reported by 12% of users. Other notable side effects include acne vulgaris (12%), mastalgia (10%), and abdominal pain (5%).

There are few medical contraindications to the use of the etonogestrel implant, with only active breast cancer noted as an absolute contraindication to use. Other conditions such as severe decompensated cirrhosis, ischemic heart disease, and liver tumors confer risks that likely outweigh the advantages of this contraceptive method [7]. Some medications lower the effectiveness of the implant, including efavirenz-based antiretroviral regimen and certain antiepileptics [40–42]. Notably, this method has not been studied in women with a BMI greater than 30 kg/m^2, but there is no evidence that effectiveness is compromised in these women [43].

Although the etonogestrel implant is solely approved for contraception, some data exist about its use in endometriosis, where it was non-inferior to depot medroxyprogesterone acetate (DMPA) in relief of pain symptoms [44]. There are no other reported noncontraceptive benefits. The implant is not approved for emergency contraception.

Short-Acting Reversible Contraceptives

Injectable

Depot medroxyprogesterone acetate (DMPA) is an injectable progestin contraceptive administered subcutaneously (104 mcg) or intramuscularly (150 mcg) every 3 months. Its mechanism of action is similar to that of the implant with dual progestin effects: cervical mucus changes and inhibition of ovulation [45]. With perfect use, DMPA is a highly effective contraceptive with a failure rate of 0.2% [46]. However, typical use failure rate is closer to 6%, thought to be due to late return for repeat injections [46]. Effectiveness is not decreased due to body weight owing to the high doses of circulating progestins [47]. Unlike the previously described methods, DMPA may cause a delay in return to fertility of several months (up to 18 months in a small subset), and women who would like to become pregnant soon after discontinuation may want to consider a different method [48, 49].

DMPA is typically administered in the office, although studies suggest self-injection with a subcutaneous formulation may improve adherence and access [50, 51]. No testing or physical examination is necessary aside from ascertaining that a woman is not pregnant. Once injected, no monitoring or follow-up is indicated until the next injection at 3 months.

Appropriate counseling about side effects of DMPA is crucial to ensure appropriate contraceptive selection and continuation [52]. All women experience menstrual changes. In the first few months of use, unscheduled bleeding is very common and progresses to amenorrhea in nearly 50% of users by one year [53]. There is some historical controversy about weight gain with DMPA, but recent data demonstrate mean weight gain is typically no more than 2 kgs in 12 months [54]. DMPA may also trigger headaches, nervousness, and abdominal pain [49]. Concern about bone demineralization prompted the FDA to issue a warning about prolonged use in adolescents and young adults, but evidence shows there is recovery of bone mineral density after cessation, and neither ACOG nor the WHO believe the evidence should limit the duration of DMPA use or prompt additional bone mineral density screening [55–58].

Like other progestin-based contraceptives, DMPA is contraindicated in breast cancer [7]. Other potential contraindications include decompensated cirrhosis, liver tumors, and ischemic heart disease.

DMPA has several noncontraceptive benefits owing to its mechanism of action [59]. Heavy menstrual bleeding and associated anemia decrease as women trend toward amenorrhea. Endometriosis-related pain and endometrial hyperplasia decrease, as well as rates of pelvic inflammatory disease and cervical cancer. DMPA is not approved for emergency contraception.

Pill

The "pill" refers to the broad category of contraceptives taken as a daily oral medication. Often the most recognizable method due to its long history and availability, patients will often use the term to refer to any one of many different formulations. These formulations can generally be broken up into two subcategories, progestin-only and combined estrogen-progestin pills.

Progestin-Only Pills (POPs)

Also known as the "minipill," progestin-only pills are taken daily by mouth. The mechanism of action is similar to the other progesterone-based methods detailed previously including cervical mucus changes and thinning of the endometrial lining, but inhibition of ovulation is less consistent [60]. Efficacy of POPs is significantly affected by user dependability as this method requires daily use within a small time window to be effective for pregnancy prevention (typically 3 h) [46]. Even delaying a dose by several hours is enough to risk contraceptive failure. As such, return to fertility is prompt after discontinuing this method.

If a patient misses a pill, she should be counseled to take it immediately upon remembering (and in addition to any dose also due at that time), and she should use a "backup" method, such as condoms, or avoid sexual intercourse for at least two days after reinitiation of the pill so that cervical mucus has a chance to thicken [6]. No physical exam or laboratory tests are indicated at the time of prescription of POPs, and no follow-up is required in the absence of side effects.

The most prevalent side effect of POPs is unscheduled bleeding and spotting [61]. There is an increased prevalence of follicular ovarian cysts, and women should be reassured that no intervention is required [62]. POPs do not lead to weight gain [54].

There are few contraindications to POPs though breast cancer is an "absolute" contraindication [7]. Similar to other progestin-based contraceptives, liver tumors and decompensated heart disease are relative contraindications. Progestin-only pills are typically used in women who have contraindications to estrogen use but desire a pill form of contraception. POPs appear to have a protective effect against endometrial cancer [63].

Combined Oral Contraceptive Pills (COCs)

Estrogen-progestin pills are also taken daily by mouth. COCs have several mechanisms of action contributing to their contraceptive effects including suppression of gonadotropin-releasing hormone and inhibition of the luteinizing hormone (LH) surge, thereby preventing ovulation [64]. In addition to these estrogen effects, COCs also benefit from the progestin-related contraceptive actions as detailed above in the POP section. COCs have a perfect-use failure rate of 0.1%; however, this number rises to 8% with typical use as efficacy relies on daily use and prompt refills [46].

In the event of missed pills, women should be counseled to take the missed dose as soon as is remembered (and in addition to any dose otherwise due) [6]. If two or more doses have been missed, she should also be counseled to use backup contraception or avoid sexual intercourse for seven days. COCs may be prescribed monthly (21 active pills followed by 7 placebo pills) or with extended cycling (84 active pills followed by 7 placebo pills) for fewer withdrawal bleeds [65]. Blood pressure should be checked before initiation and then at routine care [6]. However, in the absence of side effects, no additional follow-up is necessary other than routine care.

There are a multitude of COC formulations, and options available to each patient may vary based on their insurance formulary. When selecting a COC, a provider must make decisions about both the estrogen and progestin components. The estrogen is typically ethinyl estradiol and can be dosed from 10 mcg to 35 mcg per day. Women experience more breakthrough bleeding at the lower end of the dosing spectrum and more estrogenic side effects such as mastalgia, nausea, and bloating at the higher end of the spectrum. Additionally, there is theoretical higher risk of venous thromboembolism (VTE) with higher estrogen doses, although the absolute risk of VTE is low for most women and far lower than the risk associated with pregnancy. Most women tolerate estradiol doses of 20–35 mcg, and pills >35 mcg are no longer used for contraception [66, 67]. Generally, it is recommended to use the lowest estradiol dose possible that is acceptable for the patient in terms of breakthrough bleeding and side effects.

Progestin components are often categorized by generation. Second-generation progestins (such as levonorgestrel and norethindrone) are the most androgenic and may cause adverse metabolic effects. Third-generation progestins (such as norgestimate) have fewer androgenic properties but may be associated with a slightly increased risk of VTE [68]. Fourth-generation progestins (most famously drospirenone) are considered antiandrogenic but have also been associated with an increased risk of VTE [69]. Without compelling reasons to push for fourth-generation progestin use, such as severe acne likely to benefit from antiandrogenic properties, most providers will select second- or third-generation progestins.

The type and frequency of side effects of COCs relate to their estrogen content and type of progestin. Early side effects including headache, mastalgia, and nausea typically improve within the first few months [70]. Breakthrough bleeding is common and expected for the first few months; after 3 months, an increase in the dose of estradiol may be considered to decrease breakthrough bleeding [66]. There is a small increase in blood pressure and incidence of myocardial infarction [71]. For this reason, women with a history of heart disease and those over 35 who smoke should not be prescribed COCs [72]. However, pregnancy also elevates these risks, so providers should consider risk-benefit counseling in women who may not be open to other, potentially safer contraceptive options. Migraines with aura are also considered contraindications to COC use as these women are at increased risk of stroke [73]. History of VTE is an absolute contraindication given the already known increased risk of VTE across all COCs. The increased risk of VTE appears to be increased severalfold in obese women [74]. Other contraindications include any pro-thrombotic states, acute liver disease, and undiagnosed vaginal bleeding [7]. As with all hormonal contraceptives, breast cancer is an absolute contraindication.

Although estrogen-containing pills are not contraindicated during lactation, they have been inconsistently implicated in decreasing milk supply [75]. As such, different contraception methods may be more appropriate in postpartum women who are breastfeeding [6].

There are many noncontraceptive benefits associated with the use of COCs [76], including reducing hirsutism, acne, menorrhagia, dysmenorrhea, endometriosis pain, and symptoms of premenstrual syndrome. While only some COCs carry a specific FDA approval for acne reduction, this benefit is mediated via estrogen's role in increasing sex-hormone-binding globulin production from the liver and so may be seen with any COC formulation. COCs may also help control bleeding secondary to fibroids. Finally, COCs use is associated with a decrease in rates of colon cancer, endometrial cancer, and ovarian cancer.

Transdermal Patch

The "patch" is a transdermal combined hormonal contraceptive containing ethinyl estradiol and norelgestromin. Its mechanism of action is the same as that of COCs. The transdermal patch is applied weekly for 3 consecutive weeks (21 days total) to the abdomen, upper arm, or buttock, followed by a patch-free week to facilitate a withdrawal bleed. Some women may be interested in extended use, where the patch-free week and withdrawal bleed are skipped. Backup method should be used if a patch is not replaced within 2 days of a scheduled switch date [6].

The efficacy, return to fertility, side effects, contraindications, and noncontraceptive benefits of the transdermal contraceptive patch are similar to those of COCs [77, 78]. Some women develop irritation at the site of the patch, particularly those with a history of sensitive skin. There is some concern about slightly increased risk of thrombosis (approximately twofold) in patch users compared to COCs [79]. Finally, obese women may have higher rates of contraceptive failure [80].

Vaginal Ring

The "ring" is a vaginal-combined contraceptive containing ethinyl estradiol and etonogestrel. The systemic estrogen absorption is lower than other combined contraceptives [81]. It is self-inserted into the vagina, left in for 3 weeks, and then removed for a withdrawal bleed for 1 week before a new one is reinserted. Some women also opt for continuous use where women replace the ring without allowing for the week of withdrawal bleeding [82]. If the ring is accidentally taken out, the US SPR has a detailed algorithm about management depending on time since removal [6].

The other characteristics of this contraceptive method (including return to fertility, efficacy, side effects, contraindications, and noncontraceptive benefits) are similar to those of COCs [78]. In addition, ring users may have an increase in vaginal discharge and vaginitis.

Of note, a new combined hormonal contraceptive ring (Annovera™) was recently approved by the FDA, although it is not yet available for prescription. Containing ethinyl estradiol and segesterone acetate, it is intended to last thirteen 28-day cycles (3 weeks inserted, 1 week removed) [83]. It is expected to carry the same risks and benefits as previously approved combined hormonal contraceptive methods, but the extended duration of use may facilitate continuation and adherence.

Nonhormonal/Barrier Methods

These methods are considered to have lower efficacy for pregnancy prevention. However, they are often easily available and may be appropriate for women whose goals or contraindications make the previously described methods less desirable. All of these methods are quickly reversible and do not cause a delay in return to fertility.

Male Condom

Male condoms are made from one of three types of material: latex, natural membrane, and synthetic (typically polyurethane). They may contain spermicide or lubricant (or neither). Almost all studies have been conducted on latex condoms. Used alone, condoms have around an 18% failure rate with typical use versus 2% with perfect use [46]. Mechanism is based on barrier protection with or without spermicidal effects depending on the type of condom used.

Male condoms are easily obtained without a prescription at any number of places including pharmacies, grocery stores, and gas stations. They are relatively inexpensive (often less than a dollar per condom) and can be easily carried by both men and women. Disadvantages of male condom use include disruption of sexual activity, decreased sensation reported by some men or women, and sometimes improper fit [84]. They may require counseling to ensure effective use. In addition, women opting to rely on male condom use for contraception must have partner cooperation and support.

The main contraindication to typical condom use is a latex sensitivity, although men can switch to synthetic material or natural membrane. In addition, latex condoms should not be paired with oil-based lubricants.

Noncontraceptive benefits of condoms include STI protection. Unlike previously described methods, condom use is the only strategy that serves as both contraception and protection against STI [85]. As such, it should be paired with any of the other methods if STI protection is desired in addition to contraception. Of note, natural membrane condoms are more porous and may not carry the same STI protection that latex and synthetic condoms do [86]. Patients should be counseled not to rely on natural membrane condoms for STI protection.

Internal Condom

The internal (or "female") condoms can be made of natural latex, synthetic latex, and polyurethane. They have an outer ring that anchors them in place and cover the cervix, vagina, and introitus. Annual failure rates are around 21% with typical use (5% with perfect use) [87]. They may be more difficult to obtain due to low prevalence of use (less than 1% of manufactured condoms are internal) and are more expensive (usually around 2 dollars per condom). Mechanism of action, contraindications, and STI protection benefits mirror those of male condoms.

Spermicide

The only spermicide available in the United States is nonoxynol-9 (N-9), a chemical that impairs sperm motility by damaging the body and flagella. Spermicide is available over the counter in many formulations including foam, gel, cream, and suppository. It costs between 60 cents and $3 per dose. Typical use failure rate is nearly 20% per year when used alone [88].

Spermicide should be applied to the vagina prior to each episode of intercourse (at least 10 min prior for the suppository to allow for dispersion). Intercourse should not be delayed longer than an hour without reapplication.

Relative contraindications include allergy to nonoxynol-9 and use in women who are at high risk of STI (particularly HIV) transmission [89]. N-9 use appears to be associated with higher rates of HIV acquisition, potentially due to spermicide-induced mucosal irritation [90]. Side effects include vaginal (and penile) irritation, increased UTI frequency, and slight increase in rates of bacterial vaginosis [88, 91, 92].

Diaphragm

This is a reusable cup-shaped device that a woman places against her cervix. It is used in conjunction with spermicide, and its mechanism of action is primarily spermicidal in addition to creating a barrier to block sperm from entering the cervix. Failure rates approach 12% per year with typical use, although the failure rate appears to be highest in multiparous women [46]. Most diaphragms must be fit to the patient, typically by a gynecologist, but at least one type (commercial name Caya) is considered single size and can be purchased directly from a pharmacy. Diaphragms are typically covered by insurance when prescribed and fitted by a provider.

Women are taught to insert their diaphragm with spermicide prior to intercourse. It should then remain in place at least 6 h from the last episode of intercourse but no more than 24 h.

Relative contraindications to diaphragm use include frequent UTIs, allergy to the components (silicone or latex), history of toxic shock syndrome, and any contraindications to spermicide use (see section on spermicide). Side effects and complications include increased risk of UTI, likely secondary to spermicide-induced changes in the vaginal flora, vaginal irritation, and toxic shock syndrome (TSS) [93, 94]. TSS is rare and almost exclusively associated with >24 h of continuous use.

Sponge

The sponge is a spermicidal-impregnated polyurethane matrix available over the counter. It contains nonoxynol-9 which is activated when the sponge is wetted. The mechanism of action is similar to that of diaphragms, although failure rates are closer to 24% for multiparous women (12% among nulliparous women) [46]. The sponge is self-inserted up to 24 h before intercourse and should be removed 6 h after the last episode of intercourse. In all, the sponge should be removed within 30 h of insertion. It is single use and should be discarded after removal. Each sponge costs approximately 5 dollars.

Relative contraindications and side effects mirror those of the diaphragm. Allergy or sensitivity to polyurethane, N-9, and sulfa should preclude use.

Fertility-Awareness-Based Method

With these methods, women track changes in the menstrual cycle to avoid pregnancy [95]. Also called "natural family planning," these methods involve identifying the date of ovulation and the associated days of fertility and abstaining from intercourse or using alternative methods of contraception during those days. Conversely, these methods can also be used to assist in conception. With perfect use, annual pregnancy rates are between 3% and 5%, but with typical use, pregnancy rates are closer to 24% annually [96]. Some described methods include standard days (SDM), 2 days (TDM), and symptothermal. For patients who desire additional information about fertility awareness methods, a number of Web-based resources including bedsider.org (https://www.bedsider.org/methods/fertility_awareness#how_to) and plannedparenthood.org (https://www.plannedparenthood.org/learn/birth-control/fertility-awareness) can provide more details [97, 98]. Smartphone applications are also available, including Natural Cycles™, which has been granted FDA approval.

Withdrawal

The withdrawal method involves the male partner pulling out his penis prior to ejaculation to keep semen out of the vagina. This method can be up to 96% effective with perfect use, but patients should be counseled that typical use results in annual pregnancy rates up to 22% [46]. In addition, this method requires trust and reliance on a woman's partner, so partner support is essential in selection of this method.

At the time of writing, the Affordable Care Act (ACA) mandates that at least one form of all FDA-approved methods (and emergency contraception) be covered by health insurance plans provided by all employers and educational institutions with no cost sharing. This excludes male birth control including male condoms and vasectomies.

Contraceptive Counseling Strategies

You prepare to counsel Jenna about her options and consider the best approach to help her in selecting the right method for her needs.

If reproductive goals counseling determines that the patient has a contraceptive desire or need, the next step is to engage in counseling to guide method selection. Similar to reproductive goals counseling, there are multiple frameworks to approach contraceptive counseling. Common counseling strategies can be broadly grouped into consumerist models (patient-driven), directive models (provider-driven), or a shared decision-making approach [99].

Within the consumerist model, there are two main approaches observed in clinical practice, both of which prioritize patient autonomy [100]. In an "informed choice" model, the provider shares objective information about various methods but does not participate in the selection itself. The downside of this model is that the provider does not necessarily help patients understand how their preferences relate to method characteristics, and the information shared is not tailored to the specific needs of the patient. In a "foreclosed" model, the provider shares information only about methods asked about by the patient. A limitation of this model is that women may not have a complete or accurate picture of the range of all available methods.

In directive counseling, providers conduct counseling with the goal of promoting a specific course of action. For example, there has been a strong push toward LARC selection given its high effectiveness, with references to these methods as "first line" by the American Academy of Pediatrics (AAP) and ACOG [101, 102]. However, in encouraging adoption of these methods, providers may be making assumptions about a patient's priorities rather than attending to the fact that women have many different goals, preferences, and needs when it comes to their contraception. "Encouragement" to select specific methods, especially when they do not align with stated preferences, can thus be perceived as pressure and be counterproductive [103–105]. This may be particularly problematic in marginalized communities, given the history of family planning abuses targeting low-income women and women of color. One recent qualitative study explored patient experiences with implicit pressure, in which providers' subtle cues appeared to favor certain contraceptive methods [106]. The young women of color included in the study had high rates of rapid discontinuation of chosen methods, with some patients curtailing future health-care visits and subsequent contraceptive use.

Family planning experts and guidelines, including the CDC's Quality in Family Planning, have promoted approaches that optimize patient centeredness, both in terms of how women prefer to make contraceptive decisions and with regard to method selection itself [107, 108]. While some patients may prefer to make fully autonomous decisions (consumerist model) and others may prefer to have their providers make strong recommendations (directive model), research has indicated that most women prefer a shared decision-making approach [109]. Shared decision-making combines features of both patient-driven and provider-driven approaches to allow a provider to guide a woman to the best method based on her individual context. Shared decision-making is a strategy that can help enhance patient centeredness when selecting a contraceptive method because it explicitly centers the discussion around a woman's preferences and priorities for method characteristics. To achieve successful shared decision-making, a number of factors must be considered to guide patients in selecting the best method for their needs.

Preferred Efficacy

Given that ambivalence is common, efficacy is not always the most important factor guiding women's contraceptive decisions. Thus, rather than assuming that all women will prioritize efficacy, providers should ask women whether this is something they value. Questions about importance of efficacy should also elicit ideal frequency of use of the method. Particularly because non-LARC methods have different efficacy based on patient adherence, it is crucial to elicit whether a woman prefers and can adhere to frequent use, such as daily pills or weekly patches. A woman who reports wanting effective contraception above all would likely benefit from a LARC method, especially if she reports difficulty in adhering to prescribed medication schedules (e.g., erratic work hours may interfere with remembering to take a daily pill at the same time every day).

Preferred Side Effect Profile

To optimize success with a selected contraceptive method, it is crucial to adequately elicit a patient's preference or tolerance regarding side effects [104, 110]. Certain side effects may be tolerable to some patients while leading to discontinuation for others. This particularly applies to menstrual changes, as can be illustrated by the levonorgestrel IUD. Some women desire amenorrhea, while others prefer monthly menses and would be better served selecting a method that does not affect their menstrual cycle [111]. Providers should make sure to assess women's understanding of the safety of amenorrhea with contraception when women state a preference for having menstrual cycles. Even if amenorrhea is desired, some women may not tolerate the unscheduled bleeding often seen in the initial months or may want to avoid it at particular times in their lives [112]. Only eliciting such preferences allows a thorough discussion regarding the experience with each method and appropriate selection.

Pattern of Sexual Activity

This information may also help a provider guide a patient's decision; a woman who is sexually active once a year may have a different view of risk/benefit profiles of various methods compared to a woman who is sexually active weekly or daily. Similarly, number of partners or relationship status may affect their preferred contraceptive profile.

Need for Privacy

Providers should also inquire about a woman's need for privacy as some women may need to select methods based on discreetness and ability to conceal use [113–116]. Reproductive coercion (behavior to control contraception and pregnancy outcomes of sexual partners) has been identified in up to 16% of relationships, with intimate partner violence co-occurring in 32% of these relationships [117] (see Chap. 35 on "Intimate Partner Violence and Sexual Trauma" for additional information). The use of discreet contraceptive methods has been identified as a potential harm reduction strategy for women in abusive relationships. If a woman voices a preference or need to keep her contraceptive use hidden, medroxyprogesterone injection may be a good option. Alternatively, an IUD can be inserted and the strings trimmed to the level of the cervical os or canal, making them nearly invisible. Depending on the exact circumstances, other methods may or may not be appropriate.

Desired Return to Fertility

Timeline to desired pregnancy may also affect the appropriateness of various methods. For example, medroxyprogesterone injection is unlikely to be an appropriate method to recommend to a patient who desires pregnancy within a year, given that the delay in return to fertility can be up to 2 years [48, 49].

Depending on the preferences elicited regarding the above factors and medical contraindications, providers should adjust the scaffolding that they offer patients for decision-making. For example, the commonly used tiered-effectiveness scaffold may not be appropriate for a patient who values avoidance of side effects over efficacy. Focusing on the methods that a woman will use successfully based on her preferences can optimize method satisfaction, adherence, and continuation.

Finally, contraception counseling should not exclude sterilization procedures, particularly in women who have completed or do not desire childbearing. Both female and male sterilization should be explored in appropriate patients as permanent contraceptive choices if desired.

Initiating Contraception and Facilitating Adherence

Jenna shares that she has trouble remembering to take medications on a daily basis. She is reluctant to have a procedure for insertion of a contraceptive device. Given that she has a history of migraines with aura, you recommend avoiding estrogen-based methods (such as the vaginal ring or transdermal patch). Based on this discussion, Jenna selects medroxyprogesterone injections.

When a woman selects a contraceptive method, the next steps are to ensure adequate initiation and help patients optimize adherence. The first step is to ensure that a woman is not currently pregnant. A set of criteria has been developed by the CDC to assist providers in ascertaining patients' pregnancy status [6] (Fig. 4.1). The use of these criteria is particularly important when initiating hormonal methods or the copper IUD.

Once pregnancy is reasonably ruled out, methods can be prescribed or inserted. Using the "quick-start" method is the current standard of care to optimize initiation and adherence [6]. "Quick-start" allows that any method can be started on any day of a woman's menstrual cycle so long as backup methods are used for 7 days after initiation. Notable exceptions to the 7-day rule include progestin-only pills which require only 2 days of a backup method and copper IUDs which are immediately effective and require no backup method.

Once a method is started, there are steps a provider can take to improve adherence and continuation. Providing the maximum number of months of contraceptive methods at a single fill (e.g., dispensing 3 or 12 months of medication at one time) has been demonstrated to improve continuation and adherence [118]. This has prompted laws in twelve states and the District of Columbia mandating that pharmacies dispense (and insurances pay for) a 12-month supply at each fill if desired by the patient. In addition, while annual visits are recommended, there is no role for refusing to prescribe contraception for a patient who is not up to date on cervical cancer screening or who has not had a pelvic examination [119]. This is highlighted in the AAFP's "Choosing Wisely" recommendations [120].

Finally, it is important that providers ensure timely access for removal of provider-controlled methods such as IUDs and subdermal implants, especially when women would like early removal of their device. Counseling regarding discontinuation and removal should be provided at the time of initiation.

Emergency Contraception and Abortion

Emergency Contraception

Emergency contraception (EC) refers to contraception used after unprotected intercourse to minimize the chance of unwanted pregnancy. There are various methods that can be used for emergency contraception. More information can be obtained through US SPR or the Princeton Emergency Contraception website [6, 121].

Copper IUD

The copper IUD is the most effective form of emergency contraception (96.9–100% effective), although it remains off-label for EC use in the United States [21]. The device should be inserted within five days of unprotected intercourse and may remain in place as long as desired (up to 10 years) for contraception.

Levonorgestrel

More commonly known as Plan B™, levonorgestrel is available with or without a prescription. It should be covered by insurance when obtained by prescription; however, insurance reimbursement is more variable when purchased over the counter (non-covered cost is approximately $40). The mechanism of action is thought to be a delay in ovulation [122]. Levonorgestrel has a failure rate of 2–3% when used within 72 h of unprotected intercourse, which equates to a theoretical decrease of 50% in expected pregnancies [123, 124]. Levonorgestrel may be taken as one dose (1.5 mg single tablet) or two doses (0.75 mg tablets taken 12 h apart), although the former is recommended due to increased convenience without compromising efficacy or increasing side effects [125]. Obese women (BMI > 30 kg/m^2) have a fourfold risk of pregnancy compared to underweight and normal weight women and should be counseled about the limitations of this method [126].

Ulipristal

Ulipristal is an antiprogestin medication available by prescription only. It is effective by delaying ovulation, even once the LH levels have begun to rise (and levonorgestrel is no longer effective) [127]. It may be taken up to 120 h after unprotected intercourse. Ulipristal has a failure rate of 1.4% or prevents approximately two-third of expected pregnancies [123, 124]. While less effective in obese women, ulipristal is more effective than levonorgestrel EC; for obese patients desiring oral EC, ulipristal is the preferred agent [128]. Of note, access to ulipristal remains limited, with one study finding less than 10% of pharmacies having the ability to immediately fill a prescription [129]. Providers prescribing ulipristal should consider verifying pharmacy availability at the time of prescription.

Yuzpe Regimen

This regimen was introduced in 1974 and allows women to take a combination of pills from standard COC prescriptions to reach a dose of 200 mcg of ethinyl estradiol and 1 mg levonorgestrel [130]. In certain areas or for privacy reasons, this method may be more accessible for patients than other EC methods. It should be initiated within 72 h of unprotected intercourse. It is less efficacious than other methods and has more side effects (nausea, vomiting, headaches, mastalgia) due to the high estrogen dose, so it is rarely recommended when other methods are available [123]. Non-levonorgestrel progestins have not been studied.

All women should be counseled about emergency contraception, regardless of whether they are using another method of contraception [131]. Some women may only need EC in the case of contraceptive failure, while some may actually prefer to rely on EC for contraception, particularly if they have infrequent intercourse or contraindications to more effective methods. As all of these methods must be initiated within 72–120 h of unprotected intercourse for efficacy, it is reasonable to counsel women about the use of EC and to make it available to them prior to needing it [6]. Exploring a woman's preferred EC method and providing advance prescriptions help improve access and use should they have unprotected intercourse [131]. This practice may also help to defray costs for those with insurance as prescription levonorgestrel EC is covered, but over-the-counter formulations may not be. Advance prescriptions do not increase the rate of unprotected intercourse.

According to ACOG, no follow-up visit is routinely required after the use of EC. A pregnancy test should be obtained if no bleeding occurs within 3–4 weeks of taking EC [131].

Abortion

Elective termination, also known as induced abortion, is an option available to women in the United States, although there is significant variability in access and options depending on the patient's location. There are two categories of elective terminations: medical and surgical abortions. Both options are safe and effective in appropriate patients, and the choice is typically made based on gestational age, availability, and patient preference [132].

Medical abortion is the termination of a pregnancy with medications alone, typically using mifepristone (an antiprogestin) combined with misoprostol for patients in the United States. Patients are given the initial dose of medication in a health-care facility and then return home for the ensuing days while the termination occurs. Medical abortion is available until a gestational age of 70 days based on the first day of the last menstrual period or ultrasound dating. Medical abortion comprises approximately 22% of abortions at ≤8 weeks and 1.2% of abortions at >8 weeks [133]. The success rate of medical abortion is 92–98%, with the other 2–8% requiring surgical evacuation [134]. Side effects include cramping, nausea, and vomiting. Significant complications are rare (0.65% of women) and include endometritis, infections, and hemorrhage (secondary to uterine atony or retained products of conceptions) [135]. Contraindications to this method include the presence of a hemorrhagic disorder or anticoagulation. Advantages of medical abortion over surgical abortion are the decreased amount of time in clinical settings and, for some patients, the feeling that they have a higher degree of control over the process [136]. Acceptability of this method is high (nearly 82% satisfaction), and 81% would choose the same method if a future abortion was required [137, 138].

Surgical abortion techniques vary depending on gestational age. In the first trimester, the procedure is typically uterine dilation and suction aspiration. The procedure is performed in a clinical setting (including outpatient or free-standing clinics), and termination is completed prior to patients returning home. Successful termination occurs in >95% of cases of surgical abortion with complication rates of approximately 9 per 1000 [134, 139]. Major complications are rare (0.71 per 1000) and include perforation, infection, cervical laceration, hemorrhage, and retained products of conception [139]. There are no true contraindications to surgical abortion; however, in women with large fibroids or other anatomic abnormalities, medical abortion may be preferred if gestation is <10 weeks given potentially complicating anatomy. Advantages of surgical abortion over medical abortion include more rapid confirmation of successful termination and higher patient satisfaction (92%) [137].

Providers should feel comfortable counseling women about where to seek abortion services if a patient wishes to learn about or desires an abortion. These services include intra-institutional resources, free-standing clinics, and/or Planned Parenthood. The local family planning division of OB/GYN may also be able to provide additional local private options.

Table 4.1 Starting specific contraceptive methods [6]

Method	Backup method	Before initiation[a]
Copper IUD	Not needed	Bimanual examination and cervical inspection
Levonorgestrel IUD	7 days	Bimanual examination and cervical inspection
Implant	7 days	None
Injectable (DMPA)	7 days	None
Combined hormonal contraception	7 days	Blood pressure measurement
Progestin-only pill	2 days	None

Adapted from Curtis et al. [6]

[a]*Must also be reasonably certain that a woman is not pregnant by meeting any one of the following criteria: is ≤7 days after the start of normal menses; has not had sexual intercourse since the start of last normal menses; has been correctly and consistently using a reliable method of contraception; is ≤7 days after spontaneous or induced abortion; is within 4 weeks postpartum; is fully or nearly fully breastfeeding (exclusively breastfeeding or the vast majority [≥85%] of feeds are breastfeeds), amenorrheic, and <6 months postpartum (CDC SPR)*

We recommend exploring acceptability of elective termination particularly for women who indicate that it is important for them to avoid pregnancy but are not using contraception or effective contraception. In addition, abortion access and acceptability should be explored among women with chronic medical conditions that would be negatively impacted by pregnancy (or vice versa) and women using teratogenic medications who decline contraception or effective methods (Table 4.1).

Summary Points

1. The use of standardized questions, such as One Key Question or the PATH questions, can help identify women's reproductive goals and need or desire for contraception and contraceptive counseling.
2. Numerous contraceptive options are available to patients, including long-acting reversible contraceptives (IUDs, implants), short-acting reversible contraceptives (pills, patches, and rings), and barrier or nonhormonal methods.
3. When counseling about contraception, patient preferences about method characteristics including effectiveness, menstrual changes, and relevant side effect profiles should guide the conversation to help patients select the most appropriate method for them.
4. The CDC MEC is a reliable resource to identify contraindicated methods of contraception in various medical comorbidities.
5. Contraceptive counseling should include counseling regarding options in the case of contraceptive failure and exploring attitudes toward and providing appropriate resources regarding EC and abortion.

Review Questions

1. A 36-year-old woman presents for her annual visit. She reports being sexually active with one male partner for the last 6 months. She is not currently using contraception. Which of the following is a patient-centered question to assess reproductive goals and preferences?
   A. "Are you trying to become pregnant?"
   B. "Would you like to become pregnant in the next year?"
   C. "Can we start you on birth control?"
   D. "Why are you not using contraception?"

   The correct answer is B. "One Key Question" is one recommended approach for eliciting reproductive goals. It is a potential first step to open conversations about reproductive desires, intentions, or concerns. It may help discern the need for preconception counseling and/or contraception counseling. "Are you trying to become pregnant?" assigns intentions to the patient that she has not expressed, and this assumption may feel judgmental to a patient who may not be actively trying to conceive despite not using regular contraception. Similarly, "why are you not using contraception?" may indicate judgment from the provider of what the patient should be doing, prior to clarifying her intentions. Finally, "can we start you on birth control?" assumes the patient is interested in preventing pregnancy at this time, which she may not yet have expressed [5].

2. A 21-year-old college student presents to clinic. She has recently become sexually active and reports that her highest priority in choosing a contraceptive method is avoiding pregnancy. She often forgets to take medications like antibiotics, so would prefer a method that she doesn't have to think about too much. She does not have any medical comorbidities and does not want to become pregnant in the next few years. Which of the following methods will likely best match her stated preferences?
   A. Levonorgestrel intrauterine implant (e.g., Mirena™)
   B. Male condoms
   C. Medroxyprogesterone injection (e.g., Depo-Provera)
   D. Etonogestrel/ethinyl estradiol vaginal ring (e.g., NuvaRing™)

   The correct answer is A. This patient is expressing preferences that match with long-acting, highly effective contraceptive. She would benefit from counseling about LARCs, either an intrauterine implant or a subdermal implant. She would be an excellent candidate for an intrauterine implant given her reported difficulty in adherence to medications. The vaginal ring and medroxyprogesterone injection are considered less effective than LARCs, and their efficacy depends on reliable timing of the medications (monthly and every 3 months, respectively). Since she endorses missed medication doses even for short-term concerns, she may have a difficult time using these methods reliably, though these options should still be explored with her. Finally, male condoms are the least effective of the above methods and thus would not be the best single method for contraception, given her priority of avoiding pregnancy. However, this patient should be counseled that condoms are the only method that prevents STI transmission and can be used in conjunction with any of the other methods [140].

3. A 27-year-old woman presents for an annual physical complaining of worsening acne. Her physical exam reveals cystic acne on her temples and chin. She is sexually active with one male partner, and they are using condoms. She reports that she would really like to get her acne under control. Menstrual history reveals irregular periods, averaging approximately five menses per year. Which of the following might be an appropriate recommendation?
   A. Medroxyprogesterone injection (e.g., Depo-Provera™)
   B. Levonorgestrel intrauterine implant (e.g., Mirena™)
   C. Norgestimate/ethinyl estradiol COCs (e.g., Sprintec)
   D. Etonogestrel subdermal implant (e.g., Nexplanon™)

   The correct answer is C. This patient seems to be suffering from hormonal acne and oligomenorrhea, which could be suggestive of PCOS. Combined oral contraceptives (COCs) have been demonstrated to have noncontraceptive benefits that include improvement of acne, and they can also regulate menses, decreasing unopposed estrogen and associated endometrial cancer risk. Levonorgestrel intrauterine implants, etonogestrel subdermal implants, and medroxyprogesterone injections have not demonstrated to have any benefits for acne or PCOS and would not be particularly beneficial in this patient [141].

4. A 38-year-old woman with a history of complex migraines presents to the office with worsening menorrhagia. Since menarche, she has had painful heavy periods, once requiring admission for a transfusion. She has been missing work due to her menses and is desperate to try something to lighten or eliminate them. She is not sexually active and does not want any more children. She is not interested in surgery as it would mean missing more work. Which option will decrease her bleeding and pain the most?
   A. Etonogestrel implant (e.g., Nexplanon)
   B. Combined oral contraceptive cycled continuously
   C. Levonorgestrel intrauterine implant (e.g., Mirena)
   D. Medroxyprogesterone injection (e.g., Depo-Provera)

   The correct answer is C. This patient's menorrhagia would best be managed with levonorgestrel intrauterine device since most women experience amenorrhea or at least a decrease in bleeding days and severity on this contraceptive. Levonorgestrel IUDs are also specifically approved for this indication. COCs cycled continuously would likely decrease her menorrhagia as well, but these are contraindicated in the setting of migraines with aura given the increased risk of stroke. Etonogestrel implant and medroxyprogesterone injections often lead to irregular bleeding without significant decrease in bleeding days or severity [142, 143].

5. A 23-year-old patient with obesity (BMI 32.1) calls in to her primary care office at 8 am on Monday morning. She reports that the condom broke the night before while she was having intercourse with her male partner. She does not use other contraceptives and does not want to get pregnant right now. She is worried about becoming pregnant and asks what to do next.
   A. Reassure her that her risk of pregnancy from one unprotected episode of intercourse is low
   B. Offer her a prescription for COCs with the recommendation to take six pills on day 1
   C. Offer her a same-day appointment for insertion of a levonorgestrel IUD
   D. Offer her a prescription for ulipristal acetate

   The correct answer is D. Of these options, ulipristal acetate has the best evidence for preventing pregnancy after unprotected intercourse, especially in obese women for whom levonorgestrel is less reliable for EC. Levonorgestrel IUD is an excellent contraceptive method but has not been established as emergency contraception after unprotected intercourse (unlike copper IUDs), and it should not be placed in women who may be pregnant. COCs can also be offered for contraception, and multiple pills may be taken off-label to achieve EC levels of levonorgestrel (1 mg), but efficacy is lower and side effects may be significant due to the high-estrogen doses. Finally, providing reassurance that pregnancy is unlikely from one episode of unprotected intercourse without offering emergency contraception is not appropriate in this situation as the patient has expressed a strong desire to avoid pregnancy [127].

References

1. Finer LB, Zolna MR. Declines in unintended pregnancy in the United States, 2008-2011. N Engl J Med. 2016;374(9):843–52. https://doi.org/10.1056/NEJMsa1506575.
2. American College of Obstetricians and Gynecologists' Committee on Health Care for Underserved Women. Committee opinion no. 654: reproductive life planning to reduce unintended pregnancy. Obstet Gynecol. 2016 Feb;127(2):e66–9. https://doi.org/10.1097/AOG.0000000000001314.
3. Johnson K, Posner SF, Biermann J, Cordero JF, Atrash HK, Parker CS, et al. Recommendations to improve preconception health and health care--United States. A report of the CDC/ATSDR Preconception Care Work Group and the Select Panel on Preconception Care. MMWR Recomm Rep. 2006;55(RR-6): 1–23.
4. Callegari LS, Aiken AR, Dehlendorf C, Cason P, Borrero S. Addressing potential pitfalls of reproductive life planning with patient-centered counseling. Am J Obstet Gynecol. 2017;216(2):129–34. https://doi.org/10.1016/j.ajog.2016.10.004.
5. Bellanca HK, Hunter MS. ONE KEY QUESTION(R): preventive reproductive health is part of high quality primary care. Contraception. 2013;88(1):3–6. https://doi.org/10.1016/j.contraception.2013.05.003.
6. Curtis, KM, Jatlaoui TC, Tepper NK, Zapata LB, Horton LG, et al. U.S. selected practice recommendations for contraceptive use, 2016. MMWR Recomm Rep. 2016;65(4):1–66, Appendices. https://doi.org/10.15585/mmwr.rr6504a1. https://www.cdc.gov/mmwr/volumes/65/rr/pdfs/rr6504.pdf
7. Curtis KM, Tepper NK, Jatlaoui TC, Berry-Bibee E, Horton LG, Zapata LB, et al. U.S. medical eligibility criteria for contraceptive use, 2016. MMWR Recomm Rep. 2016;65(3):1–103. https://doi.org/10.15585/mmwr.rr6503a1.
8. Birth Control. 2019. Available from: https://www.plannedparenthood.org/learn/birth-control.
9. Method Explorer. Birth Control Methods-Method Explorer. https://www.bedsider.org/methods
10. Heinemann K, Reed S, Moehner S, Minh TD. Comparative contraceptive effectiveness of levonorgestrel-releasing and copper intrauterine devices: the European Active Surveillance Study for Intrauterine Devices. Contraception. 2015 Apr;91(4):280–3. https://doi.org/10.1016/j.contraception.2015.01.011.
11. Cramer DW, Schiff I, Schoenbaum SC, Gibson M, Belisle S, Albrecht B, et al. Tubal infertility and the intrauterine device. N Engl J Med. 1985;312(15):941–7.
12. Payne JB, Sundstrom B, DeMaria AL. A qualitative study of young women's beliefs about intrauterine devices: fear of infertility. J Midwifery Womens Health. 2016;61(4):482–8. https://doi.org/10.1111/jmwh.12425.
13. American College of Obstetricians and Gynecologists. ACOG practice bulletin no. 121: Long-acting reversible contraception: implants and intrauterine devices. Obstet Gynecol. 2011;118(1): 184–96. https://doi.org/10.1097/AOG.0b013e318227f05e.
14. Hardeman J, Weiss BD. Intrauterine devices: an update. Am Fam Physician. 2014;89(6):445–50.
15. Caddy S, Yudin MH, Hakim J, Money DM; Infectious Disease Committee; Special Contributor. Best practices to minimize risk of infection with intrauterine device insertion. J Obstet Gynaecol Can. 2014;36(3):266–74. https://doi.org/10.1016/S1701-2163(15)30636-8.
16. Vessey MP, Lawless M, McPherson K, Yeates D. Fertility after stopping use of intrauterine contraceptive device. Br Med J (Clin Res Ed). 1983;286(6359):106.
17. Mansour D, Gemzell-Danielsson K, Inki P, Jensen JT. Fertility after discontinuation of contraception: a comprehensive review of the literature. Contraception. 2011;84(5):465–77. https://doi.org/10.1016/j.contraception.2011.04.002.
18. Stanford JB, Mikolajczyk RT. Mechanisms of action of intrauterine devices: update and estimation of postfertilization effects. Am J Obstet Gynecol. 2002;187(6):1699–708.
19. Ortiz ME, Croxatto HB, Bardin CW. Mechanisms of action of intrauterine devices. Obstet Gynecol Surv. 1996;51(12 Suppl):S42–51.
20. Long-term reversible contraception. Twelve years of experience with the TCu380A and TCu220C. Contraception. 1997;56(6):341–52.

21. Wu S, Godfrey EM, Wojdyla D, Dong J, Cong J, et al. Copper T380A intrauterine device for emergency contraception: a prospective, multicentre, cohort clinical trial. BJOG. 2010;117(10):1205–10. https://doi.org/10.1111/j.1471-0528.2010.02652.x.
22. Turok DK, Godfrey EM, Wojdyla D, Dermish A, Torres L, Wu SC. Copper T380 intrauterine device for emergency contraception: highly effective at any time in the menstrual cycle. Hum Reprod. 2013;28(10):2672–6. https://doi.org/10.1093/humrep/det330.
23. Diedrich JT, Desai S, Zhao Q, Secura G, Madden T, Peipert JF. Association of short-term bleeding and cramping patterns with long-acting reversible contraceptive method satisfaction. Am J Obstet Gynecol. 2015;212(1):50.e1–8. https://doi.org/10.1016/j.ajog.2014.07.025.
24. Lowe RF, Prata N. Hemoglobin and serum ferritin levels in women using copper-releasing or levonorgestrel-releasing intrauterine devices: a systematic review. Contraception. 2013;87(4):486–96. https://doi.org/10.1016/j.contraception.2012.09.025.
25. Lewis RA, Taylor D, Natavio MF, Melamed A, Felix J, Mishell D Jr. Effects of the levonorgestrel-releasing intrauterine system on cervical mucus quality and sperm penetrability. Contraception. 2010;82(6):491–6. https://doi.org/10.1016/j.contraception.2010.06.006.
26. Wu JP, Pickle S. Extended use of the intrauterine device: a literature review and recommendations for clinical practice. Contraception. 2014;89(6):495–503. https://doi.org/10.1016/j.contraception.2014.02.011.
27. Fan G, Kang S, Ren M, Weisberg E, Lukkari-Lax E, et al. A single-arm phase III study exploring the efficacy and safety of LNG-IUS 8, a low-dose levonorgestrel intrauterine contraceptive system (total content 13.5 mg), in an Asia-Pacific population. Contraception. 2017;95(4):371–7. https://doi.org/10.1016/j.contraception.2016.11.005.
28. Darney PD, Stuart GS, Thomas MA, Cwiak C, Olariu A, Creinin MD. Amenorrhea rates and predictors during 1 year of levonorgestrel 52 mg intrauterine system use. Contraception. 2018;97(3):210–4. https://doi.org/10.1016/j.contraception.2017.10.005.
29. Sivin I, Stern J. Health during prolonged use of levonorgestrel 20 micrograms/d and the copper TCu 380Ag intrauterine contraceptive devices: a multicenter study. International Committee for Contraception Research (ICCR). Fertil Steril. 1994;61(1):70–7.
30. Cortessis VK, Barrett M, Brown Wade N, Enebish T, Perrigo JL, Tobin J, Zhong C, et al. Intrauterine device use and cervical cancer risk: a systematic review and meta-analysis. Obstet Gynecol. 2017;130(6):1226–36. https://doi.org/10.1097/AOG.0000000000002307.
31. Lethaby AE, Cooke I, Rees M. Progesterone or progestogen-releasing intrauterine systems for heavy menstrual bleeding. Cochrane Database Syst Rev. 2005;4:CD002126.
32. Abou-Setta AM, Al-Inany HG, Farquhar CM. Levonorgestrel-releasing intrauterine device (LNG-IUD) for symptomatic endometriosis following surgery. Cochrane Database Syst Rev. 2006;4:CD005072.
33. Kaunitz AM, Bissonnette F, Monteiro I, Lukkari-Lax E, Muysers C, Jensen JT. Levonorgestrel-releasing intrauterine system or medroxyprogesterone for heavy menstrual bleeding: a randomized controlled trial. Obstet Gynecol. 2010;116(3):625–32. https://doi.org/10.1097/AOG.0b013e3181ec622b.
34. Croxatto HB. Mechanisms that explain the contraceptive action of progestin implants for women. Contraception. 2002;65(1):21–7.
35. Darney P, Patel A, Rosen K, Shapiro LS, Kaunitz AM. Safety and efficacy of a single-rod etonogestrel implant (Implanon): results from 11 international clinical trials. Fertil Steril. 2009;91(5):1646–53. https://doi.org/10.1016/j.fertnstert.2008.02.140.
36. McNicholas C, Maddipati R, Zhao Q, Swor E, Peipert JF. Use of the etonogestrel implant and levonorgestrel intrauterine device beyond the U.S. Food and Drug Administration-approved duration. Obstet Gynecol. 2015;125(3):599–604. https://doi.org/10.1097/AOG.0000000000000690.
37. Davies GC, Feng LX, Newton JR, Van Beek A, Coelingh-Bennink HJ. Release characteristics, ovarian activity and menstrual bleeding pattern with a single contraceptive implant releasing 3-ketodesogestrel. Contraception. 1993;47(3):251–61.
38. Croxatto HB, Urbancsek J, Massai R, Coelingh Bennink H, van Beek A. A multicentre efficacy and safety study of the single contraceptive implant Implanon. Hum Reprod. 1999;14(4):976–81.!!!!!!!!!!Implanon Group not in replacement text.
39. Creinin MD, Kaunitz AM, Darney PD, Schwartz L, Hampton T, et al. The US etonogestrel implant mandatory clinical training and active monitoring programs: 6-year experience. Contraception. 2017;95(2):205–10. https://doi.org/10.1016/j.contraception.2016.07.012.
40. Leticee N, Viard JP, Yamgnane A, Karmochkine M, Benachi A. Contraceptive failure of etonogestrel implant in patients treated with antiretrovirals including efavirenz. Contraception. 2012;85(4):425–7. https://doi.org/10.1016/j.contraception.2011.09.005.
41. Vieira CS, Bahamondes MV, de Souza RM, Brito MB, Rocha Prandini TR, Amaral E, et al. Effect of antiretroviral therapy including lopinavir/ritonavir or efavirenz on etonogestrel-releasing implant pharmacokinetics in HIV-positive women. J Acquir Immune Defic Syndr. 2014;66(4):378–85. https://doi.org/10.1097/QAI.0000000000000189.
42. Lazorwitz A, Davis A, Swartz M, Guiahi M. The effect of carbamazepine on etonogestrel concentrations in contraceptive implant users. Contraception. 2017;95(6):571–7. https://doi.org/10.1016/j.contraception.2017.03.004.
43. Morrell KM, Cremers S, Westhoff CL, Davis AR. Relationship between etonogestrel level and BMI in women using the contraceptive implant for more than 1 year. Contraception. 2016;93(3):263–5. https://doi.org/10.1016/j.contraception.2015.11.005.
44. Walch K, Unfried G, Huber J, Kurz C, van Trotsenburg M, et al. Implanon versus medroxyprogesterone acetate: effects on pain scores in patients with symptomatic endometriosis--a pilot study. Contraception. 2009;79(1):29–34. https://doi.org/10.1016/j.contraception.2008.07.017.
45. Kaunitz AM. Long-acting injectable contraception with depot medroxyprogesterone acetate. Am J Obstet Gynecol. 1994;170(5 Pt 2):1543–9.
46. Trussell J. Contraceptive failure in the United States. Contraception. 2011;83(5):397–404. https://doi.org/10.1016/j.contraception.2011.01.021.
47. Segall-Gutierrez P, Taylor D, Liu X, Stanzcyk F, Azen S, Mishell DR Jr. Follicular development and ovulation in extremely obese women receiving depo-medroxyprogesterone acetate subcutaneously. Contraception. 2010;81(6):487–95. https://doi.org/10.1016/j.contraception.2010.01.021.
48. Schwallie PC, Assenzo JR. The effect of depo-medroxyprogesterone acetate on pituitary and ovarian function, and the return of fertility following its discontinuation: a review. Contraception. 1974;10(2):181–202.
49. Kaunitz AM. Injectable depot medroxyprogesterone acetate contraception: an update for U.S. clinicians. Int J Fertil Womens Med. 1998;43(2):73–83.
50. Kohn JE, Simons HR, Della Badia L, Draper E, Morfesis J, Talmont E, et al. Increased 1-year continuation of DMPA among women randomized to self-administration: results from a randomized controlled trial at Planned Parenthood.

Contraception. 2018;97(3):198–204. https://doi.org/10.1016/j.contraception.2017.11.009.
51. Prabhakaran S, Sweet A. Self-administration of subcutaneous depot medroxyprogesterone acetate for contraception: feasibility and acceptability. Contraception. 2012;85(5):453–7. https://doi.org/10.1016/j.contraception.2011.09.015.
52. Hubacher D, Goco N, Gonzalez B, Taylor D. Factors affecting continuation rates of DMPA. Contraception. 1999;60(6):345–51.
53. Hubacher D, Lopez L, Steiner MJ, Dorflinger L. Menstrual pattern changes from levonorgestrel subdermal implants and DMPA: systematic review and evidence-based comparisons. Contraception. 2009;80(2):113–8. https://doi.org/10.1016/j.contraception.2009.02.008.
54. Lopez LM, Ramesh S, Chen M, Edelman A, Otterness C, et al. Progestin-only contraceptives: effects on weight. Cochrane Database Syst Rev. 2016;8:CD008815. https://doi.org/10.1002/14651858.CD008815.pub4.
55. Kaunitz AM, Arias R, McClung M. Bone density recovery after depot medroxyprogesterone acetate injectable contraception use. Contraception. 2008;77(2):67–76. https://doi.org/10.1016/j.contraception.2007.10.005.
56. American College of Obstetricians and Gynecologists. Committee Opinion No. 602: depot medroxyprogesterone acetate and bone effects. Obstet Gynecol. 2014;123(6):1398–402. https://doi.org/10.1097/01.AOG.0000450758.95422.c8.
57. d'Arcangues C. WHO statement on hormonal contraception and bone health. Contraception. 2006;73(5):443–4.
58. Depo-Provera information. LAB-0148-5.1. Pharmacia and Upjohn Company, Division of Pfizer, Inc., New York. https://www.accessdata.fda.gov/drugsatfda_docs/label/2010/020246s036lbl.pdf
59. Cullins VE. Noncontraceptive benefits and therapeutic uses of depot medroxyprogesterone acetate. J Reprod Med. 1996;41(5 Suppl):428–33.
60. Milsom I, Korver T. Ovulation incidence with oral contraceptives: a literature review. J Fam Plann Reprod Health Care. 2008;34(4):237–46. https://doi.org/10.1783/147118908786000451.
61. Belsey EM. Vaginal bleeding patterns among women using one natural and eight hormonal methods of contraception. Contraception. 1988;38(2):181–206.
62. Tayob Y, Adams J, Jacobs HS, Guillebaud J. Ultrasound demonstration of increased frequency of functional ovarian cysts in women using progestogen-only oral contraception. Br J Obstet Gynaecol. 1985;92(10):1003–9.
63. McCann MF, Potter LS. Progestin-only oral contraception: a comprehensive review. Contraception. 1994;50(6 Suppl 1):S1–195.
64. Rivera R, Yacobson I, Grimes D. The mechanism of action of hormonal contraceptives and intrauterine contraceptive devices. Am J Obstet Gynecol. 1999;181(5 Pt 1):1263–9.
65. Edelman A, Gallo MF, Nichols MD, Jensen JT, Schulz KF, Grimes DA. Continuous versus cyclic use of combined oral contraceptives for contraception: systematic Cochrane review of randomized controlled trials. Hum Reprod. 2006;21(3):573–8.
66. Gallo MF, Nanda K, Grimes DA, Lopez LM, Schulz KF. 20 microg versus >20 microg estrogen combined oral contraceptives for contraception. Cochrane Database Syst Rev. 2011;1:CD003989. https://doi.org/10.1002/14651858.CD003989.pub4.
67. Lidegaard Ø, Edström B, Kreiner S. Oral contraceptives and venous thromboembolism: a five-year national case-control study. Contraception. 2002;65(3):187–96.
68. Stegeman BH, de Bastos M, Rosendaal FR, van Hylckama VA, Helmerhorst FM, et al. Different combined oral contraceptives and the risk of venous thrombosis: systematic review and network meta-analysis. BMJ. 2013;347:f5298. https://doi.org/10.1136/bmj.f5298.
69. Vasilakis-Scaramozza C, Jick H. Risk of venous thromboembolism with cyproterone or levonorgestrel contraceptives. Lancet. 2001;358(9291):1427–9.
70. Rosenberg MJ, Waugh MS, Meehan TE. Use and misuse of oral contraceptives: risk indicators for poor pill taking and discontinuation. Contraception. 1995;51(5):283–8.
71. Lidegaard Ø, Løkkegaard E, Jensen A, Skovlund CW, Keiding N. Thrombotic stroke and myocardial infarction with hormonal contraception. N Engl J Med. 2012;366(24):2257–66. https://doi.org/10.1056/NEJMoa1111840.
72. Chasan-Taber L, Stampfer MJ. Epidemiology of oral contraceptives and cardiovascular disease. Ann Intern Med. 1998;128(6):467–77.
73. Etminan M, Takkouche B, Isorna FC, Samii A. Risk of ischaemic stroke in people with migraine: systematic review and meta-analysis of observational studies. BMJ. 2005;330(7482):63. Epub 2004 Dec 13.
74. Sidney S, Petitti DB, Soff GA, Cundiff DL, Tolan KK, Quesenberry CP Jr. Venous thromboembolic disease in users of low-estrogen combined estrogen-progestin oral contraceptives. Contraception. 2004;70(1):3–10.
75. Truitt ST, Fraser AB, Grimes DA, Gallo MF, Schulz KF. Combined hormonal versus nonhormonal versus progestin-only contraception in lactation. Cochrane Database Syst Rev. 2003;2:CD003988.
76. ACOG practice bulletin no. 110: noncontraceptive uses of hormonal contraceptives. Obstet Gynecol. 2010;115(1):206–18. https://doi.org/10.1097/AOG.0b013e3181cb50b5.
77. Audet MC, Moreau M, Koltun WD, Waldbaum AS, Shangold G, Fisher AC, et al. Evaluation of contraceptive efficacy and cycle control of a transdermal contraceptive patch vs an oral contraceptive: a randomized controlled trial. JAMA. 2001;285(18):2347–54.
78. Gallo MF, Grimes DA, Schulz KF. Skin patch and vaginal ring versus combined oral contraceptives for contraception. Cochrane Database Syst Rev. 2003;1:CD003552.
79. Dore DD, Norman H, Loughlin J, Seeger JD. Extended case-control study results on thromboembolic outcomes among transdermal contraceptive users. Contraception. 2010;81(5):408–13. https://doi.org/10.1016/j.contraception.2009.12.009.
80. Zieman M, Guillebaud J, Weisberg E, Shangold GA, Fisher AC, Creasy GW. Contraceptive efficacy and cycle control with the Ortho Evra/Evra transdermal system: the analysis of pooled data. Fertil Steril. 2002;77(2 Suppl 2):S13–8.
81. van den Heuvel MW, van Bragt AJ, Alnabawy AK, Kaptein MC. Comparison of ethinylestradiol pharmacokinetics in three hormonal contraceptive formulations: the vaginal ring, the transdermal patch and an oral contraceptive. Contraception. 2005;72(3):168–74.
82. Miller L, Verhoeven CH, Hout JI. Extended regimens of the contraceptive vaginal ring: a randomized trial. Obstet Gynecol. 2005;106(3):473–82.
83. Weisberg E, Fraser IS, Lacarra M, Mishell DR Jr, Alvarez F, et al. Efficacy, bleeding patterns, and side effects of a 1-year contraceptive vaginal ring. Contraception. 1999;59(5):311–8.
84. Reece M, Herbenick D, Dodge B. Penile dimensions and men's perceptions of condom fit and feel. Sex Transm Infect. 2009;85(2):127–31. https://doi.org/10.1136/sti.2008.033050.
85. Holmes KK, Levine R, Weaver M. Effectiveness of condoms in preventing sexually transmitted infections. Bull World Health Organ. 2004;82(6):454–61.
86. Lytle CD, Routson LB, Seaborn GB, Dixon LG, Bushar HF, Cyr WH. An in vitro evaluation of condoms as barriers to a small virus. Sex Transm Dis. 1997;24(3):161–4.
87. Farr G, Gabelnick H, Sturgen K, Dorflinger L. Contraceptive efficacy and acceptability of the female condom. Am J Public Health. 1994;84(12):1960–4.

88. Burke AE, Barnhart K, Jensen JT, Creinin MD, Walsh TL, Wan LS, et al. Contraceptive efficacy, acceptability, and safety of C31G and nonoxynol-9 spermicidal gels: a randomized controlled trial. Obstet Gynecol. 2010;116(6):1265–73. https://doi.org/10.1097/AOG.0b013e3181fc3b1a.
89. Centers for Disease Control and Prevention (CDC). Nonoxynol-9 spermicide contraception use--United States, 1999. MMWR Morb Mortal Wkly Rep. 2002;51(18):389–92.
90. Kreiss J, Ngugi E, Holmes K, Ndinya-Achola J, Waiyaki P, Roberts PL, et al. Efficacy of nonoxynol 9 contraceptive sponge use in preventing heterosexual acquisition of HIV in Nairobi prostitutes. JAMA. 1992;268(4):477–82.
91. Handley MA, Reingold AL, Shiboski S, Padian NS. Incidence of acute urinary tract infection in young women and use of male condoms with and without nonoxynol-9 spermicides. Epidemiology. 2002;13(4):431–6.
92. Schreiber CA, Meyn LA, Creinin MD, Barnhart KT, Hillier SL. Effects of long-term use of nonoxynol-9 on vaginal flora. Obstet Gynecol. 2006;107(1):136–43.
93. Fihn SD, Latham RH, Roberts P, Running K, Stamm WE. Association between diaphragm use and urinary tract infection. JAMA. 1985;254(2):240–5.
94. Schwartz B, Gaventa S, Broome CV, Reingold AL, Hightower AW, et al. Nonmenstrual toxic shock syndrome associated with barrier contraceptives: report of a case-control study. Rev Infect Dis. 1989;11 Suppl 1:S43–8; discussion S48–9.
95. Grimes DA, Gallo MF, Grigorieva V, Nanda K, Schulz KF. Fertility awareness-based methods for contraception. Cochrane Database Syst Rev. 2004;4:CD004860.
96. Trussell J, Grummer-Strawn L. Further analysis of contraceptive failure of the ovulation method. Am J Obstet Gynecol. 1991;165(6 Pt 2):2054–9.
97. Planned Parenthood: Fertility Awareness.
98. Bedsider: Fertility Awareness.
99. Dehlendorf C, Krajewski C, Borrero S. Contraceptive counseling: best practices to ensure quality communication and enable effective contraceptive use. Clin Obstet Gynecol. 2014;57(4):659–73. https://doi.org/10.1097/GRF.0000000000000059.
100. Dehlendorf C, Kimport K, Levy K, Steinauer J. A qualitative analysis of approaches to contraceptive counseling. Perspect Sex Reprod Health. 2014;46(4):233–40. https://doi.org/10.1363/46e2114.
101. Ott MA, Sucato GS; Committee on Adolescence. Contraception for adolescents. Pediatrics. 2014;134(4):e1257–81. https://doi.org/10.1542/peds.2014-2300.
102. Committee on Gynecologic Practice Long-Acting Reversible Contraception Working Group. Committee opinion no. 642: increasing access to contraceptive implants and intrauterine devices to reduce unintended pregnancy. Obstet Gynecol. 2015;126(4):e44–8. https://doi.org/10.1097/AOG.0000000000001106.
103. Lessard LN, Karasek D, Ma S, Darney P, Deardorff J, Lahiff M, et al. Contraceptive features preferred by women at high risk of unintended pregnancy. Perspect Sex Reprod Health. 2012;44(3):194–200. https://doi.org/10.1363/4419412.
104. Kalmuss D, Davidson AR, Cushman LF, Heartwell S, Rulin M. Determinants of early implant discontinuation among low-income women. Fam Plan Perspect. 1996;28(6):256–60.
105. Callegari LS, Zhao X, Schwarz EB, Rosenfeld E, Mor MK, Borrero S. Racial/ethnic differences in contraceptive preferences, beliefs, and self-efficacy among women veterans. Am J Obstet Gynecol. 2017;216(5):504.e1–504.e10. https://doi.org/10.1016/j.ajog.2016.12.178.
106. Gomez AM, Wapman M. Under (implicit) pressure: young Black and Latina women's perceptions of contraceptive care. Contraception. 2017;96(4):221–6. https://doi.org/10.1016/j.contraception.2017.07.007.
107. Dehlendorf C, Fox E, Sobel L, Borrero S. Patient-centered contraceptive counseling: evidence to inform practice. Curr Obstet Gynecol Rep. 2016;5(1):55–63.
108. Gavin L, Moskosky S, Carter M, Curtis K, Glass E, Godfrey E, et al. Providing quality family planning services: recommendations of CDC and the U.S. Office of Population Affairs. MMWR Recomm Rep. 2014;63(RR-04):1–54.
109. Dehlendorf C, Grumbach K, Schmittdiel JA, Steinauer J. Shared decision making in contraceptive counseling. Contraception. 2017;95(5):452–5. https://doi.org/10.1016/j.contraception.2016.12.010.
110. Yee LM, Simon MA. Perceptions of coercion, discrimination and other negative experiences in postpartum contraceptive counseling for low-income minority women. J Health Care Poor Underserved. 2011;22(4):1387–400. https://doi.org/10.1353/hpu.2011.0144.
111. Baldaszti E, Wimmer-Puchinger B, Löschke K. Acceptability of the long-term contraceptive levonorgestrel-releasing intrauterine system (Mirena): a 3-year follow-up study. Contraception. 2003;67(2):87–91.
112. Backman T, Huhtala S, Blom T, Luoto R, Rauramo I, Koskenvuo M. Length of use and symptoms associated with premature removal of the levonorgestrel intrauterine system: a nation-wide study of 17,360 users. BJOG. 2000;107(3):335–9.
113. Gee RE, Mitra N, Wan F, Chavkin DE, Long JA. Power over parity: intimate partner violence and issues of fertility control. Am J Obstet Gynecol. 2009;201(2):148.e1–7. https://doi.org/10.1016/j.ajog.2009.04.048.
114. Coggins M, Bullock LF. The wavering line in the sand: the effects of domestic violence and sexual coercion. Issues Ment Health Nurs. 2003;24(6–7):723–38.
115. Thiel de Bocanegra H, Rostovtseva DP, Khera S, Godhwani N. Birth control sabotage and forced sex: experiences reported by women in domestic violence shelters. Violence Against Women. 2010;16(5):601–12. https://doi.org/10.1177/1077801210366965.
116. Cromer BA, Smith RD, Blair JM, Dwyer J, Brown RT. A prospective study of adolescents who choose among levonorgestrel implant (Norplant), medroxyprogesterone acetate (Depo-Provera), or the combined oral contraceptive pill as contraception. Pediatrics. 1994;94(5):687–94.
117. Clark LE, Allen RH, Goyal V, Raker C, Gottlieb AS. Reproductive coercion and co-occurring intimate partner violence in obstetrics and gynecology patients. Am J Obstet Gynecol. 2014;210(1):42.e1–8. https://doi.org/10.1016/j.ajog.2013.09.019.
118. Steenland MW, Rodriguez MI, Marchbanks PA, Curtis KM. How does the number of oral contraceptive pill packs dispensed or prescribed affect continuation and other measures of consistent and correct use? A systematic review. Contraception. 2013;87(5):605–10. https://doi.org/10.1016/j.contraception.2012.08.004.
119. Stewart FH, Harper CC, Ellertson CE, Grimes DA, Sawaya GF, Trussell J. Clinical breast and pelvic examination requirements for hormonal contraception: current practice vs evidence. JAMA. 2001;285(17):2232–9.
120. American Academy of Family Physicians. Choosing wisely: don't require a pelvic exam or other physical exam to prescribe oral contraceptive medications. 2013.
121. Princeton Emergency Contraception Website.
122. Gemzell-Danielsson K. Mechanism of action of emergency contraception. Contraception. 2010;82(5):404–9. https://doi.org/10.1016/j.contraception.2010.05.004.
123. Cheng L, Gülmezoglu AM, Piaggio G, Ezcurra E, Van Look PF. Interventions for emergency contraception. Cochrane Database Syst Rev. 2008;2:CD001324. https://doi.org/10.1002/14651858.CD001324.pub3.
124. Glasier A. Emergency contraception: clinical outcomes. Contraception. 2013;87(3):309–13. https://doi.org/10.1016/j.contraception.2012.08.027.

125. Festin MP, Bahamondes L, Nguyen TM, Habib N, Thamkhantho M, Singh K, et al. A prospective, open-label, single arm, multicentre study to evaluate efficacy, safety and acceptability of pericoital oral contraception using levonorgestrel 1.5 mg. Hum Reprod. 2016;31(3):530–40. https://doi.org/10.1093/humrep/dev341.
126. Kapp N, Abitbol JL, Mathé H, Scherrer B, Guillard H, et al. Effect of body weight and BMI on the efficacy of levonorgestrel emergency contraception. Contraception. 2015;91(2):97–104. https://doi.org/10.1016/j.contraception.2014.11.001.
127. Gemzell-Danielsson K, Berger C, Lalitkumar PG. Emergency contraception -- mechanisms of action. Contraception. 2013;87(3):300–8. https://doi.org/10.1016/j.contraception.2012.08.021.
128. Moreau C, Trussell J. Results from pooled Phase III studies of ulipristal acetate for emergency contraception. Contraception. 2012;86(6):673–80. https://doi.org/10.1016/j.contraception.2012.05.012.
129. Shigesato M, Elia J, Tschann M, Bullock H, Hurwitz E, et al. Pharmacy access to Ulipristal acetate in major cities throughout the United States. Contraception. 2018;97(3):264–9. https://doi.org/10.1016/j.contraception.2017.10.009.
130. Yuzpe AA, Thurlow HJ, Ramzy I, Leyshon JI. Post coital contraception--a pilot study. J Reprod Med. 1974;13(2):53–8.
131. Practice bulletin no. 152: emergency contraception. Obstet Gynecol. 2015;126(3):e1–11. https://doi.org/10.1097/AOG.0000000000001047.
132. American College of Obstetricians and Gynecologists. ACOG practice bulletin: clinical management guidelines for obstetrician-gynecologists number 76, October 2006: postpartum hemorrhage. Obstet Gynecol. 2006;108(4):1039–47.
133. Jatlaoui TC, Ewing A, Mandel MG, Simmons KB, Suchdev DB, et al. Abortion surveillance - United States, 2013. MMWR Surveill Summ. 2016;65(12):1–44. https://doi.org/10.15585/mmwr.ss6512a1.
134. Henshaw RC, Naji SA, Russell IT, Templeton AA. A comparison of medical abortion (using mifepristone and gemeprost) with surgical vacuum aspiration: efficacy and early medical sequelae. Hum Reprod. 1994;9(11):2167–72.
135. Cleland K, Creinin MD, Nucatola D, Nshom M, Trussell J. Significant adverse events and outcomes after medical abortion. Obstet Gynecol. 2013;121(1):166–71. https://doi.org/10.1097/AOG.0b013e3182755763.
136. Robson SC, Kelly T, Howel D, Deverill M, Hewison J, Lie ML, et al. Randomised preference trial of medical versus surgical termination of pregnancy less than 14 weeks' gestation (TOPS). Health Technol Assess. 2009;13(53):1–124, iii–iv. https://doi.org/10.3310/hta13530.
137. Rørbye C, Nørgaard M, Nilas L. Medical versus surgical abortion: comparing satisfaction and potential confounders in a partly randomized study. Hum Reprod. 2005;20(3):834–8.
138. Jensen JT, Harvey SM, Beckman LJ. Acceptability of suction curettage and mifepristone abortion in the United States: a prospective comparison study. Am J Obstet Gynecol. 2000;182(6):1292–9.
139. Hakim-Elahi E, Tovell HM, Burnhill MS. Complications of first-trimester abortion: a report of 170,000 cases. Obstet Gynecol. 1990;76(1):129–35.
140. https://www.cdc.gov/reproductivehealth/contraception/unintendedpregnancy/pdf/Contraceptive_methods_508.pdf
141. Arowojolu AO, Gallo MF, Lopez LM, Grimes DA. Combined oral contraceptive pills for treatment of acne. Cochrane Database Syst Rev. 2012;7:CD004425. https://doi.org/10.1002/14651858.CD004425.pub6.
142. Hidalgo M, Bahamondes L, Perrotti M, Diaz J, Dantas-Monteiro C, Petta C. Bleeding patterns and clinical performance of the levonorgestrel-releasing intrauterine system (Mirena) up to two years. Contraception. 2002;65(2):129–32.
143. Tepper NK, Krashin JW, Curtis KM, Cox S, Whiteman MK. Update to CDC's U.S. medical eligibility criteria for contraceptive use, 2016: revised recommendations for the use of hormonal contraception among women at high risk for HIV infection. MMWR Morb Mortal Wkly Rep. 2017;66(37):990–4. https://doi.org/10.15585/mmwr.mm6637a6.

Menstruation and Secondary Amenorrhea

5

Rachel S. Casas and Cynthia H. Chuang

Learning Objectives

1. Differentiate the clinical presentations of physiologic, hypothalamic/pituitary, ovarian, and structural causes of amenorrhea.
2. Describe an approach to diagnostic testing in a patient with secondary amenorrhea based upon suspected etiology.
3. Formulate a treatment plan to manage secondary amenorrhea and associated health risks based upon diagnosis.
4. Identify when a patient with amenorrhea should be referred to a subspecialist for advanced diagnostic testing or treatment.

Rosalia is a 35-year-old woman who presents to primary care clinic with no menses for the past 6 months. She underwent menarche at age 14 with regular menses until a year ago when her cycles started to occur less frequently.

Secondary amenorrhea is defined as the absence of menses for three cycles or 3 to 6 months in previously menstruating women [1]. Primary amenorrhea is the absence of onset of menses at age 15 for women with secondary sexual characteristics (breast enlargement, body hair, hip widening) or at age 13 in women without secondary sexual characteristics [1]. Important causes of primary amenorrhea are congenital, leading to hormonal dysregulation and anatomical dysgenesis at the level of the hypothalamus (Kallmann syndrome), gonads (Turner syndrome), uterus (Mayer-Rokitansky-Kuster-Hauser syndrome, androgen insensitivity syndrome), outflow tract (transverse vaginal septum, imperforate hymen), or entire reproductive tract (5-alpha reductase deficiency). As it is unusual for women to present to adult primary care with a new diagnosis of primary amenorrhea, the remainder of this chapter will focus on secondary amenorrhea.

Epidemiology

The prevalence of secondary amenorrhea is approximately 3–5% of women worldwide [2–4]. After excluding pregnancy, the most common causes of secondary amenorrhea are hypothalamic suppression (34%), polycystic ovary syndrome (PCOS) (28–73%), hyperprolactinemia (13–15%), primary ovarian insufficiency (POI) (12%), thyroid dysfunction (2–15%), and Asherman syndrome (7%) [3, 5, 6]. About 1% of women are affected by POI before age 40, with incidence rates of about 10 per 10,000 person-years in women ages 15–29 and 76 per 10,000 person-years in women ages 30–39 years [7].

R. S. Casas (✉) · C. H. Chuang
Division of General Internal Medicine, Penn State Milton S. Hershey Medical Center, Hershey, PA, USA
e-mail: rcasas@pennstatehealth.psu.edu

S. A. Tilstra et al. (eds.), *Sex- and Gender-Based Women's Health*, https://doi.org/10.1007/978-3-030-50695-7_5

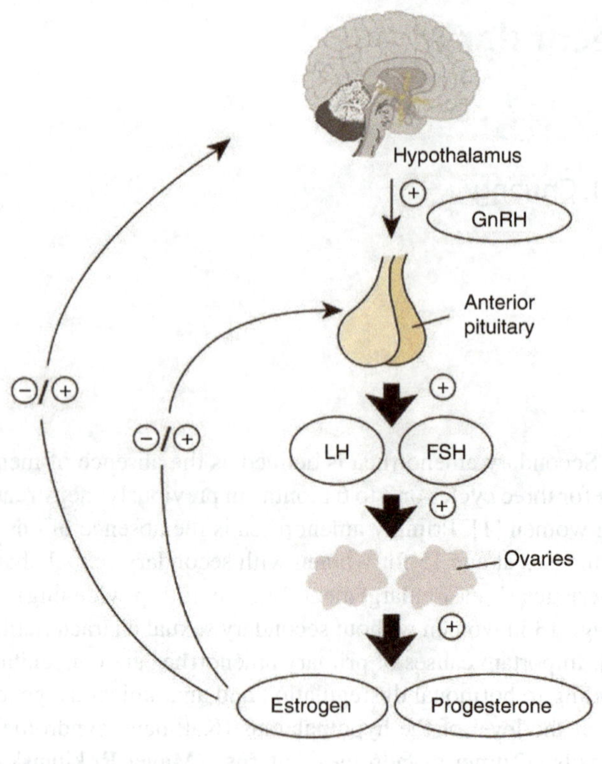

Fig. 5.1 Hypothalamic-pituitary-gonadal (HPG) axis in women (Reprinted from Hiller-Sturmhofel and Bartke [8])

Physiology

The majority of secondary amenorrhea is caused by hormonal dysregulation of the hypothalamic-pituitary-gonadal (HPG) axis (Fig. 5.1). Normally, gonadotropic-releasing hormone (GNRH) released by the hypothalamus stimulates release of FSH and luteinizing hormone (LH) from the anterior pituitary, which then stimulate estrogen and progesterone release from the ovaries. Estrogen and progesterone provide regulatory feedback to the HPG axis at the levels of the hypothalamus and pituitary.

Hormones of the HPG axis regulate menstruation (Fig. 5.2). In the early follicular phase, a rise in FSH stimulates recruitment of ovarian follicles and increased estrogen production. Estrogen at first stimulates follicle growth and endometrial proliferation and suppresses LH release in the follicular phase. Once estrogen rises to higher levels, it triggers an LH surge and release of an oocyte from the follicle (ovulation). In the luteal phase, the follicle transforms into a corpus luteum which produces estrogen and progesterone, preparing the endometrial lining for potential implantation. The corpus luteum atrophies if not fertilized, and the subsequent decrease in progesterone stimulates menstruation.

Hormonal dysfunction leading to disruption of the menstrual cycle can occur at any level of the HPG pathway.

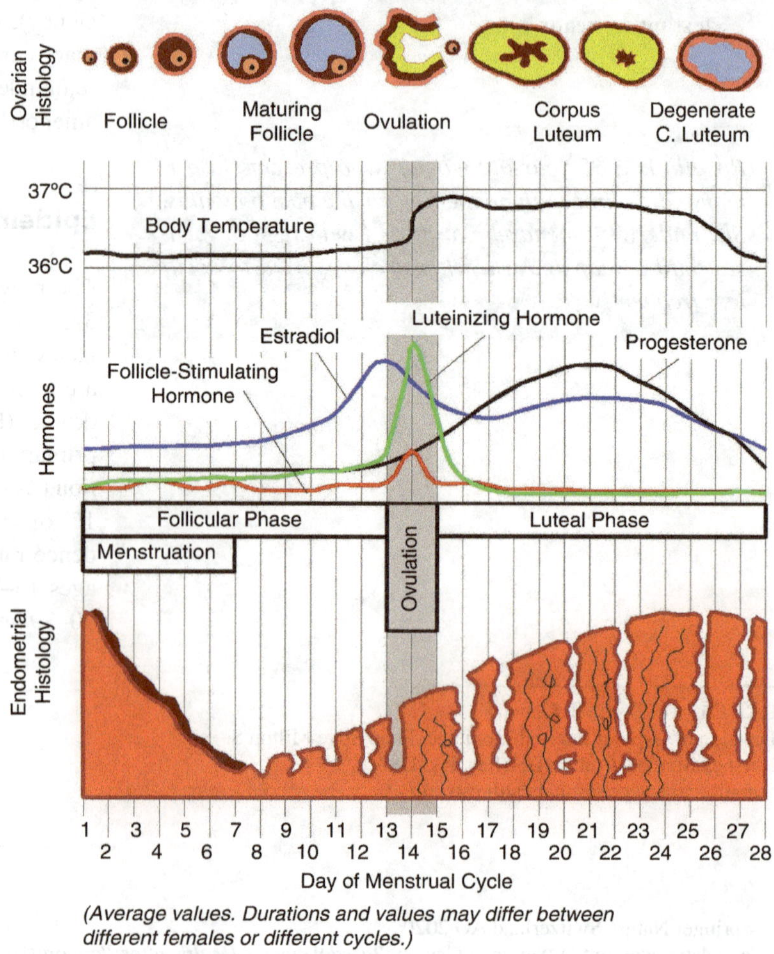

Fig. 5.2 The normal menstrual cycle [9] (Source: This Wikipedia and Wikimedia Commons image is from the user Chris 73 and is freely available at //commons.wikimedia.org/wiki/File:MenstrualCycle.png under the creative commons cc-by-sa 3.0 license)

Pathophysiology

This chapter is organized into sections that discuss the physiologic, structural, pharmacologic, hypothalamic/pituitary (low FSH), ovarian (high FSH), and other endocrine causes of amenorrhea. Notably, many of the above conditions (including POI, breastfeeding, and other chronic diseases) are not reliable inducers of anovulation and amenorrhea; patients who do not desire pregnancy should be offered contraceptive counseling (please see Chap. 4, Patient-Centered Contraceptive Counseling).

Physiologic

Pregnancy and menopause are important causes of amenorrhea and are described further in Chap. 39, Obstetric Medicine, and Chap. 8, Menopause, respectively. Regular breastfeeding causes amenorrhea through secretion of prolactin by the pituitary, which inhibits GNRH and subsequently suppresses the menstrual cycle.

Structural

Uterine procedures and operations including dilation and curettage, or infections like endometritis, can cause cervical stenosis and/or intrauterine scarring known as Asherman syndrome. Both of these conditions can lead to outflow obstruction of menses.

Pharmacologic

Contraceptives, including continuous or extended combined oral contraceptives (COC), hormonal intrauterine devices (IUDs), and intramuscular medroxyprogesterone acetate, commonly induce amenorrhea. There is no physiologic requirement for regular menses in women using these forms of contraception [10]. With each of these methods, amenorrhea is due to constant progestin levels in the uterus that thin the endometrium. COCs and medroxyprogesterone acetate additionally prevent cyclical thickening of the endometrium through hormonal suppression of the HPG axis [10].

Other medications affect prolactin release through inhibition by dopamine or stimulation by serotonin (antipsychotics, antidepressants, prokinetics, antihypertensives) and GNRH suppression (opioids and glucocorticoids) [11–13]. Elevated prolactin leads to feedback inhibition of GNRH with resulting HPG axis suppression (Table 5.1).

Table 5.1 Medications associated with hyperprolactinemia [11]

Psychiatric medications	Antipsychotics (typical and atypical) Tricyclic antidepressants SSRIs MAO-I Others: trazodone, buspirone, alprazolam
Estrogens	Combined oral contraceptives
Gastrointestinal medications	Antiemetics: prochlorperazine, metoclopramide H2 antagonists: cimetidine, ranitidine
Antihypertensives	Methyldopa, reserpine, verapamil
Other	Opiates Cocaine

Hypothalamic/Pituitary (Low FSH/LH)

Hypothalamic or functional amenorrhea is due to a decrease in GNRH secretion, which can occur in the setting of weight loss, excessive exercise, disordered eating, poor nutrition, and chronic disease. Hypothalamic amenorrhea is a diagnosis of exclusion [14]. Chronic disease such as advanced kidney and liver disease, malignancy, and malabsorption with associated malnutrition and weight fluctuations can lead to hypothalamic amenorrhea and alterations in hormone metabolism. Women with low body mass index (BMI) and disordered eating can present with thin body habitus, enlarged parotid glands, and lanugo. The female athlete triad (amenorrhea/oligomenorrhea, low energy availability with or without disordered eating, and decreased bone density) is further detailed in Chap. 34, Eating Disorders and the Female Athlete Triad.

Pituitary tumors can cause excess or deficient hormone secretion. Tumor compression through mass effect can lead to panhypopituitarism, including deficiency of LH, FSH, and thyroid-stimulating hormone (TSH), with resulting menstrual dysfunction. Patients with prolactinomas can present with galactorrhea, headaches, and vision changes.

Central hypogonadism can result from infiltration or destruction of the hypothalamus and/or pituitary. Infiltrative causes can include hemochromatosis, amyloidosis, inflammatory disorders (sarcoidosis, lymphocytic hypophysitis, Wegener's granulomatosis), infectious diseases (tuberculosis, syphilis, meningitis), or malignancy (carcinoma, lymphoma, leukemia) [15]. Other causes of damage to these structures include traumatic brain injury, radiation, and ischemia. Pituitary ischemia in the setting of postpartum hemorrhage (Sheehan syndrome) generally presents with difficulty breastfeeding and other symptoms of panhypopituitarism such as fatigue, weight change, cold intolerance, decreased appetite, decreased libido, hair loss, and constipation.

In addition to pituitary tumors, hyperprolactinemia occurs with physiologic conditions (stress, breast stimulation), endocrine disorders (Cushing's disease, acromegaly, hypothyroidism, PCOS), neurologic disorders (seizures), systemic disease (chronic renal or liver disease), and medications (as discussed in the pharmacologic section) [11, 12].

Ovarian (High FSH)

Primary ovarian insufficiency, POI, also previously called premature menopause and primary ovarian failure, is defined as dysfunction or depletion of ovarian follicles with cessation of menses before age 40 years [16, 17]. Patients may present with hot flashes, sleep disturbance, depression, sexual dysfunction, and night sweats.

Various conditions are associated with POI, including congenital disorders (Turner syndrome, fragile X, and Bloom syndrome), signal defects (FSH/LH receptor or G protein mutation), enzyme deficiency (aromatase or 17/20-lyase), iatrogenic causes (chemotherapy, radiation), endocrine/autoimmune diseases (Hashimoto's thyroiditis, Graves' disease, diabetes mellitus type 1, autoimmune adrenal insufficiency), and infection (mumps) [16, 17]. Other tumors that can disrupt ovarian function include granulosa, theca, teratoma, metastatic, and androgen-producing tumors.

Other Endocrine Disorders

Hyperandrogenism

Hyperandrogenic anovulation occurs through multiple endocrinologic conditions. PCOS is the most common cause of mildly elevated androgens and menstrual dysfunction, with mechanisms detailed further in Chap. 6, Polycystic Ovary Syndrome. Obesity, independent from PCOS, can also lead to menstrual anomalies due to dysregulation of metabolic, endocrine, and inflammatory pathways, including increased peripheral conversion of androgens to estrogen by aromatase in adipose tissue [18]. In Cushing's syndrome, excess adrenocorticotropic hormone (ACTH) production by the pituitary increases secretion of both cortisol and androgens from the adrenals [19]. Direct glucocorticoid suppression of GNRH secretion and feedback inhibition by hyperandrogenemia may also result in hypogonadotropic hypogonadism and menstrual dysfunction [19]. Nonclassical adrenal hyperplasia due to 21-hydroxylase deficiency can present with secondary amenorrhea and symptoms and physical exam findings of hirsutism in adult women [20]. With acromegaly, pituitary compression can occur along with direct growth hormone effects on gonadal function [13]. Exogenous androgens and androgen-secreting ovarian or adrenal tumors are important to exclude.

Thyroid Dysfunction

Both hyper- and hypothyroidism influence menses through effects on GNRH secretion, prolactin, steroid metabolism, and sex hormone-binding globulin [19]. In hyperthyroidism, associated weight loss can lead to hypothalamic amenorrhea; autoimmune thyroid disease is also associated with POI [19].

Clinical Manifestations

Rosalia is sexually active with one male partner and uses condoms intermittently. She has been pregnant twice, with one cesarean section and one spontaneous miscarriage. She takes ibuprofen as needed for menstrual cramps and otherwise denies medication and substance use. There are no known gynecologic or endocrine issues in her family.

The evaluation of amenorrhea should include a detailed medical, surgical, and social history. A complete review of systems should be documented particularly targeting menstruation, sex, pregnancy, intrauterine procedures, and medications (Table 5.2) [21, 22]. History questions should focus on a potential neurologic, endocrine, or gynecologic etiology for amenorrhea. Family history should include menstrual history of first-degree family members, puberty delay (delayed or incomplete sexual maturation, primary amenorrhea), genetic disorders (Turner syndrome, Bloom syndrome, fragile X), chronic illness (especially autoimmune and endocrine), and infertility. Physical exam should include BMI, cranial nerves (especially II, VI, VI), visual fields, thyroid (enlargement, tenderness, nodules), skin (dryness, lanugo, hirsutism, acne), breast (tenderness, enlargement, nipple discharge), and a pelvic exam (vaginal dryness, cliteromegaly, adnexal mass, uterine enlargement).

Rosalia has experienced episodes of feeling hot, flushed, and sweaty lasting a few hours. Her review of systems is otherwise negative. On exam, her BMI is 26.6 kg/m^2, and she is in no distress with unremarkable visual field, thyroid, breast, abdominal, pelvic, and skin exams.

Evaluation

All women with amenorrhea should first have pregnancy testing with a urine or serum hCG test. Pregnancy remains the most common cause of secondary amenorrhea and should always be excluded in the evaluation of menstrual changes.

In nonpregnant women, initial evaluation should focus on the most common endocrinologic causes of amenorrhea with a serum prolactin and TSH [21, 23].

Table 5.2 Clinical manifestations of secondary amenorrhea [19]

Etiology	Symptoms and relevant history	Physical exam findings
Physiologic		
Pregnancy	Breast tenderness, nausea, vomiting, abdominal pain, increased urinary frequency, weight gain	Breast tenderness and/or enlargement, abdominal distension
Outflow tract		
Asherman syndrome/cervical stenosis	Cyclical pelvic pain, prior uterine or cervical procedures, recurrent pregnancy loss, prior chemotherapy or radiation	Enlarged, tender uterus (not always present)
Hypothalamic/pituitary		
Hypothalamic amenorrhea	Weight loss, excessive exercise, disordered eating, poor nutrition, psychosocial stressors	Thin body habitus, enlarged parotid glands, lanugo
Pituitary tumor	Galactorrhea, headaches, vision changes	Visual field deficits, nipple discharge
Sheehan syndrome	Significant blood loss during birth, difficulty breastfeeding, fatigue, weight change, cold intolerance	Hypotension
Ovarian		
Primary ovarian insufficiency and menopause	Hot flashes, sleep disturbance, depression, sexual dysfunction, night sweats	Vaginal dryness
Ovarian tumor (or androgen-producing tumor)	Abdominal pain, rapid-onset hirsutism	Abdominal mass, cliteromegaly, male pattern baldness, acne, facial hair
Other endocrine disorders		
PCOS	Weight gain, acne, hirsutism	Male pattern baldness, acne on back/trunk, facial hair, acanthosis nigricans
Thyroid dysfunction	Heat or cold intolerance, palpitations, diarrhea, constipation, hair loss, fatigue, depression	Dry skin, brittle nails, thyroid enlargement/ tenderness
Hypercortisolism	Weight gain, acne, hirsutism, weakness, headache, fatigue, depression, easy bruising	Hypertension, buffalo hump, rounded face, purple striae, central obesity, muscle atrophy, thin skin

Prolactin elevated to >100 ng/mL is usually due to a pituitary adenoma and should prompt a brain MRI [12, 21]. Prolactin levels >200 ng/mL are diagnostic of pituitary adenoma, while medications rarely cause prolactinemia >100 ng/mL [12]. If the serum prolactin is elevated but <100 ng/mL, evaluate for contributing medications (Table 5.1) or medical conditions such as primary hypothyroidism. Next steps would include discontinuing these medications if feasible, in collaboration with prescribing specialists as appropriate. The prolactin level should be repeated in the early morning, or consider a pituitary MRI if potentially contributing medication cannot be discontinued [13].

Obtaining an initial FSH level can also be considered [13, 22, 24]. While elevated FSH can suggest ovarian failure and low/normal FSH can suggest hypothalamic/pituitary disease, this hormone level fluctuates with the menstrual cycle (Fig. 5.2). The FSH level should ideally be checked within the first 5 days following onset of menses, which can be challenging in the setting of amenorrhea.

If these initial tests are unrevealing, further evaluation of hypothalamic/pituitary or ovarian causes should occur as discussed below.

Additional Testing

Progesterone Withdrawal

In women with amenorrhea, progesterone (medroxyprogesterone acetate 10 mg or norethindrone acetate 5 mg orally daily for 7–10 days) will induce a withdrawal bleed in women who have sufficient endogenous estrogen to build an endometrial lining and who do not have outflow obstruction. Low estrogen can occur in patients due to POI or gonadotropin deficiency (hypothalamic amenorrhea, Sheehan syndrome, hyperprolactinemia, hypothyroidism, pituitary tumors, Cushing's syndrome). The utility of progesterone withdrawal testing, or "challenge" as it is known clinically, has been questioned in women with amenorrhea. For example, about 50% of women with POI may have withdrawal bleeding due to varied ovarian function [22, 25].

If possible, obtain lab tests (FSH, LH, estradiol) 1–5 days after withdrawal bleeding starts [23]. Low or inappropriately normal FSH and LH with low estradiol suggests hypothalamic/pituitary disease, and high FSH (with or without elevated LH) and low estradiol suggest POI (Table 5.3). In POI, FSH levels are in the menopausal range (30–40 mIU/mL) with estradiol less than 50 pg/mL [16]. As ovarian function can fluctuate in POI, FSH and estradiol should be checked on at least two occasions at least 1 month apart [17, 24]. An increased LH: FSH ratio can be observed in PCOS but is often not present with this condition and is not part of the diagnostic criteria for PCOS (please see Chap. 6, Polycystic Ovary Syndrome, for further discussion).

Table 5.3 Expected hormone responses in conditions causing secondary amenorrhea

Disorder	GNRH	FSH/LH	Estrogen	Androgens
Hypothalamic amenorrhea	↓	↓	↓	→
Hyperprolactinemia	↓	↓	↓	→
Sheehan syndrome	↑	↓	↓	→
Primary ovarian insufficiency	↑	↑	↓	→
Polycystic ovary syndrome	→[a]	LH: ↑→ FSH:→	↑→	↑

[a]GNRH levels may be normal, but with increased pulse frequency [26]

Testing for Androgen Excess

In patients with symptoms or physical exam findings of androgen excess, total testosterone and dehydroepiandrosterone-sulfate (DHEA-S) should be checked. DHEA-S is preferred to DHEA due to its longer half-life and lower variability [23]. Marked elevations in total testosterone (>200 ng/dL) or DHEA-S (>700 ng/dL) suggest an androgen-producing tumor from the ovaries or adrenals, respectively. More mildly elevated androgen values should prompt an evaluation for other causes of hyperandrogenic anovulation, for example, nonclassical adrenal hyperplasia (morning serum 17-OH hydroxyprogesterone), hypercortisolism (24-hour urine cortisol or dexamethasone suppression test), and acromegaly (serum IGF-1).

Imaging and Procedures

Obtain a transvaginal ultrasound in the setting of an abnormal pelvic exam, suspicion for anatomical anomaly, history of prior intrauterine procedures or infection, or highly elevated testosterone. Consider an MRI brain if symptoms, exam, or laboratory workup suggests an intracranial process. Adrenal CT should be completed in the setting of highly elevated DHEA-S. Women with Asherman syndrome should be referred for hysteroscopy, which is considered the most accurate method for diagnosis of this condition in comparison to transvaginal ultrasound, hysterosalpingography, and transcervical sounding [27–29].

Rosalia has a negative urine hCG, normal TSH and prolactin, and elevated FSH. A progesterone withdrawal test does not result in vaginal bleeding, a repeat FSH and LH is elevated, and estradiol is low. A transvaginal ultrasound shows normal uterine and ovarian size and position.

Additional Testing for Primary Ovarian Insufficiency

In a patient diagnosed with POI not associated with a known syndrome, consider screening for fragile X (FMR1 premutation), autoimmune thyroid disease (TPO), diabetes (fasting glucose or hemoglobin A1c), and autoimmune adrenal disease (indirect immunofluorescence or 21-hydroxylase [CYP21] immunoprecipitation) [17]. In one study of women with secondary amenorrhea due to POI, 32% were found to have autoantibodies, with 10% having clinically evident autoimmune disease (hypothyroidism, Graves' disease, diabetes mellitus, Addison's disease) [30]. Additional studies in women with POI showed that 24–25% had anti-TPO antibodies, 6% had FMR1 permutations, and 3% had adrenal autoimmunity [30–33].

Additional workup for systemic and autoimmune disease can be based upon symptoms and signs of these conditions, including free T4, erythrocyte sedimentation rate, serum protein, BMP, CBC, antinuclear antibody, rheumatoid factor, and corticotropin stimulation tests [17, 21]. Consider karyotyping to identify chromosomal abnormalities, especially in women less than 30 years, as 13% of these younger women may have an abnormal karyotype [24, 34]. Evaluate for enlarged, polycystic ovaries which can be seen with autoimmune oophoritis and 17,20 desmolase insufficiency with a pelvic ultrasound [35]. Testing for ovarian antibodies and ovarian biopsy are not currently recommended [36].

You diagnose Rosalia with primary ovarian insufficiency. Rosalia asks you about the health implications of this condition and if she can become pregnant again.

Treatment

Treatment of secondary amenorrhea can be challenging and depends on the etiology and concomitant medical conditions. Most often, primary care providers work closely with specialists and subspecialists to diagnose and manage these patients. All conditions with amenorrhea may lead to infertility and other health risks based upon underlying hormone status (Table 5.4). Women with a diagnosis known to cause infertility who desire pregnancy should be referred to a reproductive endocrinologist without delay. Timing of referral to specialists depends upon the diagnosed condition and expertise of the primary care provider (Table 5.4).

The following references provide more detailed clinical guidelines for management of the conditions in Table 5.4:

Table 5.4 Treatment of causes of secondary amenorrhea

Etiology	Health implications	Treatment	Where/when to refer
Hypothalamic/pituitary			
Hypothalamic amenorrhea	Bone density loss	Nutrition Exercise modification Stress reduction Cognitive behavioral therapy Calcium and vitamin D supplementation Combined oral contraceptives	Nutritionist Psychologist/psychiatrist as needed
Pituitary tumor	Dependent on size and functionality of tumor	Surgery Radiation Medication suppression (e.g., dopamine agonists for hyperprolactinemia)	Endocrinology and neurosurgery upon diagnosis
Sheehan syndrome	Panhypopituitarism	Corticosteroid, thyroid, sex hormones, and growth hormone supplementation	Endocrinology upon diagnosis
Ovarian			
Primary ovarian insufficiency	Urogenital atrophy Vasomotor symptoms Osteoporosis Cardiovascular disease Increased all-cause mortality	Combined oral contraceptive Combined cyclical hormone therapy Calcium and vitamin D supplementation Reproductive technology	Consider endocrinology, rheumatology, and genetics during initial evaluation of etiology. Gynecology if persistent sexual dysfunction beyond expertise Endocrinology if osteoporosis with first-line treatments
Ovarian tumor	Virilization	Surgery	Gynecology or gynecology-oncology upon diagnosis
Outflow tract			
Asherman syndrome/ cervical stenosis	Chronic pelvic pain	Hysteroscopic lysis of adhesions	Gynecology for diagnosis and management
Multifactorial			
PCOS	Endometrial hyperplasia Metabolic syndrome	Combined oral contraceptives Metformin Antiandrogens Fertility treatment	Nutritionist Endocrinology as needed
Thyroid dysfunction	Cardiovascular risk Hypothyroidism: Myxedema Hyperthyroidism: thyrotoxicosis	Hypothyroidism: thyroid hormone replacement Hyperthyroidism: surgery, iodine ablation, medication suppression	Endocrinology as needed
Cushing's syndrome	Metabolic syndrome Hypertension	Surgery and/or radiation (if tumor present) Medication suppression of corticosteroid production (e.g., metyrapone) or receptors (e.g., mifepristone)	Endocrinology at diagnosis Neurosurgery if intracranial tumor present

hypothalamic amenorrhea [37, 38], hyperprolactinemia/pituitary tumor [39, 40], hypopituitarism [41], POI [42], ovarian tumor [43], Asherman syndrome [29], PCOS [44, 45], thyroid dysfunction [46, 47], and Cushing's syndrome [48].

Hypothalamic Amenorrhea

The mainstay of treatment for hypothalamic amenorrhea includes treatment of the underlying chronic condition if present. Multidisciplinary teams involving primary care, nutrition, and psychiatry may be most effective in the setting of an underlying eating disorder. Pharmacologic treatments can include calcium and vitamin D supplementation for prevention of bone loss and combined oral contraceptives (COCs) for regulation of menses, endometrial protection, and pregnancy prevention. Generally, use of low-dose (0.02 mg) ethinyl estradiol and a second-generation progestin (e.g., levonorgestrel 0.01 mg/day) is considered first-line treatment. Additional information for this condition can be found in the cited clinical practice guidelines and in Chap. 34, Eating Disorders and the Female Athlete Triad, in the section on the female athlete triad [37, 38].

Polycystic Ovary Syndrome

In women with PCOS that do not desire pregnancy, COCs are typically used to regulate menses and provide contraception. Symptoms of excess androgen, particularly acne, are most often managed with COCs, specifically those containing third- or fourth-generation progestins with higher relative antiandrogenic activity compared to early generation progestins. Antiandrogen medications, such as spironolactone, can also help with hair growth and acne but can cause hypotension and electrolyte imbalance. Topical creams and cosmetic routes, like hair plucking and electrolysis, are often used by patients for hirsutism. Women with PCOS who have amenorrhea for over 3 months should have induced menses with a progesterone withdrawal bleed. Providers should have a low threshold to obtain an endometrial biopsy in the setting of prolonged amenorrhea or abnormal uterine bleeding given the increased risk for endometrial hyperplasia and malignancy with this disorder. Metformin can improve weight loss, insulin resistance, and fertility in women with PCOS. Women with PCOS who desire pregnancy should be managed in coordination with an infertility specialist. Additional information for this condition can be found in the cited clinical practice guidelines and in Chap. 6 on Polycystic Ovary Syndrome [44, 45].

Primary Ovarian Insufficiency

Treatment of POI should focus on minimizing associated cardiovascular disease, bone density loss, mortality, sexual dysfunction, and psychosocial stress [16, 49–56]. Women with POI may benefit from a multidisciplinary team to address their complex medical and psychosocial care, especially if a primary cause of POI is identified [55–57].

If the cause of POI is idiopathic and not treatable or amenorrhea continues with treatment, cyclical combined hormone therapy (HT) or COCs are recommended to prevent bone density loss and increase quality of life [42, 58, 59]. Women should be evaluated for contraindications to hormones (please see Chap. 4 on Patient-Centered Contraceptive Counseling and Chap. 8 on Menopause for more details), although the findings of the Women's Health Initiative may not apply to younger women with POI [42]. Examples of cyclical combined HT include estrogen (estradiol 100 μg/day transdermal, conjugated equine estrogen 0.625–1.25 mg oral/day, or micronized estradiol 1–2 mg oral/day) and progesterone, which can be dosed daily (100 mg micronized progesterone oral/day or medroxyprogesterone acetate 2.5–5.0 mg/day) or at higher dosing for 12 days per month (200 mg micronized progesterone oral/day or medroxyprogesterone acetate 10 mg oral/day) [42]. Current recommendations are to continue hormonal treatment until the age of natural menopause (50–51 years) [42].

Women with POI have a 5–10% chance of spontaneous pregnancy due to varied ovarian function [60]. For this reason, women with POI not desiring pregnancy should use contraception. COCs provide more hormone than needed for physiologic replacement but have the added benefit of contraception. However, the effectiveness of COCs for contraception in this population is uncertain due to potentially inadequate suppression of FSH [17, 61]. HT provides lower hormone doses and can be used in conjunction with other contraceptive methods such as IUDs and barrier methods. If pregnancy is desired, options include awaiting spontaneous conception, oocyte donation, and embryo donation [57, 62].

To optimize bone health, women with POI should also strive for regular weight-bearing exercise; 1200 mg of calcium per day, preferably through diet than supplements; and 1000 IU of vitamin D per day [63]. Bisphosphonates are not currently recommended for reproductive age women due to the long half-life of this medication, teratogenicity, and uncertain safety profile in this population [16, 64].

Monitoring of women with POI should focus on cardiovascular risk factors, with regular blood pressure and weight measures, screening for dyslipidemia and diabetes, and counseling on lifestyle modification if appropriate. Dual energy X-ray absorptiometry (DEXA) is recommended to evaluate for bone density loss in women with POI, but there is a lack of consensus about timing of testing, testing intervals, and appropriate treatment [16, 17, 52–54].

Tumors and Endocrinopathies

While some endocrinopathies such as thyroid disorders or PCOS are managed in primary care, many other causes of secondary amenorrhea discussed in this chapter are co-managed with specialists. Primary care providers should initiate an evaluation of patients with secondary amenorrhea and facilitate referral as needed to endocrinologists, gynecologists, rheumatologists, geneticists, or neurosurgeons who may play a role in managing patients with these conditions.

Following a discussion about the health risks associated with POI, Rosalia would like to attempt another pregnancy. You start a prenatal vitamin and refer her to reproductive endocrinology.

Summary Points

1. The history and physical exam in women with amenorrhea should focus on signs of intracranial, uterine, ovarian, and endocrine anomalies to guide the differential and diagnostic workup.
2. Pregnancy is the first diagnosis of exclusion in all presentations of amenorrhea, with TSH, FSH, and prolactin as the next initial testing in nonpregnant women.
3. Amenorrhea can be associated with health risks including infertility, osteoporosis, and endometrial hyperplasia

depending upon the etiology, with treatment individualized to minimize these risks.

4. Patients should be referred to subspecialists if the workup reveals neurologic, endocrinologic, or gynecologic abnormalities beyond the scope of your practice.

Review Questions

1. A 35-year-old woman with a history of dysmenorrhea presents to clinic with pelvic pain and amenorrhea. She has not had a period in 4 months and has experienced a few days of bilateral cramping pelvic pain each month. Her history is notable for three prior pregnancies, one elective dilation and curettage, and two cesarean sections. She had a copper intrauterine device placed for contraception 2 years ago. On pelvic exam, the patient has a non-tender uterus of normal size. Which of the following tests is most likely to diagnose this patient's underlying condition?
   A. Hysteroscopy
   B. Transvaginal ultrasound
   C. CT abdomen and pelvis
   D. MRI brain
   The correct answer is A. This patient's history of cyclical pelvic pain with multiple intrauterine procedures is suggestive of amenorrhea due to uterine adhesions (Asherman syndrome). Uterine anomalies in women with uterine adhesions are not always detected on physical exam. Transvaginal ultrasound has been found to have a sensitivity of 0 to 52% in the diagnosis of uterine adhesions compared to hysteroscopy (gold standard) [27, 28]. In the primary care setting, transvaginal ultrasound may be a reasonable first diagnostic imaging study, especially in a patient with a palpable uterine or adnexal anomaly on pelvic exam. In patients with suspected uterine adhesions, however, a normal transvaginal ultrasound should not preclude a referral for hysteroscopy, which has a higher sensitivity for diagnosing this disorder. Hysteroscopy also has the added benefit of providing an opportunity for treatment (lysis of adhesion) upon diagnosis.
   This patient does not have symptoms or physical exam findings of an intracranial process to prompt an MRI brain. A CT abdomen could be considered if the patient had physical exam, symptoms, or laboratory findings of hyperandrogenism of a suspected adrenal source.
2. A 28-year-old woman with a history of obesity and prediabetes presents to clinic with amenorrhea for the past 6 months. She is sexually active with a male partner and uses condoms regularly. She feels fatigued at times but denies weight change, heat/cold intolerance, diarrhea, constipation, palpitations, abdominal pain, galactorrhea, and hair or skin changes. Her BMI is 38, and skin, abdominal, thyroid, and pelvic exams are normal. Her medications include metformin. Testing includes a negative urine pregnancy test, normal TSH and prolactin, and a slightly elevated FSH. A progesterone withdrawal test results in vaginal bleeding. What is the next best step in evaluating this patient's amenorrhea?
   A. Androgen testing
   B. Repeat FSH and estrogen
   C. Karyotype
   D. Transvaginal ultrasound
   The correct answer is B. While this patient does have risk factors associated with PCOS (obesity and insulin resistance), her elevated FSH is not consistent with this diagnosis and more suggestive of POI. Progestin withdrawal testing generally results in withdrawal bleeding in women with sufficient endogenous estrogen to build an endometrial lining, including PCOS, and no outflow tract obstruction. While women with POI typically have reduced production of estrogen, ovarian function can vary with as many as 50% of women with POI having a withdrawal bleed [25]. The next best step would be to repeat an FSH and estrogen 1 to 5 days following the onset of menses from the progestin withdrawal. If FSH is again elevated, this would confirm a diagnosis of POI.
   It can be reasonable to check androgens when there is a high clinical suspicion for PCOS, but this patient does not have any symptoms or physical exam findings of androgen excess. A karyotype should be checked in this patient if POI is confirmed with an additional high FSH given her age of less than 30 years. This patient does not have any abnormalities on pelvic exam to prompt transvaginal ultrasound as a next step, but if POI is confirmed, this study can be considered to evaluate for enlarged, multicystic ovaries which can be seen with autoimmune oophoritis and 17,20 desmolase insufficiency.
3. A 38-year-old woman with a history of Graves' disease treated with iodine ablation with resulting hypothyroidism presents to clinic with 5 months of amenorrhea. She otherwise feels well and review of systems is negative. She is sexually active with a male partner and does not desire pregnancy. She takes levothyroxine daily and does not currently use contraception. Her vitals and physical exam are normal and a pregnancy test is negative. Initial workup shows a normal TSH and prolactin with an elevated FSH. A progesterone withdrawal test did not produce a withdrawal bleed, with repeat labs showing an elevated FSH and low estrogen. What is the next best step in management of this patient?
   A. Combined cyclic hormone therapy
   B. Bisphosphonate
   C. Levonorgestrel intrauterine device
   D. Combined oral contraceptive

The correct answer is D. Women with POI are at risk for cardiovascular disease, bone density loss, higher mortality, sexual dysfunction, and psychosocial stress. Either COC or combined HT can be considered for management of vasomotor symptoms and preservation of bone density in women with POI. It is important to counsel patients with POI that they have a 5–10% chance of spontaneous pregnancy due to varied ovarian function [60]. COC have the added benefit of contraception, but their contraceptive effectiveness in women with POI is uncertain due to potentially inadequate suppression of FSH [17, 61]. Combined cyclic hormone therapy would not be recommended in this patient who does not desire pregnancy without an additional contraceptive.

Bisphosphonates are not currently recommended for reproductive age women due to the long half-life of this medication, teratogenicity, and uncertain safety profile in this population [16, 64]. While a levonorgestrel intrauterine device would provide effective contraception, hormone from this method is minimally systemically absorbed and would not be expected to mitigate the systemic side effects of POI.

4. A 33-year-old woman with a history of idiopathic primary ovarian insufficiency presents to clinic because she desires pregnancy. She was regularly taking a combined oral contraceptive pill until 2 months ago, and she has not had a period since stopping this medication. She is sexually active with her husband twice weekly. She currently takes a prenatal vitamin. A pregnancy test is negative. What is the next best step in management of this patient?
   A. Encourage more regular sexual activity
   B. Counsel that pregnancy is not possible
   C. Refer to infertility specialist
   D. Prescribe course of progesterone

   The correct answer is C. Because POI is a known risk factor for infertility, women with POI who desire pregnancy should be referred to an infertility specialist without delay. Women with POI have a 5–10% chance of spontaneous pregnancy due to varied ovarian function and should be counseled that spontaneous pregnancy without fertility treatment is possible but less likely compared to women without POI [60]. Progesterone may induce a withdrawal bleed but would not influence the underlying ovarian insufficiency that is the source of infertility.

References

1. Beckmann C, Ling F, Herbert W, Laube D, Smith R, Casanova R, et al. Obstetrics and Gynecology. Seventh ed. Baltimore: Lippincott Williams & Wilkins; 2014.
2. Munster K, Helm P, Schmidt L. Secondary amenorrhoea: prevalence and medical contact–a cross-sectional study from a Danish county. Br J Obstet Gynaecol. 1992;99(5):430–3.
3. Hernandez I, Cervera-Aguilar R, Vergara MD, Ayala AR. Prevalence and etiology of secondary amenorrhea in a selected Mexican population. Ginecol Obstet Mex. 1999;67:374–6.
4. Bachmann GA, Kemmann E. Prevalence of oligomenorrhea and amenorrhea in a college population. Am J Obstet Gynecol. 1982;144(1):98–102.
5. Reindollar RH, Novak M, Tho SP, McDonough PG. Adult-onset amenorrhea: a study of 262 patients. Am J Obstet Gynecol. 1986;155(3):531–43.
6. Chandeying P, Pantasri T. Prevalence of conditions causing chronic anovulation and the proposed algorithm for anovulation evaluation. J Obstet Gynaecol Res. 2015;41(7):1074–9.
7. Coulam CB, Adamson SC, Annegers JF. Incidence of premature ovarian failure. Obstet Gynecol. 1986;67(4):604–6.
8. Hiller-Sturmhofel S, Bartke A. The endocrine system: an overview. Alcohol Health Res World. 1998;22(3):153–64.
9. Chris 73. Wikimedia Commons. File:MenstrualCycle.png. 29 Nov 2004. //commons.wikimedia.org/wiki/File:MenstrualCycle.png under the creative commons cc-by-sa 3.0 licens, Accessed March 29, 2018.
10. Lin K, Barnhart K. The clinical rationale for menses-free contraception. J Womens Health (Larchmt). 2007;16(8):1171–80.
11. Torre DL, Falorni A. Pharmacological causes of hyperprolactinemia. Ther Clin Risk Manag. 2007;3(5):929–51.
12. Pickett CA. Diagnosis and management of pituitary tumors: recent advances. Prim Care. 2003;30(4):765–89.
13. Fourman LT, Fazeli PK. Neuroendocrine causes of amenorrhea--an update. J Clin Endocrinol Metab. 2015;100(3):812–24.
14. Marshall JC, Eagleson CA, McCartney CR. Hypothalamic dysfunction. Mol Cell Endocrinol. 2001;183(1–2):29–32.
15. McDermott MT. Infiltrative diseases of the pituitary gland. Diseases of the pituitary: diagnosis and treatment. Totowa: Humana Press; 1997. p. 305–22.
16. Committee opinion no. 605: primary ovarian insufficiency in adolescents and young women. Obstet Gynecol. 2014;124(1):193–7.
17. Nelson LM. Clinical practice. Primary ovarian insufficiency. N Engl J Med. 2009;360(6):606–14.
18. Seif MW, Diamond K, Nickkho-Amiry M. Obesity and menstrual disorders. Best Pract Res Clin Obstet Gynaecol. 2015;29(4):516–27.
19. Gardner D, Shoback D. Greenspan's basic & clinical endocrinology. Ninth ed. China: McGraw-Hill Companies, Inc.; 2011.
20. Witchel SF, Azziz R. Nonclassic congenital adrenal hyperplasia. Int J Pediatr Endocrinol. 2010;2010:1–11.
21. Heiman DL. Amenorrhea. Prim Care. 2009;36(1):1–17, vii.
22. Klein DA, Poth MA. Amenorrhea: an approach to diagnosis and management. Am Fam Physician. 2013;87(11):781–8.
23. Rothman MS, Wierman ME. Female hypogonadism: evaluation of the hypothalamic-pituitary-ovarian axis. Pituitary. 2008;11(2):163–9.
24. Practice Committee of American Society for Reproductive Medicine. Current evaluation of amenorrhea. Fertil Steril. 2008;90(5 Suppl):S219–25.
25. Rebar RW, Connolly HV. Clinical features of young women with hypergonadotropic amenorrhea. Fertil Steril. 1990;53(5):804–10.
26. Tsutsumi R, Webster NJG. GnRH pulsatility, the pituitary response and reproductive dysfunction. Endocr J. 2009;56(6):729–37.
27. Soares SR, Barbosa dos Reis MM, Camargos AF. Diagnostic accuracy of sonohysterography, transvaginal sonography, and hysterosalpingography in patients with uterine cavity diseases. Fertil Steril. 2000;73(2):406–11.
28. Salle B, Gaucherand P, de Saint HP, Rudigoz RC. Transvaginal sonohysterographic evaluation of intrauterine adhesions. J Clin Ultrasound. 1999;27(3):131–4.
29. AAGL Elevating Gynecologic Surgery. AAGL practice report: practice guidelines on intrauterine adhesions developed in collaboration with the European Society of Gynaecological Endoscopy (ESGE). Gynecol Surg. 2017;14(1):6.

30. Conway GS, Kaltsas G, Patel A, Davies MC, Jacobs HS. Characterization of idiopathic premature ovarian failure. Fertil Steril. 1996;65(2):337–41.
31. Bakalov VK, Vanderhoof VH, Bondy CA, Nelson LM. Adrenal antibodies detect asymptomatic auto-immune adrenal insufficiency in young women with spontaneous premature ovarian failure. Hum Reprod. 2002;17(8):2096–100.
32. Marozzi A, Vegetti W, Manfredini E, Tibiletti MG, Testa G, Crosignani PG, et al. Association between idiopathic premature ovarian failure and fragile X premutation. Hum Reprod. 2000;15(1):197–202.
33. Goswami R, Marwaha RK, Goswami D, Gupta N, Ray D, Tomar N, Singh S. Prevalence of thyroid autoimmunity in sporadic idiopathic hypoparathyroidism in comparison to type 1 diabetes and premature ovarian failure. J Clin Endocrinol Metab. 2006;91(11):4256–9.
34. Rebar RW, Erickson GF, Yen SS. Idiopathic premature ovarian failure: clinical and endocrine characteristics. Fertil Steril. 1982;37(1):35–41.
35. Bakalov VK, Anasti JN, Calis KA, Vanderhoof VH, Premkumar A, Chen S, et al. Autoimmune oophoritis as a mechanism of follicular dysfunction in women with 46,XX spontaneous premature ovarian failure. Fertil Steril. 2005;84(4):958–65.
36. Novosad JA, Kalantaridou SN, Tong ZB, Nelson LM. Ovarian antibodies as detected by indirect immunofluorescence are unreliable in the diagnosis of autoimmune premature ovarian failure: a controlled evaluation. BMC Womens Health. 2003;3(1):2.
37. Committee opinion no.702: female athlete triad. Obstet Gynecol. 2017;129(6):e160–e7.
38. Gordon CM, Ackerman KE, Berga SL, Kaplan JR, Mastorakos G, Misra M, et al. Functional hypothalamic amenorrhea: an Endocrine Society clinical practice guideline. J Clin Endocrinol Metab. 2017;102(5):1413–39.
39. Melmed S, Casanueva FF, Hoffman AR, Kleinberg DL, Montori VM, Schlechte JA, et al. Diagnosis and treatment of hyperprolactinemia: an Endocrine Society clinical practice guideline. J Clin Endocrinol Metab. 2011;96(2):273–88.
40. Freda PU, Beckers AM, Katznelson L, Molitch ME, Montori VM, Post KD, et al. Pituitary incidentaloma: an endocrine society clinical practice guideline. J Clin Endocrinol Metab. 2011;96(4):894–904.
41. Fleseriu M, Hashim IA, Karavitaki N, Melmed S, Murad MH, Salvatori R, et al. Hormonal replacement in hypopituitarism in adults: an Endocrine Society clinical practice guideline. J Clin Endocrinol Metab. 2016;101(11):3888–921.
42. Committee opinion no. 698: hormone therapy in primary ovarian insufficiency. Obstet Gynecol. 2017;129(5):e134–e41.
43. American College of Obstetricians and Gynecologists. ACOG Practice Bulletin. Management of adnexal masses. Obstet Gynecol. 2007;110(1):201–14.
44. ACOG Committee on Practice Bulletins—Gynecology. ACOG practice bulletin no. 108: polycystic ovary syndrome. Obstet Gynecol. 2009;114(4):936–49.
45. Legro RS, Arslanian SA, Ehrmann DA, Hoeger KM, Murad MH, Pasquali R, et al. Diagnosis and treatment of polycystic ovary syndrome: an Endocrine Society clinical practice guideline. J Clin Endocrinol Metab. 2013;98(12):4565–92.
46. Garber JR, Cobin RH, Gharib H, Hennessey JV, Klein I, Mechanick JI, et al. Clinical practice guidelines for hypothyroidism in adults: cosponsored by the American Association of Clinical Endocrinologists and the American Thyroid Association. Endocr Pract. 2012;18(6):988–1028.
47. Bahn RS, Burch HB, Cooper DS, Garber JR, Greenlee MC, Klein I, et al. Hyperthyroidism and other causes of thyrotoxicosis: management guidelines of the American Thyroid Association and American Association of Clinical Endocrinologists. Endocr Pract. 2011;17(3):456–520.
48. Nieman LK, Biller BM, Findling JW, Murad MH, Newell-Price J, Savage MO, et al. Treatment of Cushing's syndrome: an Endocrine Society clinical practice guideline. J Clin Endocrinol Metab. 2015;100(8):2807–31.
49. Atsma F, Bartelink ML, Grobbee DE, van der Schouw YT. Postmenopausal status and early menopause as independent risk factors for cardiovascular disease: a meta-analysis. Menopause. 2006;13(2):265–79.
50. Jacobsen BK, Knutsen SF, Fraser GE. Age at natural menopause and total mortality and mortality from ischemic heart disease: the Adventist Health Study. J Clin Epidemiol. 1999;52(4):303–7.
51. de Kleijn MJ, van der Schouw YT, Verbeek AL, Peeters PH, Banga JD, van der Graaf Y. Endogenous estrogen exposure and cardiovascular mortality risk in postmenopausal women. Am J Epidemiol. 2002;155(4):339–45.
52. Anasti JN, Kalantaridou SN, Kimzey LM, Defensor RA, Nelson LM. Bone loss in young women with karyotypically normal spontaneous premature ovarian failure. Obstet Gynecol. 1998;91(1):12–5.
53. Gallagher JC. Effect of early menopause on bone mineral density and fractures. Menopause. 2007;14(3 Pt 2):567–71.
54. Leite-Silva P, Bedone A, Pinto-Neto AM, Costa JV, Costa-Paiva L. Factors associated with bone density in young women with karyotypically normal spontaneous premature ovarian failure. Arch Gynecol Obstet. 2009;280(2):177–81.
55. van der Stege JG, Groen H, van Zadelhoff SJ, Lambalk CB, Braat DD, van Kasteren YM, et al. Decreased androgen concentrations and diminished general and sexual well-being in women with premature ovarian failure. Menopause. 2008;15(1):23–31.
56. Schmidt PJ, Cardoso GM, Ross JL, Haq N, Rubinow DR, Bondy CA. Shyness, social anxiety, and impaired self-esteem in Turner syndrome and premature ovarian failure. JAMA. 2006;295:1374–6.
57. Rafique S, Sterling EW, Nelson LM. A new approach to primary ovarian insufficiency. Obstet Gynecol Clin N Am. 2012;39(4):567–86.
58. Benetti-Pinto CL, Ferreira VB, Yela DA. Long-term follow-up of bone density in women with primary ovarian insufficiency. Menopause. 2015;22(9):946–9.
59. Popat VB, Calis KA, Kalantaridou SN, Vanderhoof VH, Koziol D, Troendle JF, et al. Bone mineral density in young women with primary ovarian insufficiency: results of a three-year randomized controlled trial of physiological transdermal estradiol and testosterone replacement. J Clin Endocrinol Metab. 2014;99(9):3418–26.
60. van Kasteren YM, Schoemaker J. Premature ovarian failure: a systematic review on therapeutic interventions to restore ovarian function and achieve pregnancy. Hum Reprod Update. 1999;5(5):483–92.
61. Alper MM, Jolly EE, Garner PR. Pregnancies after premature ovarian failure. Obstet Gynecol. 1986;67(3 Suppl):59s–62s.
62. Baker V. Life plans and family-building options for women with primary ovarian insufficiency. Semin Reprod Med. 2011;29(4):362–72.
63. Camacho PM, Petak SM, Binkley N, Clarke BL, Harris ST, Hurley DL, et al. American Association of Clinical Endocrinologists and American College of Endocrinology clinical practice guidelines for the diagnosis and treatment of postmenopausal osteoporosis - 2016. Endocr Pract. 2016;22(Suppl 4):1–42.
64. Drake MT, Clarke BL, Khosla S. Bisphosphonates: mechanism of action and role in clinical practice. Mayo Clin Proc. 2008;83(9):1032–45.

Polycystic Ovary Syndrome

6

Azadeh Nasseh and Jenna Sarvaideo

Learning Objectives

1. List the diagnostic criteria for PCOS.
2. Discuss the diagnostic work-up for PCOS.
3. Describe the underlying pathophysiology of PCOS.
4. Demonstrate knowledge of metabolic abnormalities in patients with PCOS such as insulin resistance, diabetes, and hyperlipidemia.
5. Describe short-term and long-term sequela associated with PCOS, including symptoms of androgen excess, endometrial cancer risk, and depression.
6. Formulate a treatment plan for a patient with PCOS that addresses weight management, symptoms of androgen excess such as acne/hirsutism, endometrial cancer prevention, and metabolic abnormalities, if present.
7. Discuss how to address infertility issues in women with PCOS.

Shazia is a 32-year-old woman here for a new annual visit who notes irregular menses. For 6 years, she has had fewer than six menses per year and her last menstrual period was 5 months ago. The irregularities worsened after she gained weight in the past few years. She is sexually active and is not using any form of contraception since she does not believe she can become pregnant. You highly suspect PCOS.

A. Nasseh
Boston Medical Center, Boston University School of Medicine, Department of Internal Medicine, Section of GIM, Boston, MA, USA

J. Sarvaideo (✉)
Medical College of Wisconsin, Department of Medicine, Division of Endocrinology, Milwaukee, WI, USA
e-mail: jsarvaideo@mcw.edu

Epidemiology

Polycystic ovary syndrome (PCOS) is the most common endocrine disorder seen in women of childbearing age [1–3] with an estimated prevalence between 5% and 16% depending on the population studied and the criteria applied [1, 4]. PCOS has been identified as a complex and heterogenous disorder that results from the interaction of diverse genetic and environmental factors and can lead to adverse reproductive and metabolic complications in affected women [5]. The syndrome was first described by Stein and Leventhal in 1935 and encompasses three cardinal features, oligo-anovulation, polycystic ovaries, and hyperandrogenism and/or hyperandrogenemia [4, 6]; further discussion of each of these features will follow below. PCOS is a common cause of infertility in women due to oligo-anovulation [2, 3] and can be associated with a wide range of metabolic abnormalities such as insulin resistance, diabetes mellitus type 2, hyperlipidemia, and increased risk of cardiovascular disease [2, 3, 7]. It can be accompanied by symptoms of androgen excess such as acne and hirsutism, increased risk of endometrial cancer, and depression [5, 7, 8]. Therefore, primary care providers must be familiar with the diagnostic criteria and basic steps in management for PCOS to identify and treat this disorder in their patients.

Diagnostic Criteria and Phenotypes

Over the past three decades, significant efforts have been made to classify PCOS. The first formal attempt was made at the National Institutes of Health (NIH) conference, April 1990 [9]; the NIH criteria served as a standard for researchers and clinicians for more than a decade. Based on NIH criteria, clinical or biochemical hyperandrogenism (HA) and chronic oligo-anovulation (OA) were considered key diagnostic features of PCOS, after exclusion of related disorders [7]. In 2003, a consensus workshop in Rotterdam, Netherlands, developed new diagnostic criteria, the

S. A. Tilstra et al. (eds.), *Sex- and Gender-Based Women's Health*, https://doi.org/10.1007/978-3-030-50695-7_6

Rotterdam criteria, which added ultrasound characteristics for polycystic ovary morphology (PCOM) to the NIH criteria definition. The 2003 Rotterdam criteria required the presence of two of the following three findings: signs of clinical or biochemical hyperandrogenism; chronic ovulatory dysfunction (OD); and the presence of polycystic ovary morphology, after exclusion of secondary causes [7, 10, 11] (Table 6.1). As a growing body of evidence supported the presence of hyperandrogenism as a key factor in the pathophysiology of PCOS and a strong predictor of the associated metabolic dysfunctions [12], a task force assembled in 2006 by the Androgen Excess and PCOS Society proposed the AE-PCOS criteria. These criteria require the diagnosis of PCOS to be based on the presence of clinical or biochemical hyperandrogenism in combination with ovarian dysfunction (i.e., OD or PCOM), excluding other causes [13]. Given the multiplicity of criteria that could cause confusion in clinical practice, the NIH sponsored an Evidence-Based Methodology PCOS Workshop in 2012 that addressed the benefits and drawbacks of existing diagnostic criteria [11]. As a result, the panel recommended the use of the broader Rotterdam 2003 criteria, while also providing detailed description of the different PCOS phenotypes defined by above criteria [7, 11].

Based on the 2012 NIH criteria, four clinical phenotypes can be defined for PCOS (Table 6.2). Phenotypes A and B are defined as "classic PCOS." This group of patients may experience more pronounced menstrual irregularities [14, 15] and is at a higher risk for metabolic dysfunction such as insulin resistance, atherogenic dyslipidemia, and obesity [7, 14, 16, 17] when compared with women diagnosed with nonclassic or non-hyperandrogenic PCOS phenotypes (phenotypes C and D). Phenotype C, "ovulatory PCOS," generally includes women with preserved ovulation who show an intermediate level of symptoms [18, 19] compared with patients with other subtypes. Phenotype D, also defined as "non-hyperandrogenic PCOS" [7], has the mildest degree of metabolic dysfunction and the lowest prevalence of metabolic syndrome of all subtypes [14, 19, 20].

Pathophysiology

The most consistent biochemical abnormality in women with PCOS is an overproduction of androgens [8]. There are two main sources of androgen production in women: the ovaries and the adrenal glands. It has been hypothesized that in most PCOS cases, intrinsic dysregulation in ovarian steroidogenesis results in functional ovarian hyperandrogenism (FOH) (Fig. 6.1). This inherent abnormality is further influenced by other hypothalamic-pituitary axis factors, including higher baseline gonadotropin-releasing hormone (GnRH)

Table 6.1 PCOS diagnostic criteria

	Hyperandrogenism (HA)	Ovulatory dysfunction (OD)	Polycystic ovarian morphology (PCOM)	Other requirements
NIH 1990 [9]	+	+ (oligo-anovulation)		Both required
Rotterdam 2003 [10]	+	+	+	Two of three required
Androgen Excess and PCOS Society 2006 [13]	+	+/–	+/–	HA + either OD or PCOM
NIH 2012 Extension of Rotterdam 2003 [11]	+	+	+	Two of three required; phenotypes added (see Table 6.2)

Reprinted from Lizneva et al. [7], with permission from Elsevier

Table 6.2 NIH 2012 PCOS phenotypes and clinical features

Clinical presentation	Phenotype A: classic PCOS	Phenotype B: classic PCOS	Phenotype C: ovulatory PCOS	Phenotype D: non-hyperandrogenic
Hyperandrogenism	+	+	+	–
Ovulatory dysfunction	+	+	–	+
Polycystic ovary morphology	+	–	+	+
Clinical features	↑ menstrual irregularities ↑ obesity, insulin resistance, metabolic syndrome ↑ risk of hepatic steatosis ↑ anti-mullerian hormone levels		Intermediate levels of insulin, androgens, atherogenic lipids, and metabolic syndrome	Mildest form: ↓↓ metabolic syndrome ↓ androgens ↓ menstrual irregularity

Reprinted from Lizneva et al. [7], with permission from Elsevier

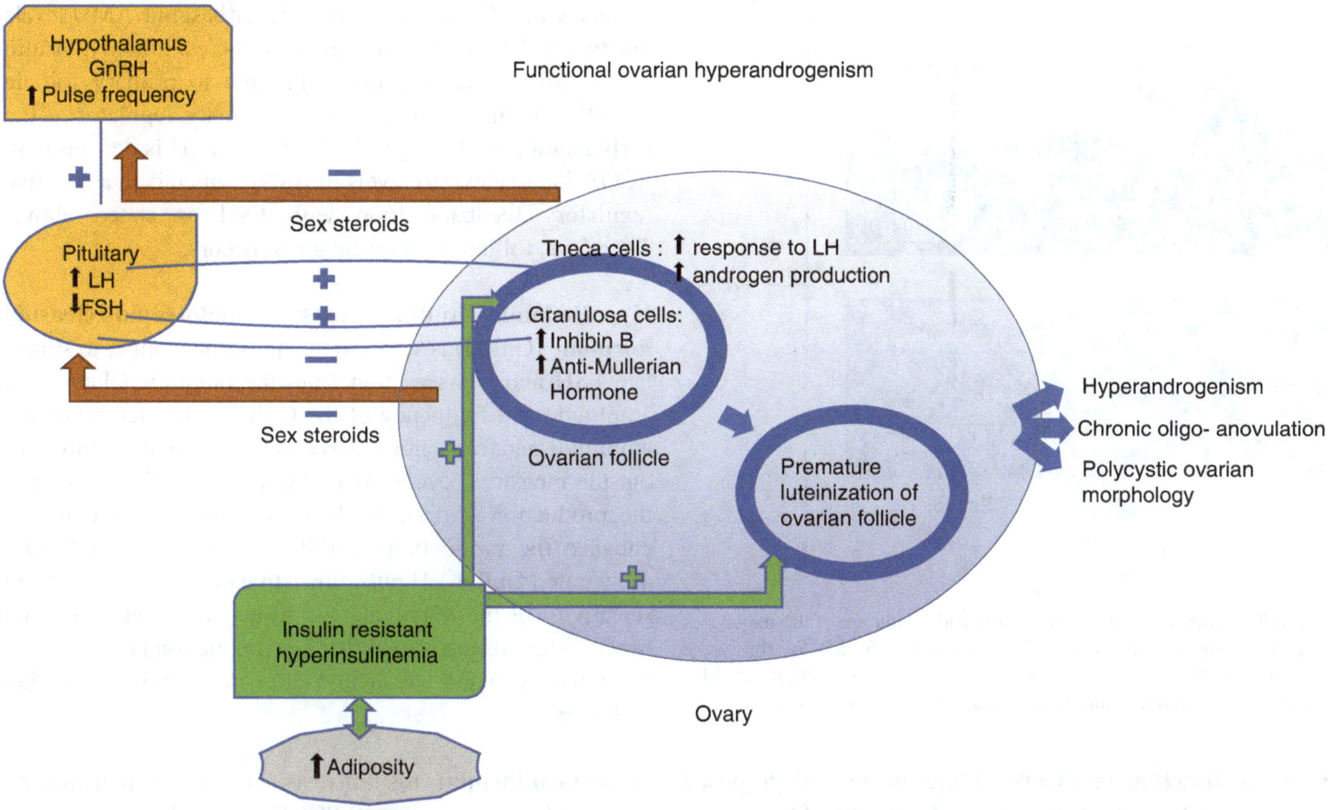

Fig. 6.1 This figure depicts the main processes involved in the pathophysiology of PCOS. Functional ovarian hyperandrogenism (FOH) is the cardinal proposed feature, and it can explain the different clinical manifestations of PCOS. LH acts on theca cells of ovarian follicles to start the process of follicle development and stimulates androgen production. Theca cells in women with PCOS have an exaggerated response to LH that leads to increase in androgens. Meanwhile, granulosa cells of antral follicles respond to FSH for further development. Inhibin-B produced by granulosa cells has an inhibitory feedback on FSH. It also increases androgen production in theca cells. Patients with PCOS have elevated levels of inhibin-B. Anti-mullerian hormone (AMH) is another key player in control of follicular growth. Its levels are increased in PCOS due to excessive number of growing follicles. It can also have a suppressing effect on FSH. Androgens accelerate luteinization of ovarian follicles (a part of normal follicular development). However, when in excess, they can cause premature luteinization and follicular growth arrest. This leads potentially to anovulation and development of polycystic ovaries. The picture also depicts contribution of the hypothalamus-pituitary axis. Patients with PCOS can have increase in pulse frequency of GnRH. This can lead to a higher LH production (compared to FSH), which at the end can contribute to enhanced androgen production by ovaries. Sex steroids produced by ovaries have negative regulatory feedback on gonadotropins. It is hypothesized that the hypothalamus-pituitary axis is less responsive to this feedback in PCOS patients as well. Insulin-resistant hyperinsulinemia can have an independent contributory role in pathophysiology of PCOS. Insulin synergizes with LH to stimulate theca cells' androgen production. Insulin also, similar to androgens, enhances luteinization of ovarian follicles. Hyperinsulinemia can trigger peripheral adiposity, and adiposity can in turn worsen insulin resistance. The figure does not depict the contribution of the adrenal glands to androgen production (functional adrenal hyperandrogenism), which is seen either alone (in a smaller number of patients) or as an adjunct to FOH

pulse frequency and reduced hypothalamic feedback response to circulating sex steroids [6, 8]. This in turn leads to hypersecretion of luteinizing hormone (LH) and subsequent enhanced ovarian androgen synthesis and folliculogenesis. Insulin-resistant hyperinsulinemia also plays an important role in PCOS. Insulin has been shown to enhance the response of androgen-producing theca cells in the ovaries to LH stimuli. In a smaller number of PCOS cases, dysregulation at the adrenal zona reticularis causes hyperandrogenism by increased production of dehydroepiandrosterone (DHEA) [1].

Functional Ovarian Hyperandrogenism (FOH)

Normal ovarian function: Ovulation takes place due to synchronized activity between the hypothalamus, pituitary, and ovarian follicles (see Chap. 5 on Menstruation and Secondary Amenorrhea). In the follicular phase, theca cells express LH receptors; LH stimulates the production of androstenedione from its precursor cholesterol [6]. Androstenedione, an androgen, is required for ovarian estrogen biosynthesis. A delicate balance exists between adequate and overproduction of androgens (Fig. 6.2).

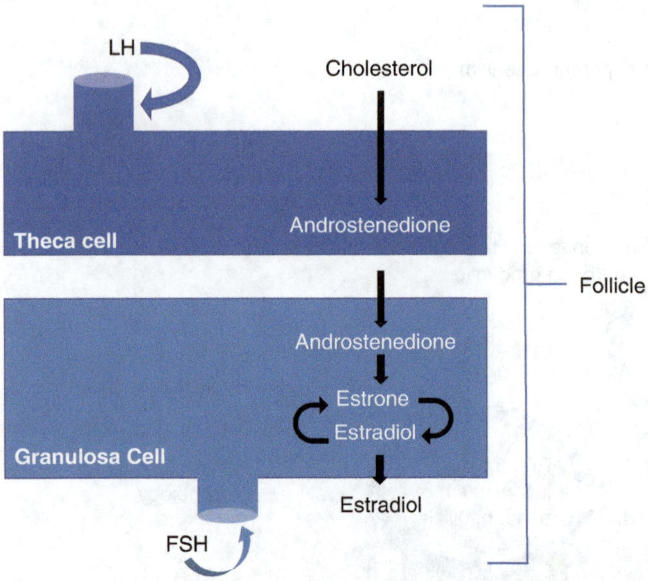

Fig. 6.2 Depiction of the organization and regulation of the major steroid biosynthetic pathways in the small antral follicle of the ovary according to the two-gonadotropin, two-cell model of ovarian steroidogenesis. LH stimulates androgen formation within theca cells

Ovarian function in PCOS: There are several proposed mechanisms to explain anovulatory cycles in PCOS.

Theca cell dysfunction: Women with PCOS are suspected to have intrinsic abnormalities in the ovarian theca cells' steroidogenesis which leads to hyperandrogenemia. In vivo and in vitro studies have shown overexpression of P450 enzymes along with LH receptors in ovaries of women with PCOS (21). This hyper-responsiveness can increase androgen production. When produced in excess, androgens cause an arrest in follicular maturation, cause follicular atresia, and hinder ovulation [5].

Granulosa cell dysfunction: Granulosa cells convert androgens coming from the thecal cells to estradiol by aromatase. In women with PCOS, there seems to be a relative aromatase deficiency likely due to inhibition by anti-mullerian hormone (AMH). Therefore, there is limited conversion of androgens to estrogens, leading to hyperandrogenemia [22]. In addition to AMH, inhibin-B is a peptide that is produced in granulosa cells and is in a reciprocal negative regulatory feedback loop with FSH. It is essential and permissive for thecal androgen production. Women with PCOS tend to have elevated serum inhibin-B as well as AMH [23].

Polycystic ovary morphology (PCOM) and role of anti-mullerian hormone (AMH): The ovaries of women with PCOS often show an excessive number of follicles. AMH is an important intrafollicular regulator of follicle growth, and women with PCOS tend to have higher baseline AMH levels due to a higher number of growing follicles. Initially, insulin and androgen promote the primordial to primary follicle transition until FSH becomes the primary regulator at the early antral follicle stage [1]. However, FSH is decreased in PCOS due to elevated levels of AMH, which is in a negative regulatory feedback loop with FSH as stated above. Therefore, follicle maturation arrest occurs.

Hypothalamic-pituitary axis: Gonadotropin-releasing hormone (GnRH) is secreted in a pulsatile manner to stimulate FSH and LH secretion from the pituitary. Changes in amplitude and frequency of the GnRH pulse determine the amplitude and frequency of LH and FSH production throughout the menstrual cycle. At higher pulses, GnRH promotes the production of LH, while lower pulsation frequencies enhance the production of FSH. In women with PCOS, accelerated GnRH-LH pulsatile activity as well as decreased sensitivity of the hypothalamus to negative feedback from ovarian steroids leads to higher LH production [1, 6]. Higher LH pulses generally lead to higher production of ovarian androgens.

Hyperinsulinemia: Insulin resistance is common in both obese and lean women with PCOS. Insulin has a direct role on ovaries and enhances androgen production from theca cells in response to an LH stimulus (Figs. 6.1 and 6.2). It is proposed that with higher insulin levels, both ovarian theca cells and adrenal zona reticularis cells have enhanced androgen production in response to LH and ACTH, respectively.

Genetics

Familial clustering of PCOS suggests a genetic basis. Heritable traits that have been identified as PCOS risk factors are maternal PCOS, polycystic ovary morphology, hyperandrogenemia, and metabolic syndrome [1]. Phenotypic features associated with PCOS such as hyperandrogenism and metabolic abnormalities can be seen in aggregate in certain families, suggesting a genetic cause. An example is sisters with hyperandrogenism and metabolic derangements, with or without menstrual irregularities. Several susceptibility genes have been implicated, especially in the region of insulin receptor genes [21]. Defects in androgen steroidogenesis as well as beta cell function have been observed in brothers of women with PCOS, manifesting itself as elevated levels of dehydroepiandrosterone-sulfate (DHEA-S) and increased risk for type 2 diabetes [21]. Furthermore, it is thought that PCOS evolved to preserve anabolism and reproductive capacity via increased androgen and insulin production in times of nutritional deprivation [1].

Clinical Manifestations

Shazia noted that she had her upper lip waxed regularly due to bothersome facial hair. She had moderate acne across her upper back as well. Based on these features and her oligomenorrhea, PCOS is highest on your differential. You discuss the diagnosis and work-up with her.

Ovulatory dysfunction with or without menstrual abnormalities: Ovulatory dysfunction typically presents with obvious disruption in menstrual flow but can present subclinically without obvious menstrual irregularity [13].

Overt dysfunction: Overt dysfunction occurs for the majority of the patients with PCOS [9, 12, 24–26] in the form of oligomenorrhea, defined as vaginal bleeding episodes occurring at greater than 35-day intervals or less than ten bleeds per year. A much smaller percentage of patients present with polymenorrhea, defined as bleeding episodes occurring frequently with less than 25 days between cycles [13, 27].

Subclinical ovulatory dysfunction: Roughly 15–40% of oligo-ovulatory patients with PCOS present with eumenorrhea (cycles every 25–35 days in length) [13, 26, 28]. In eumenorrheic patients for whom there is a high suspicion of PCOS, day 18–24 progesterone levels can clarify the diagnosis. Levels below 3 to 4 ng/mL may suggest an anovulatory cycle but should be checked on at least two different occasions as the presence of one anovulatory cycle may not indicate chronic anovulation [13].

Hyperandrogenemia or hyperandrogenism: Hyperandrogenemia refers to higher than normal levels of circulating endogenous androgens, including testosterone (T), androstenedione (A4), and DHEA-S [13]. Clinical features of elevated androgens (known as hyperandrogenism) include hirsutism, acne, and androgenic alopecia [8, 13].

Hirsutism: Hirsutism refers to the presence of course, pigmented hair on the face and/or body in a male pattern distribution, including the upper lip, chin, chest, upper back and shoulders, lower back, abdomen, upper arms, and thighs. While the degree of hirsutism can vary based on race and ethnicity [13], hirsutism affects approximately 65–75% of patients with PCOS [16], including women of White, Black, and Southeast Asian backgrounds. If a clinician is uncertain regarding the presence of hirsutism, the Ferriman-Gallwey score can be used to further quantify the degree of hirsutism present [29, 30]. This score, originally introduced in 1961, assesses terminal hair growth in nine body areas. The degree of hirsutism can be assessed by assigning a score of 0–4 based on the density of terminal hairs [13, 21, 29, 30]. A total score of 8 or greater based on the 95th percentile of the data originally collected by Ferriman and Gallwey may suggest hirsutism. Race and ethnicity specific normative ranges are not well established. Figure 6.3 depicts the visual scoring method used for assessing hirsutism.

Acne: The prevalence of acne varies by ethnicity but is estimated to affect 15–25% of patients with PCOS [10]. There is no consistent scoring for assessment, and it is unclear how much PCOS raises the prevalence of acne over that in the general population given a general prevalence of 5–20% [13].

Androgenic alopecia: Women with PCOS who experience androgenic alopecia tend to lose hair in the anterior midvertex area extending to the crown. The anterior hairline remains intact in women with PCOS, and significant bitemporal scalp hair recession is unusual except in virilizing syndromes [32, 33]. The prevalence of androgenic alopecia is reported to be as high as 22% in some studies [34].

Polycystic ovaries: Polycystic ovaries are defined by three features: ovarian size and volume, stromal volume, and follicle size and number. Based on the Rotterdam criteria, polycystic ovaries contain 12 or more follicles measuring 2–9 mm in diameter and/or increased ovarian volume >10 mL in at least 1 ovary [35]. It should be noted that this definition cannot be used for women on oral contraceptives. The prevalence of polycystic ovaries in patients with PCOS is high: in one study, 60% of women met size criteria, while another 35% met follicular criteria [36–38].

Other Features Associated with PCOS

While the clinical criteria for diagnosing PCOS include ovulatory dysfunction, hyperandrogenemia or its clinical findings, or polycystic ovary features on ultrasound, a number of other clinical features may accompany this syndrome (Fig. 6.4).

Insulin resistance, hyperinsulinemia, and the metabolic syndrome: Impaired glucose tolerance or diabetes mellitus type 2 develops in about 40% of women with 1990 NIH-defined PCOS by the fourth decade of life. Glycemic control worsens with age and weight gain [8, 39]. Women with PCOS can also have dyslipidemia, which manifests as lower levels of high-density lipoprotein (HDL) cholesterol, increased levels of triglycerides, and increased low-density lipoprotein (LDL) cholesterol [40–42]. Metabolic syndrome is also highly prevalent in patients with PCOS compared to BMI-matched

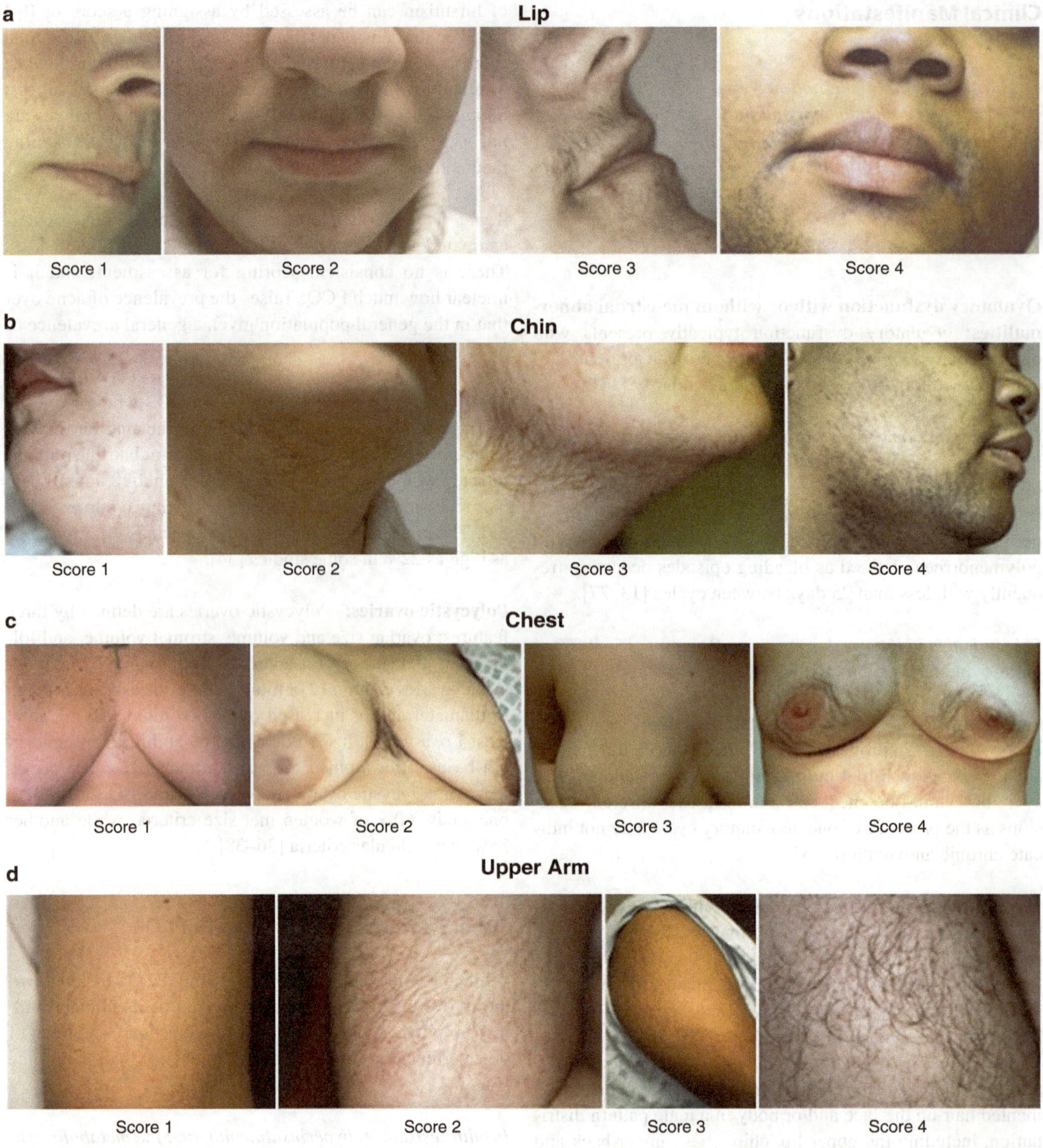

Fig. 6.3 Facial and body terminal hair growth scored according to the modified Ferriman-Gallwey method. All were taken on women who had not used laser or electrolysis for at least 3 months, not depilated or waxed for at least 4 weeks, and not shaved or plucked for at least 5 days before the photograph. The photographs depict scores of 1 through 4 for the upper lip (**a**), chin (**b**), chest (**c**), arm (**d**), upper abdomen (**e**), lower abdomen (**f**), upper back (**g**), lower back (**h**), and thighs (**i**). The areas were photographed with a standard single-lens reflex camera (Nikon N50, Nikon Corp, Melville, NY, USA) equipped with a macro lens (Vivitar 50 or 100 mm Auto Focus Macro, Vivitar Corp, Newbury Park, Calif) and ring flash (Vivitar Macroflash 5000, Vivitar Corp). For film, Kodacolor VR 200 ISO film (Eastman Kodak Co, Rochester, NY, USA) was used. Representative areas were selected. All photographs of hair were anonymized and all identifying information removed, meeting current Institutional Review Board for Human Use and Health Insurance Portability and Accountability Act of 1996
A score of 0–4 based on the density of hair is given in each region; scores >8 are suggestive of hirsutism (Reprinted from Yildiz et al. [31], by permission of Oxford University Press)

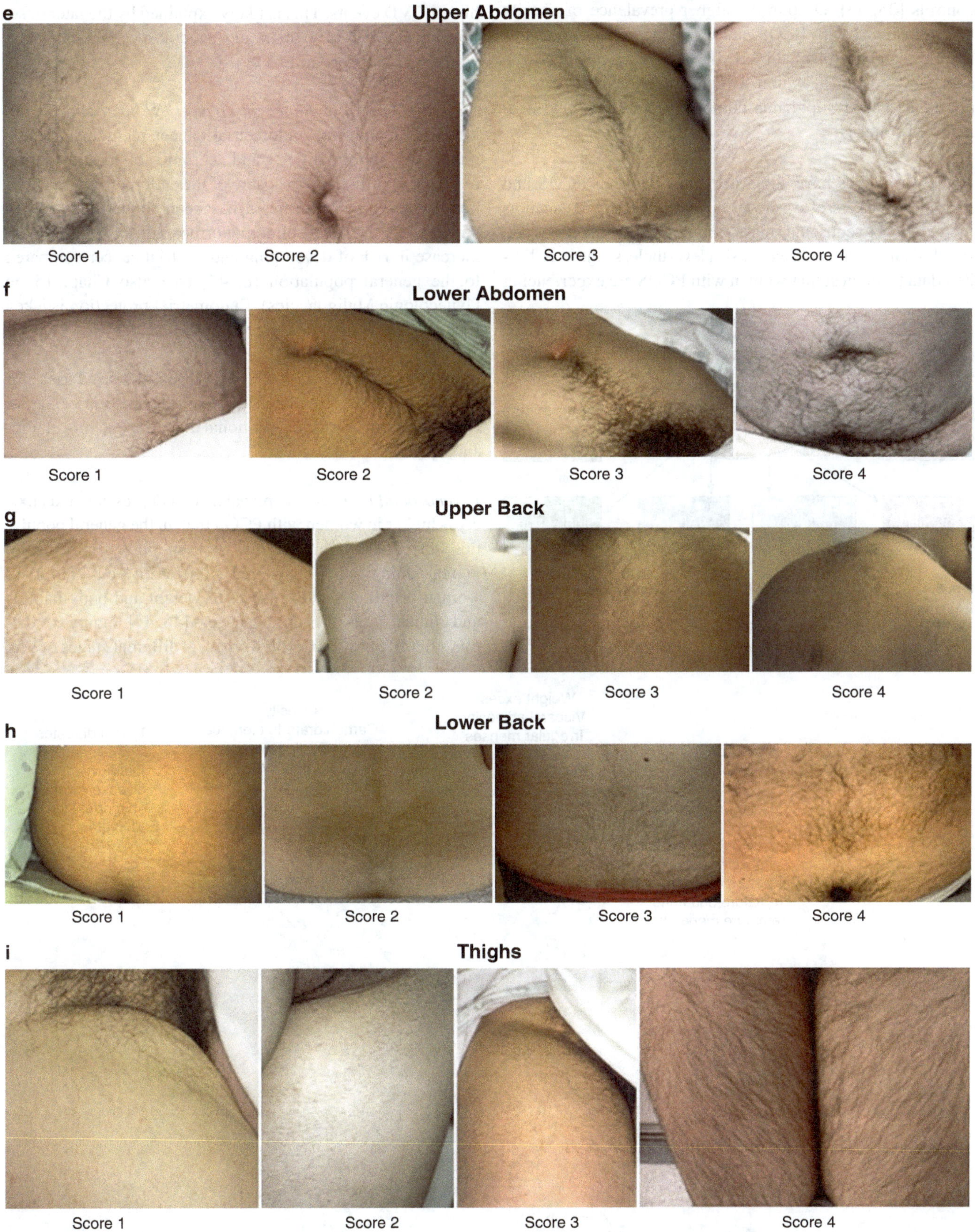

Fig. 6.3 (continued)

controls [25, 43]. Despite the higher prevalence of obesity among patients with PCOS, not all of the metabolic abnormalities can be explained by BMI. Studies suggest that even lean PCOS women exhibit a higher prevalence of insulin resistance and dyslipidemia compared to weight- and age-matched controls.

Newer studies have suggested links between PCOS and surrogate markers of cardiovascular disease (CVD) such as increased left ventricular mass, endothelial dysfunction, and subclinical vascular disease [8]. Nevertheless, there is limited data to suggest that women with PCOS are experiencing higher CVD events. This is likely explained by the later onset of clinical CVD in women and paucity of studies in older women with history of PCOS [8].

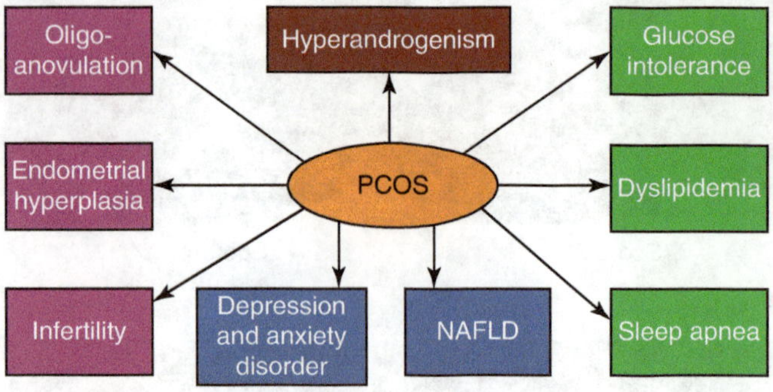

Fig. 6.4 Clinical components of PCOS. This figure illustrates the clinical features of PCOS that need to be carefully assessed and addressed. NAFLD refers to nonalcoholic fatty liver disease (Reprinted from Trikudanathan [21], with permission from Elsevier)

Increased risk of endometrial cancer: Women with PCOS have risk factors for endometrial cancer including obesity, metabolic abnormalities, and chronic oligo-anovulation resulting in prolonged exposure of the endometrium to unopposed estrogen. Therefore, it has been shown that women with PCOS that have oligomenorrhea can have a 2.7-fold increase in risk of developing endometrial cancer compared to the general population [8, 44] (see also Chap. 15 on Gynecologic Malignancies). Endometrial protection is a key focus of PCOS treatment (see below).

Infertility: Women with PCOS are at increased risk for infertility due to anovulatory cycles. They also have higher risk of preterm delivery, gestational diabetes, and preeclampsia [8].

Psychosocial issues: The prevalence of depression and anxiety is higher in women with PCOS than in the general population [45]. These symptoms may be even more pronounced in young adult women concerned with fertility but can affect women of all ages with respect to weight and body habitus and clinical signs of androgen excess [46, 47]. Figure 6.5 displays the effect of PCOS on women, at different stages of life.

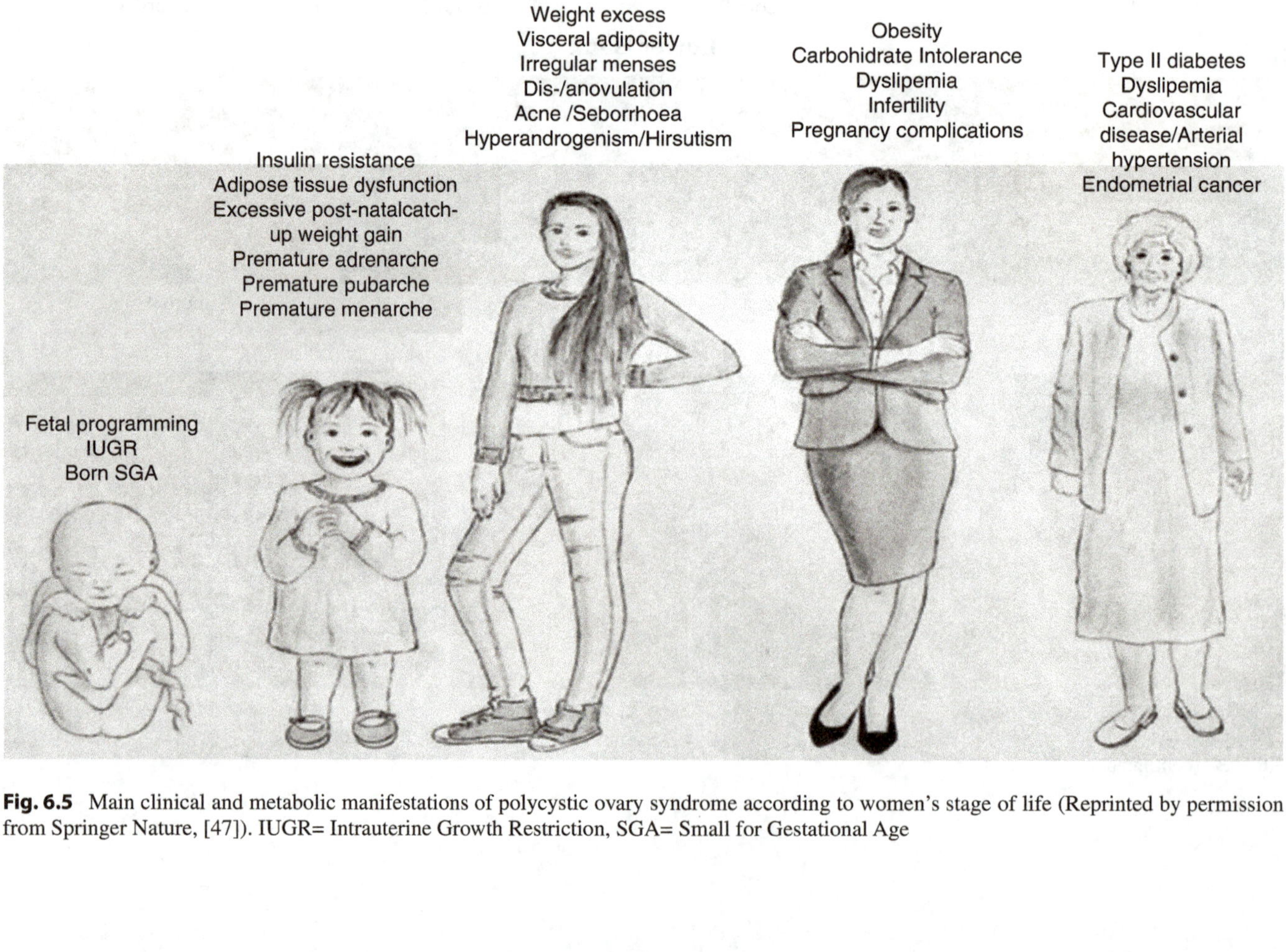

Fig. 6.5 Main clinical and metabolic manifestations of polycystic ovary syndrome according to women's stage of life (Reprinted by permission from Springer Nature, [47]). IUGR= Intrauterine Growth Restriction, SGA= Small for Gestational Age

Diagnostic Evaluation

It is essential to start with a detailed history and physical exam when evaluating a patient for PCOS. The history should include questions about (1) onset of menses and menstrual patterns; (2) hirsutism, specifically on the chin, jawline, chest, back, breasts, and stomach; (3) acne; (4) weight gain or the inability to lose weight; (5) the presence of galactorrhea; (6) behaviors and practices to offset symptoms such as plucking/waxing hair, acne treatments, excessive exercise/dieting, and taking medications that may mask or induce symptoms like hormones or steroids; and (7) family history, specifically regarding the presence of endocrinopathies, PCOS, cardiovascular disease, lipid disorders, and diabetes. The exam should focus on the skin looking for acne, alopecia, striae, and hirsutism; the presence of a goiter or thyroid nodule; adiposity; virilization which may result from an androgen-producing tumor; and the genitourinary tract, evaluating for clitoromegaly and uterine and ovarian abnormalities.

It is important to consider other possible diagnoses that can mimic PCOS and to evaluate for these conditions. For example, in women presenting with hyperandrogenism, consideration should be given to nonclassic congenital adrenal hyperplasia (NCCAH) and/or androgen-secreting tumors. For a woman with oligomenorrhea as her presenting feature, pregnancy, hypothyroidism, hyperprolactinemia, primary ovarian insufficiency, and Cushing syndrome should be considered (see Chap. 5 on Menstruation and Secondary Amenorrhea).

According to the 2003 Rotterdam criteria, a diagnosis of PCOS is made when two of the following are present: signs of hyperandrogenism, including clinical features like hirsutism or acne, or biochemical features such as elevated testosterone or DHEA-S; chronic ovulatory dysfunction; and/or the presence of polycystic ovaries on imaging, preferably on transvaginal ultrasound. Once the diagnosis of PCOS is secured, patients should be screened for diabetes, hyperlipidemia, and metabolic syndrome. Diabetes screening options include fasting blood glucose, hemoglobin A1c and 2-hour oral glucose tolerance test (OGTT). Hemoglobin A1c is often used instead of OGTT for patient convenience, though A1c alone may miss patients with isolated postprandial hyperglycemia. A fasting blood glucose or A1c may also underestimate the degree of insulin resistance for these patients. Screening every 3 years for those with normal results and annual screening for those with impaired results is recommended.

It is also important to note that assessments of free testosterone levels are more sensitive than the measurement of total testosterone for the diagnosis of hyperandrogenic disorders [1, 13, 21]. Table 6.3 provides an outline of the recommended evaluation for different features associated with PCOS.

Shazia had mild elevation of her testosterone and normal thyroid function tests, prolactin, and FSH. Her ultrasound did not have features of polycystic ovaries. She asks how best to manage her symptoms and if she is at risk of any other conditions—she read that PCOS can lead to infertility and endometrial cancer and is worried.

Table 6.3 Differential diagnosis and diagnostic evaluation by clinical feature of PCOS

Clinical feature	Differential diagnosis	Diagnostic evaluation
Ovulatory dysfunction	Pregnancy Thyroid disorders Hyperprolactinemia Primary ovarian insufficiency Cushing syndrome Structural gynecologic disease	Urine HCG TSH, free T4 Prolactin FSH, estradiol Salivary cortisols, 24-hour urine cortisol, dexamethasone suppression test Pelvic ultrasound Hysteroscopy
Hyperandrogenism	Nonclassic congenital adrenal hyperplasia (NCCAH) Androgen-secreting tumors	Morning 17-OH progesterone Testosterone, free and total DHEA-S
Metabolic complications: Obesity, insulin resistance, metabolic syndrome, dyslipidemia, hepatic steatosis	Thyroid disease Diabetes Physical inactivity and/or diet Primary lipid disorder Other familial disorders of metabolism	TSH, free T4 OGTT, A1c, and/or fasting glucose Liver function tests, lipid panel
Endometrial hyperplasia	Structural causes of AUB (polyps, adenomyosis, leiomyoma) Endometrial cancer	Transvaginal ultrasound Endometrial biopsy
Infertility	Includes all of the above conditions	Work-up for ovulatory dysfunction and/or hyperandrogenism Referral to fertility specialist for additional evaluation

PCOS Treatment

The goals of treatment for PCOS are to restore menses and/or ovulation, reduce hyperandrogenism, and/or reduce the risk of developing associated complications such as diabetes (Table 6.4). Treatment of PCOS should target the patient's most bothersome symptoms (i.e., hirsutism) and/or complications that can cause harm (i.e., anovulatory cycles, metabolic syndrome). Not all treatments recommended for PCOS will treat *all* complications of PCOS; therefore, patient and provider together must outline a management plan based on patient preferences, clinical manifestations, and medical comorbidities.

One key goal of PCOS treatment includes reducing insulin resistance. Weight loss, medications, and bariatric surgery are all employed to achieve this goal with improvement in ovulation and hyperandrogenemia as the final outcome [48]. A weight reduction of as little as 5% can restore ovulation in up to 60% of patients with PCOS [49]. The Endocrine Society Clinical Practice Guideline suggests the use of exercise therapy along with diet modification as first-line treatment to manage obesity in women with PCOS [50]. Based on studies on rodent models, it is suggested that early intervention with dietary restrictions and exercise in young adolescents with PCOS as well as in prepubertal children at risk of PCOS may improve metabolic, reproductive, and endocrine parameters. This improvement is caused by regulation of the neuropeptides in the hypothalamic-pituitary-gonadal axis [50, 51]. Pretreatment weight loss has also been studied as infertility treatment in PCOS. Pretreatment lifestyle modification and weight loss for 16 weeks, with or without concurrent oral contraceptive therapy, is associated with a significant improvement in the ovulation rate and an even greater increase in live birth rates as compared to immediate fertility treatment without lifestyle modification [49, 52].

The following sections will be organized by treatment modalities that target specific symptoms and manifestations of PCOS.

Menstrual Regulation and Endometrial Protection

Oral contraceptive pills (OCPs): OCPs are useful for women with oligomenorrhea, hirsutism, and acne and/or those who desire contraceptive benefit [53]. The most commonly used OCPs contain both estrogen and progestin, also known as combined oral contraceptive pills (COCs) (Table 6.4). The estrogen component increases sex hormone-binding globulin (SHBG), which binds testosterone and helps reduce hirsutism. One specific combination shown to have benefit in patients with PCOS includes both ethinyl estradiol and a low-androgenic progestin such as norgestimate; in general, any COC is fine. Patients need to be counseled that there is an increased risk of venous thromboembolism, along with potential increase in blood pressure, triglycerides, and HDL cholesterol levels [53] (see Chap. 4 on Patient-Centered Contraceptive Counseling).

Progestin therapy: Women may choose to take progestin-only therapy for endometrial protection. Examples include medroxyprogesterone acetate 5–10 mg or micronized progesterone 200 mg for 10–14 days monthly or continuous therapy with norethindrone 0.35 mg daily. The latter also provides contraception. Unlike COCs, progestin-only therapy will not reduce symptoms of acne or hirsutism as estrogen is required for SHBG to increase and subsequently bind testosterone.

Intrauterine device (IUD): COCs are recommended as first-line therapy given the multiple potential benefits described above. For women who cannot or choose not to take COCs, IUDs can provide endometrial protection and contraception for a woman with oligomenorrhea. While IUDs can be either hormonal (levonorgestrel-releasing) or nonhormonal, only the levonorgestrel-releasing hormone has endometrial protective effect. For primary care providers who do not place IUDs, referral to a gynecologist can facilitate IUD placement, particularly for patients who desire highly effective contraception.

Table 6.4 Specific therapies to address PCOS symptoms or complications

	Restore menses	Reduce hyperandrogenism	Improve metabolic syndrome	Reduce endometrial cancer risk	Improve fertility
Weight loss	√	√	√	√	√
Combined oral contraceptives	√	√		√	
Levonorgestrel IUD				√	
Metformin[a]	√		√		√
Spironolactone		√			
Topical acne medications or hair removal		√			
Clomiphene or letrozole					√

Adapted from McCartney and Marshall [48]
[a] May have modest (3%) impact on weight loss

Metformin: Metformin can be useful for women who do not want to take OCPs but have oligomenorrhea. Recall that insulin resistance and hyperinsulinemia are part of the pathophysiology of PCOS. By acting to improve insulin resistance, metformin can both impact patients' glucose metabolism and oligomenorrhea. A recent study found that metformin, at a dose of at least 1000 mg daily, restored menses in at least 42% of women within 6 months of treatment [58].

Metformin has been available for use for many years and has a mostly tolerable adverse effect profile. The most common adverse effect is GI distress such as bloating and diarrhea, which occasionally resolves after a few weeks of use. Metformin does not seem to have a significant effect on hirsutism, and it may increase pregnancy risk given its effect to restore menses and ovulation; patients who do not desire pregnancy require effective contraception.

Hyperandrogenism

Spironolactone: If a patient is bothered by hirsutism and acne, spironolactone, an anti-androgen, is an option. Spironolactone works by competing with dihydrotestosterone (DHT) for binding to the androgen receptor and inhibits enzymes involved in androgen biosynthesis. In general, it is recommended to start patients on a COC for 6 months, and if desired reduction in hirsutism is not attained, spironolactone can be started [50]. There is danger that a male fetus could be feminized by spironolactone therapy, so women desiring treatment with spironolactone also require adequate contraception. The typical effective dose is 50–100 mg twice daily and the clinical effect is dose-dependent. Despite these high doses, patients with normal blood pressure tend to tolerate spironolactone quite well. It is also important to be mindful that spironolactone could cause adverse effects including, but not limited to, hypotension, hyperkalemia, kidney injury, GI discomfort, and headache.

Other treatment options: In addition to COCs and spironolactone, topical agents can be used to treat bothersome acne. Commonly used topical therapies include, but are not limited to, benzoyl peroxide, retinoids, sulfone agents, and salicylic acid. Both oral and topical antibiotics are often used in conjunction with these therapies. Benzoyl peroxide is an antibacterial agent that kills *P. acnes* and is mildly comedolytic. Strengths available for acne treatment range from 2.5% to 10%. Topical retinoids are vitamin A derivatives and are both comedolytic and anti-inflammatory. Examples are tretinoin (0.025–0.1% in cream or gel), adapalene (0.1%, 0.3% cream or 0.1% lotion), and tazarotene (0.05%, 0.1% cream, gel, foam). The sulfone agent, dapsone 5% gel, is available as a twice-daily agent. It works primarily for inflammatory lesions. Combination with topical retinoids may be indicated if comedones are also present. Finally, salicylic acid is a comedolytic agent that is available over the counter in 0.5% to 2% strengths. If acne is treatment-resistant, scarring, or causing severe distress, oral isotretinoin may be appropriate, and referral to a dermatologist should be made [54].

Metabolic Complications

Weight loss and exercise can help to improve the metabolic profile in patients with PCOS. Metformin can be used for treatment of prediabetes and diabetes. Newer treatments such as liraglutide, a GLP-1 agonist, can help treat diabetes mellitus type 2 in women with PCOS while also mediating weight loss.

Infertility

It is important for women with PCOS to know that they are indeed fertile but that it may be more challenging to conceive due to anovulation. Some women with PCOS conceive naturally; when they do not, ovulation induction is possible with medical management and/or assisted reproduction techniques. As stated earlier, metformin can restore ovulation in some patients, but referral to a reproductive endocrinologist is encouraged if patients do not conceive after 6 months to 1 year of unprotected and frequent intercourse.

Clomiphene, a selective estrogen receptor modulator (SERM), and letrozole, an aromatase inhibitor (AI), have been studied for use in ovulation induction (Fig. 6.6). Both inhibit the negative feedback of estrogen at the hypothalamus with a consequent increase in ovarian stimulation by endogenous gonadotropin [55]. A randomized trial of ovulation induction involving women with PCOS and infertility showed a higher live-birth rate among women who received clomiphene than among women who received metformin

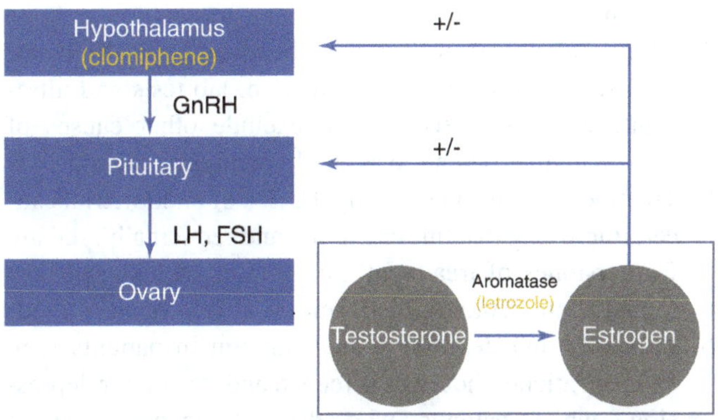

Fig. 6.6 Mechanisms of actions of clomiphene, a selective estrogen receptor modulator (SERM), and letrozole, an aromatase inhibitor

alone (22.5% vs. 7.2%). There was an even greater live-birth rate in the combination therapy group (26.8%) [56]. However, a subsequent randomized trial from 2014 compared clomiphene 50 mg daily to letrozole 2.5 mg daily and found more live births in the group that took letrozole (27.5% to 19.1%). There was also significantly more ovulation, conception, and pregnancy. This effect was most significantly seen in women with a BMI >30.3 to <=39.4 kg/m² [57].

Mental Health

As noted above, depression is more common in patients with PCOS than in those without. Patients with PCOS should be screened using common primary care depression screening tools like the PHQ-2 and PHQ-9. If positive, standard treatments should be offered (see Chap. 33 on Depressive and Anxiety Disorders).

Addressing patients' concerns in regard to their signs and symptoms of hirsutism, as well as providing appropriate counseling and timely referral to specialists when it comes to their concerns about fertility, can be important in managing patients with PCOS.

Summary Points

1. PCOS is a common disorder in women of childbearing age. It is important to ask about each woman's menstrual pattern and consider PCOS in women who report oligomenorrhea or other menstrual changes.
2. The main clinical features of PCOS are oligo-anovulation, androgen excess, and polycystic ovaries. Two of these three features are necessary to diagnose PCOS according to the currently used Rotterdam criteria.
3. PCOS can be associated with a spectrum of metabolic abnormalities such as impaired glucose tolerance and diabetes. Guidelines often recommend screening every 3 years. Those with abnormal test results should be screened annually.
4. While a diagnosis of PCOS can be made clinically based on history and physical examination, lab tests and ultrasound are often necessary to exclude other causes of oligo-anovulation and to assess hyperandrogenism.
5. Treatments focus on reducing the risk of endometrial cancer, improving insulin sensitivity, and reducing hirsutism. Cornerstones of treatment include weight loss and hormonal contraceptives; metformin is also frequently used.
6. Infertility and depression are common in patients with PCOS. Patients should be screened and treated for depression, while patients who do not conceive within 6–12 months should be promptly referred to a reproductive endocrinologist.

Review Questions

1. Jane is a 30-year-old woman who visits in your office for her annual exam. She has recently gained 15 pounds. Her BMI is now 29. One of her friends who had a recent weight gain was diagnosed with a condition called "polycystic ovarian syndrome" or (PCOS). She is worried that she also has this condition. Which of the following would be needed so that you can make the same diagnosis for her?
   A. Menstrual cycles between 24 and 28 days, mild acne, mildly elevated insulin levels
   B. Prolonged episodes of amenorrhea, A1c in 6 range, low normal FSH
   C. Menstrual cycles generally >35 days apart, increased hair growth under chin area, normal range A1c
   D. Transvaginal ultrasound showing enlarged ovaries with multiple cysts, normal testosterone level, and impaired glucose tolerance test

   The correct answer is C. Although most of the features described in the answer choices above can be associated with PCOS, the criteria for diagnosis require generally two out of the three characteristics of chronic oligo-anovulation, signs and symptoms of hyperandrogenism or hyperandrogenemia, and polycystic ovarian morphology on ultrasound [4, 6]. This is based on the most recent and agreed-upon criteria for diagnosis of PCOS (2012 extension of Rotterdam criteria) [7, 10]. Oligo-anovulatory cycles are generally defined as vaginal bleeding episodes occurring at greater than 35-day intervals or less than ten bleeds per year. A much smaller percentage of patients present with polymenorrhea, defined as bleeding episodes occurring frequently with less than 25 days between cycles [13, 27]. Hyperandrogenemia refers to higher than normal levels of circulating endogenous androgens, including testosterone (T), androstenedione (A4), and DHEA-S [13]. Clinical features of elevated androgens (known as hyperandrogenism) include hirsutism, acne, and androgenic alopecia [8, 13].

   Although PCOS can be associated with hyperinsulinemia and increased risk of diabetes (manifesting itself as elevation in A1C or abnormalities in the glucose tolerance test) [8, 39], these endocrine abnormalities are not a part of criteria for diagnosis of PCOS. FSH and other hormone levels are only used to rule out other endocrine abnormalities causing oligo-anovulatory pictures (i.e., primary ovarian insufficiency). They are not a part of criteria for diagnosis of PCOS.
2. Tina is 35 years old. She is in your office to discuss her new onset of amenorrhea for almost 6 months. She used to have cycles every 26–28 days. She has noticed new hair growth under her chin area; she is embarrassed to

go out with her friends. What are the best next steps in her care?

A. You explain to her that she is a typical case of a condition called “polycystic ovarian syndrome or PCOS” and you think since she makes two out of three Rotterdam criteria, no further work-up is necessary.
B. You explain to her that she is a typical case of a condition called PCOS, but to further confirm the diagnosis, you order a transvaginal ultrasound to assess her ovaries as well.
C. You explain to her that although you suspect that her symptoms can be suggestive of PCOS, however given new prolonged amenorrhea and new onset of hirsutism, you think further work-up including TSH, prolactin, FSH, and testosterone levels are necessary to rule out secondary causes of amenorrhea and testosterone-secreting ovarian tumors.
D. You explain to her that although you suspect that her symptoms can be suggestive of PCOS, however to further confirm the diagnosis, you need to order an insulin level and a glucose tolerance test.

The correct answer is C. Your patient seems to have two out of three criteria for PCOS based on the Rotterdam criteria (chronic anovulatory cycles based on her prolonged amenorrhea episode and hyperandrogenism manifesting itself as increased hair growth under her chin area) [7]. Meanwhile, generally when making the diagnosis of PCOS, one needs to rule out other causes of amenorrhea (especially a new onset of amenorrhea in this case). These can include but are not limited to hypothyroidism, hyperprolactinemia, primary ovarian insufficiency, and Cushing syndrome (please see Table 6.3 in the text). Also, given the new onset of signs of hyperandrogenism, androgen levels need to be checked. Mild elevation is expected in PCOS.

3. You make the diagnosis of PCOS for one of your patients Leslie, who had come to you with new onset of hair growth in her upper lip area, and finding of polycystic ovaries on her pelvic ultrasound for evaluation of intermittent heavy cycles. She informs you that she had been a biology major while she was in college and is particularly interested to understand the underlying mechanism for her syndrome. What are the cardinal features that contribute to the pathophysiology of polycystic ovary syndrome that are responsible for her symptoms?
   A. Functional ovarian hyperandrogenism is the cardinal feature in most patients and can be worsened by insulin-resistant hyperinsulinemia.
   B. Functional ovarian hyperandrogenism is the cardinal feature in most patients but is only seen in obese patients.
   C. Overproduction of androgens from the ovaries is mainly due to abnormalities of LH and FSH production from the pituitary.
   D. Overproduction of testosterone from ovaries is always the primary cause.

The correct answer is A. Functional ovarian hyperandrogenism is considered the cardinal feature leading to symptoms of PCOS [1]. Women with PCOS are suspected to have intrinsic abnormalities in the ovarian theca cells’ steroidogenesis which leads to hyperandrogenemia [21]. This hyper-responsiveness can increase androgen production and excess androgens can ultimately hinder ovulation [5]. Hyperinsulinemia plays a direct role on ovaries and enhances androgen production from theca cells in response to LH stimulus. Insulin resistance is common in both obese and lean women with PCOS.

LH and FSH production are mediated by GnRH secreted from the hypothalamus. GnRH is generally secreted in a pulsatile manner. At higher pulses, GnRH promotes the production of LH in the pituitary gland, while lower pulsation frequencies enhance the production of FSH. In women with PCOS, accelerated GnRH-LH pulsatile activity as well as decreased sensitivity of the hypothalamus to negative feedback from ovarian steroids leads to higher LH production [1, 48]. Higher LH pulses generally lead to higher production of ovarian androgens. That being said, the ovarian androgen production abnormalities are considered largely an inherent characteristic of the ovaries in patients with PCOS. In a smaller number of PCOS cases, dysregulation at the adrenal zona reticularis causes hyperandrogenism by increased production of DHEA [1].

4. Eleanor is a 35-year-old female patient presenting with a 6-month history of amenorrhea. You have confirmed she is not pregnant. Her TSH, prolactin, and FSH levels are normal. She has mild hirsutism and her testosterone levels are in the 40 range. At this point you make the diagnosis of PCOS for her. What are some of the concerns that you make sure you should address with her?
   A. You counsel her for weight loss, but given she has no family history of diabetes, you don’t feel it is necessary to check her for metabolic abnormalities.
   B. You assess her family planning goals, and if she is not planning to get pregnant, you start her only on a norgestimate containing birth control.
   C. Given her hirsutism is mild, there is no indication for her to get started on any specific treatment.
   D. You screen her for depressive symptoms and you refer her to specialist as indicated.

The correct answer is D. The cornerstones of treatment in patients with PCOS are weight loss, protection of the endometrium against prolonged unopposed exposure to estrogen (which can increase the risk of future endometrial cancer), screening and treatment for metabolic abnormalities such as diabetes and hypercholesterolemia, treating hirsutism or other signs of hyperandrogenism (based on patient's preferences), treatments to address infertility and/or to increase chance of ovulation, and screening and providing appropriate treatments for depression and other psychosocial conditions associated with PCOS [49, 50, 53–55]. When addressing endometrial protection, all the different contraceptive options are potentially acceptable treatments. The choice depends on the patients' comorbid conditions, as well as their personal preferences. Treatment for signs of hyperandrogenism largely depends on patients' preferences and can be offered at any stage of hirsutism. Screening patients for depression and other psychosocial consequences is an important part of evaluation and treatment of patients with PCOS and can also include referral to behavioral health specialists.

5. Rose, a patient that you recently diagnosed with PCOS, returns to your office 6 months after her initial visit and states that she is interested in getting pregnant. What available treatments for ovulation induction could you recommend?
   A. Metformin only
   B. Metformin and clomiphene
   C. Clomiphene and letrozole
   D. Metformin, clomiphene, and letrozole

   The correct answer is D. Metformin, clomiphene, and letrozole are all acceptable treatments for ovulation induction and treatment of infertility in PCOS patients. The choice of medication can depend on how long the couple has been trying to get pregnant, patient's age, BMI, and personal preferences. Trials have suggested higher rates of pregnancy and live births with addition of clomiphene compared to metformin alone [55, 56]. Another study found that letrozole was associated with higher live birth and ovulation rates compared with clomiphene [55, 57]. In general, if the patient is not able to conceive after 6–12 months of unprotected and frequent intercourse and other treatments directed toward increased chance of ovulation (weight loss, metformin), referral to an infertility specialist is recommended.

References

1. Rosenfield R, Ehrmann D. The pathogenesis of polycystic ovary syndrome (PCOS): the hypothesis of PCOS as functional ovarian hyperandrogenism revisited. Endocr Rev. 2016;37(5):467–520.
2. Carvalho L, Ferreira C, Sóter M, Sales M, Rodrigues K, Martins S, et al. Microparticles: inflammatory and haemostatic biomarkers in polycystic ovary syndrome. Mol Cell Endocrinol. 2017;443:155–62.
3. Palomba S, Santagni S, Falbo A, La Sala G. Complications and challenges associated with polycystic ovary syndrome: current perspectives. Int J Women's Health. 2015;7:745–63.
4. Lauritsen M, Bentzen J, Pinborg A, Loft A, Forman J, Thuesen L, et al. The prevalence of polycystic ovary syndrome in a normal population according to the Rotterdam criteria versus revised criteria including anti-Mullerian hormone. Hum Reprod. 2014;29(4):791–801.
5. Baskind N, Balen A. Hypothalamic–pituitary, ovarian and adrenal contributions to polycystic ovary syndrome. Best Pract Res Clin Obstet Gynaecol. 2016;37:80–97.
6. Stein IF, Leventhal ML. Amenorrhea associated with bilateral polycystic ovaries. Am J Obstet Gynecol. 1935;29(2):181–91.
7. Lizneva D, Suturina L, Walker W, Brakta S, Gavrilova-Jordan L, Azziz R. Criteria, prevalence, and phenotypes of polycystic ovary syndrome. Fertil Steril. 2016;106(1):6–15.
8. Dumesic D, Oberfield S, Stener-Victorin E, Marshall J, Laven J, Legro R. Scientific statement on the diagnostic criteria, epidemiology, pathophysiology, and molecular genetics of polycystic ovary syndrome. Endocr Rev. 2015;36(5):487–525.
9. Zawadzki JK, Dunaif A. Diagnostic criteria for polycystic ovary syndrome; towards a rational approach. In: Dunaif A, Givens JR, Haseltine F, Merriam G, editors. Polycystic ovary syndrome. Boston: Blackwell Scientific; 1992.
10. Rotterdam ESHRE/ASRM-Sponsored PCOS Consensus Workshop Group. Revised 2003 consensus on diagnostic criteria and long-term health risks related to polycystic ovary syndrome. Fertil Steril. 2004;81(1):19–25.
11. National Institutes of Health. Evidence-based methodology workshop on polycystic ovary syndrome, December 3–5, 2012. Executive summary. Available at: https://prevention.nih.gov/docs/programs/pcos/FinalReport.pdf. Accessed March 1, 2016.
12. Georgopoulos NA, Papadakis E, Armeni AK, Katsikis I, Roupas ND, Panidis D. Elevated serum androstenedione is associated with a more severe phenotype in women with polycystic ovary syndrome (PCOS). Hormones. 2014;13(2):213–21.
13. Azziz R, Carmina E, Dewailly D, Diamanti-Kandarakis E, Escobar-Morreale HF, Futterweit W, et al. The Androgen Excess and PCOS Society criteria for the polycystic ovary syndrome: the complete task force report. Fertil Steril. 2009;91(2):456–88.
14. Kim J, Hwang K, Choi Y, Moon S, Chae S, Park C, et al. Complete phenotypic and metabolic profiles of a large consecutive cohort of untreated Korean women with polycystic ovary syndrome. Fertil Steril. 2014;101(5):1424–30.e3.
15. Panidis D, Tziomalos K, Papadakis E, Chatzis P, Kandaraki E, Tsourdi E, et al. Associations of menstrual cycle irregularities with age, obesity and phenotype in patients with polycystic ovary syndrome. Hormones. 2015;14:431–7.
16. Diamanti-Kandarakis E, Panidis D. Unravelling the phenotypic map of polycystic ovary syndrome (PCOS): a prospective study of 634 women with PCOS. Clin Endocrinol. 2007;67(5):735–42.
17. Moran L, Teede H. Metabolic features of the reproductive phenotypes of polycystic ovary syndrome. Hum Reprod Update. 2009;15(4):477–88.
18. Rizzo M, Berneis K, Hersberger M, Pepe I, Di Fede G, Rini G, et al. Milder forms of atherogenic dyslipidemia in ovulatory versus anovulatory polycystic ovary syndrome phenotype. Hum Reprod. 2009;24(9):2286–92.
19. Guastella E, Longo R, Carmina E. Clinical and endocrine characteristics of the main polycystic ovary syndrome phenotypes. Fertil Steril. 2010;94(6):2197–201.
20. Goverde A, van Koert A, Eijkemans M, Knauff E, Westerveld H, Fauser B, et al. Indicators for metabolic disturbances in anovulatory women with polycystic ovary syndrome diagnosed according to the Rotterdam consensus criteria. Hum Reprod. 2008;24(3):710–7.
21. Trikudanathan S. Polycystic ovarian syndrome. Med Clin North Am. 2015;99(1):221–35.
22. Jakimiuk A. Aromatase mRNA expression in individual follicles from polycystic ovaries. Mol Hum Reprod. 1998;4(1):1–8.
23. Balen A. The pathophysiology of polycystic ovary syndrome: trying to understand PCOS and its endocrinology. Best Pract Res Clin Obstet Gynaecol. 2004;18(5):685–706.

24. Williamson K, Gunn AJ, Johnson N, Milsom SR. The impact of ethnicity on the presentation of polycystic ovarian syndrome. Aust N Z J Obstet Gynaecol. 2001;41(2):202–6.
25. Glueck CJ, Papanna R, Wang P, Goldenberg N, Sieve-Smith L. Incidence and treatment of metabolic syndrome in newly referred women with confirmed polycystic ovarian syndrome. Metab Clin Exp. 2003;52(7):908–15.
26. Chang WY, Knochenhauer ES, Bartolucci AA, Azziz R. Phenotypic spectrum of polycystic ovary syndrome: clinical and biochemical characterization of the three major clinical subgroups. Fertil Steril. 2005;83(6):1717–23.
27. Azziz R, Sanchez LA, Knochenhauer ES, Moran C, Lazenby J, Stephens KC, et al. Androgen excess in women: experience with over 1000 consecutive patients. J Clin Endocrinol Metab. 2004;89(2):453–62.
28. Carmina E, Lobo RA. Do hyperandrogenic women with normal menses have polycystic ovary syndrome? Fertil Steril. 1999;71(2):319–22.
29. Ferriman D, Gallwey JD. Clinical assessment of body hair growth in women. J Clin Endocrinol Metab. 1961;21(11):1440–7.149.
30. Hatch R, Rosenfield RL, Kim MH, Tredway D. Hirsutism: implications, etiology, and management. Am J Obstet Gynecol. 1981;140:815–30.
31. Yildiz B, Bolour S, Woods K, Moore A, Azziz R. Visually scoring hirsutism. Hum Reprod Update. 2009;16(1):51–64.
32. O'Driscoll JB, Mamtora H, Higginson J, Pollock A, Kane J, Anderson DC. A prospective study of the prevalence of clear-cut endocrine disorders and polycystic ovaries in 350 patients presenting with hirsutism or androgenic alopecia. Clin Endocrinol. 1994;41(2):231–6.
33. Ludwig E. Classification of the types of androgenetic alopecia (common baldness) occurring in the female sex. Br J Dermatol. 1977;97(3):247–54.
34. Quinn M, Shinkai K, Pasch L, Kuzmich L, Cedars M, Huddleston H. Prevalence of androgenic alopecia in patients with polycystic ovary syndrome and characterization of associated clinical and biochemical features. Fertil Steril. 2014;101(4):1129–34.
35. Jonard S, Robert Y, Cortet-Rudelli C, Pigny P, Decanter C, Dewailly D. Ultrasound examination of polycystic ovaries: is it worth counting the follicles? Hum Reprod. 2003;18(3):598–603.
36. Adams J, Polson DW, Franks S. Prevalence of polycystic ovaries in women with anovulation and idiopathic hirsutism. Br Med J. 1986;293(6543):355–9.
37. Carmina E, Orio F, Palomba S, Longo RA, Lombardi G, Lobo RA. Ovarian size and blood flow in women with polycystic ovary syndrome and their correlations with endocrine parameters. Fertil Steril. 2005;84(2):413–9.
38. Tehrani F, Simbar M, Tohidi M, Hosseinpanah F, Azizi F. The prevalence of polycystic ovary syndrome in a community sample of Iranian population: Iranian PCOS prevalence study. Reprod Biol Endocrinol. 2011;9(1):39.
39. Boudreaux MY, Talbott EO, Kip KE, Brooks MM, Witchel SF. Risk of T2DM and impaired fasting glucose among PCOS subjects: results of an 8-year follow-up. Curr Diab Rep. 2006;6(1):77–83.
40. Valkenburg O, Steegers-Theunissen RP, Smedts HP, et al. A more atherogenic serum lipoprotein profile is present in women with polycystic ovary syndrome: a case-control study. J Clin Endocrinol Metab. 2008;93(2):470–6.
41. Wild RA, Carmina E, Diamanti-Kandarakis E, et al. Assessment of cardiovascular risk and prevention of cardiovascular disease in women with the polycystic ovary syndrome: a consensus statement by the Androgen Excess and Polycystic Ovary Syndrome (AE-PCOS) Society. J Clin Endocrinol Metab. 2010;95(5):2038–49.
42. Valkenburg O, Steegers-Theunissen R, Smedts H, Dallinga-Thie G, Fauser B, Westerveld E, et al. A more atherogenic serum lipoprotein profile is present in women with polycystic ovary syndrome: a case-control study. J Clin Endocrinol Metab. 2008;93(2):470–6.
43. Dokras A, Bochner M, Hollinrake E, Markham S, Vanvoorhis B, Jagasia DH. Screening women with polycystic ovary syndrome for metabolic syndrome. Obstet Gynecol. 2005;106(1):131–7.
44. Haoula Z, Salman M, Atiomo W. Evaluating the association between endometrial cancer and polycystic ovary syndrome. Hum Reprod. 2012;27(5):1327–31.
45. Cooney L, Lee I, Sammel M, Dokras A. High prevalence of moderate and severe depressive and anxiety symptoms in polycystic ovary syndrome: a systematic review and meta-analysis. Hum Reprod. 2017;32(5):1075–91.
46. Elsenbruch S, Hahn S, Kowalsky D, Öffner A, Schedlowski M, Mann K, et al. Quality of life, psychosocial well-being, and sexual satisfaction in women with polycystic ovary syndrome. J Clin Endocrinol Metab. 2003;88(12):5801–7.
47. Bellver J, Rodríguez-Tabernero L, Robles A, Muñoz E, Martínez F, Landeras J, et al. Polycystic ovary syndrome throughout a woman's life. J Assist Reprod Genet. 2018;35(1):25–39.
48. McCartney CR, Marshall JC. Clinical practice. Polycystic ovary syndrome. N Engl J Med. 2016;375(1):54–64.
49. Palomba S. Infertility in women with polycystic ovary syndrome: pathogenesis and management. Cham: Springer; 2018.
50. Legro R, Arslanian S, Ehrmann D, Hoeger K, Murad M, Pasquali R, et al. Diagnosis and treatment of polycystic ovary syndrome: an Endocrine Society clinical practice guideline. J Clin Endocrinol Metab. 2013;98(12):4565–92.
51. Diane A, Kupreeva M, Borthwick F, Proctor S, Pierce W, Vine D. Cardiometabolic and reproductive benefits of early dietary energy restriction and voluntary exercise in an obese PCOS-prone rodent model. J Endocrinol. 2015;226(3):193–206.
52. Legro R, Dodson W, Kunselman A, Stetter C, Kris-Etherton P, Williams N, et al. Benefit of delayed fertility therapy with preconception weight loss over immediate therapy in obese women with PCOS. J Clin Endocrinol Metab. 2016;101(7):2658–66.
53. Dokras A. Noncontraceptive use of oral combined hormonal contraceptives in polycystic ovary syndrome—risks versus benefits. Fertil Steril. 2016;106(7):1572–9.
54. Descamps V. Clinical guidelines for management of acne vulgaris. JAMA. 2017;317(2):213.
55. Legro R. Ovulation induction in polycystic ovary syndrome: current options. Best Pract Res Clin Obstet Gynaecol. 2016;37:152–9.
56. Legro RS, et al. "Clomiphene, metformin, or both for infertility in the polycystic ovary syndrome." N Engl J Med. 2007;356(6):551–6.
57. Legro RS, et al. "Letrozole versus clomiphene for infertility in the polycystic ovary syndrome." N Engl J Med. 2014;371(2):119–29.
58. Yang P-K, Hsu C-Y, Chen M-J, et al. The efficacy of 24-month metformin for improving menses, hormones, and metabolic profiles in polycystic ovary syndrome. J Clin Endocrinol Metab. 2018;103(3):890–9.

Abnormal Uterine Bleeding

7

Raj Narayan and Benjamin D. Beran

Learning Objectives

1. Discuss the burden of abnormal uterine bleeding (AUB).
2. Define current terminology used to describe AUB including heavy menstrual bleeding and intermenstrual bleeding.
3. Compare the clinical presentations of abnormal uterine bleeding across the lifespan.
4. Describe the steps used to evaluate AUB.
5. Identify indications for treatment and referral to gynecologists when managing AUB and postmenopausal bleeding.

Background

Tamara is a 46-year-old woman, G3P3003, who presents for an episode of heavy vaginal bleeding. She has been changing an overnight pad every 2 to 3 hours for 2 to 3 days during her last three regular menstrual periods. She reports frustration with her symptoms; she has a long flight next week and is worried the bleeding will worsen while she is traveling.

Abnormal uterine bleeding (AUB) is one of the most common presenting complaints of reproductive age women and results in a third of all outpatient gynecologic visits [1]. Studies have shown that AUB significantly decreases quality of life for women aged 18–54 years; women with AUB scored below the 25th percentile of national norms on six of the eight subscales in the validated quality of life assessment: the SF-36 scale [2]. Further, AUB is associated with sexual dysfunction [3, 4], psychological effects [3, 5, 6], and decreased quality of life in the domains of social, professional, and family life [3, 7]. Sexual function assessed by the Medical Outcomes Study Sexual Problems Index showed that women who failed medical management of AUB scored well below the typical age-adjusted mean [4]. Given the degree to which AUB impacts women's quality of life, many argue that the main outcome measure to determine effectiveness of any intervention should be improvement in quality of life rather than merely the actual blood loss [8]. Additionally, the annual direct cost to society (in the United States) associated with heavy menstrual bleeding is estimated to be as high as $1.55 billion with annual indirect costs as high as $36 billion [2].

Table 7.1 Parameters of normal and abnormal uterine bleeding [11].

Descriptive term	Definition
Irregular menstrual bleeding	>20 days in individual cycle lengths in a year
Absent menstrual bleeding	No bleeding in a 90-day period
Infrequent menstrual bleeding	≤2 episodes in a 90-day period
Frequent menstrual bleeding	>4 episodes in a 90-day period
Prolonged menstrual bleeding	>8 days in duration on a regular basis
Shortened menstrual bleeding	≤2 days in duration

Adapted from Fraser et al. [11]

AUB refers to uterine bleeding patterns that differ from normal, established patterns (Table 7.1) or which negatively impact a patient's quality of life [8]. The FIGO Menstrual Disorders Working Group further divides AUB into two categories: acute and chronic. Acute AUB is a clinical diagnosis based on a perceived need for immediate intervention in the setting of an episode of heavy menstrual bleeding. Chronic AUB is defined by the FIGO Menstrual Disorders Working Group as "bleeding from the uterine corpus that is abnormal in volume, regularity, and/or timing that has been present for the majority of the last 6 months" [9].

R. Narayan (✉) · B. D. Beran
Froedtert & Medical College of Wisconsin, Department of Obstetrics and Gynecology, Wauwatosa, WI, USA
e-mail: rnarayan@mcw.edu

S. A. Tilstra et al. (eds.), *Sex- and Gender-Based Women's Health*, https://doi.org/10.1007/978-3-030-50695-7_7

PALM		COEIN
Polyp		Coagulopathy
Adenomyosis		Ovulatory dysfunction
Leiomyomas →	Submucous / Other	Endometrial
Malignancy & hyperplasia		Iatrogenic
		Not otherwise classified

Leiomyomas subclassification system

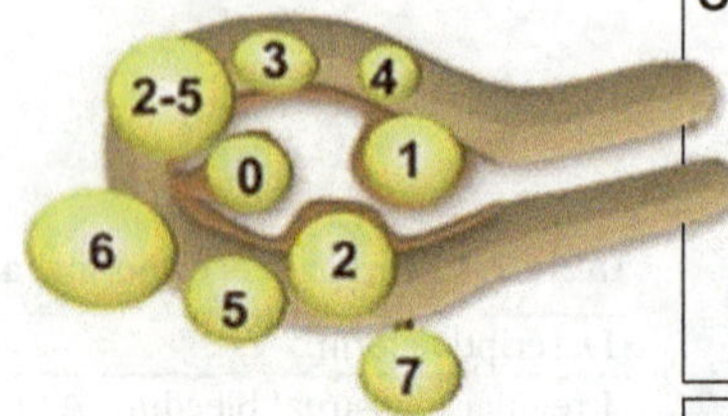

SM - Submucous	0	Pedunculated intracavitary
	1	<50% intramural
	2	≥50% intramural
O - Other	3	Contacts endometrium; 100% intramural
	4	Intramural
	5	Subserous ≥50% intramural
	6	Subserous <50% intramural
	7	Subserous pedunculated
	8	other (specify e.g. cervical, parasitic)
Hybrid leiomyomas (impact both endometrium and serosa)		Two numbers are listed separated by a hyphen, By convention, the first refers to the relationship with the endometrium while the second refers to the relationship to the serosa. One example is below
	2-5	Submucous and subserous, each with less than half the diameter in the endometrial and peritoneal cavities, respectively.

Fig. 7.1 PALM-COEIN classification of abnormal uterine bleeding [13]. (Reprinted from Best Practice and Research Clinical Obstetrics and Gynaecology, Munro [13], © 2017, with permission from Elsevier)

Traditional descriptions of patterns of abnormal uterine bleeding are based on abnormal frequency, duration, and quantity of flow and include such terms as menorrhagia, metrorrhagia, menometrorrhagia, hypermenorrhea, hypomenorrhea, polymenorrhea, polymenorrhagia, epimenorrhea, epimenorrhagia, metropathia hemorrhagica, dysfunctional uterine hemorrhage, and functional uterine hemorrhage [10]. However, these terms are often subjective, and studies have shown that these descriptions are inaccurate [11]. Instead, terms such as abnormal uterine bleeding (AUB), heavy menstrual bleeding (HMB), prolonged menstrual bleeding (PMB), heavy and prolonged menstrual bleeding (HPMB), and intermenstrual bleeding (IMB) are recommended to describe specific symptoms [11].

Notably, AUB refers to women who are premenopausal; any bleeding in women who are postmenopausal is abnormal and requires prompt evaluation (see section below and Chap. 15 on Gynecologic Malignancies).

Classification of Causes of Abnormal Uterine Bleeding (PALM-COEIN)

In 2011, the FIGO Working Group on Menstrual Disorders proposed a new classification system for causes of abnormal uterine bleeding [12, 13]. In this system, the causes of AUB are broadly divided into structural causes and nonstructural causes. The acronym PALM-COEIN was created to aid memory and recall (Fig. 7.1) [13–15].

Leiomyomas, which patients commonly refer to as fibroids, are further classified because of their high prevalence. Subserous fibroids typically cause pressure symptoms when they are large but do not lead to menstrual abnormalities. Intramural and submucous fibroids often cause heavy menstrual bleeding. Submucosal fibroids which protrude into the cavity of the uterus cause intermenstrual or irregular bleeding. The diagnoses are not mutually exclusive. Many women will have incidental structural findings with nonstructural causes of abnormal uterine bleeding. This is particularly true of leiomyomas that often coexist with other conditions such as endometrial hyperplasia, cancer, or polyps.

> *Tamara reports that she had normal periods until age 44. Since then, her periods have been irregular, occurring every 1–3 months. She endorses intermittent hot flashes at night.*

Pathophysiology

Normal Menstrual Cycle

The normal menstrual cycle relies on a complex and intricate relationship between the hypothalamus, pituitary gland, ovaries, and uterus. Hormonal signals are sent bidirectionally from the hypothalamus and pituitary gland to the ovaries, some with agonistic effects and others with antagonistic effects. When all feedback loops function properly, the menstrual cycle occurs in a predictable nature every 24–35 days [16]. The cycle is typically divided into three phases: follicular, ovulatory, and luteal (see also Chap. 5 Menstruation and Secondary Amenorrhea, Fig. 5.2).

Follicular Phase

The follicular phase represents the initial 10–14 days of the normal menstrual cycle. During this phase, a dominant follicle is recruited for ovulation from a pool of antral follicles. Follicle-stimulating hormone (FSH) from the pituitary gland stimulates estrogen production in ovarian granulosa cells, which in turn inhibits further FSH secretion. The dominant follicle survives the decreasing FSH levels as local effects of estradiol enhance FSH action for this follicle selected for ovulation. The continued rise in estradiol stimulates endometrial proliferation and eventually leads to a surge in release of luteinizing hormone (LH) from the pituitary gland [16].

Ovulatory Phase

The ovulatory phase is a brief phase occurring at the end of the follicular phase, typically during the 10th–14th day of the menstrual cycle. The beginning of the LH surge precedes ovulation by approximately 34–36 hours [10]. LH stimulates progesterone production in the granulosa and theca cells, which facilitates ovulation of a mature oocyte.

Luteal Phase

While the follicular phase is dominated by estrogen production, the luteal phase is dominated by progesterone secretion produced by the corpus luteum, a temporary endocrine tissue from the remnant of the dominant ovulatory follicle. Progesterone promotes a transition to a secretory endometrium [16] in preparation for possible implantation of a fertilized embryo. In the absence of a pregnancy, the luteal phase is consistently 14 ± 1 days in length following ovulation [16]. In the absence of human chorionic gonadotropin (hCG) from a pregnancy, the corpus luteum undergoes attrition, and levels of progesterone and estradiol fall. This withdrawal of progesterone and estradiol leads to shedding of the endometrium and resultant menstrual bleeding. The first day of bleeding represents the first day of the follicular phase of a new menstrual cycle. The normal length of bleeding is 4.5–7 days with a majority of the menstrual blood flow occurring in the first 3 days [16].

Menstrual Bleeding and Endometrial Hemostasis

Just as prostaglandins and hemostatic factors such as platelet aggregation and thrombus formation are critical to bleeding and hemostatic processes throughout the body, these factors also play a role in menstrual bleeding patterns and endometrial hemostasis. Endometrial prostaglandin production plays a significant role in endometrial shedding and regeneration [17, 18]. Activity of COX-2, an enzyme essential in prostaglandin synthesis, is elevated in the endometrium of women with heavy menstrual bleeding providing evidence of increased inflammation and prostaglandin activity in women with heavy menstrual bleeding [19].

Endometrial hemostasis facilitates the end of menstrual bleeding and is achieved through the effects of local endocrine, immunological, and hemostatic factors. Tissue factor and thrombin control menstrual bleeding via the activation of coagulation factors, while fibrinolysis prevents clot organization within the uterine cavity. Plasminogen activator inhibitors and fibrinolysis inhibitors that control plasminogen activators and plasmin activity maintain this balance [20]. Platelet aggregation, fibrin deposition, and thrombus formation occur in sequence. Abnormalities of uterine bleeding can result from imbalance of the hemostatic factors.

A systematic review [21] found no variation in von Willebrand factor (VWF), factor VIII, factor XI, factor XIII, fibrinolytic factors, or fibrinogen levels throughout the menstrual cycle in most of the studies. However, in studies where cyclic variation was noted, the lowest levels occurred during the menstrual and early follicular phases, especially for VWF, factor VIII, and platelet function tests. Given these findings, menstruation and the early follicular phase are the optimal times to pursue hemostatic testing (see Laboratory Testing, below) [21].

Abnormal Uterine Bleeding: Structural Causes -(PALM)

Tamara stopped using combined hormonal contraception at age 35 after tubal sterilization. She had a normal, HPV negative Pap smear 2 years ago. There is no history of breast, endometrial, or ovarian cancer in her family.

The FIGO classification system of AUB, "PALM-COEIN," relegates structural causes of AUB to the initial portion, "PALM." Polyps, adenomyosis, leiomyomas, and malignancy are considered structural etiologies and require visualization with imaging or histopathology for diagnosis [14].

Polyps

Endometrial and endocervical polyps are epithelial proliferations comprised of glandular, vascular, fibromuscular, and connective tissue [14, 22]. Prevalence of polyps is unknown since the majority are asymptomatic. However, in a Danish population study, when 622 randomly selected women were evaluated using ultrasound and sonohysterography, 7.8% had polyps, and the prevalence rose from 0.9% in 20–29-year age group to 9.3% in ≥30-year age group and from 5.8% in premenopausal to 11.8% in postmenopausal women [23]. Polyps may demonstrate fewer hormone receptors than typical endometrium, making them less responsive to the cyclic changes of the menstrual cycle [24]. Some polyps protrude from the cervical os and are visible on physical exam with a speculum. In other cases, polyps are diagnosed with transvaginal ultrasonography (especially saline-infusion sonography), hysteroscopy, or endometrial biopsy. Polyps frequently coexist with submucosal leiomyomas; they may also be misdiagnosed as submucosal leiomyomas on ultrasound [22]. Endometrial and endocervical polyps are usually benign, but a minority of polyps may have atypical or malignant cells [14]. For this reason, polyps are often removed and sent to pathology for diagnosis [24].

Adenomyosis

One of the best descriptions of adenomyosis dates back to 1972: "adenomyosis may be defined as the benign invasion of endometrium into the myometrium, producing a diffusely enlarged uterus which microscopically exhibits ectopic non-neoplastic, endometrial glands and stroma surrounded by the hypertrophic and hyperplastic myometrium" [25]. This often leads to painful heavy menstrual bleeding, though adenomyosis may also be asymptomatic [26]. Reported risk factors for the development of adenomyosis include multiparity and uterine procedures such as endometrial curettage, termination of pregnancy, or cesarean delivery [26]. Many studies report a 20–35% population prevalence, with some reports suggesting a range of 5– 70% [14, 26]. Patients with adenomyosis often report painful or heavy, regular menstrual bleeding. However, clinical symptoms are neither sensitive nor specific [26]. Adenomyosis may be focal or diffuse. Diagnosis can be made with ultrasonography or magnetic resonance imaging (MRI), although diagnostic criteria may vary [26, 27]. Histologic diagnosis is usually made only after removal of the uterus; endometrial biopsy is not useful [14, 22, 26].

Leiomyoma

Leiomyomas (also known as "myomas" and "fibroids") of the uterus are benign fibromuscular tumors, with each lesion arising from a single smooth muscle cell [14, 28]. Nearly 70% of Caucasian women and 80% of African-American women develop leiomyoma by age 50 [14, 28, 29]. While highly prevalent, only 20–50% of women develop AUB as a result of the leiomyoma [14, 30]. Given that the location of a leiomyoma frequently determines a patient's symptoms, a secondary classification system requires evaluating the relationship of the leiomyoma to the endometrium, myometrium, and uterine serosa [14, 29]. Submucosal leiomyomas. contact or deviate the endometrium and are most likely to cause AUB regardless of size [14, 29]. The initial leiomyoma diagnosis can be made by ultrasonography or MRI. When needed, clarification of submucosal location can be performed using saline-infusion sonography, MRI, or hysteroscopy [14, 27]. Gynecologists planning myomectomy, uterine fibroid embolization, or ablation often obtain MRI for surgical planning; primary care providers will usually defer ordering MR imaging to colleagues in gynecology.

Malignancy and Premalignant Lesions

Malignancies that lead to abnormal uterine bleeding include cervical cancer, endometrial cancer, and sarcomas, while ovarian cancer rarely presents with AUB [22, 31]. The main risk factor for cervical cancer development is human papillomavirus (HPV) infection acquired via sexual activity (Chap. 14 on Cervical Cancer and Human Papillomavirus) [32]. Endometrial hyperplasia is more common than uterine cancer, and the WHO 2015 classification separates this diagnosis into two groups: hyperplasia without atypia and atypical hyperplasia/endometrial intraepithelial neoplasia [33]. Unopposed estrogen exposure leads to higher risk for most common types of endometrial cancer. Conditions with chronic anovulation such as polycystic ovary syndrome (PCOS), obesity, or improper administration of exogenous hormonal therapy are some sources of unopposed estrogen [34]. Uterine sarcomas are rare with risk factors such as increasing age, long-term use of tamoxifen, and previous pelvic radiation [22]. No imaging technique alone can diagnose these conditions definitively, though ultrasound or MRI may be pursued when there is a high clinical suspicion [22]. Endometrial biopsy, endometrial curettage, or hysterectomy allow a definitive tissue diagnosis [22, 35]. See Chap. 15 on Gynecologic Malignancies for more information.

Nonstructural Causes of AUB-COEIN

Coagulopathy

As many as 13% of women affected by AUB may have a coagulopathy, the most common of which is von Willebrand disease (vWD) [14, 22]. Most coagulopathies are inherited, and other examples include hemophilia type A (factor VIII deficiency) and type B (factor IX deficiency), platelet dysfunction, and various other factor deficiencies [36]. A detailed history will accurately identify up to 90% of women with coagulopathies. Evaluation for coagulopathy is indicated if there is a positive history (Fig. 7.2) [37].

Ovulatory Disorders

Failure of ovulation contributes to AUB through prolonged endometrial proliferation, and the lack of progesterone leads to instability of the endometrium and causes irregular ripening and shedding of the endometrium. This leads to unpredictable erratic bleeding [12, 14, 22, 35, 37, 38]. This is a common occurrence in the first 2–3 years following menarche because the hypothalamic-pituitary-ovarian (HPO) axis is immature and is also common in the perimenopausal years – up to 8 years preceding menopause [36].

Numerous endocrinopathies also contribute to ovulatory dysfunction including polycystic ovary syndrome (see Chap. 6 on Polycystic Ovary Syndrome), uncontrolled diabetes mellitus, and thyroid dysfunction [12, 14, 22, 35]. Additional risk factors for abnormal uterine bleeding include obesity, anorexia, weight loss, mental stress, and extreme levels of exercise [14, 22]. Diagnosis of ovulatory dysfunction should be suspected with a history of amenorrhea or when menstrual cycles are spaced more than 38 days apart (see Chap. 5 on Menstruation and Secondary Amenorrhea) [14, 22, 35].

1. Structured history— positive screen if:
   a. Excessive menstrual bleeding since menarche, or
   b. History of one of the following—postpartum hemorrhage, surgery-related bleeding, or bleeding associated with dental work, or
   c. History of two or more of the following— bruising greater than 5 cm once or twice/ month, epistaxis once or twice/month, frequent gum bleeding, family history of bleeding symptoms.
2. Initial laboratory evaluation: Complete blood cell count

Fig. 7.2 Primary evaluation for an underlying disorder of hemostasis in females with excessive menstrual bleeding [37]. (Reprinted from Fertility and Sterility, Kouides et al. [37], © 2005; with permission from Elsevier)

Endometrial Causes

Endometrial causes of AUB are based on molecular level abnormalities that affect proper vasoconstriction and lead to increased fibrinolysis and vasodilation [39, 20]. Clinical testing of these changes is not currently available; thus, this classification remains one of exclusion when a patient is shown to have a structurally normal uterus, normal menstrual cycle, and lack of coagulopathy [39, 20]. For example, women presenting with intermenstrual bleeding without any obvious structural causes or iatrogenic causes such as hormonal treatment may have endometrial causes.

Iatrogenic Causes

Iatrogenic causes of AUB include all pharmacologic therapies prescribed for other purposes but result in unscheduled or heavy menstrual bleeding (see Table 7.2) [13, 14, 22]. Exogenous estrogens and/or progestins, especially those dosed in a continuous fashion, can lead to AUB based on the progestin component inducing a gradual atrophy and eventual fragility of the endometrium. Progestin-containing intrauterine devices (IUDs) and progestin-only contraceptives such as depot medroxyprogesterone acetate and etonorgestrel contraceptive implant (Nexplanon™) commonly cause AUB during the initial months of therapy [13, 14]. Anticoagulant or antiplatelet therapies (e.g., warfarin, low-molecular-weight heparin, and heparin) often contribute to AUB through their desired interference with proper coagulation pathways [13]. Antidepressants and other medications

Table 7.2 Common causes of medication-induced AUB

Class	Medications
Hormonal contraceptives	Combined oral contraceptive pills, combined hormonal vaginal ring, depot medroxyprogesterone acetate, etonorgestrel implant, levonorgestrel intrauterine device
Hormonal medications	Androgens, danazol, tamoxifen, selective progesterone receptor modulators, gonadotrophin-releasing hormone agonist and antagonist, menopausal hormone replacement therapy
Anticoagulants	Warfarin, heparin, low-molecular-weight heparins, rivaroxaban, apixaban, clopidogrel
Anticonvulsant	Valproic acid
Antibiotics	Rifampin, griseofulvin
Antidepressants	SSRI, SNRI, tricyclic antidepressants
Antipsychotic	Typical and atypical classes

that affect serotonin or dopamine levels can contribute to AUB by altering prolactin release, leading to infrequent menstruation [13, 14].

AUB Not Otherwise Classified

This classification is reserved for conditions that are poorly defined or rare. Current examples include arteriovenous malformations, cesarean scar defects, myometrial hypertrophy, and chronic endometritis not related to an IUD [13, 14, 22, 40, 41]. As these conditions become better understood, they may be reclassified.

Evaluation

History and Physical Examination

> *On exam, Tamara's vitals show a BP of 126/76, HR 80, and a BMI of 30. Her abdominal exam is nontender without hepatosplenomegaly, and her pelvic exam is normal other than moderate vaginal bleeding.*

An appropriate evaluation for AUB begins with a thorough history and physical examination tailored to the patient's age. While details of menstrual flow are helpful, with excessive amounts defined as changing pads or tampons every 1–2 hours or bleeding longer than 7 days [35], it is important to recall that the definition of AUB is bleeding that negatively impacts a patient's quality of life [8, 13].

Adolescence

While the hypothalamic-pituitary-ovarian (HPO) axis coordinates to initiate menarche, it often takes 12–18 months, sometimes even up to 36 months, to fully mature [36, 38]. During this maturation process, ovulatory dysfunction is common and is the leading cause of AUB in the adolescent girl [36, 38]. The simplest measure of ovulation is a menstrual cycle length within the normal 24- to 35-day range but can also be suggested by presence of premenstrual breast tenderness, cyclic mood changes, and cramping [38]. A careful sexual history will provide insight toward possible sexually transmitted infection (STI) or pregnancy. Additionally, especially in adolescents with anemia from AUB, screening for coagulopathy should be undertaken using a structured process (Fig. 7.2).

Physical exam should focus upon height, weight, body mass index (BMI), and Tanner staging of breasts and pubic hair [36]. Pelvic examination including the use of speculum is rarely required in adolescence as STI testing can be obtained noninvasively, structural abnormalities can be identified with imaging, and cervical cancer screening is not indicated until 21 years of age [36].

Mid-reproductive Years

Even after the HPO axis has attained maturity, anovulation can occur due to obesity, polycystic ovary syndrome (PCOS), or hypothyroidism [38]. The work-up of suspected ovulatory dysfunction is similar to that in the adolescent and focuses on identifying patients with menstrual cycle lengths outside the normal range of 24–35 days. The presence of intermenstrual bleeding may suggest a structural abnormality such as a polyp or submucosal leiomyoma [41]. Pelvic pressure or urinary frequency may suggest an enlarged uterus from leiomyoma or adenomyosis. Medication list should be carefully reviewed (Table 7.2).

Concern for malignancy or hyperplasia should be based first on BMI and then on age, as BMI greater than 30 kg/m^2 has been shown to increase risk of endometrial hyperplasia or malignancy fourfold [42]. Age greater than 45 and BMI over 30 in a younger woman are often used as criteria for endometrial biopsy (see below and Chap. 15 on Gynecologic Malignancies). Physical exam may reveal a pelvic mass suggestive of a fibroid uterus. Features of hyperinsulinemia such as acanthosis nigricans or hyperandrogenism evidenced by excessive facial hair and acne suggest PCOS. Speculum examination should be performed to look for vaginal or cervical abnormalities, and bimanual examination for uterine irregularities or adnexal masses.

Perimenopause

Ovulatory dysfunction is the leading cause of AUB in the perimenopause and can occur up to 8 years prior to actual menopause [35]. The evaluation of these patients is otherwise similar to the mid-reproductive years. Adenomyosis is one of the most common causes of AUB in this time period, though it is often a diagnosis of exclusion given the limitations of current imaging modalities in its detection [25, 26].

Postmenopausal Patients

Postmenopausal bleeding (PMB) is not typically considered a subtype of AUB. The high prevalence of endometrial hyperplasia and malignancy in patients who present with PMB requires a different approach than for the groups discussed above. Prompt evaluation of postmenopausal bleeding is imperative since as many as 1–14% of women will be diagnosed with endometrial cancer [43]. Ninety percent of women with endometrial cancer present with vaginal bleeding [43]. A thorough evaluation is needed before any treatment is initiated.

The evaluation of postmenopausal bleeding begins with an appropriate assessment of menopausal status. Diagnosis of menopause is based primarily on history of amenorrhea for 12 months [44]. However, many women have infrequent cycles during the perimenopause, making it difficult to diagnose postmenopausal bleeding. Although there is significant intra- and intersubject variability in hormone levels, use of laboratory testing for follicle-stimulating hormone (FSH) and estradiol can help identify presence or absence of ovarian function in patients with abnormal bleeding in women under 45 years of age. Persistently elevated FSH and low estradiol in the presence of amenorrhea for more than 12 months would be consistent with postmenopausal status.

The most common cause of postmenopausal bleeding is atrophic endometrium in 60–80% of patients [45]. Hormone replacement therapy accounts for another 15–25%, and benign endometrial or endocervical polyps in 2–12% [45]. Other causes are leiomyomas, cervicitis, vaginitis, trauma, or anticoagulation [45].

Endometrial cancer occurs in up to 14% of patients with postmenopausal bleeding and warrants investigations for early diagnosis [43]. Risk factors for endometrial cancer in the postmenopausal state include elevated estrogen from peripheral aromatization of androgens in obesity, exogenous estrogen in the form of prescribed or over-the-counter medications or supplements, or an estrogen-secreting neoplasm [44]. Women with hereditary nonpolyposis colon cancer have a lifetime risk of endometrial cancer in the range of 42–60% [44]. Medical comorbidities such as history of polycystic ovary disease, type 2 diabetes mellitus, family history of gynecologic malignancy, or history of atypical endometrial cells on cervical cytologic screening are additional risk factors for endometrial cancer [43]. Use of tamoxifen as adjuvant therapy for breast cancer carries a 3–6 times risk of endometrial cancer compared to nonusers [44].

A thorough history and physical examination are essential to determine the cause of postmenopausal bleeding and distinguish between uterine, cervical, vaginal, vulvar, urethral, and rectal bleeding [44]. Appropriate consultation with a gynecologist is required for further evaluation.

The next step in evaluation of uterine bleeding includes endometrial sampling or transvaginal ultrasonography [44]. Transvaginal ultrasonography is the most cost-effective approach in the initial evaluation of postmenopausal bleeding [46, 47]. Transvaginal ultrasonography effectively assesses endometrial thickness. The American College of Obstetricians and Gynecologists recommends that any endometrial thickness >4 mm requires further evaluation with endometrial sampling [43]. Endometrial thickness ≤4 mm has a greater than 99% negative predictive value for endometrial cancer. Women with an endometrial stripe ≤4 mm need no further evaluation unless bleeding persists [43]. Of note, an incidental finding of an endometrial stripe >4 mm in a postmenopausal woman who does not have vaginal bleeding does not need further evaluation, though an individualized approach based on risk factors is reasonable [43].

In patients who require endometrial sampling, an office biopsy is indicated. Office endometrial biopsy is accurate but may yield inadequate tissue in 10% of women. In another 10% of women, an attempt at office biopsy fails due to inability to visualize the cervix, cervical stenosis, or a distorted uterus [44]. Focal abnormalities such as endometrial polyps can be missed in up to 18% of women [45]. An abnormal endometrial stripe and persistent vaginal bleeding are indications for referral to a gynecologist for further evaluation with saline-infusion sonohysterography or hysteroscopy [45]. Please see Chap. 15 on Gynecologic Malignancies for more information.

Laboratory Testing

Given the duration and severity of bleeding, a CBC is obtained which shows a hemoglobin of 11 gm/dL. A urine pregnancy test was negative.

Figure 7.3 describes additional laboratory evaluation for patients presenting with AUB. In all patients, a pregnancy test should be performed as the initial step in the evaluation of abnormal uterine bleeding. Additional tests to consider are complete blood counts (CBC) to evaluate severity of bleeding and thyroid-stimulating hormone testing to assess for thyroid-induced abnormal bleeding [12, 35, 41]. When interpreting test results, hemoglobin and/or hematocrit levels may not accurately reflect the degree of menstrual blood loss in some women. Leiomyomas often have higher erythropoietin activity and are occasionally associated with erythrocytosis [48]. The UK's National Institute for Health and Care Excellence (NICE) recommends thyroid function screening only in the presence of signs and symptoms of thyroid disease [8]. The healthcare provider must always ensure cervical cancer screening is up to date and give consideration to testing for *Chlamydia trachomatis*, especially in high-risk populations [12, 41].

Coagulopathy should be considered as the cause of AUB based on a thorough history, particularly in adolescents or adult patients with concerning features. One approach to

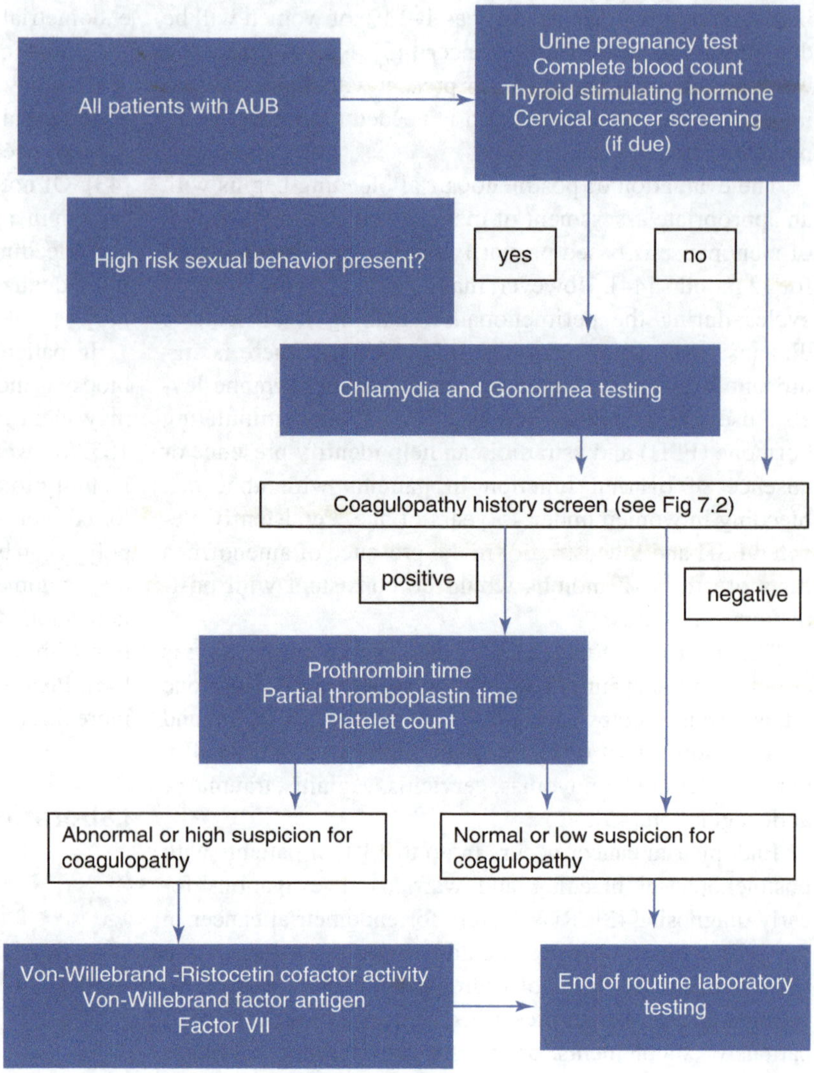

Fig. 7.3 Suggested workflow for laboratory evaluation of AUB

assessing a patient's risk for coagulopathy is presented in Fig. 7.3. Patients who meet criteria should be evaluated with complete blood count (to rule out thrombocytopenia), prothrombin time (PT), and partial thromboplastin time (PTT). If these tests are abnormal or in patients with a history otherwise suggestive of von Willebrand disease, further testing with von Willebrand ristocetin cofactor activity, von Willebrand factor (vWF) antigen, and factor VIII is appropriate [49].

Imaging

A pelvic ultrasound is obtained; the uterus measures 8 cm × 5 cm × 3 cm and the ovaries are normal.

An imaging study is indicated whenever pelvic examination is unsatisfactory or suggests an abnormality and when initial noninvasive medical management fails. Additionally, intermenstrual bleeding is suggestive of a structural abnormality that may be identified primarily through imaging [8, 12, 22, 38, 41]. Imaging of the uterus using two-dimensional ultrasonography with color-flow Doppler interrogation is commonplace as an adjunct to pelvic examination. Gynecologists may also perform saline sonohysterography, which can further enhance the capability to distinguish subtle abnormalities, diagnose AV malformations [40], and increase accuracy to distinguish benign from malignant conditions especially with leiomyomas [50]. MRI can be used to diagnose adenomyosis or to map leiomyomas prior to ablation or surgical removal.

Ultrasonography

Ultrasonography of the female pelvis may be performed via a transabdominal and/or transvaginal approach. Transabdominal images give a global view of pelvic structures but sacrifice detail. Transvaginal ultrasonography increases the resolution of images, allowing improved evaluation of the endometrium and ovaries. However, transvaginal imaging is not recommended for the adolescent or virginal patient.

If identifiable menstrual cycles are present, performance of ultrasonography on days 4–6 of the cycle improves evaluation of the endometrium for structural abnormalities as it is the thinnest during these days [38]. Although in postmenopausal women, the correlation between endometrial thickness and pathologic abnormality has been standardized, in premenopausal patients there is no accepted normal maximal thickness of the endometrium. However, measurements above 15 mm may raise suspicion of abnormality [38]. Sensitivity and specificity of transvaginal ultrasonography for endometrial pathology are only 56% and 73%, respectively [12], and it has been shown that this imaging technique alone may miss one out of every six intracavitary lesions [38, 41]. For this reason, additional imaging with sonohysterography and/or endometrial biopsy is also needed.

Sonohysterography

Sonohysterography, also known as hysterosonography or saline-infusion sonography, involves instilling saline through a transcervical catheter to distend the endometrial cavity during transvaginal ultrasonography. It is well established that sonohysterography improves evaluation for intracavitary pathology with sensitivities ranging from 96 to 100% and negative predictive values of 94–100% [22, 35, 38, 41]. However, there is controversy regarding the recommendations for performing sonohysterography or routine transvaginal ultrasonography as the first-line imaging test for evaluation of AUB [8, 41].

Magnetic Resonance Imaging (MRI)

MRI is not recommended as a first-line imaging modality for AUB evaluation [8, 12]. However, MRI does offer advantages for localizing leiomyomas with precision especially in the enlarged uterus [12], and adenomyosis is more easily diagnosed using MRI. Ultrasonography alone provides 72% sensitivity and 81% specificity, while MRI provides 77% sensitivity and 89% specificity for diagnosis of adenomyosis [26].

Invasive Testing

Tamara is referred to a gynecologist for an endometrial biopsy. The results show fragments of an endometrial polyp and proliferative endometrium. There was no evidence of hyperplasia or malignancy.

Endometrial Biopsy

The American College of Obstetricians and Gynecologists recommends endometrial biopsy for all women with AUB over the age of 45. In women under the age of 45, endometrial biopsy should be performed when significant risk factors for exposure to unopposed estrogen are present or if the patient does not respond to medical therapy, especially if intermenstrual bleeding is present [12, 38, 41]. Adolescent patients almost never need a biopsy except when there is a lack of response to medical therapies [38]. The UK NICE Guidelines suggest endometrial biopsy for persistent intermenstrual bleeding or nonresponsive AUB in women over age 45 [8]. While patient age dominates these clinical guidelines to determine when to perform a biopsy, there is new data suggesting that BMI should be given higher priority, with an indication for endometrial biopsy in any patient with AUB and a BMI greater than 30 kg/m^2 [42].

Diagnostic Hysteroscopy

Hysteroscopy involves the insertion of an endoscope through the cervical canal and using a medium (most commonly normal saline) to distend the uterine cavity. This allows full visualization of the cavity and has a 94% sensitivity and 89% specificity for detecting intracavitary pathology [35]. This procedure can be performed on a conscious patient in the office or in the operating room on a sedated or anesthetized patient. It is not recommended as a first-line test for AUB evaluation [8] but is reserved for women with inconclusive imaging or endometrial biopsy or those with persistent treatment failure. The "see-and-treat" principle is preferred by many as abnormalities can be diagnosed and immediately treated with targeted biopsy or removal [22, 38].

Diagnostic Laparoscopy

AUB alone is not an indication for diagnostic laparoscopy. As most structural causes of AUB are intracavitary, evaluation should focus on the endometrial cavity, such as hysteroscopy or sonohysterography. Laparoscopy only allows examination of the external uterine contour, fallopian tubes, and ovaries. While endometriosis may be diagnosed with laparoscopy, it is not a recognized cause of AUB, but rather a cause of dysmenorrhea, dyspareunia, and infertility which often coexist with AUB.

Treatment

Tamara follows up with the gynecologist, where her treatment options are discussed and include hysteroscopy, endometrial polypectomy, hormonal therapy options with levonorgestrel IUD, or other progestin therapies.

Medical Management

Management of acute severe uterine bleeding is addressed in Chap. 11 on Gynecologic Emergencies. Fortunately, a majority of patients will present without acute, severe features and can be managed as discussed below.

Expectant Management

Treatment is tailored to the patient's need by taking a detailed assessment of presenting symptoms, their impact on quality of life, and their potential for worsening. Since there is no reliable way to objectively measure menstrual blood loss, and there is poor correlation between actual blood loss and women's perception of bleeding, hematocrit is often indicated to determine severity of blood loss [8, 51]. However, in the absence of premalignant or malignant conditions, patient's symptoms often dictate the appropriateness of expectant management. Since obesity and low BMI can both be associated with AUB, weight management is an essential component. Healthy diet and iron supplementation can help delay onset of iron deficiency anemia.

Nonhormonal Options

Nonsteroidal Anti-inflammatory Drugs (NSAIDs)

The anti-inflammatory effect of NSAIDs occurs through inhibition of cyclooxygenase (COX), the enzyme that catalyzes the transformation of arachidonic acid to prostaglandins and thromboxanes [16]. This results in inhibition of prostaglandin synthesis. NSAIDs are effective first-line therapies for abnormal uterine bleeding [52]. NSAIDs are particularly useful in women trying to conceive or have other contraindications to hormonal therapy.

Oral mefenamic acid 500 mg three times a day for 5 days from day 1 of menses resulted in a 20% reduction of mean blood loss compared to placebo [53]. In another double-blind crossover study, naproxen and mefenamic acid were compared and found to reduce menstrual blood loss by 46% and 47%, respectively [54]. Adverse effects include nausea, vomiting, and abdominal pain. NSAIDs are contraindicated if there is a coexisting bleeding disorder, platelet dysfunction, severe gastroesophageal reflux disease, or other known contraindications to NSAID use.

Tranexamic Acid

The fibrinolytic system plays an important role in menstruation. Heavy menstrual bleeding is associated with increased levels of tissue plasminogen activator and reduced levels of plasminogen activator inhibitor 1 [55]. Tranexamic acid is a synthetic lysine that acts as an antifibrinolytic agent, reducing tissue plasminogen activator activity in the endometrium and elsewhere in the body. A randomized controlled trial (RCT) showed that tranexamic acid 1 gram, every 6 hours, for 5 days reduced menstrual bleeding by 54% compared to placebo [53]. Another RCT found a significant reduction in menstrual blood loss (40.4%) with significant improvement in limitations to activities with tranexamic acid 3.9 g/ day for 5 days when compared with placebo [56]. Although there is a theoretical risk of thromboembolic complications with tranexamic acid, population studies have not shown an association [57, 58]. Caution is advised when combining tranexamic acid and estrogen-containing oral medications due to the concern for thrombosis [59].

Other Specific Nonhormonal Therapies

In women with associated comorbidities complicating abnormal uterine bleeding, appropriate treatment is necessary, usually in consultation with a hematologist. Women with hemophilia A with factor VIII levels greater than 5%, vWD type 1, and some patients with vWD type 2 can be effectively treated with desmopressin [60]. Administered as an injection (0.3 microgram/kg IV) or as a nasal spray (150 microgram), it is particularly effective in acute hemorrhage or prior to invasive procedures [60]. Factor VIII concentrate containing vW factor is indicated specifically for treatment of vWD type 3, vWD type 2B, when there is a poor response to desmopressin in vWD types 1 and 2A, and for severe acute hemorrhage when a patient is in need of emergent surgery [60]. The FDA approved recombinant vWF concentrate in 2015 for use in adults with vWD. Although NSAIDs are not effective, tranexamic acid and hormonal treatments are effective in women with vWD [60].

Evaluation and treatment of pelvic infections such as cervicitis, endometritis, and pelvic inflammatory disease is indicated if history is suggestive of these conditions. (See Chap. 13 on Sexually Transmitted Infections.) Endometriosis and pelvic congestion syndrome may also be associated with abnormal uterine bleeding and dysmenorrhea. Individualized treatment is necessary to treat these conditions. (See Chap. 31 on Chronic Pelvic Pain.)

Hormonal Options

During the secretory phase of the menstrual cycle, progesterone – with its potent anti- inflammatory property – prevents endometrial shedding. In the absence of a pregnancy, the corpus luteum regresses and progesterone levels decline. There is a sudden release of inflammatory mediators and endometrial breakdown ensues [61]. Progesterone is therefore an effective way to combat anovulatory bleeding. Both estrogen and progesterone are highly effective in modifying endometrial shedding. The choice of hormones to treat abnormal uterine bleeding is determined less by the etiology and more by patient preference, ability to comply, side effect profile, and cost-effectiveness. It is notable that a majority of hormonal treatments for abnormal uterine bleeding also preclude pregnancy [62].

Combined Hormonal Treatment

Combined hormonal contraceptives contain estrogen and progesterone and are available in oral and parenteral routes (vaginal ring and transdermal patch). Although the use of combined estrogen-progesterone formulations for treatment of heavy menstrual bleeding is considered a class effect, only the combination of oral estradiol valerate with dienogest has been approved by the US Food and Drug Administration (FDA) and the European Union for treatment of abnormal uterine bleeding. A pooled analysis of two randomized controlled studies showed that after 6 months of treatment, median menstrual blood loss decreased by 88% with this formulation compared with 24% with placebo [63]. The combined formulations are used either in cyclic or continuous regimens depending on patient preference, the etiology of AUB being treated, and the presence of comorbidities. Extended cycle regimens that reduce the frequency of menstruation are particularly useful in patients with anemia, coagulopathy, menstrual migraine, dysmenorrhea, or for occupational reasons (i.e., women soldiers with limited ability to manage irregular bleeding). Cycle control can be achieved with all types of monophasic or triphasic oral contraceptive pills [64–66]. Triphasic combined contraceptive pills containing the newer progestins (desogestrel, gestodene, and norgestimate) have better cycle control compared with those with norethindrone or levonorgestrel [64].

High-dose combined oral contraceptive pills are also useful in acute heavy uterine bleeding, and this is addressed in Chap. 11 on Gynecologic Emergencies [65].

The side effects include mood changes, headaches, nausea, fluid retention, breast tenderness and, rarely, venous thromboembolism, stroke, or myocardial infarction [8]. The thromboembolic risk is estrogen dose-dependent and also varies with type of progestin. For example, when compared to nonusers, odds ratio (OR) for thromboembolic events are: levonorgestrel formulations OR 3.6, gestodene OR 5.6, desogestrel OR 7.3, and drospirenone OR 6.3. Despite the elevated risk, the absolute risk remains quite low for all formulations in women without additional thromboembolic risk factors [67]. The transdermal combined contraceptive patch has a twofold higher thromboembolic risk compared to norgestimate-containing oral contraceptive pill [68]. Norgestimate is a third-generation progestin, like desogestrel, and is less androgenic and a weaker progestin than levonorgestrel [60]. An additional benefit of combined hormonal formulations is the contraceptive effect. Contraindications to the use of estrogen-containing formulations include a history of deep vein thrombosis, presence of cardiovascular risk factors, and a history of smoking in women over 35 years of age. Please see Chap. 4 on Patient-Centered Contraceptive Counseling for more information [69, 70].

Progestational Agents

Progesterone and its synthetic derivatives induce secretory change and endometrial atrophy and can be used in AUB especially in women where estrogen is contraindicated [71].

Oral progestogens have been studied in randomized controlled trials. Norethindrone acetate and medroxyprogesterone acetate, two commonly used progestogens, were assessed as a short 2-week course as well as a long course lasting at least 21 days per cycle. Trials of the 2-week course of progestogen (used from day 15 or 19 to day 26 of the cycle) showed low effectiveness when compared to danazol, tranexamic acid, nonsteroidal anti-inflammatory drugs (NSAIDs), or levonorgestrel IUD in the treatment of AUB [71]. The results for the longer course of progestogens were more positive. When used for 21 days of the cycle, progestogens led to a significant reduction in menstrual blood loss, though levonorgestrel IUD remained more effective than oral progestogens [71]. A 21-day course of progestogen use is more effective than the 14-day course: the former led to a 63–78% reduction in menstrual blood loss, while the short course of progestogens resulted in only a 2–30% reduction in menstrual blood loss [72, 73]. Oral progestogens are associated with adverse effects such as headaches, bloating, breast tenderness, weight gain, and acne [69].

Long- acting injectable progestin Treatment with depot medroxyprogesterone acetate (DMPA) every 3 months given intramuscularly or subcutaneously leads to amenorrhea in 50% of women [74]. However, the side effects such as irregular bleeding, weight gain, acne, and bloating affect the acceptability of this intervention [70]. Irregular bleeding from DMPA use can be controlled temporarily with short courses of COX2 inhibitors [75] or estrogen [76]. There is an association of thromboembolism with the use of injectable progestins [77] with odds ratio ranging from 2.2 to 3 compared to nonusers, although this risk may translate to few women in absolute numbers [78]. There is also an increased risk of decreased bone mineral density with injectable medroxyprogesterone acetate [79], but this appears to be reversible over a few years after stopping therapy [80].

The levonorgestrel intrauterine device (LNG IUD) is a highly effective treatment for women with nonstructural AUB as well as structural causes such as adenomyosis and small leiomyomas. The progestin component leads to inhibition of endometrial proliferation and eventual atrophy of the endometrial tissue. As noted above, the LNG IUD is more effective than other medical therapies for heavy menstrual bleeding [81]. Patients experienced consistent reduction in vaginal bleeding of greater than 72% in the first 3 months of treatment with further reduction of bleeding during the first year of use that was maintained for up to 4 years of use [81].

When compared to endometrial ablation, satisfaction rates and quality of life measures were similar [82]. While both treatments improved quality of life, the LNG IUD appeared more cost-effective than hysterectomy for up to 10 years after treatment [82].

Levonorgestrel IUD is associated with minor adverse effects such as irregular vaginal bleeding compared with oral therapy. There was a 7% expulsion rate mainly in the first 6 weeks and a 1:1000 risk of uterine perforation during insertion [72]. Although it is also likely to suppress ovulation especially in the first year of use, LNG IUD causes less systemic side effects compared to oral or injectable progestins [73]. Other side effects of levonorgestrel IUD include breast tenderness, ovarian cyst, acne, and pain [72].

Gonadotrophin-releasing hormone agonists as well as antagonists suppress the pituitary-ovarian axis and decrease follicle-stimulating hormone as well as luteinizing hormone. This results in a hypogonadal-menopause-like state. The resulting endometrial atrophy causes amenorrhea, with rates of 90% reported [83]. There is also a temporary decrease in size of leiomyomas. However, side effects such as vasomotor symptoms, vaginal atrophy, bone loss, and depression are common and preclude its prolonged use [61]. This therapy is most useful preoperatively in patients with leiomyomas and in patients with endometriosis associated with AUB.

Danazol is a weak androgen that inhibits follicle-stimulating hormone and luteinizing hormone. It is found to reduce menstrual blood loss more effectively than placebo, progestins, NSAIDs, or combined oral contraceptive pills [84]. Significant androgenic side effects such as hot flashes, myalgia, acne, and weight gain limit its use. It is an FDA-approved medication for heavy menstrual bleeding but is only used when other hormonal methods, NSAIDs, tranexamic acid, and surgery are contraindicated.

Selective progesterone receptor modulators (SPRMs) inhibit proliferation in the endometrium resulting in amenorrhea [30, 85]. Two landmark randomized controlled trials [86, 87] have studied the use of oral ulipristal acetate in women with heavy menstrual bleeding associated with fibroid uterus. Approximately 50% of the patients in the 5-mg daily ulipristal acetate group and 70% of the patients in the 10-mg daily group became amenorrheic within the first 10 days. Headache and breast discomfort were the most common adverse events in the ulipristal acetate groups. Both doses of ulipristal were non-inferior to once-monthly leuprolide acetate in controlling uterine bleeding and were significantly less likely to cause hot flashes. SPRMs cause benign endometrial changes that are not precancerous [88]. Although the use of ulipristal for leiomyoma is not approved by the FDA, it is approved in the European Union for this indication. Reports of elevated liver enzymes in a few patients have resulted in a recommendation to closely monitor liver function in patients taking ulipristal for more than 3–6 months [88].

Medical treatment of specific conditions Endometrial hyperplasia without atypia is best managed by referral to gynecologists where it can be managed with continuous progestin therapy. Typically, patients and gynecologists will choose between depot medroxyprogesterone acetate (DMPA), continuous oral norethindrone acetate (5 mg daily), megestrol (10 mg daily), and levonorgestrel IUD [89]. Biopsies should be repeated periodically to ensure resolution of endometrial hyperplasia.

Surgical Management

Surgical management of AUB is indicated when the patient exhausts trials of medical management and continues to have bothersome bleeding [8]. The precise procedure should be based upon findings from the evaluation. Newer technologies such as uterine fibroid embolization, magnetic resonance-guided focused ultrasound ablation of leiomyomas, and myolysis (destruction of leiomyoma) using radiofrequency energy provide multiple minimally invasive uterus-preserving options for women. Similar advances in operative hysteroscopy techniques for removal of intrauterine pathology, global endometrial ablation using different energy sources, and minimally invasive hysterectomy have radically transformed the choices available to treat AUB.

Minimally Invasive Options

Most surgical therapies for AUB can be performed in a minimally invasive fashion, allowing faster recovery, shorter hospitalization, and quicker return to normal daily activities.

Hysteroscopy

Polypectomy

Detection of endometrial polyps during evaluation of AUB should prompt referral for hysteroscopic removal. Hysteroscopy allows complete visualization of the endometrial polyp and ensures complete removal. Endometrial curettage without concurrent hysteroscopy does not ensure complete removal of the polyp [90]. Similar to diagnostic hysteroscopy, this procedure can be performed safely in the office, which reduces costs and increases patient satisfaction due to convenience and reduced recovery time [8, 12]. Polypectomy has been shown to reduce 75–100% of AUB symptoms when endometrial polyps are diagnosed [35].

Myomectomy

Submucosal leiomyomas are candidates for removal via hysteroscopy when they measure less than 4–5 cm in largest diameter [91]. Larger size and increased depth of leiomyoma penetration into the myometrium increase the need for multiple procedures for complete removal [92]. If the leiomyoma completely traverses the myometrium and contacts or distorts the uterine serosa, hysteroscopic approaches are contraindicated due to the risk of uterine perforation. This can be assessed well with transvaginal ultrasonography, but MRI is the best modality to identify the proximity of leiomyoma to the uterine serosa [92]. Hysteroscopic resection of leiomyoma allows a patient to retain fertility and may reduce the incidence of recurrent pregnancy loss [93]. Hysteroscopic myomectomy is an outpatient procedure with a short recovery time for the patient. Risks of this procedure include uterine perforation, fluid and electrolyte disturbances from intravasation of distension medium into the blood vessels, hemorrhage, and intrauterine adhesions which can negatively impact fertility [92].

Endometrial Ablation

Endometrial ablation is a procedure where the endometrium, down to its basal layer, is either resected or destroyed permanently in order to decrease uterine bleeding. The procedure is often performed in the gynecologist's office or an outpatient surgery center under local anesthesia along with oral, intramuscular, or intravenous pain relief and sedation. It can only be considered in women who no longer desire fertility. As endometrial ablation itself does not act as an effective contraception, the provider must ensure the patient has reliable contraception in place or combine the ablation procedure with permanent sterilization.

Endometrial ablation is generally accepted as appropriate for patients with a uterus less than 10 weeks' gravid size and having a regular uterine cavity. Some endometrial ablation devices have shown success in the presence of <3 cm submucosal leiomyomas [8, 94]. Rates of amenorrhea vary in reports from 15 to 72%, but 85–98% of women report satisfaction with the reduction in bleeding [94]. However, levonorgestrel IUDs have been shown to have similar efficacy in reducing menstrual blood loss compared to endometrial ablation for at least 2 years following initiation of therapy [94].

Short-term complications of endometrial ablation include endometritis (2.0%), urinary tract infection (1.67%), and hematometra (1.48%) [94]. If future pregnancy occurs, increased rates of ectopic pregnancy (7.5%), preterm birth (25%), and morbidly adherent placenta (7.5%) may occur [94]. Lastly, up to 20–25% of women report pain after endometrial ablation, and many proceed to a hysterectomy at a later date [94]. This is most common when leiomyoma, adenomyosis, or pelvic endometriosis are present and is more probable if the patient has also undergone bilateral tubal occlusion at any time [26, 94].

Uterine Fibroid Embolization

Uterine fibroid embolization is performed by interventional radiologists with the patient under conscious sedation. Under fluoroscopic guidance, embolic material is targeted to occlude the blood vessels supplying symptomatic fibroids [95]. Relative contraindications include solitary fibroids measuring greater than 10 cm in diameter or a multi-fibroid uterus greater than 20 weeks' gravid size [95]. Although desire for fertility is considered a contraindication, reports of healthy pregnancies after uterine fibroid embolization exist. The main concern in pregnancy after uterine fibroid embolization is a morbidly adherent placenta [95]. Recovery is faster than surgical treatments and there is a lower rate of major complications [95]. However, at 5 years post-procedure, there is a 28% reintervention rate after uterine fibroid embolization compared to 9% after non-hysteroscopic myomectomy or hysterectomy [95].

Magnetic Resonance-Guided Focused Ultrasound Ablation (MRgFUS)

MRgFUS uses high-intensity ultrasound waves to destroy fibroids in order to improve symptoms of bulk pressure or AUB. This procedure is also performed under conscious sedation by interventional radiologists. Pain is typically mild, but treatment sessions last several hours and occasionally require additional sessions [95]. A patient lies in prone fashion on a specially designed bed while real-time MRI guides ultrasound beams to focus into a fibroid and cause coagulative necrosis. The FDA has approved its use in women desiring future pregnancy [95]. Contraindications are similar to those for MRI such as the presence of shrapnel, metal implants, or defibrillators [95]. Patient satisfaction remains high, with a similar reintervention rate (23% over 4 years) to uterine fibroid embolization in a non-comparative study [95].

Myolysis: Radiofrequency Thermal Ablation

Myolysis is also known as radiofrequency thermal ablation and is available in a laparoscopic or hysteroscopic platform for use by trained gynecologists. Under intraoperative ultrasound guidance, electrode arrays are deployed into fibroids to cause coagulative necrosis via radiofrequency ablation. Compared to laparoscopic myomectomy, laparoscopic myolysis showed the ability to treat more fibroids (98.6% versus 80.3%) while incurring less blood loss and shorter hospitalization [95]. Pregnancy appears safe following myolysis, but data is limited. There is limited availability of this procedure in the USA.

Other Surgical Options

Abdominal Myomectomy

Large submucosal, any intramural, and any subserosal leiomyoma thought to be causing AUB or bulk symptoms can be removed through abdominal myomectomy. Some consider it the gold standard procedure for patients desiring preservation of fertility with pregnancy rates of 57–69% following the procedure [96, 97]. Shorter recoveries are seen with minimally invasive options, including laparoscopy and minilaparotomy, compared to laparotomy. Complication rates of abdominal myomectomy are between 8% and 11% and include infection and blood loss with a need for transfusion [96]. Recurrence of leiomyomas is common following myomectomy with rates of 11.7% after 1 year and 84.4% at 8 years. However, reoperation rates remain low with only 16% of patients needing it over 8 years [96].

Hysterectomy

Hysterectomy involves the complete removal of the uterus and is the only definitive therapy of AUB [97]. Quality of life is typically improved within 3 months of surgery [97]. Similar to abdominal myomectomy, hysterectomy can be accomplished with shorter recovery times if a laparoscopic or vaginal approach is used, while laparotomic route needs a longer recovery period. One randomized controlled trial allocated 63 women aged 30–50 years with at least 2 months of AUB to medical management or hysterectomy [98]. The hysterectomy group had significantly more improvement in multiple quality of life domains and sexual functioning but used more healthcare resources in the first 12 months following randomization. Within 24 months of randomization, 16 of the 30 women allocated to medical management underwent hysterectomy. The authors concluded that with AUB refractory to medical management at 6 months, better symptom improvement was seen with hysterectomy than continued medical management [98].

Tamara opts for the placement of a levonorgestrel IUD. At her follow-up primary care visit 4 months later, she notes resolution of her abnormal uterine bleeding. While she continues to endorse hot flashes, they are minimally bothersome at this point, and she is happy with her treatment.

Summary Points

Pathophysiology

1. Abnormal uterine bleeding is defined as bleeding that creates a bothersome negative effect on quality of life; there are no specific duration, frequency, and quantity of bleeding limits to the diagnosis.
2. The FIGO classification system of AUB, "PALM-COEIN," is a useful mnemonic to remember structural causes (polyps, adenomyosis, leiomyomas, and malignancy) and nonstructural causes (coagulopathy, ovulatory dysfunction, endometrial, iatrogenic, and not otherwise classified). Many patients will have AUB from more than one cause.

Evaluation

1. A thorough history and physical exam should be performed in all patients, including menstrual history, sexual history, and a structured screening history for coagulopathy.
2. Evaluation will vary based on age and comorbidities.
3. The preferred method of imaging for AUB is ultrasonography of the pelvis, especially transvaginal sonography.
4. Endometrial biopsy should be performed in all women over age 45, considered in all women with BMI > 30 kg/m^2, and in those women failing to respond to therapies.
5. Postmenopausal bleeding is never normal; the approach differs from that of AUB in that all patients with postmenopausal bleeding require immediate evaluation in conjunction with a gynecologist.

Medical Management

6. Nonhormonal options such as NSAIDs and tranexamic acid are first-line therapies.
7. Hormonal therapies are more cost-effective when administered parenterally (depot medroxyprogesterone injections, levonorgestrel intrauterine device), but a combination of estrogen and progesterone via either combined oral contraceptive pill or vaginal ring may provide a more acceptable bleeding profile.

Surgical Management

1. Surgical management is often the preferred management for structural causes of AUB and may be a component of therapy for nonstructural causes as well.
2. There are numerous surgical options for managing AUB which can often be performed in noninvasive or minimally invasive fashion; patients may retain the ability to safely conceive pregnancies after some surgical interventions.

Review Questions

1. A 40-year-old woman with a BMI of 42 kg/m^2 presents with irregular heavy menstrual bleeding that occurs two to three times a year. The next step in the evaluation must rule out the following condition:
   A. Idiopathic thrombocytopenic purpura
   B. Atypical endometrial hyperplasia

C. Polycystic ovary syndrome
D. Coagulation disorder
E. Menopause

The correct answer is B. This patient has a history of irregular periods that suggests anovulatory bleeding. In addition, her obesity results in excessive peripheral aromatization of androgens to estrogen. The endometrium is therefore exposed to unopposed estrogen. The most important condition to rule out, with an endometrial biopsy, would be endometrial hyperplasia, atypical hyperplasia, or endometrial cancer [12]. Idiopathic thrombocytopenic purpura and coagulation disorder present with regular heavy menstruation along with history of other bleeding sites such as petechiae, epistaxis, and bleeding gums [44]. Menopause results in absence of menstrual bleeding.

2. A 30-year-old nulliparous woman, who is trying to conceive, complains of regular, monthly, heavy menstrual bleeding. Her BMI is 28, and her hemoglobin measures 10gm/dL. Her last normal period started 4 days ago. The next step in the evaluation most likely to determine the cause of heavy menstrual bleeding is:
A. Serum iron panel
B. Pelvic ultrasonography
C. Serum quantitative hCG
D. von Willebrand panel

The correct answer is B. Common causes of heavy regular menstrual bleeding in a 30-year-old woman include leiomyomas and adenomyosis [15]. Thyroid dysfunction and coagulation disorders are less common causes. Serum iron is not indicated in most women unless oral iron therapy fails to correct the anemia even after control of heavy menstrual bleeding [8]. While a urine pregnancy test is cost-effective and indicated, a quantitative hCG assay is not indicated.

3. A 35-year-old nulliparous woman, who is trying to conceive, complains of regular monthly heavy menstrual bleeding. She desires treatment to reduce the 7 days of heavy bleeding. The best option for management would be:
A. Clomiphene citrate
B. Levonorgestrel IUD
C. Mefenamic acid
D. Combined oral contraceptive pill
E. Progesterone-only pill

The correct answer is C. NSAIDs are the first line for treatment of heavy menstrual bleeding in ovulatory cycles as well as anovulatory cycles [8, 41, 57] and do not preclude pregnancy. Since the patient is actively trying to conceive, levonorgestrel IUD and combined oral contraceptive pill are not indicated although they are effective in treating heavy menstrual bleeding [8]. The progesterone-only pill is not effective in controlling menstrual bleeding and is a contraceptive. Clomiphene citrate is a selective estrogen receptor modulator used to induce ovulation and is not indicated in a patient with regular cycles who is likely to be ovulating.

4. A 56-year-old multiparous woman reports that she had a 3-day episode of light vaginal bleeding 2 months earlier. Her past episode of menstrual bleeding was 2 years earlier. Pelvic examination is normal and cervical cancer screening is up to date. The next step in evaluation is:
A. Reassurance that sometimes ovulation can occur sporadically during the first few years of menopause.
B. Discuss the importance of continuing contraception to prevent unplanned pregnancy.
C. Discuss the need for further evaluation with pelvic sonography to evaluate the endometrial thickness.
D. Explain that she will need endometrial biopsy if she has another episode of vaginal bleeding.

The correct answer is C. Postmenopausal bleeding needs appropriate evaluation to rule out endometrial cancer and hyperplasia. Other causes of postmenopausal bleeding in this patient include endometrial polyp or genital atrophy. The initial approach to a woman with postmenopausal bleeding is to evaluate the endometrium with transvaginal ultrasonography. Depending on the thickness of the endometrium, she may need office endometrial biopsy [43]. Reassurance without further evaluation or waiting for recurrent bleeding is not appropriate and may lead to delayed diagnosis of endometrial cancer. Follicle-stimulating hormone is not indicated and does not help in the evaluation of postmenopausal bleeding. Although there is a small possibility that this patient is not in menopause, likelihood of pregnancy in a 56-year-old who has not had a spontaneous period for 2 years is very low.

5. An 18-year-old nulliparous woman presents with irregular vaginal bleeding over the last 2 weeks. Based on your office records, she is compliant with depot medroxyprogesterone injections for contraception. The next step in the evaluation of her AUB is:
A. Urine pregnancy test
B. TSH, LH, and FSH
C. von Willebrand panel
D. Testing for chlamydia

The correct answer is D. Cervicitis, salpingitis, and pelvic inflammatory disease can present with irregular vaginal bleeding and are common in sexually active women under the age of 25 [12, 36]. Abnormal uterine bleeding in a young woman on progestin-only contraception of short duration does not need any other evaluation since breakthrough bleeding is a common side effect of any hormonal contraception, particularly progestin-only types. The perfect use of depot medroxyprogesterone injections is a very effective birth control, and the risk of pregnancy is too low to be a concern. Polycystic ovary disease and von Willebrand disease typically present a pattern of AUB over a longer period of time than the 2 weeks in this case.

References

1. Awwad JT, Toth TL, Schiff I. Abnormal uterine bleeding in the perimenopause. Int J Fertil Menopausal Stud. 1993;38(5):261–9.
2. Liu Z, Doan QV, Blumenthal P, et al. A systematic review evaluating health- related quality of life, work impairment, and health- care costs and utilization in abnormal uterine bleeding. Value Health. 2007;10:183–94.
3. Coulter A, Peto V, Jenkinson C. Quality of life and patient satisfaction following treatment for Menorrhagia. Fam Pract. 1994;11(4):394–401. https://doi.org/10.1093/fampra/11.4.394.
4. Kuppermann M, Varner RE, Summitt RL, et al. Effect of hysterectomy vs medical treatment on health-related quality of life and sexual functioning: the medicine or surgery (Ms) randomized trial. JAMA. 2004;291:1447–55.
5. Gath D, Osborn M, Bungay G, et al. Psychiatric disorder and gynecological symptoms in middle aged women: a community survey. Br Med J (Clin Res Ed). 1987;294:213–8.
6. Shapley M, Jordan K, Croft PR. Increased vaginal bleeding and psychological distress: a longitudinal study of their relationship in the community. BJOG. 2003;110:548–54.
7. Shaw RW, Brickley MR, Evans L, Edwards MJ. Perceptions of women on the impact of menorrhagia on their health using multi-attribute utility assessment. Br J Obstet Gynaecol. 1998;105: 1155–9.
8. Heavy menstrual bleeding: assessment and management. National Institute for Health and Care Excellence Clinical Guideline 88. March 2018 updated November 2018; Available at: nice.org.uk/guidance/ng88. Accessed 25 Nov 2018.
9. Munro MG, Critchley HO, Fraser IS, Group FMDW. The FIGO classification of causes of abnormal uterine bleeding in the reproductive years. Fertil Steril. 2011;95(7):2204–8, 8.e1-3.
10. Fritz MA, Speroff L. Regulation of the menstrual cycle. In: Fritz MA, Speroff L, editors. Clinical gynecologic endocrinology and infertility. 8th ed. Philadelphia: Lippincott Williams & Wilkins; 2011. p. 199–242.
11. Fraser IS, Critchley HO, Broder M, Munro MG. The FIGO recommendations on terminologies and definitions for normal and abnormal uterine bleeding. Semin Reprod Med. 2011;29(5):383–90.
12. Diagnosis of abnormal uterine bleeding in reproductive-aged women. American College of Obstetricians and Gynecologists Practice Bulletin 128. Obstet Gynecol. 2012;120(1):197–206.
13. Munro MG. Practical aspect of the two FIGO systems for management o0f abnormal uterine bleeding in the reproductive years. Best Pract Res Clin Obstet Gynecol. 2017;40:3–22.
14. Munro MG, Critchley HOD, Broder MS, Fraser IS. FIGO classification system (PALM-COEIN) for causes of abnormal uterine bleeding in nongravid women of reproductive age. Int J Gynecol Obstet. 2011;113:3–13.
15. Munro MG, Critchley H, Fraser IS. Research and clinical management for women with abnormal uterine bleeding in the reproductive years: more than PALM-COEIN. BJOG. 2017;124(2):185–9.
16. Hoffman BL, Schorge JO, Bradshaw KD, Halvorson LM, Schaffer JI, Corton MM, editors. Williams gynecology. 3rd ed. New York: McGraw-Hill. http://accessmedicine.mhmedical.com.proxy.lib.mcw.edu/content.aspx?bookid=1758&sectionid=118165489. Accessed 24 Nov 2018.
17. Maybin JA, Barcroft J, Thiruchelvam U, Hirani N, Jabbour HN, Critchley HOD. The presence and regulation of connective tissue growth factor in the human endometrium. Hum Reprod. 2012;27(4):1112–21.
18. Rakhila H, Carli C, Daris M, Lemyre M, Leboeuf M, Akoum A. Identification of multiple and distinct defects in prostaglandin biosynthetic pathways in eutopic and ectopic endometrium of women with endometriosis. Fertil Steril. 2013;100(6):1650–9.
19. Milling Smith OP, Jabbour HN, Critchley HOD. Cyclooxygenase enzyme expression and E series prostaglandin receptor signaling are enhanced in heavy menstruation. Hum Reprod. 2007;22(5):1450.
20. Davies J, Kadir RA. Endometrial haemostasis and menstruation. Rev Endocr Metab Disord. 2012;13(4):289–99.
21. Knol HM, Kemperman RFJ, Henneke CKN, Mulder AB, Meijer K. Haemostatic variables during normal menstrual cycle. Thromb Haemost. 2012;107:22–9.
22. Whitaker L, Critchley HOD. Abnormal uterine bleeding. Best Pract Res Clin Obstetr Gynaecol. 2016;34:54–65.
23. Dreisler E, Stampe Sorensen S, Ibsen PH, Lose G. Prevalence of endometrial polyps and abnormal uterine bleeding in a Danish population aged 20-74 years. Ultrasound Obstet Gynecol. 2009;33(1):102–8.
24. Clark TJ, Stevenson H. Endometrial Polyps and Abnormal Uterine Bleeding (AUB-P): what is the relationship, how are they diagnosed and how are they treated? Best Pract Res Clin Obstetr Gynaecol. 2017;40:89–104.
25. Benagiano G, Brosens I. History of adenomyosis. Best Pract Res Clin Obstet Gynaecol. 2006;20:449–63.
26. Abbott JA. Adenomyosis and Abnormal Uterine Bleeding (AUB-A)- pathogenesis, diagnosis, and management. Best Pract Res Clin Obstet Gynaecol. 2017;40:68–81.
27. Dueholm M, Hjorth IM. Structured imaging technique in the gynecologic office for the diagnosis of abnormal uterine bleeding. Best Pract Res Clin Obstet Gynaecol. 2017;40:23–43.
28. Moroni RM, Vieira CS, Ferriani RA, RMd R, Nogueira AA, Brito LGO. Presentation and treatment of uterine leiomyoma in adolescence: a systematic review. BMC Womens Health. 2015;15:4.
29. Lasmar RB, Lasmar BP. The role of leiomyomas in the genesis of abnormal uterine bleeding (AUB). Best Pract Res Clin Obstet Gynaecol. 2017;40:82–8.
30. Singh SS, Belland L, Leyland N, von Riedemann S, Murji A. The past, present, and future of selective progesterone receptor modulators in the management of uterine fibroids. Am J Obstet Gynecol. 2018;218(6):563–572.e1.
31. Adams T, Denny L. Abnormal vaginal bleeding in women with gynaecological malignancies. Best Pract Res Clin Obstet Gynaecol. 2017;40:134–47.
32. Management of abnormal cervical cancer screening test results and cervical cancer precursors. American College of Obstetricians & Gynecologists Practice Bulletin 140. Obstet Gynecol. 2013;122(6):1338–66.
33. Emons G, Beckmann MW, Schmidt D, Mallmann P. New WHO classification of endometrial hyperplasias. Geburtshilfe Frauenheilkd. 2015;75(2):135–6.
34. Endometrial cancer. American College of Obstetricians and Gynecologists Practice Bulletin 149. Obstet Gynecol. 2015;125(4):1006–26.
35. Sweet MG, Schmidt-Dalton TA, Weiss PM, Madsen KP. Evaluation and management of abnormal uterine bleeding in premenopausal women. Am Fam Physician. 2012;85(1):35–43.
36. Jamieson MA. Disorders of menstruation in adolescent girls. Pediatr Clin N Am. 2015;62(4):943–61.
37. Kouides PA, Conard J, Peyvandi F, Lukes A, Kadir R. Hemostasis and menstruation: appropriate investigation for underlying disor-

ders of hemostasis in women with excessive menstrual bleeding. Fertil Steril. 2005;84(5):1345–51.

38. Management of Abnormal Uterine Bleeding Associated with Ovulatory Dysfunction. Practice Bulletin 136. American College of Obstetricians and Gynecologists. Obstet Gynecol. 2013;122(1):176–85.
39. Fraser IS, Critchley HO, Munro MG. Abnormal uterine bleeding: getting our terminology straight. Curr Opin Obstet Gynecol. 2007;19:591–5.
40. Timor-Tritsch IE, Haynes MC, Monteagudo A, et al. Ultrasound diagnosis and management of acquired uterine enhanced myometrial vascularity arteriovenous malformations. Am J Obstet Gynecol. 2016;214:731.e1–10.
41. Bradley LD, Gueye N. The medical management of abnormal uterine bleeding in reproductive-aged women. Am J Obstetr Gynecol. 2016;214(1):31–44.
42. Wise MR, Gill P, Lensen S, et al. Body mass index trumps age in decision for endometrial biopsy: cohort study of symptomatic premenopausal women. Am J Obstet Gynecol. 2016;215:598.e1–8.
43. The role of transvaginal ultrasonography in evaluating the endometrium of women with postmenopausal bleeding. American College of Obstetricians and Gynecologists Committee opinion 734. Obstet Gynecol. 2018;131(5):e124–9.
44. Munro MG. Investigation of women with postmenopausal uterine bleeding: clinical practice recommendations. The Southern California Permanente Medical Group's Abnormal Uterine Bleeding Working Group. Perm J. 2014;18(1):55–70.
45. Null DB, Weiland CM, Camlibel AR. Postmenopausal bleeding: first steps in the workup. J Fam Pract. 2012;61(10):597–604.
46. Weber AM, Belinson JL, Bradley LD, Piedmonte MR. Vaginal ultrasonography versus endometrial biopsy in women with postmenopausal bleeding. Am J Obstet Gynecol. 1997;177(4):924–9.
47. Medverd JR, Dubinsky TJ. Cost analysis model: US versus endometrial biopsy in evaluation of peri- and postmenopausal abnormal vaginal bleeding. Radiology. 2002;222(3):619–27.
48. Asano R, Asai-Sato M, Miyagi Y, et al. Aberrant expression of erythropoietin in uterine leiomyoma: implications in tumor growth. Am J Obstet Gynecol. 2015;213:199.e1–8.
49. Heijdra JM, Cnossen MH, Leebeek FW. Current and emerging options for the management of inherited von Willebrand disease. Drugs. 2017;77:1531–47.
50. Exacoustos C, Romanini ME, Amadio A, Amoroso C, Szabolcs B, Zupi E, Arduini D. Can gray-scale and color Doppler sonography differentiate between uterine leiomyosarcoma and leiomyoma? J Clin Ultrasound. 2007;35(8):449–57.
51. Fraser IS, Warner P, Marantos PA. Estimating menstrual blood loss in women with normal and excessive menstrual fluid volume. Obstet Gynecol. 2001;98:5.1):806–14.
52. Cashman JN. The mechanisms of action of NSAIDs in analgesia. Drugs. 1996;52(Suppl 5):13–23.
53. Bonnar J, Sheppard BL. Treatment of menorrhagia during menstruation: randomised controlled trial of ethamsylate, mefenamic acid, and tranexamic acid. BMJ. 1996;313:579.
54. Hall P, MacLachlan N, Thorn N, Nudd MWE, Taylor CG, Garrioch DB. Control of menorrhagia by the cyclo-oxygenase inhibitors naproxen sodium and Mefenamic acid. BJOG. 1987;94(6):554–6.
55. Gleeson NC, Buggy F, Sheppard BL, Bonnar J. The effect of tranexamic acid on measured menstrual loss and endometrial fibrinolytic enzymes in dysfunctional uterine bleeding. Acta Obstet Gynecol Scand. 1994;73(3):274–7.
56. Lukes AS, Moore KA, Muse KN, Gersten JK, Hecht BR, Edlund M, Richter HE, Elder SE, Attia GR, Patrick DL, Rubib A, Shangold GA. Tranexamic acid treatment for heavy menstrual bleeding a randomized controlled trial. Obstet Gynecol. 2010;116(4):865–75.
57. Sundstrom A, Seaman H, Kieler H, Alfredsson L. The risk of venous thromboembolism associated with the use of tranexamic acid and other drugs used to treat menorrhagia: a case–control study using the General Practice Research Database. BJOG. 2009;116(1):91–7.
58. Wellington K, Wagstaff AJ. Tranexamic acid: a review of its use in the management of menorrhagia. Drugs. 2003;63(13):1417–33.
59. Sriprasert I, Pakrashi T, Kimble T, Archer DF. Heavy menstrual bleeding diagnosis and medical management. Contracept Reprod Med. 2017;2:20.
60. Swami A, Kaur V. von Willebrand disease: a concise review and update for the practicing physician. Clin Appl Thromb Hemost. 2017;23(8):900–10.
61. Maybin JA, Critchley HOD. Medical management of heavy menstrual bleeding. Womens Health. 2017;12(1):27–34.
62. Heikinheimo O, Fraser I. The current status of hormone therapies for heavy menstrual bleeding. Best Pract Res Clin Obstet Gynaecol. 2017;40:111–20.
63. Fraser IS, Parke S, et al. Effective treatment of heavy and/or prolonged menstrual bleeding without organic causes: pooled analysis of two multinational, randomized, double-blind, placebo-controlled trials of oestradiol valerate and dienogest. Eur J Contracep Reprod Health Care. 2011;16:258–69.
64. Cedars MI. Triphasic oral contraceptives: review and comparison of various regimens. Fertil Steril. 2002;77(1):1–14.
65. ACOG committee opinion no. 557. Management of acute abnormal uterine bleeding in nonpregnant reproductive-aged women. Obstet Gynecol. 2013;121(4):891–6.
66. Kaunitz AM, Burkman RT, Fisher AC, LaGuardia KD. Cycle control with a 21- day compared with a 24-day oral contraceptive pill: a randomized controlled trial. Obstet Gynecol. 2009;114:1205–12.
67. van Hylckama VA, Helmerhorst FM, Vandenbroucke JP, Doggen CJ, Rosendaal FR. The venous thrombotic risk of oral contraceptives, effects of Oestrogen dose and progesterone type: results of the MEGA case-control study. BMJ. 2009;339:b2921. https://doi.org/10.1136/bmj.b2921.
68. Dore DD, Norman H, Loughlin J, Seager JD. Extended case-control study results on thromboembolic outcomes among transdermal contraceptive users. Contraception. 2010;81:408–13.
69. Pinkerton J. Pharmacological therapy for abnormal uterine bleeding. Menopause. 2011;18(4):453–61.
70. Curtis KM, Tepper NK, Jatlaoui TC, Berry-Bibee E, Horton LG, Zapata LB, Simmons KB, Pagano HP, Jamieson DJ, Whiteman MK. U.S. Medical eligibility criteria for contraceptive use, 2016. MMWR Recomm Rep. 2016;65(3):1–103. https://doi.org/10.15585/mmwr.rr6503a1.
71. Lethaby A, Irvine GA, Cameron IT. Cyclical progestogens for heavy menstrual bleeding (review). Cochrane Database Syst Rev. 2008;(1):CD001016.
72. Bitzer J, Heikinjeimo O, Nelson AL, Calaf-Alsina J, Fraser IS. Medical management of heavy menstrual bleeding: a comprehensive review of the literature. Obstet Gynecol Survey. 2015;70(2):115–30.
73. Irvine GA, Campbell-Brown MB, Lumsden MA, Heikkilä A, Walker JJ, Cameron IT. Randomised comparative trial of the levonorgestrel intrauterine system and norethisterone for treatment of idiopathic menorrhagia. Br J Obstet Gynaecol. 1998;105(6):592–8.
74. Said S, Omar K, Koetsawang S, Kiriwat O, Srisatayapan Y, Kazi A, Ajmal F, Wynter HH, Pretnar-Darovec A, Benitez IB. World Health Organization, Task Force on long-acting systemic agents for fertility regulation, special programme of research, development and research training in human reproduction. A multicentered phase III comparative clinical trial of depot-medroxyprogesterone acetate given three-monthly at doses of 100 mg or 150 mg: II. The comparison of bleeding patterns. Contraception. 1987;35:591–610.
75. Nathirojanakun P, Taneepanichskul S, Sappakitkumjorn N. Efficacy of a selective COX-2 inhibitor for controlling irregular uterine bleeding in DMPA users. Contraception. 2006;73:584–7.

76. Abdel-Aleem H, d'Arcangues C, Vogelsong KM, Gaffield ML, Gülmezoglu AM. Treatment of vaginal bleeding irregularities induced by progestin only contraceptives. Cochrane Database Syst Rev. 2013;(10):CD003449. https://doi.org/10.1002/14651858.CD003449.pub5.
77. Barsoum MK, Heit JA, Ashrani AA, Leibson CL, Petterson TM, Bailey KR. Is progestin an independent risk factor for incident venous thromboembolism? A population-based case-control study. Thromb Res. 2010;126:373–8.
78. Tepper NK, Whiteman MK, Marchbanks PA, James AH, Curtis KM. Progestin- only contraception and thromboembolism: a systematic review. Contraception. 2016;94:678–700.
79. Kaunitz AM, Darney PD, Ross D, Wolter KD, Speroff L. Subcutaneous DMPA vs. intramuscular DMPA: a 2-year randomized study of contraceptive efficacy and bone mineral density. Contraception. 2009;80(1):7–17.
80. Rosenberg L, Zhang Y, Constant D, Cooper D, Kalla AA, Micklesfield L, Hoffman M. Bone status after cessation of use of injectable progestin contraceptives. Contraception. 2007;76:425–31.
81. Gupta J, Kai J, Middleton L, Pattison H, Gray R, Daniels J. Levonorgestrel intrauterine system versus medical therapy for menorrhagia. N Engl J Med. 2013;368:128–37.
82. Lethaby A, Hussain M, Rishworth JR, Rees MC. Progesterone or progestogen- releasing intrauterine systems for heavy menstrual bleeding. Cochrane Database Syst Rev. 2015;(4). Art. No.: CD002126 https://doi.org/10.1002/14651858.CD002126.pub3.
83. Friedman AJ, Hoffman DI, Comite F, Browneller RW, Miller JD. Treatment of leiomyomata uteri with leuprolide acetate depot: a double blind, placebo- controlled, multicenter study. Obstet Gynecol. 1991;77(5):720–5.
84. Beaumont HH, Augood C, Duckitt K, Lethaby A. Danazol for heavy menstrual bleeding. Cochrane Database Syst Rev. 2007;(3). Art. No.: CD001017 https://doi.org/10.1002/14651858.CD001017.pub2.
85. Spitz I. Clinical utility of progesterone receptor modulators and their effect on the endometrium. Curr Opin Obstet Gynecol. 2009;21(4):318–24.
86. Donnez J, Tatarchuk TF, Philippe Bouchard P, Puscasiu L, Zakharenko NF, Ivanova T, et al. for the PEARL I Study Group. Ulipristal acetate versus placebo for fibroid treatment before surgery. N Engl J Med. 2012;366:409–20.
87. Donnez J, Tomaszewski J, Vázquez F, Bouchard P, Lemieszczuk B, Baró F, et al. for the PEARL II Study Group. Ulipristal acetate versus leuprolide acetate for uterine fibroids. N Engl J Med. 2012;366:421–32.
88. Murji A, Whitaker L, Chow TL, Sobel ML. Selective progesterone receptor modulators (SPRMs) for uterine fibroids (review). Cochrane Database Syst Rev. 2017;4:CD010770. https://doi.org/10.1002/14651858.CD010770.pub2.
89. Haimovich S, Checa MA, Mancebo G, Fuste P, Carreras R. Treatment of endometrial hyperplasia without atypia in peri- and postmenopausal women with a levonorgestrel intrauterine device. Menopause. 2008;15:1002–4.
90. Gebauer G, Hafner A, Siebzehnrubl E, Lang N. Role of hysteroscopy in detection and extraction of endometrial polyps: results of a prospective study. Am J Obstet Gynecol. 2001;184(2):59–63.
91. Emanuel MH, Wamsteker K, Hart AA, Metz G, Lammes FB. Long term results of hysteroscopic myomectomy for abnormal uterine bleeding. Obstet Gynecol. 1999;93:743–748 (II-2).
92. AAGL practice report: practice guidelines for the diagnosis and management of submucous leiomyomas. J Minim Invasive Gyn. 2012;19(2):152–71.
93. Pritts EA, Parker WH, Olive DL. Fibroids and infertility: an updated systematic review of the evidence. Fertil Steril. 2009;91:1215–23.
94. Famuyide A. Endometrial ablation. J Minim Invasive Gynecol. 2018;25(2):299–307.
95. Laughlin-Tommaso SK. Alternatives to hysterectomy: management of uterine fibroids. Obstetr Gynecol Clin North Am. 2016;43(3):397–413.
96. Alternatives to hysterectomy in the management of leiomyomas. American College of Obstetricians and Gynecologists Practice Bulletin Number 96. Obstet Gynecol. 2008;112(2):387–400.
97. Fortin C, Flyckt R, Falcone T. Alternatives to hysterectomy: the burden of fibroids and the quality of life. Best Pract Res Clin Obstet Gynaecol. 2018;46:31–42.
98. Showstack J, Lin F, Learman LA, Vittinghoff E, Kuppermann M, Varner RE, et al. Randomized trial of medical treatment versus hysterectomy for abnormal uterine bleeding: resource use in the Medicine or Surgery (Ms) trial. Am J Obstet Gynecol. 2006;194:332–8.

Menopause

8

Molly Ainsman Fisher, Akeira L. Johnson, and Rachel A. Bonnema

Learning Objectives

1. Define menopause and describe the related changes in hormones.
2. Describe the clinical manifestations of menopause.
3. Compare and contrast the hormonal and nonhormonal medications used to treat the symptoms of menopause.
4. Examine the evidence behind the safety of hormonal therapy and counsel a patient about the risks and benefits.

Sasha is a 53-year-old female who presents to your clinic for worsening symptoms of vaginal irritation and intermittent hot flashes. She has had no vaginal bleeding for 18 months; prior to that her menses were irregular for 2 years. She describes five to six hot flashes per day, lasting less than 30 minutes each, and has developed drenching night sweats. She describes her vaginal symptoms as very dry in between episodes of discharge. She is happily married to her husband of 28 years. Recently when they have tried to engage in vaginal penetrative intercourse, it feels as if her genital skin is "ripping." She sometimes wears a panty liner because of thin vaginal discharge and she is worried she may have an infection. She also wonders if the infection has caused her night sweats.

Definition

Change in the menstrual cycle is the defining feature of menopause. During the late reproductive years, women often experience subtle changes in flow and length of their cycles. During perimenopause, women undergo marked fluctuations in sex hormone levels; cycles become more variable typically with lengthening cycles, followed by skipped cycles and episodes of amenorrhea, with increasing frequency of anovulatory cycles [1]. The hormonal fluctuations at this time, including declining estrogen levels, contribute to neurochemical changes within the central nervous system and lead to vasomotor menopausal symptoms [2].

Menopause is a clinical diagnosis defined retrospectively as 12 months without a menstrual cycle. For women over 45 years of age, this change in menses can be expected and further testing is often not necessary. The average age of menopause is 51, though it can normally occur between ages 45 and 55 (or even later) [3]. Though likelihood of pregnancy does significantly decrease at this age, pregnancy is in the differential diagnosis of amenorrhea after age 45, and a pregnancy test is warranted if the patient is having sex without contraception. If other symptoms are present, consideration of thyroid testing is reasonable. Though elevated FSH is expected in a postmenopausal woman, an elevated FSH is **not** required to make the diagnosis, and checking an FSH level can be misleading. Therefore, clinicians should make a clinical diagnosis of menopause in a woman over age 45 with 12 months of amenorrhea in the absence of other causes.

Clinical Manifestations

The most common manifestation of both perimenopause and menopause is vasomotor instability, occurring in approximately 75% of women [2]. Vasomotor symptoms (VMS) are described as hot flashes and sweating that last for less than 5 minutes and are often followed by a chill. Hot flashes are referred to as night sweats when they occur at night. VMS

M. A. Fisher
Allegheny Health Network, Pittsburgh, PA, USA

A. L. Johnson
Clement Zablocki VA, Department of General Internal Medicine, Milwaukee, WI, USA

R. A. Bonnema (✉)
University of Texas Southwestern Medical Center, Dallas, TX, USA
e-mail: rachel.bonnema@utsouthwestern.edu

S. A. Tilstra et al. (eds.), *Sex- and Gender-Based Women's Health*, https://doi.org/10.1007/978-3-030-50695-7_8

are regulated by the anterior hypothalamus [4]. Increased cutaneous blood flow from inappropriate peripheral vasodilation leads to the feeling of warmth. There is evidence that cigarette smoking may worsen VMS, but evidence that other factors (obesity, inactivity, and socioeconomic) contribute has been inconclusive [5]. The duration of VMS is variable: half of women experience resolution within 5 years, but about 10% women will report VMS for 10–12 years after menopause. Women who experience VMS earlier in the perimenopausal transition tend to experience them longer into postmenopause [2].

Genitourinary syndrome of menopause (GSM) is caused by a hypoestrogenic state and is characterized by an increase in the vaginal pH, vaginal dryness, loss of labial fullness, and loss of vaginal rugae and elasticity. Second to vasomotor symptoms, GSM is one of the most common complaints of menopausal women. Unlike vasomotor symptoms that improve with time, symptoms of GSM typically worsen throughout a woman's life with progressive decline in estrogen levels.

GSM should be evaluated clinically with a pelvic exam. The exam should begin with full inspection of the vulva, assessing for evidence of vulvar agglutination and clitoral phimosis, in addition to inspection for any lesions or skin changes. A small or pediatric speculum can be used with adequate lubrication for the internal exam. Inspection of the vaginal tissue should include examining for any evidence of loss of rugae, petechiae, or cervical lesions. Normal vaginal tissue may be replaced with less elastic tissue that appears thinner, shinier, and easily friable. Measuring vaginal pH can assist in the diagnosis; due to loss of estrogen, menopausal vaginal pH is >4.5. A bimanual exam is not required unless there is a necessity to evaluate for pelvic pain or pelvic floor dysfunction.

Many perimenopausal and menopausal women will experience a multitude of other symptoms including sleep disturbances, mood changes, cognitive complaints, and musculoskeletal issues. Sleep disturbances can be secondary to hot flashes or night sweats and may be compounded by anxiety and depression symptoms. Sleep issues may also be exacerbated by obstructive sleep apnea, which affects more women in postmenopause than premenopause [2].

Multiple studies have shown that women in the menopausal transition are more likely to report a depressed mood than premenopausal women. One study demonstrated that women were significantly more likely to report depressive symptoms during early perimenopause, late perimenopause, and postmenopause [6], and women with a personal history of depression are at risk of relapse during the menopausal transition [7]. Data also shows that anxiety levels may be increased during perimenopause, independent of a prior history of anxiety disorder, thus making the menopausal transition a critical time for women who may be vulnerable to anxiety disorders [2].

It is extremely common for women to complain of forgetfulness and issues with concentration during perimenopause, and while female sex hormones are important in cognitive function [8], longitudinal studies have not confirmed cognitive decline in menopause [9]. Perimenopausal women with increased anxiety or depression are at higher risk for memory problems. Additionally, sleep disturbance can also contribute to cognitive complaints. Further research is needed to better define the relationship between menopause and cognitive dysfunction. Currently, there is no known association between timing of menopause, change in hormones, and risk for dementia [9].

Women often note back and joint pain during perimenopause/menopause, independent of associated osteoarthritis. Unfortunately, many of the issues already outlined as occurring during menopause can contribute to pain, such as sleep disturbance or depression. The complaint of pain in menopausal women can be related to endogenous hormone changes, medications that alter hormone effects (such as aromatase inhibitors), situational stress, or concomitant menopausal symptoms [10].

Sasha's general exam is normal. Her vulva is erythematous without any lesions or ulcerations. Upon insertion of a Pederson speculum, you see that her vaginal mucosa has a pale and shiny appearance with a loss of vaginal rugae. There are petechiae and her vaginal pH is 6. She does not have any evidence of bowel or bladder prolapse. The cervix appears grossly normal. Sasha is very interested in potential treatments to help improve her sexual health, decrease her vaginal discharge, and get rid of her disturbing night sweats.

Treatment

The initial approach to women with menopausal symptoms, specifically vasomotor symptoms, is to start with lifestyle modifications. Suggestions such as lowering room temperatures, using fans, dressing in layers, and avoiding triggers such as spicy foods or alcohol may be helpful. If those do not alleviate symptoms or if women have severe VMS, it is appropriate to consider pharmacologic therapy.

Menopausal hormone therapy (MHT) is the mainstay of symptom management. It is defined as estrogen or combined estrogen-progestin therapy to treat menopausal symptoms [11]. MHT has been the topic of much debate over the past several decades. Several large clinical trials have caused the pendulum of best practices in MHT prescribing to swing back and forth. It is important for prescribers to understand the history and scientific literature of MHT in order to best provide patient-centered counseling on its use. Current consensus is that in healthy, recently menopausal women with symptoms, the benefits of MHT outweigh its risks [11].

The Women's Health Initiative (WHI) was designed to evaluate longitudinal hormone use for the prevention of heart disease in postmenopausal women, as was common practice at the time [12]. This randomized clinical trial examined the use of conjugated equine estrogens (CEE) combined with medroxyprogesterone acetate (MPA) in over 27,000 women aged 50–79 years. The trial was ended early due to safety concerns; results demonstrated an increased risk of cardiovascular disease, stroke, venous thromboembolism, and breast cancer among women who used hormones compared with placebo [12]. Multiple studies have since been published reexamining these data by age and time since menopause leading to development of the timing theory, which is that MHT is safer in younger menopausal women. Since the WHI, much of the relevant scientific exploration tested this theory.

Deciding which patients are good candidates for MHT requires a stepwise process that weighs the risks and benefits of the treatment. MHT is extremely effective in managing symptoms and has been approved by the Food and Drug Administration (FDA) for bothersome vasomotor symptoms, premature ovarian insufficiency, and genitourinary symptoms [11]. However there are risks associated with this treatment, which are influenced by patient age, number of years since menopause, comorbidities, and family history. MHT is considered to be safest in women who are less than 60 years of age or within 10 years of menopause onset [11]. Risks include potentially higher rates of breast cancer, coronary heart disease (CHD), and venous thromboembolic (VTE) disease. These are discussed in detail below. Absolute contraindications include unexplained vaginal bleeding, prior estrogen-sensitive breast or endometrial cancer, coronary heart disease, stroke, dementia, personal history or inherited high risk of thromboembolic disease, severe active liver disease, porphyria cutanea tarda, or hypertriglyceridemia [11].

For women who have an intact uterus, unopposed estrogen therapy carries a high risk of endometrial hyperplasia and cancer [13]. Therefore, women with a uterus must be on either progestin or bazedoxifene to protect the uterus from the negative effects of estrogen. It is important to note the estrogen alone carries different risks than combined estrogen and progestin. These risks are discussed in detail below.

Risk of Breast Cancer with MHT

There is a complicated relationship between MHT and the risk for breast cancer. Theoretically, since prolonged exposure to higher concentrations of endogenous estrogen increases a woman's risk of breast cancer, exogenous estrogen may do the same. A large meta-analysis suggested that for each year a woman uses MHT, her risk of breast cancer increases by 2.3% [14]. It is important to note that most of these women were using CEE/MPA, which are no longer the recommended first-line MHT formulations. The WHI demonstrated an increased risk for breast cancer with CEE/MPA therapy, although these women were older than most who would benefit from MHT for symptom control, and increased age is an important risk factor for breast cancer [12, 15]. The attributable risk of breast cancer in the WHI CEE/MPA group, where the average age was 63 years, is less than 1 additional case of breast cancer diagnosed per 1000 users annually. To put this in perspective, this risk is less than the risk associated with two daily glasses of wine and similar to the risk associated with obesity or low physical activity [16]. Please see Chap. 20 on Care of the Breast Cancer Survivor for treatment of hot flashes in breast cancer survivors.

Risk of Coronary Heart Disease, VTE, and Stroke with MHT

Age appears to play a strong role in the effects of MHT on cardiovascular disease. A 2015 Cochrane review found that MHT initiated fewer than 10 years after menopause lowered CHD in postmenopausal women, reduced all-cause mortality, and showed no increase in stroke, though there was an increased risk of VTE [17]. Further studies have shown that the formulation of estrogen and progesterone may have an impact on this VTE risk. For estrogens, lower oral doses or transdermal doses may have a lower risk, and vaginal estrogen carries no increased risk at all [18]. For progestins, micronized progesterone may carry a lower risk for thrombosis. Medroxyprogesterone acetate (MPA) has been associated with an excess risk of CHD and breast cancer when administered with conjugated estrogen. The WHI did demonstrate an increased risk in CHD in women who started MHT more than 10 years postmenopause [12]. A meta-analysis of 19 randomized controlled trials, including the WHI, demonstrated that for women of *all* ages, MHT was associated with an extra 6 strokes, 8 cases of VTE including pulmonary embolism (PE), and 4 cases of pulmonary embolism (PE) per 10,000 women; the risk of CHD was not significant [17].

Benefits of MHT

MHT has been demonstrated to have significant health benefits beyond improving quality of life by alleviating menopausal symptoms, although it is not recommended to use

MHT for the prevention of any disease [11]. MHT prevents bone loss in postmenopausal women by inhibiting osteoclast-driven bone resorption and reducing the rate of bone remodeling. It therefore prevents osteoporosis and fractures [19]. In addition, MHT has been shown to decrease the risk of type 2 diabetes mellitus, decrease the accumulation of abdominal adipose tissue, as well as decrease the incidence of colorectal cancer [15].

Prescribing MHT

The first step of initiating MHT is deciding if a woman is a good candidate. Women who are less than 60 years old or less than 10 years postmenopause, and do not have absolute contraindications or excess cardiovascular or breast cancer risks, are eligible for MHT [20]. The algorithm depicted in Fig. 8.1 outlines how to determine a patient's candidacy for

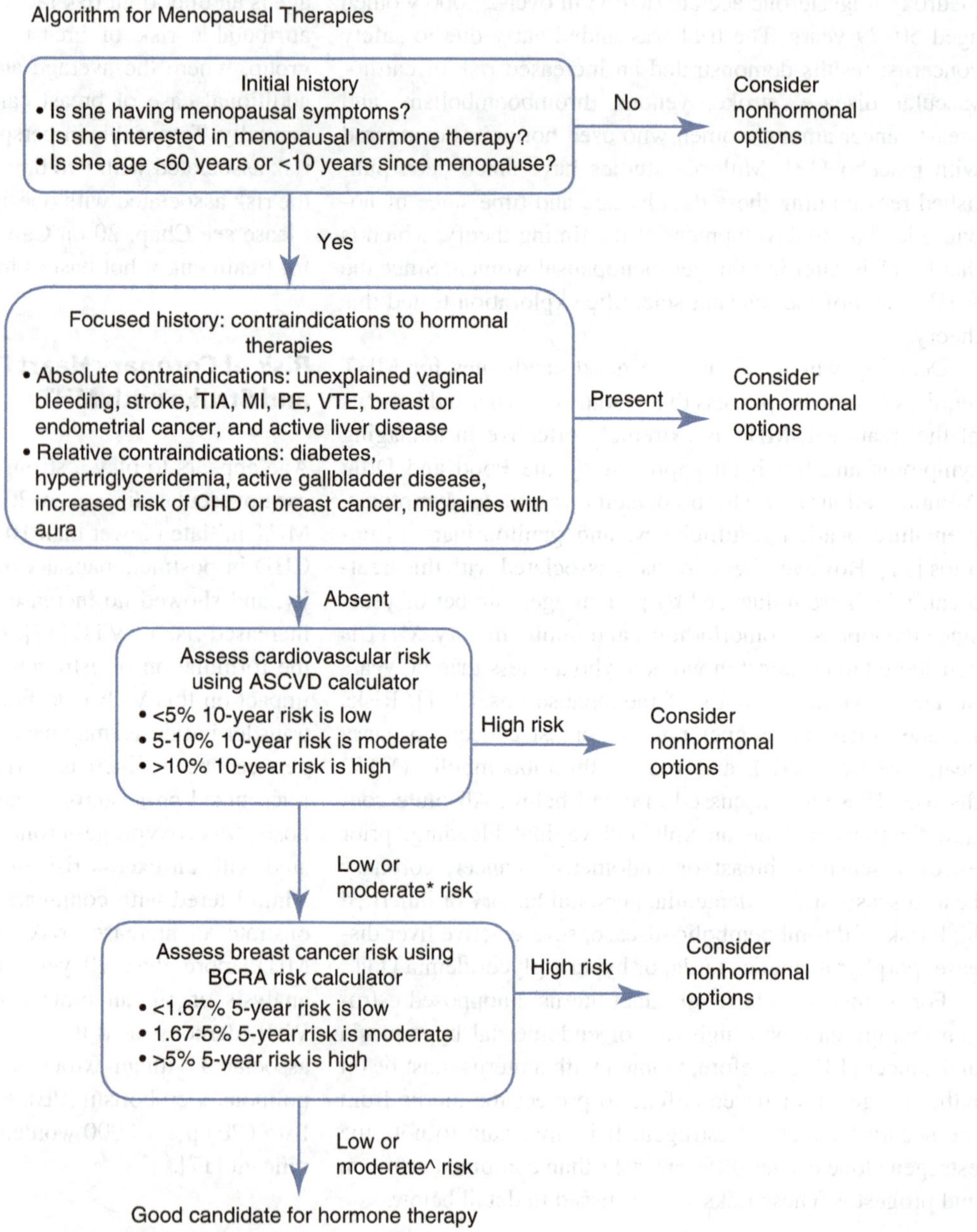

Fig. 8.1 Algorithm for menopausal therapies (Reprinted from Stuenkel et al. [20], by permission of Oxford University Press)

* For moderate cardiovascular risk, use transdermal estrogen and add micronized progesterone if she has a uterus
^ For moderate breast cancer risk, use with caution
TIA = transient ischemic attack; MI = myocardial infarction; PE = pulmonary embolism; VTE = venous thromboembolism; CHD = coronary heart disease

hormonal therapy. Examples of hormonal formulations are seen in Table 8.1.

Once a patient has decided to initiate MHT, the first step is choosing an estrogen. Estrogen comes in multiple forms and all systemic forms are equivalent for treating symptoms. The initial recommendation is to start with transdermal 17-beta estradiol. A large meta-analysis has shown no increased risk of VTE with transdermal estrogen [22]. There may also be a decreased risk of stroke with transdermal as opposed to oral, but the data are conflicting [20]. If the

Table 8.1 Selected hormonal options for menopausal symptoms

Commonly prescribed estrogens				
Mode of delivery	Preparation	Example products and typical doses	Cost[a]	Comments
Oral	Micronized estradiol	Estrace 0.5–2.0 mg/d	$18	Structurally identical to estrogen made by premenopausal ovary
	Conjugated equine estrogen (CEE)	Premarin 0.3–1.25 mg/d	$200	Used in the Women's health initiative (WHI) trial
	Esterified estrogen	Menest 0.3–1.25 mg/d	$100	
	Estropipate	Ogen 0.75–3 mg/d	$20	
Transdermal	Twice-weekly estradiol patch	Vivelle-dot 0.025–0.1 mg/d	$85	
	Weekly estradiol patch	Climara 0.025–0.1 mg/d	$75	
	Topical estradiol gel	Elestrin 0.06% (dosing varies based on brand and product)	$105	Can be transferred to other people or pets by skin contact
	Topical estradiol spray	Evamist 1.53 mg/spray	$160	Can be transferred to other people or pets by skin contact
Vaginal	Estradiol ring – *with systemic effects*	Femring 0.05–0.1 mg/d	$530	Cost/unit, lasts for 90 days
	Estradiol ring – *with only local effects*	Estring 7.5 mcg/d	$500	Cost/unit, lasts for 90 days Only for genitourinary symptoms
	Estradiol tablet	Vagifem 10 mcg/tab, 2–3 times per week	$170	Only for genitourinary symptoms
	Estradiol or CEE cream	Estrace 0.1 mg/g, 2–3 times per week Premarin 0.625 mg CEE/g, 2–3 times per week	$100	Only for genitourinary symptoms

Commonly prescribed progestins (often used in conjunction with systemic estrogen formulations)					
Mode of delivery	Preparation	Product names	Doses	Cost	Comments
Oral	Medroxyprogesterone acetate (MPA)	Provera	Cyclic: 5–10 mg/d for 12 days each calendar month Continuous: 1.25–2.5 mg/d	$12	Most common, used in WHI
	Micronized progesterone	Prometrium	Cyclic: 200 mg/d for 12 days each calendar month Continuous: 100 mg/d	$50	Avoid brand name if peanut allergy, generic is safe
Intrauterine	Levonorgestrel-releasing	Mirena			Change every 5 years

Commonly prescribed combined estrogen/progestins					
Mode of delivery	Preparation	Example products	Doses	Cost	Comments
Oral	CEE/MPA	Prempro	0.3 mg/1.50 mg 0.625/5 mg	$220	Continuous
	Estradiol/norgestimate	Prefest	1 mg/0.09 mg	$160	Cyclic
	Estradiol/norethindrone acetate	Activella, Mimvey	0.5 mg/0.1 mg 1 mg/0.5 mg	$110	Continuous
	Ethinylestradiol/norethindrone acetate	Jevantique Lo	0.5 mg/2.5 mcg	$105	Continuous
		Jinteli	1 mg/5 mcg	$115	Continuous
	Estradiol/drospirenone	Angeliq	0.5 mg/0.25 mg 1 mg/0.5 mg	$220	Continuous
Transdermal	Estradiol/norethindrone	CombiPatch	0.05 mg/0.14 mg 0.05 mg/0.25 mg	$190	Twice weekly
	Estradiol/levonorgestrel	Climara pro	0.045 mg/0.015 mg	$220	Weekly

(continued)

Table 8.1 (continued)

Combined estrogen/selective estrogen receptor modulator (SERM)					
Mode of delivery	Preparation	Product names	Doses	Cost	Comments
Oral	CEE/bazedoxifene	Duavee	0.45 mg/20 mg	$210	Continuous

SERM					
Mode of delivery	Preparation	Product names	Doses	Cost	Comments
Oral	Ospemifene	Osphena	60 mg daily	$250	FDA approved for dyspareunia and genitourinary syndrome of menopause; No increased risk of venous thromboembolism or breast cancer

[a]Lowest estimated retail cash price calculated per month (note insurance may have different pricing) [21]

patient prefers the oral route, either oral 17-beta estradiol or conjugated estrogen can be used. The downside of oral estrogen is that it results in a procoagulant effect and increases sex hormone-binding globulin (SHBG), thyroid-binding globulin, cortisol-binding globulin, triglycerides, and markers of inflammation such as C-reactive protein [20]. It is advisable to start with the lowest dose and titrate the dose based on symptoms.

Medication interactions must be considered when initiating estrogen therapy. For women who are taking anticonvulsants such as phenytoin and carbamazepine, an increased dose of estrogen may be necessary due to increased hepatic clearance of estrogen [23]. In women receiving T4 replacement, oral estrogen may increase T4 requirements since there is an increase in thyroid-binding globulin.

For women with a uterus, estrogen must be combined with a progestin or a selective estrogen receptor modulator (SERM) known as bazedoxifene to protect against endometrial proliferation and the development of endometrial cancer. If progestins are not included in combination with the provided estrogen formulation, women most commonly take oral micronized progesterone. While a continuous method is favored (100 mg daily), women who are perimenopausal (or within 2 years of menopause) may benefit from a cyclic method if they have irregular bleeding. Some women have difficulty tolerating oral progesterone due to bloating and mood changes. These women can consider using a levonorgestrel-releasing intrauterine device (IUD).

For women who do not tolerate oral progesterone or a levonorgestrel-releasing IUD, a conjugated estrogen/bazedoxifene combination can be considered. One caution is that there is an increased risk of VTE in patients using bazedoxifene when compared with placebo [24]. There are no available data comparing the VTE risk of estrogen/bazedoxifene vs. estrogen/progesterone.

Deciding on the duration of MHT can be challenging. When women first initiate MHT, they should be seen within 1–3 months to evaluate efficacy and side effects [20]. Once on a stable dose, they should be seen every 6–12 months for symptom monitoring. The decision to continue MHT should be reevaluated annually, targeting the shortest duration of hormonal treatment and strongly weighing the risks and benefits of continuing beyond 5 years [11]. Once a woman has decided to stop MHT, there are no data suggesting a difference between a gradual taper and an abrupt stop [25]. One reasonable approach would be to counsel a woman to stop MHT, but if she develops symptoms, provide instruction on a gradual taper over weeks to months. The taper may be customized to patient routines. For example, a woman could initially stop taking the hormones only on weekends and gradually taper during the week, making sure to avoid dose changes and tapering during times of stress.

Nonhormonal Options

Nonhormonal medications can be considered for women who have contraindications to MHT or prefer not to take hormones. These primarily include antidepressants and gabapentinoids. First-line therapy includes SSRIs and SNRIs, which seem to reduce vasomotor symptoms by 25–69% [26]. Low-dose paroxetine is the only antidepressant that is FDA approved for this indication. There are no head-to-head trials comparing SSRIs and SNRIs. Table 8.2 outlines specific nonhormonal medications options to treat menopausal symptoms.

Gabapentin and pregabalin can also be used to treat VMS [27]. Gabapentin has shown similar efficacy to SNRIs and works particularly well for women with night sweats [28]. Clonidine has historically been used to manage VMS, but not as effectively as those outlined above, and has more side effects. Since hot flash symptomatology gradually wanes with time, revisiting the need for non-pharmacological therapy every year is necessary.

Genitourinary Syndrome of Menopause

Since some women begin to experience symptoms of the genitourinary syndrome of menopause (GSM) in the perimenopausal state, it is important to discuss the treatment options available early in the midlife transition. As women

Table 8.2 Nonhormonal options for menopausal symptom management

Medication class		Formulations	Comments
Antidepressants	SSRI	Paroxetine	Only nonhormonal agent FDA approved for VMS; inhibits CYP2D6 so should be avoided in tamoxifen users (different class recommended)
		Citalopram	
		Escitalopram	
	SNRI	Venlafaxine	No benefit seen beyond 75 mg/d SR
		Desvenlafaxine	
Gabapentinoids		Gabapentin	Start with 300 mg qhs and uptitrate; BID dosing can also be used if needed
		Pregabalin	Effective, less well studied
Anticholinergics		Oxybutynin	Dosage varies; watch for typical anticholinergic side effects (dry mouth, constipation)

SSRI selective serotonin reuptake inhibitor, *SNRI* serotonin and norepinephrine reuptake inhibitor, *VMS* vasomotor symptoms

progress into menopause and the postmenopausal state, symptoms may worsen resulting in painful vaginal intercourse and genitourinary (GU) symptoms such as burning and dryness. Due to the difficulty in achieving and sustaining adequate lubrication for comfortable vaginal penetration in women who suffer from GSM, treatment discussions should include long-term goals. Painful vaginal intercourse can result in decreased sexual desire, distress, and avoidance of vaginal sexual intercourse altogether. Depending on mutual decision-making, longer treatment options may be discussed as long as risks do not outweigh benefits.

Treatments for GSM include nonhormonal and hormonal treatment options. Vaginal moisturizers can be purchased over the counter and used two to three times weekly for maintenance therapy in mild to moderate cases of symptoms of GSM [29]. Many vaginal moisturizers are water-based and treat GSM symptoms by replenishing moisture to the vaginal tissue. This is a good option for women who are opposed to, have contraindications to, or have an intolerance to local estrogen therapy. Patients should be counseled that vaginal moisturizers require continual adherence for symptom improvement and maintenance therapy.

Vaginal lubricants are for as needed use, typically for improvement in sexual symptoms, and can be combined with vaginal moisturizers and local estrogen therapy. There are many types of vaginal lubricants that can be found over the counter. Women should be counseled on the options of silicone, water-based, and hybrid lubricants. Water-based lubricants are typically thinner in consistency and may not provide adequate relief for vaginal intercourse if GSM symptoms are severe. Silicone-based lubricants are typically thicker in consistency but may produce an oily residue if copious amounts are used in one setting. Hybrids are a blend of both water and silicone and typically have a consistency that is thicker than water, but thinner than silicone-only lubricants. Patients should be advised to sample a few brands to find the product that works best [30].

Hormonal treatment for GSM includes local estrogen creams, vaginal and oral estrogen tablets, and a vaginal ring. FDA-approved vaginal treatments available in the United States all deliver estrogen that may treat GSM, but patient preference may determine decision-making. When first initiating treatment for severe GSM, a vaginal cream is recommended; a vaginal tablet may not be able to be inserted comfortably or absorbed adequately, and a vaginal ring may also be difficult to insert due to vaginal atrophy or stenosis. Later, one can transition from one form of local estrogen therapy to another, and these switches occur commonly based on change in symptoms, treatment goals, and individual preference [29].

Local estrogen preparations have not been shown to have an increased risk of breast or endometrial cancer. Patients should be instructed on appropriate use; if local estrogen cream is used more frequently than prescribed, systemic levels can be detected. Duration of treatment varies with individual goals and response to treatment; however, many women will have return of symptoms with cessation of local estrogen. Explaining long-term safety at initiation of treatment may help patients achieve treatment goals.

Sasha opted to start vaginal estrogen treatments but preferred not to use a systemic treatment for her night sweats. At a 6-month follow-up visit, her vaginal symptoms and dyspareunia have improved, but she is still having night sweats that are now causing significant disruption to her sleep. She also has developed multiple hot flashes during the day. Sasha would also like to revisit possible treatments for her vasomotor symptoms, in particular wondering if there is something "natural" that she can use.

Women frequently request information on the effect of complementary and alternative medicine (CAM) on VMS and menopausal symptoms in general. These types of treatment are easily accessible without visiting a physician and generally acceptable to women who may otherwise be confused or hesitant about menopausal symptoms and treatments. Most studies of CAM for menopausal symptoms have demonstrated CAM to be ineffective or are comprised of limited, biased data [31]. Cognitive behavioral therapy (CBT) and hypnosis are two therapies that have shown statistically significant efficacy in decreasing VMS [31]. Phytoestrogens may have some effect on VMS as compared with placebo but have no demonstrated effect on night sweats [32]. However, questions remain regarding optimal phytoestrogen type, dosing, and whether certain types of women may respond better to phytoestrogens than others [31].

Other options with only limited data showing benefit include weight loss, mindfulness, and stellate ganglion block. Weight loss has been shown to be helpful in decreasing VMS but is difficult and takes time to achieve. Mindfulness can help women manage the stress of VMS and menopausal symptoms without changing their severity. Stellate ganglion block, injection of local anesthetic in the sympathetic nerve region of the neck, has previously been used for pain management. Initial studies have been promising; a sham-controlled trial demonstrated improvement in moderate to severe VMS and intensity of VMS [33] with stellate ganglion block.

Many lifestyle changes or mind-body techniques can have overall health benefits but haven't shown specific improvement in VMS including regular exercise, yoga, and paced respiration. Acupuncture has been shown to be beneficial for VMS as well as quality of life when compared with no treatment. However, when acupuncture is compared with sham acupuncture, there is no significant difference in outcomes [31]. Delaying effective treatments for menopause for patients to solely work on these methods is not recommended, though they may have positive effects on health overall. Ineffective therapies that should *not* be routinely recommended include over-the-counter supplements and herbal remedies (i.e., black cohosh, evening primrose oil, dong quai, flaxseed, hops, vitamins) [31].

Understanding a patient's treatment goals and providing supportive, patient-centered care plans remains the cornerstone in managing menopause. Helping patients understand treatment options, and why they are effective or recommended, assists women in navigating a challenging life change. It is important to revisit treatment options as symptoms develop or if treatments fail. Some patients may not be initially interested in systemic therapies, but as symptoms progress and wear on overall well-being, women may feel differently about medications or effective mind-body therapies.

Special Populations

Patients with spontaneous primary ovarian insufficiency (formerly called premature ovarian failure) are diagnosed based on amenorrhea and estrogen deficiency in women less than age 40. Etiology can be chemotherapy, surgery, or autoimmune disease or may remain unknown. Typically, these women have secondary amenorrhea and FSH levels >40 IU/l (drawn twice, at least 4 weeks apart) and may be experiencing typical menopausal symptoms as outlined above [34]. These women are at significant risk for osteoporosis and cardiovascular disease. Thus, true hormone replacement should be initiated to maintain health and avoid increased risk for heart disease and increased mortality [34]. In these women, because they may still require reliable protection from pregnancy, using oral contraceptive pills is appropriate.

Pre- and postmenopausal women with breast cancer typically experience significant menopausal symptoms particularly while on endocrine therapy. Unfortunately, many women report adverse impacts of endocrine therapy on quality of life, and these symptoms can result in early treatment discontinuation, in turn affecting treatment outcomes [35]. Though data is not conclusive, available information has led the majority of guideline committees to consider MHT to be contraindicated in breast cancer survivors [36]. Nonhormonal agents as seen in Table 8.2 are recommended for women with VMS. SSRIs may lead to inhibition of CYP2D6 enzyme which can negatively affect the activity of tamoxifen. Paroxetine is a particularly potent inhibitor of CYP2D6 and should be avoided in women taking tamoxifen; the authors recommend SNRIs or gabapentinoids as safer options in in breast cancer survivors with hot flashes on tamoxifen [36].

GSM is quite common in breast cancer survivors, and women should initiate treatment with vaginal moisturizers and add lubricants for dyspareunia. Use of low-dose vaginal estrogen in breast cancer survivors does not have robust safety data. One observational study looked at low-dose vaginal estrogen and found no increased breast cancer recurrence risk during a 3.5-year mean follow-up. In general, the use of vaginal estrogen in breast cancer survivors has been discouraged; only in consultation with the oncologist should a vaginal ring, which provides a daily fixed dose of hormone and has low risk of systemic absorption, be considered [36].

Summary Points

1. Menopause is a clinical diagnosis defined retrospectively as 12 months without menses.
2. Women going through the menopausal transition may experience a range of symptoms including vasomotor, genitourinary, mood, and sleep. These symptoms are the result of hormonal fluctuations.
3. Optimal care of menopausal women requires understanding the differences between local and systemic hormonal therapy, the utility of nonhormonal therapy, and when to use either alone or in combination, to manage symptoms.

4. Hormonal therapy is the most effective treatment for menopausal symptoms. Counseling on systemic hormonal therapy should include a small attributable risk of breast cancer and VTE. While there are favored methods, choice of a specific formulation will depend on multiple patient factors, and shared decision-making is critical.

Review Questions

1. A 48-year-old female with no significant past medical history presents to discuss her periods. Over the past 6 months, her periods have become more irregular and she has had difficulty sleeping. She is currently sexually active with her husband of 25 years and is not using contraception. She is on no medications.

   Which of the following is the next best step in diagnostic workup?

   A. Endometrial biopsy
   B. FSH
   C. TSH
   D. Urine pregnancy test
   E. CBC

   The correct answer is D. This patient is likely perimenopausal; however she is still having menstrual cycles and is sexually active without contraception. Therefore, pregnancy must be ruled out prior to a workup for menopause. If her pregnancy test is negative, she can be diagnosed with perimenopause based on clinical history. Endometrial biopsy is not indicated as she is not having heavy bleeding. FSH and LH levels vary and are therefore not used routinely for diagnosis. TSH would be reasonable if she were showing other signs of a thyroid disorder. CBC would only be necessary if you are worried that her menstrual bleeding is leading to an anemia.

2. A 54-year-old female with past medical history of hypertension had her last menstrual period 10 months ago, and since then she has had no vaginal bleeding. She is suffering from debilitating hot flashes and has started missing work and social activities due to her discomfort. She has no family history of breast cancer, and her annual mammograms have all been normal. She denies any personal history of DVT or stroke, and her uterus is intact. Her ASCVD risk score shows a 3% risk of a cardiovascular event. Her BP is 128/84 on medication. She is interested in hormonal therapy but is worried about the associated risks.

   Which is the best next step for therapy?

   A. Daily estrogen and cyclic dosing of progesterone
   B. Daily estrogen and daily progesterone
   C. Daily estrogen without progesterone
   D. Follow-up visit to ensure hypertension control
   E. Nonhormonal options

   The correct answer is A. This patient is perimenopausal and a good candidate for hormonal therapy. In patients like Paula, with moderate to severe symptoms and no risk factors, hormonal therapy is considered to be first-line treatment. This should include daily oral or transdermal estrogen. Since this patient has an intact uterus, she also requires progesterone to prevent endometrial hyperplasia. In perimenopausal or newly menopausal (<2 years) women, cyclic progesterone is better tolerated than continuous progesterone because there is less breakthrough bleeding. Women who are more than 2 years out from menopause should be on continuous progesterone.

3. A 57-year-old woman presents for evaluation of insomnia. She has had severe night sweats for the last 3 years. She doesn't complain of significant hot flashes during the day. She never feels she gets restful sleep due to her drenching night sweats requiring a change of clothes and constant adjustments of her bed covers. She has a past medical history of venous thromboembolism, and she is currently on no medications and does not smoke. Her exam, including vital signs, is normal.

   Which of the following is the best treatment for this patient's night sweats?

   A. Amitriptyline
   B. Gabapentin
   C. Mirtazapine
   D. Sertraline
   E. Zolpidem

   The correct answer is B. This patient is experiencing night sweats as the most problematic symptom of menopause. Gabapentin is a medication that particularly targets night sweats and can be dosed every night with minimal daytime effects. Selective serotonin receptor inhibitors (SSRIs) can be effective for hot flashes, but are not more effective for night sweats. However, sertraline is not particularly known to have beneficial effects for hot flashes and should not be the first nonhormonal agent chosen to manage hot flashes. Amitriptyline and mirtazapine are not known to have any effect on hot flashes or night sweats. Zolpidem, while effective for short-term management of insomnia, is not known to have any effect on night sweats. A safer method of managing this patient's insomnia is to target the underlying cause, which is her night sweats, rather than initiate zolpidem treatment.

References

1. Harlow SD, Gass M, Hall JE, Lobo R, Maki P, Rebar RW, et al..; STRAW+ 10 Collaborative Group. Executive summary of the stages of reproductive aging workshop+ 10: addressing the unfinished agenda of staging reproductive aging. J Clin Endocrinol Metab. 2012;97(4):1159–68.

2. Monteleone P, Mascagni G, Giannini A, Genazzani AR, Simoncini T. Symptoms of menopause—global prevalence, physiology and implications. Nat Rev Endocrinol. 2018;14:199–215.
3. McKinlay SM, Brambilla DJ, Posner JG. The normal menopause transition. Maturitas. 1992;14(2):103.
4. Grady D. Management of menopausal symptoms. N Engl J Med. 2006;355(22):2338–47.
5. Casper RF, Yen SS. Neuroendocrinology of menopausal flushes: an hypothesis of flush mechanism. Clin Endocrinol. 1985;22(3):293–312.
6. Bromberger JT, Matthews KA, Schott LL, Brockwell S, Avis NE, Kravitz HM, et al. Depressive symptoms during the menopausal transition: the Study of Women's Health Across the Nation (SWAN). J Affect Disord. 2007;103(1):267–72.
7. Freeman EW, Sammel MD, Lin H, Nelson DB. Associations of hormones and menopausal status with depressed mood in women with no history of depression. Arch Gen Psychiatry. 2006;63(4):375–82.
8. Weber MT, Maki PM, McEermott MP. Cognition and mood in perimenopause: a systematic review and meta-analysis. J Steroid Biochem Mol Biol. 2014;142:90–8.
9. Georgakis MK, Kalogirou EI, Diamantaras AA, Daskalopoulou SS, Munro CA, Lyketsos CG, et al. Age at menopause and duration of reproductive period in association with dementia and cognitive function: a systematic review and meta-analysis. Psychoneuroendocrinology. 2016;73:224–43.
10. Mitchell ES, Woods NF. Pain symptoms during the menopausal transition and early postmenopause. Climacteric. 2010;13:467–78.
11. Pinkerton JA, Aguirre FS, Blake J, Cosman F, Hodis H, Hoffstetter S, et al. The 2017 hormone therapy position statement of the North American Menopause Society. Menopause. 2017;24(7):728–53.
12. Rossouw JE, Prentice RL, Manson JE, Wu L, Barad D, Barnabei VM, et al. Postmenopausal hormone therapy and risk of cardiovascular disease by age and years since menopause. JAMA. 2007;297(13):1465–77.
13. Furness S, Roberts H, Marjoribanks J, Lethaby A. Hormone therapy in postmenopausal women and risk of endometrial hyperplasia. Cochrane Database Syst Rev. 2012;(8):CD000402.
14. Collaborative Group on Hormonal Factors in Breast Cancer. Breast cancer and hormone replacement therapy: collaborative reanalysis of data from 51 epidemiological studies of 52,705 women with breast cancer and 108,411 women without breast cancer. Lancet. 1997;350(9084):1047–59.
15. Manson JE, Chlebowski RT, Stefanick ML, Aragaki AK, Rossouw JE, Prentice RL, et al. Menopausal hormone therapy and health outcomes during the intervention and extended poststopping phases of the Women's Health Initiative randomized trials. JAMA. 2013;310(13):1353–68.
16. Chen WY, Manson JE, Hankinson SE, Rosner B, Holmes MD, Willett WC, Colditz GA. Unopposed estrogen therapy and the risk of invasive breast cancer. Arch Intern Med. 2006;166(9):1027–32.
17. Boardman HM, Hartley L, Eisinga A, Main C, Roqué i Figuls M, Bonfill Cosp X, et al. Hormone therapy for preventing cardiovascular disease in post-menopausal women. Cochrane Database Syst Rev. 2015;(3):CD002229.
18. Canonico M, Oger E, Plu-Bureau G, Conard J, Meyer G, Lévesque H, et al. Hormone therapy and venous thromboembolism among postmenopausal women: impact of the route of estrogen administration and progestogens: the ESTHER study. Circulation. 2007;115(7):840–5.
19. Bush TL, Wells HB, James MK, Marcus R, Greendale G, Hunsberger S, McGowan J. Effects of hormone therapy on bone mineral density-results from the postmenopausal estrogen/progestin interventions (PEPI) trial. JAMA. 1996;276(17):1389–96.
20. Stuenkel CA, Davis SR, Gompel A, Lumsden MA, Murad MH, Pinkerton JV, Santen RJ. Treatment of symptoms of the menopause: an endocrine society clinical practice guideline. J Clin Endocrinol Metab. 2015;100(11):3975–4011.
21. Good RX. www.goodrx.com. Accessed October 29, 2018.
22. Mohammed K, Abu Dabrh AM, Benkhadra K, Al Nofal A, Carranza Leon BG, Prokop LJ, et al. Oral vs transdermal estrogen therapy and vascular events: a systematic review and meta-analysis. J Clin Endocrinol Metab. 2015;100(11):4012–20.
23. Mattson RH, Cramer JA, Darney PD, Naftolin F. Use of oral contraceptives by women with epilepsy. JAMA. 1986;256(2):238–40.
24. De Villiers TJ, Chines AA, Palacios S, Lips PT, Sawicki AZ, Levine AB, et al. Safety and tolerability of bazedoxifene in postmenopausal women with osteoporosis: results of a 5-year, randomized, placebo-controlled phase 3 trial. Osteoporos Int. 2011;22(2):567–76.
25. Haskell SG, Bean-Mayberry B, Gordon K. Discontinuing postmenopausal hormone therapy: an observational study of tapering versus quitting cold Turkey: is there a difference in recurrence of menopausal symptoms? Menopause. 2009;16(3):494–9.
26. Rada G, Capurro D, Pantoja T, Corbalán J, Moreno G, Letelier LM, Vera C. Non-hormonal interventions for hot flushes in women with a history of breast cancer. Cochrane Database Syst Rev. 2004;(9):CD004923.
27. Guttuso T Jr, Kurlan R, McDermott MP, Kieburtz K. Gabapentin's effects on hot flashes in postmenopausal women: a randomized controlled trial. Obstet Gynecol. 2003;101(2):337–45.
28. Bordeleau L, Pritchard KI, Loprinzi CL, Ennis M, Jugovic O, Warr D, et al. Multicenter, randomized, cross-over clinical trial of venlafaxine versus gabapentin for the management of hot flashes in breast cancer survivors. J Clin Oncol. 2010;28(35):5147–52.
29. Faubion SS, Sood R, Kapoor E. Genitourinary syndrome of menopause: management strategies for the clinician. Mayo Clinic Proc. 2017;92(12):1842–9.
30. Edwards D, Panay N. Treating vulvovaginal atrophy/genitourinary syndrome of menopause: how important is vaginal lubricant and moisturizer composition? Climacteric. 2016;19(2):151–61.
31. Nonhormonal management of menopause-associated vasomotor symptoms: 2015 position statement of The North American Menopause Society. Menopause. 2015;22(11):1155–74.
32. Franco OH, Chowdhury R, Troup J, Voortman T, Kunutsor S, Kavousi M, et al. Use of plant-based therapies and menopausal symptoms a systematic review and meta-analysis. JAMA. 2016;315(23):2554–63.
33. Walega DR, Rubin LH, Banuvar S, Shulman LP, Maki PM. Effects of stellate ganglion block on VMS: findings from a randomized controlled clinical trial in postmenopausal women. Menopause. 2014;21:807–14.
34. Nippita TA, Baber RJ. Premature ovarian failure: a review. Climacteric. 2007;10:11–22.
35. Leon-Ferre RA, Majitha N, Loprinzi CL. Management of hot flashes in women with breast cancer receiving ovarian function suppression. Cancer Treat Rev. 2017;52:82–90.
36. Santen RJ, Stuenkel CA, Davis SR, Pinkerton JV, Gompel A, Lumsden MA. Managing menopausal symptoms and associated clinical issues in breast cancer survivors. J Clin Endocrinol Metab. 2017;102:3647–61.

Female Sexual Function and Dysfunction

9

Juliana M. Kling and Holly N. Thomas

Learning Objectives
1. Define healthy female sexual function and frameworks for understanding female sexual response.
2. Discuss the impact of female sexual dysfunction (FSD).
3. Screen for and diagnose FSD.
4. Use a biopsychosocial approach in the evaluation and treatment of FSD.

Susan is a 58-year-old female who has been happily married for 30 years with previously healthy sexual function. For the last year, she has noticed distressing sexual function issues and is wondering if anything may help.

Female Sexual Function: Definition, Impact, and Framework

Healthy sexual function is a vital part of many women's lives. Women report that sexual enjoyment is important for their overall health [1], and studies have found that impaired sexual function is associated with decreased relationship satisfaction, decreased quality of life, and other negative health outcomes such as depression and low self-image [2–6]. Sexual health is defined by the World Health Organization (WHO) and Pan American Health Organization (PAHO) as "a state of physical, emotional, mental, and social well-being in relationship to sexuality; it is not merely the absence of disease, dysfunction or infirmary. Sexual health requires a positive and respectful approach to sexuality and sexual relationships, as well as the possibility of having pleasurable and safe sexual experiences, free of coercion, discrimination and violence" [7]. According to the WHO, a woman's physician should play a key role in maintaining sexual health.

Sexual dysfunction imparts a major negative impact. Women with sexual dysfunction have significantly lower quality of life scores compared to women without sexual dysfunction [4, 5, 8]. The quality of life scores of women with hypoactive sexual desire disorder are similar to those of individuals with chronic back pain and diabetes [5]. Women with sexual dysfunction have 3–5 times higher odds of low general happiness [9], 11 times higher odds of sexual dissatisfaction, and 2–3 times higher odds of relationship dissatisfaction [4]. Ninety-six percent of women with hypoactive sexual desire disorder feel that they are "letting their partner down" [4].

Several models of female sexual response have been proposed and provide a framework for evaluating and diagnosing female sexual dysfunction (FSD). The most commonly discussed models are the Masters and Johnson model and the Basson model (Figs. 9.1 and 9.2) [10–12]. The Masters and Johnson model was developed in the 1960s and applies to both women and men. This model is linear and illustrates sexual response progressing from excitement to plateau, orgasm, and then resolution. Helen Singer Kaplan, recognizing that sexual desire is an important component of sexual response, subsequently created a three-phase model with desire, excitement, and orgasm, called the Masters-Johnson-Kaplan model [13]. Dr. Paul Robinson believed the Masters and Johnson model did not adequately distinguish between the excitement phase and plateau phase, so he presented a modification as well [14].

Further critique of the linear model as it pertains to female sexual functioning led to the development of an alternative framework. In 2000, Dr. Rosemary Basson proposed a circular model that is believed to better explain women's sexual

J. M. Kling (✉)
Mayo Clinic, Department of Women's Health Internal Medicine, Rochester, NY, USA
e-mail: kling.juliana@mayo.edu

H. N. Thomas
University of Pittsburgh, Department of Medicine, Pittsburgh, PA, USA

S. A. Tilstra et al. (eds.), *Sex- and Gender-Based Women's Health*, https://doi.org/10.1007/978-3-030-50695-7_9

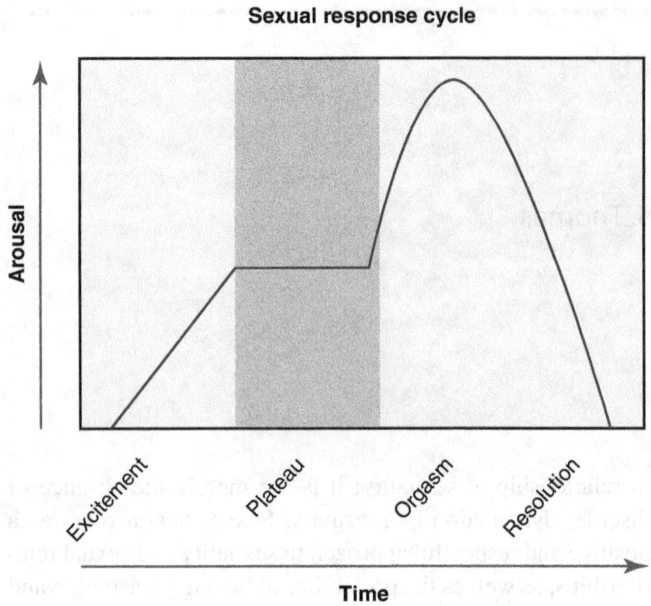

Fig. 9.1 Masters-Johnson model of sexual response (Adapted from Masters and Johnson [10])

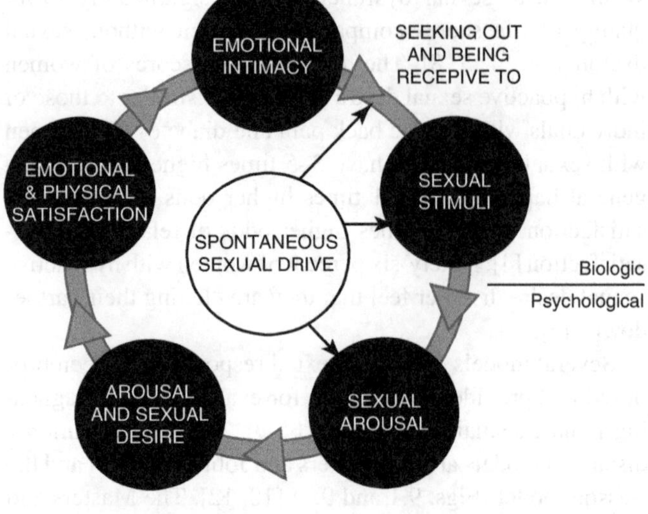

Fig. 9.2 Basson model of female sexual response (Adapted from [11, 12]. Adapted with permission from Thomas and Thurston [12], with permission from Elsevier)

response, especially for those in long-term relationships [11]. The model includes both physical *and* emotional satisfaction as important outcomes of sexual activity, such that these two factors may lead to higher emotional intimacy and subsequently greater receptivity and interest in sexual stimuli, creating a circular feedback loop. Furthermore, sexual activity is not always prompted by desire and instead could result from feelings of emotional intimacy with one's partner that may lead her to be more receptive to sexual stimulation. Sexual arousal and desire often co-occur and may be the *result* of sexual stimuli and not the impetus that leads to sexual stimuli. Hence, desire does not always need to precede arousal, as it does in the previous frameworks. This important distinction is supported by research demonstrating significant overlap in women's conceptualization of desire and arousal [15–17].

There is disagreement about which model most accurately aligns with women's experiences. A systematic review in 2011 found 13 original studies and 1 review article that evaluated aspects of these models, with only 2 directly comparing the 2 models [18]. There was limited evidence that most women identified with the linear model, although these studies utilized the Female Sexual Function Index (FSFI) to assess sexual function, which is based on the Masters-Johnson-Kaplan model. It may be that aspects of each model are applicable to different women at different stages in their lives. For example, one study showed women were more likely to agree with the Basson model if they were postmenopausal or if they were found to have sexual dysfunction as defined by the FSFI [19]. Incorporating aspects of each framework can be helpful when evaluating women with sexual health concerns.

Prevalence and Epidemiology of FSD

Prior research indicates that sexual problems are highly prevalent among women. One of the largest US studies found that 43% of women will report a sexual problem, the most common being low desire [9]. Notably, this study found that sexual problems are more prevalent in women than men. However, a sexual problem does not cross the threshold to sexual dysfunction unless it causes significant personal distress. One of the only studies to assess distress found that while 43% of US women report sexual problems, 12% of women have sexual problems causing significant distress [6]. This is still a significant proportion of women. While reporting of sexual problems increases with older age, *distress* associated with sexual problems peaks at midlife.

There are differences in sexual function across racial and ethnic groups. Studies are mixed regarding Black women, with some studies [6, 20] showing they have lower odds of sexual dysfunction compared to White women and others [9, 21, 22] showing higher odds. Studies are more consistent regarding Hispanic and Asian American women; they have higher odds of sexual dysfunction compared to White women [21, 23, 24].

Less is known about sexual function in sexual minorities. Despite a popular misconception that many lesbian couples cease sexual activity over time, most studies report that lesbian women have better sexual function and satisfaction compared to heterosexual women [25–27]. The risk factors for sexual dysfunction are similar in lesbian women and heterosexual women, including aging, relationship dissatisfaction, and mood symptoms [28, 29]. However, dyadic desire discrepancies (when partners have discordant desires) and internalized homophobia have been associated with sexual dysfunction among lesbian women as well [29, 30]. There are fewer studies among transgender individuals, and sample sizes are small. For both male-to-female and female-to-male transgender individuals, sexual function is typically worse than in cisgender individuals [31, 32], but hormone treatment and gender-affirming surgery appear to improve sexual function [32–34]. These latter studies are limited by lack of control groups.

Female Sexual Function Changes with Aging and Menopause

Both aging and menopause lead to physiologic changes in women that may impact sexual function. Up to half of postmenopausal women experience vaginal dryness due to declining estrogen levels [35], referred to as the genitourinary syndrome of menopause (GSM), previously known as atrophic vaginitis or vulvovaginal atrophy [36]. Dryness can lead to dyspareunia, which can in turn decrease sexual desire and contribute to pelvic floor muscle hypertonicity and deep pelvic pain. Vaginal dryness negatively impacts sexual function during menopause [37, 38]. Although a few smaller longitudinal studies found stable reports of desire and sexual activity during midlife [19, 39–41], most large age-adjusted studies have demonstrated worsening sexual function during the menopausal transition [19, 39, 40, 42–44]. Interpretation of these studies can be challenging; the contributing biopsychosocial factors are complex, there is not one standard sexual function instrument used, and most studies do not assess distress. (See Chap. 8 on Menopause for a discussion of general management of menopause.)

Importance of a Biopsychosocial Approach

Generally, these longitudinal studies of menopausal women highlight a common theme [12]: menopausal factors are only a part of the picture, and other important aspects of a woman's life impact sexual function. These aspects include many psychosocial as well as health variables including partner loss or absence of a sexual partner, changes in the quality of relationships with partners, lower socioeconomic status, insomnia, depression, stress, anxiety or other mood symptoms, children living at home, and declining overall health [19, 37–41, 44–46]. Many of these aspects can impact women's sexual function at any stage. Hence, it makes most sense to view female sexual function through a biopsychosocial model which takes into consideration biologic as well as psychological, interpersonal, and sociocultural factors independently and as they interact with each other over time.

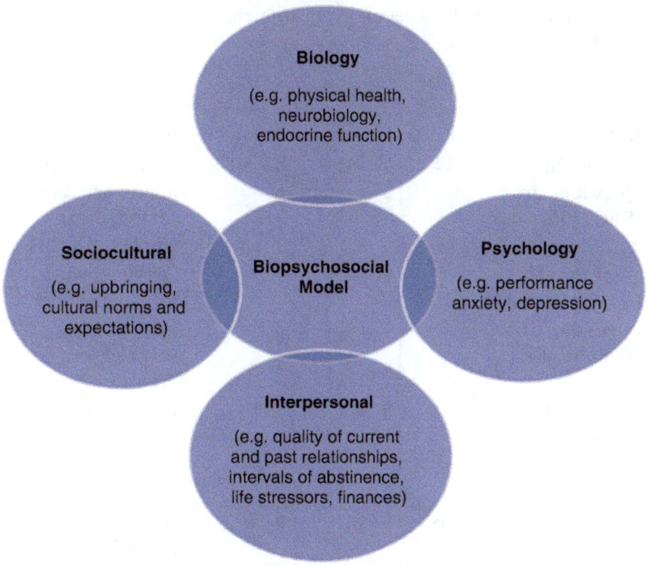

Fig. 9.3 Biopsychosocial mode of female sexual function [47, 48] (Adapted from Rosen and Barsky [47] and Levine [48])

Figure 9.3 illustrates each of these areas, as well as examples of factors within each area. For the patient in the case, starting with an assessment of her menopause status, symptoms including presence or absence of vaginal dryness or dyspareunia, is important. Then, inquiring about interpersonal, psychological, and sociocultural factors will provide a full picture of possible culprits to her symptoms and assist in next steps in the evaluation.

Screening for FSD

Given that the prevalence of sexual problems among women is high and has a significant negative impact on quality of life and relationships, it is reasonable to routinely screen for sexual problems during preventative visits. The vast majority of patients want their primary care providers to discuss sexual problems [49–51], but only a very small proportion of providers actually do [49, 50], and patients are hesitant to bring it up themselves [51]. Screening rates are even low among specialty providers, such as urogynecologists [52, 53]. Providers cite concerns about time constraints, lack of training, sociocultural differences, and lack of treatment options as reasons for failure to screen [53–55]. Brief screening instruments can assist primary care providers in screening for sexual dysfunction among their female patients (Table 9.1). Tips for screening in the primary care setting include [62]:

- Establish a good rapport.
- Normalize screening for sexual problems.
- Avoid assumptions about patients' sexual behavior (i.e., number of partners, sexual orientation).

Table 9.1 Selected screening instruments for female sexual dysfunction

Instrument	No. of items	Sensitivity	Specificity	Notes
Sexual Function Questionnaire (SFQ) [56]	34	70–83%	62–80%	Low feasibility in primary care setting given number of items
Brief Profile of Female Sexual Function (B-PFSF) [57]	7	96%	97%	Only validated for women with hypoactive sexual desire disorder
Decreased Sexual Desire Screener (DSDS) [58]	4	84%	88%	Focuses on desire only
Female Sexual Function Index-6 (FSFI-6) [59]	6	93%	94%	Assesses multiple domains, good performance
Kriston et al. single item [60]	1	76%	77%	Very brief, but lower sensitivity and specificity
Sexual Complaints Screener for Women (SCS-W) [61]	10	Not available	Not available	No validation data published

- Screen for sexual problems with patients clothed to avoid vulnerability.

A positive screen indicates that the provider should move on to a full sexual health assessment.

Susan started noticing a decreased libido about a year ago, and she's tried various strategies including a special date night once a week, but to no avail. She denies any vaginal dryness or dyspareunia since starting vaginal estrogen 3 years ago. She is still able to reach orgasm, but it takes her much longer than before.

Female Sexual Dysfunction: Domains and Definitions

Female sexual function is complex and multifactorial, so diagnosing sexual dysfunction requires familiarity with these complexities. There are validated instruments available that help to characterize and define female sexual function [12, 63]. The most common instrument is the Female Sexual Function Index (FSFI), which includes six domains of sexual function including desire, arousal, lubrication, orgasm, pain, and satisfaction, and has been validated in multiple languages and age groups and for multiple sexual disorders [64]. It is a 19-item questionnaire with scores ranging from 2.0 to 36.0, with a lower score indicating worse sexual function. A total FSFI score of less than 26.55 identifies women with sexual dysfunction [65]. Although studies have shown that midlife and older women tend to have lower scores [66], no widely accepted scoring adjustments have been made for this population. The FSFI does not include questions about sexual distress. The Female Sexual Distress Scale-Revised (FSDS-R) is a 13-item scale with scores ranging from 0 to 52 that measures sexual distress, and a score higher than 11 indicates clinically significant sexual distress [67].

The *Diagnostic and Statistical Manual* (DSM-5) has defined four distinct types of female sexual dysfunction: Female Orgasmic Disorder, Female Sexual Interest/Arousal Disorder (FSIAD, previously known as two entities – Hypoactive Sexual Desire Disorder (HSDD) and Female Sexual Arousal Disorder (FSAD) in the DSM IV), Genito-Pelvic Pain/Penetration Disorder (previously referred to as vaginismus and dyspareunia), and Substance/Medication-Induced Sexual Dysfunction [68]. They are described overall as a "heterogeneous group of disorders that are typically characterized by a clinically significant disturbance in a person's ability to respond sexually or to experience sexual pleasure." As such, diagnosis requires that symptoms have been present for at least 6 months, cause clinically significant distress in the patient (not just her partner), and are not explained by another factor, such as GSM or a relationship issue (Table 9.2 includes DSM-5 components for diagnosis). Each disorder should be specified as lifelong or acquired and include the degree of severity (mild, moderate, or severe) as well as if it is generalized or situational.

Since desire disorders are the most prevalent sexual health problems in women [6], it is important to note that the diagnostic category replacing HSDD in the DSM-5, Female Sexual Interest/Arousal Disorder, has not been validated in clinical research studies [69, 70]. It is not uniformly accepted by experts in the area, and HSDD is still recognized by certain groups including the International Society for the Study of Women's Sexual Health [71].

Evaluation of FSD

As with any medical concern, the assessment of a sexual problem should begin with a comprehensive history and physical examination. Keeping in mind the biopsychosocial model (Fig. 9.3), the history should include discussion of medical, psychological, emotional, interpersonal, and sociocultural factors that may be contributors, including asking about a history or current evidence of emotional, physical, or sexual abuse, and their beliefs toward sex, aging, menopause, and their body image. Both adverse childhood experiences and more recent trauma can play a role in FSD. Previous

Table 9.2 Four types of female sexual dysfunction by *Diagnostic and Statistical Manual* (DSM-5)

Disorder	Components for diagnosis
Female Orgasmic Disorder	Significant change in orgasm occurring most of the time (75–100%) with either (1) reduced orgasm intensity or (2) absence, infrequency, or delay of orgasm
Female Sexual Interest/ Arousal Disorder (FSIAD)[a]	Complete lack of or significant reduction in sexual interest or sexual arousal with three out of six of the following either absent or decreased: (1) sexual interest, (2) erotic fantasies or thoughts, (3) initiation of sexual activity or responsiveness to a partner's attempts to initiate sex, (4) pleasure and excitement, (5) sensations during sexual activity, and (6) response to sexual cues
Genito-Pelvic Pain/ Penetration Disorder[b]	Includes difficulties with one or more of the following symptom dimensions that is persistent or recurrent: (1) tightening of the pelvic floor muscle when vaginal penetration is attempted; (2) pain, burning, or tension during or when vaginal penetration is attempted; (3) decrease in or no desire for intercourse; and (4) anxiety or fear of pain, pelvic or vulvovaginal, as a result of, during penetration, or in anticipation of penetration
Substance/ Medication-Induced Sexual Dysfunction	A clinically significant sexual dysfunction developed soon after or during intoxication with or withdrawal of a substance capable of producing sexual dysfunction or after exposure to such a medication And the dysfunction does not only occur during a course of delirium

Adapted from the American Psychiatric Association [68]
[a]Previously known as two entities – Hypoactive Sexual Desire Disorder (HSDD) and Female Sexual Arousal Disorder (FSAD) in the DSM IV
[b]Previously referred to as vaginismus and dyspareunia

gynecologic history including surgery or trauma during childbirth should be elicited. Other factors common during midlife and menopause that may impact sexual function and should be discussed include sleep problems, depression, anxiety, and substance use [12, 46, 72]. If a relationship issue is identified, consider referral to a therapist certified by the American Association of Sexuality Educators Counselors and Therapists (AASECT). If an abuse issue is identified, please see Chap. 35 on Intimate Partner Violence and Sexual Trauma.

A detailed sexual history is also critical and should be completed in a nonjudgmental manner that is culturally sensitive and considers the patient's background and lifestyle [73, 74]. Providing a safe space and time for a woman to share will improve the ability to identify the true culprit(s) for the complaint [12]. For example, a woman may report a primary issue with orgasm, but upon further questioning, the provider learns that the patient's partner has erectile dysfunction, and the patient does not want to ask him about non-penetrative activities that could improve her ability to orgasm out of fear of upsetting him. This example also highlights the importance of asking if her partner is experiencing any sexual health issues (e.g., low libido, erectile dysfunction), as that can be a factor affecting them both.

After a thorough history, a physical examination including a pelvic examination is essential. Attention should be paid to blood pressure, heart rate, peripheral pulses, and sensation [75], as abnormalities in these areas may explain underlying pathophysiology contributing to sexual dysfunction. On the pelvic examination, particular attention should be paid to vulvovaginal conditions such as GSM, vaginitis, dermatoses, and neoplasia. An assessment of the pelvic floor should also be performed, looking for hypo- or hypertonicity or prolapse [74]. Pelvic floor dysfunction is generally described as a deep pelvic pain associated with penetrative sex that can radiate to the inner thigh or low back and often times persists after penetration [76]. Generally, laboratory testing and ultrasound evaluation is unnecessary unless a secondary issue is suspected. Assessing hormone levels is typically not necessary, since estrogen and testosterone levels do not consistently correlate with sexual dysfunction [77, 78]. Based on the history and physical examination, providers may consider testing for sexually transmitted infections, vaginal infections, thyroid testing, blood counts, or pelvic ultrasound if the primary concern is pelvic pain.

On further questioning, it turns out that Susan had started a selective serotonin reuptake inhibitor (SSRI) just prior to the onset of her symptoms for situational depression related to the loss of a parent. She has been feeling well from a mood perspective and asks if stopping the medication will help her sexual function.

Antidepressant-Associated Sexual Dysfunction

Susan's scenario is a good example of why a thorough medical history, including reviewing all medications, is pertinent to evaluating and treating FSD. Medications and medical disorders that are associated with sexual problems are discussed in Table 9.3. Since depression and sexual dysfunction are closely correlated [117], it is not uncommon to see women with FSD on antidepressant medications [117, 118]. The risk of a sexual side effect on an antidepressant is approximately 40%, and sexual side effects can occur with SSRIs, serotonin norepinephrine reuptake inhibitors (SNRIs), and tricyclic antidepressants (TCAs) alike. Among those who experience sexual side effects, 83% report problems with arousal, 72% report problems with desire, and 42% report problems with orgasm [79–82].

When starting an antidepressant for a patient at risk of FSD, bupropion or mirtazapine may be preferred options, as

Table 9.3 Medical and psychiatric issues that may impact sexual function

Medical	Genitourinary syndrome of menopause [37, 38]
	Cardiovascular disease [87]
	Diabetes mellitus [91, 92]
	Neurologic disease (stroke, spinal cord injury, multiple sclerosis) [94, 95]
	Hypertension [93]
	Breast, ovarian, uterine, and cervical cancer [96–100]
	History of gynecologic surgery [101]
	Chronic renal failure [102–104]
	Urinary incontinence [105, 106]
Psychiatric	Major depressive disorder [88, 89]
	Generalized anxiety [88, 89]
	History of emotional, physical, or sexual abuse [9, 90]
Medications	Antidepressants (selective serotonin reuptake inhibitors, serotonin norepinephrine reuptake inhibitors, tricyclic antidepressants, monoamine oxidase inhibitors), antipsychotics, benzodiazepines [79–86]
	Opiates/narcotics [71]
	Cancer therapies (for breast and gynecologic cancer) [96, 107–109]
	Antihypertensives (beta-blockers, alpha-blockers, diuretics)[a] [110–112]
	Antiepileptics (particularly gabapentin, topiramate, and phenytoin) [113–115]
	Hormones (oral contraceptives, estrogens, progestins, antiandrogens, GnRH agonists) [116]
	Amphetamines [116]
	Steroids [75]

[a]Data on antihypertensives and sexual dysfunction in women are mixed

they have fewer sexual side effects [83–86, 119, 120]. Since almost half of patients with untreated depression may experience sexual dysfunction [121], it is important to assess sexual function prior to starting the antidepressant and then in follow-up. It is important to counsel patients starting antidepressant medication that sexual side effects are common, but often improve after the first 1–2 weeks using the medication. For patients that develop sexual dysfunction while on an antidepressant, first-line options include:

- Augmentation therapy by adding another drug to counteract the adverse sexual effects, such as mirtazapine or higher doses of bupropion (150 mg twice daily) [122, 123].
- Behavioral therapies (exercise, scheduling sexual activity, psychotherapy, vibratory stimulation) [124–128].

Other options in selected situations include:

- Sildenafil (specifically for arousal dysfunction) [129].
- Testosterone [130] or acupuncture [131], although only evaluated in small, limited studies.
- Watchful waiting for 4–8 weeks, mixed results [123, 132].
- Dose reduction or a brief drug holiday, mixed results [123, 133].
- Switching antidepressants, with preference to antidepressant without adverse sexual effects, also mixed results [123, 134].

It is important to take into consideration the degree of distress related to the sexual side effect, as well as the risk of relapse of depression, when deciding on an appropriate strategy. For our patient's scenario, it is appropriate to facilitate titration off of her antidepressant and then arrange short-interval follow-up to reassess her mood and sexual function.

One of her friends was just started on flibanserin, and she's wondering if that's appropriate for her. If not, she wants to know what will work for her.

General Approach to the Treatment of FSD

All women with FSD can be counseled on general lifestyle recommendations including regular exercise, adequate sleep, maintenance of a healthy weight, stress management, dedicating time to connect with her partner, and increasing her exposure to sexual stimuli [12]. Encouraging women to use open communication with their partners about their sexual needs, as well as exploring new types of sexual activity or positions, can be helpful. Discussing normative sexual behaviors is also important, such as the fact that orgasm from vaginal penetration is unusual and most women require clitoral stimulation. Referring her to resources such as books or websites with additional information may help. Book examples include *Come as You Are* [135], *Becoming Orgasmic* [136], *Getting the Sex You Want* [137], and *Naked at Our Age* [138], and websites include the North American Menopause Society (menopause.org) [139].

Given its complexity, female sexual dysfunction is often best treated using a multidisciplinary team that includes a medical provider, a pelvic floor physical therapist, and a sex therapist. Pelvic floor physical therapist uses common physical therapy techniques, such as stretching and biofeedback, while focusing on the pelvic floor either to relax or strengthen the muscle. Working with a trained sex therapist can particularly be helpful for those experiencing relationship issues. Patients may be referred to the American Association of Sexuality Educators, Counselors, and Therapists (ASSECT) website (https://www.aasect.org) to identify trained therapists in their area [140].

After a thorough biopsychosocial approach has been utilized to evaluate and diagnose FSD, treatment should focus on the specific disorder identified (Female Orgasmic Disorder (FOD), Female Sexual Interest/Arousal Disorder (FSIAD), Genito-Pelvic Pain/Penetration Disorder, and Substance/Medication-Induced Sexual Dysfunction) and the

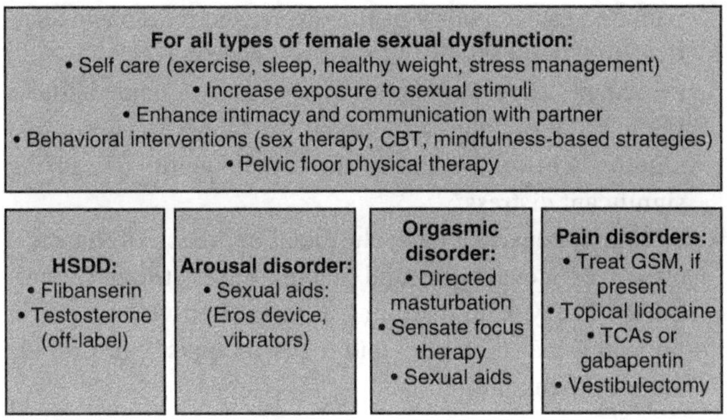

Fig. 9.4 Treatment approach to female sexual dysfunction disorders

identified causes contributing to this disorder (biologic, psychological, interpersonal, or sociocultural factors) (Fig. 9.4).

Treatments for HSDD and Non-pain Disorders

Flibanserin is the first FDA-approved treatment for HSDD in the United States and is indicated for premenopausal women so it would not be indicated for the patient described above. It has been studied and found to be effective in postmenopausal women, but use in postmenopausal women would be off-label. Flibanserin is taken daily, not on an as needed basis, since it acts centrally as a 5-HT1A agonist and 5-HT2A antagonist [141]. Candidates for flibanserin should not have any other medical, psychological, or relationship issues identified as their root cause of FSD. Since alcohol increases the risk of hypotension and syncope with flibanserin [142], women must be counseled and sign an agreement that they will not drink alcohol while taking the medication. Additional common adverse events include dizziness, nausea, fatigue, and somnolence [142]. Studies have demonstrated improvement in satisfying sexual events, sexual desire scores, and FSFI desire domain scores with flibanserin [143], but some point to an unfavorable risk-benefit profile [144]. If after an 8-week trial there is no improvement, it should be discontinued. Prescribers and pharmacies must be certified to prescribe and dispense flibanserin.

There is no FDA-approved formulation of testosterone for use in women available in the United States. Despite this, it is widely used off-label for the treatment of HSDD, since increasing research has shown its efficacy for this condition [145, 146]. Of note, most research has been done on postmenopausal women, many surgically menopausal, who were on testosterone in combination with estrogen. Androgen levels are not used to define an androgen deficiency syndrome in women: testosterone levels do not consistently correlate with female sexual function [78], in part because of the difficulty in accurately measuring testosterone, but also since female sexual function is complex and androgen status likely only plays a modest role [147]. Testosterone treatment has been associated with improvements in many aspects of sexual functioning including subjective arousal, desire, and orgasm, as well as decreases in distress related to HSDD/FSAID [148–150]. The Endocrine Society guideline suggests a 3- to 6-month trial for women meeting criteria for HSDD/FSAID with close clinical and laboratory evaluation monitoring for signs of hyperandrogenism such as acne, hirsutism, and dyslipidemia [151]. Testosterone can be converted to estrogens, so potential risks also include venous thromboembolism as well as dysplasia of the breast and endometrium. It should not be used in women with a history of VTE or hormone-responsive cancer [152]. Despite the rise of the use of compounded testosterone, there remains a lack of regulation, and concentrations of testosterone in compounded products can vary widely [153]. Long-term safety and efficacy data on testosterone are lacking.

There are also non-pharmaceutical options that are effective for HSDD, including sex therapy, cognitive behavioral therapy, or mindfulness-based strategies [154–156]. Cognitive behavioral therapy, which focuses on altering behaviors and thoughts that distract or inhibit sexual thoughts, has been found to be effective in as many as 44% of women with sexual health concerns [154]. Sensate focus, a strategy involving the partner with graded non-demand sensual touching, can help reduce anxiety and decrease avoidance of sensual touching to help improve communication and reintroduce intimacy between couples. Psychotherapy, a recognized treatment strategy for HSDD, focuses on modifying emotions, behaviors, beliefs, and thoughts, as well as relationship communication and behaviors that interfere with desire [71].

Female arousal and orgasmic disorders can be improved with directed masturbation and sensate focus [157]. Manual stimulation with vibrators or the Eros device, a small, handheld medical device for clitoral application, may increase sensation and lubrication and enhance orgasm [158, 159].

Susan titrates off of her SSRI and notices improvement in her libido, but now reports deep dyspareunia. On exam, she has pelvic floor hypertonicity. After a few weeks of successful pelvic floor physical therapy, she is happy to report a healthy sexual relationship.

Treatments for Sexual Pain Disorders

Genital sexual pain disorders are most effectively managed by a multidisciplinary team including a physician, pelvic floor physical therapist, and sex therapist [160, 161]. It is important to advise patients to stop engaging in painful sexual activity and seek treatment, as continued painful experiences can increase situational anxiety and result in increased pelvic floor tension and pain [161]. If GSM is present, vaginal moisturizers, vaginal estrogen, ospemifene, or physical therapy may be offered (see Chap. 8 on Menopause for further discussion).

Cognitive behavioral therapy, biofeedback, and mindfulness-based approaches have been shown to be helpful for pain disorders [162–168]. Additional targeted therapies for *genito-pelvic pain or penetration disorders* that have been tried with mixed results include topical lidocaine [169, 170], antidepressants such as tricyclic antidepressants [171], anticonvulsants such as gabapentin [172], or vestibulectomy [172–175], although the latter is reserved for women who have failed less invasive treatments first.

The case vignette highlights that many factors may contribute to FSD, and a multidisciplinary team approach is the best way to assure adequate treatment of all biopsychosocial contributors. In addition, this case demonstrates the concept that FSD symptoms and contributors may overlap and evolve over time, reinforcing the importance of an ongoing, trusting relationship with a primary care professional. Regular follow-up with patients with FSD allows for identification and proper referral for other issues that may arise or be contributing to their sexual health.

Conclusion

Sexual function is an important part of most women's lives. FSD is under-identified and undertreated and should be screened for during routine preventative examinations. Untreated sexual dysfunction is associated with decreased relationship satisfaction, decreased quality of life, depression, and low self-image. A comprehensive, biopsychosocial approach to evaluation, diagnosis, and treatment exploring all psychological, emotional, interpersonal, and sociocultural contributing factors is best. Treatment of FSD should focus on the underlying diagnosis. General recommendations for all patients with FSD include increasing exposure to sexual stimuli such as erotic literature, scheduling sex, decreasing stressors, as well as focusing on overall general health such as adequate sleep, exercise, and a healthy diet.

Summary Points

1. Sexual health is an important part of many women's lives and is defined as "a state of physical, emotional, mental and social well-being in relationship to sexuality."
2. Female sexual dysfunction is common, estimated to affect 22–43% of women worldwide. FSD is associated with decreased quality of life, decreased relationship satisfaction, depression, and poor self-image.
3. Providers should regularly screen for and address FSD. FSD is diagnosed based on DSM-5 criteria and requires a history of persistent sexual symptoms causing significant distress.
4. A comprehensive biopsychosocial approach is the most effective for evaluating and treating FSD. Utilizing a multidisciplinary team including a medical provider, a pelvic floor physical therapist, and a sex therapist can provide the most benefit.

Review Questions

1. Female sexual response has been described by various models. The model which includes both physical and emotional satisfaction as important outcomes of sexual activity is called the:
   A. Masters-Johnson model
   B. Basson model
   C. Masters-Johnson-Kaplan model
   D. Robinson model
   The correct answer is B. Several models of female sexual response have been proposed and provide a framework for evaluating and diagnosing female sexual dysfunction (FSD). The most commonly discussed models are the Masters and Johnson model and the Basson model. The Masters and Johnson model was developed in the 1960s and applies to both women and men. This model is linear and illustrates sexual response progressing from excitement to plateau, orgasm, and then resolution. The Basson model includes both physical *and* emotional satisfaction as important outcomes of sexual activity. These two factors may lead to higher emotional intimacy and subsequently greater receptivity and interest in sexual stimuli, creating a circular feedback loop. Furthermore, the Basson model highlights that sexual activity is not always prompted by desire, and instead feelings of emotional intimacy with one's partner may lead her to be more receptive to sexual stimulation. Sexual arousal and desire often co-occur and may be the *result* of sexual stimuli and not the impetus that leads to sexual stimuli.
2. Female sexual problems are prevalent, with rates as high as 43%. The most common female sexual problem reported is with:
   A. Lubrication
   B. Orgasm
   C. Desire
   D. Arousal
   The correct answer is C. The most commonly reported female sexual problem is low sexual desire. Although 43% of US women report sexual problems, 12% of

women have sexual problems causing significant distress. Reporting of sexual problems consistently increases with older age, but reporting of sexual problems causing distress peaks at midlife.

3. Female sexual dysfunction is defined as a sexual problem accompanied by:
   A. Vaginal dryness
   B. Clinically significant distress
   C. Decreased frequency of intercourse
   D. Pain

   The correct answer is B. It is only when women express clinically significant distress that a sexual health problem becomes a dysfunction. Importantly, distress to the partner does not qualify for the diagnosis. Although vaginal dryness, pain, and decreased intercourse frequency are common sexual problems, they would only be considered a dysfunction if the woman was distressed by the symptom.
4. The only FDA-approved medication that specifically addresses low libido and hypoactive sexual desire disorder (HSDD) in premenopausal women is:
   A. Testosterone
   B. Sildenafil
   C. Flibanserin
   D. Bupropion

   The correct answer is C. Flibanserin is the only FDA-approved treatment for HSDD in premenopausal women. Testosterone is frequently used off-label to treat HSDD, especially in postmenopausal women. Sildenafil can improve antidepressant-induced FSD. Bupropion is an antidepressant with lower risk for sexual side effects and can be used as augmentation therapy to improve antidepressant-induced FSD.
5. A 54-year-old female presents with decreased libido and no other sexual function problems after starting citalopram 2 months ago. She has tried lowering the dose of citalopram and took a drug holiday without significant improvement. She noticed worsening depression on the drug holiday. Which next treatment recommendation is best to help with her probable antidepressant-induced FSD?
   A. Augmentation therapy with bupropion.
   B. Lower the dose of the antidepressant further.
   C. Add sildenafil.
   D. All of the above.

   The correct answer is A. Sildenafil, a phosphodiesterase type 5 inhibitor FDA-approved for male erectile dysfunction, has been shown in one small randomized, double-blind, placebo-controlled study to improve orgasm functioning in women with antidepressant-induced FSD effects. The patient in the case has libido issues but is not reporting orgasm issues, so sildenafil would not be as helpful in her case. Since she has already tried lowering her antidepressant with a flare of her depression, this is not a good option. Augmentation therapy with higher doses of bupropion (150 mg twice daily) has been shown to improve antidepressant-induced FSD.

References

1. Mott G, Hinchliff S. How important is sex in later life? The views of older people. Soc Sci Med. 2003;56:1617–28.
2. Kingsberg SA, Rezaee RL. Hypoactive sexual desire in women. Menopause. 2013;20:1284–300.
3. Kingsberg SA. Attitudinal survey of women living with low sexual desire. J Women's Health. 2014;23(10):817–23.
4. Leiblum SR, Koochaki PE, Rodenberg CA, Baron IP, Rosen RC. Hypoactive sexual desire disorder in postmenopausal women: US results from the Women's International Study of Health and Sexuality (WISHes). Menopause. 2006;13(1):46–56.
5. Biddle AK, West SL, D'Aloisio AA, Wheeler SB, Borisov NN, Thorp J. Hypoactive sexual desire disorder in postmenopausal women: quality of life and health burden. Value Health. 2009;12(5):763–72.
6. Shifren JL, Monz BU, Russo PA, Segreti A, Johannes CB. Sexual problems and distress in United States women: prevalence and correlates. Obstet Gynecol. 2008;112(5):970–8.
7. World Health Organization. Defining sexual health: report of a technical consultation on sexual health. Geneva: World Health Organization; 2006.
8. Ventegodt S. Sex and the quality of life in Denmark. Arch Sex Behav. 1998;27(3):295–307.
9. Laumann EO, Paik A, Rosen RC. Sexual dysfunction in the United States: prevalence and predictors. JAMA. 1999;281(6):537–44.
10. Masters WH, Johnson VE. Human Sexual Response. Boston: Little, Brown & Co; 1966.
11. Basson R. The female sexual response: a different model. J Sex Marital Ther. 2000;26(1):51–65.
12. Thomas HN, Thurston RC. A biopsychosocial approach to women's sexual function and dysfunction at midlife: a narrative review. Maturitas. 2016;87:49–60.
13. Kaplan HS. Disorders of sexual desire. New York: Simon and Schuster; 1979.
14. Robinson P. The modernization of sex: Havelock Ellis, Alfred Kinsey, William Masters and Virginia Johnson. New York: Harper & Row, Publishers; 1976.
15. Laan E, Both S. What makes women experience desire? Fem Psychol. 2008;18(4):505–14.
16. Brotto LA, Heiman JR, Tolman DL. Narratives of desire in mid-age women with and without arousal difficulties. J Sex Res. 2009;46(5):387–98.
17. Graham CA, Sanders SA, Milhausen RR, McBride KR. Turning on and turning off: a focus group study of the factors that affect women's sexual arousal. Arch Sx Behav. 2004;33(6):527–38.
18. Hayes RD. Circular and linear modeling of female sexual desire and arousal. J Sex Res. 2011;48(2–3):130–41.
19. Sand M, Fisher WA. Women's endorsement of models of female sexual response: the nurses' sexuality study. J Sex Med. 2009;6(10):2761–71.
20. Addis IB, Van Den Eeden SK, Wassel-Fyr CL, Vittinghoff E, Brown JS, Thorn DH. Sexual activity and function in middle-aged and older women. Obstet Gynecol. 2006;107(4):755–64.
21. Avis NE, Brockwell S, Randolph JF Jr, et al. Longitudinal changes in sexual functioning as women transition through menopause: results from the Study of Women's Health Across the Nation. Menopause. 2009;16(3):442–52.

22. Avis NE, Colvin A, Karlamangla AS, Crawford S, Hess R, Waetjen LE, et al. Change in sexual functioning over the menopausal transition: results from the Study of Women's Health Across the Nation. Menopause. 2017;24(4):379–90.
23. Avis NE, Zhao X, Johannes CB, Ory M, Brockwell S, Greendale GA. Correlates of sexual function among multi-ethnic middle-ages women: results from the Study of Women's Health Across the Nation (SWAN). Menopause. 2005;12(4):385–98.
24. Laumann EO, Das A, Waite LJ. Sexual dysfunction among older adults: prevalence and risk factors from a nationally representative U.S. probability sample of men and women 57–85 years of age. J Sex Med. 2008;5(10):2300–11.
25. Coleman EM, Hoon PW, Hoon EF. Arousability and sexual satisfaction in lesbian and heterosexual women. J Sex Res. 1983;19(1):58–73.
26. Beaber TE, Werner PD. The relationship between anxiety and sexual functioning in lesbians and heterosexual women. J Homosex. 2009;56:639–54.
27. Breyer BN, Smith JF, Eisenberg ML, Ando KA, Rowen TS, Shindel AW. The impact of sexual orientation on sexuality and sexual practices in north American medical students. J Sex Med. 2010;7(7):2391–400.
28. Tracy JK, Junginger J. Correlates of lesbian sexual functioning. J Women's Health. 2007;16(4):499–509.
29. Henderson AW, Lehavot K, Simoni JM. Ecological models of sexual satisfaction among lesbian/bisexual and heterosexual women. Arch Sex Behav. 2009;38(1):50–65.
30. Bridges SK, Horne SG. Sexual satisfaction and desire discrepancy in same sex women's relationships. J Sex Marital Ther. 2007;33(1):41–53.
31. Weyers S, Elaut E, De Sutter P, Gerris J, T'Sjoen G, Heylens G, et al. Long-term assessment of the physical, mental, and sexual health among transsexual women. J Sex Med. 2009;6(3):752–60.
32. Bouman WP, Clae L, Marshall E, Pinner GT, Longworth J, Maddox V, et al. Sociodemographic variables, clinical features and the role of preassessment cross-sex hormones in older trans people. J Sex Med. 2016;13(4):711–9.
33. Constantino A, Cerpolini S, Alvisi S, Morselli PG, Venturoli S, Meriggiola MC. A prospective study on sexual function and mood in female-to-male transsexuals during testosterone administration and after sex reassignment surgery. J Sex Marital Ther. 2013;39(4):321–35.
34. Wierckx K, Van Caenegem E, Elaut E, Dedecker D, Van de Peer F, Toye K, et al. Quality of life and sexual health after sex reassignment surgery in transsexual men. J Sex Med. 2011;8(12):3379–88.
35. Management of symptomatic vulvovaginal atrophy: 2013 position statement of the North American Menopause Society. Menopause. 2013;20(9):888–902.
36. Portman DJ, Gass ML. Vulvovaginal atrophy terminology consensus conference panel. Genitourinary syndrome of menopause: new terminology for vulvovaginal atrophy from the International Society for the Study of Women's Sexual Health and The North American Menopause Society. Maturitas. 2014;79(3):349–54.
37. Gracia CR, Freeman EW, Sammel MD, Lin H, Modul M. Hormones and sexuality during transition to menopause. Obstet Gynecol. 2007;109(4):831–90.
38. Mishra G, Kuh D. Sexual functioning throughout menopause: the perceptions of women in a British cohort. Menopause. 2006;13(6):880–90.
39. Avis NE, Stellato R, Crawford S, Johannes C, Longcope C. Is there an association between menopause status and sexual functioning. Menopause. 2000;7(5):297–309.
40. Guthrie JR, Dennerstein L, Taffe JR, Lehert P, Burger HG. The menopausal transition: a 9-year prospective population-based study. The Melbourne Women's Midlife Health Project. Climacteric. 2004;7(4):375–89.
41. Woods NF, Mitchell ES, Smith-Di JK. Sexual desire during the menopausal transition and early postmenopause: observations from the Seattle Midlife Women's Health Study. J Women's Health. 2010;19(2):209–18.
42. George LK, Weiler SJ. Sexuality in middle and late life. The effects of age, cohort and gender. Arch Gen Psychiatry. 1981;38(8):919–23.
43. Hallstrom T, Samuelsson S. Changes in women's sexual desire in middle life: the longitudinal study of women in Gothenburg. Arch Sex Behav. 1990;19(3):259–68.
44. Koster A, Garde K. Sexual desire and menopausal development. A prospective study of Danish women born in 1936. Maturitas. 1993;16(1):49–60.
45. Prairie BA, Scheier MF, Matthews KA, Chang CC, Hess R. A higher sense of purpose in life is associated with sexual enjoyment in midlife women. Menopause. 2011;18(8):839–944.
46. Kling JM, Manson JE, Naughton MH, Temkit M, Sullivan SD, Gower EW, et al. Association of sleep disturbance and sexual function in postmenopausal women. Menopause. 2017;24(6):604–12.
47. Rosen RC, Barsky JL. Normal sexual response in women. Obstet Gynecol Clin N Am. 2006;33(4):515–26.
48. Levine SB. An essay on the nature of sexual drive. J Sex Marital Ther. 1984;10:83–96.
49. Read S, King M, Watson J. Sexual dysfunction in primary medical care: prevalence, characteristics and detection by the general practitioner. J Public Health Med. 1997;19(4):387–91.
50. Ende J, Rockwell S, Glasgow M. The sexual history in general medicine practice. Arch Intern Med. 1984;144(3):558–61.
51. Gott M, Hinchliff S. Barriers to seeking treatment for sexual problems in primary care: a qualitative study with older people. Fam Pract. 2003;20(6):690–5.
52. Pauls RN, Kleeman SD, Segal JL, Silva WA, Goldenhar LM, Karram MM. Practice patterns of physical members of the American Urogynecologic Society regarding female sexual dysfunction: results of a national survey. Int Urogynecol J Pelvic Floor Dysfunct. 2005;16(6):460–7.
53. Roos AM, Thaker R, Sultan AH, Scheer I. Female sexual dysfunction: are urogynecologists ready for it? Int Urogynecol J Pelvic Floor Dysfunct. 2008;20:89–101.
54. Bachmann G. Female sexuality and sexual dysfunction: are we stuck on the learning curve. J Sex Med. 2006;3(4):639–45.
55. Gott M, Galena E, Hinchliff S, Elford H. "Opening a can of worms": GP and practice nurse barriers to talking about sexual health in primary care. Fam Pract. 2004;21(5):528–36.
56. Quirk F, Haughie S, Symonds T. The use of the sexual function questionnaire as a screening tool for women with sexual dysfunction. J Sex Med. 2005;2(4):469–77.
57. Rust J, Derogatis L, Rodenberg C, Koochaki P, Schmidt S, Golombok S. Development and validation of a new screening tool for hypoactive sexual desire disorder: the brief profile of female sexual function (B-PFSF). Gynecol Endocrinol. 2007;23(11):638–44.
58. Clayton AH, Goldfischer ER, Goldstein I, Derogatis L, Lewis-D'Agostino DJ, Pyke R. Validation of the decreased sexual desire screener (DSDS): a brief diagnostic instrument for generalized acquired female hypoactive sexual desire disorder (HSDD). J Sex Med. 2009;6(3):730–8.
59. Isidori AM, Pozza C, Esposito K, Giugliano D, Morano S, Vignozzi L, et al. Development and validation of a 6-item version of the female sexual function index (FSFI) as a diagnostic tool for female sexual dysfunction. J Sex Med. 2010;7(3):1139–46.
60. Kriston L, Gunzler C, Rohde A, Berner MM. Is one question enough to detect female sexual dysfunctions? A diagnostic accuracy study in 6,194 women. J Sex Med. 2010;7(5):1831–41.
61. Giraldi A, Rellini A, Pfaus JG, Bitzer J, Laan E, Jannini EA, Fugi-Meyer AR. Questionnaires for assessment of female sexual dys-

function: a review and proposal for a standardized screener. J Sex Med. 2011;8(10):2681–706.
62. Kingsberg S, Althof SE. Evaluation and treatment of female sexual disorders. Int Urogynecol J. 2009;20(Suppl 1):S33–43.
63. Jeffery DD, Tzeng JP, Keefe FJ, et al. Initial report of the cancer patient-reported outcomes measurement information system (PROMIS) sexual function committee: review of sexual function measures and domains used in oncology. Cancer. 2009;115(6):1142–53.
64. Rosen R, Brown C, Heiman J, Leiblum S, Meston C, Shabsigh R, et al. The female sexual function index (FSFI): a multidimensional self-report instrument for the assessment of female sexual function. J Sex Marital Ther. 2000;26:191–208.
65. Wiegel M, Meston C, Rosen R. The female sexual function index (FSFI): cross-validation and development of clinical cutoff scores. J Sex Marital Ther. 2005;31(1):1–20.
66. Thomas HN, Chang CC, Dillon S, Hess R. Sexual activity in midlife women: importance of sex matters. JAMA Intern Med. 2014;174(4):631–3.
67. Derogatis L, Clayton A, Lewis-D'Agostino D, Wunderlich G, Fu Y. Validation of the female sexual distress scale-revised for assessing distress in women with hypoactive sexual desire disorder. J Sex Med. 2008;5(2):357–64.
68. American Psychiatric Association. Diagnostic and Statistical Manual of Mental Disorders: DSM-5. In: DSM-5 task force. 5th ed. Washington DC: American Psychiatric Association; 2013.
69. Clayton AH, DeRogatis LR, Rosen RC, Pyke R. Intended or unintended consequences? The likely implications of raising the bar for sexual dysfunction diagnosis in the proposed DSM-5 revisions: 2. For women with loss of subjective sexual arousal. J Sex Med. 2012;9(8):2040–6.
70. DeRogatis LR, Clayton AH, Rosen RC, Sand M, Pyke RE. Should sexual desire and arousal disorders in women be merged? Arch Sex Behav. 2011;40(2):217–9.
71. Goldstein I, Kim NN, Clayton AH, et al. Hypoactive sexual desire disorder: International Society for the Study of Women's Sexual Health (ISSWSH) expert consensus panel review. Mayo Clin Proc. 2017;92(1):114–28.
72. Peugh J, Belenko S. Alcohol, drugs and sexual function: a review. J Psychoactive Drugs. 2001;33(3):223–32.
73. Althof SE, Rosen RC, Perelman MA, Rubio-Aurioles E. Standard operating procedures for taking a sexual history. J Sex Med. 2013;10:26–35.
74. Vegunta S, Kling JM, Faubion SS. Sexual health matters: management of female sexual dysfunction. J Women's Health. 2016;25(9):952–4.
75. Kingsberg SA. Taking a sexual history. Obstet Gynecol Clin N Am. 2006;33:535–47.
76. Faubion SS, Shuster LT, Bharucha AE. Recognition and management of nonrelaxing pelvic floor dysfunction. Mayo Clin Proc. 2012;87(2):187–93.
77. Krapf JM, Simon JA. The role of testosterone in the management of hypoactive sexual desire disorder in postmenopausal women. Maturitas. 2009;63:213–9.
78. Davis SR, Davison SL, Donath S, Bell RJ. Circulating androgen levels and self-reported sexual function in women. JAMA. 2005;294:91–6.
79. Serretti A, Chiesa A. Treatment-emergent sexual dysfunction related to antidepressants: a meta-analysis. J Clin Psychopharmacol. 2009;29(3):259–66.
80. Reichenpfader U, Garlehner G, Morgan LC, et al. Sexual dysfunction associated with second-generation antidepressants in patients with major depressive disorder: results from a systemic review with network meta-analysis. Drug Saf. 2014;37(1):19–31.
81. Garlehner G, Hansen RA, Morgan LC, et al. Comparative benefits and harms of second-generation antidepressants for treatment major depressive disorder: an updated meta-analysis. Ann Intern Med. 2011;155(11):772–85.
82. Clayton A, Keller A, McGarvey EL. Burden of phase-specific sexual dysfunction with SSRIs. J Affect Disord. 2006;91(1):27–32.
83. Modell JG, Katholi CR, Modell JD, De Palma RL. Comparative sexual side effects of bupropion, fluoxetine, paroxetine and sertraline. Clin Pharmacol Ther. 1997;61(4):467–87.
84. Croft H, Settle E Jr, Houser T, Batey SR, Donahue RM, Ascher JA. A placebo-controlled comparison of the antidepressant efficacy and effects on sexual functioning of sustained-release bupropion and sertraline. Clin Ther. 1999;21(4):643–58.
85. Coleman CC, King BR, Bolden-Watson C, et al. A placebo-controlled comparison of the effects on sexual functioning of bupropion sustained release and fluoxetine. Clin Ther. 2001;23(7):1040–58.
86. Clayton AH, Croft HA, Horrigan JP, et al. Bupropion extended release compared with escitalopram: effects on sexual functioning and antidepressant efficacy in 2 randomized double-blind, placebo-controlled studies. J Clin Psychiatry. 2006;67(5):736–46.
87. Lewis RW, Fugl-Meyer KS, Bosch R, et al. Epidemiology/risk factors of sexual dysfunction. J Sex Med. 2004;1(1):35–9.
88. Van Lankveld JJ, Grotjohann Y. Psychiatric comorbidity in heterosexual couples with sexual dysfunction assessed with the composite international diagnostic interview. Arch Sex Behav. 2000;29(5):479–98.
89. Mitchell KR, Mercer CH, Ploubidis GB, et al. Sexual function in Britain: findings from the third National Survey of Sexual Attitudes and Lifestyles (Natsal-3). Lancet. 2013;382(9907):1817–29.
90. Lutfey KE, Link CL, Litman HJ, Rosen RC, McKinlay JB. An examination of the association of abuse (physical, sexual, or emotional) and female sexual dysfunctions: results from the Boston Area Community Health Survey. Fertil Steril. 2008;90(4):957–64.
91. Erol B, Tefekli A, Ozbey I, et al. Sexual dysfunction in type II diabetic females: a comparative study. J Sex Marital Ther. 2002;28(Supp. 1):55–62.
92. Enzlin P, Mathieu C, Van den Bruel A, Bosteels J, Vanderschueren D, Demyttenaere K. Sexual dysfunction in women with type 1 diabetes: a controlled study. Diabetes Care. 2002;25(4):672–7.
93. Manolis A, Doumas M. Sexual dysfunction: the 'prima ballerina' of hypertension-related quality-of-life complications. J Hypertens. 2008;26(11):2074–84.
94. Rees PM, Fowler CJ, Maas CP. Sexual function in men and women with neurological disorders. Lancet. 2016;369(9560):512–25.
95. Hulter BM, Lundberg PO. Sexual function in women with advanced multiple sclerosis. J Neurol Neurosurg Psychiatry. 1995;59(1):83–6.
96. Falk SJ, Dizon DS. Sexual dysfunction in women with cancer. Fertil Steril. 2013;100(4):916–21.
97. Gilbert E, Ussher JM, Perz J. Sexuality after breast cancer: a review. Maturitas. 2010;66(4):397–407.
98. Bodurka DC, Sun CC. Sexual function after gynecologic cancer. Obstet Gynecol Clin N Am. 2006;33(4):621–30.
99. Jensen PT, Groenvold M, Klee MC, Thranov I, Petersen MA, Machin D. Longitudinal study of sexual function and vaginal changes after radiotherapy for cervical cancer. Int J Radiat Oncol Biol Phys. 2003;56(4):937–49.
100. Bergmark K, Avall-Lundqvist E, Dickman PW, Henningsohn L, Steineck G. Vaginal changes and sexuality in women with a history of cervical cancer. N Engl J Med. 1999;340(18):1383–9.
101. Thaker R, Manyonda I, Stanton SL, Clarkson P, Robinson G. Bladder, bowel and sexual function after hysterectomy for benign conditions. Br J Obstet Gynaecol. 1997;104(9):983–7.
102. Stippoli GF, Vecchio M, Palmer S, et al. Sexual dysfunction in women with ERSD requiring hemodialysis. Clin J Am Soc Nephrol. 2012;7(6):974–81.

103. Palmer BF. Sexual dysfunction in men and women with chronic kidney disease and end-stage kidney disease. Adv Res Replace Ther. 2003;10(1):48–60.
104. Peng YS, Chiang CK, Kao TW, et al. Sexual dysfunction in female hemodialysis patients: a multicenter study. Kidney Int. 2005;68(2):760–5.
105. Salonia A, Zanni G, Nappi RE, et al. Sexual dysfunction is common in women with lower urinary tract symptoms and urinary incontinence: results of a cross-sectional study. Eur Urol. 2004;45(5):642–8.
106. Handa VL, Harvey L, Cundiff GW, Siddique SA, Kjerulff KH. Sexual function among women with urinary incontinence and pelvic organ prolapse. Am J Obstet Gynecol. 2004;191(3):751–6.
107. Baumgart J, Nilsson K, Evers AJ, Kallak TK, Poromaa LS. Sexual dysfunction in women on adjuvant endocrine therapy after breast cancer. Menopause. 2013;20(2):162–8.
108. Mok K, Juraskova I, Friedlander M. The impact of aromatase inhibitors on sexual functioning: current knowledge and future research directions. Breast. 2008;17(5):436–40.
109. Schover LR. Premature ovarian failure and its consequences: vasomotor symptoms, sexuality, and fertility. J Clin Oncol. 2008;26(5):753–8.
110. Thomas H, Evans GW, Berlowitz DR, et al. Antihypertensive medications and sexual function in women: baseline data from the SBP intervention trial (SPRINT). J Hypertens. 2016;34(6):1224–31.
111. A randomized trial of propranolol in patients with acute myocardial infarction. I. Mortality results. JAMA. 1982;247(12):1707–14.
112. Fogari R, Preti P, Zoppi A, et al. Effect of valsartan and atenolol on sexual behavior in hypertensive postmenopausal women. Am J Hypertens. 2004;17(1):77–81.
113. Clark JD, Elliott J. Gabapentin-induced anorgasmia. Neurology. 1999;53(9):2209.
114. Newman LC, Broner SW, Lay CL. Reversible anorgasmia with topiramate therapy for migraine. Neurology. 2005;65(8):1333–4.
115. Morrell MJ, Flynn KL, Done S, Flaster E, Kalayjian L, Pack AM. Sexual dysfunction, sex steroid hormone abnormalities, and depression in women with epilepsy treated with antiepileptic drugs. Epilepsy Behav. 2005;6(3):36–365.
116. Buster JE. Managing female sexual dysfunction. Fertil Steril. 2013;100(4):905–15.
117. Bonierbale M, Lancon C, Tinol J. The ELIXIR study: evaluation of sexual dysfunction in 4557 depressed patients in France. Curr Med Res Opin. 2003;19(2):114–24.
118. Lorenz T, Rullo J, Faubion S. Antidepressant-induced female sexual dysfunction. Mayo Clin Proc. 2016;91(9):1280–6.
119. Gelenberg AJ, McGahuey C, Laukes C, Okayli G, Moreno F, Zentner L, et al. Mirtazapine substitution in SSRI-induced sexual dysfunction. J Clin Psychiatry. 2000;61:356–60.
120. Koutouvidis N, Pratikakis M, Fotiadou A. The use of mirtazapine in a group of 11 patients following poor compliance to selective serotonin reuptake inhibitor treatment due to sexual dysfunction. Int Clin Psychopharmacol. 1999;14:253–5.
121. Johannes CB, Clayton AH, Odom DM, et al. Distressing sexual problems in the United States women revisited: prevalence after accounting for depression. J Clin Psychiatry. 2009;70(12):1698–706.
122. Ozmenler NK, Karlidere T, Bozkurt A, Yetkin S, Doruk A, Sutcigil L, et al. Mirtazapine augmentation in depressed patients with sexual dysfunction due to selective serotonin reuptake inhibitors. Hum Psychopharmacol. 2008;23:321–6.
123. Taylor MJ, Rudkin L, Bullemor-Day P, Lubin J, Chukwujekwu C, Hawton K. Strategies for managing sexual dysfunction induced by antidepressant medication. Cochrane Database Syst Rev. 2013;(5):CD003382.
124. Lorenz TA, Mston CM. Exercise improves sexual function in women taking antidepressants: results from a randomized crossover trial. Depress Anxiety. 2014;31(3):188–95.
125. Lorenz TA, Meston CM. Acute exercise improves physical sexual arousal in women taking antidepressants. Ann Behav Med. 2012;43(3):352–61.
126. Khamba B, Aucoin M, Lytle M, et al. Efficacy of acupuncture treatment of sexual dysfunction secondary to antidepressants. J Altern Complement Med. 2013;19(11):862–9.
127. McElroy SL, Keck PE Jr, Friedman LM. Minimizing and managing antidepressant side effects. J Clin Psychiatry. 1995;56(suppl 2):49–55.
128. King VL Jr, Horowitz IR. Vaginal anesthesia associated with fluoxetine use. Am J Psychiatry. 1993;150(6):984–5.
129. Numberg HG, Hensley PL, Heiman JR, Croft HA, Debattista C, Pain S. Sildenafil treatment of women with antidepressant associated sexual dysfunction: a randomized controlled trial. JAMA. 2008;300(4):395–404.
130. Fooladi E, Bell RJ, Jane R, Robinson PJ, Kulkami J, Davis SR. Testosterone improves antidepressant-emergent loss of libido in women: findings from a randomized, double-blind, placebo-controlled trial. J Sex Med. 2014;11(3):831–9.
131. O'Mulla C, Doherty M, Coates R, Matt Tilley PJ. 'Accepting what is': an approach for managing the long-term sexual side effects of selective serotonin reuptake inhibitors (SSRs) in women. Sex Relation Ther. 2015;30(3):325–37.
132. Gelenberg AJ, Dunner DL, Rothschild AJ, Pedersen R, Dorries KM, Ninan PT. Sexual functioning in patients with recurrent major depressive disorder enrolled in the PREVENT study. J Nerv Ment Dis. 2013;201(4):266–73.
133. Rothschild AJ. Selective serotonin reuptake inhibitor-induced sexual dysfunction: efficacy of a drug holiday. Am J Psychiatry. 1995;152(10):1514–6.
134. Hirschfeld RM. Management of sexual side effects of antidepressant therapy. J Clin Psychiatry. 1999;60(suppl 14):27–30.
135. Nagoski E. Come as you are: the surprising new science that will transform your sex life. New York: Simon and Schuster; 2015.
136. Heiman J, LoPiccolo J. Becoming orgasmic: a sexual and personal growth program for women. New York: Simon and Schuster; 1987.
137. Leiblum S, Sachs J. Getting the sex you want: a woman's guide to becoming proud, passionate, and pleased in bed. Lincoln, Nebraska: ASJA Press; 2002.
138. Price J. Naked at our age: talking out loud about senior sex. Berkeley: Seal Press; 2011.
139. North American Menopause Society: For Women. Retrieved May 14, 2018, from https://www.menopause.org/for-women.
140. American Association of Sexuality Educators, Counselors, and Therapists (ASSECT): Locate a Professional. Retrieved May 14, 2018, from https://www.aasect.org/referral-directory.
141. Croft HA. Understanding the role of serotonin in female hypoactive sexual desire disorder and treatment options. J Sex Med. 2017;14(12):1575–84.
142. Jaspers L, Feys F, Bramer WM, Franco OH, Leusink P, Laan ET. Efficacy and safety of flibanserin for the treatment of hypoactive sexual desire disorder in women: a systematic review and meta-analysis. JAMA Intern Med. 2016;176(4):453–62.
143. Gao Z, Yang D, Yu L, Cui Y. Efficacy and safety of flibanserin in women with hypoactive desire disorder: a systematic review and meta-analysis. J Sex Med. 2015;12(11):2095–104.
144. Gellad WF, Flynn KE, Alexander GC. Evaluation of flibanserin science and advocacy at the FDA. JAMA. 2015;314(9):869–70.
145. Davis SR, Braunstein GD. Efficacy and safety of testosterone in the management of hypoactive sexual desire disorder in postmenopausal women. J Sex Med. 2012;9(4):1134–48.

146. American College of Obstetricians and Gynecologists Committee on practice bulletins-gynecology, ACOG practice bulletin no. 119: female sexual dysfunction. Obstet Gynecol. 2011;117(4):996–1007.
147. Shifren JL, Davis SR. Androgens in postmenopausal women: a review. Menopause. 2017;24:970–9.
148. Davis SR, Moreau M, Kross R, et al. Testosterone for low libido in postmenopausal women not taking estrogen. N Engl J Med. 2008;359(19):2005–17.
149. Davis SR, Worsley R. Androgen treatment of postmenopausal women. J Steroid Biochem Mol Biol. 2014;142:107–14.
150. Panay N, Al-Azzawi F, Bouchard C, et al. Testosterone treatment of HSDD in naturally menopausal women: the ADORE study. Climacteric. 2010;13(2):121–31.
151. Wierman ME, Arlt W, Basson R, et al. Androgen therapy in women: a reappraisal: an Endocrine Society clinical practice guideline. J Clin Endocrinol Metab. 2014;99(10):3489–510.
152. Braunstein GD. Management of female sexual dysfunction in postmenopausal women by testosterone administration: safety issues and controversies. J Sex Med. 2007;4(4 pt 1):859–66.
153. Gass ML, Stuenkel CA, Utian WH, LaCrois A, Liu JH, Shifren JL. Use of compounded hormone therapy in the United States: report of The North American Menopause Society Survey. Menopause. 2015;22(12):1276–84.
154. McCabe MP. Evaluation of a cognitive behavior therapy program for people with sexual dysfunction. J Sex Marital Ther. 2001;27(3):259–71.
155. Trudel G, Marchand A, Ravart M, Aubin S, Turgeon L, Fortier P. The effect of a cognitive-behavioral group treatment program on hypoactive sexual desire in women. Sex Relatsh Ther. 2001;16(2):145–64.
156. Brotto LA, Basson R, Luria M. A mindfulness-based group psychoeducational intervention targeting sexual arousal disorder in women. J Sex Med. 2008;5(7):1646–59.
157. McMullen S, Rosen RC. Self-administered masturbation training in the treatment of primary orgasmic dysfunction. J Consult Clin Psychol. 1979;47(5):912–8.
158. Billups KL. The role of mechanical devices in treating female sexual dysfunction and enhancing the female sexual response. World J Urol. 2002;20(2):137–41.
159. Wilson SK, Delk JR 2nd, Bilups KL. Treating symptoms of female sexual arousal disorder with the Eros-Clitoral Therapy Device. J Gend Specif Med. 2001;4(2):54–8.
160. Faubion SS, Rullo JE. Sexual dysfunction in women: a practical approach. Am Family Physician. 2015;92(4):281–8.
161. Fugl-Meyer KS, Bohm-Starke N, Damsted Petersen C, Fugl-Meyer A, Parish S, Giraldi A. Standard operating procedures for female genital sexual pain. J Sex Med. 2013;10(1):83–93.
162. Brotto LA, Bitzer J, Laan E, Leiblum S, Luria M. Women's sexual desire and arousal disorders. J Sex Med. 2010;7(1 Pt 2):586–614.
163. Brotto LA, Basson R. Group mindfulness-based therapy significantly improves sexual desire in women. Behav Res Ther. 2014;57:43–54.
164. Brotto LA, Erskine Y, Carey M, et al. A brief mindfulness-based cognitive behavioral intervention improves sexual functioning versus waitlist control in women treated for gynecologic cancer. Gynecol Oncol. 2012;125(2):320–5.
165. Brotto LA, Basson R, Carlson M, Zhu C. Impact of an integrated mindfulness and cognitive behavioral treatment for provoked vestibulodynia (IMPROVED): a qualitative study. Sex Relatsh Ther. 2013;28(1–2):1–16.
166. Glazer HI, Rodke G, Swencionis C, Hertz R, Young AW. Treatment of vulvar vestibulitis syndrome with electromyographic biofeedback of pelvic floor musculature. J Reprod Med. 1995;40(4):283–90.
167. Bergeron S, Binik YM, Khalife S, et al. A randomized comparison group cognitive-behavioral therapy, surface electromyographic biofeedback, and vestibulectomy in the treatment of dyspareunia resulting from vulvar vestibulitis. Pain. 2001;91(3):297–306.
168. Goldstein AT, Pukall CF, Brown C, Bergeron S, Stein A, Kellogg-Spadt S. Vulvodynia: assessment and treatment. J Sex Med. 2016;13(4):572–90.
169. Danielsson L, Torstensson T, Brodda-Jansen G, Bohm-Starke N. EMG biofeedback versus topical lidocaine gel: a randomized study for the treatment of women with vulvar vestibulitis. Acta Obstet Gynecol Scand. 2006;85(11):1360–7.
170. Goetsch MF, Lim JY, Caughey AB. A practical solution for dyspareunia in breast cancer survivors: a randomized controlled trial. J Clin Oncol. 2015;33(30):3394–400.
171. Reed BD, Haefner HK, Cantor L. Vulvar dysesthesia (vulvodynia). A follow-up study. J Reprod Med. 2003;48(6):409–16.
172. Leo RJ. A systematic review of the utility of anticonvulsant pharmacotherapy in the treatment of vulvodynia pain. J Sex Med. 2013;10(8):2000–8.
173. Goldstein AT, Klingman D, Christopher K, Johnson C, Marinoff SC. Surgical treatment of vulvar vestibulitis syndrome: outcome assessment derived from a postoperative questionnaire. J Sex Med. 2006;3(5):923–31.
174. Bergeron S, Bouchard C, Fortier M, Binik YM, Khalife S. The surgical treatment of vulvar vestibulitis syndrome: a follow up study. J Sex Marital Ther. 1997;23(4):147–52.
175. Kehoe S, Luesley D. Vulvar vestibulitis treated by modified vestibulectomy. Int J Gynaecol Obstet. 1999;64(2):147–52.

Fibroids, Endometriosis, and Ovarian Cysts

10

Amy H. Farkas, Sarah A. Tilstra, and Alda Maria R. Gonzaga

Learning Objectives

1. Describe the clinical presentation and diagnostic evaluation related to uterine fibroids.
2. Counsel women on the management options available to treat bleeding and/or bulk symptoms secondary to fibroids.
3. Explain the clinical presentation and treatment of endometriosis.
4. List the differential diagnosis, diagnostic work-up, and management of ovarian cysts.
5. Assess the risk for ovarian cancer in women with an ovarian cyst and determine when referral to gynecology oncologist is appropriate.

Fibroids (Leiomyomas)

Georgette is a 46-year-old woman who presents to clinic complaining of fatigue and increasingly heavy menses. While manageable in her 30s, her menstrual cycles are now heavier and occasionally she passes clots. Her hemoglobin is 7.2 g/dl.

A. H. Farkas
Department of Internal Medicine, Medical College of Wisconsin, Clement Zablocki VA, Milwaukee, WI, USA

S. A. Tilstra
University of Pittsburgh School of Medicine, Division of General Internal Medicine, Department of Medicine, Pittsburgh, PA, USA

A. M. R. Gonzaga (✉)
University of Pittsburgh School of Medicine, Departments of Medicine and Pediatrics, Pittsburgh, PA, USA
e-mail: gonzagaa@upmc.edu

Epidemiology

Fibroids, also known as leiomyomas, are benign tumors of smooth muscle in the uterus. Fibroids are the most common benign tumor in reproductive age women with a cumulative incidence of up to 70% in White women and up to 80% in Black women by age 50 [1]. One-third of women affected by fibroids will be symptomatic [2], and roughly one-quarter of these women will have symptoms severe enough to require treatment [3]. The two strongest risk factors for developing fibroids are age (until menopause) and Black race [4], though the reasons why Black women experience more symptoms and complications from fibroids than White women are unknown and require further study [3]. Other risk factors include nulliparity, use of oral contraceptives prior to age 16, and obesity [5, 6]; genetics may also play a role given that chromosomal abnormalities in fibroids have been documented [6]. Increasing parity, diets rich in fruits and vegetables, and the use of injectable progesterone contraception serve as protective factors against the development of fibroids [6].

Physiology and Pathophysiology

Fibroids grow from the myometrium and are classified by their location in the uterus [7]. The International Federation of Gynecology and Obstetrics has developed a detailed classification system which assigns fibroids a number 0–9 based on their relation to the endometrium (lower number) and serosal surface (higher number) [8]. In general, submucosal fibroids arise from the myometrium nearest the uterine cavity and often extend into the cavity itself; intramural fibroids are located completely within the myometrium, and subserosal fibroids are derived from the myometrium nearest the visceral surface of the uterus and can grow on the external surface of the uterus. Both submucosal and subserosal fibroids can be pedunculated, i.e., can grow on a stalk [7, 8].

S. A. Tilstra et al. (eds.), *Sex- and Gender-Based Women's Health*, https://doi.org/10.1007/978-3-030-50695-7_10

The location of the fibroid impacts the symptoms that a woman may experience [9].

There is limited data regarding the natural history of fibroids and both substantial growth and regression are common [10]. Hormones were initially hypothesized to play a role in fibroid growth because fibroids are not found before puberty and tend to regress in size following menopause. Additionally, smooth muscle cells in fibroids express higher rates of steroid hormone receptors, growth factors, and growth factor receptors relative to normal myometrium. These receptors make fibroid tissue exquisitely sensitive to estrogen, progesterone, and growth factors such as vascular endothelial growth factor (VEGF), which helps to facilitate aberrant growth [6].

Given Georgette's low hemoglobin and heavy menstrual cycles, you suspect an intrauterine lesion. A transvaginal ultrasound demonstrates a large submucosal fibroid.

Clinical Manifestations

The most common presenting symptoms of fibroids are heavy vaginal bleeding and bulk symptoms [11, 12]. Submucosal fibroids, because they are located close to the endometrium, often present with dysmenorrhea, heavy menses, or abnormal uterine bleeding (see Chap. 7 on Abnormal Uterine Bleeding). Some of these women may not recognize their bleeding as abnormal and may present with symptoms related to iron deficiency anemia such as fatigue, pallor, dyspnea, or pica, which refers to cravings for soil, raw starches, or ice. Large fibroids in any location can produce bulk symptoms, which can be vague in nature and hard for patients to describe. Women may complain of heaviness or pain in their pelvic region [12]. If the fibroid is pushing on or obstructing the bladder, they may have urinary symptoms such as retention or urge incontinence or may experience problems with defecation if the fibroid is obstructing the colon. Fibroids can also cause bloating, impact sexual function, and cause dyspareunia in some women [9, 12].

While women may present with abnormal uterine bleeding or bulk symptoms, many women with one or more fibroids are asymptomatic. In this case, fibroids may be first apparent on physical examination. Providers may feel a pelvic mass or an enlarged or abnormally contoured uterus during the bimanual exam. Subserosal fibroids can be palpated as a distinct mass on abdominal exam. In addition to detection on physical examination, some fibroids are incidentally noted on abdominal and pelvic imaging obtained for other indications [1].

Data are inconclusive regarding the role that fibroids play in infertility and miscarriage. While both submucosal fibroids and intramural fibroids have been associated with infertility, it is difficult to determine causality [13]. Fibroids are present in approximately one-quarter of women seeking treatment for infertility, but are only thought to cause infertility in 13% of infertile women [14]. A 2009 systematic review found that the benefit of myomectomy in infertile women varied based on the location of the fibroid; myomectomy in women with submucosal fibroids may improve fertility rates, while women with intramural fibroids had no change in conception rate or pregnancy after myomectomy [13]. However, a Cochrane review conducted in 2012 found insufficient evidence from randomized controlled trials to support myomectomy for women with infertility regardless of fibroid location [15]. Couples with infertility require a complete assessment for both partners before concluding that fibroids are the cause of infertility. At the time of publication, experts recommend offering myomectomy to women struggling with infertility thought to be due to fibroids, but only to those with submucosal fibroids [16].

With regard to miscarriage rates, previous literature has found an increased risk of spontaneous abortion among women with fibroids; however, the most recent meta-analysis conducted in 2017 found no such association in an analysis of more than 20,000 pregnant women in the general obstetric population [17].

Differential Diagnosis

Women will either present with the incidental finding of a fibroid or with a symptom for which fibroids can be on the differential diagnosis. As described earlier in the chapter, abnormal uterine bleeding (AUB) and dysmenorrhea are common; it is critical to consider the full differential for AUB even in the setting of a known fibroid [9]. While fibroids are one cause of AUB, other causes include endometrial polyps, endometrial hyperplasia or carcinoma, adenomyosis, thyroid disease, coagulopathies, and medications. It is important to consider the risk for endometrial hyperplasia or carcinoma and indications for endometrial biopsy in these women [10]. Risk factors for endometrial cancer fall under the umbrella of exposure to unopposed estrogen and include early menarche, late menopause, chronic anovulation, and obesity. Women with a family history of genetic cancer syndromes such as Lynch syndrome are also at increased risk [18]. Please see Chap. 7 on Abnormal Uterine Bleeding and Chap. 15 on Gynecological Malignancies for more information.

Since bulk symptoms are hard to describe for some women, fibroids should be on the differential diagnosis for any woman presenting with pelvic pressure, urinary incontinence, bloating, constipation, sexual dysfunction, and dyspareunia as women may present with any of these symptoms [7]. Pelvic pain is less common with fibroids but may represent torsion or degeneration of the fibroid [7]; therefore, one should consider a wide differential in women presenting with pelvic pain including endometriosis, adenomyosis, prior pelvic inflammatory disease, adhesions, myofascial pelvic pain syndrome, as well as urologic and gastrointestinal causes of chronic pelvic pain. While fibroids can cause urinary symptoms due to mass effect on the bladder, neurogenic causes of urinary retention, incontinence, and difficulty with defecation must also be explored [19]. Bloating in the abdomen in women with a pelvic mass should raise concern for a malignancy, particularly if it is associated with early satiety or ascites [20]. Keep in mind that fibroids are common and their presence on exam or imaging does not ensure causation of clinical complaints [21]. History, physical exam findings, and diagnostic work-up must be thorough to exclude other disease processes occurring concomitantly.

Once a diagnosis of fibroids has been made, one must also consider uterine sarcoma in the differential diagnosis of fibroids. Albeit a rare gynecologic malignancy, uterine sarcomas and benign leiomyomas can be indistinguishable in clinical presentation and imaging [7]. Unfortunately, there are currently no definitive means to diagnose uterine sarcoma among women presenting for fibroid treatment; however, patients who present with growth of a suspected fibroid, have excessive bleeding, or have progressive symptoms in the postmenopausal period should prompt consideration for malignancy [7]. Risk factors such as advanced age, history of pelvic irradiation, genetic cancer syndromes, and tamoxifen use can also be taken into account when choosing to pursue a cancer evaluation [22]. Endometrial biopsy and MR imaging may indicate the presence of a uterine sarcoma, but normal studies do not rule it out [23, 24] . Please see Chap. 15 on Gynecologic Malignancies for more information.

Diagnostic Strategies

When fibroids are suspected, transvaginal ultrasound is the preferred imaging modality to confirm diagnosis. If an abdominal mass is palpated on exam, an abdominal ultrasound should also be ordered.

It is important to complete appropriate testing for women presenting for bleeding and bulk symptoms even after fibroids are confirmed on imaging. For women with heavy menstrual bleeding or intermenstrual bleeding, testing for pregnancy, thyroid disease, and coagulation disorders should be done [10]. Coagulation defects in platelets and the coagulation cascade can cause menorrhagia; thus, checking a CBC with platelets, PT/INR/PTT, and von Willebrand disease screen is appropriate in this population. Chronic heavy bleeding should also trigger an evaluation for anemia and iron deficiency as young women can be asymptomatic even at very low hemoglobin levels. Additionally, an endometrial biopsy may be appropriate for certain women at higher risk for endometrial hyperplasia and carcinoma and considered for any woman greater than 45 that presents with heavy vaginal bleeding [25]. See Chap. 7 on Abnormal Uterine Bleeding for a detailed review of the evaluation for vaginal bleeding.

Additional imaging should be obtained if a provider suspects that gastrointestinal or urologic conditions are contributing to bulk symptoms, especially if there is concern for an abdominal mass or ascites on exam.

Georgette is seen by gynecologist and an endometrial biopsy is obtained, which is normal. After discussing her management options with gynecologist, she chooses to undergo endometrial ablation to reduce her bleeding.

Treatment Strategies

Only women with symptomatic fibroids need to be treated [7]; it is appropriate to monitor women clinically who present with minor symptoms. There is no evidence to support routine imaging of these women [7] as most often, fibroids regress in size and cause fewer symptoms over time, particularly after the menopause [26]. For symptomatic women, the treatment options are divided into women who are experiencing bleeding symptoms versus those who have bulk symptoms.

Managing Bleeding Symptoms

Medications are considered the first line of therapies to control bleeding and improve quality of life for women who are experiencing heavy bleeding. Nonsteroidal anti-inflammatory medications (NSAIDs) have been shown to help reduce heavy bleeding and pain associated with menstruation, but there are no studies that document these effects for women with symptoms thought to be secondary to fibroids. Despite this, moderate to high doses (600–800 mg 2–3 times per day of ibuprofen) are used either just before or at the first sign of menstruation to help with symptoms [9]. Oral contraceptive pills, both combination and progesterone-only pills, can help to reduce bleeding in women with fibroids [7, 9]. A Cochrane review conducted in 2013 found that progesterone intrauterine devices (IUDs) were effective at reducing heavy vaginal bleeding secondary to fibroids and are considered an excellent management option by both the American College of Obstetricians and Gynecologists (ACOG) and the Society of Obstetricians and Gynaecologists of Canada (SOGC) [7, 9]. There are concerns that women with fibroids may have higher expulsion rates of IUDs than women without [9, 25] due to the irregular contour of the uterine cavity or malposition; however, these rates are very low and women should not be deterred from considering IUD placement. While there is some evidence demonstrating that tranexamic acid, an antifibrinolytic that works by inhibiting plasmin, can reduce menorrhagia in women with fibroids [27], it is not currently recommended as a treatment strategy by either ACOG or SOGC [7, 9].

When medications do not adequately address bleeding symptoms, hysteroscopic myomectomy (surgical removal of the fibroid) or endometrial ablation can be considered. For women who desire fertility preservation, hysteroscopic myomectomy is the first-line option for women with submucosal fibroids [7]. Hysteroscopic myomectomy, where the fibroid is surgically resected, improves bleeding symptoms and potentially improves pregnancy rates by restoring the shape of the uterine cavity, which may have been distorted by the fibroid [13]. For women who do not desire future fertility, endometrial ablation may be an option. Ablation is accomplished by insertion of a probe into the uterine cavity via the cervix; heat (most commonly radiofrequency), cold, or mechanical means is/are used to destroy the endometrial lining [10]. It is important to remember that women who have undergone ablation still require contraception as ablation does not necessarily cause infertility and pregnancy complications can increase following the procedure [10].

Managing Bulk Symptoms

For women who are experiencing bulk symptoms, gonadotropin-releasing hormone (GnRH) agonists can reduce the size of fibroids; however, they are not considered a long-term option given their significant side effect profile including hot flashes, vaginal dryness, and bone health concerns. Use should be limited to 6 months [9]. GnRH agonists can be helpful as a short-term bridge to menopause or used prior to a planned surgical intervention to help reduce the size of the fibroids preoperatively [9].

Three uterine-sparing options for management of bulk symptoms include myomectomy, uterine artery embolization, and MRI-assisted ultrasound therapy. Myomectomy (as described above) is the preferred option for women who wish to preserve their fertility. It has similar complications and risks as hysterectomy. Uterine artery embolization is an interventional radiology procedure which treats the entire uterus by injecting embolizing particles into the uterine arteries. While there have been reports of successful pregnancies following uterine artery embolization, it is not the preferred method for women who desire future pregnancy as limited data suggest that pregnancy rates may be better among women who undergo myomectomy [21]. There is some concern for loss of ovarian function following embolization, but a recent systematic review found no difference in fertility between surgery and embolization [28]. When compared to myomectomy, women who underwent uterine artery embolization have higher rates of re-intervention and future hysterectomies but have lower rates of procedural complications [21, 28, 29]. MRI-guided focused ultrasound therapy uses ultrasound thermal ablation to treat bulk symptoms from fibroids. It is a well-tolerated treatment with improvement in both fibroid size and quality of life [30], though little data exist regarding how ultrasound therapy compares to alternative treatments [29]. There are documented cases of successful pregnancy following ultrasound therapy but the data remains limited [30]. Despite their success, many women who choose uterine-sparing options will often require a second procedure, with estimates as high as 15–17% [29].

Hysterectomy is the most common procedure for women experiencing bulk symptoms and is the most definitive treatment for either bleeding or bulk symptoms [16, 29]. Hysterectomy is only appropriate for women who no longer desire fertility. There are surgical risks associated with hysterectomy [10], and new data suggest that women who undergo hysterectomy, even with ovarian preservation, have an increased risk of cardiovascular disease [31]. There is also data to suggest that women who choose hysterectomy have higher quality of life following the procedure [2].

When to Refer

Women with persistent bleeding despite optimal medical therapy should be referred to gynecologist to consider additional evaluation and procedural management. Additionally, women with abnormal uterine bleeding in the setting of fibroids who are over 45 years of age require endometrial biopsy; biopsy should also be considered for younger women with BMI >30 [25, 32].

Endometriosis

Lynda is a 34-year-old woman who presents to clinic to discuss painful menstrual cycles. She mentions that she finds sex painful and that she and her husband have been attempting to conceive for the past year without success.

Epidemiology

Endometriosis, the presence of endometrial gland tissue implanted on peritoneal surfaces outside the uterus, occurs conservatively in 10–11% of women [33, 34]. In women diagnosed with infertility, the estimated prevalence lies between 25% and 50% [35, 36], while 40–80% of women with chronic pelvic pain have been reported to have endometriosis [36–38]. As endometriosis is definitively diagnosed by laparoscopic tissue biopsy, prevalence and incidence rates vary widely between studies. As a result, women are often older than 30 years of age when they are diagnosed with endometriosis [33].

Non-Hispanic White women are diagnosed with endometriosis more commonly than women of other racial and ethnic backgrounds [33]. Risk factors for endometriosis include early menarche and late menopause (which allows for increased exposure to estrogen over time), menstrual outflow obstruction, and short menstrual cycles [34]. Protective factors include multiple pregnancies and prolonged lactation [34].

Table 10.1 Symptoms and corresponding odds ratios present in women with endometriosis vs. women without endometriosis [37]

Symptom	Odds ratio (95% CI)
Subfertility	8.2 (6.9–9.9)
Dysmenorrhea	8.1 (7.2–9.3)
Ovarian cysts (endometriomas)	7.3 (5.7–9.4)
Dyspareunia and/or postcoital bleeding	6.8 (5.7–8.2)
Abdominopelvic pain	5.2 (4.7–5.7)
Menorrhagia	4.0 (3.5–4.5)

Physiology and Pathophysiology

The pathophysiology of endometriosis is not well understood but may be secondary to implantation of endometrial tissue outside of the uterus as a result of retrograde menstruation [39]. Implantation of this estrogen-sensitive tissue onto the peritoneal surface of the abdomen elicits a local inflammatory response. This pathogenic inflammatory response can lead to debilitating pain at or near the sites of endometrial implants due to local scarring, development of adhesions, distortion of the pelvic anatomy, and alterations in the neuronal pathways that process pain [39]. Implantation on ovarian tissue is common and results in endometrial lined ovarian cysts (chocolate cysts or endometriomas) that are seen in 55% of affected women. Endometrial implants are found on the peritoneum of the pelvic floor (35% of affected women), uterus (11%), fallopian tubes (1–4%), bladder (1%), and rectum (0.5%) [40]. There are rare case reports of more distant endometrial tissue implants, such as on the liver [38], within the bowel wall [41], and within the pleural space [42]. All endometrial tissue is hormone sensitive; thus women tend to be relatively more symptomatic at the time of the menses. When hormones are altered by medication or by menopause, symptoms often improve [43].

Clinical Manifestations

Women with endometriosis experience a wide array of symptoms. Most commonly, patients describe chronic dysmenorrhea; dyspareunia; abdominal, back, or pelvic pain; and fatigue (Table 10.1). The pain of endometriosis is variable and often occurs with menses, usually starting a few days before and lasting until the cycle is complete. The pain often feels "crampy" but can be sharp and stabbing at times. As the disease progresses, patients often develop chronic, occasionally debilitating, pelvic pain. Sexual activity, particularly deep vaginal penetration, can trigger pain as the anterior and posterior cul-de-sacs and the pouch of Douglas are common sites for endometrial implants [40]. Patients can also struggle with bowel and bladder symptoms such as nausea, abdominal distention, tenesmus, dysuria, or hematuria due to inflammation associated with endometrial implants within the bowel wall, bladder, genitourinary tract, and abdominal wall [41].

Up to half of women with infertility will be diagnosed with endometriosis [35, 36], and patients may be unaware that they are affected until they try to conceive. The exact mechanism and extent as to how endometriosis affects fertility is unknown; researchers postulate that inflammation, cytokine activity, macrophage activation, and mechanical obstruction affect hormone concentrations, oocyte development and release, sperm motility, embryo transport, endometrium receptivity, and implantation [44]. Patients with endometriosis often experience significant debility due to chronic pain and decreased fertility. Additionally, women with endometriosis may suffer from concomitant depression and/or anxiety related to their endometriosis [45].

The diagnosis of endometriosis can lag by months or years as clinical symptoms can be vague and nonspecific. In one study of American women with surgically confirmed endometriosis, symptom onset occurred an average of 11.73 ± 9.05 years before diagnosis [46]. In that study, women with chronic pain due to endometriosis had a delay in diagnosis of 9.21 ± 6.21 years between 1979 and 1984, which decreased to 4.63 ± 4.62 years between 1990 and 1995; in women with infertility due to endometriosis, the delay in diagnosis decreased from 3.52 ± 2.53 to 2.93 ± 2.57 years, respectively [47]. Increased physician awareness of endometriosis has likely contributed to improvements in time to diagnosis [47].

Most women will have a normal pelvic exam, but some patients will have rectovaginal nodularity, limited motion of the uterus or ovaries, an adnexal mass, or tenderness in the posterior fornix on exam. A rectovaginal exam may be indicated in order to allow palpation of the uterosacral ligament and rectovaginal septum that can harbor painful nodules rep-

Table 10.2 Differential diagnosis of chronic pelvic pain

Gynecologic	Non-gynecologic
Endometriosis	Irritable bowel syndrome
Pelvic inflammatory disease	Inflammatory bowel disease
Pelvic adhesions	Interstitial cystitis
Ovarian cysts or masses	Myofascial pain syndrome
Fibroids	Pelvic floor dysfunction
Adenomyosis	Depression
Vulvovaginal atrophy	Trauma and sexual abuse
Pelvic congestion syndrome	

Table 10.3 Differential diagnosis of female infertility

Structural/tubal factors	Ovulatory dysfunction	Others
Pelvic inflammatory disease	Polycystic ovary syndrome	Antiphospholipid syndrome
Endometriosis	Primary ovarian failure	Genetic factors
Adhesions from pelvic surgery	Functional hypothalamic amenorrhea	Unexplained
Cervical stenosis	Hyperprolactinemia	
Uterine anomalies (e.g., septate uterus)	Medical illness (e.g, uncontrolled diabetes mellitus)	
Uterine fibroids	Thyroid disease	
	Advanced maternal age	

resenting endometrial implants. Additionally, examination during menstruation may provide a better assessment of pain and help detect deeply infiltrating disease [48].

Differential Diagnosis

Given the vague symptoms associated with endometriosis, a lengthy differential diagnosis should be considered for the two most common manifestations: chronic pelvic pain (Table 10.2) and infertility (Table 10.3). A careful history and physical exam can help differentiate disorders associated with chronic pelvic pain. See Chap. 31 on Chronic Pelvic Pain to appreciate how patients with endometriosis present differently than patients with other causes of pelvic pain. There are also full chapters dedicated to Irritable Bowel Syndrome (Chap. 27), Sexually Transmitted Infections (Chap. 13), Interstitial Cystitis (Chap. 30), Chronic Pelvic Pain (Chap. 31), and Intimate Partner Violence and Sexual Trauma (Chap. 35).

Diagnostic Strategies

Most providers err on the side of making a "presumed" diagnosis of endometriosis based on history, physical exam findings, and the absence of objective findings for other causes of symptoms; this is the preferred path of evaluation and treatment by the Society of Obstetricians and Gynaecologists of Canada (SOGC) [48]. This is because the gold standard of diagnosis is direct visualization and tissue biopsy, often completed during diagnostic laparoscopy, or cystoscopy, colonoscopy, or speculum exam if there are endometrial implants outside of the peritoneal cavity. Laparoscopy is indicated when medical management fails, with a goal of both confirming the presumed diagnosis and treating symptoms via debulking [48]. Endometriosis can be staged at laparoscopy using the Revised Classification of Endometriosis Staging system form by the American Society for Reproductive Medicine [49], ranging from Stage I, minimal disease, to Stage IV, severe disease. Disease staging is the standard approach for reporting surgical findings; however, it does not correlate with severity of pain or predict responsiveness to treatment [50].

Prior to a laparoscopy, providers can obtain imaging studies to aid in diagnosis. Transvaginal ultrasonography (TVUS) reliably detects endometriomas, which are cystic masses arising from ectopic endometrial tissue within or on the ovary [51]. TVUS has a sensitivity and specificity of 89% and 91%, respectively, for endometriomas when an ovarian mass is adequately visualized; however, it can miss smaller lesions [51]. TVUS can also reliably detect deeply infiltrating endometriosis (serosal/muscular layer) in the rectal region with a sensitivity and specificity of 98% and 99% but may miss more superficial lesions [52]. The use of magnetic resonance imaging (MRI) to aid in detection of endometriosis has been studied but performs less accurately than ultrasonography [53]. However, MRI can be used to evaluate for other structural lesions in the pelvis if there are questionable findings on TVUS. Given the lower cost of ultrasonography and higher detection rates, it is the preferred initial imaging modality in patients suspected to have endometriosis. If no lesions are found on TVUS, this does not exclude a diagnosis of endometriosis. CA-125, a cancer marker for ovarian cancer, has been studied extensively but has limited utility in the diagnosis of endometriosis given its poor sensitivity and specificity [54].

Treatment Strategies

Approaches to treating endometriosis are best organized by symptom management.

Treatments for Chronic Pelvic Pain Due to Endometriosis

Nonsteroidal anti-inflammatory drugs (NSAIDs) are the most common first-line treatment for pain, as they have been shown to reduce symptoms of dysmenorrhea. However, there is inconclusive evidence that NSAIDs are more effective than placebo in treating endometriosis [55].

Hormonal treatments that suppress ovarian function reduce disease activity and pain associated with endometriosis. Ovarian suppression limits the hormonal exposure to endometrial tissue outside of the uterine cavity, which in turn limits the local inflammatory response, chronic scarring, and neuronal dysfunction. Evidence supports the use of combined hormonal oral contraceptives, administered either cyclically or continuously, and continuous progestins (e.g., medroxyprogesterone acetate, norethindrone, cyproterone acetate, or dienogest) [56]. The most effective treatment for pain relief from ovarian suppression is gonadotrophin-releasing hormone analogues (GnRHa) such as leuprolide or goserelin, which are associated with relief of pelvic tenderness and painful menstrual cycles when compared with placebo or no treatment [57]. However, these agents are often poorly tolerated due to clinical manifestations of the "medical menopause" they induce, such as hot flashes and vaginal dryness [57]. Low-dose estrogen-progestin add-back therapies can minimize these side effects [56]. Moderate-quality evidence demonstrates that levonorgestrel intrauterine system controls pain better than expectant management [58]. This is likely due to the local effect of progestin on the pelvic tissues and not due to ovarian suppression though the exact mechanism is unclear [58].

Laparoscopic ablation or excision of lesions reduces pain at 6 months when compared with diagnostic laparoscopy. Excision of endometrioma cyst walls appears more effective at controlling pain than ablation. However, surgical resection of endometriomas does reduce ovarian reserve and can negatively impact fertility. Strategies should be taken during such surgeries to minimize the damage to the normal ovary to optimize future fertility, and patients should be informed of these risks before proceeding [58, 59].

Endometriosis recurs after surgery, with rates ranging from 10% to 50%. Regardless of the amount of endometriosis visualized and removed during laparoscopy, patients' pain may progress or remain unchanged. Expectations of treatments should be discussed with patients, and realistic goals should be set, especially prior to any invasive intervention. Additional therapies include the FDA-approved oral GnRH antagonist elagolix, and the potential use of immunotherapy or aromatase inhibitors [60, 61].

Treatments for Infertility Due to Endometriosis

As noted above, endometriosis frequently leads to infertility. Patients with endometriosis and infertility should undergo a work-up to identify reversible causes; this work-up may be initiated by the primary care provider but is ideally performed in conjunction with the patient's gynecologic care provider and/or a reproductive endocrinologist. Once endometriosis is established as the cause of the infertility, treatment focuses on attempting to restore normal ovulation and anatomy by removing endometrial tissue and adhesions in the pelvic cavity. Two main types of surgical interventions have been studied, laparoscopic excision of endometrioma cyst walls and ablation of endometrial implants. Overall, these interventions are similar in improving pregnancy and live birth rates but this is based on low-quality data [59]. Patients should be counseled that laparoscopic surgical intervention could be a promising modality for women with mild or moderate disease in reducing pain and improving fertility, but decisions about the efficacy, type, and timing of procedure must be made in consultation with their surgeon [59, 62].

If surgical resection of endometrial tissue is unsuccessful, referral for assisted reproductive technology (ART) is indicated. In vitro fertilization (IVF) is also recommended as first-line treatment for women with advanced disease due to the risk of decreasing ovarian reserve during surgery [63]. There is no role for ovarian suppression with combined oral contraceptive, GnRHa, medroxyprogesterone acetate, or diazole in the treatment of infertility [64]. However, some data suggest using GnRHa prior to IVF for women with infertility secondary to endometriosis to increase pregnancy rates [63].

There is no evidence that complementary medicine treatments of acupuncture and Chinese herbal medicine are effective in managing the pain or infertility associated with endometriosis [65, 66]. However, patients should be encouraged to seek treatments that they feel minimize their pain and increase their quality of life.

When to Refer

Primary care providers should be comfortable identifying and treating women with presumed endometriosis. If symptom control cannot be achieved with hormonal methods (continuous progestins or combined oral contraceptives) or supportive care (NSAIDs), then referral to gynecologist for medical (i.e., GnRHa) and/or surgical evaluation and treatment is appropriate. Any couple who has been attempting to conceive for greater than 1 year should be referred for an infertility assessment, especially if the woman has chronic pelvic pain. When a woman is unsuccessful in conceiving after 6 months and she is over 35 years old, referral to gynecologist or reproductive endocrinologist is recommended [67].

Ovarian Cysts

Juliana is a 32-year-old woman who presents to you for follow-up after a visit to the emergency department for right-sided abdominal pain. While she was in the emergency department, she had a CT scan and was told that she has an ovarian cyst.

Epidemiology

Ovarian cysts are common in women of all ages. Reproductive age women develop a functional cyst every month as the ovary prepares for ovulation. The prevalence of ovarian cysts in premenopausal women is variable, anywhere from 7% in healthy women [68] to 35% in first- or second-degree relatives of patients with ovarian cancer [69]. Despite the cessation of menses, postmenopausal women develop ovarian cysts as well. Data from the Prostate, Lung, Colorectal, and Ovarian Cancer Screening Trial found that among postmenopausal women, 14% had a simple unilocular cyst detected on initial transvaginal ultrasound with a 1-year incidence of new cysts of 8% [70]; however other studies have documented the prevalence in postmenopausal women as low as 2.5% [71]. The vast majority of cysts are asymptomatic and discovered incidentally on imaging or during physical exam [72]. The difficult job that providers face is determining which cysts are likely benign and which are more concerning for ovarian malignancy.

Physiology and Pathophysiology

There are several different types of ovarian cysts including functional or simple cysts, hemorrhagic cysts, endometriomas, and mature teratomas (dermoid cyst). A functional or simple cyst occurs as a follicle develops and fails to rupture or after a follicle ovulates but the corpus luteum continues to increase in size instead of involuting. Hemorrhagic cysts occur when there is bleeding into a functional cyst or corpus luteum [73]. As discussed above, endometriomas result when endometrial tissue is located inside an ovarian cyst and may present with symptoms of endometriosis. Mature teratomas, the most common type of ovarian germ cell tumor, appear as complex cysts. They are derived from all three germ cell layers and generally made up of different types of tissue including hair, teeth, skin, muscle, and connective tissue [74].

The majority of cysts are benign, even in postmenopausal women, and will resolve over time. In 1 study of pre- and postmenopausal women, 3511 adnexal masses were identified, of which 1148 were classified as unilocular cysts. In the group of unilocular cysts, only 11 were malignant on pathological exam for a malignancy rate of <1%; however, on pathology reports, 7 of the 11 unilocular cysts had solid components; thus they had been misclassified as benign on ultrasound prior to surgical resection [75]. In another study, 15,106 women over the age of 50 were screened with transvaginal ultrasound, and 18% (2763) of participants were diagnosed with a simple cyst, all of which were less than 10 cm in diameter. After 6.3 years of follow-up, two-thirds of these simple cysts resolved, and none of these 2763 women developed ovarian cancer [76]. The rest of this chapter will focus on evaluation and management of simple ovarian cysts.

With regard to other cyst types, endometriomas and mature teratomas can be managed expectantly with serial imaging [72]. Surgical removal of endometriomas can negatively affect ovarian reserve [77] and therefore should be avoided when possible.

Clinical Manifestations

Ovarian cysts often produce no symptoms; however, for women who do experience symptoms, pelvic or abdominal pain is the most common presenting complaint [78]. Ovarian cysts cause abdominal or pelvic pain by mass effect on the surrounding structures in the pelvis, acute stretching of the ovarian cortex during rupture, or from peritoneal irritation from a ruptured or slowly leaking cyst that causes a local inflammatory reaction. Women presenting with increased abdominal girth and bloating should raise the concern for ovarian cancer compared to a benign ovarian cyst [78]. The presence of an ovarian cyst in a woman with abdominal or pelvic pain may not be the cause of her pain, and additional work-up is indicated depending on presenting symptoms.

Juliana has noticed the pain on the right side of her lower abdomen for about a month. It is worse with her menstrual cycles. She reports pain with sexual intercourse, particularly deep penetration. On exam, there is tenderness in the right adnexa; however, there is no enlargement or nodularity and the exam is otherwise normal.

Differential Diagnosis

The differential diagnosis of an adnexal mass includes both benign and malignant etiologies (Table 10.4) [72].

A thorough history informs the differential diagnosis of an adnexal mass, with particular focus on ovarian cancer risk factors. Age is the number one risk factor for ovarian cancer; the average age at diagnosis is 63 years, and risk continues to rise with age [79]. Providers also need to take a detailed family history, including breast cancer, ovarian cancer, and familial cancer syndromes, such as BRCA 1&2. Women with a family history of ovarian cancer but without a BRCA history have a lifetime risk of ovarian cancer of 5–8.1% [80, 81], whereas women who have the BRCA gene have a life-

Table 10.4 Differential diagnosis of adnexal mass [72]

Benign	Malignant
Functional cysts	Epithelial carcinoma
Endometrioma	Germ cell tumor
Hemorrhagic cysts	Sex cord or stromal tumor
Mature teratoma (dermoid)	Metastatic cancer
Cystadenoma (mucinous or serous)	
Hydrosalpinx	
Paratubal cysts	
Fibroid	
Mullerian anomalies	
Medical emergencies Tubo-ovarian abscess Ectopic pregnancy	

time risk of ovarian cancer of up to 46% [82]. Additional risk factors for ovarian cancer include nulliparity, early menarche, late menopause, and obesity [79]. See Chap. 15 on Gynecologic Malignancies for additional information.

Beyond assessing the risk for malignancy, it is also important to evaluate for any gynecological complaints that may require more urgent management in the setting of adnexal tenderness or a pelvic mass. While a cyst may cause pain, one should consider evaluation for ovarian torsion, pelvic inflammatory disease (PID), tubo-ovarian abscess (TOA), acute hemorrhage into a cyst or rupture, or an ectopic pregnancy, particularly if the pain is acute in nature [83]. Patients with infectious etiologies like PID and TOA may have fevers, chills, nausea, vomiting, peritonitis, vaginal discharge, and a history of unprotected sex or new sexual partner(s). The pain from ovarian torsion is often described as unilateral and "colicky," as the ovary twists upon itself and the blood supply to the gonad is compromised. Patients can have sharp unrelenting pain from an ectopic pregnancy and, if ruptured, signs of hemodynamic instability and peritonitis [83]. Acute rupture of the cyst can cause severe pain that may mimic an abdominal catastrophe. Rupture can be triggered by sexual activity and tends to occur late in the menstrual cycle, between days 20 and 26. While hemorrhage from a ruptured ovarian cyst can occur, hemodynamic compromise from this is rare [84]. Gastrointestinal and urological causes of pain such as appendicitis, diverticulitis, and nephrolithiasis can also mimic pain caused by an ovarian cyst and must be ruled out. A complete history and review of systems can help guide the differential diagnosis.

Diagnostic Strategies

All women with pelvic pain or an asymptomatic, incidentally discovered ovarian mass should undergo a complete abdominal and gynecological exam. The provider should be assessing for (1) the size, shape, mobility, tenderness, and position of the ovaries and uterus, (2) cervical motion tenderness and characteristics of the vaginal discharge to help evaluate for infection, (3) pain with palpation in the anterior or posterior vaginal fornix or "studding" along the pelvic floor or rectovaginal wall that may indicate endometrial implants or malignancy, and (4) peritonitis, abdominal masses, and costovertebral tenderness that may reflect GI and GU pathology. Patients often have pain with manipulation of the ovaries and/or uterus when infection (PID or TOA), torsion, or an ectopic pregnancy is present. (See Chap. 11 on Gynecologic Emergencies.) Peritonitis is nonspecific but indicative of an acute, inflammatory issue (PID, TOA, torsion, ruptured ectopic, GI pathology, malignancy) that needs immediate evaluation. A fixed, firm, or irregular mass; bilateral masses; and/or the presences of ascites should raise concern for ovarian malignancy [72]. In asymptomatic women, a normal pelvic exam is not uncommon as data suggest that even in ideal settings with experienced providers, the pelvic exam is insensitive in detecting adnexal pathology [85–88].

Every patient must have a pregnancy test. If the pregnancy test is positive and the patient is having abdominal pain, she must be immediately evaluated for an ectopic pregnancy. If untreated, patients have an 18% chance of rupture, which can lead to life-threatening hemorrhage [89].

Transvaginal ultrasound with Doppler is the preferred imaging modality for adnexal masses [72]. If patients present after ovarian cysts are noted on non-ultrasound imaging, transvaginal ultrasound should be performed next as neither CT nor MRI are first-line modalities to evaluate the adnexa [72]. Ideally, the ultrasound should be performed by an experienced technician and interpreted by a radiologist with expertise in pelvic ultrasound. As cysts grow, it is possible that ultrasound imaging can be incomplete. When an ultrasound report indicates that all of the borders of a large cyst are not visible, due to patient anatomy or body habitus, a follow-up pelvic MRI can assess for septations and/or solid components [90].

In 2010, the Society of Radiologists in Ultrasound produced consensus guidelines for the interpretation of ovarian cysts. Per these guidelines, simple cysts measuring <3 cm in diameter in premenopausal women and <1 cm in postmenopausal women are considered normal and do not need to be described in an ultrasound report. Any cyst larger than these thresholds should be characterized in an ultrasound report [73]. The ultrasound report should describe the size and laterality of the adnexal mass, the components of the mass (cystic versus solid), any septations (thin versus thick and single versus multiple), and any papillary or nodular projections in the mass. Doppler flow assesses vascular flow to the cyst [72]. These guidelines also provide descriptions and recommendations for follow-up of other common adnexal cysts including hemorrhagic cysts, endometriomas, and dermoids, all of which have distinctive appearances on ultrasound. Recommendations are largely based on size of the cyst,

Table 10.5 Ultrasound findings for ovarian cysts [72]

Reassuring ultrasound findings	Concerning ultrasound findings
Size up to 10 cm in diameter	Cysts larger than 10 cm in diameter
Thin smooth walls	Thick/multiple septations
Absence of septations	Papillary projections/solid components
Absence of papillary projections/ solid components	Doppler flow
Absence of Doppler flow	Presences of ascites

menopausal state, and any concerning findings on ultrasound [73]. The American College of Obstetricians and Gynecologists (ACOG) published a practice bulletin in 2016 on the management of adnexal masses. This bulletin encourages providers to focus on ultrasound *findings* of the cyst as opposed to the size of the cyst at presentation. The biggest change in these guidelines when compared to previous recommendations is the "10-cm rule" – stable asymptomatic simple cysts in pre- or postmenopausal women can be followed until they reach 10 cm in size without surgical intervention, as the risk of malignancy is extremely low. Table 10.5 includes descriptions of reassuring and concerning ultrasound findings [72].

After ultrasonography, laboratory evaluation may be appropriate based on a patient's other presenting symptoms and signs. Providers should obtain urine HCG testing in all women of reproductive age. A complete blood count and STI testing should be considered for an infectious etiology of an adnexal mass such as a tubo-ovarian abscess [72, 91].

The most studied biomarker for ovarian malignancy is CA-125; however, providers must understand the limitations to its use. CA-125 will be elevated in about 80% of patients with epithelial ovarian cancer but is only elevated in 50% of patients with Stage 1 disease [92]. It is also not the primary cancer marker in ovarian cancers that present in premenopausal women, such as germ cell tumors and sex cord stromal tumors. CA-125 can be elevated by any process which irritates the perineum such as normal menses, pelvic inflammatory disease, and endometriosis [92]. Given these limitations in specificity, CA-125 is less predictive of malignancy in premenopausal woman and should not be used to distinguish between a benign and malignant adnexal mass [72].

For premenopausal women, it is reasonable to check a CA-125 if an ovarian mass has concerning features on ultrasound, but note that it is not recommended to check a CA-125 in every premenopausal female with an ovarian mass without discretion, especially in the setting of a simple cyst on imaging. Guidelines do not recommend a specific cutoff or range of CA-125 that would make an ovarian mass in a premenopausal woman more concerning for malignancy, but based on expert opinion, a level of >200 U/ml should prompt referral to gynecology oncologists for further evaluation [72].

For postmenopausal women presenting with an adnexal mass, a CA-125 should be checked near the time of the first ultrasound. The ACOG guidelines recommend referral to gynecologic oncologist when a patient's CA-125 level is greater than 35 U/ml in the presence of an adnexal mass [72]. A low CA-125 in the setting of an ovarian mass at any age, especially with concerning features, does not rule out malignancy, and further work-up should be pursued.

Beyond CA-125, other tumor markers associated with germ cell tumors include b-hCG, L-lactate dehydrogenase, and alpha-fetoprotein [72]. While there has been research assessing the use of biomarker panels and multivariate assays, these are not first-line diagnostic tests [72]. A Risk of Ovarian Malignancy Algorithm (ROMA) has been developed to risk stratify women with ovarian cysts into groups at either low or high risk for ovarian malignancy prior to undergoing surgical intervention for ovarian cysts that have already been identified as needing surgical intervention based on imaging or clinical findings. Most often used by the surgical team, this algorithm includes CA-125, menopausal status, and epididymis protein 4 [93]. In a meta-analysis epididymis protein 4 had a pooled sensitivity of 81% and a pooled specificity of 91% for the detection of ovarian malignancy [94].

Juliana's pregnancy test is negative. You suspect she may have endometriosis. You send her for a transvaginal ultrasound that demonstrates a 4-cm endometrioma in her right ovary.

Treatment Strategies

Treatment is based on the patient's symptoms, ultrasound characteristics, and risk for malignancy. When a woman is asymptomatic, a simple cyst up to 10 cm in diameter can be followed with expectant management regardless of menopausal status *if the cyst has been adequately imaged* [76]. Benign disease, such as endometriomas or mature teratomas, can also be managed expectantly [72]. While oral contraceptive pills have been recommended in the past for the suppression and treatment of functional ovarian cysts, a 2014 systematic review found them to be of no benefit [95]. In symptomatic women, gynecology referral for possible surgical excision is reasonable for a cyst of any size. However, in young women, it is important to consider future fertility and preservation of normal ovarian tissue should be emphasized [72]. When concerned that the cyst may represent an ovarian malignancy, the patient should be referred for immediate gynecologic oncology evaluation [72].

Monitoring

The interval between initial and repeat imaging has not been well established for patients presenting with benign cysts [72]. The American Academy of Family Physicians suggests repeating a transvaginal ultrasound 4–12 weeks after the initial test; this interval is often practiced clinically [91]. Repeat imaging serves two functions: (1) to judge growth or recession and (2) to confirm the findings of the first ultrasound. Many adnexal masses will exhibit intermediate findings that are often benign but not obvious enough to establish a clear diagnosis with one evaluation. For example, a fluid-filled simple cyst may have a single thin septation or a small amount of calcium in the wall. Similarly, features consistent with a hemorrhagic cyst, endometrioma, or dermoid cyst are often not obvious on the first imaging study but become clearer as time progresses [91].

With regard to the timing and duration of monitoring, some experts recommend monitoring stable cysts without solid components for 1 year and stable cysts with solid components for 2 years [96]. The rationale behind this recommendation stems from a study in which women over 50 years old with ultrasound-detected complex adnexal masses were followed with serial ultrasounds prior to surgical resection. Masses diagnosed as epithelial tumors at surgical resection had all demonstrated growth on or before 7 months of follow-up [76], inferring that cancers will see growth most often within the first year of ultrasound follow-up. Because the studies that evaluated surveillance of ovarian cysts used both ultrasound and CA-125 levels, it is recommended that in postmenopausal women with cysts, a CA-125 level is drawn at each follow-up ultrasound [97, 98]. Should the CA-125 level trend above 35 U/ml in the presence of an adnexal mass in a postmenopausal woman, a referral to gynecology oncologist is recommended [72].

When to Refer

For symptomatic women, referral to gynecologist for possible surgical removal of a cyst is appropriate. It is important to emphasize that if there is any concern for malignancy, such as elevated CA-125, ultrasound findings suggestive of malignancy, nodular or fixed pelvic mass, ascites, or evidence of metastasis, then a woman should be referred to gynecology oncologist as opposed to a general gynecologist. Evidence suggests that women with ovarian cancer have increased survival when managed by gynecologic oncologists [72].

Summary Points

1. Uterine fibroids are common and can be asymptomatic; when symptomatic, women present with heavy vaginal bleeding and/or bulk symptoms such as heaviness, pain, or problems with urination or defecation.
2. Medical and surgical management options for fibroids vary based on which symptoms predominate and include NSAIDs, hormonal methods, IUDs, myomectomy, endometrial ablation, uterine artery embolization, MRI-guided ultrasound therapy, and hysterectomy.
3. Endometriosis often presents with dysmenorrhea, dyspareunia, and menorrhagia but can also be asymptomatic, with the diagnosis determined only during infertility evaluation.
4. Numerous options can alleviate pain secondary to endometriosis: NSAIDs, combined oral contraceptive pills, levonorgestrel IUD, medroxyprogesterone acetate, and GnRH agonists.
5. Patients with infertility secondary to endometriosis should be referred for consideration of surgical intervention to remove endometrial implants or in vitro fertilization (IVF).
6. When evaluating an ovarian cyst, consider both benign etiologies such as simple cysts, endometriomas, hemorrhagic cysts, and mature teratomas and malignant etiologies such as ovarian cancer. Assessment includes a transvaginal ultrasound, obtaining a CA-125 level, and a risk assessment for ovarian cancer.
7. Indications for early referral to gynecology oncologist include an elevated CA-125 (>35 U/ml in postmenopausal woman), ultrasound findings concerning for malignancy, a fixed or nodular pelvic mass, ascites, or evidence of distance metastasis.

Review Questions

1. A 31-year-old woman presents to your office with menorrhagia and anemia. Her transvaginal ultrasound demonstrates a large submucosal fibroid. She is considering having a third child. What is the best management option?
   A. Hysteroscopic myomectomy to remove the fibroid
   B. IUD insertion to manage bleeding until she is ready to have her third child
   C. Uterine artery embolization
   D. Endometrial ablation

   The correct answer is A. Myomectomy should be the first-line treatment for women considering additional children because there is evidence that it may improve pregnancy rates. A progesterone IUD could help manage bleeding symptoms and if she is opposed to procedural options could be considered appropriate. Both uterine artery embolization and endometrial ablation should be reserved for women who have completed childbearing [7, 9].

2. A 54-year-old postmenopausal woman presents to your office with a complaint of heaviness in her pelvis and urinary incontinence for the last several years. On exam, her uterus is enlarged. A transvaginal ultrasound demonstrates a large subserosal fibroid that abuts her bladder. What is the best management option for her symptoms?
   A. GnRH agonist
   B. Hysterectomy
   C. Endometrial ablation
   D. Hysteroscopic myomectomy

   The correct answer is B. A GnRH agonist would not be appropriate as she is already postmenopausal. Endometrial ablation and hysteroscopic myomectomy would not address her bulk symptoms [7, 9].
3. A 26-year-old woman presents with dyspareunia and dysmenorrhea. She has tenderness with her gynecological exam particularly with deep palpation in the posterior fornix. She denies any bowel or bladder symptoms. You suspect endometriosis and obtain a transvaginal ultrasound to exclude other pathology; it is normal. What would be the best next step?
   A. Empiric treatment with combined oral contraceptive pills.
   B. Refer to gynecologist for diagnostic laparoscopy.
   C. Trial of NSAIDs for relief of her dysmenorrhea.
   D. Start GnRH agonist.

   The correct answer is A. While NSAID therapy is often used to treat dysmenorrhea, combined oral contraceptive pills are more effective. While endometriosis can only be definitely diagnosed via laparoscopy, empiric treatment is recommended for most patients [48].
4. Which woman would benefit from referral to gynecology oncologist?
   A. A 36-year-old woman with a 4-cm hemorrhagic cyst on ultrasound and CA-125 of 3 U/ml
   B. A 27-year-old woman with a 5-cm endometrioma on ultrasound and CA-125 of 40 U/ml
   C. A 56-year-old woman with a 4-cm cyst with multiple thick septations and CA-125 of 30 U/ml
   D. A 66-year-old woman with an 8-cm simple cyst on ultrasound and CA-125 of 2 U/ml

   The correct answer is C. Even though her CA-125 is less than 35 U/ml in a postmenopausal woman, her cyst has multiple thick septations which is concerning for malignancy. All the other women have benign-appearing cysts on ultrasound, and in premenopausal women there is no definitive cutoff for CA-125 [72].
5. A 35-year-old woman presents after a transvaginal ultrasound obtained for heavy menstrual bleeding demonstrated a 6-cm simple cyst without septations or solid components. She has no risk factors for ovarian cancer and no family history of breast or ovarian malignancy. She asks if this could be ovarian cancer. How would you advise her?
   A. You recommend referral to gynecology oncologist for consideration of surgical excision of the cyst.
   B. You recommend a repeat ultrasound in 6–12 weeks and reassure her that the risk of malignancy is low.
   C. You recommend a repeat ultrasound in 6–12 weeks with a CA-125 and reassure her that the risk of malignancy is low.
   D. You recommend she obtain a MRI to better categorize the cyst before making a decision on referral to gynecology oncologist.

   The correct answer is B. Her cyst is simple appearing on ultrasound. She is premenopausal, and given that she has no concerning features on ultrasound, she does not need to have a CA-125 drawn. It would be appropriate to reimage her in 6–12 weeks to assess for resolution or stability of the cyst. Should the cyst change and become more concerning for malignancy, a CA-125 would be indicated [72].

References

1. Baird DD, Dunson DB, Hill MC, Cousins D, Schectman JM. High cumulative incidence of uterine leiomyoma in black and white women: ultrasound evidence. Am J Obstet Gynecol. 2003;188(1):100–7.
2. Fortin C, Flyckt R, Falcone T. Alternatives to hysterectomy: the burden of fibroids and the quality of life. Best Pract Res Clin Obstet Gynaecol. 2018;46:31–42. https://doi.org/10.1016/j.bpobgyn.2017.10.001.
3. Borah BJ, Nicholson WK, Bradley L, Stewart EA. The impact of uterine leiomyomas: a national survey of affected women. Am J Obstet Gynecol. 2013;209(4):319 e1–e20.
4. Marshall LM, Spiegelman D, Barbieri RL, Goldman MB, Manson JE, Colditz GA, et al. Variation in the incidence of uterine leiomyoma among premenopausal women by age and race. Obstet Gynecol. 1997;90(6):967–73.
5. Marshall LM, Spiegelman D, Goldman MB, Manson JE, Colditz GA, Barbieri RL, et al. A prospective study of reproductive factors and oral contraceptive use in relation to the risk of uterine leiomyomata. Fertil Steril. 1998;70(3):432–9.
6. Wise LA, Laughlin-Tommaso SK. Epidemiology of uterine fibroids: from menarche to menopause. Clin Obstet Gynecol. 2016;59(1):2–24.
7. Vilos GA, Allaire C, Laberge PY, Leyland N. The management of uterine leiomyomas. J Obstet Gynaecol Can. 2015;37(2):157–78. https://doi.org/10.1016/S1701-2163(15)30338-8.
8. Munro MG, Critchley HO, Broder MS, Fraser IS. FIGO classification system (PALM-COEIN) for causes of abnormal uterine bleeding in nongravid women of reproductive age. Int J Gynaecol Obstet. 2011;113(1):3–13.

9. American College of Obstetricians Gynecologists. ACOG practice bulletin. Alternatives to hysterectomy in the management of leiomyomas. Obstet Gynecol. 2008;112(2 Pt 1):387–400.
10. Stewart EA. Clinical practice. Uterine fibroids. N Engl J Med. 2015;372(17):1646–55.
11. Wegienka G, Baird DD, Hertz-Picciotto I, Harlow SD, Steege JF, Hill MC, et al. Self-reported heavy bleeding associated with uterine leiomyomata. Obstet Gynecol. 2003;101(3):431–7.
12. Zimmermann A, Bernuit D, Gerlinger C, Schaefers M, Geppert K. Prevalence, symptoms and management of uterine fibroids: an international internet-based survey of 21,746 women. BMC Womens Health. 2012;12(1):6.
13. Pritts EA, Parker WH, Olive DL. Fibroids and infertility: an updated systematic review of the evidence. Fertil Steril. 2009;91(4):1215–23.
14. Whynott RM, Vaught KCC, Segars JH. The effect of uterine fibroids on infertility: a systematic review. Sem Reprod Med. 2017;35(6):523–32.
15. Metwally M, Cheong YC, Horne AW. Surgical treatment of fibroids for subfertility. Cochrane Database Syst Rev. 2012;(11):CD003857.
16. Carranza-Mamane B, Havelock J, Hemmings R. The management of uterine fibroids in women with otherwise unexplained infertility. J Obstet Gynaecol Can. 2015;37(3):277–85.
17. Sundermann AC, Velez Edwards DR, Bray MJ, Jones SH, Latham SM, Hartmann KE. Leiomyomas in pregnancy and spontaneous abortion: a systematic review and meta-analysis. Obstet Gynecol. 2017;130(5):1065–72.
18. American Cancer Society. Endometrial cancer risk factors [updated February 29, 2016]. Available from: https://www.cancer.org/cancer/endometrial-cancer/causes-risks-prevention/risk-factors.html#written_by. Accessed March 18, 2019.
19. Lumsden MA, Wallace EM. Clinical presentation of uterine fibroids. Baillieres Clin Obstet Gynaecol. 1998;12(2):177–95.
20. American College of Obstetricians and Gynecologists. Committee opinion no. 477: the role of the obstetrician-gynecologist in the early detection of epithelial ovarian cancer. Obstet Gynecol. 2011;117(3):742–6.
21. Gupta JK, Sinha A, Lumsden MA, Hickey M. Uterine artery embolization for symptomatic uterine fibroids. Cochrane Database Syst Rev. 2014;(12):CD005073.
22. Stewart EA, Morton CC. The genetics of uterine leiomyomata: what clinicians need to know. Obstet Gynecol. 2006;107(4):917–21.
23. Tanaka YO, Nishida M, Tsunoda H, Okamoto Y, Yoshikawa H. Smooth muscle tumors of uncertain malignant potential and leiomyosarcomas of the uterus: MR findings. J Magn Reson Imaging. 2004;20(6):998–1007.
24. Schwartz LB, Diamond MP, Schwartz PE. Leiomyosarcomas: clinical presentation. Am J Obstet Gynecol. 1993;168(1 Pt 1):180–3.
25. American College of Obstetricians and Gynecologists. Committee opinion no. 557: management of acute abnormal uterine bleeding in nonpregnant reproductive-aged women. Obstet Gynecol. 2013;121(4):891–6.
26. De La Cruz MS, Buchanan EM. Uterine fibroids: diagnosis and treatment. Am Fam Physician. 2017;95(2):100–7.
27. Peitsidis P, Koukoulomati A. Tranexamic acid for the management of uterine fibroid tumors: a systematic review of the current evidence. World J Clin Cases. 2014;2(12):893–8.
28. Fonseca MCM, Castro R, Machado M, Conte T, Girao M. Uterine artery embolization and surgical methods for the treatment of symptomatic uterine leiomyomas: a systemic review and meta-analysis followed by indirect treatment comparison. Clin Ther. 2017;39(7):1438–55.e2.
29. Borah BJ, Yao X, Laughlin-Tommaso SK, Heien HC, Stewart EA. Comparative effectiveness of uterine leiomyoma procedures using a large insurance claims database. Obstet Gynecol. 2017;130(5):1047–56.
30. Clark NA, Mumford SL, Segars JH. Reproductive impact of MRI-guided focused ultrasound surgery for fibroids: a systematic review of the evidence. Curr Opin Obstet Gynecol. 2014;26(3):151–61.
31. Laughlin-Tommaso SK, Khan Z, Weaver AL, Smith CY, Rocca WA, Stewart EA. Cardiovascular and metabolic morbidity after hysterectomy with ovarian conservation: a cohort study. Menopause (New York). 2018;25(5):483–92.
32. Wise MR, Gill P, Lensen S, Thompson JM, Farquhar CM. Body mass index trumps age in decision for endometrial biopsy: cohort study of symptomatic premenopausal women. Am J Obstet Gynecol. 2016;215(5):598.e1–8.
33. Buck Louis GM, Hediger ML, Peterson CM, Croughan M, Sundaram R, Stanford J, et al. Incidence of endometriosis by study population and diagnostic method: the ENDO study. Fertil Steril. 2011;96(2):360–5.
34. Giudice LC. Clinical practice. Endometriosis. N Engl J Med. 2010;362(25):2389–98.
35. Houston DE, Noller KL, Melton LJ 3rd, Selwyn BJ, Hardy RJ. Incidence of pelvic endometriosis in Rochester, Minnesota, 1970-1979. Am J Epidemiol. 1987;125(6):959–69.
36. Balasch J, Creus M, Fabregues F, Carmona F, Ordi J, Martinez-Roman S, et al. Visible and non-visible endometriosis at laparoscopy in fertile and infertile women and in patients with chronic pelvic pain: a prospective study. Hum Reprod. 1996;11(2):387–91.
37. Ballard KD, Seaman HE, de Vries CS, Wright JT. Can symptomatology help in the diagnosis of endometriosis? Findings from a national case-control study--part 1. BJOG. 2008;115(11):1382–91.
38. Carter JE. Combined hysteroscopic and laparoscopic findings in patients with chronic pelvic pain. J Am Assoc Gynecol Laparosc. 1994;2(1):43–7.
39. American College of Obstetricians and Gynecologists. Practice bulletin no. 114: management of endometriosis. Obstet Gynecol. 2010;116(1):223–36.
40. Jenkins S, Olive DL, Haney AF. Endometriosis: pathogenetic implications of the anatomic distribution. Obstet Gynecol. 1986;67(3):335–8.
41. Lee HJ, Park YM, Jee BC, Kim YB, Suh CS. Various anatomic locations of surgically proven endometriosis: a single-center experience. Obstet Gynecol Sci. 2015;58(1):53–8.
42. Athwal P, Patel K, Hassani C, Bahadori S, Nardi P. A case of multisystem endometriosis. J Radiol Case Rep. 2013;7(10):1–6.
43. Practice Committee of the American Society for Reproductive Medicine. Treatment of pelvic pain associated with endometriosis. Fertil Steril. 2008;90(5 Suppl):S260–9.
44. Holoch KJ, Lessey BA. Endometriosis and infertility. Clin Obstet Gynecol. 2010;53(2):429–38.
45. Laganà AS, Condemi I, Retto G, Muscatello MRA, Bruno A, Zoccali RA, et al. Analysis of psychopathological comorbidity behind the common symptoms and signs of endometriosis. Eur J Obstet Gynecol Reprod Biol. 2015;194:30–3.
46. Hadfield R, Mardon H, Barlow D, Kennedy S. Delay in the diagnosis of endometriosis: a survey of women from the USA and the UK. Hum Reprod. 1996;11(4):878–80.
47. Dmowski WP, Lesniewicz R, Rana N, Pepping P, Noursalehi M. Changing trends in the diagnosis of endometriosis: a comparative study of women with pelvic endometriosis presenting with chronic pelvic pain or infertility. Fertil Steril. 1997;67(2):238–43.
48. Leyland N, Casper R, Laberge P, Singh SS, SOGC. Endometriosis: diagnosis and management. J Obstet Gynaecol Can. 2010;32(7 Suppl 2):S1–32.
49. Revised American Society for Reproductive Medicine classification of endometriosis: 1996. Fertil Steril. 1997;67(5):817–21.
50. Vercellini P, Fedele L, Aimi G, Pietropaolo G, Consonni D, Crosignani PG. Association between endometriosis stage, lesion type, patient characteristics and severity of pelvic pain symp-

toms: a multivariate analysis of over 1000 patients. Hum Reprod. 2007;22(1):266–71.
51. Alcazar JL, Laparte C, Jurado M, Lopez-Garcia G. The role of transvaginal ultrasonography combined with color velocity imaging and pulsed Doppler in the diagnosis of endometrioma. Fertil Steril. 1997;67(3):487–91.
52. Hudelist G, Tuttlies F, Rauter G, Pucher S, Keckstein J. Can transvaginal sonography predict infiltration depth in patients with deep infiltrating endometriosis of the rectum? Hum Reprod. 2009;24(5):1012–7.
53. Abrao MS, Goncalves MO, Dias JA Jr, Podgaec S, Chamie LP, Blasbalg R. Comparison between clinical examination, transvaginal sonography and magnetic resonance imaging for the diagnosis of deep endometriosis. Hum Reprod. 2007;22(12):3092–7.
54. Mol BW, Bayram N, Lijmer JG, Wiegerinck MA, Bongers MY, van der Veen F, et al. The performance of CA-125 measurement in the detection of endometriosis: a meta-analysis. Fertil Steril. 1998;70(6):1101–8.
55. Brown J, Crawford TJ, Allen C, Hopewell S, Prentice A. Nonsteroidal anti-inflammatory drugs for pain in women with endometriosis. Cochrane Database Syst Rev. 2017;(1):CD004753.
56. Al Kadri H, Hassan S, Al-Fozan HM, Hajeer A. Hormone therapy for endometriosis and surgical menopause. Cochrane Database Syst Rev. 2009;(1):CD005997.
57. Brown J, Pan A, Hart RJ. Gonadotrophin-releasing hormone analogues for pain associated with endometriosis. Cochrane Database Syst Rev. 2010;(12):CD008475.
58. Abou-Setta AM, Houston B, Al-Inany HG, Farquhar C. Levonorgestrel-releasing intrauterine device (LNG-IUD) for symptomatic endometriosis following surgery. Cochrane Database Syst Rev. 2013;(1):CD005072.
59. Hart RJ, Hickey M, Maouris P, Buckett W. Excisional surgery versus ablative surgery for ovarian endometriomata. Cochrane Database Syst Rev. 2008;(2):CD004992.
60. Hickey M, Ballard K, Farquhar C. Endometriosis. BMJ (Clinical research ed). 2014;348:g1752.
61. Taylor HS, Giudice LC, Lessey BA, Abrao MS, Kotarski J, Archer DF, et al. Treatment of endometriosis-associated pain with elagolix, an Oral GnRH antagonist. N Engl J Med. 2017;377(1):28–40.
62. Duffy JM, Arambage K, Correa FJ, Olive D, Farquhar C, Garry R, et al. Laparoscopic surgery for endometriosis. Cochrane Database Syst Rev. 2014;(4):CD011031.
63. Sallam HN, Garcia-Velasco JA, Dias S, Arici A, Abou-Setta AM. Long-term pituitary down-regulation before in vitro fertilization (IVF) for women with endometriosis. Cochrane Database Syst Rev. 2006;(1):CD004635.
64. Hughes E, Brown J, Collins JJ, Farquhar C, Fedorkow DM, Vanderkerchove P. Ovulation suppression for endometriosis for women with subfertility. Cochrane Database Syst Rev. 2007;(3).
65. Zhu X, Hamilton KD, McNicol ED. Acupuncture for pain in endometriosis. Cochrane Database Syst Rev. 2011;(9):CD007864.
66. Flower A, Liu JP, Chen S, Lewith G, Little P. Chinese herbal medicine for endometriosis. Cochrane Database Syst Rev. 2009;(3):CD006568.
67. American College of Obstetricians and Gynecologists. Female age-related fertility decline. Committee opinion no. 589. Fertil Steril. 2014;101(3):633–4.
68. Christensen JT, Boldsen JL, Westergaard JG. Functional ovarian cysts in premenopausal and gynecologically healthy women. Contraception. 2002;66(3):153–7.
69. Pavlik EJ, Ueland FR, Miller RW, Ubellacker JM, DeSimone CP, Elder J, et al. Frequency and disposition of ovarian abnormalities followed with serial transvaginal ultrasonography. Obstet Gynecol. 2013;122(2 Pt 1):210–7.
70. Greenlee RT, Kessel B, Williams CR, Riley TL, Ragard LR, Hartge P, et al. Prevalence, incidence, and natural history of simple ovarian cysts among women >55 years old in a large cancer screening trial. Am J Obstet Gynecol. 2010;202(4):373.e1–9.
71. Castillo G, Alcazar JL, Jurado M. Natural history of sonographically detected simple unilocular adnexal cysts in asymptomatic postmenopausal women. Gynecol Oncol. 2004;92(3):965–9.
72. American College of Obstetricians and Gynecologists' Committee on Practice B-G. Practice bulletin no. 174: evaluation and management of adnexal masses. Obstet Gynecol. 2016;128(5):e210–e26.
73. Levine D, Brown DL, Andreotti RF, Benacerraf B, Benson CB, Brewster WR, et al. Management of asymptomatic ovarian and other adnexal cysts imaged at US Society of radiologists in ultrasound consensus conference statement. Ultrasound Q. 2010;26(3):121–31.
74. Fabiola Medeiros KCS. Germ cell tumors of the ovary. In: Diagnostic gynecologic and obstetric pathology. New York: Elsevier; 2018. p. 949–1010.
75. Valentin L, Ameye L, Franchi D, Guerriero S, Jurkovic D, Savelli L, et al. Risk of malignancy in unilocular cysts: a study of 1148 adnexal masses classified as unilocular cysts at transvaginal ultrasound and review of the literature. Ultrasound Obstet Gynecol. 2013;41(1):80–9.
76. Modesitt SC, Pavlik EJ, Ueland FR, DePriest PD, Kryscio RJ, van Nagell JR Jr. Risk of malignancy in unilocular ovarian cystic tumors less than 10 centimeters in diameter. Obstet Gynecol. 2003;102(3):594–9.
77. Somigliana E, Berlanda N, Benaglia L, Vigano P, Vercellini P, Fedele L. Surgical excision of endometriomas and ovarian reserve: a systematic review on serum antimullerian hormone level modifications. Fertil Steril. 2012;98(6):1531–8.
78. Goff BA, Mandel LS, Melancon CH, Muntz HG. Frequency of symptoms of ovarian cancer in women presenting to primary care clinics. JAMA. 2004;291(22):2705–12.
79. American Cancer Society. What are the risk factors for ovarian cancer 2016 [updated February 4, 2016]. Available from: https://www.cancer.org/cancer/ovarian-cancer/causes-risks-prevention/risk-factors.html. Accessed March 14, 2019.
80. Kerlikowske K, Brown JS, Grady DG. Should women with familial ovarian cancer undergo prophylactic oophorectomy? Obstet Gynecol. 1992;80(4):700–7.
81. Piver MS. Prophylactic oophorectomy: reducing the U.S. death rate from epithelial ovarian cancer. A continuing debate. Oncologist. 1996;1(5):326–30.
82. Lancaster JM, Powell CB, Chen LM, Richardson DL. Society of Gynecologic Oncology statement on risk assessment for inherited gynecologic cancer predispositions. Gynecol Oncol. 2015;136(1):3–7.
83. Givens V, Mitchell GE, Harraway-Smith C, Reddy A, Maness DL. Diagnosis and management of adnexal masses. Am Fam Physician. 2009;80(8):815–20.
84. Bottomley C, Bourne T. Diagnosis and management of ovarian cyst accidents. Best Pract Res Clin Obstet Gynaecol. 2009;23(5):711–24.
85. Guirguis-Blake JM, Henderson JT, Perdue LA. Periodic screening pelvic examination: evidence report and systematic review for the US preventive services task force. JAMA. 2017;317(9):954–66.
86. Qaseem A, Humphrey LL, Harris R, Starkey M, Denberg TD. Screening pelvic examination in adult women: a clinical practice guideline from the American College of Physicians. Ann Intern Med. 2014;161(1):67–72.
87. Padilla LA, Radosevich DM, Milad MP. Limitations of the pelvic examination for evaluation of the female pelvic organs. Int J Gynaecol Obstet. 2005;88(1):84–8.
88. Padilla LA, Radosevich DM, Milad MP. Accuracy of the pelvic examination in detecting adnexal masses. Obstet Gynecol. 2000;96(4):593–8.

89. Job-Spira N, Fernandez H, Bouyer J, Pouly JL, Germain E, Coste J. Ruptured tubal ectopic pregnancy: risk factors and reproductive outcome: results of a population-based study in France. Am J Obstet Gynecol. 1999;180(4):938–44.
90. Patel MD. Practical approach to the adnexal mass. Radiol Clin N Am. 2006;44(6):879–99.
91. Biggs WS, Marks ST. Diagnosis and management of adnexal masses. Am Fam Physician. 2016;93(8):676–81.
92. Soletormos G, Duffy MJ, Othman Abu Hassan S, Verheijen RH, Tholander B, Bast RC Jr, et al. Clinical use of cancer biomarkers in epithelial ovarian cancer: updated guidelines from the European Group on Tumor Markers. Int J Gynaecol Obstet. 2016;26(1): 43–51.
93. Karlsen MA, Sandhu N, Hogdall C, Christensen IJ, Nedergaard L, Lundvall L, et al. Evaluation of HE4, CA125, risk of ovarian malignancy algorithm (ROMA) and risk of malignancy index (RMI) as diagnostic tools of epithelial ovarian cancer in patients with a pelvic mass. Gynecol Oncol. 2012;127(2):379–83.
94. Huang J, Chen J, Huang Q. Diagnostic value of HE4 in ovarian cancer: a meta-analysis. Eur J Obstet Gynecol Reprod Biol. 2018;231:35–42.
95. Grimes DA, Jones LB, Lopez LM, Schulz KF. Oral contraceptives for functional ovarian cysts. Cochrane Database Syst Rev. 2014;(4):CD006134.
96. Suh-Burgmann E, Kinney W. Potential harms outweigh benefits of indefinite monitoring of stable adnexal masses. Am J Obstet Gynecol. 2015;213(6):816.e1–4.
97. Maggino T, Gadducci A, D'Addario V, Pecorelli S, Lissoni A, Stella M, et al. Prospective multicenter study on CA 125 in postmenopausal pelvic masses. Gynecol Oncol. 1994;54(2):117–23.
98. Schutter EM, Kenemans P, Sohn C, Kristen P, Crombach G, Westermann R, et al. Diagnostic value of pelvic examination, ultrasound, and serum CA 125 in postmenopausal women with a pelvic mass. An international multicenter study. Cancer. 1994;74(4):1398–406.

11 Gynecologic Emergencies

Michael Lund and Jill C. Costello

Learning Objectives

1. Describe the evaluation of vaginal bleeding in early pregnancy and refer appropriately.
2. Distinguish the most common causes of acute pelvic pain in the reproductive-age female patient and identify emergency situations.
3. Compare the presentations and management of ovarian emergencies, including ovarian torsion, ruptured cysts, and cyst hemorrhage.
4. Diagnose acute, heavy vaginal bleeding in the non-pregnant patient and identify emergencies.

Sophia is a 29-year-old female patient who presents to your office complaining of new-onset left lower quadrant pain. She is uncertain of the exact date of her last menstrual period but has been spotting for the past few days. Because she is a reproductive-age woman having new pelvic pain, you order a urine pregnancy test in your office, which is positive.

Maintain High Suspicion for the Possibility of Pregnancy

First-trimester bleeding is one of the most common complications of pregnancy. The diagnosis can be more challenging because many patients do not realize they are pregnant. For this reason, all primary care providers should be familiar with early recognition of pregnancy, as well as emergencies that can occur early in pregnancy.

Pregnancy Testing and Differential Diagnosis

There have been tremendous advances in pregnancy testing over the past several decades. Point-of-care urine pregnancy tests, both at home and in clinics, have improved to the point that a negative test will exclude pregnancy with high sensitivity when used for pregnancies advanced enough to result in complications. All pregnancy tests rely on the detection of human chorionic gonadotropin (hCG) in serum or urine. While there are several forms of hCG, the relevant subunit is the "beta"-molecule. This can be measured *qualitatively* in urine or serum or *quantitatively* in serum [1].

Pregnancy is by far the most common cause of secondary amenorrhea in the reproductive-age patient. Any woman of reproductive age who gives a history of a prolonged menstrual interval (the number of days between the first day of consecutive cycles), especially when associated with other symptoms such as bleeding or abdominal pain, should undergo urine pregnancy testing even when she does not consider herself at risk for pregnancy. Obtaining pregnancy tests in women of child-bearing age, as a routine habit, will prevent the occasional missed pregnancy which could result in life-threatening complications such as ruptured ectopic pregnancy.

The differential diagnosis of bleeding in early pregnancy can be limited to three major entities: spontaneous abortion, ectopic pregnancy, and threatened abortion (but ultimately viable pregnancy). As noted earlier, keeping a high suspicion for ectopic pregnancy will result in work-up of more patients but should prevent important misses in diagnoses.

Ectopic pregnancy occurs in 2–3% of recognized pregnancies. The cardinal symptoms are abdominal pain, bleeding, and a positive pregnancy test. It is difficult to define a "typical" description of abdominal pain or bleeding that

M. Lund (✉)
Department of Obstetrics and Gynecology, Medical College of Wisconsin, Milwaukee, WI, USA
e-mail: mlund@mcw.edu

J. C. Costello
Department of Medicine/Division of Rheumatology, Medical College of Wisconsin, Milwaukee, WI, USA

S. A. Tilstra et al. (eds.), *Sex- and Gender-Based Women's Health*, https://doi.org/10.1007/978-3-030-50695-7_11

should prompt one to consider this diagnosis. Risk factors include anything that can cause dysfunction of the fallopian tubes: previous history of sexually transmitted infection (especially *Chlamydia trachomatis*), endometriosis, previous tubal ligation, known pelvic adhesions, or previous pelvic surgery [2, 3].

As the early gestation implants into the lumen of the fallopian tube in cases of ectopic pregnancy, there can be pain associated from distension of this very sensitive organ as well as bleeding that results initially from muscular invasion of the tube and eventually from rupture of the tube itself. While initially pain tends to be unilateral, by the time of tubal rupture it can be diffuse and severe. Pain from an ectopic pregnancy may be described as "cramping" or "sharp."

Transvaginal ultrasound performed the same day reveals a normal uterus (without obvious pregnancy), a 2-cm cyst in the left ovary, and a small amount of free pelvic fluid. You order a serum hCG which is 3425 IU.

Diagnosing Ectopic Pregnancy

When the urine or serum pregnancy test is positive in a patient presenting with abdominal pain or bleeding, the diagnostic approach relies on immediate quantitative measurement of hCG combined with prompt transvaginal ultrasonography. Normally, the hCG level is obtained first to avoid unnecessary imaging (e.g., if the hCG level is very low, the ultrasound will likely be normal). When the hCG level is significantly elevated (>100 mIU/mL) and ultrasound cannot be performed at the site of initial patient evaluation, the patient should be transferred to a facility where imaging can be accomplished on the same day; this may often be the emergency department. Ultrasonography serves two practical purposes here: first, if an intrauterine pregnancy can be documented, ectopic pregnancy is almost excluded – except for the rare but increasingly frequent heterotopic pregnancy [4], where both intrauterine and ectopic pregnancy occur in the same patient. Second, in some cases the ectopic gestation can be visualized as either an obvious gestational sac outside of the uterus (sometimes with cardiac activity) or, more commonly, as an adnexal mass separate from the normal ovary and with or without free fluid, which suggests bleeding in the pelvis. The presence of free fluid in the pelvis of the patient from our vignette should be a red flag to the care team that the patient may be experiencing ectopic pregnancy.

The quantitative hCG level is useful only in the circumstance of early pregnancy, before an intrauterine pregnancy with cardiac activity has been documented. When ordered after cardiac activity has been documented on ultrasound, the results will not affect management and therefore do not provide value. The hCG level for patients in early pregnancy serves two main purposes: first, the trend over time can be used to predict normal or abnormal outcome, and second, the level is associated with an expectation of when an intrauterine pregnancy should be visualized by ultrasound (the concept of the "discriminatory zone" discussed below).

In a normally progressing, viable pregnancy, the hCG level will rise in a characteristic manner. Though the common mnemonic is "the level should double every two days," this is an oversimplification; in reality, the level should rise by only 53% every 48 hours [5, 6]. If this more conservative rule is used, 99% of normal intrauterine pregnancies will follow the rule; using an expected rise of 35% increases this to 99.9% of normal pregnancies [7]. In general, the level should be followed over at least two 48-hour intervals before any management decisions are made. If the level does not rise by the expected amount, ectopic pregnancy or spontaneous abortion is much more likely. If the level falls, it should be checked regularly until negative, unless an intrauterine pregnancy had previously been confirmed by ultrasound. This is done to reduce concern for retained tissue after spontaneous abortion or chronic ectopic pregnancy.

An intrauterine pregnancy is normally seen by transvaginal ultrasonography at a quantitative hCG level of 1500–3500 mIU/mL [6], with the wide range depending on both patient characteristics (e.g. body habitus) and operator characteristics (e.g. skill of the ultrasonographer and quality of the equipment being used). Each ultrasonography unit typically uses a standardized level referred to as the *discriminatory zone*. The practical use of this is as follows: if the hCG level is well above the discriminatory zone and no intrauterine pregnancy is seen, there is high suspicion for ectopic pregnancy, especially if the patient has not passed tissue vaginally or the hCG level is known to be rising; if the hCG level is below this discriminatory zone, the level is typically followed every 48 hours until it is above the zone, at which time ultrasound is repeated. If an intrauterine pregnancy is then seen, suspicion for ectopic pregnancy is markedly reduced, whereas concern remains high if it is not seen.

You repeat the quantitative HCG level 48 hours later and it is now 4251 IU/mL. You have already arranged for the patient to be seen in obstetrics/gynecology clinic today. After checking other labwork, the obstetrician discusses medical management and surgical management with your patient.

Management of Confirmed Ectopic Pregnancy

Options for management of ectopic pregnancy are medical and surgical. Expectant management is rarely recommended as it can have life-threatening consequences, with the exception being the rapidly falling hCG level in a pregnancy of unknown location.

Medical management has become much more popular over the past two decades. Methotrexate can be administered intramuscularly in a single-dose, two-dose, or multiple-dose protocol (with increasing success rate but increasing side effects, respectively). The single-dose protocol is the most common because of ease of administration and low side effect burden – the initial dose is 50 mg methotrexate per meter squared body surface area. The hCG level is then followed weekly until negative. Any rise or plateau in the hCG level (as opposed to falling) should prompt repeat dosing or surgical intervention [6, 8]. Contraindications to medical management include hematologic, hepatic, or renal dysfunction; a complete blood count, hepatic function panel, and creatinine are evaluated prior to administration to ensure patient safety. Adverse effects of systemic methotrexate used for ectopic pregnancy are fortunately rare, with stomatitis and transient elevations in transaminases being most common.

Surgical management includes either the removal of the tube containing the ectopic pregnancy (i.e. salpingectomy) or removal of only the gestation through a small slit in the fallopian tube (i.e. salpingostomy) [6, 9]. The decision depends on the condition of the tube, whether rupture has already occurred, the woman's desire for future fertility, and her history of previous tubal surgery or ectopic pregnancy. Future fertility appears to be similar when comparing methotrexate protocols and salpingostomy [10].

Recurrence rates for ectopic pregnancy average 10–25% with a history of one or two ectopic pregnancies, respectively [3].

The patient chooses medical management and is given methotrexate on the day of diagnosis. She is compliant with follow-up and has her hCG level monitored weekly with appropriate drop each week until the level reaches zero. Six months later, she attempts pregnancy again and conceives a normal intrauterine pregnancy.

In summary, the role of the primary care provider is to recognize bleeding complications early by always including pregnancy in the differential diagnosis of any reproductive-age patient from menarche to menopause who presents with abnormal vaginal bleeding or acute abdominal pain. Prompt referral to a gynecologist can improve future fertility, reduce complications, and in many cases, be life-saving, as ectopic pregnancy is still responsible for 1 out of 16 maternal deaths in the United States [11].

Maria is a 15-year-old female patient who comes to urgent care today complaining of severe right lower quadrant pain. The pain has been intermittent over the past few days, but today has become constant and more severe (she rates it 9/10). Though the triage nurse reported to you that she appeared to be in distress, she appears relatively comfortable when you interview her. Urine pregnancy test is negative.

Adnexal Torsion

As noted early in this chapter, one of the challenges for the busy primary care provider is distinguishing true emergencies from nonemergencies when symptoms and signs can be similar. Among the gynecologic emergencies, adnexal torsion is one of the key "can't miss" diagnoses, because the consequence of delayed recognition is potential loss of one ovary, fallopian tube, or both. This can have dramatic effects on the patient's future fertility and gonadal function.

Adnexal torsion is defined as the twisting of the ovary, and usually the fallopian tube, around its own supportive pedicle, which contains the ovarian artery and vein. Torsion can be intermittent or complete and can involve one or many twists. Interestingly, the right ovary is more at risk for torsion than is the left ovary, likely due to the longer length of the right utero-ovarian ligament or the presence of the sigmoid colon in the left pelvic space, which restricts left ovarian movement.

Adnexal torsion can occur in any age group but is most common during the reproductive years. It is a frequent cause of abdominal pain in adolescents as well as a frequent indication for surgery in adolescents. However, it can also occur in premenarchal or postmenopausal females (accounting for about 17% of torsions).

The most common risk factor for adnexal torsion is the presence of an adnexal mass. It is believed that the increased size and weight of the adnexal mass predisposes the organ to twist, though torsion can be seen in adnexae without any abnormal mass [12]. In most cases, the ovaries are enlarged, even if there is not a discrete ovarian cyst or mass [13].

On examination, temperature 97.8, heart rate 88, respiratory rate 20, and blood pressure 102/65. Abdomen is soft, nondistended, with mild tenderness in right lower quadrant but without rebound and without guarding. Pelvic examination is remarkable for mild-moderate right adnexal tenderness.

Clinical Manifestations of Adnexal Torsion

There is no "typical" presentation of adnexal torsion. However, patients may present with a similar progression of symptoms. Pain generally begins unilaterally and is often initially described as mild and crampy. Patients rarely present for care at this point due to the mild nature of the pain. The pain may become colicky, with increased frequency and duration of the episodes; between episodes, the pain may resolve almost completely. In most cases, pain will eventually become severe and constant, and at this stage patients generally seek emergency care. When pain becomes constant, the character can vary from cramping to sharp, stabbing, or gnawing pain, and the location can be more diffuse, potentially radiating to the back, and is often associated with peritoneal signs such as rebound tenderness. Commonly, nausea and vomiting accompany the pain at this stage. Pelvic examination becomes challenging because of significant tenderness; if a patient allows a bimanual examination at this point, the exam typically reveals a unilateral adnexal mass.

Physiologically, pain occurs due to intermittent obstruction of inflow and outflow of blood to the ovary and tube. Because of lower pressure relative to the ovarian artery, the ovarian vein is almost always obstructed first; this leads to worsening edema (and mass) within the ovary and the initial pain. The ovary may undergo hemorrhage and increasing size as it distends with blood that enters but cannot exit. The ovary may rupture at some point or may continue to twist until eventual obstruction of arterial flow, at which point necrosis occurs.

Colicky, but steadily worsening, unilateral pain can be the most helpful symptom to suspect torsion in many cases. In general, signs suggesting infection are not present until necrosis begins to occur.

Differential Diagnosis

The differential diagnosis of abdominal or pelvic pain in female patients is extensive; history remains the first and most important diagnostic step. Ultrasound consistent with adnexal masses suggests a possible gynecologic etiology, but functional ovarian cysts are ubiquitous and may be unrelated to her pain. Hemorrhagic ovarian cysts typically occur in the luteal phase of the menstrual cycle and cause more constant, localized, pain than adnexal torsion. These generally resolve with time. Ruptured ovarian cysts are typically identified on ultrasound, occurring from mid-cycle to menses, and can cause more diffuse pain because the cystic fluid or blood leaks into the peritoneum, causing significant irritation. The presence of significant free fluid in the pelvis suggests rupture of a cyst. Pelvic inflammatory disease must also be considered in the differential diagnosis (Please see Chap. 13 on Sexually Transmitted Infections).

Other causes of abdominal pain, such as acute appendicitis, can also occur in female patients with similar symptoms and findings. For example, a patient with acute appendicitis may experience cervical motion tenderness on examination because of local peritoneal inflammation. A thorough abdominal and pelvic examination should be performed in any female patient with pelvic pain.

Maria's ultrasound reveals a 6 cm right adnexal mass. The radiologist cannot specifically identify vascular flow in the mass.

Unfortunately, history and examination findings have low predictive value for diagnosing adnexal torsion. Transvaginal ultrasound is the most useful tool for diagnosis, though the sensitivity and specificity have varied across studies. Ultrasound is most useful for determining whether an adnexal mass is present on the same side of unilateral pain – if there is no adnexal mass and the ovaries appear normal in size, torsion is less likely. In addition, color flow doppler of the ovarian artery and vein can show obstructed flow. Results must be interpreted with caution, as torsion can occur despite the presence of bidirectional vascular flow; conversely, torsion may not be present even in the case of suspected absent vascular flow [12].

Management and Referral

Given limitations of testing, clinicians must maintain a high suspicion for adnexal torsion and a low threshold for referral to a gynecologist. Torsion can only be definitively diagnosed via surgery (usually laparoscopy). While in the past treatment necessitated removal of the affected ovary and tube, modern practice calls for simple untwisting of the adnexa and removal (either immediately or delayed) of any adnexal pathology. Some believe removing the cystic mass later may lead to less bleeding or destruction of the ovary, which may be edematous or even necrotic at the initial surgery. There is ongoing debate about whether the ovary should be fixed (sutured) to the uterus or pelvic sidewall to prevent recurrence.

You refer Maria to a gynecologist in your practice and express your concern for adnexal torsion. The gynecologist agrees and operates a short while later. Operative findings include a right ovarian cyst, and the tube and ovary are both twisted three times. After untwisting, the ovary and tube appear normal. The cyst is left for removal at a future date.

In summary, adnexal torsion typically occurs in the presence of a unilateral adnexal mass, can occur in young or old patients, and often follows a pattern of worsening, colicky, unilateral pain. While ultrasound can be helpful establishing the diagnosis, sensitivity and specificity are suboptimal necessitating early gynecology referral. Maintaining this "better safe than sorry" approach can potentially result in the preservation of a patient's ovary and/or fallopian tube.

Audrey is a 32-year-old G0 female patient with a history of irregular menses. She does not have a history of abnormal Pap tests (Pap was normal last year) or other gynecologic problems. Over the past 12 months, she has had only five menstrual cycles and has not been able to predict when the next will begin. Her last menses started ~90 days ago. Today, she started bleeding very heavily.

Acute, Heavy Vaginal Bleeding

The diagnosis and management of abnormal vaginal bleeding – usually, but not always uterine in origin – can be quite complicated and is described in detail in Chap. 7 on Abnormal Uterine Bleeding. It is important for the primary care provider to recognize when bleeding becomes severe enough to be considered a gynecologic emergency. A primary care provider can manage initial steps in treatment to help patients avoid significant consequences.

Most episodes of acute, very heavy vaginal bleeding will occur during the reproductive years. The first step in management for women presenting with heavy bleeding is to exclude pregnancy with a point-of-care urine pregnancy test. The management of pregnancy-associated bleeding after the first trimester is beyond the scope of this textbook. Next, vital signs should be reviewed to determine patient stability, and patients should be assessed for tachycardia or hypotension, symptoms of dizziness or orthostasis, and active or profuse ongoing bleeding. Obtaining vascular access and readying blood products are key steps if the patient has already lost significant blood. If a patient's vital signs are unstable or if she endorses worrisome symptoms, she should be immediately transferred to a facility or location that can transfuse blood, observe the patient, and potentially perform surgery, typically an emergency department.

As discussed in Chap. 7 on Abnormal Uterine Bleeding, the major etiologies of bleeding are classified by the PALM-COEIN system: Polyps, Adenomyosis, Leiomyoma, Malignancy; Coagulopathy, Ovulatory, Endometrial, Iatrogenic, Not Otherwise Classified [14–16]. Think of the first four etiologies (PALM) as *structural* causes and the second five as *nonstructural* causes (COEIN). Structural causes are typically identified by ultrasound.

The most likely causes of bleeding that require emergency department evaluation are nonstructural causes, especially coagulopathy and ovulatory dysfunction (also known as anovulatory bleeding). Coagulopathy (e.g. von Willebrand disease) should be suspected in young women with heavy menstrual bleeding since menarche, women with a history of surgical or significant obstetric bleeding, women with frequent bruising, epistaxis, or gum bleeding, and women with a family history of bleeding disorder. Recommended testing includes partial thromboplastin time, prothrombin time, von Willebrand panel including ristocetin cofactor, and platelet function [15]. A suggested workup is discussed in Chap. 7 on Abnormal Uterine Bleeding.

Once bleeding disorders and structural disorders are excluded, the most likely diagnosis is anovulatory bleeding, which is also the most likely overall cause of acute, heavy vaginal bleeding. Normally, follicle-stimulating hormone (FSH) leads to the development of several follicles in each ovary. Estradiol levels increase causing proliferation of the endometrial lining. Ovulation occurs after the luteinizing hormone (LH) surge, and the corpus luteum (ovulation cyst) secretes progesterone, which converts the endometrial lining to a secretory, stable histology. When progesterone levels drop 14 days later, an organized withdrawal menses will occur. For details, see Chap. 5 on Menstruation and Secondary Amenorrhea.

If ovulation does not occur for any reason, the endometrium will continue to proliferate under the influence of estradiol, and can become dyssynchronous and disorganized, eventually leading to unpredictable and potentially very heavy bleeding. Additionally, ongoing proliferation is a significant risk factor for the development of endometrial hyperplasia and eventually carcinoma; risk for endometrial hyperplasia and carcinoma increases with age as well as body-mass index.

Urine pregnancy test is negative. On examination, you are unable to see her cervix because of bright red blood filling the vagina. After removing as much of the blood as possible, you note that there is active, brisk bright red bleeding from the cervix. Blood pressure is 98/70, heart rate 95. Upon completing your examination, your patient complains of dizziness.

Approach to Management

After pregnancy has been ruled out, a careful examination should be performed. The provider should look for systemic signs of illness and evidence of coagulopathy. The primary purpose of the pelvic examination is to assess the volume and degree of bleeding and to determine whether the uterus feels "normal" in size and shape. Active bleeding from the cervix that requires multiple swabs to evacuate for visualization is considered heavy. Similarly, when a patient endorses syncope, near-syncope, passage of large clots, or bleeding for prolonged periods of time, she requires careful evaluation, as these symptoms suggest high-volume bleeding.

Consideration should be given to endometrial sampling to evaluate for hyperplasia or carcinoma. Patients at higher risk include women >35 years old, women with a prolonged history of anovulation, obesity, or polycystic ovary syndrome. This can be done using a simple suction device such as the Pipelle. Often, the degree of vaginal bleeding will make this challenging (because only blood is obtained), and, in those cases, sampling should occur once bleeding is stabilized. Typically, endometrial biopsy is performed by gynecologists though some primary care providers may do this testing as well.

Because of her significant bleeding, Audrey is transferred to the emergency department where she receives two 14-gauge IVs and fluids. Her hemoglobin is 9; her other labwork including coagulation studies is normal.

Treatment

The fastest and most effective therapy for anovulatory bleeding is hormonal. Treatment can be instituted with estrogen alone, progestin alone, or a combination of the two. The simplest therapy is to start combination oral contraceptives at an estrogen dose of 30–35 micrograms two or three times daily until bleeding slows or stops. For patients who cannot take estrogen—such as those with a personal history of estrogen responsive malignancy, thromboembolic disease, or smoking—progestin therapy can be started with either medroxyprogesterone acetate (10–20 mg PO three times daily) or norethindrone therapy (5–10 mg three times daily).

Alternately, intravenous estrogen therapy (25 mg every 4 hours) can be used to stop acute bleeding. It is important to note that there is little to no difference in onset of action; however, both oral and IV estrogen can lead to significant nausea and the IV route avoids loss of medication due to vomiting [15].

Tranexamic acid, a fibrinolysis inhibitor, can also reduce heavy menstrual bleeding by up to 50%. The typical dosing is 1300 mg every 8 hours for up to 5 days. While there was theoretical concern for thrombosis with this class of medications, multiple studies have not demonstrated this when used for acute heavy vaginal bleeding.

If bleeding continues after several days of IV or oral high-dose estrogen therapy, gynecologic consultation is recommended for consideration of surgical therapy. The treatment of choice will depend on the patient's age and fertility status; hysterectomy is incompatible with future fertility, and endometrial ablation and uterine artery embolization are relatively contraindicated. Simple uterine curettage (D&C) will be effective in many patients, but its effects are only temporary. Hysteroscopy is useful for identifying structural, focal lesions but can be challenging in cases of active bleeding.

Following hormonal manipulation of very heavy uterine bleeding, it is recommended to continue hormones at the "usual" daily dose (i.e. one combined oral contraceptive pill daily or a standard low dose of progestin) for several cycles (taken continuously). This prevents further withdrawal bleeding for several cycles and permits repletion of red blood cells and recovery from the episode. A withdrawal period should then be allowed, and discussion should occur with the patient regarding long-term plans for continuing or discontinuing the medication.

Audrey feels better after IV fluids and her hemoglobin remains stable over 4 hours. You advise her to take a 30-microgram pill three times daily until bleeding stops completely, then decrease to one pill daily. You emphasize the need for further evaluation with ultrasound and endometrial biopsy (if she has any risk factors for endometrial hyperplasia).

Conclusion

All primary care providers should be aware of the initial diagnosis and management of gynecologic emergencies such as ectopic pregnancy, adnexal torsion, and abnormal uterine bleeding that lead to significant blood loss. It is important to recognize the severity of the concerns, so patients may receive necessary emergency care when appropriate. Through a standardized approach, the risk of delaying therapy can be minimized.

Summary Points

1. The differential diagnosis of acute abdominopelvic pain in the female patient includes gynecologic and nongynecologic causes and relies on a thorough menstrual and sexual history.
2. The most common cause of secondary amenorrhea in the reproductive-aged patient is pregnancy; any patient who is late for regular menses or presents with undiagnosed abdominopelvic pain should have a point-of-care urine pregnancy test.
3. The diagnosis of adnexal torsion is challenging and remains a clinical diagnosis. While ultrasound can be helpful, a high suspicion and low threshold for surgical consultation are key to early diagnosis and treatment.
4. Acute vaginal hemorrhage in the nonpregnant patient is generally best managed with aggressive hormonal therapy, sometimes requiring hospitalization until initial effect is noted. Diagnostic tests should be performed to rule out malignancy or pre-malignancy when suspected. Surgical management in the acute phase is rarely necessary.

Review Questions

1. A 37-year-old comes to your office complaining of irregular menses and the gradual onset of lower abdominal pain. Upon further questioning, she states that her last menstrual period was exactly 5 weeks ago and she is not using contraception. Her menses are normally very regular (every 29 days). The abdominal pain started 4–5 days ago, was vague in character and location, but is now sharper and more left-sided than right. Neither acetaminophen nor ibuprofen has relieved her discomfort. A urine pregnancy test was positive in your office today. Vitals are as follows: T 37.6 C, HR 68, RR 12, BP 108/64. Pain is 3/10.

   What is your next best management step?

   A. Transfer the patient by ambulance to the nearest emergency department for evaluation
   B. Arrange for her to have a pelvic ultrasound at the nearest hospital
   C. Draw a stat serum hCG level in your office or lab
   D. Ask the patient to return to your office in 48 hours to determine whether her pain is worse or better

   The correct answer is C. Bleeding in the first trimester requires immediate evaluation. However, the stable patient does not necessarily need to be evaluated in the emergency setting. Because spontaneous abortion and ectopic pregnancy can lead to significant bleeding or other complications, expectant management is not a reasonable option in most cases. While ultrasound is normally part of the evaluation, in most cases having the hCG result first is more useful. A very low hCG level negates the need for ultrasound in stable patients as the ultrasound likely wouldn't provide useful information (neither a normal pregnancy nor ectopic pregnancy would be expected to be seen), whereas a very high hCG level suggests that the ultrasound may be more useful in making a diagnosis.

2. An 18-year-old patient being seen in your urgent care clinic. She complains of gradually worsening abdominal pain that started on the right and occurs in episodes that last several hours each with near-total resolution of pain between episodes. However, she has been in much more pain over the past 8 hours and notes that ibuprofen no longer controls her pain. Vitals are: T 38.1C, HR 96, RR 20, BP 124/80. Pain 9/10. On examination, you note normoactive bowel sounds but significant tenderness with rebound in the right lower quadrant. She is unable to cooperate with pelvic examination.

   Which of the following is true regarding her presentation?

   A. Adnexal torsion occurs most commonly in the prepubertal female.
   B. If ultrasound is performed and flow is seen to both ovaries, ovarian torsion should be considered excluded from the differential diagnosis.
   C. The sign most suggestive of adnexal torsion would be the presence of an adnexal mass on ultrasound.
   D. If adnexal torsion is confirmed, standard of care is unilateral oophorectomy as the ovary has likely undergone necrosis.

   The correct answer is C. Though there are many causes of acute pelvic pain in the female patient, adnexal torsion is one of the most important to consider, as failure to diagnose early can lead to necrosis of the ovary, tube, or both. Adnexal torsion can occur at any age, but is most common during the reproductive years. Pain is typically unilateral and gradually grows more severe; pain can also occur in a colicky pattern. Adnexal mass is usually (not always) appreciated on pelvic examination or ultrasound. Ultrasound findings can include changes in the Doppler flow to or from the ovary, but the sensitivity and specificity of this finding are limited [12]. Adnexal torsion is treated surgically, but conservation of the adnexa (and simple untwisting of the twisted pedicle is now standard of care).

3. A 44-year-old is in the emergency department complaining of heavy vaginal bleeding. She has type II diabetes and polycystic ovary syndrome. Her menses have been irregular over the past year, every 35–65 days. Her last normal menses was approximately 55 days ago. She then started bleeding 14 days ago and it has been progressively heavier. Today, she has been passing lemon-size clots and changing pads every 30–40 minutes. She is lightheaded when standing. Vitals are: T 36.5C, HR 104, RR 18, BP 88/48. Pain 2/10 (described as intermittent cramps). Urine pregnancy test is negative.

   Which of the following is true regarding her management?

   A. Endometrial biopsy is not indicated to rule out endometrial hyperplasia or carcinoma as she is not yet menopausal.
   B. After ordering labs, it would be reasonable to discharge the patient to complete the full workup as an outpatient.
   C. Because it is critical to the diagnosis, no treatment should be initiated until pelvic ultrasound has been performed.
   D. The irregular cycles suggest that the most likely diagnosis is anovulatory bleeding.

   The correct answer is D. Often, patients who present to the emergency department with heavy vaginal bleeding have avoided seeking help for an extended period of time, so this complaint should always be taken very seriously. In this case, the vital signs and description of bleeding call for rapid labwork, hemodynamic stabilization (including transfusion as necessary), and immediate treatment to slow her bleeding, generally requiring at least a short hospitalization [15]. Her history of polycystic ovary syndrome and progressively more irregular cycles do suggest that anovulatory bleeding is the most likely cause and should respond well to hormonal therapy. Endometrial biopsy is an essential step in the workup of any patient at risk for endometrial hyperplasia or cancer, generally considered to be any patient over age 35 and patients younger than 35 with particular risk factors, including significant obesity or long-term anovulation. While pelvic ultrasound may be useful to evaluate nonhormonal causes of bleeding, treatment should not be delayed for those results.

References

1. Cole LA. The hCG assay or pregnancy test. Clin Chem Lab Med. 2012;50(4):617–30.
2. Ankum WM, Mol BW, Van der Veen F, Bossuyt PM. Risk factors for ectopic pregnancy: a meta-analysis. Fertil Steril. 1996;65(6):1093–9.
3. Barnhart KT, Sammel MD, Gracia CR, Chittams J, Hummel AC, Shaunik A. Risk factors for ectopic pregnancy in women with symptomatic first-trimester pregnancies. Fertil Steril. 2006;86(1):36–43.
4. Clayton HB, Schieve LA, Peterson HB, Jamieson DJ, Reynolds MA, Wright VC. Ectopic pregnancy risk with assisted reproductive technology procedures. Obstet Gynecol. 2006;107(3):595–604.
5. Barnhart KT. Clinical practice. Ectopic pregnancy. N Engl J Med. 2009;361(4):379–87.
6. Seeber BE, Barnhart KT. Suspected ectopic pregnancy. Obstet Gynecol. 2006;107(2 Pt 1):399–413.
7. Seeber BE, Sammel MD, Guo W, Zhou L, Hummel A, Barnhart KT. Application of redefined human chorionic gonadotropin curves for the diagnosis of women at risk for ectopic pregnancy. Fertil Steril. 2006;86(2):454–9.
8. Lipscomb GH, Stovall TG, Ling FW. Nonsurgical treatment of ectopic pregnancy. N Engl J Med. 2000;343(18):1325–9.
9. Rabischong B, Larraín D, Pouly J-L, Jaffeux P, Aublet-Cuvelier B, Fernandez H. Predicting success of laparoscopic salpingostomy for ectopic pregnancy. Obstet Gynecol. 2010;116(3):701–7.
10. Hajenius PJ, Mol F, Mol BWJ, Bossuyt PM, Ankum WM, Van der Veen F. Interventions for tubal ectopic pregnancy. Cochrane Gynaecology and Fertility Group, editor. Cochrane Database Syst Rev [Internet]. 2007 [cited 2018 Mar 23]; Available from: http://doi.wiley.com/10.1002/14651858.CD000324.pub2.
11. Creanga AA, Syverson C, Seed K, Callaghan WM. Pregnancy-related mortality in the United States, 2011–2013. Obstet Gynecol. 2017;130(2):366–73.
12. Sasaki KJ, Miller CE. Adnexal torsion: review of the literature. J Minim Invasive Gynecol. 2014;21(2):196–202.
13. Geimanaite L, Trainavicius K. Ovarian torsion in children: management and outcomes. J Pediatr Surg. 2013;48(9):1946–53.
14. Munro MG, Critchley HOD, Fraser IS. The FIGO classification of causes of abnormal uterine bleeding: Malcolm G. Munro, Hilary O.D. Crithcley, Ian S. Fraser, for the FIGO Working Group on Menstrual Disorders. Int J Gynaecol Obstet. 2011;113(1):1–2.
15. American College of Obstetricians and Gynecologists. ACOG committee opinion no. 557: management of acute abnormal uterine bleeding in nonpregnant reproductive-aged women. Obstet Gynecol. 2013;121(4):891–6.
16. Committee on Practice Bulletins—Gynecology. Practice bulletin no. 128: diagnosis of abnormal uterine bleeding in reproductive-aged women. Obstet Gynecol. 2012;120(1):197–206.

12 Vaginitis and Vulvar Conditions

Swati Shroff and Janice Ryden

Learning Objectives

1. Discuss the differential diagnosis of vaginal discharge.
2. Compare and contrast the signs and symptoms of the three common types of vaginitis, i.e., bacterial vaginosis, vulvovaginal candidiasis, and trichomoniasis.
3. List the management options for the three common types of vaginitis.
4. Identify when recurrent vaginitis warrants chronic management.
5. Describe management strategies for contact vaginitis.
6. Describe general therapeutic measures for patients with vulvar problems.
7. Discuss the importance of prescribing ointments rather than creams for vulvar conditions.
8. Identify the risks of untreated lichen sclerosus and vulvar lichen planus.
9. Compare the varied and subtle presentation of vulvar malignancies and the importance of timely biopsy of any undiagnosed lesions.
10. Describe the presentation and management strategies of vulvodynia, including provoked vestibulodynia and generalized unprovoked vulvodynia.

S. Shroff (✉)
Sidney Kimmel Medical College, Thomas Jefferson University, Department of Medicine, Philadelphia, PA, USA

J. Ryden
Johns Hopkins University School of Medicine, Johns Hopkins Community Physicians, Department of Internal Medicine (*retired*), Baltimore, MD, USA

Maureen is a 32-year-old woman who calls your office complaining of a one-week history of vaginal discharge.

Vaginitis

Introduction

By definition, vaginitis is inflammation of the vagina, most commonly caused by an infection. Bacterial vaginosis (BV), vulvovaginal candidiasis (VC), and trichomoniasis account for a majority of vaginal infections. In a review of studies evaluating women presenting to primary care, BV was the most common etiology followed by VC and lastly trichomoniasis [1]. Less commonly vaginitis has a noninfectious etiology, as in the case of vaginitis associated with menopause (discussed in Chap. 8 on "Menopause"), contact dermatitis, and desquamative inflammatory vaginitis.

Infectious Vaginitis

Epidemiology

BV is the most common cause of vaginitis in women of child-bearing age, affecting almost one-third of women in the United States (U.S.) at any given time [2]. BV is caused by an alteration in the normal vaginal flora, where high concentrations of anaerobic bacterial species such as *Gardnerella vaginalis* replace the protective *Lactobacillus* species in the vagina. Many studies show douching and cigarette smoking are risk factors for BV acquisition [3–6]. While studies consistently show an association between sexual activity and BV, it remains unclear whether this is caused directly by sexual transmission or the impact of sexual activity on

S. A. Tilstra et al. (eds.), *Sex- and Gender-Based Women's Health*, https://doi.org/10.1007/978-3-030-50695-7_12

Lactobacillus vaginal colonization [7–9]. Therefore, BV is not classified as a sexually transmitted infection (STI).

Vulvovaginal candidiasis is the second most common infectious cause of vaginitis, affecting an estimated 75% of women during their lifetime [10]. *Candida albicans* is responsible for 85–95% of VC infections while *Candida glabrata* accounts for most of the remaining infections [10]. Candida primarily enters the vagina from the surrounding perianal area but does not necessarily result in symptomatic vaginitis [10], as up to 30% of asymptomatic women are colonized with *Candida* as part of their normal vaginal flora [11]. Yeast infections occur in celibate women; however, risk is increased with sexual activity, particularly receptive orogenital sex [10]. Uncontrolled diabetes; immunosuppression; estrogen exposure from pregnancy, estrogen-containing contraception, or postmenopausal hormone treatment; recent antibiotic or corticosteroid use; and douching are other important risk factors as well [10, 12].

Trichomoniasis is caused by the flagellated protozoan *Trichomonas vaginalis* (*T. vaginalis*) and is the most prevalent nonviral STI in the U.S. [13] and worldwide. Trichomoniasis is transmitted exclusively through sexual contact. Risk factors for trichomoniasis and STIs more generally include unprotected sex and multiple sexual partners (For more details on STIs see Chap. 13 on "Sexually Transmitted Infections").

Maureen describes the discharge as thin, white, and associated with pruritus. She denies fevers, chills, abdominal pain, and dysuria. She has only had sex with her husband in the last 5 years. She has an intrauterine device in place for contraception and does not use condoms.

Clinical Manifestations

Vaginitis caused by BV, VC, or trichomoniasis may be asymptomatic. When symptomatic, the most common symptom of vaginitis is vaginal discharge. Odor and pruritus are two other possible symptoms, and these are particularly helpful in distinguishing the cause of vaginitis. It is also important to characterize the volume, consistency, and color of the vaginal discharge, as well as evaluate for any associated symptoms. Since dysuria commonly occurs with vulvar irritation resulting from vaginal discharge, the differential diagnosis for women reporting dysuria extends beyond the urinary tract.

BV classically presents with a thin, homogenous, white discharge with a fishy odor, caused by the release of amines from anaerobic bacterial overgrowth. The volume of discharge can be minimal, and sometimes disagreeable odor is the sole complaint. A lack of perceived odor makes BV less likely (LR, 0.07 [95% confidence interval (CI), 0.01–0.51]) [1].

VC usually presents with a thick, curd-like, white discharge without any odor; however, at times the discharge may be yellow or thin or even absent. Describing a "cheesy" discharge increases the likelihood of VC (likelihood ratio [LR], 2.4; 95% CI, 1.4–4.2) [1]. VC is often associated with pruritus, burning, dyspareunia, and dysuria. Pruritus is frequently the dominant, and at times the only, symptom of VC. A lack of itching makes the diagnosis of VC less likely (range of LRs, 0.18 [95% CI, 0.05–0.70] to 0.79 [95% CI, 0.72–0.87]) [1]. On exam, women infected with VC may have accompanying vulvar erythema and edema; the presence of inflammatory signs is more commonly associated with VC (range of LRs, 2.1 [95% CI, 1.5–2.8] to 8.4 [95% CI, 2.3–3.1]) [1].

Women with trichomoniasis characteristically complain of vaginal discharge that may be associated with burning, dysuria, dyspareunia, and less commonly pruritus. Exam typically reveals copious, thin, malodorous, green-yellow discharge that pools in the posterior fornix, although a less "classic" thick discharge of different color is present nearly half the time. When present, bubbles in the discharge are fairly specific for trichomoniasis.

Despite these generalizations, the features of the three common types of vaginitis overlap significantly and variation in presentation is common. Moreover, coinfection with more than one type of vaginitis is not unusual. One should therefore not rely solely on history and exam to make the diagnosis.

Maureen says her symptoms remind her of a bacterial vaginosis infection in the past, and she requests a prescription for oral metronidazole.

Diagnosis and Differential Diagnosis

While over-the-counter treatments for vaginitis are commonly purchased, studies indicate that patient self-diagnosis is frequently incorrect [14]. Moreover, in addition to the three common infectious agents, the differential diagnosis of vaginal discharge includes physiologic discharge, noninfectious vaginitis, cervicitis, and pelvic inflammatory disease (PID).

Physiologic or normal vaginal discharge is typically transparent or white (although it may turn yellow upon drying) and varies with the menstrual cycle. It is flocculent, meaning it is a liquid base containing flecks of solid material, and it does not adhere to the vaginal walls but rather pools in the posterior fornix when the patient is recumbent.

Young women are often unaware that physiologic discharge is normal; patient education is facilitated by asking, "Is your current vaginal discharge different from your usual vaginal discharge?" Leukorrhea, a thick, whitish or yellowish discharge, results from estrogen exposure and is often seen in pregnancy and with use of the contraceptive vaginal ring.

Excluding PID (and cervicitis as well, since this can progress to PID) is critical in the evaluation of any woman complaining of vaginal discharge, as, unlike vaginitis, PID is commonly associated with significant morbidity and, albeit rarely, mortality. (See Chap. 13 on "Sexually Transmitted Infections".) All patients complaining about vaginal discharge should be questioned regarding abdominal pain, deep dyspareunia, intermenstrual bleeding, subjective fevers or chills, and nausea/vomiting. The sexual history should assess for multiple partners, new partners (defined as contact beginning within 2 months) and unprotected sex.

Evaluation: Examination and Testing

Women presenting with vaginal discharge require a full evaluation that includes pelvic examination, the whiff test, pH testing and office microscopy (or point-of-care testing or laboratory microsopy). A specimen for gonorrhea/chlamydia testing is also usually collected. The pelvic examination provides valuable information in a patient with vaginitis and is essential to exclude an upper tract infection (PID). Cervicitis is also a concern, and while most often the cervix appears normal in the setting of cervicitis, subtle visible abnormalities are occasionally evident, such as cervical edema or scant discharge from the cervical os. PID sometimes presents with cervical discharge, but the more reliable finding is tenderness on bimanual exam—either cervical motion tenderness or uterine or adnexal tenderness (covered in Chap. 13 on "Sexually Transmitted Infections").

Vaginal or cervical specimens for chlamydia and gonorrhea testing are usually collected at the time of the exam when possible infection with STIs is a concern. This swab can be discarded if ultimately deemed unnecessary but is used in certain presentations; for instance, if the bimanual exam raises concern for PID, if the wet mount exam shows excess leukocytes but no culprit organism (suggesting possible cervicitis or PID), or if the wet mount examination uncovers *Trichomonas* (an STI).

Urinary symptoms such as dysuria commonly accompany vaginitis and can stem from possible etiologies that range from inflamed vulvar mucosa, urethritis from a sexually transmitted infection or a urinary tract infection. Likewise, pyuria on urine testing may originate from contamination of the specimen with an inflammatory vaginal discharge rather than the urinary tract itself, and therefore must be interpreted carefully. Urine specimens are helpful for office pregnancy testing, which should be performed for women at risk.

Vaginal pH testing is an underutilized but helpful test. A sample of vaginal discharge from the lateral vaginal wall can be tested with narrow range pH paper, although lubricating gel can alter the pH and should not contaminate the tested sample. Vaginal pH in a premenopausal woman ranges from 4 to 4.5, because estrogen promotes glycogen production by the vaginal epithelium, which acts as a substrate for lactic acid production by inhabitant lactobacilli. An elevated pH in a premenopausal woman suggests BV or trichomoniasis (or a mixed infection) and helps exclude yeast, but is less useful in postmenopausal women, who lack this estrogen effect and whose vaginal pH is normally greater than 5 [15].

To prepare a wet mount, a small amount of discharge should be obtained from the lateral vaginal wall and placed on two slides. One drop of saline should be added to one slide and one drop of 10% potassium hydroxide (KOH) should be added to the other and a cover slip should be placed over each sample. Providers should "whiff" the KOH slide to assess for the presence of a fishy odor. A positive "whiff test" is predictive of BV (LR, 3.2 [95% CI, 2.1–4.7]), while lack of odor is associated with VC (LR, 2.9 [95% CI, 2.4–5]) [1]. However, a positive "whiff test" is also commonly found with trichomoniasis, due to overgrowth of anaerobes following oxygen consumption by trichomonads.

The saline slide should be viewed first (Fig. 12.1) [16], while the KOH slide is allowed to sit for one to two minutes to allow lysis of the cell membranes of vaginal epithelial cells to enable easier detection of budding yeast and hyphae. Slides should be viewed at low power 10x setting first, but optimal viewing occurs at the higher 40x setting. When examining a saline wet mount, the appearance of the squamous cells should be assessed, the leukocyte presence should be roughly quantified to determine if excessive, and several high power fields should be carefully scanned in search of trichomonads and fungal elements—although the latter are more easily detected on the KOH slide. The saline wet mount should be reviewed promptly (within 15 minutes of collection), while trichomonads are still motile.

The saline wet prep may demonstrate clue cells, which are epithelial cells coated with coccobacilli (best appreciated at the margins of the cells) (Fig. 12.2) [17] or motile trichomonads (Fig. 12.3) [17]. The presence of increased leukocytes (defined as >10 per high-powered field or a ratio of leukocytes to epithelial cells exceeding 1:1) (Fig. 12.3) may indicate infection with *Trichomonas* or suggest the diagnosis of cervicitis or PID – especially if a culprit organism is not seen on microscopy. Excess leukocytes can also be seen with noninfectious forms of vaginitis.

The KOH slide is next reviewed for budding yeast and hyphae (Fig. 12.4) [17]; several (approximately twenty)

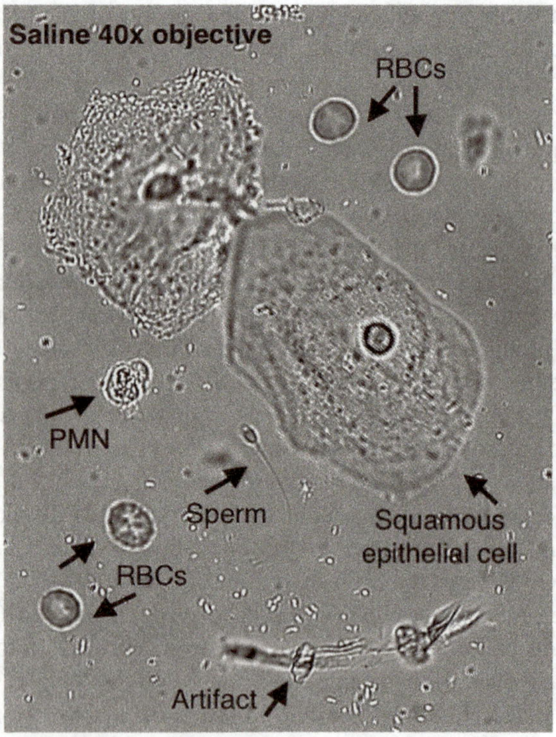

Fig. 12.1 Saline Wet Mount ("Wet Prep"). This saline wet mount of vaginal sampling from an asymptomatic woman depicts normal findings. The vaginal epithelial cells ("squamous cells") appear smooth, leukocytes are not increased, and no trichomonads or fungal elements are seen. Close inspection also reveals numerous tiny rod-shaped bacteria (*Lactobacillus*) throughout the field. Image from the University of Washington STD Prevention Training Center [16]. Used with permission

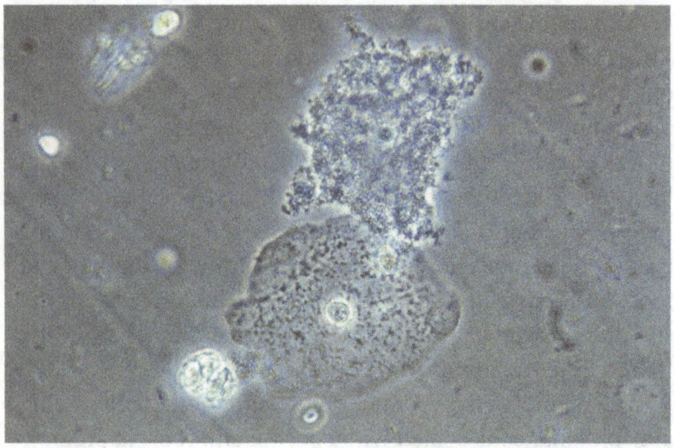

Fig. 12.2 Bacterial Vaginosis. This saline wet mount of vaginal sampling depicts two vaginal epithelial cells, the lower one appearing fairly normal and the upper one studded with bacteria --a "clue cell." The clue cell's roughened, speckled appearance is best appreciated at the cell margins. Diagnostic criteria for BV require that at least 20% of the epithelial cells be "clue cells." Note that leukocyte numbers are not increased. Image from CDC Public Image Library, CDC/Credit M. Rein [17]

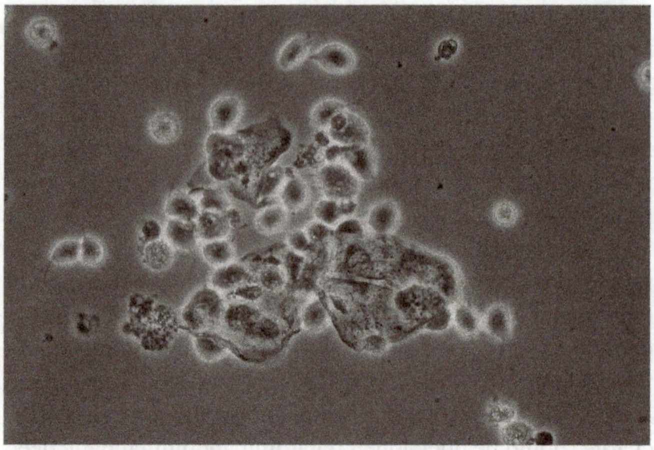

Fig. 12.3 Trichomoniasis. This saline wet mount of vaginal sampling shows numerous Trichomonads, which appear pear shaped, oval, or round and similar in size to the surrounding leukocytes, which are present in increased numbers. Detection of this protozoan is aided by its wriggling motion and the whipping action of its rotatory flagellae. Image from CDC Public Image Library, CDC/Credit Joe Miller [17]

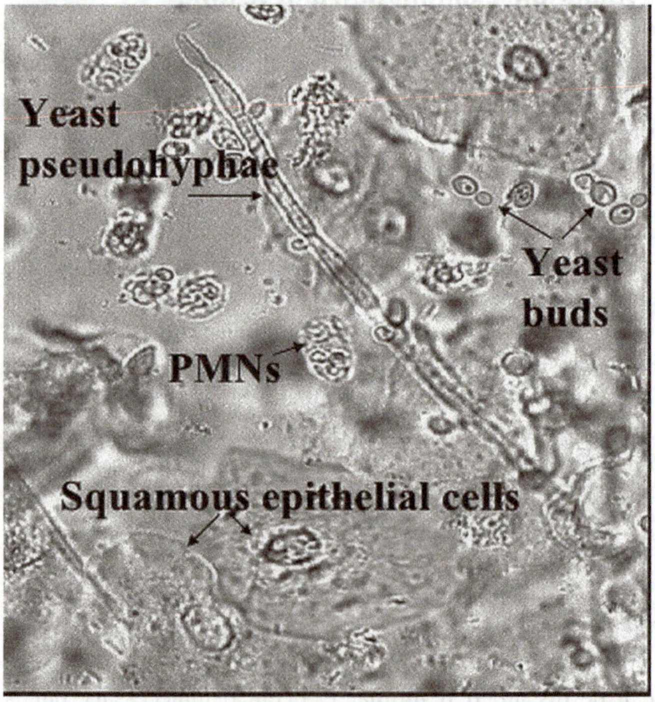

Fig. 12.4 Vulvovaginal Candidiasis. This saline wet mount depicts the two possible microscopic findings of yeast, namely the pseudohyphae/hyphae (nonbranching/branching) filamentous structures and spores, which are round or oval bodies that are smaller than erythrocytes and identifiable by their thick cell walls. The KOH slide is preferred, as lysis of surrounding cellular material aids in detecting these fungal elements, which are nonetheless often elusive. Saline: 40x objective. Image from the University of Washington STD Prevention Training Center [16]. Used with permission

high-power fields should be examined, as the sensitivity of this test is poor. Sometimes the diagnosis of vulvovaginal candidiasis must be made without observing yeast buds or hyphae. In such situations one should also consider the possibility of contact dermatitis, as the two entities share a number of clinical features.

BV is diagnosed by the presence of three out of four of Amsel criteria, which include the presence of a thin, homogenous vaginal discharge; vaginal pH > 4.5; a positive whiff test; and clue cells on wet prep. The sensitivity and specificity of Amsel criteria are 69% and 93%, respectively [18]. Recall also that leukocyte numbers are not increased in the setting of BV, in contrast to trichomoniasis [19].

The sensitivity of the wet mount for detecting trichomonads is only fair (51–65%) [5] and therefore when the organism is not seen on office microscopy yet there is continued concern for this infection, additional testing should be pursued, typically by adding *Trichomonas* NAAT testing to the vaginal swab specimen collected for chlamydia and gonorrhea testing.

Of note, trichomonads are sometimes reported incidentally on cervical cytology reports. While liquid-based Pap testing is not sensitive for diagnosing trichomoniasis, its specificity is as high as 99% and treatment is indicated without further testing [20]. On the other hand, conventional Pap smear testing is neither sensitive nor specific, and therefore should not be used to diagnose trichomoniasis, although such a report should trigger patient evaluation [21].

Newer point-of-care rapid antigen and DNA-amplification tests may be useful when offices lack a microscope, providers lack experience in examining wet mounts, or administrative protocols do not permit point-of-care microscopy. The wet mount, as a provider-performed microscopy procedure, is subject to regulations under CLIA (Clinical Laboratory Improvement Amendments) and thus even interested, trained primary care providers may not be able to perform microscopy depending on the protocols at their clinic sites. Studies indicate the BD Affirm VPIII test, a DNA probe assay, is more sensitive for diagnosing BV (sensitivity 95–100%), VC (90–100%), and trichomoniasis (90 to 100%) compared to office microscopy [18, 22], and the CDC encourages its wider use [5]. However, disadvantages of this newer semi-automated office-based technology are its cost and the time required to run some of the tests (approximately 45 min). Also, this technology fails to provide additional information that is evident on microscopy, such as the presence of inflammation, the number of lactobacilli or the degree of estrogen effect on the squamous epithelial cells. A second option when office microscopy is unavailable is to submit a specimen for wet mount evaluation to be performed by a lab. Some labs also include rapid antigen or DNA-amplification tests as a routine component of wet mount processing and interpretation.

Cultures are generally unhelpful for diagnosing vaginitis due to the polymicrobial nature of the vagina and because many culprit organisms represent normal flora that can be cultured from asymptomatic women. In addition, cultures are costly and delay diagnosis and treatment. Rarely, cultures play a role when the diagnosis is unclear, such as symptomatic women with repeatedly negative testing, or in women whose symptoms persist after treatment.

Maureen comes to the office for evaluation. Her examination is notable for white curd-like discharge, with erythema and swelling noted both in the vagina and vulva. The whiff test is negative and her vaginal pH is 4.5. Bimanual exam reveals no tenderness. The wet mount is notable for normal-appearing epithelial cells and no trichomonads. The KOH slide reveals budding yeast and hyphae. You diagnose her with a yeast infection. She asks about treatment and how to prevent future infections.

Treatment

Bacterial Vaginosis (BV) The Centers for Disease Control and Prevention (CDC) recommends treating symptomatic women diagnosed with BV [5]. Recommended and alternative oral and topical treatment regimens are listed in Table 12.1. A Cochrane review found clindamycin and metronidazole had equivalent rates of clinical cure (91% and 92%, respectively) [23]. The review also confirmed oral and topical preparations had comparable effectiveness. Topical treatments are associated with fewer adverse effects than oral metronidazole, which causes a transient metallic taste and

Table 12.1 Bacterial vaginosis: treatment regimens [5]

Recommended	Alternative
Metronidazole 500 mg orally twice daily for 7 days[a]	Tinidazole 2 g orally once daily for 2 days[a]
Metronidazole vaginal gel 0.75%, one applicatorful (5 g) intravaginally once daily at bedtime for 5 day[a]	Tinidazole 1 g orally once daily for 5 days[a]
Clindamycin cream[b] 2%, one applicatorful (5 g) intravaginally once daily at bedtime for 7 days	Clindamycin ovules[b] 100 mg intravaginally once daily at bedtime for 3 days
	Clindamycin 300 mg orally twice daily for 7 days[c]

Adapted using data from Workowski and Bolan [5]

[a]Patients taking metronidazole and tinidazole should be advised to avoid consuming alcohol during use and for 24 and 72 h thereafter, respectively, due to a possible risk of disulfiram-like reaction

[b]Topical clindamycin is oil-based and may weaken latex or rubber products (i.e. condoms and diaphragms)

[c]Oral clindamycin is not FDA-approved for this indication

sometimes nausea and vomiting. However, oral preparations may be more convenient for patients, and topical preparations are often more expensive.

Importantly, alcohol consumption should be avoided during treatment with oral or vaginal metronidazole until 24 h after completion of therapy to avoid a disulfiram-like reaction (e.g. flushing, nausea, vomiting, headaches). Tinidazole is an alternative treatment that carries similar risk, and due to this medication's longer half-life, alcohol must be avoided for 72 h after ingestion. Pregnant women with symptomatic BV may be treated with the same oral and topical treatment regimens recommended for nonpregnant women with BV, with the exception that tinidazole should be avoided in pregnancy [5].

Partner therapy is currently not recommended for male or female partners of women diagnosed with BV. A recent systematic review concluded that high quality evidence shows antibiotic treatment for male sexual partners of women with BV does not increase the rate of clinical or symptomatic improvement, and low-quality evidence suggests that male partner treatment does not decrease recurrence rates [24], while another systematic review concluded that six randomized controlled trials (RCT) had significant flaws and insufficient power to detect a reasonable effect size [25]. There have not been any RCTs specifically evaluating the treatment of female sexual partners. However, for women who have sex with women, studies consistently indicate high rates of concordant BV infections. Therefore, some experts recommend providing education on proper cleaning of sex toys as well as avoiding sexual activity during active infections, though no studies to date show these behaviors reduce BV recurrence rates [26].

Vaginal Candidiasis (VC) Since *Candida* can be a constituent of the normal vaginal flora, women found to have yeast on wet mount should be treated only if symptomatic. If symptomatic, it is important to differentiate between uncomplicated and complicated VC infections [10] (See Table 12.2). Uncomplicated VC infections can be treated with a 1-, 3-, or 7-day course of a topical azole or a single dose of an oral azole, whereas complicated VC infections require a regimen of longer duration, typically a 7- to 14-day course of a topical azole or three doses of an oral azole separated by 72 h. Oral azoles (e.g. fluconazole) and topical azoles (e.g. butoconazole, clotrimazole, miconazole, etc.) have comparable cure rates. While adverse effects and drug interactions are less of a concern with topical azoles, women typically prefer the convenience of the oral formulation, and oral fluconazole 150 mg is commonly prescribed [27].

The optimal treatment for non-*Candida albicans* VC is unclear, but first-line therapy is treatment with a topical or oral non-fluconazole azole drug (e.g., itraconazole) for 7–14 days [5, 28]. For azole-refractory *Candida glabrata* vaginitis, a two-week course of intravaginal boric acid or topical flucytosine may be effective [5, 29]. For women with severe vulvar inflammation, a low potency topical corticosteroid ointment may be applied for up to 48 h until the antifungal medication can take effect. For treatment of VC in pregnancy, only topical azole therapies are recommended, typically for a 7-day duration [5, 28]. Partner therapy is not indicated for VC infections.

Table 12.2 Characteristics of uncomplicated vs. complicated vulvovaginal candidiasis[a] [10]

Uncomplicated	Complicated
≤3 episodes per year *AND*	Recurrent VC (≥4 episodes per year) *OR*
Mild to moderate symptoms *AND*	Moderate to severe symptoms *OR*
Probable infection with *C. albicans AND*	Candida species other than *C. albicans OR*
Healthy, nonpregnant woman	Adverse risk factors (e.g. pregnancy, poorly controlled diabetes, immunosuppression)

Reprinted from The Lancet, Vol. 69/Number 9577, Sobel JD, Vulvovaginal candidosis; pgs 1961–1971, © 2007, with permission from Elsevier

[a]The distinction between Uncomplicated and Complicated VC has management implications, as complicated VC infections require a longer course of treatment (see text). See text also for chronic suppressive regimen for recurrent VC

Occasionally VC treatment failures using topical regimens result from patients mistakenly choosing to apply topical therapy to the vulva only and not the vagina. In certain settings it may be beneficial to emphasize the need for intravaginal treatment to eradicate the source of infection.

Trichomoniasis In contrast to BV and VC, treatment for trichomoniasis is indicated in both asymptomatic and symptomatic women and partner therapy is indicated as well, since trichomoniasis is sexually transmitted (see Chap. 13 on "Sexually Transmitted Infections" for further detail regarding partner therapy). Both metronidazole and tinidazole are FDA-approved for the treatment of trichomoniasis, and standard therapy is 2 g orally of either drug. Topical antimicrobials are not recommended because they are unlikely to achieve therapeutic levels in the urethra and perivaginal glands where the protozoan can also live [28]. An alternative regimen is metronidazole 500 mg orally twice daily for 7 days. The recommended regimen for treatment of trichomoniasis in pregnancy is oral metronidazole as a single 2 g dose. Both metronidazole and tinidazole have similar efficacy, but tinidazole is significantly more expensive [5]. Recall that during and following ingestion of metronidazole and tinidazole, alcohol must be avoided for 24 and 72 h, respectively. Women treated for trichomoniasis should be assigned an appointment within 3 months to screen for reinfection. (For details see section on Recurrent Vaginitis, Follow Up and Sequelae.)

Table 12.3 Summary of evaluation and treatment of infectious vaginitis

Type (% prevalence)[a]	Etiology	Symptoms and signs[b]	Office testing[c]	Treatment
Bacterial vaginosis (22–50%)	*Gardnerella vaginalis*, anaerobic bacteria	Odor Sometimes mild pain or pruritus Homogenous, thin, clear/white/gray, malodorous discharge	Whiff test positive pH > 4.5 Clue cells on microscopy, comprise ≥20% of epithelial cells	Metronidazole, oral or topical Clindamycin, topical
Vulvovaginal candidiasis (17–39%)	*Candida albicans*; Less commonly *C. krusei* or *C. glabrata*	Pruritus or "burning" Dysuria and dyspareunia also common White, thick, odorless discharge, but sometimes gray and thin, sometimes absent Vulvar and vaginal inflammation evident	Whiff test negative Normal pH (3.8–4.5) Budding yeast and hyphae on microscopy (best seen on KOH slide); no excess leukocytes (saline slide)	Azoles, oral or topical
Trichomoniasis (4–35%)	*Trichomonas vaginalis*	Discomfort (irritation, soreness, etc.) Dyspareunia, dysuria, Pruritus Green-yellow, frothy discharge Vaginal inflammation evident	Whiff test often positive pH > 4.5 Motile trichomonads on microscopy along with excess leukocytes; clue cells often present as well	Metronidazole, oral Tinidazole, oral
Normal physiologic discharge		No disagreeable odor or other symptom Clear or white flocculent discharge that does not adhere to vaginal walls	Whiff test negative pH 3.8–4.5 (premenopausal); pH 5–7 (postmenopausal) Smooth-appearing epithelial cells with few clue cells (<20%) on microscopy, only occasional leukocyte	Reassurance if needed

Data from Anderson et al. [1]

[a]Prevalence per review of studies of symptomatic women presenting in primary care

[b]Patient symptoms and vaginal discharge characteristics may vary from the "classic" disease presentation as listed above, and there is overlap in the features of the three types of infectious vaginitis. Coinfection is also common. These caveats underscore the importance of complete office evaluation.

[c]Point-of-care testing is an alternative to microscopy

A persistent trichomoniasis infection usually represents reinfection from an untreated sex partner, since treatment resistance is uncommon. (See Chap. 13 on "Sexually Transmitted Infections" section on expedited partner therapy.) If a true treatment failure is suspected after a single dose of a nitroimidazole, metronidazole 500 mg orally twice daily for 7 days is recommended [5]. If this regimen also fails, clinicians should consider treatment with metronidazole or tinidazole at 2 g orally once daily for 7 days [5]. If several 1-week regimens fail and both nonadherence and reinfection are unlikely, the CDC can provide assistance with susceptibility testing and treatment of nitroimidazole-resistant *T. vaginalis* (telephone: 404-718-4141; website: http://www.cdc.gov/std) [30]. Chronic *Trichomonas* carriage is also possible (see next section). Table 12.3 summarizes the etiology, symptoms, diagnosis, and treatment of infectious vaginitis.

In the next year, Maureen has three more episodes of vulvovaginal candidiasis, and today you diagnose her with another yeast infection. She wonders how to avoid another infection.

Recurrent Vaginitis, Follow-Up, and Sequelae

Recurrent vaginitis is common. However, persistent symptoms occasionally stem from misdiagnosis, thus repeat evaluation should first be performed to exclude this possibility. Patients confirmed to have recurrent vaginitis are often candidates for chronic management, and sometimes benefit from addressing potential risk factors.

More than half of patients diagnosed with BV experience a recurrence within 1 year [31]. For women with multiple recurrences despite completion of recommended treatment regimens, the only approved suppressive therapy is topical metronidazole (nocturnal application two nights per week for 6 months) [26]. Alternatively, a small, randomized trial found that monthly oral metronidazole 2 g plus oral fluconazole 150 mg also reduced the incidence of BV and in addition promoted colonization with normal vaginal flora [32]. Patients with recurrent BV should also be advised that the use of condoms and estrogen-containing contraceptives may reduce recurrences [31, 33, 34]. (See Chap. 4 on "Patient-Centered Contraceptive Counseling" for safe prescribing of estrogen-containing contraception.) Smokers should be informed that cigarette smoking is associated with an increased risk of BV in a dose-dependent manner [35], and some patients benefit from a reminder that douching should be avoided [36].

Approximately half of women diagnosed with VC will experience a recurrence, and 5 to 8% will suffer recurrent VC, defined as ≥4 episodes in 1 year [10]. Although most sufferers of recurrent VC are healthy women, one should screen for symptoms of uncontrolled diabetes, and testing for diabetes should certainly be performed for postmenopausal women [10]. Also, women with recurrent VC can be made aware of modifiable risk factors such as the use of estrogen-containing contraceptives and unprotected sexual activity – especially receptive orogenital sex, as well as douching and the use of panty hose and panty liners [37]. Others may benefit from learning that some women suffer recurrent VC while ingesting a diet high in refined sugars (despite having normal serum glucose levels) and enjoy resolution of the problem upon adoption of a healthier diet [38].

Women with recurrent VC can be offered a 6-month course of chronic treatment. Since non-*Candida albicans* species may be responsible a vaginal culture should first be obtained. Women should be made aware that treatment is suppressive, not curative, and that typically episodes of VC recur following completion of the regimen. Most women choose to continue episodic treatment, but for those who desire chronic therapy the Infectious Diseases Society of America (IDSA) recommends treating recurrent VC with 10–14 days of induction therapy using a topical or oral azole followed by oral fluconazole at 150 mg once per week for 6 months [39]. Other beneficial measures for recurrent VC include the use of the injectable contraceptive medroxyprogesterone acetate (Depo Provera) [40] and possibly daily oral ingestion of yogurt that contains live cultures (confirmatory trials are needed) [41].

One study found that up to 17% of women treated for trichomoniasis were reinfected within 3 months [42]. Because of high rates of reinfection, the CDC recommends rescreening for trichomoniasis in all sexually active women within 3 months of treatment [5]. Nucleic acid amplification testing should be deferred for at least 2 weeks following treatment due to concern for false positive results from persistent dead organisms. Also of note, a recent study suggests that while *T. vaginalis* may be undetectable months after treatment, it can nonetheless be present and persist in a dormant state, only to become evident on testing months to years later in asymptomatic women reporting no new sexual activity [43]. Chronic asymptomatic carriage would explain the unusual older age distribution of trichomoniasis, as rates of trichomoniasis are highest in women over 40 years of age [44, 45]. The possibility of chronic asymptomatic *T. vaginalis* carriage may be important to include as part of patient counseling, particularly for patients who are abstinent or report long-term monogamous relationships and are uncertain of how they acquired the infection.

Primary care physicians should not underestimate the importance of their work in diagnosing and treating infectious vaginitis, as both bacterial vaginosis and trichomoniasis are sometimes associated with serious morbidity. BV appears to increase susceptibility to infection with certain STIs such as *Trichomonas*, chlamydia, and gonorrhea [46, 47], while trichomoniasis appears to possibly increase the risk of PID [48]. Even more concerning, both BV and trichomoniasis increase a woman's risk of acquiring HIV [49, 50] as well as her risk of transmitting the HIV infection to others [51, 52]. Consequently, some have advocated treating asymptomatic BV to reduce the spread of HIV; however, there is insufficient evidence to support this strategy at the current time. BV and trichomoniasis are also associated with pregnancy complications such as preterm births [53, 54]; however, treatment has not proved beneficial. Despite these potential complications, vaginitis is usually not associated with significant long-term sequelae, and patients should be appropriately reassured.

Maureen meets the defined criteria for recurrent vulvovaginal candidiasis. You screen her for diabetes and testing is negative. You offer her induction therapy followed by 6 months of suppressive therapy. However, today Maureen admits that, despite previous office discussions regarding lifestyle factors, she has continued her habit of drinking multiple glasses of sugary soda throughout the day. Maureen states she would first prefer a trial of following a diet that is lower in refined sugars and agrees to an appointment in 3 months. At her follow-up visit Maureen is happy to report that she has had no further vaginal yeast infections.

Noninfectious Vaginitis

The genitourinary syndrome of menopause (previously termed atrophic vaginitis and covered in Chap. 8 on "Menopause"), contact vulvovaginitis, and desquamative inflammatory vaginitis are noninfectious causes of vaginitis. Since contact dermatitis typically involves the vulva more than the vagina, it is covered in the Common Vulvar Problems section of this chapter (see below).

Desquamative Inflammatory Vaginitis

Desquamative inflammatory vaginitis (DIV) is an uncommon chronic vaginitis of unknown cause, although an immune etiology is suspected. It occurs mainly in

Caucasian women, and while half of sufferers are of reproductive age, peak incidence occurs in peri-menopausal women [55].

Nearly all patients describe three symptoms: a purulent vaginal discharge, severe dyspareunia, and vaginal discomfort [56]. Patients typically have symptoms for more than 1 year before being diagnosed [57]. On exam, purulent discharge is seen. Evidence of vaginal inflammation is always present, either in the form of a spotted vaginal rash (either petechial or ecchymotic), diffuse vaginal erythema, or linear erosions. Occasionally the cervix is involved with papules having a pale center (resembling donuts) [57]. The vestibule is often also erythematous and in extreme cases, an erythematous macular rash may be evident on the vulva [56].

The vaginal pH is always greater than 4.5. Saline wet mount shows an increase in parabasal cells, which are small, round immature epithelial cells that have a large nucleus and little cytoplasm. Inflammation is also evident, defined as the leukocyte to epithelial cell ratio exceeding 1:1. Careful inspection also reveals an absence of lactobacilli [58].

Because of overlap in clinical presentation, it is sometimes reasonable to exclude other diagnoses before making a diagnosis of DIV, such as trichomoniasis (using PCR testing), Group A *Streptococcus* (with vaginal culture) [56] and lichen planus (by performing careful examination of the oral cavity and skin). Of note, some clinicians suspect DIV may be a variant of erosive lichen planus [59].

Retrospective studies suggest similar efficacy with either topical clindamycin or vaginal corticosteroids. Both act via anti-inflammatory effects. Clindamycin is known to have such properties, and substitution with antibiotics having similar antimicrobial activity is ineffective. In fact, clinical response to any antibiotic other than clindamycin (or response to estrogen therapy) excludes the diagnosis of DIV.

Initial treatment consists of either nightly intravaginal clindamycin or corticosteroids plus medication applied to the vestibule for 4 weeks [58]. Nearly all patients demonstrate remarkable initial improvement and after 4 weeks the regimen is usually tapered to twice weekly maintenance therapy. Thereafter progress slows and the majority of women must continue maintenance treatment for longer than 1 year [58]. In addition to monitoring symptoms and physical exam, follow-up wet mount examination helps assess progress. Assessment of vaginal pH, however, is not useful in the setting of clindamycin use. Since treatment predisposes to yeast vaginitis, some providers prescribe suppressive therapy using fluconazole 150 mg weekly or, for women suspected of having DIV plus symptomatic vaginal atrophy, topical estrogen.

Common Vulvar Problems

Overview

The vulva consists of the labia majora, labia minora, clitoris, vaginal vestibule, vaginal introitus, urethral meatus, and the openings of the ducts of the greater vestibular glands (Fig. 12.5). The vulva serves to direct urine flow, prevent admission of foreign bodies into the vagina, and contribute to sexual pleasure [60].

Although vulvar symptoms most commonly result from discharge originating from the vagina or cervix, primary processes specific to the vulva also occur. These include contact dermatitis (both irritant and allergic), dermatoses (e.g. psoriasis, lichen sclerosus, lichen planus, and lichen simplex chronicus), vulvar neoplasms, and vulvodynia. Although genital *Candida* infections are a common cause of vulvitis, this topic is discussed in the Infectious Vaginitis section of this chapter. Likewise, those sexually transmitted infections (i.e. herpes simplex virus, syphilis and low-risk human papillomavirus (HPV) that can cause vulvar lesions are covered in Chap. 13 on "Sexually Transmitted Infections".

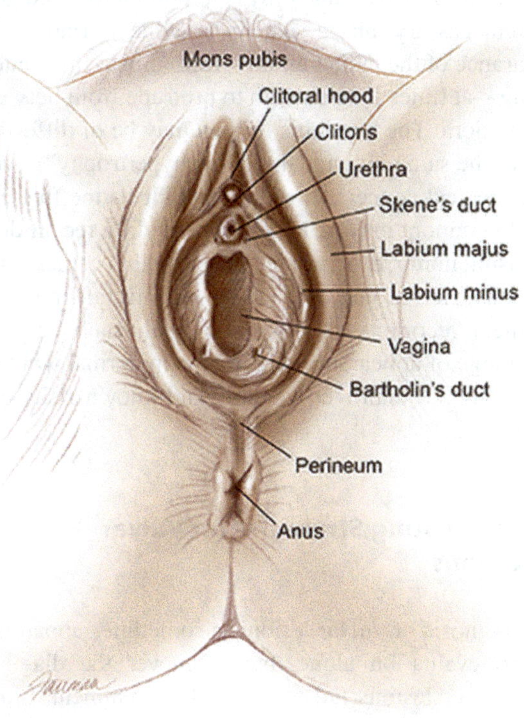

Fig. 12.5 Anatomy of the Vulva. The vulva consists of the labia majora, labia minora, clitoris, clitoral hood, and vaginal vestibule. The vaginal vestibule encompasses the space between the two labia minora and contains the openings of the urethra, vagina, and ducts of the greater vestibular glands. Illustration © 2019, Jennifer E. Fairman, CMI, FAMI. Johns Hopkins University. Used with permission

History

Most women do not recognize the vulva as an anatomic entity and are also unfamiliar with the term "vulva," and therefore typically refer to the area as the "vagina" or with vague terminology. Using a term such as "external genital area" when eliciting history can help clarify location. Studies indicate that patients with vulvar complaints delay seeking evaluation for months or even years due to embarrassment or anxiety. Clinicians should therefore be attentive to providing care in a nonjudgmental and supportive fashion. In addition to the usual medical, surgical, gynecological, sexual, social, and family history and medication list, evaluation of vulvar problems sometimes requires obtaining an extensive history of all vaginal and vulvar contactants.

Physical Examination

A proper pelvic examination includes thorough inspection of the vulva using adequate lighting—which in some settings is aided by the light source contained within the illuminated plastic speculum held before the vulva. Familiarity with normal variants in vulvar anatomy is important to avoid generating unnecessary alarm. There is wide variation in the appearance of the labia minora—from thin to thick and short to long—at times long enough to protrude from between the labia majora. The two labia minora may be of differing size even in the same individual ("labial hypertrophy"), which is of no medical concern. In some individuals the free edge of the labia minora may be hyperpigmented. In recent decades, increasing numbers of women have sought cosmetic surgery for their external genitalia, and a recently affirmed ACOG statement recommends discussing with such patients the wide range of appearance of genitalia in normal women [61] as well as the unproven benefits and known risks of such surgery [62].

General Testing Strategies for Vulvar Conditions

The diagnosis of vulvar lesions is sometimes apparent from clinical evaluation alone, but whenever the diagnosis is uncertain or lesions fail to respond to treatment, biopsy or referral is indicated. The importance of promptly biopsying undiagnosed vulvar lesions cannot be overemphasized given that vulvar malignancies assume a wide range of appearances. Primary care physicians adept at performing skin biopsies can perform biopsies of the vulva; however, referral to gynecology or dermatology is often warranted. Some tertiary centers have specialized vulvovaginal clinics staffed by either gynecologists or dermatologists, preferably both, and sometimes infectious disease specialists as well. Familiarity with the available local expertise can benefit one's patients with vulvar conditions.

General Therapeutic Measures for Vulvar Dermatitis

For patients with vulvar problems, a number of measures can promote vulvar health, alleviate discomfort, and speed healing. Underpants should be loose-fitting and made of absorbent material (such as cotton). Women may also benefit from avoiding tight pants, lycra garments and pantyhose, and wearing no underpants while sleeping. To avoid allergen exposure, underwear should be laundered with fragrance-free detergent without fabric softener. Patients with acute vulvar conditions often benefit from a daily warm bath (without soap or bubble bath), plus tap water compresses twice daily for 20 min. Wipes, deodorants, and douches contain common irritants and/or allergens and their use should be avoided. When washing, a bar of moisturizing rather than a deodorant or liquid soap should be used, if soap is used at all. Daily panty liners should also be avoided, and tampons are less irritating to the vulva than pads.

Several barrier options can provide symptomatic relief from vulvar discomfort. Zinc oxide ointment serves as an excellent barrier that prevents irritating discharge or urine from contacting inflamed mucosa and can be applied on top of medication if needed. Olive oil and petroleum jelly are moisturizers and skin protectants that are unlikely to cause allergy. In contrast, powders are best avoided on the vulva.

Rubbing and scratching often exacerbate vulvar problems and should be discouraged and the pruritus treated. Cool Sitz baths or cool packs applied to the vulva are helpful. Antihistamines such as hydroxyzine (25–50 mg) or the tricyclic antidepressant doxepin (10–25 mg) dosed once daily at bedtime can relieve nighttime itching. Cetirizine (5–10 mg) may be dosed in the daytime, although a minority of patients will experience sedation. Topical antihistamine preparations should be avoided due to the risks of contact dermatitis and sensitizing the patient to the antihistamine [63] as well as poor efficacy [64].

When prescribing topical treatment, ointments are preferred over creams, which contain alcohols or preservatives that can cause irritant or contact dermatitis. Mid-potency topical steroids, such as triamcinolone ointment 0.1% for up to 10–14 days, treat most acute problems. Prolonged use of topical steroids on the vulva can cause permanent skin changes such as striae or atrophy on the medial thighs or buttocks, although usually not on the vulva itself. Most primary care physicians seek consultation from either a dermatologist or gynecologist if either ultrapotent or long-term use of topical corticosteroids is needed.

Lidocaine ointment 5% is effective for temporary local pain control for patients with mucosal ulcers or for some types of vulvodynia. Over-the-counter benzocaine (Vagisil) should be avoided, as it is a common cause of allergic contact dermatitis.

Specific Conditions of the Vulva

Contact Vulvovaginitis

Cady is a 19-year-old who presents with "a yeast infection that just won't go away." She states she began suffering itching "down there" approximately 1 month ago, and trials of two different over-the-counter yeast treatments "just made it worse." She has had difficulty sleeping the past two nights due to the itching and discomfort.

Contact vulvovaginitis is a common cause of vulvar symptoms and accounts for approximately half of patients presenting to vulvar clinics [65]. The peaks in prevalence occur between the ages of 10–20 years and 40–50 years [66]. Contact dermatitis may result from irritants (irritant contact dermatitis) or, less commonly, allergens (allergic contact dermatitis).

Irritant contact dermatitis results from exposure to agents that cause direct injury to the skin cells or lipid barrier. By contrast, allergic dermatitis develops only in susceptible individuals following exposure to an antigen that triggers an immunologic reaction. Irritant vulvovaginitis appears quickly, within minutes to hours of exposure, while the allergic dermatitis is a form of delayed type hypersensitivity and onset is 24–48 h after exposure. Because of the anatomical location of the vulva, allergic contact dermatitis may result from allergen exposure via several routes, including direct application of topical products, inadvertent manual transfer from other body sites, exposure to allergen in urine or feces following oral consumption, or systemic contact reactions.

Common causes of irritant vulvovaginitis include prolonged exposure to urine, sweat, feces, semen, and abnormal vaginal discharge. Spermicides, lubricants, irritants found in douches and other feminine hygiene products, harsh soaps and detergents, and simply overzealous hygiene are other causes. Daily use of pads and panty liners can also cause an irritant dermatitis due to friction. Topical medications containing alcohols or certain acids are common culprits. Feminine wipes and moist toileting wipes contain both irritants and a common allergen.

Common causes of allergic vulvovaginitis include (1) fragrances (and therefore soaps, body washes, laundry detergents, and pads and tampons that contain deodorant), (2) preservatives in topical medications, (3) topical medications themselves—especially topical anesthetics (i.e. benzocaine in Vagisil), topical antibiotics (i.e. neomycin and aminoglycosides), topical anti-fungals, and even topical corticosteroids, (4) propylene glycol and (5) lanolin. Other relatively common causes of allergic contact dermatitis include the chemicals in the rubber and natural latex used in condoms and diaphragms. Chemicals such as rosin or acrylates that are in feminine hygiene or incontinence pads have also been implicated. Over-the-counter topical formulations containing botanical agents are becoming increasingly popular, and these are important potential allergens. In patients with anogenital complaints, ingestion of spices and peppermint oil are common culprits [67].

History

Most women with irritant vulvovaginitis report burning or irritation, while those with allergic vulvovaginitis complain of itching [68], but symptom overlap occurs. Vaginal discharge is not often present.

When searching for the cause of contact dermatitis, an exhaustive history regarding potential exposures is frequently required, and occasionally, the exposures of the sex partner as well.

On pelvic exam, Cady's vulva is diffusely erythematous and swollen, and scattered erythematous papules are seen. Her vaginal mucosa appears normal, and there is no vaginal discharge. Her vaginal pH is normal, the whiff test is negative and no fungal elements or increased leukocytes are seen on microscopic examination of the wet mount and KOH prep.

Examination

Examination of the patient with contact dermatitis commonly reveals vulvar erythema and swelling and well-demarcated edematous papules and vesicles, which can ulcerate [69]. Occasionally the vaginal mucosa is also involved, as in the setting of contact dermatitis from douches, deodorant-containing tampons, spermicides, etc. Contact dermatitis can easily be mistaken for candida vulvovaginitis; however, the lack of vaginal discharge or fungal elements on microscopy help distinguish the two. Mild irritants may not always produce physical findings to accompany a patient's symptoms.

Management

The treatment of either form of contact vulvovaginitis entails permanent avoidance or elimination of the trigger plus temporary use of topical low- to mid-potency steroid ointments such as desonide ointment 0.05% or triamcinolone ointment 0.1% for 2–4 weeks. Patients with severe pruritus should also be treated with oral antihistamines or doxepin (see above). If an allergic contact dermatitis is suspected, referral to a dermatologist for patch testing is often helpful.

When there are bullae or erosions on the vulva and the diagnosis is unclear, biopsy may be needed to rule out an immunobullous disorder [68]. Irritant vulvovaginitis may complicate an underlying vulvar dermatosis, in which case the diagnosis may be challenging. Sometimes contact dermatitis may become infected with yeast or bacteria, in which case systemic antibiotics are preferred over topical.

Although Cady suspected a yeast infection, the physical exam and microscopy findings are consistent with contact dermatitis. An extensive history uncovers her new habit of using moist toileting wipes beginning 1 month ago. You recommend immediate and permanent avoidance of all moist toileting wipes. You also advise temporary use of cool Sitz baths and cool compresses and prescribe desonide ointment 0.05% to be applied sparingly to the vulva twice daily for 14 days. Given the severity of her itching you also prescribe cetirizine 10 mg daily in the morning and hydroxyzine 25 mg at bedtime.

Dermatoses

The four important dermatoses that affect the vulva are lichen sclerosus, lichen planus, psoriasis, and lichen simplex chronicus.

Your next patient of the morning is Luisa, a 55-year-old healthy woman who presents for a "routine Pap smear." She complains of worsening vulvar itching and entrance dyspareunia that began approximately 1 year ago.

Lichen Sclerosus

Lichen sclerosus (LS, previously termed lichen sclerosus et atrophicus) is an inflammatory, likely autoimmune, disease that causes pigment and texture changes of the vulvar mucosa and, left untreated, eventual destruction of vulvar structures. The disease is also associated with risk of malignant transformation to squamous cell carcinoma. Affected patients are usually older than 50 years; however, the condition occurs in women of all ages and even girls; in one large study the mean age at diagnosis was 55 years (range 18–86 years) [70].

On pelvic examination, Luisa's vulva appears abnormal: the mucosa is diffusely thickened and pale, and the mucosa of the perineum and perianal areas is affected as well. Her labia minora appear shrunken and her introitus is narrowed.

History and Examination

Patients with LS usually complain of itching, burning, and introital dyspareunia; if anal involvement is present, patients can experience painful defecation and anal fissures. Examination reveals pallor and initially abnormal thickening of the vulva mucosa, which is usually diffuse but sometimes focal. When involvement is diffuse and includes the perineum and perianal areas, it can resemble a "figure 8." Over time the mucosa becomes abnormally thin and wrinkled ("cigarette paper appearance") and bruises can result from scratching the fragile mucosa. In the absence of trauma, vulvar ecchymoses are virtually pathognomonic for LS [71, 72]. Adhesions, tissue resorption, and scarring affect the architecture of the vulva: the clitoris may become sealed under the clitoral hood, the labia minora may shrink and even disappear altogether, and the introitus may narrow significantly [72] (Fig. 12.6). Biopsy findings help distinguish the condition from lichen planus and malignant transformation [73].

A vulvar biopsy confirms the diagnosis of LS and you refer Luisa to a gynecologist for management. You emphasize that even after the condition comes under control, she will need lifelong treatment with topical steroids and monitoring every 6–12 months, due to the increased risk of SCC.

Management

Ultrapotent topical corticosteroid ointments (i.e. clobetasol ointment 0.05%) are the mainstay of treatment. At diagnosis, the ointment is applied once daily for 1 month, followed by every other day for 1 month, and then twice weekly for 1 month. Thereafter regimens are less well defined and vary; common regimens include twice weekly clobetasol or substitution of a less-potent corticosteroid. Symptoms resolve within days or

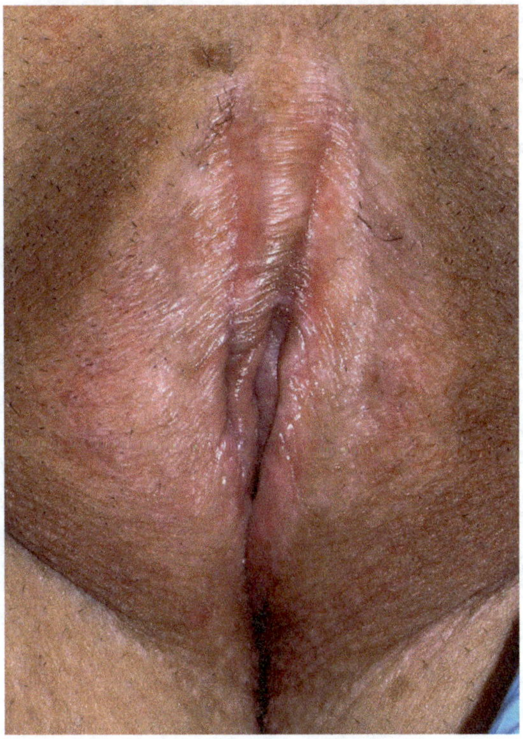

Fig. 12.6 Lichen sclerosus (later stage). The vulvar mucosa is pale, thin, and wrinkled. The right labium minus is markedly shrunken, the left labium minus is completely resorbed and the clitoris is buried under a stenotic clitoral hood. In addition to destruction of her vulvar anatomy, untreated LS places this patient at higher risk for vulvar carcinoma. Untreated vulvar lichen planus carries these same risks. Used with permission

weeks of initiating treatment but pallor and atrophy take longer to respond. Spontaneous resolution can occur; however, most recommend continuing topical steroid treatment indefinitely. Some women require alternative therapies such as immunomodulators, and surgery is sometimes needed to treat adhesions. Most women diagnosed with LS are managed by either a gynecologist or dermatologist, since management requires the use of ultrapotent topical corticosteroids and close monitoring for the possible development of vulvar cancer.

Women with LS have a 3–5% risk of developing vulvar SCC, and thus even once the condition is stable patients require lifelong monitoring at least every 6–12 months, with prompt biopsy of suspicious areas. Scarring is not expected to reverse, however, the mucosal thickening and pigment changes of LS are highly responsive to therapy. Any areas of mucosa that appear "unresponsive" likely represent either vulvar intraepithelial neoplasia (VIN) or squamous cell carcinoma (SCC)—especially if they appear as a pink patch or a white raised lesion. Patients should also be counseled to report any lump, ulcer, or hardening of the skin [74].

Cessation of therapy commonly leads to relapse and attendant risks for destruction of vulvar structures and vulvar cancer. Although a controlled trial would now be unethical, a large longitudinal study following affected women for 5 years suggested that continued corticosteroid treatment is likely effective in preventing vulvar cancer, as no cases were seen among the compliant patients yet 4.7% of the noncompliant patients were affected [70]. Since patients are often tempted to quit treatment when they are no longer symptomatic, the importance of continuing long-term topical steroids should be emphasized. Patients with LS also have a higher likelihood of other autoimmune disorders such as thyroid disease (incidence 16.3%) [75] and pernicious anemia, and should be appropriately screened.

Because of the association of LS with thyroid disease and pernicious anemia, you ask Luisa to obtain lab work after today's visit. You employ the teach-back method to confirm she understands the importance of long-term treatment and regular follow-up of this condition.

Lichen Planus

Margaret is a 57-year-old woman who presents for routine follow-up of her hypertension and arthritis, for which she has taken metoprolol and ibuprofen for years. She reports 3 years of worsening pain and soreness "in my private area" and reveals she quit having intercourse 1 year ago due to entrance as well as deep dyspareunia. She states she finally mustered enough courage to see her gynecologist last month and was diagnosed with lichen planus. She is now under the care of a dermatologist.

As with lichen sclerosus, lichen planus (LP) is an inflammatory, likely autoimmune, disorder that can lead to destruction of the normal architecture of the vulva, but LP can also involve the vagina as well. There are three main types: erosive, papulosquamous, and hyperkeratotic disease. Genital LP can occur in isolation or as part of a systemic disease involving skin, hair, nails, or other mucosa. Women with the erosive form usually also have oral involvement, most commonly in the form of ulcers on the buccal mucosa.

Margaret brings with her the dermatologist's note, which describes her vulva as brightly erythematous and having erosions on the labia minora that are surrounded by a white rim. Her vagina is described as brightly erythematous, shortened and coated with an adherent film. She also has ulcers on her buccal mucosa.

History and Objective Findings

Genital LP can be asymptomatic or cause itching, burning, post-coital bleeding, dyspareunia, or yellow vaginal discharge. The appearance of the vulva depends on which of the three LP variants is present. Erosive LP, the most common and most destructive form, manifests as bright erythema and erosions on the labia minora that are surrounded by a white reticular rim. Left untreated, erosions can lead to scarring with strictures, such as phimosis of the clitoris and stenosis of the urethra or vaginal introitus. In advanced disease the introitus may be reduced to a very small opening or the vulva may lose all landmarks and become "featureless." In the vagina, erosions and internal synechiae can cause eventual stenosis and loss of length of the vagina. The less common papulosquamous variant presents with polygonal, flat-topped papules with white reticulated borders (Wickhams's striae) on the vulva that are reminiscent of the violaceous LP papules found elsewhere on the body. The third form of LP, hyperkeratotic, exhibits hyperkeratotic lesions of the perineum and perianal areas.

Biopsy is often nondiagnostic but helps exclude a neoplastic disorder. Diagnosis usually rests on vulvar examination and extravulvar manifestations of LP; formal diagnostic criteria have been established [76].

Management

As with lichen sclerosus, ultrapotent topical corticosteroid ointments (e.g., clobetasol ointment 0.05%) are the first-line treatment for LP of the vulva and are important to prevent destruction of the vulvar architecture and reduce the risk of vulvar cancer [74]. In addition, measures must also be undertaken to manage vaginal involvement. Hydrocortisone 25 mg rectal suppositories should be placed intravaginally twice daily, then reduced to twice weekly once symptoms improve. Alternatively, hydrocortisone enema foam (Colifoam) delivered directly from the aerosol can [77] or placed in a vaginal applicator [74] can be used. To prevent vaginal stenosis, patients either should also use dilators coated with corticosteroid ointment or engage in vaginal intercourse at regular intervals.

Often monotherapy with topical corticosteroids is inadequate for treating the vulva. In such cases a calcineurin inhibitor (tacrolimus ointment) or systemic therapies [74] may be required. Surgical lysis of adhesions on the vulva or in the vagina is also sometimes necessary. Patients with genital LP are usually managed by a dermatologist in conjunction with a gynecologist.

Lichen planus also increases the risk of vulvar cancer, and therefore affected women should undergo monitoring at least every 12 months [73]. Of note, a large population study indicates an unexplained association of vulvar LP with NSAID and beta-blocker use, and experts recommend that consideration be given to discontinuing these medications in women diagnosed with LP. The same study found that ACE-inhibitors may be protective [78].

You inform Margaret of the unexplained association of LP with beta-blockers and NSAIDs, and she agrees to discontinue the metoprolol and ibuprofen and begin a trial of lisinopril and acetaminophen. You emphasize the importance of adhering to the dermatologist's treatment plan in order to prevent further destruction of the vulvar and vaginal anatomy. You point out that even once her symptoms resolve, continued treatment is important to prevent both destruction of her vulva as well as cancer, and regular follow-up with the dermatologist at least once yearly allows for monitoring.

Psoriasis

Approximately half of patients with psoriasis have involvement of the genital area [79]. On the other hand, in 2–5% of patients with psoriasis, the condition is confined to the genital area, which can present more of a diagnostic challenge. In such instances, full body skin exam (particularly of the gluteal crease, umbilicus, scalp, fingernails, and toenails) can sometimes uncover unrecognized psoriasis and aid in establishing the diagnosis.

Women with vulvar psoriasis experience pruritus but also often report pain or burning of the vulva due to friction, perspiration, and maceration of lesions. On examination, the mons pubis, the cutaneous vulva (the hair-bearing areas of the labia majora) and the perianal areas are more often affected [80]. Psoriasis on the vulva can manifest as symmetric, brightly erythematous, shiny, thin plaques, sometimes with satellite erythematous papules. If scale is scraped off it leads to punctate bleeding (Auspitz's sign), which helps confirm the diagnosis. However, on the vulva, scale is frequently absent [81]. A biopsy is usually not needed except when the clinical diagnosis is uncertain or when lesions fail to respond to treatment.

Management

Treatment of genital psoriasis initially consists of low- to mid-potency topical steroid ointments for 2–4 weeks or less, followed by topical vitamin D analogues or topical calcineurin inhibitors (e.g. tacrolimus ointment). These latter agents are often poorly tolerated on the vulva due to stinging, however, and systemic therapies must often be employed. Unless the condition is easily controlled primary care providers usually refer patients with vulvar psoriasis to a dermatologist.

Lichen Simplex Chronicus

Lichen simplex chronicus (LSC) is not a specific entity but rather a term that describes lichenification – thickening and hardening—of the skin caused by scratching. Lichen simplex chronicus of the vulva usually develops in mid- to late-adult life and is common, occurring in 0.5% of the American population [73]. Patients experience intense pruritus, especially in the evening or during sleep, and consciously or unconsciously scratch the area leading to an itch-scratch cycle. A hallmark of the condition is that scratching provides temporary improvement in symptoms. LSC may begin in normal skin in atopic individuals or arise secondary to an inciting condition such as psoriasis or an episode of vulvovaginal candidiasis. In atopic individuals important triggers include psychological distress arising from anxiety, depression or worsening symptoms of obsessive-compulsive disorder, or environmental factors such as heat, sweating or friction [82]. Iron deficiency may sometimes contribute to the compulsion to scratch and should be excluded for women at risk (e.g. vegetarians, those with menorrhagia, etc.) [83].

On exam, one or more erythematous or hyperpigmented, scaling plaques with overlying excoriations can be found and broken off hairs may be seen [84]. The labia majora are mostly affected, and the condition is usually bilateral, but sometimes asymmetric or even unilateral, likely due to a preference for scratching with the dominant hand. The affected skin usually appears erythematous (ranging from pink if mild to bright or dusky red), but sometimes the erythema is masked by post-inflammatory hyperpigmentation [82]. If the condition is longstanding, the skin of the vulva appears thick and leathery (Fig. 12.7). The combination of lichenification and excoriations makes the condition easy to identify. Exam findings and diagnoses are more challenging when LSC is superimposed on another disorder, but biopsy is usually unnecessary.

Initial treatment entails ultra-potent topical corticosteroid, such as halobetasol propionate ointment 0.05% once daily for a few weeks, followed by a mid-potency topical corticosteroid (such as triamcinolone acetonide ointment 0.01%) once or twice daily. Thick lesions that fail to respond to topical therapy may require intralesional corticosteroid injection. Tacrolimus ointment 0.1% has also been used. Nonsedating antihistamines (e.g., cetirizine) are dosed in the daytime, and sedating antihistamines (e.g. hydroxyzine) are dosed at bedtime. If pruritus is refractory, nightly doxepin 10–25 mg can be substituted. Short fingernails are also recommended [85]. Some patients benefit from cognitive behavioral therapy while others respond to treatment with SSRI medications such as citalopram 20 mg once daily, increasing gradually to 60 mg if needed [82]. Treatment is important as irreversible destruction and scarring of the vulva can occur.

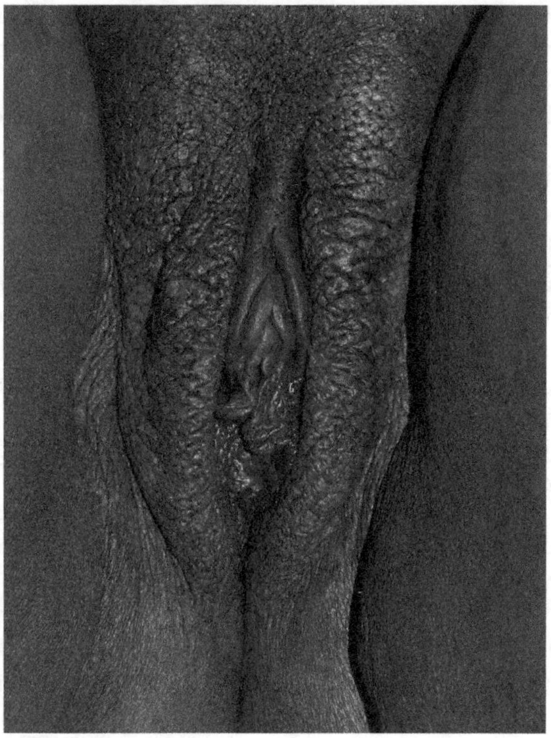

Fig. 12.7 Lichen simplex chronicus Lichen simplex chronicus describes skin that is thickened and hardened as a result of chronic scratching. The condition is evident in this image by the thick and leathery appearance of the labia minora and labia majora. When excoriations are also present the diagnosis is particularly straightforward. The root cause of the pruritus can be any of a variety of possible conditions, some of which are psychologic. Used with permission

Women affected by LSC should take particular care to avoid any potential irritants or allergens. In addition to the usual measures some also recommend that affected patients wash only with water and use washable fabric feminine pads and diapers [85]. Application of petroleum jelly throughout the day serves as an emollient and protectant.

Malignant Vulvar Neoplasms

Malignant lesions of the vulva are uncommon, representing only 5% of all gynecologic malignancies. Squamous cell carcinoma is the most common of the vulvar malignancies (90%), with malignant melanoma, sarcoma, basalioma, extramammary Paget disease, Bartholin gland cancer, and verrucous carcinoma possible but rare [60].

The most common presentation of vulvar cancer is either a lump that the patient has noted herself or mild pruritus. Bleeding, pain, and discharge are indicative of advanced disease. Very often, vulvar cancer is asymptomatic and recognized only on careful exam.

Vulvar malignancies can assume a wide range of appearances: they may be ulcerative, hyperkeratotic or warty, present in almost any color, and can at times be multifocal. Primary care providers should have a low threshold to refer for biopsy given the good prognosis when vulvar cancer is treated early [60]. Unfortunately, studies indicate that patients with vulvar cancer usually delay office presentation for 6 months [86] and providers fail to biopsy promptly. (Vulvar malignancies are discussed further in Chap. 15 on "Gynecologic Malignancies".)

Vulvodynia

Vulvodynia, defined as idiopathic vulvar pain of at least 3 months' duration, is a common chronic pain disorder. Approximately 4% of U.S. reproductive-aged women are affected at any given time and the lifetime prevalence is 9.9% [87]. The direct health care costs of vulvodynia are calculated to be enormous [88] and the psychological toll immeasurable.

Per the 2015 nomenclature and classification, vestibulodynia is defined as pain limited to the vestibule, and contrasts with generalized vulvodynia, which indicates pain affecting the entire vulvar area (but which more often is "mixed" and includes vestibulodynia as well). A second distinction is made between pain that is provoked (i.e. by intercourse, tampon insertion, gynecologic exams, riding a bicycle, the sitting position) or unprovoked.

Histologic studies reveal an increased density of nociceptors at the vestibule of affected women [89]. Numerous diverse triggers have been identified as likely leading to the neuropathic changes. Sequelae from a resolved *Candida* vulvitis [90] and disruption of the hormonal environment from combined hormonal contraceptive (COC) use –particularly when used prior to age 17 [91, 92]—appear to be possible causes of vulvodynia. Pelvic floor disorders resulting from a singular event such as trauma, surgery, or childbirth have also been implicated [88]. In general, any acute, painful surgical or medical condition (including an infection) involving the vulva, urinary tract, or anus, may lead to vulvodynia—especially if the event occurred in a setting of emotional distress [83]. In clinical settings the trigger is not always obvious nor sought.

Population studies show that at least half of vulvodynia sufferers have at least one other pain condition, most commonly fibromyalgia or irritable bowel syndrome [93]. Population studies also reveal that affected women have higher rates of childhood physical or sexual abuse [94] as well as higher rates of depression and anxiety prior to the onset of symptoms [95]. Not surprisingly, since vulvodynia frequently causes dyspareunia and can have a significant negative impact on relationships, vulvodynia frequently *causes* depression and anxiety as well. (See Chap. 9 on "Female Sexual Function and Dysfunction" for a discussion of sexual pain disorders.)

Affected patients usually present with a complaint of burning, tingling, stinging, rawness or irritation. Pruritus is not a prominent complaint. Most patients suffer symptoms for 2 years before the diagnosis is made [96]. The intensity of pain may fluctuate over time, and improvement may occur either spontaneously or following treatment [97]. Physical exam is normal, with the exception that for a patient with provoked vestibulodynia, gentle application of a cotton-tipped applicator to the vestibule causes tenderness. A careful neurologic exam of the pelvic region is important to exclude another neurologic source.

Treatment for provoked vestibulodynia generally entails topical anesthetics for introital dyspareunia [83]. Lidocaine 5% ointment or lidocaine 2% gel can be applied 15–20 min prior to intercourse and washed off immediately prior to penetration. Generalized unprovoked vulvodynia is managed with a variety of different modalities including chronic oral pain medications such as amitriptyline 5–25 mg nightly [96] or gabapentin begun at 300 mg nightly and increased to as high as 1200 mg total dose per day [98]. TENS units have also been used [99] as well as physical therapy when a pelvic floor disorder is diagnosed. Individual or group cognitive-behavior therapy [100] appears helpful for some. Surgical intervention with vestibulectomy is a last resort, since efficacy appears no better than cognitive behavioral therapy [101] and the risk of aggravating pain with surgery is considerable [83]. When generalized unprovoked vulvodynia is resistant to treatment, pelvic and lumbosacral MRI should be performed [83] to exclude another neurologic problem.

Women experiencing vulvodynia often experience dismissive behaviors from providers. Studies indicate that women with vulvodynia typically consult three physicians and are told their pain is "all in their head" before a diagnosis is made [88]. Empathic communication is a critical component of patient care in this setting. An oral explanation of vulvodynia followed by a written description of the diagnosis can perform many functions, including helping to restore a patient's self-esteem. In addition, the patient benefits when the physician expresses understanding and empathy regarding the impact that vulvodynia symptoms have had on the patient's life as this helps validate her experience [83].

Summary Points

1. Bacterial vaginosis (BV), vulvovaginal candidiasis (VC), and trichomoniasis are the most common causes of vaginitis in pre-menopausal women.
2. When evaluating a patient with vaginal discharge, it is important to include PID and cervicitis in the differential diagnosis. History taking should include a sexual history as well as questions regarding possible fever, pelvic pain, dyspareunia, changes in bleeding, and dysuria.
3. When a woman presents with vaginal discharge, a thorough evaluation is needed. This includes history, pelvic exam, whiff test, pH testing, and office microscopy (or point-of-care testing or laboratory microscopy).
4. Women require treatment for bacterial vaginosis and vulvovaginal candidiasis only if symptomatic.
5. Trichomoniasis is a sexually transmitted infection that requires treatment, screening for other STIs and reevaluation within 3 months to exclude reinfection. Partner management is essential as well.
6. When a woman presents with recurrent BV or VC, she should first undergo reevaluation to confirm the original diagnosis was correct. Risk factors should be assessed and she can be offered maintenance therapy or adjunctive measures.
7. Irritant and allergic contact dermatitis are noninfectious causes of vulvovaginitis. Patients report burning or pruritus and exam findings may resemble candida vulvovaginitis. Distinction can often be made by the lack of vaginal discharge on exam or fungal elements on microscopy.
8. There are several general measures that support vulvovaginal health and provide comfort in the setting of vulvar inflammation, such as wearing loose-fitting cotton undergarments, taking warm water baths, using zinc oxide protectant, and avoiding panty liners, douches, harsh soaps, wipes, and other irritants.
9. Since topical creams often contain alcohols or preservatives that may be irritating to mucosal tissues, ointments are preferred for treating vulvar conditions.
10. Lichen sclerosus and vulvar lichen planus are inflammatory dermatoses that share two important possible sequelae: Left untreated, they can both cause destruction of genital structures and increase the risk of vulvar cancer.
11. Vulvar cancers are rare but they can assume many appearances – ulcerative, hyperkeratotic or warty, appear in almost any color and sometimes have a multifocal presentation. Any undiagnosed vulvar lesion that fails to respond to therapy should be biopsied promptly.
12. Patients with provoked vestibulodynia complain of entrance dyspareunia, and the diagnosis can be made be during the pelvic exam, when gentle application of a cotton-tipped swab to the vestibule reproduces the pain. Treatment includes appropriately timed topical anesthetics as well as patient education.
13. Generalized unprovoked vulvodynia is often treated with psychotropic pain medications such as tricyclic anti-depressants or gabapentin, but other beneficial treatment options can be offered.

Review Questions

1. Tamara is a 34-year-old woman who calls your office complaining of vaginal discharge that started 2 days ago. She tells you the discharge is thin, yellow, and malodorous. She denies dysuria and dyspareunia, but notes mild associated pruritus. She tells you she is sexually active with only her husband, and they do not use condoms. She also says that her symptoms are similar to when she had a bacterial vaginosis infection earlier this year, and you confirm in the medical record that she was diagnosed with bacterial vaginosis 6 months ago. She requests a prescription for oral metronidazole. What do you advise?
   A. An office visit is not required; prescribe metronidazole 500 mg orally twice daily for 7 days
   B. An office visit is not required; prescribe metronidazole vaginal gel 0.75%, 5 g intravaginally once nightly for 5 days
   C. An office visit is not required; prescribe clindamycin 2% cream, 1 applicatorful once nightly for 7 days
   D. Advise her to come to the office to be evaluated

   The correct answer is D: Advise her to come to the office to be evaluated [1]. Bacterial vaginosis (BV) is typically associated with a thin, homogenous, malodorous discharge. It is not usually associated with any pain or pruritus. However, none of these symptoms are diagnostic of BV. While choices A and B are recommended treatment regimens for a confirmed diagnosis of BV, a proper evaluation that includes history, pelvic exam, and office microscopy is required to confirm the diagnosis and rule out cervicitis and PID. Choice C is an alternative treatment regimen for BV.

2. Sweta is a 37-year-old woman presenting for vaginal discharge. She complains of thick, white discharge associated with pruritus. She is not sexually active. She reports having three "yeast infections" in the last year and believes this is another one. You perform a pelvic exam and prepare a wet mount, confirming a diagnosis of

vulvovaginal candidiasis. Sweta is frustrated by the recurrent infections and wants to know what can be done. What do you advise?

A. Prescribe a single dose of oral fluconazole 150 mg; suppressive therapy is not indicated
B. Prescribe three doses of oral fluconazole 150 mg separated by 72 h; suppressive therapy is not indicated
C. Prescribe 10 days of a topical azole or oral fluconazole 150 mg, followed by oral fluconazole 150 mg once per week for 6 months
D. Prescribe a single dose of oral fluconazole 150 mg, followed by oral fluconazole 150 mg once per week for 6 weeks

The correct answer is choice C. Prescribe 10 days of a topical azole or oral fluconazole 150 mg, followed by oral fluconazole 150 mg once per week for 6 months. This woman has complicated and recurrent VC, defined as ≥4 episodes per year. Given that she is frustrated by the frequent symptoms she should be offered a course of chronic therapy. For the management of recurrent VC, the Infectious Diseases Society of America recommends 10–14 days of induction therapy with a topical azole or oral fluconazole followed by 6 months of maintenance therapy consisting of oral fluconazole 150 mg once weekly [44]. A single dose of oral fluconazole (Choice A) would be the correct choice if this was an uncomplicated vulvovaginal candidiasis (VC) infection (e.g. ≤3 episodes per year, mild to moderate symptoms), and choice B would be the correct answer if this was only complicated VC and Sweta was not bothered by her symptoms.

3. A 20-year-old woman presents complaining of 5 days of severe vulvar pruritus. Following full evaluation, the two of you determine that it is from an allergic dermatitis resulting from an allergy to the deodorant in her feminine pads, which she used for the first time beginning 1 week ago. What do you recommend?

A. She should soak in very warm baths for relief
B. She should use a strong liquid soap to remove any residual antigen
C. She should immediately cease and permanently avoid using this product (and perhaps all feminine products that contain deodorant)
D. She should take diphenhydramine around-the-clock for relief of pruritus

The correct answer is C. Immediate and permanent avoidance of the culprit antigen is the cornerstone of treating allergic contact dermatitis. In addition, topical steroid ointments and, if needed, oral antihistamines are used. Warm baths would aggravate the pruritus; cool Sitz baths and compresses are helpful. Harsh soaps are never recommended on the vulva. Diphenhydramine would be too sedating for daytime use; the preferred antihistamines for pruritus are cetirizine in the daytime and hydroxyzine at night.

4. A 55-year-old woman presents for a "routine Pap smear." She reports mild vulvar itching for the past year or two. Her vulva appears abnormal with diffuse pallor and thinning, and her labia minora appear markedly shrunken. You recommend:

A. Referral to dermatology or gynecology
B. Waiting for the results of her cervical cytology to determine the next step
C. A trial of watchful waiting
D. A trial of topical estrogen

The correct answer is A. This presentation is classic for lichen sclerosus, which presents with focal or diffusely pale vulvar mucosa that is either abnormally thick (early stage) or thin (later stage). LS requires treatment using ultrapotent topical corticosteroids plus close monitoring for the possible development of vulvar cancer. For this reason, patients with LS are usually managed by dermatologists or gynecologists. Cervical cytology has no bearing on the patient's vulvar problem. Watchful waiting is inappropriate since without treatment the destruction of her vulvar anatomy will progress and the risk of vulvar cancer is increased. The patient's exam findings, particularly the changes to her labia minora, are too dramatic to be consistent with the genitourinary syndrome of menopause.

5. A 75-year-old healthy woman presents complaining of several months of progressive burning "in my private parts." Her exam is notable for erosions with white borders on her labia minora as well as in her vagina. The most likely etiology is:

A. Genital psoriasis
B. Lichen sclerosus
C. Lichen simplex chronicus
D. Lichen planus

The correct answer is D. The erosive form of lichen planus is the only chronic dermatosis of the vulva that also involves the vagina, and erosions with surrounding white reticular borders are characteristic. Psoriasis involves plaques (not erosions). Lichen sclerosus presents with pale mucosa that is either abnormally thick or thin. Lichen simplex chronicus presents with plaques, lichenification, excoriations, and broken-off hairs that all result from excessive scratching.

6. A 50-year-old healthy woman presents with vulvar pruritus. Her pelvic exam reveals several symmetric erythematous plaques with rounded borders on the outer (hair-bearing) aspects of the labia majora. No scale is seen. Which of the following is true?

A. Examination of the scalp, gluteal cleft, umbilicus, and nails might uncover findings that support the diagnosis

B. This cannot be psoriasis since no silvery scale is present
C. Biopsy is needed to confirm the diagnosis
D. These lesions are most likely malignant

The correct answer is A. The findings described are classic for psoriasis on the vulva; uncovering psoriasis elsewhere on the body would be supportive of the diagnosis. Due to the apposition of the skin and overall moist environment of the vulva, scale is frequently absent at this location. Biopsy is rarely needed to make the diagnosis of psoriasis, even when isolated to the vulva. Although malignancies on the vulva may present in any of a myriad of presentations, the symmetry of lesions makes this unlikely.

7. Your next patient is a 24-year-old woman who is new to you. In eliciting her medical history, you learn that she quit using contraception because she and her husband have not had intercourse in nearly a year due to entrance dyspareunia. She tearfully explains that she has seen two physicians for this problem but was told "everything is normal." She has no other genital complaints and she is healthy overall. You advise:
A. A referral for individual psychotherapy
B. Couple's counseling
C. Diagnostic pelvic exam
D. A trial of amitriptyline or gabapentin

The correct answer is C. This patient describes provoked vestibulodynia. Although the mucosa of the vaginal vestibule appears normal in women with this condition, gentle application of a cotton-tipped applicator to the vestibule may reproduce the patient's pain, and this maneuver should be performed during the pelvic exam to make the diagnosis. Histologic studies indicate an increased number of nociceptors at the vestibule of affected women, and an important component of patient counseling is communicating that the condition is real. Treatment includes topical anesthetics applied to the vestibule 15–20 min before intercourse then washed off immediately prior to penetration. Referral for individual or couples' counseling is premature given that any mood or relationship problems might promptly resolve with treatment of her vestibulodynia. Chronic pain medications are used for *unprovoked* vulvar pain, typically generalized unprovoked vulvodynia.

References

1. Anderson MR, Klink K, Cohrssen A. Evaluation of vaginal complaints. JAMA. 2004;291(11):1368–79.
2. Allsworth JE, Peipert JF. Prevalence of bacterial vaginosis: 2001-2004 National Health and Nutrition Examination Survey data. Obstet Gynecol. 2007;109(1):114–20.
3. Klebanoff MA, Nansel TR, Brotman RM, Zhang J, Yu KF, Schwebke JR, et al. Personal hygienic behaviors and bacterial vaginosis. Sex Transm Dis. 2010;37(2):94–9.
4. Bradshaw CS, Walker SM, Vodstrcil LA, Bilardi JE, Law M, Hocking JS, et al. The influence of behaviors and relationships on the vaginal microbiota of women and their female partners: the WOW Health Study. J Infect Dis. 2014;209(10):1562–72.
5. Workowski KA, Bolan GA. Sexually transmitted diseases treatment guidelines, 2015. MMWR Recomm Rep. 2015;64(Rr-03):1–137.
6. Smart S, Singal A, Mindel A. Social and sexual risk factors for bacterial vaginosis. Sex Transm Infect. 2004;80(1):58–62.
7. Fethers KA, Fairley CK, Hocking JS, Gurrin LC, Bradshaw CS. Sexual risk factors and bacterial vaginosis: a systematic review and meta-analysis. Clin Infect Dis. 2008;47(11):1426–35.
8. Schwebke JR, Rivers C, Lee J. Prevalence of Gardnerella vaginalis in male sexual partners of women with and without bacterial vaginosis. Sex Transm Dis. 2009;36(2):92–4.
9. Mitchell C, Manhart LE, Thomas KK, Agnew K, Marrazzo JM. Effect of sexual activity on vaginal colonization with hydrogen peroxide-producing lactobacilli and Gardnerella vaginalis. Sex Transm Dis. 2011;38(12):1137–44.
10. Sobel JD. Vulvovaginal candidosis. Lancet (London, England). 2007;369(9577):1961–71.
11. Giraldo P, von Nowaskonski A, Gomes FA, Linhares I, Neves NA, Witkin SS. Vaginal colonization by Candida in asymptomatic women with and without a history of recurrent vulvovaginal candidiasis. Obstet Gynecol. 2000;95(3):413–6.
12. Wilson JF. In the clinic. Vaginitis and cervicitis. Ann Intern Med. 2009;151(5):ITC3-1–ITC3-15; Quiz ITC3-6.
13. Satterwhite CL, Torrone E, Meites E, Dunne EF, Mahajan R, Ocfemia MC, et al. Sexually transmitted infections among US women and men: prevalence and incidence estimates, 2008. Sex Transm Dis. 2013;40(3):187–93.
14. Ferris DG, Nyirjesy P, Sobel JD, Soper D, Pavletic A, Litaker MS. Over-the-counter antifungal drug misuse associated with patient-diagnosed vulvovaginal candidiasis. Obstet Gynecol. 2002;99(3):419–25.
15. Gandhi J, Chen A, Dagur G, Suh Y, Smith N, et al. Genitourinary syndrome of menopause: an overview of clinical manifestations, pathophysiology, etiology, evaluation, and management. Am J Obstet Gynecol. 2016;215(6):704–11. https://doi.org/10.1016/j.ajog.2016.07.045.
16. University of Washington STD Prevention Training Center. UWPTC.org
17. CDC Image Library Centers for Disease Control (CDC) Public Health Image Library (PHIL). https://phil.cdc.gov/QuickSearch.aspx?key=true
18. Hainer BL, Gibson MV. Vaginitis. Am Family Physician. 2011;83(7):807–15.21.
19. Frobenius W, Bogdan C. Diagnostic value of vaginal discharge, wet mount and vaginal pH – an update on the basics of gynecologic infectiology. Geburtshilfe Frauenheilkd. 2015;75(4):355–66.
20. Lara-Torre E, Pinkerton JS. Accuracy of detection of trichomonas vaginalis organisms on a liquid-based papanicolaou smear. Am J Obstet Gynecol. 2003;188(2):354–6.
21. Wiese W, Patel SR, Patel SC, Ohl CA, Estrada CA. A meta-analysis of the Papanicolaou smear and wet mount for the diagnosis of vaginal trichomoniasis. Am J Med. 2000;108(4):301–8.
22. Brown HL, Fuller DD, Jasper LT, Davis TE, Wright JD. Clinical evaluation of affirm VPIII in the detection and identification of Trichomonas vaginalis, Gardnerella vaginalis, and Candida species in vaginitis/vaginosis. Infect Dis Obstet Gynecol. 2004;12(1):17–21.
23. Oduyebo OO, Anorlu RI, Ogunsola FT. The effects of antimicrobial therapy on bacterial vaginosis in non-pregnant women. Cochrane Database Syst Rev. 2009;3:Cd006055.

24. Amaya-Guio J, Viveros-Carreno DA, Sierra-Barrios EM, Martinez-Velasquez MY, Grillo-Ardila CF. Antibiotic treatment for the sexual partners of women with bacterial vaginosis. Cochrane Database Syst Rev. 2016;10:Cd011701.
25. Mehta SD. Systematic review of randomized trials of treatment of male sexual partners for improved bacteria vaginosis outcomes in women. Sex Transm Dis. 2012;39(10):822–30.
26. Marshall AO. Managing recurrent bacterial vaginosis: insights for busy providers. Sex Med Rev. 2015;3(2):88–92.29.
27. Watson MC, Grimshaw JM, Bond CM, Mollison J, Ludbrook A. Oral versus intra-vaginal imidazole and triazole anti-fungal treatment of uncomplicated vulvovaginal candidiasis (thrush). Cochrane Database Syst Rev. 2001;4:Cd002845.
28. Gioia-Flynt L. Vaginitis. In: Stovall TL, Ling F, Zite N, Chuang A, Tillmanns T, editors. Gynecology for the primary care physician. Philadelphia, PA: Springer; Current Medicine Group LLC a division of Springer Science+Business Media LLC. 2nd ed; 2008.
29. Sobel JD, Chaim W, Nagappan V, Leaman D. Treatment of vaginitis caused by Candida glabrata: use of topical boric acid and flucytosine. Am J Obstet Gynecol. 2003;189(5):1297–300.
30. CDC phone and website to obtain assistance with nitroimidazole-resistant *T. vaginalis* (*i.e. susceptibility testing* and treatment of infected persons); 404–718–4141. https://www.cdc.gov/laboratory/specimensubmission/detail.html?CDCTestCode=CDC-10239
31. Bradshaw CS, Morton AN, Hocking J, Garland SM, Morris MB, Moss LM, et al. High recurrence rates of bacterial vaginosis over the course of 12 months after oral metronidazole therapy and factors associated with recurrence. J Infect Dis. 2006;193(11):1478–86.
32. McClelland RS, Richardson BA, Hassan WM, Chohan V, Lavreys L, Mandaliya K, et al. Improvement of vaginal health for Kenyan women at risk for acquisition of human immunodeficiency virus type 1: results of a randomized trial. J Infect Dis. 2008;197(10):1361–8.
33. Bradshaw CS, Vodstrcil LA, Hocking JS, Law M, Pirotta M, Garland SM, et al. Recurrence of bacterial vaginosis is significantly associated with posttreatment sexual activities and hormonal contraceptive use. Clin Infect Dis. 2013;56(6):777–86.
34. Brooks JP, Edwards DJ, Blithe DL, et al. Effects of combined oral contraceptives, depot medroxyprogesterone acetate and the levonorgestrel-releasing intrauterine system on the vaginal microbiome. Contraception. 2017;95(4):405–13. https://doi.org/10.1016/j.contraception.2016.11.006.
35. Hellberg D, Nilsson S, Mårdh PA. Bacterial vaginosis and smoking. Int J STD AIDS. 2000;11(9):603–6.
36. Brotman RM, Klebanoff MA, Nansel TR, et al. A longitudinal study of vaginal douching and bacterial vaginosis--a marginal structural modeling analysis. Am J Epidemiol. 2008;168(2):188–96. https://doi.org/10.1093/aje/kwn103.
37. Gonçalves B, Ferreira C, Alves CT, Henriques M, Azeredo J, Silva S. Vulvovaginal candidiasis: epidemiology, microbiology and risk factors. Crit Rev Microbiol. 2016;42(6):905–27. https://doi.org/10.3109/1040841X.2015.1091805. Review.
38. Donders GG, Prenen H, Verbeke G, Reybrouck R. Impaired tolerance for glucose in women with recurrent vaginal candidiasis. Am J Obstet Gynecol. 2002;187(4):989–93.
39. Pappas PG, Kauffman CA, Andes D, Benjamin DK Jr, Calandra TF, Edwards JE Jr, et al. Clinical practice guidelines for the management of candidiasis: 2009 update by the Infectious Diseases Society of America. Clin Infect Dis. 2009;48(5):503–35.
40. Dennerstein GJ. Depo-Provera in the treatment of recurrent vulvovaginal candidiasis. J Reprod Med. 1986;31(9):801–3.
41. Hu H, Merenstein DJ, Wang C, et al. Impact of eating probiotic yogurt on colonization by Candida species of the oral and vaginal mucosa in HIV-infected and HIV-uninfected women. Mycopathologia. 2013;176(3–4):175–81. https://doi.org/10.1007/s11046-013-9678-4. Epub 2013 Aug 8.
42. Peterman TA, Tian LH, Metcalf CA, Satterwhite CL, Malotte CK, DeAugustine N, et al. High incidence of new sexually transmitted infections in the year following a sexually transmitted infection: a case for rescreening. Ann Intern Med. 2006;145(8):564–72.
43. Peterman TA, Tian LH, Metcalf CA, Malotte CK, Paul SM, Douglas JM Jr. Persistent, undetected Trichomonas vaginalis infections? Clin Infect Dis. 2009;48(2):259–60.
44. Stemmer SM, Mordechai E, Adelson ME, Gygax SE, Hilbert DW. Trichomonas vaginalis is most frequently detected in women at the age of peri−/premenopause: an unusual pattern for a sexually transmitted pathogen. Am J Obstet Gynecol. 2018;218(3):328.e1–e13.
45. Ginocchio CC, Chapin K, Smith JS, Aslanzadeh J, Snook J, Hill CS, et al. Prevalence of Trichomonas vaginalis and coinfection with Chlamydia trachomatis and Neisseria gonorrhoeae in the United States as determined by the Aptima Trichomonas vaginalis nucleic acid amplification assay. J Clin Microbiol. 2012;50(8):2601–8.
46. Martin HL, Richardson BA, Nyange PM, Lavreys L, Hillier SL, Chohan B, et al. Vaginal lactobacilli, microbial flora, and risk of human immunodeficiency virus type 1 and sexually transmitted disease acquisition. J Infect Dis. 1999;180(6):1863–8.
47. Bautista CT, Wurapa EK, Sateren WB, et al. Association of bacterial vaginosis with chlamydia and gonorrhea among women in the U.S. Army. Am J Prev Med. 2017;52(5):632–9. https://doi.org/10.1016/j.amepre.2016.09.016.
48. Moodley P, Wilkinson D, Connolly C, et al. *Trichomonas vaginalis* is associated with pelvic inflammatory disease in women infected with human immunodeficiency virus. Clin Infect Dis. 2002;34:519–22.
49. Atashili J, Poole C, Ndumbe PM, Adimora AA, Smith JS. Bacterial vaginosis and HIV acquisition: a meta-analysis of published studies. AIDS. 2008;22(12):1493–501. https://doi.org/10.1097/QAD.0b013e3283021a37.
50. McClelland RS, Sangare L, Hassan WM, et al. Infection with Trichomonas vaginalis increases the risk of HIV-1 acquisition. J Infect Dis. 2007;195(5):698–702.
51. Cohen CR, Lingappa JR, Baeten JM, et al. Bacterial vaginosis associated with increased risk of female-to-male HIV-1 transmission: a prospective cohort analysis among African couples. PLoS Med. 2012;9(6):e1001251. https://doi.org/10.1371/journal.pmed.1001251.
52. Sorvillo F, Smith L, Kerndt P, Ash L. Trichomonas vaginalis, HIV, and African-Americans. Emerg Infect Dis. 2001;7(6):927–32. https://doi.org/10.3201/eid0706.010603.
53. Hay PE, Lamont RF, Taylor-Robinson D, et al. Abnormal bacterial colonisation of the genital tract and subsequent preterm delivery and late miscarriage. BMJ. 1994;308(6924):295–8.
54. Cotch MF, Pastorek JG 2nd, Nugent RP, Hillier SL, Gibbs RS, et al. Trichomonas vaginalis associated with low birth weight and preterm delivery. The Vaginal Infections and Prematurity Study Group. Sex Transm Dis. 1997;24(6):353–60.
55. Nyirjesy P, Peyton C, Weitz MV, Mathew L, Culhane JF. Causes of chronic vaginitis: analysis of a prospective database of affected women. Obstet Gynecol. 2006;108(5):1185–91.
56. Reichman O, Sobel J. Desquamative inflammatory vaginitis. Best Pract Res Clin Obstet Gynaecol. 2014;28(7):1042–50. https://doi.org/10.1016/j.bpobgyn.2014.07.003.
57. Sobel JD. Desquamative inflammatory vaginitis: a new subgroup of purulent vaginitis responsive to topical 2% clindamycin therapy. Am J Obstet Gynecol. 1994;171(5):1215–20.

58. Sobel JD, Reichman O, Misra D, Yoo W. Prognosis and treatment of desquamative inflammatory vaginitis. Obstet Gynecol. 2011;117(4):850–5. https://doi.org/10.1097/AOG.0b013e3182117c9e.
59. Murphy R, Edwards L. Desquamative inflammatory vaginitis: what is it? J Reprod Med. 2008;53(2):124–8.
60. Alkatout I, Schubert M, Garbrecht N, Weigel MT, Jonat W, Mundhenke C, Günther V. Vulvar cancer: epidemiology, clinical presentation, and management options. Int J Women's Health. 2015;7:305–13. https://doi.org/10.2147/IJWH.S68979. eCollection 2015. Review.
61. Lloyd J, Crouch NS, Minto CL, Liao LM, Creighton SM. Female genital appearance: "normality" unfolds. BJOG. 2005;112:643–6.
62. ACOG. Vaginal "rejuvenation" and cosmetic vaginal procedures. ACOG committee opinion no. 378. American College of Obstetricians and Gynecologists. Obstet Gynecol. 2007;110:737–8. (Reaffirmed 2017).
63. Lew BL, Haw CR, Lee MH. Cutaneous drug eruption from cetirizine and hydroxyzine. J Am Acad Dermatol. 2004;50(6):953–6.
64. Eschler DC, Klein PA. An evidence-based review of the efficacy of topical antihistamines in the relief of pruritus. J Drugs Dermatol. 2010;9(8):992–7.
65. Fischer GO. The commonest causes of symptomatic vulvar disease: a dermatologist's perspective. Australas J Dermatol. 1996;37(1):12–8.
66. Farage MA. Vulvar susceptibility to contact irritants and allergens: a review. Arch Gynecol Obstet. 2005;272(2):167–72.
67. Woodruff CM, Trivedi MK, Botto N, Kornik R. Allergic contact dermatitis of the vulva. Dermatitis. 2018;29(5):233–43. https://doi.org/10.1097/DER.0000000000000339. Review.
68. Pichardo-Geisinger R. Atopic and contact dermatitis of the vulva. Obstet Gynecol Clin N Am. 2017;44(3):371–8. https://doi.org/10.1016/j.ogc.2017.05.003. Review.
69. Bauer A, Rodiger C, Greif C, Kaatz M, Elsner P. Vulvar dermatoses--irritant and allergic contact dermatitis of the vulva. Dermatology. 2005;210(2):143–9. Review.
70. Lee A, Bradford J, Fischer G. Long-term management of adult vulvar lichen sclerosus: a prospective cohort study of 507 women. JAMA Dermatol. 2015;151(10):1061–7. https://doi.org/10.1001/jamadermatol.2015.0643.
71. Meffert JJ, Davis BM, Grimwood RE. Lichen sclerosus. J Am Acad Dermatol. 1995;32(3):393–416; quiz 417–8. Review.
72. Thomas RH, Ridley CM, McGibbon DH, Black MM. Anogenital lichen sclerosus in women. J R Soc Med. 1996;89(12):694–8.
73. Simonetta C, Burns EK, Guo MA. Vulvar dermatoses: a review and update. Mo Med. 2015;112(4):301–7.
74. Bradford J, Fischer G. Management of vulvovaginal lichen planus: a new approach. J Low Genit Tract Dis. 2013;17(1):28–32. https://doi.org/10.1097/LGT.0b013e318258bf5b.
75. Cooper SM, Ali I, Baldo M, Wojnarowska F. The association of lichen sclerosus and erosive lichen planus of the vulva with autoimmune disease: a case-control study. Arch Dermatol. 2008;144(11):1432–5. https://doi.org/10.1001/archderm.144.11.1432.
76. Simpson RC, Thomas KS, Leighton P, Murphy R. Diagnostic criteria for erosive lichen planus affecting the vulva: an international electronic-Delphi consensus exercise. Br J Dermatol. 2013;169(2):337–43. https://doi.org/10.1111/bjd.12334.
77. Machin SE, McConnell DT, Adams JD. Vaginal lichen planus: preservation of sexual function in severe disease. BMJ Case Rep. 2010;2010:bcr08.2009.2208.84.
78. Clayton R, Chaudhry S, Ali I, Cooper S, Hodgson T, Wojnarowska F. Mucosal (oral and vulval) lichen planus in women: are angiotensin-converting enzyme inhibitors protective, and beta-blockers and non-steroidal anti-inflammatory drugs associated with the condition? Clin Exp Dermatol. 2010;35(4):384–7. https://doi.org/10.1111/j.1365-2230.2009.03581.x. Epub 2009 Oct 23.85.
79. Meeuwis KAP, Potts Bleakman A, van de Kerkhof PCM, Dutronc Y, Henneges C, Kornberg LJ, Menter A. Prevalence of genital psoriasis in patients with psoriasis. J Dermatolog Treat. 2018;29(8):754–60. https://doi.org/10.1080/09546634.2018.1453125.
80. Meeuwis KA, de Hullu JA, Massuger LF, van de Kerkhof PC, van Rossum MM. Genital psoriasis: a systematic literature review on this hidden skin disease. Acta Derm Venereol. 2011;91(1):5–11. https://doi.org/10.2340/00015555-0988.87.
81. Sand FL, Thomsen SF. Off-label use of TNF-alpha inhibitors in a dermatological university department: retrospective evaluation of 118 patients. Dermatol Ther. 2015;28(3):158–65. https://doi.org/10.1111/dth.12222.
82. Lynch PJ. Lichen simplex chronicus (atopic/neurodermatitis) of the anogenital region. Dermatol Ther. 2004;17:8–19.
83. van der Meijden WI, Boffa MJ, Ter Harmsel WA, Kirtschig G, Lewis FM, et al. 2016 European guideline for the management of vulval conditions. J Eur Acad Dermatol Venereol. 2017;31(6):925–41. https://doi.org/10.1111/jdv.14096.
84. O'Connell TX, Nathan LS, Satmary WA, Goldstein AT. Non-neoplastic epithelial disorders of the vulva. Am Fam Physician. 2008;77(3):321–6. Review.
85. Chibnall R. Vulvar pruritus and lichen simplex chronicus. Obstet Gynecol Clin N Am. 2017;44(3):379–88. https://doi.org/10.1016/j.ogc.2017.04.003.
86. Creasman WT. New gynecologic cancer staging. Obstet Gynecol. 1990;75(2):287–8.
87. Arnold LD, Bachmann GA, Rosen R, Kelly S, Rhoads GG. Vulvodynia: characteristics and associations with comorbidities and quality of life. Obstet Gynecol. 2006;107(3):617–24.
88. Pukall CF, Goldstein AT, Bergeron S, Foster D, Stein A, et al. Vulvodynia: definition, prevalence, impact, and pathophysiological factors. J Sex Med. 2016;13(3):291–304. https://doi.org/10.1016/j.jsxm.2015.12.021. Review.
89. Weström LV, Willén R. Vestibular nerve fiber proliferation in vulvar vestibulitis syndrome. Obstet Gynecol. 1998;91(4):572–6.
90. Farmer MA, Taylor AM, Bailey AL, Tuttle AH, MacIntyre LC, et al. Repeated vulvovaginal fungal infections cause persistent pain in a mouse model of vulvodynia. Sci Transl Med. 2011;3(101):101ra91. https://doi.org/10.1126/scitranslmed.3002613.
91. Bazin S, Bouchard C, Brisson J, Morin C, Meisels A, Fortier M. Vulvar vestibulitis syndrome: an exploratory case-control study. Obstet Gynecol. 1994;83(1):47–50.
92. Bouchard C, Brisson J, Fortier M, Morin C, Blanchette C. Use of oral contraceptive pills and vulvar vestibulitis: a case-control study. Am J Epidemiol. 2002;156(3):254–61.
93. Reed BD, Harlow SD, Sen A, Edwards RM, Chen D, Haefner HK. Relationship between vulvodynia and chronic comorbid pain conditions. Obstet Gynecol. 2012;120(1):145–51. https://doi.org/10.1097/AOG.0b013e31825957cf.
94. Harlow BL, Stewart EG. Adult-onset vulvodynia in relation to childhood violence victimization. Am J Epidemiol. 2005;161(9):871–80.
95. Khandker M, Brady SS, Vitonis AF, Maclehose RF, Stewart EG, Harlow BL. The influence of depression and anxiety on risk of adult onset vulvodynia. J Womens Health (Larchmt). 2011;20(10):1445–51. https://doi.org/10.1089/jwh.2010.2661.
96. van Beekhuizen HJ, Oost J, van der Meijden WI. Generalized unprovoked vulvodynia; a retrospective study on the efficacy of treatment with amitriptyline, gabapentin or pregabalin. Eur J Obstet Gynecol Reprod Biol. 2018;220:118–21. https://doi.org/10.1016/j.ejogrb.2017.10.026.
97. Reed BD, Haefner HK, Sen A, Gorenflo DW. Vulvodynia incidence and remission rates among adult women: a 2-year follow-

up study. Obstet Gynecol. 2008;112(2 Pt 1):231–7. https://doi.org/10.1097/AOG.0b013e318180965b.

98. Spoelstra SK, Borg C, Weijmar Schultz WC. Anticonvulsant pharmacotherapy for generalized and localized vulvodynia: a critical review of the literature. J Psychosom Obstet Gynaecol. 2013;34(3):133–8. https://doi.org/10.3109/0167482X.2013.823942.
99. Murina F, Graziottin A, Felice R, Radici G, Tognocchi C. Vestibulodynia: synergy between palmitoylethanolamide + transpolydatin and transcutaneous electrical nerve stimulation. J Low Genit Tract Dis. 2013;17(2):111–6. https://doi.org/10.1097/LGT.0b013e3182652316.
100. ter Kuile MM, Weijenborg PT. A cognitive-behavioral group program for women with vulvar vestibulitis syndrome (VVS): factors associated with treatment success. J Sex Marital Ther. 2006;32(3):199–213.
101. De Andres J, Sanchis-Lopez N, Asensio-Samper JM, Fabregat-Cid G, Villanueva-Perez VL, et al. Vulvodynia--an evidence-based literature review and proposed treatment algorithm. Pain Pract. 2016;16(2):204–36. https://doi.org/10.1111/papr.12274. Review.

13 Sexually Transmitted Infections

Janice Ryden

Learning Objectives

1. Describe the health impact of sexually transmitted infections and list measures that providers can embrace to reduce the incidence of sexually transmitted infections (STIs).
2. Perform an appropriate medical evaluation of a woman reporting documented exposure to an STI, including history, physical examination, testing, empiric treatment, and screening for other STIs.
3. Contrast the management of cervicitis caused by chlamydia or gonorrhea to the management of women presenting with symptoms concerning for pelvic inflammatory disease (PID).
4. Differentiate the characteristics of new genital ulcers caused by herpes simplex virus (HSV), syphilis, and human immunodeficiency virus (HIV) and discuss the best approach to diagnostic testing.
5. Provide appropriate antiviral treatment for an initial HSV infection and contrast this with treatment options for recurrent episodes.
6. Counsel a patient regarding the natural history of low-grade human papilloma virus (HPV) infection and the management options for genital warts.
7. Identify patients who would benefit from pre- or post-exposure prophylaxis for human immunodeficiency virus (HIV).

J. Ryden (✉)
Johns Hopkins University School of Medicine, Johns Hopkins Community Physicians, Department of Internal Medicine (*retired*), Baltimore, MD, USA
e-mail: jryden@jhmi.edu

Your first patient of the day is Carol, a 21-year-old woman who had unprotected sex 1 week ago when she encountered her old high school boyfriend at a party. He texted her yesterday that she might have caught an STI; his doctor just treated him for Chlamydia.

Sexually transmitted infections (STIs) are common and carry significant negative impact on health. Even seemingly benign infections can facilitate HIV transmission and susceptibility in women. Many STIs can be associated with serious long-term sequelae, such as infertility, ectopic pregnancy, spontaneous abortion, chronic pelvic pain, seronegative arthritis, neurologic disease, cardiovascular disease, and malignancy. STIs may also affect offspring by increasing the risk of low birth weight, neonatal infection, and congenital anomalies.

Appropriate screening starts with an understanding of risk factors. First, adolescents are at particularly high risk for acquiring STIs; about half of the STIs in the United States are diagnosed in 15- to 24-year-olds [1]. Other identified risk factors include unmarried status, new sex partner within the past 60 days, multiple partners, history of a previous STI, illicit drug use, admission to a correctional facility, meeting partners on the Internet, contact with sex workers, women having sex with women, and inconsistent condom use. Regional and racial disparities in acquisition of STIs are also present in the United States.

Providers can help optimize their patients' health as well as stem the STI epidemic by providing prevention counseling, STI screening, accurate diagnosis, prompt treatment, and management of partners. In addition, vaccination can prevent Hepatitis B and HPV infection. Chronic suppressive therapy for HSV-discordant couples and pre- and post-exposure prophylaxis for those at high risk for HIV acquisition are other effective, targeted strategies.

S. A. Tilstra et al. (eds.), *Sex- and Gender-Based Women's Health*, https://doi.org/10.1007/978-3-030-50695-7_13

Counseling on STI Prevention

Prevention counseling is most effective when delivered respectfully, in a nonjudgmental manner, and using language appropriate for each patient. A thoughtful sexual history allows counseling to be tailored to specific behaviors. The CDC notes that abstinence from oral, vaginal, and anal sex or involvement in a long-term, mutually monogamous relationship with a partner known to be uninfected are the two most reliable ways to avoid STI transmission. For patients who are sexually active in relationships that are either not long-term or not mutually monogamous, providing counseling regarding the use of condoms and advising STI testing of both persons prior to initiating sexual activity with a new partner can help prevent STI transmission [2].

When used correctly and consistently, male condoms are highly effective in preventing the transmission of HIV, chlamydia, gonorrhea, and Trichomonas. (For discussion of Trichomonas please see Chap. 12 on Vaginitis and Vulvar Conditions). Condoms are less effective in preventing certain STIs like herpes, syphilis, or HPV, since skin-to-skin contact outside the area where condoms provide barrier protection can enable transmission. The failure of condoms to prevent STI transmission (and pregnancy) most often relates to incorrect or inconsistent use, but studies indicate that male latex condoms do break during 2% of vaginal intercourse encounters [2]. Polyurethane condoms are more resistant to deterioration and can be used with oil-based lubricants and vaginal medications, but they have not been as extensively studied regarding reduction in STI transmission and for this reason are currently FDA-recommended solely for latex-allergic persons. Natural membrane condoms ("lambskins") block passage of sperm but their large pore size permits passage of viral STIs.

Studies of the female condom lack data regarding STI prevention, but it may be equivalent or superior to the male condom since its design provides barrier protection over much of the vulva. The female condom is more expensive ($2 per condom) but offers the advantage of allowing women control of the decision to use a condom. Its effectiveness with receptive anal intercourse has not been studied. The male condom should not be used in conjunction with the female condom [2].

Although it may seem obvious, patients should be advised that other forms of contraception offer no protection against HIV or other STIs. One should also inform patients that the spermicide nonoxynol-9 has been associated with an increased risk of HIV acquisition, likely through disruption of the genital epithelium [3], and therefore its use in pregnancy prevention should be limited to monogamous couples known to be HIV negative. On the brighter side, prior concern regarding possible increased risk of HIV acquisition with the use of injectable medroxyprogesterone contraception has been allayed by a large randomized trial [4].

As counseling regarding condom use and safe-sex practices can be time-consuming in a busy practice setting, patients can also be directed to view a brief video on safer sex on their cell phone during an office visit (e.g., Safer Sex video: https://www.plannedparenthood.org/learn/stds-hiv-safer-sex/safer-sex). Studies show these videos are effective educational tools [2]. Practices can also be designed to use appropriate team members for education (See Chap. 2 on High-Value Health Care).

STI Screening and Treatment: General Principles

After discussing condom use, Carol decides to keep a female condom in her purse from now on. She is confident she did not "catch" any STIs since she has no symptoms and asks you just to "double-check" for the infection her partner reported. However, you suggest a different plan….

Universal Screening of Asymptomatic Individuals

Since STIs are often asymptomatic, particularly in women, screening represents a valuable strategy to interrupt transmission networks. Because chlamydia and gonorrhea are prevalent, often asymptomatic, and carry significant risks if untreated, the United States Preventive Services Task Force (USPSTF) recommends annual screening for these two infections in all sexually active women age 24 and younger, as well as in older women felt to be at increased risk [5]. For asymptomatic women not needing a pelvic exam, self-collected vaginal swabs are best for specimen procurement. The diagnostic yield of self-collected swabs is comparable to physician-collected specimens and is associated with reduced time and patient barriers. Urine specimens have a reduced sensitivity for detecting chlamydia and gonorrhea in females [6] but would be the specimen of choice in a woman who has undergone hysterectomy including removal of the cervix. Optimal urine specimens are collected without using a perineal wipe beforehand and include the initial portion of the urine stream ("first-catch"), both steps different than for urinary tract infection testing.

The US Centers for Disease Control (CDC) also recommends universal "opt-out" HIV screening for all Americans age 13–64 [2] with inclusion of older persons felt to be at increased risk [7]. At the present time, the CDC recommends annual Trichomonas screening only for HIV-infected women.

The USPSTF specifically recommends *against* routine universal screening of sexually active persons for herpes simplex virus (HSV) and Hepatitis B [8].

STI Testing Following Potential Exposure

> *You talk with Carol about receiving empiric treatment today and explain that the standard of care after known STI exposure also includes a comprehensive evaluation with history, physical exam, and testing for all common STIs.*

Patients often present to the primary care setting after unprotected sex requesting STI screening. Women with this chief complaint should be screened for symptoms, and if none are present, they are managed with STI testing alone. As previously mentioned, the optimal method to screen for chlamydia, gonorrhea, and Trichomonas in an asymptomatic woman is a self-collected vaginal swab specimen.

On the other hand, when a patient reports a recent *known* exposure to a curable STI (e.g. chlamydia, gonorrhea, Trichomonas, or syphilis), she undergoes testing but is also examined and empirically treated at that visit. The appropriate evaluation includes a pelvic exam and, ideally, an oral exam and brief skin survey as well. A wet mount and collection of specimens for STI testing is obtained and empiric treatment for the reported STI is prescribed. When treating STIs, the CDC recommends optimizing adherence by choosing single dose therapy whenever possible with onsite administration using directly observed therapy when feasible [2]. Testing for the reported infection is included for verification purposes, as a confirmatory result allows notification of her respective sexual partners—namely persons exposed within the past 60 days for most infections—as well as the local health department. Coinfection with another STI is common and is the reason for screening for other common or important STIs. Testing in a patient with a known exposure to an STI therefore includes chlamydia, gonorrhea, *Trichomonas*, HIV, and syphilis (and for the unvaccinated patient, Hepatitis B). Due to the time required for seroconversion, patients should be assigned an appointment to return in 3–4 weeks for repeat HIV and syphilis testing when there is significant concern. In situations where there is substantial risk of acquisition of HIV and the patient presents within 72 hours, nonoccupational post-exposure prophylaxis for HIV can be offered (see section on "HIV Postexposure Prophylaxis"). Chlamydia, gonorrhea, syphilis (including congenital syphilis), HIV infection, AIDS, and chancroid are reportable diseases in every state, and other STIs may be reportable in some states.

Partner Services and Expedited Partner Therapy

From a public health perspective, the diagnosis of a new STI in one patient necessitates attention to their sexual partner(s) as well. The term "partner services" includes the process of ensuring that sexual partners of a patient diagnosed with an STI are informed, educated, tested, empirically treated, and screened for other STIs. Most local health departments have large caseloads and therefore may only be able to provide partner services for new diagnoses of HIV [2], thus the responsibility often falls to individual providers. The treating provider should encourage patients to notify their partners or patients can authorize their provider or public health department to do so. The CDC recommends providers invite partners into the office for evaluation and treatment and also suggests a joint appointment for simultaneous treatment when feasible [2].

Expedited partner therapy (EPT) is an alternative practice of treating the STI in sexual partners without evaluating them. This practice has been validated for chlamydia and gonorrhea infections in heterosexual couples. Studies show EPT is associated with a significant decrease (as high as 29%) in the recurrence of infection in the index patient, although studies were performed with provision of medication, not a written prescription [2]. Caveats include the need to clarify possible drug allergies and pregnancy status, provide medication instructions, and provide written warnings to seek medical evaluation if symptoms—particularly symptoms of pelvic inflammatory disease (PID)—are present. EPT appears particularly effective for treating male partners of women patients. There are several drawbacks to EPT, including the inability both to test partners for other STIs and to track their respective partners. Also, when using EPT for gonorrhea, the preferred intramuscular treatment regimen is not possible and an alternative regimen consisting of two oral medications must be substituted. EPT is legal in most but not all states; further state-specific information is available from the CDC at https://www.cdc.gov/std/ept/legal/default.htm [9].

STIs and Pregnancy

> *You note that Carol's last menstrual period was 4 weeks ago and advise office urine pregnancy testing.*

Women presenting with STI concerns are often also at risk for pregnancy. Assessment for possible pregnancy with menstrual history and point-of-care urine pregnancy testing is appropriate, as pregnancy may influence antibiotic choice or overall management. Also, although counseling for STI prevention emphasizes condom use, some women presenting with STIs may benefit from more reliable contraception in addition to condoms.

STIs and Comprehensive Care

Patients presenting with STI concerns may derive benefit from more comprehensive care. In addition to addressing contraceptive needs, providers can offer the HPV vaccine to eligible patients (i.e., women age 26 and younger who have not already completed the series). (See Chap. 14 on Cervical Cancer and Human Papillomavirus.) Also, counseling regarding STI risk reduction through condom use may have particular impact in the context of the patient's presenting concern.

Specific Sexually Transmitted Infections

Carol's pregnancy test comes back negative and she declines other contraceptive methods. She heard that there is a urine test for chlamydia and requests this as she is in a hurry to get back to work.

Chlamydia and Gonorrhea General Overview

Chlamydia and gonorrhea are the first and second most common notifiable STIs in the U.S., with the incidence of chlamydia exceeding that of gonorrhea by a factor of 10. These two infections share a particular importance in that each has the ability to cause pelvic inflammatory disease (PID). Unfortunately, the incidence of both infections has been rising since 2010 [2].

Misconceptions regarding chlamydia and gonorrhea are common. Recent studies indicate that gonorrhea, like chlamydia, is most often asymptomatic in both men (60–80%) and women (>85%) [10]. Also, in addition to the columnar cells of the cervix, urogenital infection of either organism in women can also involve the urethra, Bartholin's glands and Skene ducts. Consequently, chlamydia and gonorrhea transmission can occur through nonpenetrative sexual contact, and infection is possible in women who have previously undergone hysterectomy. When sexually active women present with UTI symptoms, the possibility of chlamydia or gonorrhea infection needs to be considered, particularly when a specimen demonstrates white blood cells with a negative urine culture, or "sterile pyuria."

Nucleic acid amplification testing (NAAT) for both chlamydia and gonorrhea can be performed on vaginal or endocervical swab specimens, on liquid cytology specimens, or on urine. Vaginal swabs are optimal [2], as sensitivity and specificity are 98.3% and 96.5% for chlamydia and 96.1% and 99.3% for gonorrhea [6]. The sensitivity of vaginal swab specimens is slightly superior to endocervical specimens, urine [6], and liquid cervical cytology specimens [11].

At the current time, treatments for both chlamydia and gonorrhea are considered curative. However, patients diagnosed with either infection should return 3 months following treatment for retesting, due to the high incidence of reinfection [2].

Chlamydia

Chlamydia trachomatis infection is most prevalent in young persons (typically 4–5%) and particularly high (13.5%) among sexually active non-Hispanic Black persons ages 14–24 [12]. The higher rates seen amongst non-Hispanic Black individuals should not be seen as related to ethnicity or heritage, instead due to social conditions that are more likely to impact individuals from minoritized groups in the United States, including but not limited to access to care. Its predilection for young people is explained partly by unprotected sex with greater numbers of partners but also attributed to the greater prevalence of cervical ectopy in girls and young women, since columnar epithelium on the surface of the external cervix may be more friable during intercourse. Chlamydial transmission is efficient, with 70% of those exposed to chlamydia acquiring a new infection [13]. While approximately 20% of infected women undergo spontaneous cure [14], asymptomatic infection can persist for over 3 years [15]. Chronic carriage, as well as the unlikely but possible false positive laboratory result (3.5%) [16], may sometimes be responsible for a new diagnosis of chlamydia in a monogamous couple; such information may impact patients' decisions regarding relationships.

The majority of women with chlamydia infection are completely asymptomatic [14], and when symptoms are present, they are frequently subtle. Women with urethral involvement sometimes report typical UTI symptoms, and some with chlamydia infection of the cervix may report a change in vaginal discharge or intermenstrual or post-coital bleeding. These latter symptoms can alternatively be associated with PID, and certainly the report of either pelvic pain or heavier menses raises concern for this possible complication.

On pelvic exam, the cervix infected with chlamydia most often appears normal; however, occasionally there can be a watery or purulent endocervical discharge, easily induced endocervical bleeding or edematous ectopy (Fig. 13.1) [17]. If examination of the infected patient reveals either cervical motion tenderness or significant uterine or adnexal tenderness, then the infection has ascended to involve the endometrium and/or salpinges, indicative of PID (see section "Pelvic Inflammatory Disease (PID)" regarding evaluation, management and counseling). At the time of the pelvic exam, NAAT testing should be procured, ideally using a vaginal swab.

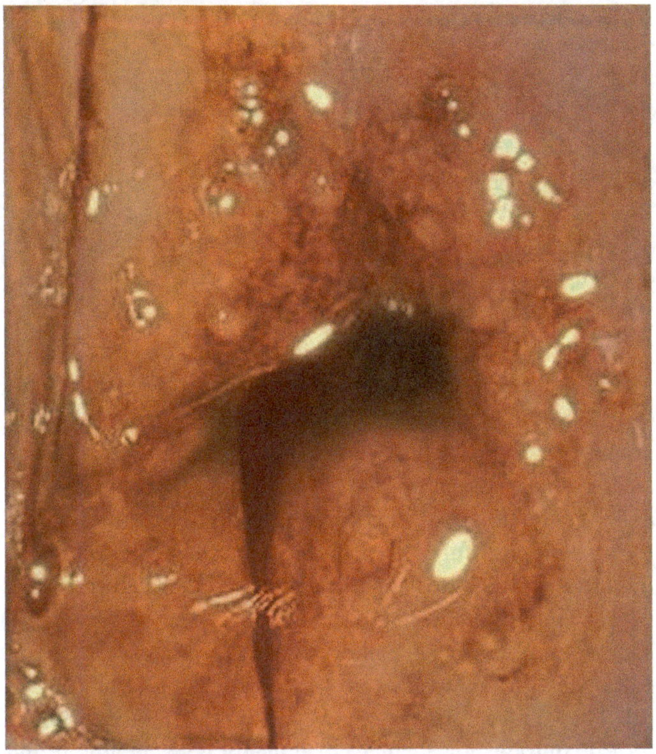

Fig. 13.1 Edematous ectopy of cervix from chlamydia infection. Other possible findings include a mucoid or watery endocervical discharge or easy bleeding; however, most often the cervix infected with chlamydia appears normal. (Image from the University of Washington STD Prevention Training Center [17]. Used with permission)

Uncomplicated chlamydial cervicitis or urethritis can be treated with either a single dose of azithromycin 1 gram or doxycycline 100 mg twice daily for 7 days (Table 13.1). Prompt treatment of chlamydia cervicitis is important in preventing PID. Studies of untreated women with chlamydia infection found that PID developed in 2–3% of women within 2 weeks of diagnosis, and 10% after 1 year [16].

Once laboratory results confirm the infection, sexual partners having had contact within 60 days of diagnosis or symptom onset should be notified, undergo evaluation, provide specimens for STI testing, and then receive empiric treatment for chlamydia. Persons remain infectious until 1 week following azithromycin administration (or until completion of the doxycycline regimen) and patients should be advised to avoid sexual contact until both parties' treatment is completed and all symptoms have resolved. Due to the high incidence of reinfection, patients should be retested in 3 months.

Table 13.1 Treatment regimens for uncomplicated chlamydia infection in nonpregnant adolescents and adults

Recommended regimens:
Azithromycin 1 g orally in a single dose
OR
Doxycycline 100 mg twice daily for 7 days[a]
Alternative regimens:
Erythromycin base 500 m orally 4 times daily for 7 days
Erythromycin ethylsuccinate 800 mg orally 4 times daily for 7 days
Levofloxacin 500 mg orally once daily for 7 days[a]
Ofloxacin 300 mg orally twice daily for 7 days[a]

Reprinted from Workowski and Bolan for the CDC [2]

[a]Doxycycline is contraindicated during the second and third trimesters of pregnancy and in lactating women. Fluoroquinolones are contraindicated in pregnant and lactating women. Erythromycin estolate is contraindicated in pregnancy

Table 13.2 Treatment regimens for uncomplicated gonococcal infection of the cervix, urethra and rectum in nonpregnant adolescents and adults

Recommended regimen:
Ceftriaxone 250 mg IM in a single dose
PLUS
Azithromycin 1 g orally in a single dose
Alternative regimen:
If ceftriaxone is not available OR for use with expedited partner therapy:
Cefixime 400 mg orally in a single dose
PLUS
Azithromycin 1 g orally in a single dose

Reprinted from Workowski and Bolan for the CDC [2]

N. Gonorrhea

Infection with *Neisseria gonorrhea* is most prevalent in persons between the ages of 15–24, non-Hispanic Blacks, and persons residing either in the southern U.S. or in a high-risk community, defined by the CDC as a zip code with high prevalence; recall from above that health disparities in STI acquisition rates often reflect social determinants of health. In addition, those having unprotected sex with multiple partners, those exchanging sex for drugs or money, incarcerated populations, military recruits, and travelers returning from outside the U.S. are considered high-risk [18].

Most infected women are asymptomatic. If present, symptoms typically begin 5–10 days following exposure [18]. Possible symptoms of cervicitis include vaginal discharge, bleeding, pruritus, and dysuria. Gonorrhea infection involving the urethra can produce classic UTI symptoms. PID occurs in 10–20% of women with untreated gonococcal cervicitis and should be suspected if a potentially infected woman reports lower abdominal (pelvic) pain, intermenstrual bleeding, or heavier menses.

Treatment of gonoccocal infection changed in 2010 due to new resistance patterns [18] and mounting concern for imminent spread of gonorrhea resistant to all available antibiotics. The sole recommended treatment regimen now includes dual antibiotic therapy using intramuscular ceftriaxone together with oral azithromycin (Table 13.2). Doxycycline is a second-line option when azithromycin use is not possible. Oral cefixime should be substituted *only* when ceftriaxone is unavailable or when expedited partner therapy is needed [2]. As with uncomplicated chlamydia infection, patients should abstain from sex until 7 days post-treatment of themselves and their partners and until symptoms have resolved. As with chlamydia, all patients treated for gonorrhea should be retested in 3 months due to high rates of reinfection.

Extragenital Chlamydia and Gonorrhea Infection

Extragenital chlamydia or gonorrhea infection may involve the rectum, pharynx, or conjunctiva. Anorectal infection with either organism in women can occur either from unprotected receptive anal intercourse or via perineal spread. While most women with anorectal infection are asymptomatic, some develop acute proctitis with symptoms such as anal pruritus, rectal pain, bleeding, mucopurulent discharge, or tenesmus. Pharyngeal infection with either organism is most often asymptomatic, but some report sore throat and benefit from treatment. Treatment of pharyngeal gonorrhea infection is associated with an approximately 10% failure rate, but test-of-cure is not recommended by the CDC unless an alternative regimen must be employed [2]. Gonococcal or chlamydia conjunctivitis is rare in adults but can result from sexual activity (usually during oral sex), autoinoculation, nonsexual interpersonal contact, or fomites. Antibiotic requirements for conjunctivitis are generally greater and ophthalmology referral is indicated as well. In addition, for gonococcal conjunctivitis, the CDC recommends a one-time eye irrigation as well as consultation with an infectious disease expert regarding treatment, as blindness can result [2]. Another rare complication is gonococcal bacteremia (disseminated gonococcal infection), which can arise 2–3 weeks following inoculation at any mucosal site and manifests as either suppurative arthritis in a single joint or the arthritis-dermatitis syndrome.

STI testing at the pharynx and rectum is performed using the larger swab typically used for vaginal testing. Rectal specimens are often self-collected; proper technique is important and proprietary instructions should be reviewed. Pharyngeal specimens are usually collected by the provider since both the tonsils and the posterior wall of the oropharynx are sampled. Testing extragenital sites is particularly helpful when the patient has symptoms concerning for infection, or if testing at the genital site alone would not adequately screen the patient (such as for women engaging in only nongenital sexual contact, or for women with more than one sexual partner and differing sites of sexual contact). Testing at the genital site is paramount in women; however, since infection at this anatomic location is associated with risk for PID.

Pelvic Inflammatory Disease (PID)

You explain why a full evaluation is needed and Carol agrees to stay for a pelvic exam. When providing history, she acknowledges lower abdominal cramping for the past few days. She assumed that it was premenstrual cramping though it is worse than her typical symptoms.

PID is relatively common, with a lifetime prevalence of 4–12% in the U.S. [19]. The typical host is a sexually active young person. PID most commonly results from the ascension of chlamydia or gonorrhea infection in the cervix to the upper genital tract, leading to complications such as endometritis, salpingitis, tubo-ovarian abscess or pelvic peritonitis. A minority of PID cases are attributable to other culprit organisms, including the sexually transmitted *Mycoplasma hominis*, bacterial vaginosis pathogens, and respiratory or enteric pathogens [20] as well as possibly cytomegalovirus (CMV) [2]. The CDC emphasizes, however, that antibiotic regimens for PID must always include coverage for both chlamydia and gonorrhea, and a negative test result at the level of the cervix does not exclude these infections in the upper tracts [2]. Although PID is initiated by chlamydia or gonorrhea cervicitis, the infection quickly becomes a polymicrobial abscess, and consequently broad-spectrum antimicrobial treatment for at least 14 days is required. PID rarely results in death, however serious sequelae sometimes result in the form of infertility, ectopic pregnancy, or chronic pelvic pain.

Uncommonly, PID is related to IUD use resulting from chlamydia or gonorrheal cervicitis present at the time of insertion; symptoms develop within the first month following placement. PID is treated without removing the IUD, unless there is inadequate progress by 3 days [2]. PID rarely occurs in postmenopausal women but when it does it usually entails tubo-ovarian abscess, and gynecologic malignancies are uncovered approximately half the time [21]. Chronic PID is also rare but can occur in untreated cases, or with unusual organisms such as Actinomyces or tuberculosis [22].

Diagnosis

PID is a clinical diagnosis. Physicians should have a low threshold to diagnose PID and initiate therapy, as prompt treatment is necessary to prevent sequelae such as infertility, ectopic pregnancy, and chronic pelvic pain [23]. Even asymptomatic PID can result in infertility [24]. Most women with PID report lower abdominal (pelvic) pain. Other women may report nonspecific symptoms such as a change in bleeding pattern (e.g.

Table 13.3 Diagnosing pelvic inflammatory disease

A clinical diagnosis of PID should be made and presumptive treatment given to appropriate hosts reporting lower abdominal pain and lacking alternative diagnosis, if they have 1 of the 3 findings on pelvic exam:
EITHER
Cervical motion tenderness
OR
Uterine tenderness
OR
Adnexal tenderness
The likelihood of PID is further increased if there is also evidence of lower tract inflammation, consisting of
EITHER:
Mucopurulent cervical discharge
OR
Excess leukocytes[a] on saline "wet prep" of vaginal fluid

Reprinted from Workowski and Bolan for the CDC [2]
[a]Excess leukocytes is defined as >1 leukocyte per epithelial cell

heavier menses or intermenstrual spotting), change in vaginal discharge, or dyspareunia. The CDC urges clinicians to promptly initiate empiric therapy when a sexually active young patient presents with pelvic pain that is not explained by other likely causes if one of the following three exam findings is evident: cervical motion tenderness, uterine tenderness, or adnexal tenderness [2]. A palpable mass or sense of fullness on bimanual exam raises concern for complication with tubo-ovarian abscess, especially when accompanied by fever or leukocytosis. Tubo-ovarian abscess rupture can be associated with life-threatening sepsis, and thus such women are admitted to hospital and undergo imaging and abscess management.

Patients with history and examination consistent with PID should also undergo a wet prep, pregnancy testing, and NAAT testing for chlamydia and gonorrhea. Excess leukocytes on a wet prep or the presence of mucoid cervical discharge on speculum exam, both signs of genital tract inflammation, increase the likelihood of PID (Table 13.3). While only half of women with PID have cervical discharge [21] and not all women have leukocytes on a wet prep, most women with PID will have one of these two findings. If neither is present, consideration should be given to alternative diagnoses [2]. A wet prep will also identify concomitant infections with trichomoniasis or bacterial vaginosis (BV), and the presence of these organisms may alter the treatment regimen (see Chap. 12 on Vaginitis and Vulvar Conditions). Pregnancy testing is performed for those at risk, as pregnant women are admitted to hospital and treated with parenteral antibiotics appropriate for pregnancy. While a positive chlamydia or gonorrhea result at the level of the cervix can help confirm the diagnosis of PID, a negative result does not exclude infection in the upper tracts [2]. Clinicians should therefore *not* rely on NAAT testing to diagnose PID, nor should they discontinue treatment for PID based on NAAT test results if the original diagnosis was made with reasonable clinical certainty.

Imaging is unnecessary in most cases of PID, though it can help to establish the diagnosis or determine its severity [21]. Transvaginal ultrasound or pelvic MRI is indicated when there is concern for possible tubo-ovarian abscess or clinically severe PID (i.e., fever, peritoneal signs on exam, nausea, or vomiting), or in the setting of an unsatisfactory pelvic examination. The presence of a tubo-ovarian abscess, thickened fluid-filled tubes, or tubal hyperemia on Doppler study confirms the diagnosis of PID. In general, MRI is more sensitive than ultrasound but more expensive and less readily available. If confirmation of endometritis is desired, endometrial biopsy is sometimes but not always helpful and typically 1 week is required for pathology results. Laparoscopy is considered the "gold standard" for diagnosing PID for research purposes; however, laparoscopy fails to detect endometritis or early salpingitis, and this invasive and expensive procedure is not often utilized for diagnostic purposes. When the diagnosis of PID is in question, an abdominopelvic CT may uncover an alternate etiology.

On pelvic examination your patient has no abnormal discharge and in fact her cervix appears completely normal. She has mild uterine tenderness on bimanual exam and significant leukocytosis on saline wet mount. You make a clinical diagnosis of PID.

Treatment

Antibiotic regimens for PID must include treatment for both chlamydia and gonorrhea as well as vaginal flora. For most patients, outpatient treatment with ceftriaxone 250 mg IM once and doxycycline 100 mg PO bid for 14 days provides appropriate treatment (Table 13.4). The CDC recommends consideration be given to adding metronidazole 500 mg PO bid to better treat anaerobes but notes that the medication's adverse effects are not always tolerated [2]. Additionally, a recent Cochrane review failed to find improved PID outcomes with the addition of metronidazole [19]. Patients treated for PID should be reassessed in the office after 48–72 hours to ensure clinical improvement.

Inpatient treatment should be considered for patients with concerning features: severe PID accompanied by high fever, nausea, or vomiting; suspected tubo-ovarian abscess; potential surgical abdomen; pregnancy; inability to tolerate or take an outpatient oral regimen; or failure to improve at 72 hours on oral therapy. Patients without clinical improvement by

Table 13.4 Treatment regimens for non-pregnant women[a] with pelvic inflammatory disease

Recommended outpatient regimens:
Ceftriaxone 250 mg IM in a single dose[b]
PLUS
Doxycycline 100 mg orally twice daily for 14 days[c]
WITH OR WITHOUT
Metronidazole 500 mg orally twice daily for 14 days
Recommended parenteral regimens[d]*:*
Cefotetan 2 g IV every 12 hours
PLUS
Doxycycline 100 mg orally (or IV) every 12 hours[c]
OR
Cefoxitin 2 g IV every 6 hours
PLUS
Doxycycline 100 mg orally (or IV) every 12 hours[c]
OR
Clindamycin 900 mg IV every 8 hours
PLUS
Gentamicin loading dose 2 mg/kg IV or IM, followed by maintenance dose (1.5 mg/kg) every 8 hours

Reprinted from Workowski and Bolan for the CDC [2]

[a]For management of pregnant women with PID please consult [2]

[b]If Ceftriaxone is unavailable then Cefoxitin 2 g IM in a single dose and Probenecid 1 g orally administered concurrently in a single dose can be substituted. Alternatively, other parenteral third –generation cephalosporins (e.g. ceftizoxime or cefotaxime) can be substituted

[c]Doxycycline is contraindicated in lactating women (and during the second and third trimesters of pregnancy)

[d]When tubo-ovarian abscess complicates PID then clindamycin (450 mg orally four times daily) or metronidazole (500 mg twice daily) should be used with the doxycycline to complete at least 14 days of therapy

72 hours should be hospitalized, have their diagnosis clarified, and transition to a parenteral regimen if PID is confirmed. Recommended parenteral regimens include cefotetan 2 g IV every 12 hours plus doxycycline 100 mg PO bid (Table 13.4). Hospitalized patients can transition to oral therapy 24–48 hours after demonstrating clinical improvement and be discharged on doxycycline 100 mg PO BID alone to complete a 14-day course.

A patient with tubo-ovarian abscess is hospitalized for a minimum of 24 hours due to the risk of abscess rupture and sepsis [2]. Transvaginal, ultrasound-guided aspiration of the abscess can avert the need for surgery in nearly all cases and should be offered at the time of diagnosis [21]. Affected patients are treated with a parenteral regimen that also includes metronidazole for anaerobic coverage. After initial therapy, patients should complete a 14-day course of clindamycin 450 mg PO QID or metronidazole 500 mg PO BID in addition to the usual doxycycline. Alternative parenteral regimens can be found at the CDC website: https://www.cdc.gov/std/tg2015/pid.htm [25].

Partner Notification and Follow-Up

As noted above, partner notification plays a crucial role in the management of PID. Empiric therapy for both chlamydia and gonorrhea is warranted for partners (regardless of the index patient's results) and partners should be tested as well [2].

You talk with Carol about her diagnosis of PID and initiate outpatient treatment with an injection of ceftriaxone in the office and a prescription for a 14-day course of oral doxycycline to begin today. You offer to help her contact her sexual partners to notify them of their exposure and offer them an appointment for testing and empiric treatment as well, but she has had no other partners in the past 2 months. She is assigned a follow-up appointment in 3 days. At her follow-up visit, her pelvic pain has resolved and she is tolerating antibiotic therapy. Carol now requests screening for herpes, since she read on the Internet that this should be done.

STIs Causing Genital Ulcers: HSV and Syphilis

In the United States, herpes and syphilis are responsible for most infectious genital ulcers. The incidence of herpes has been falling in recent decades while that of syphilis has been rising; however, herpes remains vastly more common [26]. Distinguishing the etiology of a genital ulcer clinically can be a challenge, thus all patients presenting with a genital ulcer should be tested for both herpes and syphilis and treated empirically for the more likely etiology. In addition to herpes and syphilis, the acute HIV syndrome can be a cause of painful oral or genital ulcers [27]. If the patient who presents with a genital ulcer appears systemically ill with symptoms typical for acute HIV syndrome, testing for acute seroconversion should also be performed using combined HIV antigen/antibody testing.

Bacterial superinfection sometimes complicates the clinical picture, and genital ulcers can also sometimes result from yeast, rare infections such as chancroid or lymphogranuloma venereum, or from noninfectious causes like aphthae, carcinoma, fixed drug eruptions, or trauma from sexual activity. For approximately one-quarter of all patients presenting with a genital ulcer, no cause is found; often this is attributed to false-negative test results, however, the above noninfectious causes are sometimes responsible. Women with persistent genital ulcers or ulcers of unknown etiology should be referred to dermatology and also ophthalmology (to help exclude Behcet's disease). Importantly, genital ulcers increase both the acquisition [28] and transmission [29] of HIV infection, and all patients with genital ulcers should undergo HIV testing for this reason.

Herpes Simplex Virus

Herpes simplex virus (HSV) is a DNA virus that causes recurrent ulcerative lesions on the oral or genital mucosa. In addition to oral and genital areas, other mucosal sites such as the ocular conjunctiva, nipple, and nose are vulnerable to infection. Genital infection can also involve the genital skin (as opposed to mucosa) and in women even the buttock or upper thigh. Primary (but not recurrent) HSV infection can also involve the skin anywhere on the body, with finger involvement (herpetic whitlow) classic in health personnel as well as occasionally accompanying genital infection in the community [30].

Following a typical incubation period lasting 3–7 days (but sometimes as long as 3 weeks), primary genital herpes classically presents as one or more clusters of painful and tender vesicles, though vulvar vesicles quickly erode and frequently present as genital ulcers instead. The vesicles crust over then clear in 10–14 days. HSV then remains dormant in nerve roots until reactivation, at which time vesicles recur at the same site. Approximately one-third of patients will have a "nonclassic" presentation consisting of fissures, cervicitis, or dysuria [31]. Other patients have no visible mucosal lesions but may have tender, bilateral, inguinal lymphadenopathy and a vaginal discharge instead. Primary perianal or anal herpes infection usually presents with a painful mucosal ulcer along with rectal pain, itching, tenesmus, and discharge. Primary infection may be accompanied by low-grade fever, malaise, and headache.

Serologic studies consistently reveal that only a small minority (10–35%) of individuals with genital HSV are aware of their infection [32]. Sexual transmission to a seronegative person is as high as 70% when lesions are active [33]; however, most transmissions occur during intervening periods of asymptomatic shedding. Importantly, the presence of genital HSV-2 infection increases the risk of HIV acquisition threefold [34].

Laboratory Testing

To confirm the diagnosis, a swab sample should be obtained from the base of an ulcer or a de-roofed vesicle and sent for either herpes cell culture or viral PCR testing; both tests utilize NAAT methods and provide type-specific results (i.e. HSV-1 or HSV-2). Because viral shedding is intermittent, false-negative results are possible, particularly when sampling healing or recurrent lesions [2]. Recall that even if considered an unlikely cause of the ulcer, serologic testing for syphilis should be ordered; HIV screening should be performed as well.

When positive, direct testing of the mucosal lesion for HSV is more helpful than HSV serologies. The CDC identifies three situations where HSV serologies are helpful: when a patient has recurrent genital symptoms but direct testing of the lesion is negative; when there is a clinical diagnosis of herpes without laboratory confirmation; and when a patient's partner has genital herpes. In the first two instances, serologic testing helps clarify diagnosis. In the last scenario it determines a patient's susceptibility to infection and may guide the couple's decisions regarding condom use or suppressive antiviral therapy. The CDC also states that screening for HSV using serologic testing can be considered for high-risk patients presenting for STI evaluation [2]. Note, however, that the USPSTF advises against screening for HSV in the general population, citing an unacceptably high rate of false-positive test results, potential for psychosocial harms, and lack of known benefit for treating asymptomatic HSV infection [35].

If serologic testing for herpes is desired, only IgG antibodies should be ordered; IgM antibodies are generally unhelpful since they are not type-specific and are associated with more error as well [2]. IgG antibodies to HSV develop a few weeks after exposure and remain positive indefinitely. Type-specific antibody tests should always be included, as clinical implications differ greatly for HSV-1 and HSV-2. Antibody to HSV-2 generally implies genital infection. Antibody to HSV-1 infection could indicate either orolabial or genital infection, but little can be concluded whether the HSV-1 antibody is relevant to the patient's recent genital concern, since IgG HSV-1 antibody could possibly result from unrecognized orolabial infection acquired in childhood. When needed, serologies are typically ordered at the follow-up visit, and sometimes retesting 6–8 weeks following initial infection is required to detect antibody.

Treatment

The CDC recommends prompt initiation of oral antiviral treatment for all patients with suspected first-episode herpes infection, without waiting for test results (Table 13.5).

Table 13.5 Treatment regimens for initial episode of genital herpes[a]

Acyclovir 400 mg orally 3 times daily for 7–10 days
Acyclovir 200 mg orally 5 times daily for 7–10 days
Valacyclovir 1 g orally twice daily for 7–10 days
Famciclovir 250 mg orally 3 times daily for 7–10 days

Reprinted from Workowski and Bolan for the CDC [2]

[a]All patients with an initial episode of genital herpes should receive antiviral treatment. Treatment duration can be extended if healing is incomplete after 10 days of therapy

Treatment is not curative nor does it impact the likelihood of recurrences. However, it can reduce the duration and extent of symptoms and reduce viral shedding, thereby decreasing the risk of transmission to others [2]. Rarely, initial HSV infection can be severe or have associated complications, such as urinary retention, disseminated disease, or meningo-encephalitis; such patients require hospitalization and IV acyclovir therapy. Topical acyclovir ointment has little benefit and is not recommended [2].

Recurrent herpes outbreaks are milder than primary infection. These outbreaks occur in 90% of patients infected with HSV-2 but far fewer patients with genital HSV-1 infection [36]. The frequency of recurrence can vary but sometimes may coincide with menses. Factors that suppress immune function, such as physical or emotional stress, sleep deprivation, and illness, contribute to recurrences.

While recurrent episodes cannot be prevented altogether, two pharmacologic strategies are available to minimize their impact: suppressive therapy with daily medication and episodic therapy initiated at symptom onset (Table 13.6). All patients diagnosed with a first episode of genital herpes should be offered suppressive therapy [2]. Suppressive therapy reduces the severity and number of recurrences and is often chosen by patients suffering frequent recurrences (>6 per year). Additionally, the use of valacyclovir 500 mg once daily showed a reduced risk of transmitting genital herpes to the uninfected partner [37]. Because the frequency of recurrences diminishes over time, a drug holiday is recommended after each 12-month period to assess the need for continued suppression [2]. Most patients choose episodic therapy instead, which shortens the course and severity of outbreak symptoms. Patients require a prescription to keep a ready supply of medication on hand in order to promptly initiate therapy at the first sign of prodromal symptoms (often "tingling" at the site), as antiviral therapy is most effective when started within 24 hours.

Table 13.6 Suppressive and episodic treatment regimens for recurrent genital herpes

Suppressive regimens:
Acyclovir 400 mg orally twice daily
Valacyclovir 500 mg orally once daily[a]
Valacyclovir 1 g orally once daily
Famciclovir 250 mg orally twice daily
Episodic regimens:
Acyclovir 400 mg orally 3 times daily for 5 days
Acyclovir 800 mg orally twice daily for 5 days
Acyclovir 800 mg orally 3 times daily for 2 days
Valacyclovir 500 mg orally twice daily for 3 days
Valacyclovir 1 g orally once daily for 5 days
Famciclovir 125 mg orally twice daily for 5 days
Famciclovir 1 g orally twice daily for 1 day
Famciclovir 500 mg once, followed by 250 mg twice daily for 2 days

Reprinted from Workowski and Bolan for the CDC [2]

[a]The Valacyclovir 500 mg once daily regimen might be a less-effective suppressive regimen for persons with very frequent recurrences (≥10/year) [2]. However, this regimen was shown to reduce transmission to seronegative partners in monogamous discordant relationships [37]

Counseling

Patients have described HSV, an incurable sexually transmitted disease, as a "devastating" diagnosis [36]. Patients should be reassured that HSV is manageable and will not severely impact their sexuality [38]. Counseling may also include information regarding the variable nature of recurrences, the risk of transmission to sex partners, and the occurrence of subclinical shedding. Patients should inform potential sex partners of the infection, abstain from intercourse during recurrences, and use condoms at other times [2]. Condoms will also protect the patient from the known increased risk of HIV acquisition.

Patients benefit from a scheduled follow-up appointment 3–4 weeks after the initial diagnosis for further supportive counseling as well as discussion of the options of episodic and suppressive therapy. Additionally, patients can be reassured that transmission of established HSV infection during vaginal delivery is rare (<1%) and that suppressive therapy during the last month of pregnancy can further reduce this risk. Patients should be counseled to inform their treating obstetrician of a history of HSV infection.

Possible concerns regarding potential infidelity should be addressed directly [36]. Patients should be advised that a partner may have had an unrecognized initial infection long ago and is shedding virus asymptomatically. Alternatively, many first episodes of clinically symptomatic genital herpes actually represent a recurrence [39]. Thus, a new diagnosis of genital herpes can occur in a monogamous couple without recent acquisition of HSV. Asymptomatic partners of a patient diagnosed with genital HSV can be offered type-specific serologic testing.

You explain to Carol that experts (USPSTF) discourage testing for herpes unless patients have evidence of the infection, partly because the test is sometimes incorrect. You advise her that she does not have any evidence of genital herpes at present but that she should contact you promptly for evaluation if she develops any painful genital "sores." You also notice that Carol forgot to go to the lab for HIV and syphilis serologies at her visit 3 days ago, and she agrees to have this testing performed today.

Syphilis

Syphilis is an acute and chronic systemic disease affecting all organ systems caused by the spirochete *Treponema pallidum*. The incidence of syphilis in the U.S. has been steadily rising following a nadir in 2000 [40]. Urban men who have sex with men, half of whom are coinfected with HIV, now comprise the majority of cases [41]. Although only 11% of syphilis infections occur in women, concern is heightened due to the recent dramatic rise in the rate of congenital syphilis.

Syphilis is most often spread through sexual contact, including oral sex, and rarely through kissing [36]. Infected persons are most contagious in early stages of the disease, when they have moist, mucocutaneous lesions [42] or spirochetes in the epidermis that can be transmitted through microabrasions created during sexual activity [43]. Syphilis can also be transmitted through transfusion of fresh blood, via placental passage, or direct inoculation (usually of the fingers of health care workers).

The incubation period varies from 3 days to 3 months (average 3 weeks), after which time an ulcer ("chancre") develops at the site of inoculation. Common locations include the external genitalia, cervix, mouth, upper lip, perianal area and anal canal, and the tongue (Fig. 13.2) [44]. Care should be exercised when evaluating a patient presenting with possible syphilis, as all mucosal and skin lesions are potentially infectious. Sometimes more than one ulcer is present but at other times no lesion develops, or the lesion goes unnoticed, as often happens with vaginal ulcers [43]. Ulcers heal spontaneously in 2 weeks to 2 months, regardless of treatment. Syphilitic ulcers differ from those from HSV in that they are usually not painful, lack any overlying mucoid material, and have "heaped up," firm borders. Also, in contrast to HSV, the regional lymphadenopathy is nontender. Despite the distinctions in clinical presentation, a patient presenting with a genital ulcer in the U.S. is nonetheless tested for both syphilis and herpes and immediately treated for the more likely etiology.

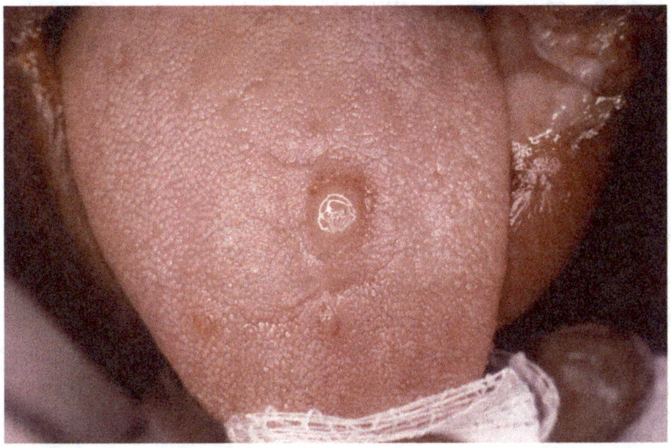

Fig. 13.2 Chancre of primary syphilis on tongue. The ulcer of primary syphilis differs from a herpes ulcer as it is painless, has "heaped-up" borders and no overlying membrane. The tongue is a common site of inoculation, as syphilis is frequently transmitted through orogenital sex [44]. (Image from CDC Public Image Library, CDC/Credit Robert E. Sumpter)

To help with diagnosis and guide management, syphilis has been divided into stages: primary, secondary, and tertiary disease. A fourth entity, neurosyphilis, can occur at any stage of infection. A patient with primary syphilis develops a papule at the site of inoculation, but this is rarely recognized as it rapidly evolves into an ulcer. Often, bilateral nontender regional (usually inguinal) lymphadenopathy is present. The second stage, beginning 2–12 weeks following exposure, reflects organism dissemination and vasculitis. This stage can present with almost any symptom including constitutional symptoms, arthralgias, various rashes, mucous patch lesions, hepatitis, and nephritis. The classic rash, which is pruritic in one-half of hosts [42], is initially macular then papular and classically involves the palms and soles. Oval mucous patches can form on any mucosal surface, and its correlates in warm intertriginous areas are gray-white to erythematous fleshy excrescences termed condyloma lata. Another key feature of secondary syphilis is diffuse, nontender lymphadenopathy; involvement of the epitrochlear nodes should suggest the diagnosis [42]. Tertiary syphilis involving cardiac lesions or gumma is now exceedingly rare in the U.S. due to antibiotic use for unrelated illnesses. Neurosyphilis can occur at any stage of infection. It can manifest in a number of ways: cranial nerve dysfunction, meningitis, stroke, acute altered mental status, auditory or ophthalmic abnormalities, or "late changes" such as tabes dorsalis and general paresis. Neurosyphilis is of particular concern for patients coinfected with HIV.

Congenital syphilis will occur in one-third of pregnant women with untreated syphilis. Possible sequelae include miscarriage, neonatal death, intrauterine growth retardation or offspring born with congenital infection—with the more common serious manifestations being bone or neurologic defects. For this reason, the USPSTF recommends screening all pregnant women for syphilis ("A" recommendation) [45]. In most states, performing this screening is mandated at the first prenatal visit. Women at higher risk for acquiring infection should be retested for syphilis throughout pregnancy and at delivery as well [41]. Antibiotic treatment is usually successful when administered prior to the middle of the second trimester. Pregnant women with syphilis are typically managed in conjunction with neonatologists, as antibiotic therapy can induce fetal distress.

Testing

The diagnosis of syphilis is established using serologies. Serologic testing consists of two types: tests that detect Treponema-specific antibodies and those that detect antibodies to nontreponemal material; results from both tests must be thoughtfully considered (and sometimes compared with previous results) before a diagnosis of current syphilis infection can be made. Treponema-specific tests detect antibodies against the organism and include the FTA-ABS, the TP-PA and the EIA-based and CIA assays. Except for a minority (12–25%) of patients treated during primary syphilis who revert to nonreactive [46], a positive Treponemal test usually remains positive indefinitely after treatment and is therefore only able to indicate lifetime exposure to syphilis. Nontreponemal tests include the RPR and the VDRL which detect antibodies directed against a cardiolipin-lecithin-cholesterol complex that arises from the interaction of host tissues with *T. pallidum*. One month may be required for antibody to become detectable, and thus when clinical suspicion of primary syphilis is high, a negative serology necessitates repeat testing in 2–4 weeks [47]. For this reason, assigning a close follow-up appointment at the time of the initial visit is warranted. Despite their poor specificity, the RPR and VDRL tests help distinguish current syphilis infection from lifetime exposure, since their antibody titers fluctuate with disease activity--although in a minority of hosts the nontreponemal test can remain reactive for a few years following treatment--the "serofast response". On the other hand, false positive RPR and VDRL results occur in 1–2% of the U.S. population [48], in such settings as advanced age, chancroid, tuberculosis, SLE, HIV infection, intravenous drug use, pregnancy, viral hepatitis, mononucleosis, and many other infections. When the results of both types of serologies are available and indicate possible current infection, it is often helpful to contact the local health department, as public health workers can provide information such as prior treatment and titer trends. Patients diagnosed with syphilis should have repeat serologies in 6 and 12 months; a response to treatment in syphilis patients is defined by resolution of symptoms and signs plus a fourfold decline in nontreponemal titers (or a change in 2 dilutions, e.g., from 1:16 to 1:4) when retested at 12 months. The same assay (RPR *or* VDRL) should be used with serial testing [2].

Since 2016, reverse screening algorithms that start with a treponemal test have been used. The reverse approach detects more cases of early syphilis, since treponemal antibodies are detectable before non-treponemal antibodies and are less prone to false-negative results [49]. However, discordant results may arise when using reverse testing, whereby a positive treponemal antibody test (e.g. positive FTA-ABS or TP-PA) triggers nontreponemal antibody (i.e. RPR or VDRL) testing that is nonreactive. This may indicate one of three possible scenarios: previously treated syphilis, untreated or incompletely treated syphilis or a false positive treponemal antibody result. If the patient was previously treated for syphilis, and currently has neither evidence of disease nor recent exposure to syphilis, then no further acute management is needed. If the previously treated patient reports recent possible exposure, then repeating the nontreponemal test in 2–4 weeks helps to exclude recent repeat infection when the titer is not rising. If the patient has no prior history of syphilis, then one should repeat testing using a different treponemal test (e.g. using FTA-ABS if TP-PA was previously used). Those with a positive confirmatory treponemal test should be evaluated and offered treatment. For those patients with a negative confirmatory test and low risk for syphilis infection, the initial treponemal test is deemed a false positive.

Evaluation of the cerebrospinal fluid (CSF) is indicated when there is concern for ocular syphilis or neurosyphilis and is also sometimes performed when titers fail to respond adequately to usual therapy, as the CSF may serve as a reservoir of untreated infection. CSF findings require careful interpretation in the setting of syphilis, and expert consultation is generally warranted. Likewise, those with possible ocular syphilis are managed in conjunction with an ophthalmologist.

Direct testing of lesions for the *Treponema pallidum* organism is typically available only at STD clinics, where clinicians perform darkfield examination of swab specimens taken from such lesions as nonoral ulcers or mucous patches, or from condyloma lata skin lesions. Such testing has limited sensitivity but is diagnostic when positive. More advanced direct testing methods (such as PCR testing of swab specimens for *Treponema pallidum*) are under development and it is anticipated that they will contribute tremendously to the diagnostic process [42].

Management

Penicillin, administered parenterally, is the preferred drug for treating persons in all stages of syphilis (Table 13.7) [2]. Earlier stages can be treated with a single injection of intramuscular benzathine penicillin (Bicillin L-A). The CDC cautions that using the proper formulation of penicillin is important, as formulations with similar names may not penetrate sequestered sites such as the CNS or aqueous humor. Late latent syphilis is treated with a series of 3 weekly intramuscular penicillin injections while tertiary syphilis, neurosyphilis, ocular syphilis, syphilis in pregnancy, and congenital syphilis all require intravenous penicillin G. Pregnant women with serious penicillin allergy require desensitization, as there is no alternative regimen in pregnancy [2].

Table 13.7 Treatment regimens for syphilis

Primary, secondary and early latent (<1 year) syphilis
Benzathine penicillin G (Bicillin L-A) 2.4 million units IM in a single dose
Late latent syphilis, latent syphilis of unknown duration and tertiary syphilis
Benzathine penicillin G (Bicillin L-A) 2.4 million units IM weekly × 3
Neurosyphilis and ocular syphilis
Recommended regimen:
Aqueous crystalline penicillin G 18–24 million units per day, administered as 3–4 million units IV every 4 hours or continuous infusion, for 10–14 days
Alternative regimen:
Procaine penicillin G 2.4 million units IM once daily
PLUS
Probenecid 500 mg orally 4 times daily, both for 10–14 days
Preferred alternative regimen for primary or secondary syphilis for nonpregnant persons with penicillin allergy or for use in expedited partner therapy
Doxycycline 100 mg PO twice daily for 14 days
Pregnant women
The penicillin regimen appropriate for their stage of infection administered by a neonatologist in a timely fashion.

Reprinted from Workowski and Bolan for the CDC [2]

Prior to treatment, patients should be warned of the possibility of the Jarisch-Herxheimer reaction, which is an acute reaction occurring within 24 hours of the initiation of treatment for syphilis. This febrile response is often accompanied by headache and myalgias. Antipyretics such as aspirin can manage symptoms; attempts to prevent the reaction are ineffective [2].

Follow-Up

Clinical and serologic follow-up is recommended at 6 and 12 months after treatment, but more frequent monitoring may be warranted if follow-up is uncertain or the potential for repeat infection a concern. A patient whose titer rises at the 6-month follow-up should have the titer repeated in 2 weeks and if confirmed, reinfection suspected and the patient re-treated. If the titer fails to decline fourfold by the 12-month follow-up the patient should receive additional clinical and serologic follow-up. The patient should be evaluated again for HIV as well as for possible CNS syphilis infection. If additional close follow-up cannot be ensured, the CDC recommends empiric retreatment, using the intramuscular benzathine penicillin regimen used for late latent syphilis (weekly injections for 3 weeks). It should be noted, however, that 15–20% of patients successfully treated do not achieve the expected fourfold decline in nontreponemal titer, especially those with low initial titers. The optimal management of such patients is unclear [2]. Latent syphilis is followed post-treatment similarly except titers are monitored at 6, 12, and 24 months, since it may take up to 2 years for the titer to decline fourfold.

Partner Management

The CDC identifies improvement in partner management as a means to reverse the recent rise in the syphilis epidemic [41]. Partners require evaluation, serologies and usually empiric treatment. Because of the long incubation period, persons who have had sexual contact within 90 days with a person diagnosed with primary syphilis should be empirically treated for early syphilis, regardless of serology results. In contrast, partners whose sexual contact occurred more than 90 days prior to the patient's diagnosis should be treated based on clinical findings or serological results, unless opportunity for follow-up is uncertain. The same is true for a person having had sexual contact within 6 months of a person diagnosed with secondary syphilis and 1 year for early latent syphilis.

Screening

In addition to all pregnant women, the CDC recommends screening for syphilis in the following groups of women: persons infected with HIV, those persons whose partners have been diagnosed with syphilis [41] and anyone diagnosed with an STI [2]. The USPSTF recognizes other high-risk groups who might also benefit from screening, namely commercial sex workers, those who have been incarcerated, and those belonging to certain racial or ethnic groups [45].

Sexually Transmitted Viruses (HIV, HBV, HCV, and HPV)

HIV

HIV is most often spread sexually, with the risk of transmission per episode of unprotected vaginal intercourse 0.1–0.2%, while that for receptive anal intercourse higher at 0.1–3% [50]. The risk of contracting HIV through oral sex is extremely low, although transmission can be facilitated by menstruation or oral lesions such as bleeding gums. Approximately 40,000 new infections occur yearly in the U.S., 20% of which are acquired by women. Disparities persist in rates of HIV acquisition in the United States due to interactions between a number of social determinants of health, with individuals from African American and Hispanic groups disproportionally affected. The highest prevalence is found in transgender women, in whom approximately one-quarter (22–28%) are infected [51]. Safe sex counseling, HIV screening, and reduction of other STIs known to promote HIV transmission and/or acquisition of HIV continue to be important. Additional strategies include prevention of HIV spread through improved recognition and prompt treatment of acute HIV infection; early referral for chronic HIV care; and for those persons at high risk of acquiring HIV, provision of nonoccupational post-exposure prophylaxis (nPEP) or preexposure prophylaxis (PrEP).

Screening

The CDC advises universal opt-out HIV screening for all persons age 13–64 in all health care settings. In addition, pregnant women [7] and patients presenting with STI concerns should be screened. Surveillance studies indicate that 16% of HIV-positive Americans are unaware of their infection [2]; intensified screening efforts, prompt disease reporting, and effective partner management are critical steps to reduce this number.

Acute HIV Syndrome

Persons with acute HIV infection are highly contagious due to high levels of virus in plasma and genital secretions. Up to one-third of people with acute infection remain asymptomatic, but the majority experience the "acute HIV syndrome" (previously called the "acute retroviral syndrome"). Symptoms typically begin 1–4 weeks following exposure and are variable and nonspecific ("flu-like") but often include fever, fatigue, sore throat, myalgias, night sweats, rash, headache, diarrhea, and vomiting [27] (Table 13.8). By contrast, nasal congestion is associated with a decreased likelihood of acute HIV infection [52]. Not surprisingly, symptoms of acute HIV syndrome are often mistakenly attributed to either influenza, "mononucleosis," severe *Streptococcal* pharyngitis or secondary syphilis. Heightened awareness to entertain the diagnosis when evaluating adults presenting with flu-like symptoms may significantly increase the number of identified cases. Also, directed effort to examine acutely ill, febrile patients for the less common but more specific findings of acute HIV syndrome--such as skin rash, painful oral or genital ulcers, and axillary or inguinal lymphadenopathy-- could potentially improve clinical recognition of acutely infected persons [27].

The rapid HIV antigen/antibody test should be used in this setting. If results are negative and one remains concerned, testing for HIV RNA (using a cut-off of >3000 copies/mL to avoid false-positive results) should be pursued. Once the diagnosis is confirmed, one should assess the patient's psychological response and offer support, making use of immediate referral when needed. One should also urgently refer to an HIV specialist to initiate antiretroviral therapy (ART, previously termed HAART) [2]. Prompt initiation of antiretroviral therapy not only improves long-term patient outcomes but also substantially reduces infectiousness and the risk of transmission. In addition, partners not known to be HIV-positive who have had contact within the 72 hours preceding the diagnosis should immediately receive post-exposure prophylaxis. One should also not overlook the critical importance of providing immediate patient education regarding safe sex to avoid transmission to others.

Table 13.8 Common symptoms, signs, and laboratory abnormalities associated with acute HIV syndrome

Symptoms and signs	Common laboratory abnormalities
Fever	Leukopenia
Malaise/fatigue	Thrombocytopenia
Night sweats	Elevated transaminases
Headache	
Myalgias	
Lymphadenopathy	
Frequent cough or shortness of breath	
Sore throat	
Rash	
Arthralgias	
Diarrhea	
Anorexia	
Meningitis	
Vomiting	
Oral or genital ulcers	
Thrush or esophageal candidiasis	

Data from Refs. [27, 52–56]

Vertical Transmission

Specific antiretroviral regimens taken throughout pregnancy can substantially reduce vertical transmission from the mother to offspring, from approximately 30% without medications to 2% with treatment [57]. Other perinatal measures include administering a brief course of antiretroviral agents to the newborn and performing elective cesarean section at 38 weeks for women with high viral loads. In the U.S. and other countries where the water supply is typically free of pathogens, HIV-positive mothers are advised not to breastfeed [2].

Postexposure Prophylaxis

Since 2005, the CDC has recommended nonoccupational post-exposure prophylaxis (nPEP) for persons exposed to potentially HIV-infected body fluids through unprotected sexual activity or needle sharing. The CDC promotes provision of nPEP by nonspecialists such as primary care providers and published updated guidelines in 2016 [58]. To be eligible for nPEP, the exposure must entail substantial risk and have occurred within 72 hours. The first step is rapid antigen/antibody HIV testing of the exposed patient to exclude established HIV infection. If results are negative or not immediately available, providers should prescribe a 28-day course of the three- or four-drug regimen (Table 13.9), after careful review of the existing medication list for drug–drug interactions and baseline ALT/AST and serum creatinine measurements. Due to risk of renal toxicity from tenofovir, patients must have a creatinine clearance ≥60 mL/min for standard nPEP. However, nPEP is commonly initiated in healthy persons before lab results are available, especially on weekends or when patients are managed by phone. Due to possible association with neural tube defects, dolutegravir should not be used in women at risk for pregnancy or in the first trimester [59]; raltegravir should be selected instead. In addition to the above testing, all should be screened for routine STIs and women at risk should be tested for pregnancy (Table 13.10). Women testing negative for pregnancy should be offered emergency contraception, and in some settings (i.e. sexual assault) offered empiric treatment for chlamydia, gonorrhea and trichomoniasis. Although nPEP appears highly effective in preventing HIV infection, patients should be counseled to use condoms or practice abstinence for the next 12 weeks to avoid potential transmission to others, and to return promptly in the event of a flu-like illness. The source individual should also be contacted to undergo HIV testing; if the source patient is found to be HIV negative then nPEP can be discontinued. Because withdrawal of ART in patients with chronic hepatitis B infection can sometimes be associated with a life-threatening hepatitis "flare," expert consultation should be sought prior to its discontinuation.

The exposed patient continuing nPEP undergoes the same battery of laboratory testing at the 4–6 week follow-up, and again at the 3-month follow-up visit. The HIV test obtained at the 3-month follow-up (8 weeks following completion of nPEP) is the final follow-up HIV serology [58]. Prevention counseling should also be provided at each visit. If there is concern for continued high-risk behavior at completion of the regimen, consideration can be given to prescribing preexposure prophylaxis (see next section). Clinicians with questions regarding post-exposure prophylaxis can access expert consultation at the national PEPline (888-448-4911/888-HIV-4911) [60]. Callers will receive a phone response within 2 hours from an experienced clinician Monday through Friday between 9:00 a.m. and 8:00 p.m. ET or between 11:00 am and 8:00 pm on weekends and holidays. A guide for clinicians is also available online at nccc.ucsf.edu [61].

Preexposure Prophylaxis

HIV-negative individuals at high risk for acquiring HIV may take chronic, daily antiretroviral medication as preexposure prophylaxis, or PrEP. The Partners PrEP Trial showed a 66% reduction in HIV acquisition when HIV-negative women with HIV-positive male partners took daily tenofovir 300 mg/emtricitabine 200 mg (Truvada). The risk reduction improved to 90% when nonadherent study subjects were excluded from analysis [62]. The FDA approved tenofovir 300 mg/emtricitabine 200 mg (Truvada) 1 tab daily for HIV prevention for men and women in 2012.

Table 13.9 CDC-recommended 28-day regimens for nonoccupational post-exposure prophylaxis (nPEP) against HIV[a]

Recommended regimen:
Tenofovir[b] 300 mg/emtricitabine 200 mg (coformulated as Truvada) once daily
PLUS
Raltegravir[c] (Isentress) 400 mg twice daily OR dolutegravir[c, d] (Tivicay) 50 mg once daily

Reprinted from Centers for Disease Control and Prevention, U.S. Department of Health and Human Service [58]

[a]Not for use in persons with chronic kidney disease. Please see CDC website for alternate regimens for these patients (www.cdc.gov/hiv/guidelines)

[b]Tenofovir can cause renal toxicity in those with existing kidney disease, and a creatinine clearance of ≥60 mL/min is required for these regimens

[c]Raltegravir and dolutegravir should not be administered with sucralfate (Carafate) or calcium, magnesium, aluminum, iron, zinc or other buffered products

[d]Dolutegravir is possibly associated with neural tube defects in offspring and should be avoided in women at risk for pregnancy and during the first trimester

Table 13.10 Laboratory monitoring with use of pre- or post-exposure prophylaxis for HIV[a] [58, 63]

HIV testing (preferably rapid Ag/Ab testing if available)
Creatinine and calculated creatinine clearance[b]
AST/ALT
Pregnancy testing
Chlamydia and gonorrhea[c]
Trichomonas[d]
Syphilis
Hepatitis B and C

[a]For nPEP (nonoccupational post-exposure prophylaxis against HIV), testing is performed at baseline, at 4–6 weeks and at 3 months; For PrEP (pre-exposure prophylaxis against HIV), testing is performed at baseline and then every 3 months indefinitely while taking medication

[b]Creatinine clearance must ≥60 mL/min (by Cockcroft formula) to use standard regimens given the risk of tenofovir toxicity

[c]For asymptomatic women, chlamydia and gonorrhea testing can be performed on self-collected vaginal swabs, or on urine if the patient has undergone hysterectomy. Self-collected rectal specimens or physician-collected oral specimens can be used when needed

[d]Trichomonas testing should only be performed at the genital site

The CDC recommends offering preexposure prophylaxis to women at substantial risk of acquiring HIV, defined as (1) any woman having had condomless vaginal or anal sex in the previous 6 months with a man who either has HIV, has sex with men, or who uses injection drugs or (2) any woman diagnosed with gonorrhea or syphilis in the previous 6 months [63]. ACOG suggests a more liberal definition of eligible women, including those "engaging in sexual activity within a high HIV-prevalence area or social network" along with a second risk factor such as inconsistent condom use, recent diagnosis of STI, drug use or alcohol dependence as well as other possible criteria [64]. The USPSTF has drafted a statement recommending PrEP for anyone at risk for HIV [65]. Others have suggested that clinicians simply trust women to assess their own increased vulnerability to HIV [66]. For women whose partners are known to be HIV-positive, one should ascertain whether the partner(s) are taking ART and if viral suppression is adequate, since HIV transmission does not occur when the HIV viral load is <400 [67], making PrEP unnecessary. Often the partners' clinical information is unknown to patients and PrEP is warranted.

Once a woman is deemed a candidate for PrEP, clinical assessment is needed to determine safety. A review of medications for drug–drug interactions is needed. Due to the risk of PrEP-induced mild bone loss, a bone health history should be taken and bone density assessment performed if osteoporosis is suspected (see Chap. 25 on Osteoporosis). A history and physical exam should also look for and exclude clinical features of existing HIV infection. Creatinine should be measured to confirm adequate renal function (≥60 mL/min). Testing should include HIV screening as well as screening for other STIs (chlamydia, gonorrhea, syphilis, Trichomonas, Hepatitis B, Hepatitis C) and pregnancy testing. These assessments are repeated at scheduled follow-up visits.

When starting PrEP, patients can be counseled on the need for follow-up visits and laboratory testing every 3 months while taking the regimen. In addition, one should emphasize the importance of strict adherence to the daily dosing schedule to ensure efficacy; patients benefit from intentional discussion regarding an adherence strategy. Adequate PrEP drug levels are reached in the rectum 7 days after initiation of medication, but 20 days are required for the vagina [63]. Experts at the national PrEP phone consultation center can answer clinicians' questions at (855-448-7737, 855-HIV-PrEP) [68] and a clinicians' guide is available at nccc.ucsf.edu [61]. If a patient contracts HIV despite taking PrEP, a specialist should be contacted to immediately convert the PrEP regimen to a full treatment regimen. The CD4 count, viral load, and viral resistance testing should be ordered but conversion of treatment should not be delayed while awaiting results.

HIV-negative women in HIV-discordant relationships attempting to achieve pregnancy have no concern regarding HIV transmission when their male partner takes ART and maintains a viral load <400 [67]. A second, slightly less safe option is for the HIV-negative woman to take PrEP while attempting conception. Sperm washing is an older strategy that removes seminal fluid and the HIV virus with it and is associated with the lowest risk of HIV transmission. However, sperm washing requires a procedure-- either intrauterine insemination (IUI) or in vitro fertilization. IUI is also the usual approach when the man is HIV-negative and woman HIV-positive [69].

Hepatitis B

Infection with Hepatitis B, a DNA virus, causes acute and chronic hepatitis. Although acute hepatitis B is fatal in 1%, most adults clear the infection and only 2–6% develop chronic hepatitis B infection. Chronic hepatitis B infection is incurable but suppressive therapy is indicated when specific disease parameters are present, and management by a specialist is appropriate.

The hepatitis B virus is found in highest concentration in blood but is also present in wound exudates, semen, vaginal secretions, saliva, tears, and bile. In the U.S. Hepatitis B is most often transmitted sexually or through injection drug use. Less commonly, HBV is transmitted perinatally or via interpersonal contact, such as sharing a toothbrush or contact with skin exudate or contaminated surfaces [70]. In addition, lapses in healthcare infection-control procedures, and settings such as facilities for the disabled are associated with infection.

The CDC identifies eventual eradication of hepatitis B from the United States as an achievable goal. All pregnant women should be screened [7]; strategies to prevent vertical transmission have been recently intensified [71]. Sexual and household contacts of infected persons are among the high-risk groups that should be screened (Table 13.11) and vaccinated. Also, any nonimmune, sexually active adult not in a mutually monogamous relationship or seeking evaluation for an STI should be offered vaccination, as should any adult that simply requests it [71]. Note that universal hepatitis B vaccination in infancy was implemented in the U.S. in 1991 with catch-up vaccinations for older children encouraged later in the 1990s, so most unvaccinated persons were born prior to then or in another country. Recently the CDC recommended identifying and screening immigrants and their offspring from at-risk countries (a color-coded map is available online [72]), particularly those persons from Asia (except Japan) and the Pacific Islands, and to vaccinate their household and sexual contacts when indicated. This effort is expected to reduce new cases [73].

When administered promptly (ideally within 24 hours) following an exposure, initiation of the hepatitis B vaccina-

Table 13.11 Screening for Hepatitis B and Hepatitis C infections [72, 78–80]

Hepatitis B
Order all 3 tests:
Surface Ag: indicates active infection
Surface Ab: indicates protection, either from resolved infection or vaccination
Core Ab: indicates current or prior infection
Hepatitis C
Screen with Hepatitis C Ab: Presence indicates past or current infection.
If Hep C Ab is positive, proceed to Hepatitis C RNA testing
Presence of Hep C RNA indicates current infection
Absence of Hep C RNA indicates resolved infection, either from spontaneous cure or from successful treatment[a]

[a]Rarely, absence of Hepatitis C RNA can alternatively indicate that the original positive Hep C Ab test was a false positive result. On the other hand, false negative Hepatitis C RNA results are possible, and testing should be repeated when this is a concern

tion series is also effective as post-exposure prophylaxis (although in particularly high-risk instances hepatitis B immunoglobulin is simultaneously administered as well, at a separate body site). In situations where it is unknown whether the patient is vulnerable, Hepatitis B serology testing is collected, followed immediately by administration of the first dose of the vaccine at the same office visit. The vaccination series is completed depending on the results of testing.

Hepatitis C

Hepatitis C virus is a cause of acute and chronic liver infection and is transmitted primarily through percutaneous exposure to infected blood, with sexual transmission a far less common cause. Heterosexual transmission of hepatitis C is rare in monogamous relationships. The HCV Partners Study followed 500 HCV-discordant monogamous heterosexual couples and found that sexual transmission in this setting was only 0.07% per year, or 1 out of every 190,000 sexual contacts [74], confirming results of prior similar studies [75, 76]. Moreover, unlike with HIV, these rare transmissions could not be attributed to specific sexual activities such as intercourse during menses or anal sex; such information is relevant for patient counseling. The CDC therefore does not recommend condoms for HCV-discordant heterosexual couples in stable, monogamous relationships. However, heterosexual transmission is higher (0.4–0.8% per year) in the setting of multiple partners or coinfection with another STI [77] and consequently, the CDC does recommend condom use for hepatitis C-infected persons engaging in heterosexual activity in nonmonogamous contexts [78]. Perinatal transmission is uncommon (4–7% of those born to infected mothers), but ideally infected women of reproductive age should undergo curative treatment prior to pregnancy. Breastfeeding by a hepatitis C infected mother is encouraged, unless complicated by cracked or bleeding nipples.

In addition to screening all persons with known risk factors for Hepatitis C [78, 79], the CDC now recommends universal screening of persons born between 1945 and 1965 [80] (Table 13.11). Effective oral treatment has been available since 2011, and now consists of either an 8- or 12-week regimen.

Genital Warts (Low-Risk Human Papilloma Virus, HPV)

Genital warts (condyloma acuminata), typically caused by low-risk HPV, affect 1% of the sexually active U.S. population at any given time with a lifetime incidence of approximately 10% [81]. HPV is the most common STI in the U.S., with approximately 75% of people infected with the virus at some point in their life, usually during the late teens or early 20s. In most cases, the HPV infection is transient and cleared by an appropriate immune response within 2 years [82]. For those who fail to clear the infection, infection may be subclinical or manifest as genital warts. Occasionally genital warts involve coinfection with high-risk strains such as HPV 16 or 18; in such instances the wart may contain foci of HSIL. Most genital warts are asymptomatic but some patients report itching or pain. Sometimes warts are large enough to interfere with toileting or intercourse [81]. Most commonly, however, it is patients' psychosocial distress related to cosmetic concerns that prompts treatment.

Warts may assume a wide range variety of appearances, from small, flat-topped or dome-shaped papules and pedunculated lesions to large cauliflower-like growths; they may be solitary or clustered. The texture may be smooth, cerebriform, or verrucous, and while frequently either skin-colored, gray, or brown, genital warts can sometimes be pink, red, purple or white [83]. Genital warts may involve any aspect of the anogenital epithelium, the anogenital tract itself or the pubic skin, where they can sometimes be extensive in the context of shaving abrasions [84]. Low-risk HPV can also cause conjunctival, nasal, oral, and laryngeal warts.

Genital warts are diagnosed using visual inspection. Biopsy is utilized only to exclude other etiologies if the lesion appears atypical or fails to respond at all to treatment, as both situations raise concern for possible malignancy [81]. Atypical findings that raise concern for verrucous carcinoma include warts that appear indurated or fixed to underlying structures, or ulcerate, grow rapidly, increase in pigmentation or otherwise change appearance [83]. Patients with warts located on the cervix, anal canal, or urethra are managed differently, however, as they require consultation with a specialist and often biopsy to exclude HSIL. Note that

HPV testing is not helpful and has no role in the diagnosis of genital warts [2].

Cauliflower-type genital warts resemble the condyloma lata of secondary syphilis, and this more serious cause should always be excluded by obtaining syphilis serologies. Seborrheic keratoses may also be mistaken for genital warts. Dermatology referral is indicated whenever the diagnosis is unclear.

Management entails observation or wart removal. Since spontaneous resolution of warts is common and treatment sometimes associated with adverse side effects, providers can offer patients a 1-year trial of observation. Smoking cessation, adequate sleep/nutrition, reduction of alcohol, and other lifestyle modifications that impact the immune system may reduce HPV infection or expression [2]. Some patients opt for treatment, and in addition the CDC recommends wart removal prior to sexual contact with a *new* sexual partner [2].

A variety of patient-applied topical therapies are available (Table 13.12). When a patient-applied therapy is prescribed, all warts should be carefully identified for the patient at the initial visit and clear instructions given regarding the treatment plan. A follow-up visit should occur several weeks later to assess the response to treatment. When successful, most warts are eliminated within 3 months of treatment, though rates of complete clearance range from 37% to 77% [81]. Lack of any response raises concern for other possible diagnoses. Because treatment only eliminates the wart and not the underlying HPV infection, it is common for warts to recur, especially in the first 3 months after completing treatment.

Provider-applied therapies include weekly application of trichloroacetic acid (TCA) or bicholoroacetic acid (BCA). These agents are caustic and extra care should be taken to prevent exposure of adjacent normal tissue. Some apply petroleum jelly to surrounding mucosa beforehand, and after application of the medication, the treated area should dry thoroughly (turn to white frost) before the patient sits or stands. Cryotherapy is effective; however, the CDC notes that providers must be trained due to concerns of over- and undertreatment of genital warts [2]. Surgical therapy using excision, electrocautery, or CO_2 laser may be optimal treatment for patients with large or extensive warts, warts failing to respond to other treatments, and intraurethral warts. Note that an appropriately ventilated room is required with laser use to prevent transmission of virus to health personnel.

Patient education should emphasize that the low-risk types of HPV responsible for genital warts differ from those that cause cancer, and women with genital warts do not need Pap smears more often the standard guidelines. Because genital warts can develop months or years after acquiring infection, the timing of HPV acquisition cannot be determined nor can the warts be attributed to the current sex part-

Table 13.12 Patient-applied therapies for the treatment of external genital warts

Agent	Medication instructions	Mechanism of action	Maximum duration	Adverse effects	Precautions
Imiquimod	Imiquimod 5% cream: Apply at bedtime 3 nights per week; wash off 6–10 hours later	Immune enhancer (stimulates interferon, other cytokines)	16 weeks	Redness, vesicles, erosions, hypopigmentation (sometimes permanent)	May worsen autoimmune conditions such as psoriasis or vitiligo Safety in pregnancy unknown
	Imiquimod 3.75% cream: Apply at bedtime each night; wash off 6–10 hours later				
Podofilox	Podfilox solution: Use cotton swab to apply to warts twice daily for 3 days followed by no treatment of 4 days	Antimitotic agent that causes wart necrosis	16 weeks	Mild to moderate pain with application	Contraindicated in pregnancy
	Podofilox gel: Same instructions except apply with finger				
Sinecatechins 15% ointment (green tea extract)	Apply 0.5 cm strand to each wart 3 times daily using finger. Do not wash off.	Anti-inflammatory, antiviral, immune stimulation	16 weeks	Erythema, pruritus, burning, pain, ulceration, edema, vesicular rash	Genital, anal and oral sexual contact must be avoided while ointment is on skin. Has not been tested in patients with HSV or HIV or other immunocompromised state Safety in pregnancy unknown

Reprinted from Workowski and Bolan for the CDC [2]

ner. Although sex partners ultimately tend to share HPV, often only one partner manifests the infection with warts. Condoms reduce the spread of HPV but offer incomplete protection since they do not cover all relevant anatomy. The HPV vaccination is highly effective in preventing genital warts; in countries with high vaccine uptake for one decade a 90% reduction in genital wart incidence has been observed [85] (see Chap. 14 on Cervical Cancer and Human Papillomavirus for more information regarding HPV vaccination).

Emerging STIs

Zika Virus

Following the Brazilian epidemic in 2015, Zika spread to 33 countries and territories in the Americas and Caribbean. In the United States, the Zika virus has been identified in mosquitos in Puerto Rico, Florida, and Brownsville, Texas. Despite the heroic achievements of the CDC to date, eventual spread of Zika in the continental U.S. is anticipated, since virtually all states have had travel-related illness introduced, and most states harbor at least one of the two species of mosquito capable of transmitting infection.

Infection with the Zika virus, when symptomatic, usually results in mild, self-limited illness. Clinical features include a pruritic macular or papular rash (90% of patients); fever, arthralgias, and conjunctivitis (most patients); and myalgias, headache, and retro-orbital pain (less than half of patients) [86]. When identified in Africa in 1953, Zika was considered benign. However, recent outbreaks have been associated with serious sequelae, such as Guillain-Barre syndrome in affected individuals and congenital defects in the offspring of women infected while pregnant, particularly microcephaly, neurologic deficits, and ocular defects [87]. Spontaneous abortion has also been noted [86].

While primarily a mosquito-borne illness, Zika can also be transmitted sexually. Male-to-female, female-to-male, and male-to-male sexual transmission have all been confirmed [88] and the virus persists in semen and vaginal secretions for months beyond resolution of illness. To prevent sexual transmission and congenital infection, the CDC recommends condom use for a prescribed duration (3 months for men and 2 months for women) following recovery of Zika illness or return from an infested area [89]. Pregnant women or women planning a pregnancy should either forego unnecessary travel to endemic areas or delay attempts at conception. Pregnant women with potentially exposed sexual partners should either avoid sex or use condoms throughout the duration of the pregnancy [90]. The CDC currently recommends that pregnant women be screened at each prenatal visit using questions regarding potential Zika exposure. Mosquito precautions are also recommended, including repellant, permethrin treatment for clothing, bed nets, window screens, and air conditioning. The CDC recommends any EPA-approved insect repellant, as all are considered safe, even in the settings of pregnancy and breastfeeding.

Zika virus has also been detected in the breast milk of infected mothers; however, there have been no reported adverse outcomes and consequently the CDC recommends breastfeeding throughout an active Zika infection, although it also advises continued monitoring of its website for updated recommendations at https://www.cdc.gov/zika/prevention/transmission-methods.html [91]. Case reports suggest that Zika is possibly transmitted through transfusion of blood products, but confirmation is needed [92].

Ebola

The West Africa epidemic of 2014–2016 demonstrated the highly contagious nature of Ebola virus. Close contact alone is sufficient to transmit the infection, though sexual transmission also occurs. The virus is found in vaginal secretions and semen, and may persist in semen long after resolution of illness; the longest documented duration is 565 days. For patients travelling to or from areas with known Ebola outbreaks, counseling should include the WHO recommendation for male Ebola survivors to practice abstinence from all types of sex or use condoms for 12 months or until two consecutive semen samples are negative for virus. Ebola has also been detected in vaginal fluid as long as 33 days following recovery [93]; however, thus far there have been no reports of female-to-male sexual transmission. Women with Ebola infection should not breastfeed because Ebola virus has been detected in breast milk.

Summary Points

1. Primary care clinicians can provide effective STI prevention counseling by directing patients to watch a brief video on their cell phone while in the exam room.
2. Annual chlamydia and gonorrhea screening is recommended for all sexually active women and girls age 24 and younger, as well as for older women at increased risk. Universal HIV screening for all Americans aged 13–64 is also recommended.
3. Although some women note subtle symptoms, most uncomplicated chlamydia and gonorrhea infections are asymptomatic and lack any signs on exam as well.
4. An asymptomatic woman reporting an unprotected sexual encounter can be screened for chlamydia, gonorrhea and *Trichomonas* using a self-collected swab specimen. Any patient reporting *documented* exposure to an STI

receives empiric treatment and also requires a full evaluation to exclude complications such as PID or coinfection with other STIs or BV.

5. Effective partner management is important to prevent reinfection. The CDC suggests that physicians seek permission from the patient to offer her sexual contact(s) appointments for evaluation and treatment.
6. PID is diagnosed in the appropriate host whenever abdominal pain is accompanied by either cervical motion tenderness, uterine tenderness, or adnexal tenderness, and there is no obvious alternative diagnosis. Only half of women with PID have cervical discharge, but such women usually have excess leukocytes on microscopic examination of the wet mount.
7. PID requires prompt treatment to help reduce the risk of sequelae, and empiric antibiotics are initiated at the time of presentation.
8. PID is a clinical diagnosis. Since negative chlamydia and gonorrhea testing does not exclude these infections in the upper tracts, one should not rely on testing to make the diagnosis, nor should a negative result lead one to discontinue therapy for a diagnosis of PID made with reasonable clinical certainty.
9. Partners of persons diagnosed with PID should be tested then empirically treated for both chlamydia and gonorrhea, regardless of the index patient's results.
10. Patients presenting with a new genital ulcer should be tested for HSV and syphilis, and then treated for the more likely etiology. A swab specimen of the ulcer should be procured for herpes testing, and serologies ordered for syphilis. HIV testing is also indicated. If the ulcer is painful and accompanied by other symptoms consistent with the acute HIV syndrome one should test using the rapid HIV Ag/Ab test. If testing is negative but concern persists then further testing using HIV RNA levels should be performed.
11. Patients diagnosed with initial genital herpes infection should be prescribed treatment at the time of presentation in order to reduce their infectiousness and to minimize the risk of complications.
12. Women with recently diagnosed genital herpes infection benefit from close follow-up to receive further education and counseling regarding their infection as well as a prescription to begin either suppressive or episodic treatment.
13. The CDC emphasizes strategies that PCPs can adopt to help curb the HIV epidemic: improved recognition and prompt treatment of acute HIV infection, and providing pre- and post-exposure prophylaxis to those at high risk for HIV infection.
14. The CDC encourages Hepatitis B screening particularly for immigrants from at-risk countries, with vaccination of household and sexual contacts of those who test positive.
15. Sexual transmission of Hepatitis C in stable, monogamous heterosexual HCV-discordant couples is exceedingly rare and no precautions are needed. However, transmission is facilitated in the settings of other STIs or multiple partners, and the CDC recommends condom use for Hepatitis C-infected persons in nonmonogamous contexts.
16. Treatment of genital warts is often ineffective and does not eliminate the underlying low-risk HPV infection. Patients not planning new sexual partnerships can be offered a 1-year trial of watchful waiting, as spontaneous resolution is common.
17. Because the Zika virus persists in genital secretions following resolution of the illness and can be spread sexually by either men or women, the CDC recommends condom use for a prescribed duration (3 months for men and 2 months for women) following recovery from illness or return from an infested area. Recommendations for pregnant women are more stringent.
18. The Ebola virus persists in semen long after resolution of the illness and male-to-female sexual transmission has been documented. The WHO recommends that male Ebola survivors abstain from all types of sex or use condoms for 12 months, or until two consecutive semen samples test negative for the virus.

Review Questions

1. A 24-year-old woman presents for routine cervical cancer screening. She and her boyfriend use latex condoms coated with nonoxynol-9, except when they occasionally use "lambskins" (natural membrane condoms). She is using injectable medroxyprogesterone acetate (Depo-Provera) for contraception as well. She is concerned about contracting HIV, since it is prevalent in her community.

   You counsel your patient that she can reduce her risk of acquiring HIV by:

   A. Continuing to use condoms coated with nonoxynol-9 spermicide.
   B. Switching to plain latex condoms.
   C. Using a male latex condom together with a female condom.
   D. Switching to natural membrane ("lambskin") condoms.
   E. Stopping the injectable contraceptive, medroxyprogesterone acetate.

   The correct answer is B. Latex condoms have been shown to be effective in preventing the spread of HIV. On the other hand, the use of nonoxynol-9 spermicide appears to increase the risk of HIV acquisition in users, likely by disrupting the genital epithelium [3]. The male and female condom should not be used together [2]. Natural membrane condoms have a large pore size that prevents the passage of sperm but not viruses [2]. Previous concern regarding the possibility that the injectable contraceptive medroxyprogesterone acetate might increase a women's risk of HIV acquisition has been laid to rest by a large randomized trial [4].

2. An 18-year-old woman presents to your office stating that she read on the Internet that since she is now sexually active, she should undergo screening for herpes infection. She and her boyfriend are healthy college students who use condoms consistently and neither of them have any relevant symptoms.

   Which of the following STI screening tests do you recommend?
   A. No STI testing is needed since she faithfully uses condoms
   B. Chlamydia, gonorrhea, and HIV
   C. Chlamydia, gonorrhea, syphilis, and HIV
   D. Chlamydia, gonorrhea, and HSV

   The correct answer is B. The CDC and USPSTF recommend annual screening for both chlamydia and gonorrhea in all sexually active women and girls age 24 and younger, as well as in older women at increased risk [2, 5]. The CDC also recommends universal HIV screening in all Americans age 13–64, at least once. Although the incidence of syphilis in the U.S. has recently increased dramatically, universal screening is not advised since infection remains unlikely in persons lacking risk factors. The USPSTF specifically recommends against routine screening for herpes in asymptomatic hosts [7].

3. A 24-year-old woman presents for an acute appointment stating that her boyfriend informed her that he was diagnosed with chlamydia yesterday. What are the next steps in management?
   A. Conduct a history; perform a pelvic exam; examine a wet mount of vaginal secretions; obtain specimens to test for gonorrhea, chlamydia, and Trichomonas; order syphilis and HIV serologies; and prescribe empiric treatment for chlamydia.
   B. Order testing for chlamydia infection and treat the patient only if the result comes back positive.
   C. Prescribe empiric treatment for chlamydia now.
   D. Take a history, perform a pelvic exam, and prescribe treatment if the patient has clinical evidence of chlamydia infection.

   The correct answer is A. The patient will be empirically treated for chlamydia based on documented exposure; however, she is evaluated as well. In addition to chlamydia infection, this patient is at risk for other STIs, since coinfection is common. Clinical evaluation is also needed to exclude PID, a serious complication that would warrant more extensive antibiotic treatment and closer monitoring [2, 21]. Confirmatory testing for the reported infection is collected prior to empiric treatment to allow notification of her other recent (within 60 days) sexual contacts if the results are positive. Uncomplicated chlamydia and gonorrhea infections are most often asymptomatic and without clinical signs.

4. A 19-year-old woman who uses condoms most of the time presents with the complaint of lower abdominal pain for 3 days. Her office pregnancy test is negative and her urine dipstick is unremarkable. Her pelvic exam is notable for uterine tenderness and cervical motion tenderness. You are concerned that your patient might have PID.

   Which additional finding is needed before you initiate treatment?
   A. Fever >101 °F orally
   B. Mucoid discharge from the cervical os
   C. Rebound tenderness on abdominal examination
   D. No additional findings are necessary before initiating treatment
   E. Positive chlamydia or gonorrhea test result

   The correct answer is D. PID is a clinical diagnosis. The CDC supports making the presumptive diagnosis and initiating treatment in a susceptible host if no other cause can be found to explain a patient's lower abdominal pain if tenderness is noted on pelvic exam (either cervical motion tenderness, uterine tenderness or adnexal tenderness). Only half of patients with PID have a cervical discharge. (However, women with PID who lack this finding usually do have evidence of inflammation in the form of excess leukocytes on wet mount). Treatment of PID should be initiated as soon as the clinical diagnosis is made, without waiting for test results. It should also be noted that a negative chlamydia or gonorrhea test result in the presence of PID is common and does not exclude this infection in the upper tracts [2].

5. A 45-year-old woman presents for urgent evaluation because of a 2-day history of a new painful "sore" on her vulva. Pelvic examination reveals a 4 mm ulcer on her vulva. Her pelvic exam is otherwise unremarkable and the patient appears well overall. The patient agrees to undergo HIV testing. Appropriate steps to diagnose her genital ulcer include:
   A. Herpes simplex virus PCR testing via ulcer swab
   B. Herpes simplex virus PCR testing via ulcer swab and serologies for syphilis
   C. PCR testing of the lesion for both herpes simplex virus and *T. pallidum.*
   D. Serologies for both syphilis and herpes simplex virus

The correct answer is B. In the U.S., infectious genital ulcers usually result from herpes or syphilis. Since the clinical features of the two infections can overlap and coinfection is possible, patients presenting with genital ulcers are always tested for both infections [2]. A swab specimen is used to obtain material from the base of the ulcer for type-specific HSV PCR testing, and serologies are ordered to diagnose syphilis. Since genital ulcers facilitate the spread of HIV, HIV testing is also recommended for all patients presenting with genital ulcers [2].

6. A 23-year-old patient recently diagnosed with genital herpes infection returns for 3-week follow-up. The PCR test of the ulcer isolated Herpes simplex virus type 2. Which of the following counseling points should be mentioned with respect to preventing future outbreaks?
   A. Once suppressive therapy is begun it is usually continued indefinitely.
   B. Chronic suppressive treatment with valacyclovir has been shown to reduce transmission of herpes to the uninfected partner in discordant couples.
   C. A recurrent outbreak will be completely prevented when episodic treatment is begun at the first sign of tingling.
   D. If PCR testing had revealed HSV type 1 then suppressive therapy would be indicated.

The correct answer is B. Chronic suppressive antiviral treatment will reduce recurrence rates of herpes outbreaks and greatly reduce viral shedding (which occurs even in the absence of outbreaks). For this reason, suppressive therapy is the first-line treatment for an HSV-discordant couple [2, 37]. Outbreaks wane over time and each year immunocompetent patients suffering few recurrences should be offered a trial off of suppressive therapy [2]. Episodic treatment shortens the duration of symptoms and reduces the intensity of outbreaks but does not affect the recurrence rate. Persons with genital HSV-1 infection are generally less prone to recurrences and are initially managed with episodic treatment.

7. A 25-year-old woman presents complaining of two growths on her vulva. Examination reveals a cluster of dome-shaped gray papules that are classic for genital warts. Appropriate management entails:
   A. Performing a Pap smear now and again in 1 year given her increased risk of cervical cancer
   B. Biopsying the lesions to first confirm the diagnosis
   C. Offering her several treatment strategies, including a trial of watchful waiting
   D. Withholding the HPV vaccine, since she already has HPV infection
   E. Performing in-office cryotherapy to destroy the wart and eliminate the HPV infection

The correct answer is C. Warts can be treated using a number of modalities; however, the success rate is only fair and wart removal likely reduces but does not eliminate the underlying HPV infection. While the CDC recommends treating warts prior to initiating a sexual relationship with a *new* partner, in most other settings a reasonable option is to withhold treatment for a year and monitor for progress, as spontaneous resolution is common [2]. Genital warts typically result from infection with benign ("low-risk") serotypes of HPV and thus the recommended frequency of cervical cancer screening remains unchanged for women with genital warts. Genital warts are diagnosed by visual inspection and biopsy is unnecessary and unhelpful unless there are atypical features or a complete lack of response to treatment--either of which raises concern for possible malignancy [81]. While it is likely that the HPV vaccine will not be therapeutic for this patient's established HPV infection, the 9-valent vaccine will likely protect her from other HPV serotypes, and women age 26 and younger are eligible for vaccination. Dedicated training in the use of cryotherapy for the treatment genital warts is recommended [2].

8. A healthy 53-year-old woman calls you on Monday in the late afternoon to report that she had unprotected sex with a friend late on Friday night. She knows he is HIV-positive and is fairly confident that he is not getting medical care. She has been trying to reach him by phone and tearfully asks if there is anything she can do for this high-risk exposure. How do you manage this patient?
   A. Prescribe a 28-day regimen of tenofovir/emtricitabine once daily and raltegravir 400 mg twice daily to begin today, and order HIV testing as well as routine chemistries and STD testing.
   B. Refer to an infectious disease physician to consider nonoccupational post-exposure HIV prophylaxis.
   C. Start once daily tenofovir/emtricitabine indefinitely
   D. Advise her that she is presenting too late for post-exposure prophylaxis

The correct answer is A. The patient should be prescribed nonoccupational post-exposure prophylaxis (nPEP) for HIV, which is effective when instituted within 72 hours of exposure [58]. Prompt initiation is critical, and thus waiting for HIV test results or referring to another clinician is inappropriate. The most common regimen in use is a 28-day course of a three-drug regimen consisting of tenofovir-emtricitabine 300 mg/200 mg (Truvada) once daily plus raltegravir (Isentress) 400 mg twice daily. Answer C is the two-drug regimen tenofovir-emtricitabine 300 mg/200 mg (Truvada), which is effective for preexposure prophylaxis [63] but inadequate for post-exposure prophylaxis.

References

1. Satterwhite CL, Torrone E, Meites E, Dunne EF, Mahajan R, et al. Sexually transmitted infections among US women and men: prevalence and incidence estimates, 2008. Sex Transm Dis. 2013;40(3):187–93. https://doi.org/10.1097/OLQ.0b013e318286bb53.
2. Workowski KA, Bolan GA for the CDC. Sexually transmitted diseases treatment guidelines, 2015. MMWR Recomm Rep. 2015;64(RR-03):1–137. Also accessible via https://www.cdc.gov/mmwr/pdf/rr/rr6403.pdf.
3. Wilkinson D, Tholandi M, Ramjee G, et al. Nonoxynol-9 spermicide for prevention of vaginally acquired HIV and other sexually transmitted infections: systematic review and meta-analysis of randomised controlled trials including more than 5000 women. Lancet Infect Dis. 2002;2:613–7.
4. Evidence for Contraceptive Options and HIV Outcomes (ECHO) Trial Consortium. HIV incidence among women using intramuscular depot medroxyprogesterone acetate, a copper intrauterine device, or a levonorgestrel implant for contraception: a randomised, multicentre, open-label trial. Lancet. 2019;394(10195):303–13. https://doi.org/10.1016/S0140-6736(19)31288-7. Epub 2019 Jun 13.
5. LeFevre for the USPSTF. Screening for chlamydia and gonorrhea: U.S. Preventive Services Task Force recommendation statement. Ann Intern Med. 2014;161(12):902–10.
6. Schachter J, Chernesky MA, Willis DE, et al. Vaginal swabs are the specimens of choice when screening for *Chlamydia trachomatis* and *Neisseria gonorrhoeae*: results from a multicenter evaluation of the APTIMA assays for both infections. Sex Transm Dis. 2005;32:725–8.
7. Meyers D, Wolff T, Gregory K, Marion L, Moyer V, et al. for the USPSTF. USPSTF recommendations for STI screening. Am Fam Physician. 2008;77(6):819–24.
8. Zakher B, Cantor AG, Pappas M, Daeges M, Nelson HD. Screening for gonorrhea and chlamydia: a systematic review for the U.S. Preventive Services Task Force. Ann Intern Med. 2014;161(12):884–93.
9. https://www.cdc.gov/std/ept/legal/default.htm. State-specific legal information regarding Expedited Partner Therapy.
10. Detels R, Green AM, Klausner JD, Katzenstein D, Gaydos C, et al. The incidence and correlates of symptomatic and asymptomatic Chlamydia trachomatis and Neisseria gonorrhoeae infections in selected populations in five countries. Sex Transm Dis. 2011;38(6):503–9.
11. Chernesky M, Freund GG, Hook E III, et al. Detection of Chlamydia trachomatis and Neisseria gonorrhoeae infections in North American women by testing SurePath liquid-based Pap specimens in APTIMA assays. J Clin Microbiol. 2007;45:2434–8.
12. Torrone E, Papp J, Weinstock H, Centers for Disease Control and Prevention (CDC). Prevalence of Chlamydia trachomatis genital infection among persons aged 14-39 years--United States, 2007-2012. MMWR Morb Mortal Wkly Rep. 2014;63(38):834–8.
13. Quinn TC, Gaydos C, Shepherd M, Bobo L, Hook EW 3rd, et al. Epidemiologic and microbiologic correlates of Chlamydia trachomatis infection in sexual partnerships. JAMA. 1996;276(21):1737–42.
14. Geisler WM, Lensing SY, Press CG, Hook EW 3rd. Spontaneous resolution of genital Chlamydia trachomatis infection in women and protection from reinfection. J Infect Dis. 2013;207(12):1850–6.
15. Geisler WM. Duration of untreated, uncomplicated Chlamydia trachomatis genital infection and factors associated with chlamydia resolution: a review of human studies. J Infect Dis. 2010;201(Suppl 2):S104–13. https://doi.org/10.1086/652402.
16. Wiesenfeld HC. Screening for Chlamydia trachomatis infections in women. N Engl J Med. 2017;376(22):2198.
17. University of Washington STD Prevention Training Center. UWPTC.org18, Morgan MK, Decker CF. Gonorrhea. Dis Mon. 2016;62(8):260–8.
18. Morgan MK, Decker CF. Gonorrhea. Dis Mon. 2016;62(8):260–8.
19. Savaris RF, Fuhrich DG, Duarte RV, Franik S, Ross J. Antibiotic therapy for pelvic inflammatory disease. Cochrane Database Syst Rev. 2017;4:CD010285.
20. Brunham RC, Gottlieb SL, Paavonen J. Pelvic inflammatory disease. N Engl J Med. 2015;372(21):2039–48.
21. Mitchell C, Prabhu M. Pelvic inflammatory disease: current concepts in pathogenesis, diagnosis and treatment. Infect Dis Clin North Am. 2013;27(4):793–809.
22. Eschenbach DA. Acute pelvic inflammatory disease. Urol Clin North Am. 1984;11(1):65–81.
23. Hillis SD, Joesoef R, Marchbanks PA, Wasserheit JN, Cates W Jr, Westrom L. Delayed care of pelvic inflammatory disease as a risk factor for impaired fertility. Am J Obstet Gynecol. 1993;168:1503–9.
24. Wiesenfeld HC, Hillier SL, Meyn LA, et al. Subclinical pelvic inflammatory disease and infertility. Obstet Gynecol. 2012;120:37–43.
25. CDC. 2015 STD treatment guidelines: PID. Includes alternative parenteral treatment regimens. https://www.cdc.gov/std/tg2015/pid.htm.
26. Centers for Disease Control and Prevention. Table 1: sexually transmitted diseases-reported cases: rates of reported cases per 100,000 population, sexually transmitted diseases surveillance 2016. https://www.cdc.gov/std/stats16/tables/1.htm. Accessed 11.14.2018.
27. Zetola NM, Pilcher CD. Diagnosis and management of acute HIV infection. Infect Dis Clin N Am. 2007;21(1):19–48, vii.
28. Wald A, Link K. Risk of human immunodeficiency virus infection in herpes simplex virus type 2-seropositive persons: a meta-analysis. J Infect Dis. 2002;185(1):45–52. Epub 2001 Dec 14.
29. Wasserheit J. Epidemiologic synergy: interrelationships between human immunodeficiency virus infection and other sexually transmitted diseases. Sex Transm Dis. 1992;19:61–77.
30. Glogau R, Hanna L, Jawetz E. Herpetic whitlow as part of genital virus infection. J Infect Dis. 1977;136(5):689–92.
31. Wald A. New therapies and prevention strategies for genital herpes. Clin Infect Dis. 1999;28(Suppl 1):S4–13.
32. Groves MJ. Genital herpes: a review. Am Fam Physician. 2016;93(11):928–34.
33. Mertz GJ. Asymptomatic shedding of herpes simplex virus 1 and 2: implications for prevention of transmission. J Infect Dis. 2008;198(8):1098–100. https://doi.org/10.1086/591914.
34. Freeman EE, Weiss HA, Glynn JR, Cross PL, Whitworth JA, et al. Herpes simplex virus 2 infection increases HIV acquisition in men and women: systematic review and meta-analysis of longitudinal studies. AIDS. 2006;20(1):73–83.
35. Feltner C, Grodensky C, Ebel C, Middleton JC, Harris RP, et al. Serologic screening for genital herpes: an updated evidence report and systematic review for the US Preventive Services Task Force. JAMA. 2016;316(23):2531–43.
36. Kimberlin DW, Rouse DJ. Clinical practice. Genital herpes. N Engl J Med. 2004;350(19):1970–7.
37. Corey L, Wald A, Patel R, Sacks SL, Tyring SK, et al. for the Valacyclovir HSV Transmission Study Group. Once-daily valacyclovir to reduce the risk of transmission of genital herpes. N Engl J Med. 2004;350(1):11–20.
38. Gnann JW Jr, Whitley RJ. Clinical practice. Genital herpes. N Engl J Med. 2016;375(7):666–74. https://doi.org/10.1056/NEJMcp1603178.
39. Diamond C, Selke S, Ashley R, Benedetti J, Corey L. Clinical course of patients with serologic evidence of recurrent genital her-

pes presenting with signs and symptoms of first episode disease. Sex Transm Dis. 1999;26(4):221–5.
40. Tuddenham S, Shah M, Ghanem KG. Syphilis and HIV: is HAART at the heart of this epidemic? Sex Transm Infect. 2017;93(5):311–2.
41. CDC. Sexually transmitted diseases: syphilis. Accessed 9/4/18 at www.cdc.gov/std/syphilis.
42. Radolf JD, Tramont EC, Salazar JC. Syphilis (Treponema pallidum). In: Mandell, Douglas and Bennett's principles and practice of infectious diseases. Updated ed. Philadelphia: Elsevier Saunders; 2015. p. 2684–2709.e5; Chap. 239.
43. Markle W, Conti T, Kad M. Sexually transmitted diseases. Prim Care. 2013;40(3):557–87.
44. CDC Public Health Image Library. https://phil.cdc.gov/Details.aspx?pid=12623
45. Draft recommendation statement: syphilis infection in pregnant women: screening. U.S. Preventive Services Task Force. April 2018. https://www.uspreventiveservicestaskforce.org/Page/Document/draft-recommendation-statement/syphilis-infection-in-pregnancy-screening1.
46. Romanowski B, Sutherland R, Fick GH Mooney D, Love EJ. Serologic response to treatment of infectious syphilis. Ann Intern Med. 1991;114:1005–9.
47. Gratzer B, Pohl D, Hotton AL. Evaluation of diagnostic serological results in cases of suspected primary syphilis infection. Sex Transm Dis. 2014;41(5):285–9.
48. Golden MR, Marra CM, Holmes KK. Update on syphilis: resurgence of an old problem. JAMA. 2003;290(11):1510–4.
49. Pillay A. CDC syphilis summit – diagnostics and laboratory issues. Sex Transm Dis. 2018;45:S13–6. https://doi.org/10.1097/OLQ.0000000000000843.
50. Mastro TD, de Vincenzi I. Probabilities of sexual HIV-1 transmission. AIDS. 1996;10(Suppl A):S75–82.
51. CDC. HIV Among transgender people, 2009–2014. CDC Fact Sheet. Accessed via https://www.cdc.gov/hiv/group/gender/transgender/index.html.
52. Daar ES, Pilcher CD, Hecht FM. Clinical presentation and diagnosis of primary HIV-1 infection. Curr Opin HIV AIDS. 2008;3(1):10–5. https://doi.org/10.1097/COH.0b013e3282f2e295.
53. Hoenigl M, Green N, Camacho M, Gianella S, Mehta SR, et al. Signs or symptoms of acute HIV infection in a cohort undergoing community-based screening. Emerg Infect Dis. 2016;22(3):532–4. https://doi.org/10.3201/eid2203.151607.
54. Henn A, Flateau C, Gallien S. Primary HIV infection: clinical presentation, testing, and treatment. Curr Infect Dis Rep. 2017;19(10):37. https://doi.org/10.1007/s11908-017-0588-3. Review. PMID: 28884279.
55. Vanhems P, Beaulieu R. Primary infection by type 1 human immunodeficiency virus: diagnosis and prognosis. Postgrad Med J. 1997;73(861):403–8.
56. Daar ES, Little S, Pitt J, Santangelo J, et al. for the Los Angeles County Primary HIV Infection Recruitment Network. Diagnosis of primary HIV-1 infection. Los Angeles County Primary HIV Infection Recruitment Network. Ann Intern Med. 2001;134(1):25–9.
57. Panel on Treatment of HIV-Infected Pregnant Women and Prevention of Perinatal Transmission. Recommendations for use of antiretroviral drugs in pregnant HIV-1-infected women for maternal health and interventions to reduce perinatal HIV transmission in the United States. Accessed 4/20/28 at https://aidsinfo.nih.gov/contentfiles/lvguidelines/perinatalgl.pdf.
58. Centers for Disease Control and Prevention, U.S. Department of Health and Human Service. Updated Guidelines for Antiretroviral Postexposure Prophylaxis After Sexual, Injection Drug Use, or Other Nonoccupational Exposure to HIV— United States, 2016. Accessed 4/20/18 via https://www.cdc.gov/hiv/pdf/programresources/cdc-hiv-npep-guidelines.pdf or via https://stacks.cdc.gov/view/cdc/38856.
59. Zash R, Makhema J, Shapiro RL. Neural-tube defects with dolutegravir treatment from the time of conception. N Engl J Med. 2018;379(10):979–81. https://doi.org/10.1056/NEJMc1807653. Epub 2018 Jul 24.
60. Post-Exposure Prophylaxis National Hotline, National Clinician Consultation Center, UCSF Medical Center, University of California, San Francisco.
61. National Clinician Consultation Center website, UCSF Medical Center, University of California, San Francisco.
62. Baeten JM, Donnell D, Ndase P, Mugo NR, Campbell JD, et al. for the Partners PrEP Study Team. Antiretroviral prophylaxis for HIV prevention in heterosexual men and women. N Engl J Med. 2012;367(5):399–410.
63. Centers for Disease Control and Prevention: US Public Health Service. Preexposure prophylaxis for the prevention of HIV infection in the United States—2017 Update: a clinical practice guideline. Published March 2018. https://www.cdc.gov/hiv/pdf/risk/prep/cdc-hiv-prep-guidelines-2017.pdf.
64. American College of Obstetricians and Gynecologists Committee on Obstetric Care. ACOG Committee Opinion No. 595: Committee on Gynecologic Practice Preexposure prophylaxis for the prevention of human immunodeficiency virus. Obstet Anesth Dig. 2015;35(2):67.
65. U.S. Preventive Services Task Force. Draft recommendation statement. Prevention of human immunodeficiency virus (HIV) infection: pre-exposure prophylaxis. https://www.uspreventiveservicestaskforce.org/Page/Document/draft-recommendation-statement/prevention-of-human-immunodeficiency-virus-hiv-infection-pre-exposure-prophylaxis. Accessed 12/5/18.
66. Seidman D, Weber S. Integrating preexposure prophylaxis for human immunodeficiency virus prevention into women's health care in the United States. Obstet Gynecol. 2016;128(1):37–43.
67. Cohen MS, Chen YQ, McCauley M, Gamble T. Hosseinipour MC et al. for the HPTN 052 Study Team. Antiretroviral therapy for the prevention of HIV-1 transmission. N Engl J Med. 2016;375(9):830–9.
68. Pre-Exposure Prophylaxis National Hotline, National Clinician Consultation Center, UCSF Medical Center, University of California, San Francisco.
69. Hanson BM, Dorais JA. Reproductive considerations in the setting of chronic viral illness. Am J Obstet Gynecol. 2017;217(1):4–10.
70. Schillie S, Vellozzi C, Reingold A, et al. Prevention of hepatitis B virus infection in the United States: recommendations of the Advisory Committee on Immunization Practices. MMWR Recomm Rep. 2018;67(No. RR-1):1–31. https://doi.org/10.15585/mmwr.rr6701a1.
71. Abara WE, Qaseem A, Schillie S, McMahon BJ, Harris AM, for the High Value Care Task Force of the American College of Physicians and the Centers for Disease Control and Prevention. Hepatitis B vaccination, screening, and linkage to care: best practice advice from the American College of Physicians and the Centers for Disease Control and Prevention. Ann Intern Med. 2017;167(11):794–804.
72. World Map: Hepatitis B prevalence at CDC. Know hepatitis B: testing Asian Americans and Pacific Islanders for hepatitis B. https://www.cdc.gov/hepatitis/hbv/pdfs/hepb-api.pdf.
73. CDC. Know hepatitis B. Professional resources. https://www.cdc.gov/knowhepatitisb/materials.htm.
74. Terrault NA, Dodge JL, Murphy EL, Tavis JE, Kiss A, Levin TR, et al. Sexual transmission of hepatitis C virus among monogamous heterosexual couples: the HCV partners study. Hepatology. 2013;57(3):881–9.
75. Vandelli C, Renzo F, Romanò L, Tisminetzky S, De Palma M, et al. Lack of evidence of sexual transmission of hepatitis C among monogamous couples: results of a 10-year prospective follow-up study. Am J Gastroenterol. 2004;99(5):855–9.

76. Tahan V, Karaca C, Yildirim B, Bozbas A, Ozaras R, et al. Sexual transmission of HCV between spouses. Am J Gastroenterol. 2005;100(4):821–4.
77. Terrault NA. Sexual activity as a risk factor for hepatitis C. Hepatology. 2002;36(5 Suppl 1):S99–105.
78. CDC: Division of Viral Hepatitis and National Center for HIV/AIDS, Viral Hepatitis, STD, and TB Prevention. Hepatitis C FAQs for health professionals. Page last updated: April 20, 2018. Accessed via https://www.cdc.gov/hepatitis/hcv/hcvfaq.htm#section4.
79. CDC. Hepatitis C questions and answers for health professionals in viral hepatitis. https://www.cdc.gov/hepatitis/hcv/hcvfaq.htm#c1.
80. Smith BD, Morgan RL, Beckett GA, Falck-Ytter Y, Holtzman D, et al. for the Centers for Disease Control and Prevention. Recommendations for the identification of chronic hepatitis C virus infection among persons born during 1945–1965. MMWR Recomm Rep. 2012;61:RR–4):1-32.
81. Karnes JB, Usatine RP. Management of external genital warts. Am Fam Physician. 2014;90(5):312–8.
82. Koshiol JE, Schroeder JC, Jamieson DJ, Marshall SW, Duerr A, et al. Time to clearance of human papillomavirus infection by type and human immunodeficiency virus serostatus. Int J Cancer. 2006;119(7):1623–9.
83. Scheinfeld N, Lehman DS. An evidence-based review of medical and surgical treatments of genital warts. Dermatol Online J. 2006;12(3):5.
84. de Vries HJ. Skin as an indicator for sexually transmitted infections. Clin Dermatol. 2014;32(2):196–208.
85. Garland SM, Kjaer SK, Muñoz N, Block SL, Brown DR, et al. Impact and effectiveness of the quadrivalent human papillomavirus vaccine: a systematic review of 10 years of real-world experience. Clin Infect Dis. 2016;63(4):519–27. Published online 2016 May 26.
86. Petersen LR, Jamieson DJ, Honein MA. Zika virus. N Engl J Med. 2016;375(3):294–5.
87. Moore CA, Staples JE, Dobyns WB, Pessoa A, Ventura CV, Fonseca EB, et al. Characterizing the pattern of anomalies in congenital Zika syndrome for pediatric clinicians. JAMA Pediatr. 2017;171(3):288–95.
88. Sakkas H, Economou V, Papadopoulou C. Zika virus infection: past and present of another emerging vector-borne disease. J Vector Borne Dis. 2016;53(4):305–11.
89. Polen KD, Gilboa SM, Hills S, Oduyebo T, Kohl KS, et al. Update: interim guidance for preconception counseling and prevention of sexual transmission of Zika virus for men with possible Zika virus exposure — United States, August 2018. MMWR Morb Mortal Wkly Rep. 2018;67(31):868–71.
90. Centers for Disease Control and Prevention, National Center for Emerging and Zoonotic Infectious Diseases (NCEZID), Division of Vector-Borne Diseases (DVBD). Zika virus: for healthcare providers. Page last updated: December 14, 2017. Accessed 4/20/18 via https://www.cdc.gov/zika/hc-providers/index.html.
91. Centers for Disease Control and Prevention, National Center for Emerging and Zoonotic Infectious Diseases (NCEZID), Division of Vector-Borne Diseases (DVBD). Zika virus: transmission methods. https://www.cdc.gov/zika/prevention/transmission-methods.html. Accessed 1/19/19.
92. Bloch EM, Ness PM, Tobian AAR, Sugarman J. Revisiting blood safety practices given emerging data about Zika virus. N Engl J Med. 2018;378:1837–41.
93. Rogstad KE, Tunbridge A. Ebola virus as a sexually transmitted infection. Curr Opin Infect Dis. 2015;28(1):83–5.

Cervical Cancer and Human Papillomavirus: Prevention and Screening

14

Nicolette A. Oleng', Halle G. Sobel, and Deborah Kwolek

Learning Objectives

1. Discuss the epidemiology and pathogenesis of cervical cancer.
2. Review current guidelines for cervical cancer screening and HPV testing.
3. Compare the recommendations for screening in special populations: HIV positive, immune-compromised, DES exposed, and post-hysterectomy patients.
4. Describe current recommendations for HPV vaccination.
5. Interpret and manage the results of an abnormal cytology or HPV test.
6. Evaluate and discuss disparities in cervical cancer prevention, screening, and treatment.

Nina is a 53-year-old woman who presents to establish care. She emigrated from the Congo one year ago. She lives with her three children and sister and works as a medical assistant at a local clinic. She has a son of age 14 and two daughters aged 18 and 21. She delivered all of her children at home in the Congo without complications. She did not have routine healthcare in her home country. She has never had a Pap or HPV test. Nina would like to know when she should bring in her two daughters for Pap tests.

Epidemiology

Cervical cancer is a leading cause of cancer death in women worldwide, but in the United States and other high-income countries (HIC), where Pap tests are routinely performed, invasive cervical cancer (ICC) deaths are uncommon. Cervical cancer ranks as the 14th cause of cancer death in the United States but as the second or third leading cause of cancer death in many low-income countries [1]. Persistent infection with high-risk strains of human papillomavirus (hrHPV or HPV) causes >99% of cervical cancer worldwide, which "implies the highest worldwide attributable fraction so far reported for a specific cause of any major human cancer" [2]. Cervical cancer can be of squamous cell (approximately 80%), glandular cell (adenocarcinoma), or mixed adenosquamous origin, all of which are associated with HPV infection. Rarely sarcoma, lymphoma, melanoma, and clear cell adenocarcinoma occur on the cervix. Squamous cell abnormalities can progress to cervical intraepithelial neoplasia (CIN), which is most common in the fourth decade of life. ICC peaks in the fifth decade of life. Mortality rates increase with age, especially in women greater than 45 years [3]. Risk factors associated with the development of cervical cancer are related to both persistent infection with high-risk HPV viral strains and host vulnerability.

N. A. Oleng' (✉)
Boston University School of Medicine, Department of General Internal Medicine, Boston Medical Center, Boston, MA, USA
e-mail: nicolette.oleng2@bmc.org

H. G. Sobel
Robert Larner MD, College of Medicine at The University of Vermont, Department of General Internal Medicine & Geriatrics, Burlington, VT, USA

D. Kwolek
Harvard Medical School, Massachusetts General Hospital, Department of Medicine, Boston, MA, USA

S. A. Tilstra et al. (eds.), *Sex- and Gender-Based Women's Health*, https://doi.org/10.1007/978-3-030-50695-7_14

Host vulnerability may include the following:

- HPV acquisition. Women with early age of sexual debut or history of multiple sexual partners have increased vulnerability to HPV acquisition.
- The cervical transformation zone. Infection of the cervical transformation zone with HPV can predispose to cervical cancer for those with: a young age of first pregnancy, a history of more than three pregnancies, STI coinfection, or oral contraceptive use for more than 5–10 years.
- Host immunity or susceptibility. Women may have increased susceptibility to HPV due to HIV infection, immunosuppression, smoking, or in utero DES exposure.
- Screening and follow-up. Women may lack appropriate screening and follow-up which can lead to inadequate screening for cervical cancer, inadequate follow-up of an abnormal screening test, or inadequate treatment of lower genital tract neoplasias [2–8].

It is estimated that over 50% of all new cases of ICC occur in women who have never been screened or have been inadequately screened for cervical cancer [6]. Women lost to follow-up after treatment for CIN or ICC are also at high risk. Worldwide, more than 80% of ICC cases occur in developing or low- and medium-income countries (LMIC) where HPV vaccination, cervical cancer screening, and cervical cancer treatment are limited [7].

In the United States, significant disparities exist in the incidence of and mortality from ICC. Between the years 2010 and 2014, the age-adjusted incidence of cervical cancer in women of all ages was 7.4 cases per 100,000 women and over 9 cases per 100,000 in Hispanic and Black women, respectively [3]. In 2014, 12,578 women in the United States were diagnosed with ICC, and 4115 women died of ICC. Mortality rates are highest in Black women in the US. Published data and statistical analyses underestimate the racial disparity by up to 44% when corrections are not made for the high rate of prior hysterectomy in Black women [9]. Low-income, minority, chronically ill, uninsured or poorly insured, lesbian, transgender, immigrant women, and those with poor healthcare access are at higher risk for morbidity and mortality due to cervical cancer, an inequity which must be addressed by healthcare providers and policy-makers [4, 9–11]. (See section on disparities below.)

Screening and Prevention

Invasive cervical cancer (ICC) is, in theory, entirely preventable. *High-risk strains of human papillomavirus (hrHPV)* are the etiologic agents of 99% of all ICC and there are highly effective vaccines to prevent the acquisition and spread of hrHPV. Low-risk strains of HPV do not cause cervical cancer, and all references to HPV testing or screening refer to screening for high-risk strains. Screening women with cervical cytology (previously referred to as the Pap test) and/or HPV testing identifies individuals at risk of ICC and detects those with abnormal cervical changes. The development of ICC from initial HPV infection takes more than 15 years in many cases, and thus the detection and treatment of precursor lesions is highly effective in preventing disease progression.

HPV is easily transmitted through contact between individuals from hand, skin, oral, vaginal, anal, penile, and scrotal contact. It is not blood-borne. HPV is also spread by autoinoculation from one part of the body to another in an individual. Women who are virgins or have sex only with women (WSW) can be HPV positive. Transgender men with a cervix are also at risk. For these reasons, it is recommended that all persons who have a cervix be screened regardless of sexual history or gender identity. Screening rates are unacceptably low in underserved populations, in those with multiple chronic illnesses, and in persons who lack or have poor access to insurance. Women under 30 and over 60 are less likely to be screened [9]. Immigrants from LMIC countries are at high risk as many have never been screened in their country of origin and may not have been screened since their arrival in the United States [12].

Cervical Anatomy: The Transformation Zone

The development of ICC begins with the infection of the transformation zone (TZ) of the cervix (Fig. 14.1). The transformation zone is the area of demarcation in which the squamous epithelium from the vagina meets the columnar epithelium from the endocervix. The TZ is also referred to as the squamocolumnar junction (SCJ). The TZ undergoes metaplasia in which columnar cells transform into squamous cells. The TZ is not visible on the cervix until puberty, but is found within the endocervix. With the onset of puberty, the TZ moves from the endocervix to the ectocervix. The ectocervix is the visible surface of the cervix. Estrogen stimulation with puberty, oral contraceptive use, and pregnancy cause the transformation zone to become more prominent, erythematous, and metabolically active with cell turnover. Increased cell replication and differentiation supports viral persistence and neoplastic changes. During the teen and young adult years, the TZ is visible on the cervix and is more exposed to possible HPV infection. In adult women over 25–30 years of age, who are not pregnant or taking OCPs, the TZ recedes into the endocervix, rendering the ectocervix more resistant to HPV infection and carcinomatous changes. The vulnerability of the TZ in the early teen years is an important argument to encourage teens to delay sexual activity, have fewer sexual partners, be selective of sexual partners, use condoms, and to be vacci-

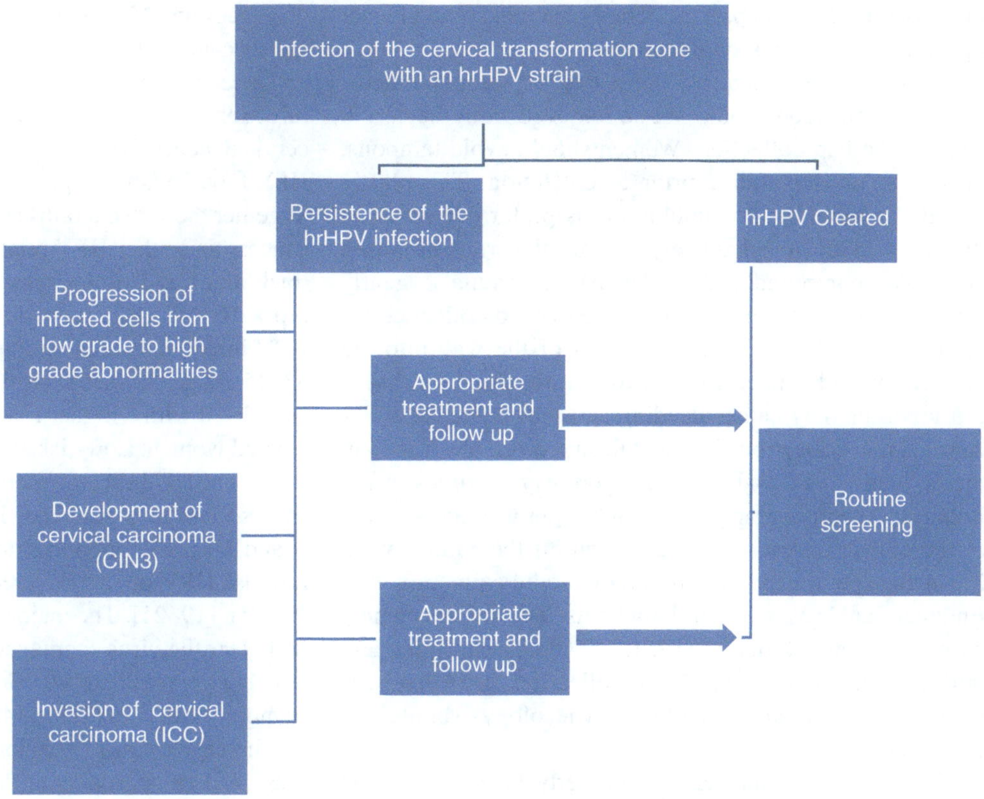

Fig. 14.1 Progression from hrHPV infection to invasive cervical cancinoma

nated against HPV. (See Chap. 13 on "Sexually Transmitted Infections".)

Screening for Cervical Cancer

The implementation of cervical cancer screening programs over the past 40+ years has successfully reduced cervical cancer incidence and mortality among women who have undergone Pap or cytology testing. Throughout this chapter, and in the literature, the term Pap test is used interchangeably with cytology testing. The incidence of cervical cancer in the United States has decreased from 14.8 per 100,000 women a year in 1975 to 6.8 per 100,000 women a year in 2014. The mortality rate from ICC in 1975 was 5.5 compared to 2.26 in 2014 per 100,000 women a year [2]. The continued mortality is thought to be due to ICC cases presenting in advanced stages in unscreened and inadequately screened women, in women who have been lost to follow-up after abnormal screening, or in woman who have received partial treatments.

There are two major components to cervical cancer screening: cytology and HPV testing. HPV testing identifies women at risk for cervical abnormalities, and cytology identifies actual cervical cell abnormalities. Neither test is 100% sensitive; however, the slow progression from HPV acquisition, to cervical cell abnormalities, to ICC allows for the detection of abnormalities on repeated sampling when screening guidelines are followed. Screening recommendations vary by age and risk category.

Cervical Cytology: The Papanicolaou (Pap) Test

The *Pap test* technique was first developed in the 1920s by George Papanicolaou who studied microscopic vaginal secretions from guinea pigs and learned to distinguish cancerous from noncancerous cells. This technique was not noticed by the medical community until the 1940s [13]. The Pap test has been the mainstay of cervical cancer screening and has evolved over the years from a yearly smear on a glass slide—the "Pap smear"—to liquid-based "thin prep" cytology specimen collection every 3–5 years. The thin prep was approved in 1996 by the FDA as the preferred option for obtaining cervical specimens, and the percentage of unsatisfactory cytology specimens has decreased since its use has become widespread. Additionally, the liquid-based test has the advantage of allowing the testing for gonorrhea, chlamydia, and trichomonas in the same vial. The Pap collection technique is as follows: the woman is asked to place her legs in foot rests in the dorsolithotomy position on an examination table, and she brings her bottom to the edge of the examination table. A speculum, moistened with water or a small amount of water-based lubricant, is gently inserted into her vagina and then opened, and the cervix is visualized using a light source. (See Chap. 3 on "The Female Sex and Gender Specific History and Examination".)

To optimize the adequacy of the Pap test sample, mucus, discharge, or blood should not be removed from the cervix prior to the Pap collection. Women should avoid tampons, douching, or intercourse prior to collection. The plastic spatula and cytobrush combination is preferred, which is the most likely to adequately sample the transformation zone. The contoured end of the plastic spatula is gently scraped against the cervix for 360 degrees to collect cervical cells. The brush is inserted most of the way into the cervical os and rotated for a ¼ to ½ turn. Rotation that is too vigorous may cause bleeding and thus decrease endocervical cell collection. The spatula and brush are placed in the collection vial and swirled vigorously 10 times in the liquid and gently scraped with each other to remove cells, or the collection ends may be broken off the endocervical brush and spatula and placed into the liquid collection vial. Endocervical brushes should not be used during pregnancy by primary care clinicians [14, 15]. If the os is stenotic and will not allow endocervical cell collection, or if there are visible cervical abnormalities, gynecology should be consulted.

The collection vial must be properly labeled with the patient's identifying information, or it will be rejected by the lab. The collection vial is sent to the laboratory with appropriate orders. The laboratory analyzes the cervical cell cytology and will also perform any additional testing that is ordered, including HPV and sexually transmitted infection screening. For a specimen to be satisfactory, sufficient squamous cells must be visible without obscuring inflammation or blood. The presence of endocervical cells and cells from the transformation zone should be present and will be commented upon by the pathologist [16].

High-Risk Human Papillomavirus (hrHPV)

HrHPV is the causative agent of cervical cancer and is the most common STI in the United States. During 2013–2014, the prevalence of genital HPV was 42.5% in the US adults aged 18–59 years. The highest prevalence was among the Black population at 64.1%, followed by the Hispanic population at 41.4% and was lowest in the Asian population at 23.8%. The prevalence was 50–60% in women aged 25–34 and twice as high in women between the ages of 25 and 29 when compared to women between the ages of 30 and 39 [17, 18]. HPV is transmitted to the anogenital region through mucosa to mucosa or skin to skin contact. HPV causes vaginal, vulvar, anal/rectal, penile, and oropharyngeal neoplasia in men and women; however, the discussion of these malignancies is beyond the scope of this chapter. (See Chap. 12 on "Vaginitis and Vulvar Conditions" and Chap. 15 on "Gynecologic Malignancies" for a discussion of vaginal and vulvar cancers.)

Once transmitted, HPV can result in acute asymptomatic infection. High-risk strains are carcinogenic and increase cervical cancer risk; low-risk strains cause genital warts. HPV type 16 is the highest risk strain, followed by type 18. Together these two strains account for about 70% of cervical cancers and other HPV-related cancers of the genitourinary tract, anus, and oropharynx. In unvaccinated women, HPV types 16 and 18 account for approximately 35.46% of the HPV infections noted on Pap tests. The HPV genotypes 31, 33, 45, 52, and 58 are classified "other high risk" and are also associated with a higher risk of high-grade lesions in unvaccinated women. Low-risk strains 6 and 11 cause most genital warts. The HPV vaccine used in the United States, Gardasil-9, covers these nine strains of HPV: 16, 18, 31, 33, 45, 52, 58, 6, and 11. Less common strains of carcinogenic HPV, and of low-risk HPV, are not covered by the currently available vaccination [19–21]. The majority of women who contract HPV will clear the virus spontaneously within 1–2 years of infection, but approximately 10% of women remain positive for 5 or more years [22] (Table 14.1).

The regression of previously positive HPV infections is presumed to be due to an adequate cell-mediated immune response, while an increased persistence of HPV is observed in immunocompromised populations. It is not clear whether HPVs are completely cleared or are maintained in a latent state in women who convert from HPV positive to HPV negative on co-testing [21].

Women with a history of CIN, cervical cancer, recent abnormal Pap tests, HIV infection, organ transplant recipients, DES exposure, and other causes of immunosuppression are at higher risk of ICC and are screened more frequently than average-risk women (discussed in section on screening guidelines). Patients with systemic lupus erythematosus or rheumatoid arthritis on biologic disease-modifying antirheu-

Table 14.1 Human papillomavirus strains [19–21]

HPV strain	Type	Causes	Covered by Gardasil-9
16	High risk	55% of cervical cancers	Yes
18	High risk	15% of cervical cancers	Yes
31, 33, 34, 52, 58	"Other high risk"		Yes
35, 39, 51, 56, 59, 68, 73, 72	"Other high risk"		No
26, 53, 66, 68, 73, 2	Probable high risk		No
6, 11	Low risk	Common genital warts	Yes
40, 42, 43, 44, 54, 61, 70, 72, 81	Low risk	Common genital warts	No

matic drug (DMARD) therapies and other biologic therapies appear to have a higher risk of cervical cancer. It is important for clinicians to be up to date on screening guidelines and HPV vaccination recommendations in these populations. Although studies are limited, annual screening is recommended for women with immunosuppression and for those on biologic therapies [23, 24].

Smokers are at higher risk of cervical cancer and have been found to obtain less frequent cervical cancer screening [8]. Tobacco use negatively impacts HPV clearance and increases the risk of persistent HPV infections. The discovery of HPV infection and ASCUS or low-grade lesions can be a strong impetus for women to stop smoking: smoking cessation is associated with increased regression of abnormal cervical lesions [25].

Cervical Cancer Screening Guidelines

Cervical cancer screening guidelines have traditionally been based on consensus by expert groups, because evidence from randomized-controlled trials is limited. Initially, Pap smears were done yearly, and then in the mid-1990s until 2012, Pap screening frequency decreased to every 2–3 years. In 2012, the US Preventive Services Task Force (USPSTF) updated the 2003 recommendation on cervical cancer screening [26]. This was an important update as it incorporated human papillomavirus (HPV) testing into the recommendations. Between 2009 and 2011, the American Cancer Society (ACS), American Society for Colposcopy and Cervical Pathology (ASCCP), and the American Society for Clinical Pathology (ASCP) developed a working group to jointly prepare cervical cancer screening guidelines. Available evidence was reviewed and updated guidelines incorporating co-testing with cytology and HPV screening were published [27].

In 2018, the USPSTF published new updated guidelines [28] on screening for cervical cancer. It commissioned a decision analysis model [29] to evaluate at which age to begin and end screening, the optimal interval for screening, the effectiveness of different screening strategies, and the related benefits and harms of different screening strategies. Screening recommendations apply to all women who possess a cervix regardless of sexual orientation, sexual history, or gender identity [30] (Table 14.2). The guidelines below *do not* apply to women with a history of precancerous cervical lesions (CIN2 or greater on biopsy), cervical cancer, HIV-positive status, immunocompromised status, or exposure to diethylstilbestrol in utero, who need more intensive screening based on expert opinion [27, 30]. Women under the age of 21 should not be routinely screened with a Pap test regardless of sexual activity.

Table 14.2 2018 USPSTF cervical cancer screening guidelines [28]

Age (years old)	Screening recommendations
Under 21	No screening
21–29	Cytology testing alone every 3 years. An HPV test should only be performed for abnormal cytology results
30–65	Co-testing with cytology and HPV testing every 5 years, or HPV testing every 5 years, or Cytology testing alone every 3 years
>65	Women who have had adequate routine screening, with normal results in the prior 10 years can exit screening[a]
History of hysterectomy	Women who have had a complete hysterectomy, with removal of the cervix, for benign reasons, do not need Pap tests[b]
History of HPV vaccination	Pap testing should still be performed in HPV-vaccinated women

[a]If a woman is over the age of 65 or with a prior hysterectomy and has a history of precancerous or cancerous cervical lesions (CIN2 or greater), Pap testing should continue for 20 years after the date of the diagnosis (interval for screening not defined)

[b]In a supracervical (also called subtotal or partial) hysterectomy, the upper part of the uterus is removed, but the cervix is left in place. Screening should follow the recommended schedule for age. If the history of hysterectomy type is unclear, a physical examination should be performed to document whether the patient has an intact cervix

The evidence for each of these recommendations is discussed below.

1. *Women under the age of 21 should not be screened with a Pap test regardless of sexual activity*

There is very little evidence to support cervical cancer screening in women under age 21 because cervical cancer is rare in this age group. Although HPV is acquired during sexual intercourse, there are multiple steps in the progression to cancer; in this age group, abnormal test results are transient as HPV tends to clear on its own. In addition, screening in this age group may increase harm associated with screening due to the pain, anxiety, and cost associated with unnecessary screening and possible cervical procedures. Multiple cervical procedures, such as Loop Electrosurgical Excision Procedure (LEEP) or conization, may also have the untoward consequence of cervical incompetence, negatively impacting future childbearing [29, 31].

2. *Women aged 21–29 years should have a Pap test every 3 years. An HPV test should only be performed for abnormal cytology results*

The evidence for screening women under the age of 30 is largely based on modeling studies. There is very little data looking at the optimal screening interval in this population. By extending screening to every 3 years, the number of colposcopies needed to evaluate abnormal Pap tests is reduced compared to annual screening [32]. When two- versus three-year screening intervals were compared, there was no difference in cervical cancer burden after a 10-year follow-up interval. Other studies have supported the conclusion that there is very little added benefit in having a two-year screening interval compared to a three-year screening interval in women aged 21–29 years [32–34]. Randomized controlled trials (RCTs) have not supported reducing the screening interval, even when a woman has a history of previous abnormal cytology results [34, 35]. (See section on management of abnormal Pap tests below.)

The prevalence of HPV is high in young women and is usually transient. Dunne et al. found that in women aged 20–24 years, the prevalence of high- and low-risk HPV was 15.2% and 17.8%, respectively. After the age of 21–29 years, the prevalence of the high-risk HPV decreases in women [35]. HPV testing either alone or as a co-test is not recommended in the 21–29 age group because there is not an added benefit over cytology alone. Women would be exposed to increased harms from overdiagnosis and overtreatment of transient infections, with increased pain, bleeding, anxiety, cervical procedures, and risks to future childbearing, similar to women under age 21 [29, 31].

Age of Initial Screening A consensus conference in Italy in 2015 addressing cervical cancer screening in women already vaccinated against HPV recommended increasing the age of first initial screening for cervical cancer to 30 years old for girls vaccinated at age 12. This is based on the assumption that at the age of 12, most girls have not had sexual intercourse and hence have not been exposed to hrHPV. It is important to note that the national rate of HPV vaccination is 71% in cohorts of 12-year-old girls in Italy [36]. As the prevalence of HPV vaccination increases in the US, an increased age for initial screening might be considered.

3. *Women aged 30–65 years should be screened with cytology alone every 3 years, with HPV testing alone every 5 years, or with co-testing every 5 years*

HPV testing alone every 5 years in women 30 and older: The USPSTF reviewed several randomized control trials comparing modalities of screening and interval between screenings to develop their 2018 recommendations. In four trials that included >250,000 women, HPV testing alone with referral to colposcopy increased the rate of detection of CIN3+ lesions and cancerous lesions compared to cytology alone. In one trial, the rate of detection of invasive cervical cancer at 5 years was higher with HPV testing alone (0.03%) compared to cytology alone (0.01%). The colposcopy rates were higher in HPV testing alone compared to cytology alone in one of the trials but comparable in the other 2 trials [28].

Cytology alone every 3 years: Modeling studies suggest that co-testing, or HPV testing every 5 years, offered comparable benefits with cytology alone every 3years with regard to the detection and prevention of ICC. Modeling studies done in 2012 and cited in the 2018 USPSTF recommendations also examined screening intervals from 1 to 5 years and have not found evidence to support the use of screening intervals longer than 3 years with cytology alone even in women with a history of negative cytology tests [29, 31]. In other words, if HPV testing is not done, Pap tests are required every 3 years.

HPV testing alone in women over 25 years as an emerging primary screening strategy: The cobas ™ hrHPV test is used for co-testing with Pap and is FDA approved [37] as a primary cervical cancer screening test for women >25 years old. The strategy of using HPV screening starting at age 25 is yet to be embraced in the US, but in Australia, HPV screening alone is recommended every 5 years to women of ages 25–74 via a national screening program [38].

Arguments in favor of HPV testing alone: HPV testing alone has a higher sensitivity for detecting CIN3 or higher lesions at 76.1% in comparison to a sensitivity of 61.7% for the hybrid strategy similar to current US screening guidelines involving reflex HPV screening for ASCUS and 47.8% for cytology alone [17]. Over a 5-year period, the probability of developing lesions of CIN3 and above is similar between primary HPV testing and co-testing. Co-testing therefore does not provide increased protection against CIN3 when compared to HPV testing alone. The concern with primary HPV testing as a screening tool for women starting at 25 years of age is that women less than 30 years have a high frequency of HPV infections that later regresses. There is the potential for overdiagnosis and overtreatment in women less than 30 years, which increases harm from cervical cancer screening.

4. *Women over the age of 65 years who have had adequate screening can exit screening*

Women who have a history of CIN2 or greater, are immunosuppressed, or have not been adequately screened in the prior 10 years, with normal results, are exceptions. Physicians may discontinue routine screening in women over the age of 65 who have been screened according to recommended guidelines for the past 10 years and have met the following criteria within the 10 years before ceasing screening:

- Three negative consecutive Pap tests (3 years apart) or
- Two negative HPV tests (5 years apart), with the last testing having occurred within the last 5 years

The acquisition of new sexual partners after age 65 does not change this approach to screening.

History of Neoplasia, Inadequate Screening, or Smoking In women over the age of 65 who have had cervical lesions CIN2 or greater, Pap screening is continued for 20 years after diagnosis. Some experts recommend continued Pap screening for women over 65 who smoke, are DES exposed, or are immunosuppressed. In women over the age of 65 who have not been adequately screened, screening for hrHPV and abnormal cytology should be undertaken and repeated at least once (editor's view). Underserved, minority, and immigrant women are at risk for inadequate, or no, screening and should be screened appropriately [14].

5. *Women who have had a total hysterectomy with removal of the cervix for benign indications do not need Pap tests*

Women who undergo a total hysterectomy with complete removal of the cervix for benign indications such as fibroids or menorrhagia no longer need screening for cervical cancer. Women who have a history of CIN2 or greater, are immunosuppressed, have a history of DES exposure, or have not been previously screened are exceptions. A Pap test in a woman without a cervix screens for vaginal cancer, which is extremely rare except as a recurrence of cervical cancer [39, 40] or as a primary cancer in a woman exposed to DES. If the cervix is left in place, as in the case of a supracervical or "partial" hysterectomy, then routine screening guidelines should be followed. In many patients, it is not clear whether the cervix was removed during hysterectomy. The patient is often unaware of the distinctions in the types of hysterectomy. Add this information to your problem list. Clues include the following:

- Why was the hysterectomy done? If possible, check or send for gynecology notes. If for cancer, the cervix was removed but continued screening is recommended.
- Was it a vaginal hysterectomy? A vaginal hysterectomy removes the cervix, but be sure it was for a benign condition before you discontinue screening.
- Was it a laparoscopic hysterectomy? It may be a partial hysterectomy which leaves the cervix intact.
- Check for abdominal wall scars which would indicate a possible abdominal "partial" hysterectomy, leaving the cervix intact.
- If not sure: Examine the woman and make a note if the cervix is present. Check hrHPV and Pap test once. If HPV is positive, and/or if unable to visualize the cervix for Pap, refer to GYN. If negative, use clinical judgment about further evaluation [40].

6. *Pap testing should still be performed in HPV-vaccinated women*

Women who have received the HPV vaccine continue to undergo cervical cancer screening according to current guidelines. Some modeling studies have looked at screening women in this population at a later age and with less frequency but this is not a currently accepted recommendation [41].

Recommendations for Specific Populations and Exceptions to Routine Guidelines

Cervical cancer screening guidelines in special populations are primarily determined by expert opinion.

Immunocompromised Women

HIV-Infected Women There is limited evidence supporting the current screening guidelines in HIV-positive women. For women under the age of 30, if a baseline Pap test is normal, annual cytology should be performed. After three consecutive normal annual screening tests, the interval is spaced to 3 years. Co-testing is not recommended in HIV-positive women under the age of 30. Women with HIV who are 30 years of age or older can be screened with cytology alone or with co-testing. If three consecutive annual tests are normal, then screening can be extended to 3 years. If co-testing is done with a normal result, the screening can extend to 3 years [42]. The incidence of invasive cervical cancer (ICC) has not been found to decrease in HIV-positive women treated with antiretroviral medications or in women who have rising CD4 counts due to treatment; therefore, increased screening intervals are recommended in these women despite adequate HIV therapy [43].

Immunosuppression from Drug Therapy Given that HPV is less likely to be transient in an immunosuppressed population, screening is recommended at closer intervals. For women with organ transplants, cervical cancer screening is recommended annually with both cytology and HPV co-testing [44]. Women exposed to chronic immunosuppression such as those on biologic therapies may have a higher rate of cervical dysplasia and/or carcinoma but guidelines based upon evidence on how to screen this population is limited. Current recommendations are for annual Pap tests [23].

Diethylstilbestrol (DES) Exposure in Utero

Between 1938 and 1971, many women used DES as it was thought to improve pregnancy outcomes. At the time, it was not known that DES would be associated with an increased risk for squamous cell carcinoma and adenocarcinoma of the cervix, clear cell adenocarcinoma of the cervix and vagina, and an increased risk of breast cancer in females who were exposed in utero. In the cohort of in utero DES-exposed women, who are now close to 50 years of age or older, screening of both the cervix and vagina is recommended with separate specimens obtained from each site [45]. The specimens can be placed in the same vial as long as there is clear labeling that samples have been obtained from both sites. A four-quadrant Pap test should be obtained, which involves sampling of all walls of the vagina. Given the increased risk of cervical neoplasia DES-exposed women, annual cytology testing is recommended [46].

After educating Nina about cervical cancer screening, she undergoes a Pap test and the result shows abnormal squamous cells of uncertain significance (ASCUS) cytology and positive HPV "other high-risk" subtypes. The results are explained to her, and she is advised that repeat cytology could be repeated in 1 year or she could be referred for colposcopy. She indicates that she would prefer to wait, but is having some family issues and may be moving soon. She is advised that she should be evaluated as soon as possible and is warned of the dangers of not following up on abnormal tests. A referral to gynecology is placed with a note indicating that there are concerns about the patient getting lost to follow-up.

Management of Abnormal Screening Results

Pap Collection - Results To be "satisfactory for evaluation," squamous cells, endocervical cells, and transformation zone (TZ) cells must be present in the cytology sample, and excess blood or inflammatory cells cannot obscure results. Generalists should be familiar with the management of abnormal Pap test results in order to determine when repeat testing or referrals are appropriate. Algorithms are available for managing abnormal Pap tests through the American Society for Colposcopy and Cervical Pathology (ASCCP) at http://www.asccp.org/asccp-guidelines. The ASCCP also has an app containing algorithms for screening, management, and follow-up that can be downloaded for a nominal fee to a smartphone from www.asccp.org algorithms [40]. Pap cytology terms are listed in Table 14.3. Low-grade and high-grade intraepithelial lesions (LGSIL and HGSIL) used in this context are distinct from the histopathology terms of low-grade and high-grade lesions which are used to describe biopsy specimens outlined in the section on colposcopy and listed in Table 14.5.

Table 14.3 Definitions and abbreviations

Cytology – Pap test, which screens for abnormal cells of cervix. Pap may also capture cells from the vagina, uterus, fallopian tubes, and ovaries
EC/TZ – Endocervical cells/transformation zone
ECC – Endocervical curettage
Colposcopy – Magnified examination of the cervix, or other genital tissues
ASCUS – Atypical squamous cells of undetermined significance
LGSIL – Low-grade squamous intraepithelial lesion
ASC-H – Atypical squamous cells, cannot exclude high-grade lesion
HGSIL – High-grade squamous intraepithelial lesion
AGC – Atypical glandular cells
AIS – Adenocarcinoma in Situ

Algorithms are complicated. In general, women who are

1. Positive for HPV 16 or 18 – refer for colposcopy regardless of cytology results.
2. Other high-risk HPV – co-test in 1 year, and refer if infection persists after 1 year.
3. Pap with a persistent unsatisfactory or ASCUS finding – refer for colposcopy.
4. Pap results of LGSIL or worse – refer for colposcopy.
5. Atypical glandular cells or worse – refer for colposcopy.

When in doubt, referral to a gynecologist is always recommended (Table 14.4).

Given the anxiety associated with abnormal test results, providers should discuss with patients the natural history of cervical cancer. HPV is usually cleared from the body in 1–2 years. Persistent HPV infection results in a small number of cases progressing to cancer. ASCUS and LGSIL on Pap are likely to regress: only 15% persist or progress. After biopsy, CIN lesions and some higher-grade lesions regress on their own. The lag time between the development of cancerous lesions from precancerous lesions is measured in years. Women at highest risk are those who were never screened, were inadequately screened, or are lost to follow-up (Table 14.5).

If the patient tests positive for HPV 16 or 18, refer for colposcopy. The rate of CIN3+ in persistent HPV 16 infection is 8.9% at 3 years, 23.8% at 5 years, and 47.4% at 12 years. Failure to treat HPV 16 has high rate of progression to malignancy. If HPV testing alone is used for screening, then only "other high-risk" HPV results need cytology to guide the referral decision. If cytology is negative, repeat co-test in 1 year. With "other hrHPV" persistent infections on two tests, the risk of CIN3+ at 12 years is 19.3% [47, 48].

Table 14.4 Pap results and suggested actions [27]

Pap result	Reflex or co-test HPV result or immediate action	Comment on follow-up
Negative for intraepithelial lesion or malignancy (NILM) with absent endocervical cells or transformation zone (EC/TZ)	21- to 29-year-old, routine screening	Early repeat testing not justified, except in high-risk women
	30- to 65-year-old, if HPV negative, routine screening	Early repeat testing not justified, except in high-risk women
	If HPV+	If 16/18+, refer for colposcopy "other high risk," co-test 1 year
	HPV unknown	HPV now or Pap in 3 years
Unsatisfactory[a]	Repeat 2–4 months	If HPV+, or if unsatisfactory on repeat Pap, refer for colposcopy
Inflammation or infection	If unsatisfactory, treat infection and repeat	
Atrophy	If unsatisfactory, treat with estrogen and repeat	
Normal cytology	HPV−	Routine screening
	HPV 16/18+	Refer for colposcopy
	Other hrHPV+	Repeat co-test 1 year
ASCUS	HPV−	Co-test 1 year If repeat co-test normal, repeat co-test 3 years If ASCUS persists, refer for colposcopy
	HPV+	Colposcopy if 16/18+, or repeat cytology in 1 year. If repeat is normal, then routine screening
Low-grade squamous intraepithelial lesion LGSIL	HPV−	Refer for colposcopy
	HPV+	Refer for colposcopy
ASCUS/LGSIL Pregnant or age 21–24	HPV−	Routine screening (cytology in 3 years)
	HPV+	Cytology 1 year
ASC-H		Refer for colposcopy
HGSIL		Refer for colposcopy
AGC	Refer GYN	Colposcopy and ECC EMB if >35 years old or risk factors
AIS	Refer GYN	
Adenocarcinoma	Refer GYN	

[a]Thick inflammation, blood, lack of squamous cells or cytolysis

Table 14.5 HrHPV-only screening results and suggested action over age 30 only (or over age 25) [40]

HPV screen test result	Subsequent cytology test	Action
Type 16/18 positive	Normal or abnormal	Refer for colposcopy
Other hrHPV+	Abnormal	Refer for colposcopy
Other hrHPV+	Normal	Repeat 12 months: if −/−, resume regular screening If HPV persists: refer for colposcopy
Negative	See section on Pap results	Routine screening if cytology results are not available. Ok to base decision on negative HPV alone

The rates of progression are the reason that evaluation, treatment, and close follow-up are essential to prevent ICC.

Colposcopy and Biopsy

A full discussion of colposcopy and biopsy is beyond the scope of this chapter. Briefly, the woman is asked to place her legs in foot rests in the dorsolithotomy position and the cervix is visualized with a speculum. The cervix is painted with acetic acid to reveal suspicious "acetowhite" lesions which reveal HPV infection or other changes. The cervix is examined with the colposcope which is basically a mounted microscope to magnify the cervix. Biopsy forceps and a tenaculum are used to take samples from the acetowhite lesions for pathology. A sampling of endocervical cells, called endocervical curettage (ECC), is obtained and sent to pathology. The designation of cervical intraepithelial neoplasia (CIN) refers to squamous cell abnormalities.

Abnormalities of glandular cells (the mucus-producing cells in the cervix) are referred to as AGC, AIS, or adenocarcinoma. The majority of cervical cancers arise from squamous cells, but adenocarcinoma has been increasing over the past few decades and comprises 20% of cervical cancers. Both types of cancers are caused by HPV and are treated in a similar manner.

The recommendations for the management of colposcopy and biopsy results are published by the ASCCP and are subject to change (see above). Principles of treatment are given in Table 14.6, for the purpose of counseling patients. Actual

Table 14.6 Histopathology results from biopsy specimens obtained during colposcopy and suggested follow-up and treatment options [40]

Biopsy: path result and relevant history	Significance[a]	Follow-up and treatment options[b] managed by gynecologic consultant
CIN 1: Pap had been HPV + ASCUS or LGSIL	Low grade – 90% will regress	Co-test in 12 months and treat according to co-test results
CIN1: Pap had been ASC-H or HGSIL	More intensive follow-up to insure that higher-grade lesions are not missed	Co-test at 12 months Or Excision: unless pregnant or patient is 21- to 24-year-old
CIN2/ CIN2+	Treated for safety 70% will regress in young women Regression is lower, at 50% for HPV16+	Treat with excision or T-zone ablation, Then 1-year follow-up with co-test If any abnormality on retesting: repeat colposcopy
CIN3/CIN3+	Precancerous: high-grade – 20–30% regress	Treat with total hysterectomy Or Excision. If margin is negative, follow-up in 1–2 years If margin is positive, re-excise or follow-up in 6 months
Invasive cancer	Treat with hysterectomy, possible radiation and chemotherapy depending on extent of spread	

[a]HPV 16+ has lower regression rate and may require more aggressive treatment
[b]Managed by gynecologic consultant

treatment and follow-up decisions are made in conjunction with gynecologic or gynecologic oncology specialist recommendations.

Nina is seen by gynecology, and a colposcopy and biopsy are performed. Her results return CIN1. She is educated about the results, and shared decision making is used to discuss her options. Although this lesion is likely to regress, and co-testing in 1 year is an option, there are concerns that she will return to the Congo and that she may get lost to follow-up. Gynecology is asked to discuss definitive treatment options with her including ablative and excisional therapies.

Treatment Options for Cervical Neoplasia

The full discussion of algorithms and treatments for CIN2/3 are beyond the scope of this chapter. (See Chap. 15 on "Gynecologic Malignancies, Cervical Cancer" section.)

In general, there are five primary treatments which are used in the treatment of precancerous lesions and carcinoma in situ (CIN3):

1. Cryotherapy – liquid nitrogen or freezing probe used to freeze acetowhite lesions from cervix. Advantage: low cost, used in "see and treat strategy" in some low-resource settings. Disadvantage: ablative, no biopsy specimen.
2. Loop electrosurgical excision procedure (LEEP) – heated semicircular wire slices off abnormal tissue or removes TZ. Advantage: biopsy specimen for pathology, can check margins. Avoid in young women.
3. Laser ablation – ablative therapy with laser.
4. Conization – LEEP or cold knife removes transformation zone. Avoid in young women.
5. Hysterectomy – avoid in young women.

Ablative therapies are rarely used in the United States. Close monitoring is preferred over ablative or excisional treatments in younger women, due to the high incidence of regression and because harm results from overscreening and overtreatment. Younger women include those who have not completed childbearing. In older women, if treatment is needed, LEEP is the most common modality. LEEP conization is preferred to cold-knife conization, as LEEP can be done in the office setting [49].

Nina asks about preventive care for her children. She is advised that her daughters should start Pap screening at the age of 21 and should be vaccinated for HPV with three doses starting as soon as possible. Her 14-year-old son should receive two doses of the HPV vaccine: one now and one in 6–12 months.

HPV Vaccination

HPV vaccination was introduced in the United States in June 2006 to prevent hrHPV infection with the intention of decreasing the incidence, morbidity, and mortality related to cervical cancer. HPV vaccination is currently recommended for all children and is best administered before sexual debut and exposure to the virus. The HPV vaccine is recommended at ages 11–12 for both girls and boys but can be initiated at age 9 (see Table 14.7 below). Gardasil™, a quad-

Table 14.7 HPV vaccination recommendations [50, 53]

Patient category	Age at initiation	Vaccine specification
Routine vaccination for all Dosing schedule by age *ACIP, CDC, ACOG*[a]	9–14 years for all persons 11–12 usual age of initiation	Two-dose schedule
	15-26 years: vaccinate all until 26	Three-dose schedule
Immunosuppressed History of sexual abuse or assault Chronic illnesses	Initiate vaccine age 9 9–26 years for all persons	Three-dose schedule if immunosuppressed, or if initiated after age 14
Selected unvaccinated individuals who would benefit from vaccination	Vaccination approved to age 45	Three-dose schedule

[a]*ACIP* Advisory Committee on Immunization Practices, *CDC* Center for Disease Control, *ACOG* American College of Obstetricians and Gynecologists

rivalent vaccine against 16, 18, 6, and 11, was approved in 2006 and was initially offered to girls. The bivalent vaccine Cervarix ™ was licensed in 2009 and covers high-risk types 16 and 18. HPV vaccination for boys was officially recommended by the Advisory Committee on Immunization Practices (ACIP) in 2011. The latest vaccine, Gardasil 9™, was approved in 2014 and is currently the only HPV vaccine available in the US. Gardasil 9™ covers hrHPV 16 and 18; it also covers "other high-risk" strains 31, 33, 45, 52, and 58 which account for 15% of cervical cancers. The addition of these other strains has the potential to increase the prevention of cervical cancer from 70 to 90% with vaccination. Gardasil-9™ also covers strains 6 and 11 which cause genital warts [50].

Based on clinical trials with the 9 valent HPV vaccine (Gardasil-9™), the Advisory Committee on Immunization Practices (ACIP) issued a recommendation to administer a two-dose series to both females and males less than 15 years, a recommendation approved by the FDA in October 2016 [50]. The second dose is administered between 6 and 12 months after the initial dose. When given at these early ages, immunogenicity is excellent with only two doses, with significantly higher titers obtained in those who received the two-dose series before age 15 as compared to those who were vaccinated with two doses at a later age. Seroconversion rates of those who receive the two-dose vaccine before age 15 and those who receive a three-dose vaccine are comparable.

The new two-dose schedule for teens less than 15 has several advantages:

- Increased completion rates: the dose schedule facilitates the completion of the vaccination series at two visits. The visits can be 12 months apart which correlates with the spacing of many annual visits.
- Patient convenience: It is convenient for adolescents receiving the vaccine, the parents, and the providers through the elimination of extra clinical visits.
- Cost reduction: Overall costs are reduced with fewer vaccine dosages, lower administration costs, savings of parent time, and fewer costs associated with bringing children to the clinic for extra visits.
- If the HPV vaccination series is initiated after the age of 15 years, however, the three-dose series at 0, 2, and 6 months is still recommended.

Approach to Previously Vaccinated Populations

For primary care providers who treat primarily adult patients, it is important to develop an approach to counseling patients who received partial HPV vaccination or who received HPV vaccination with non-Gardasil-9 immunizations. The basic principles are as follows:

1. If a person initiated vaccination for HPV prior to age 15 and received two doses of any of the three approved vaccinations at the recommended schedule, a third vaccine is not needed.
2. The 9 valent HPV vaccine can be used to complete a vaccination series that was started with either a bivalent or tetravalent vaccine.
3. For persons who have previously completed an earlier HPV vaccine series, there is no recommendation for additional vaccination with the new 9 valent HPV vaccine.
4. For interrupted vaccination series, continuation is recommended with no need to restart the series unless one or more of the intervals between doses was *shorter* than recommended.

Since the introduction of the HPV vaccine, there has been a decline in hrHPV infections and a decrease in high-risk lesions. In the US, data from the HPV-IMPACT Project demonstrated that cervical intraepithelial neoplasia (CIN2) lesions and higher attributed to hrHPV 16/18 decreased from 53.6% in 2008 to 28.45 in 2012 among women 18 years or older who had received at least one dose of the vaccine. Rates of initiation and completion of HPV vaccination had been suboptimal in the United States at that time. As of the year 2017, 66% of girls between 13 and 17 had received at least one dose of the vaccine, and only 49% were up to date on the HPV vaccine. Fortunately, vaccination rates have been increasing by 5% per year in the United States and there is a movement to provide HPV vaccination worldwide, including low- and middle-income countries (LMICs) [51, 52]. As vaccination rates improve, the effectiveness of the HPV vaccine for preventing HPV infections and subsequent cellular changes in the cervix will be more fully realized.

Vaccination is recommended for all persons age 9–26, ideally at age 9–12. Catch-up vaccination for those not previously vaccinated for HPV is recommended for all persons through age 26, regardless of sexual activity or gender. In 2018, the FDA approved Gardasil-9™ use until age 45. Clinical judgment and shared decision making should be used to make vaccination decisions in adults aged 27–45 until guidelines are updated. Vaccination in adults over age 45 is not currently recommended. Further study is needed to fully understand the risks and benefits of vaccination in the older cohort [53, 54].

HPV Vaccination in Specific Populations

The following recommendations are given for specific populations:

- Children with a history of sexual abuse or assault: initiate vaccine at age 9, sooner than the normal 11–12 years of age.
- Medical conditions: for primary and secondary immunocompromising conditions, the ACIP recommends the three-dose HPV vaccination in those aged 9–26 due to the potential for reduction in cell-mediated or humoral immunity. Examples include patients with HIV or autoimmune disease, patients taking immunosuppressive therapy, patients who have had a transplant, or those receiving treatment for malignant neoplasms.

Disparities in Cervical Cancer Prevention and Mortality

There are significant disparities in the prevention, incidence, treatment, and mortality from cervical cancer in the United States and around the world. Patient, physician, social, economic, and system issues contribute to the discrepancy. Race, structural racism, socioeconomic status, access to healthcare, geographic isolation, educational level, insurance, poverty, and other chronic medical illness adversely affect outcomes.

Disparities in Incidence

Between 2011 and 2015, the Hispanic population had the highest *incidence* of cervical cancer at a rate of 9.4 cases per 100,000, 95% CI (9.1–9.9), compared to the Black population at 9.0 cases per 100,000, 95% CI (8.8–9.2); the White population at 7.4 cases per 100,000, 95% CI (7.4–7.7); and the Alaskan and Indian Native population at 6.5 cases per 100,000, 95% CI (5.3–7.6) [17].

Disparities in Mortality

Race For the reasons noted above, the Black (African-American non-Hispanic) population in the United States has the highest *mortality rate* from cervical cancer (per 100,000 women) at 3.7 deaths, compared to Hispanic women at 2.6 deaths, White women at 2.2 deaths, and Alaskan Indian and Pacific Islander both at 1.8 deaths [3, 10, 11]. The mortality among Black women is significantly *underestimated* for the following reason: women who have had a total hysterectomy for benign reasons are no longer at risk for cervical cancer. Data that does not correct for hysterectomy status underestimates the mortality rate for cervical cancer in all races. Between 2000 and 2012, the unadjusted overall mortality rate for all women was 3.4 deaths per 100,000 women, compared to a higher rate of 5.0 deaths per 100,000 women when adjusted for hysterectomy status. This underestimation is greatest among Black women. When stratified by race, Black women had a higher correction factor due to the higher rates of hysterectomy in this population, with rates increasing from 5.7 to 10.1 per 100,000 women, compared to a change from 3.2 to 4.7 per 100,000 White women [55].

Socioeconomic status and differential access to care appear to be major factors contributing to disparities in cancer mortality. Studies show higher mortality rates from cervical cancer in women of lower socioeconomic status. Women in isolated geographic areas and those in medically underserved areas, e.g., Appalachian women, have higher mortality rates compared to other White women and to the US average [55].

Disparities in Screening

Age Women of all races and socioeconomic status at the extreme ends of the screening age recommendations between the ages of 23 and 29 and between 60 and 65 were less likely to be screened than women ages 30–59 [6].

Race American Indian and Alaska natives are least likely to receive a Pap within the previous 3 years according to the CDC [56] at a rate of 60.9%. Native Hawaiians and Pacific Islanders were screened at 64.9%, Hispanic at 68.6%, White women at 68.4%, and Black women at 74.6%.

Insurance Uninsured and underinsured women were most likely not to be screened. In the 2015 survey data referenced above, there was an 80.5% Pap screening rate within 3 years for those with insurance compared to 59.3% among those without insurance.

Chronic Disease Women with one or more chronic diseases (e.g., kidney disease, arthritis, depression) are less likely to be screened [9, 56].

Disparities: Follow-Up of Abnormal Pap Test

Inadequate follow-up of abnormal results in women who have been screened is a significant risk to women and is caused by poor or inadequate access to care, nonexistent or inadequate insurance coverage, inadequate surveillance systems to track abnormal results and follow-up, and clinician failure to adhere to recommended guidelines for the follow-up of abnormal Pap test results causing delays in care.

It is estimated that about 50 million women undergo Pap tests per year, and 3.5% of these have cytological abnormalities requiring further follow-up. An analysis of data from a program whose goal is to increase access to screening, diagnostic, and follow-up services among low-income and uninsured women between 1991 and 2000 showed poor adherence to guidelines for follow-up of abnormal tests in medically underserved areas. Only 44% of women with two abnormal tests were followed in accordance with the guidelines at the time. Black or African-American women had the lowest percentage of follow-up compared to other ethnic groups, and Alaskan Natives and Native Americans had the highest number of third Pap tests performed instead of a colposcopy [57].

In a New Zealand study, among women with CIN3 who have had punch or wedge biopsies with no subsequent treatment, the rate of cancer was 31.3% within 30 years. Of these women in whom CIN3 persisted for 2 years, and punch or wedge biopsy had been the only treatment modality, 50.3% developed cancer within 30 years. The failure to receive adequate treatment results in an extreme risk of progression to cervical cancer. However, when treated and followed appropriately, the development of cervical cancer after 30 years was 0.7% [48].

HPV Prevalence

Between 2013 and 2014, the prevalence of any genital HPV in the United States in individuals between the ages of 18 and 59 according to the National Health and Nutrition Examination Survey (NHANES) was highest among the Black population (64.1%). The Hispanic population had a prevalence of 41.4%, the White non-Hispanic population had a prevalence of 40.0%, and the Asian population a prevalence of 23.8% [18].

HPV Vaccination

In the HPV Vaccine Impact Monitoring (HPV-IMPACT) Project [58], a significant difference in vaccination rates was observed based on race/ethnicity and insurance coverage. Of the vaccinated women in the study, non-Hispanic White women had a vaccination rate of 67.45% compared to 18% vaccination rate in non-Hispanic Black women and 10.3% vaccination rate in Hispanic women. Women with private insurance were more likely to be vaccinated (65.1%) compared to those with public insurance (27.9%) and those without insurance (2.3%).

In the National Immunization Survey Teen (NIS-Teen) for adolescents aged 13–17 years, Black or Hispanic adolescents and adolescents living below the federal poverty level were significantly less likely to complete vaccination series [59].

In addition to access to care and cost, research has demonstrated mistrust in vaccination, which stems from a legacy of unethical medical research, patients lived experiences of racism in medical settings, and lack of accessible healthcare. Specifically regarding HPV vaccination, vaccine acceptance is lower amongst parents who expressed mistrust in government health agencies, though trust in health information from a physician or healthcare professional was not predictive of vaccine acceptance [60]. Ongoing efforts by healthcare systems and government agencies to repair this trust are needed.

Private insurances generally cover the cost of HPV vaccination. The National Vaccine Program, Vaccines for Children (VFC), provides free vaccination for children and adolescents through 18 years of age for people who would otherwise not be able to afford the vaccine [61]. Barriers to completion among low-income groups – lack of transportation, limited healthcare access, and work schedules – can result in incomplete vaccination series even when vaccine programs pay for the initial dose.

A higher level of maternal education, having continuous insurance coverage from age 11, and living in the Northeast were all associated with higher rates of vaccine completion [59].

Disparities Among Foreign-Born Women

Data from the 2013 National Health Interview Survey (NHIS) conducted by the National Center for Health Statistics reveal that HPV vaccination initiation was higher among American-born women aged less than 26 years compared to foreign-born women (27.1% verses 17.2%) [12]. Even when controlling for confounders in a multivariate logistic analysis (demographic, economic, and healthcare variables), the difference remained unchanged. Regardless of the place of birth, females were more likely to initiate vaccination compared to males. Overall, younger foreign-born males had the lowest access to healthcare compared to all other groups.

Insurance status and access to healthcare account for most of the differential rates in HPV vaccination. This is most evident in the undocumented foreign-born persons who are not eligible for public health insurance and may not have valid social security numbers or funds to pay for private insurance. This is also supported in part by the finding that foreign-born women in the higher-income group had similar HPV vaccination rates compared to their American-born high-income group counterparts [12].

A Potential Solution: Vaginal Sample Collection

This strategy is aimed at improving screening rates in unscreened, high-risk women who have barriers to regular screening including discomfort, costs, and clinical accessibility. Patients may collect vaginal samples at home and send them in, with positive results necessitating a clinical visit and follow-up. It is not clear how this test compares to the accuracy of office-based screening, or whether follow-up of positive results would be adequate. Vaginal sample collection is not currently approved by the FDA. It is however endorsed by the World Health Organization (WHO) and is currently being studied in the United States [62, 63].

Conclusion

Cervical cancer continues to be a major public health burden throughout the world and among underserved populations in the United States. HPV vaccination, cervical cancer screening, precursor lesion treatment, and adequate follow-up of all women will advance the goal of saving the lives of women who die needlessly from invasive cervical cancer each year, a largely preventable disease.

Summary Points

1. Ninety-nine percent of cervical cancer is caused by persistent high-risk HPV strains that infect the transformation zone of the cervix and lead to precancerous and cancerous changes.
2. Routine cervical cancer screening guidelines call for Pap testing alone every 3 years from age 21 to 29. Women ages 30–65 should be screened with either co-testing every 5 years, hrHPV testing every 5 years, or Pap testing alone every 3 years. With some exceptions, women who have undergone a complete hysterectomy for benign conditions and women over 65 may exit screening assuming they have received adequate recommended testing in the prior 10 years.
3. HIV-positive, immune-compromised, DES-exposed, and women with a history of CIN2 or greater are at higher risk of cervical cancer and are screened more intensely than those outlined in the routine guidelines.
4. HPV vaccination with Gardasil-9™ is approved for use in persons aged 9–45. Current recommendations are for most children to be vaccinated with two doses at ages 11 and 12. Persons who start immunization older than 15 years of age should receive three doses at 0, 2, and 6 months. Immunocompromised persons should receive three doses, even if started at the younger age.
5. Algorithms for the management of abnormal Pap smears and biopsy results are available online via a downloadable app from the ASCCP. Persons positive for HPV 16 or 18, with persistent "other high-risk strains," with cytology of ASC-H or greater, or with ASCUS/LGSIL with HPV+ should be referred for colposcopy. CIN1 is low grade and often regresses, whereas CIN2/3 are high-grade changes which need increased monitoring and/or treatment by gynecologists.
6. Significant disparities exist among certain populations in the United States and also in low and middle income countries including differences in HPV vaccination, cervical cancer screening, follow-up and treatment of abnormal results, and mortality. These disparities are particularly notable for low-income, minority, chronically ill, immigrant, poorly insured women and those with poor access to healthcare. Continued effort to reach a goal of universal HPV vaccination and universal cervical cancer screening will help close these gaps in care.

Review Questions

1. A 19-year-old woman presents to the clinic to establish care with a doctor for adults. She had routine care with her pediatrician and completed the HPV vaccine series. She has been sexually active for 2 years and is on oral contraceptives. She was recently diagnosed with chlamydia and treated. Her mother told her that she needs a Pap smear. Which of the following is recommended?
   A. She should be tested for high-risk HPV now.
   B. She should have a Pap test with HPV co-testing now.
   C. She should have a Pap test at age 21.
   D. HPV testing should be performed at age 21.
   The correct answer is C. Pap testing should not start prior to age 21, even in sexually active women. HPV testing is not recommended for screening in women under age 30 (25 in some countries) except as a reflex test for abnormal Pap results. Her recent chlamydia

diagnosis does not change these recommendations [17, 30].

2. A 66-year-old woman, who moved to the United States from India 1 year ago, comes in to establish care. She does not believe she has ever had a Pap test. She has stopped menstruating and denies any postmenopausal vaginal bleeding or discharge. Which of the following is correct?
   A. She is asymptomatic and over age 65. Pap screening is not needed.
   B. She should be tested with yearly Pap smears for the next 20 years because of her unknown history.
   C. She should receive the three-dose HPV vaccination series.
   D. She should undergo Pap and HPV co-testing today.

   The correct answer is D. Women over 65 may exit screening if they have been screened adequately in the past 10 years, with the most recent test in the last 5 years. Clinical judgment should be used in recommendations for her screening, but she should be screened now for HPV and cervical cancer and again in 3–5 years since she has not been adequately screened in the past 10 years. Yearly Pap smears are recommended for some high-risk women, but would not apply unless she was DES exposed, infected with HIV, immunosuppressed, or had a history of cervical or vaginal malignancy within the last 20 years. HPV vaccination is not approved for persons over 45 years of age [17, 30].

3. An undocumented 40-year-old Hispanic woman, G1P1, presents to the free mobile clinic for a Pap test. She and her family move frequently to find work. She does not remember how long ago she had her last Pap, but thinks it may have been abnormal. She is unsure if she has ever had a colposcopy. She undergoes Pap and HPV co-testing today and the clinic social worker meets with her to discuss ways to get insurance and housing for her family, because they are homeless.

   Which of the following is the most important next step before the patient leaves the clinic today?
   A. Tell her that she is high risk for cervical cancer and refer her to gynecology.
   B. Have her sign a release of information to get old records from all the prior healthcare facilities where she received care.
   C. Determine how she should be contacted to receive her Pap test results, and fully explain why follow-up is very important.
   D. Discuss that colon cancer screening starts at age 45 if she does not have a prior history of colorectal cancer.

   The correct answer is C. Healthcare disparities should be considered when seeing patients, and lack of follow-up for abnormal results is a serious issue in certain populations. Hispanic patients are an ethnic group that often has poor follow-up for abnormal test results, and undocumented persons are at particularly high risk. There must be a secure plan to reach the patient and arrange for follow-up if the Pap test is abnormal. Telling her that she is high risk for cervical cancer is premature and may cause unnecessary anxiety. Obtaining prior medical records should be attempted, but the ability to follow-up on the current testing is more important at this visit. Colon cancer screening is important, but will not be needed for 5 years [57].

4. A 30-year-old woman presents with 9-year-old twins, a girl and a boy. She asks if her daughter should get the HPV vaccine. What are the current recommendations for HPV vaccination?
   A. Both children should be vaccinated at age 11 with two doses.
   B. The daughter should be vaccinated at age 11, the son at age 9.
   C. The daughter should be vaccinated with three doses, the son with two doses.
   D. Both children should be vaccinated now with two doses.

   The correct answer is A. For children aged 9–14, the ACIP recommends a two-dose schedule for male and female patients, usually at ages 11–12. Children are vaccinated at age 9 in cases of immunosuppression or sexual abuse. The vaccination is approved for persons age 9–45, so clinical judgment can be used when making vaccination recommendations for adults [50].

5. A 31-year-old woman with HIV comes in to establish primary care. She was diagnosed with HIV at age 27 and has had three normal annual Pap smears. Her most recent testing at age 30 was normal cytology and HPV negative. How often should she receive a Pap test in the future?
   A. Every 3 years for life.
   B. Every 5 years with HPV co-testing until age 65.
   C. Annually, may discontinue at age 65.
   D. Biannually for life.

   The correct answer is A. The current guidelines for HIV-positive women, which is based on limited data, recommend annual Pap starting at the time of diagnosis. At age 30, co-testing should be done. If co-testing is normal, the next testing can be delayed for 3 years. Screening does not end at age 65. These recommendations do not change based on the use of antiretroviral therapy, CD4 counts, or viral load [64].

6. A 32-year-old woman presents for care. She states that she is a virgin and is refusing a pelvic examination or Pap test. She said that she was told by her last physician that she was at very low risk for cancer, and therefore, Paps

were not needed. Which of the following statements is correct according to current guidelines?

A. She is at risk of cervical cancer despite her sexual history, and she should be made to sign an "against medical advice" form if she refuses testing.
B. All women should be screened for cervical cancer despite sexual history starting at age 21.
C. She should self-test for HPV and only get a Pap if the results are positive.
D. Women who have sex with women, nuns, and virgins do not need Pap tests.

The correct answer is B. All persons with a cervix should be screened for cervical cancer between the ages of 21 and 65, regardless of sexual history, sexual orientation, or gender identity. Although persons who have never had penetrating sexual intercourse with a man may be at lower risk, HPV is spread through other forms of contact. A prior history of sexual contact or sexual assault may be denied or not remembered by the patient. The idea of self-collection of a vaginal collection for HPV screening has merit and is being suggested for screening in some lower-resource settings, but there are no current guidelines to guide its use. If she refuses pelvic examination, she should not be pressured or traumatized, but relationship building and patient education may, in time, change her mind about the screening. Refusals of recommended care, and discussions of the risks to the patient of not screening, should be clearly documented in the medical record [17].

References

1. Group USCSW. United States cancer statistics: 1999–2014 incidence and mortality web-based report 2017 cited 2017. Available from: http://www.cdc.gov/uscs
2. Walboomers JM, Jacobs MV, Manos MM. Human papillomavirus is a necessary cause of invasive cervical cancer worldwide. J Pathol. 1999;189(1):12–9.
3. Cancer Stat Facts: Cervical Cancer: NIH: National Cancer Institute Surveillance, Epidemiology, and End Results Program. Available from: https://seer.cancer.gov/statfacts/html/cervix.html.
4. Hillemanns P, Soergel P, Hertel H, Jentschke M. Epidemiology and early detection of cervical cancer. Oncol Res Treat. 2016;39:501–6.
5. Chelimo C, Wouldes TA, Cameron LD, Elwood JM. Risk factors for and prevention of human papillomaviruses (HPV), genital warts and cervical cancer. J Infect. 2013;66:207–17.
6. Benard VB, Thomas CC, King J, Massetti GM, Doria-Rose VP, Saraiya M, et al. Vital signs: cervical cancer incidence, mortality, and screening - United States, 2007-2012. MMWR Morb Mortal Wkly Rep. 2014;63(44):1004–9.
7. Castellsague X. Natural history and epidemiology of HPV infection and cervical cancer. Gynecol Oncol. 2008;110(3 Suppl 2):S4–7.
8. Fonseca-Moutinho JA. Smoking and cervical cancer. Obstet Gynecol. 2011;2011:847684. https://doi.org/10.5402/2011/847684.
9. Crawford A, Benard V, King J, Thomas CC. Understanding barriers to cervical cancer screening in women with access to care, behavioral risk factor surveillance system, 2014. Prev Chronic Dis. 2016;13:E154.
10. Cervical Cancer Rates by Race and Ethnicity Centers for Disease Control and Prevention: Division of Cancer Prevention and Control. Centers for Disease Control and Prevention; 2017 updated June 19. Available from: https://www.cdc.gov/cancer/cervical/statistics/race.htm
11. Viens LJHS, Watson M, Markowitz LE, Thomas CC, Thompson TD, Razzaghi H, Saraiya M, Centers for Disease Control and Prevention (CDC). Human papillomavirus–associated cancers—United States, 2008–2012. MMWR Morb Mortal Wkly Rep. 2016;65:661–6. https://doi.org/10.15585/mmwr.mm6526a1
12. De P, Budhwani H. Human papillomavirus (HPV) vaccine initiation in minority Americans. Public Health. 2017;144:86–91.
13. Tan SY, Tatsumura Y. George Papanicolaou (1883–1962): discoverer of the Pap smear. Singap Med J. 2015;56(10):586–7. https://doi.org/10.11622/smedj.2015155.
14. https://www.cytopathology.org/specimen-collection-adequacy-requisition/. Accessed 23 May 2018.
15. Tibbs RF, Wong JY, Logrono R. Enhancing recovery of endocervical component on gynecologic cytology specimens processed by thin-layer technology. Acta Cytol. 2003;47:172–6.
16. Elumir-Tanner L, Doraty M, for the Southern Alberta Primary Care Research Network (SAPCReN). Management of Papanicolaou test results that lack endocervical cells. CMAJ. 2011;183(5):563–8.
17. Wright TC, Stoler MH, Behrens CM, Sharma A, Zhang G, Wright TL. Primary cervical cancer screening with human papillomavirus: end of study results from the ATHENA study using HPV as the first-line screening test. Gynecol Oncol. 2015;136(2):189–97.
18. McQuillan G, Kruszon-Moran D, Markowitz LE, Unger ER, Paulose-Ram R. Prevalence of HPV in Adults Aged 18–69: United States, 2011–2014. NCHS data brief. 2017(280):1–8.
19. Paz-Zulueta M, Alvarez-Paredes L, Rodriguez Diaz JC, Paras-Bravo P, Andrada Becerra ME, Rodriguez Ingelmo JM, et al. Prevalence of high-risk HPV genotypes, categorized by their quadrivalent and nine-valent HPV vaccination coverage, and the genotype association with high-grade lesions. BMC Cancer. 2018;18(1):112.
20. Stanley M. Immunobiology of HPV and HPV vaccines. Gynecol Oncol. 2008;109:S15–21.
21. Schiffman M, Castle PE, Jeronimo J, Rodriguez AC, Wacholder S. Human papillomavirus and cervical cancer. Lancet. 2007;370(9590):890–907.
22. Rodriguez A, Schiffman M, Wacholder HR, et al. Rapid clearance of human papillomavirus and implications for clinical focus on persistent infections. J Natl Cancer Inst. 2008;100(7):513–7. https://doi.org/10.1093/jnci/djn044.
23. Allegretti JR, Barnes EL, Cameron A. Are patients with inflammatory bowel disease on chronic immunosuppressive therapy at increased risk of cervical high-grade dysplasia/cancer? A meta-analysis. Inflamm Bowel Dis. 2015;21(5):1089–97. https://doi.org/10.1097/MIB.0000000000000338.
24. Kim SC, Schneeweiss S, Liu J, et al. Biologic disease-modifying antirheumatic drugs and risk of high-grade cervical dysplasia and cervical cancer in rheumatoid arthritis: a cohort study. Arthritis Rheumatol. 2016;68(9):2106–13. https://doi.org/10.1002/art.39689.
25. Matsumoto K, Oki A, Furuta R, Maeda H, Yasugi T, et al. Tobacco smoking and regression of low-grade cervical abnormalities. Cancer Sci. 2010;101:2065–73.
26. Moyer VA. Screening for cervical cancer: U.S. Preventive Services Task Force recommendation statement. Ann Intern Med. 2012;156(12):880–91, w312.
27. Saslow D, Solomon D, Lawson HW, Killackey M, Kulasingam SL, Cain J, et al. American Cancer Society, American Society for Colposcopy and Cervical Pathology, and American Society for Clinical Pathology screening guidelines for the prevention and early detection of cervical cancer. Am J Clin Pathol. 2012;137(4):516–42.

28. US Preventive Services Task force. Screening for cervical cancer. US Preventive Services Task Force recommendation statement. JAMA. 2018;320(7):674–86.
29. Kulasingam SL, Havrilesky LJ, Ghebre R, Myers ER. Screening for cervical cancer: a modeling study for the US Preventive Services Task Force. J Low Genit Tract Dis. 2013;17(2):193–202.
30. Agenor M, Muzny CA, Schick V, Austin EL, Potter J. Sexual orientation and sexual health services utilization among women in the United States. Prev Med. 2017;95:74–81.
31. Stout NK, Goldhaber-Fiebert JD, Ortendahl JD, Goldie SJ. Trade-offs in cervical cancer prevention: balancing benefits and risks. Arch Intern Med. 2008;168(17):1881–9.
32. Sasieni P, Adams J, Cuzick J. Benefit of cervical screening at different ages: evidence from the UK audit of screening histories. Br J Cancer. 2003;89(1):88–93.
33. Miller MG, Sung HY, Sawaya GF, Kearney KA, Kinney W, Hiatt RA. Screening interval and risk of invasive squamous cell cervical cancer. Obstet Gynecol. 2003;101(1):29–37.
34. Sawaya GF, McConnell KJ, Kulasingam SL, Lawson HW, Kerlikowske K, Melnikow J, et al. Risk of cervical cancer associated with extending the interval between cervical-cancer screenings. N Engl J Med. 2003;349(16):1501–9.
35. Dunne EF, Unger ER, Sternberg M, McQuillan G, Swan DC, Patel SS, et al. Prevalence of HPV infection among females in the United States. JAMA. 2007;297(8):813–9.
36. Giorgi Rossi P, Carozzi F, Federici A, Ronco G, Zappa M, Franceschi S, et al. Cervical cancer screening in women vaccinated against human papillomavirus infection: recommendations from a consensus conference. Prev Med. 2017;98:21–30.
37. http://www.ascopost.com/issues/august-10-2018/fda-approves-hpv-test/. Accessed 16 Oct 2018.
38. http://www.cancerscreening.gov.au/internet/screening/publishing.nsf/Content/cervical-screening-1. Accessed 15 Oct 2018.
39. Pearce KF, Haefner HK, Sarwar SF, Nolan TE. Cytopathological findings on vaginal Papanicolaou smears after hysterectomy for benign gynecologic disease. N Engl J Med. 1996;335(21):1559–62.
40. American Society for Colposcopy and Cervical Pathology (ASCCP) guidelines for managing abnormal PAP tests. http://www.asccp.org/asccp-guidelines
41. Kim JJ, Burger EA, Sy S, Campos NG. Optimal cervical cancer screening in women vaccinated against human papillomavirus. J Natl Cancer Inst. 2017;109(2):djw216.
42. (ACOG) TACoOaG. Gynecologic care of women and adolescents with human immunodeficiency virus. Washington, DC: Lippincott Williams & Wilkins; 2016. Available from: https://www.acog.org/Clinical-Guidance-and-Publications/Practice-Bulletins/Committee-on-Practice-Bulletins-Gynecology/Gynecologic-Care-for-Women-and-Adolescents-With-Human-Immunodeficiency-Virus.
43. Heard I. Prevention of cervical cancer in women with HIV. Curr Opin HIV AIDS. 2009;4(1):68–73.
44. Inamoto Y, Shah NN, Savani BN, Shaw BE, Abraham AA, Ahmed IA, et al. Secondary solid cancer screening following hematopoietic cell transplantation. Bone Marrow Transplant. 2015;50(8):1013–23.
45. Herbst AL. The current status of the DES-exposed population. Obstet Gynecol Annu. 1981;10:267–78.
46. Troisi R, Hatch EE, Palmer JR, et al. Prenatal diethylstilbestrol exposure and high-grade squamous cell neoplasia of the lower genital tract. Am J Obstetr Gynecol. 2016;215(3):322.e1–8. https://doi.org/10.1016/j.ajog.2016.03.007.
47. Gynecologists ACoOa. Abnormal cervical cancer screening test results. Washington, DC: Lippincott Williams & Wilkins; 2016. Available from: https://www.acog.org/Patients/FAQs/Abnormal-Cervical-Cancer-Screening-Test-Results
48. McCredie MR, Sharples KJ, Paul C, Baranyai J, Medley G, Jones RW, et al. Natural history of cervical neoplasia and risk of invasive cancer in women with cervical intraepithelial neoplasia 3: a retrospective cohort study. Lancet Oncol. 2008;9(5):425–34.
49. Martin-Hirsch PL, Paraskevaidis E, Kitchener H. Surgery for cervical intraepithelial neoplasia. Cochrane Database Syst Rev. 2013;12:CD001318.
50. Meites E, Kempe A, Markowitz LE. Use of a 2-dose schedule for human papillomavirus vaccination - updated recommendations of the advisory committee on immunization practices. MMWR Morb Mortal Wkly Rep. 2016;65(49):1405–8.
51. HPV Vaccination coverage data. https://www.cdc.gov/hpv/hcp/vacc-coverage/index.html. Accessed 14 Oct 2018.
52. WHO recommendations for routine immunizations. Updated August 2018. https://www.who.int/immunization/policy/Immunization_routine_table1.pdf?ua=1. Accessed 16 Oct 2018.
53. https://www.acog.org/Clinical-Guidance-and-Publications/Committee-Opinions/Committee-on-Adolescent-Health-Care/Human-Papillomavirus-Vaccination. Accessed 12 Sept 2018.
54. Meites E, Szilagyi PG, Chesson HW, Unger ER, Romero JR, Markowitz, LE. Human Papillomavirus Vaccination for Adults: Updated Recommendations of the Advisory Committee on Immunization Practices. MMWR Morb Mortal Wkly Rep. 2019;68:698–702.
55. Beavis AL, Gravitt PE, Rositch AF. Hysterectomy-corrected cervical cancer mortality rates reveal a larger racial disparity in the United States. Cancer. 2017;123(6):1044–50.
56. National Center for Health Statistics. Use of Pap smears among women aged 18 and over, by selected characteristics: United States, selected years 1987–2015. Available from: https://www.cdc.gov/nchs/fastats/pap-tests.htm
57. Benard VB, Lawson HW, Eheman CR, Anderson C, Helsel W. Adherence to guidelines for follow-up of low-grade cytologic abnormalities among medically underserved women. Obstet Gynecol. 2005;105(6):1323–8.
58. Hariri S, Bennett NM, Niccolai LM, Schafer S, Park IU, Bloch KC, et al. Reduction in HPV 16/18-associated high grade cervical lesions following HPV vaccine introduction in the United States - 2008-2012. Vaccine. 2015;33(13):1608–13.
59. Niccolai LM, Mehta NR, Hadler JL. Racial/Ethnic and poverty disparities in human papillomavirus vaccination completion. Am J Prev Med. 2011;41(4):428–33.
60. Nan X, Daily K, Richards A, Holt C, Wang MQ, Tracy K, Qin Y. The role of trust in health information from medical authorities in accepting the HPV vaccine among African American parents. Hum Vaccin Immunother. 2019;15(7–8):1723–31. https://doi.org/10.1080/21645515.2018.1540825. Epub 2018 Nov 5. PMID: 30396312; PMCID: PMC6746524.
61. Vaccines for Children (VCF) Program. Available from: https://www.cdc.gov/features/vfcprogram/#vfclist
62. WHO. Comprehensive cervical cancer control: a guide to essential practice Second edition. Department of Reproductive Health and Research. Switzerland; 2014.
63. Des Marais A, ZhaoHome Y, Hobbs M, et al. Self-collection by mail to test for human papillomavirus and sexually transmitted infections. Obstet Gynecol. 2018;132(6):1412–20. https://doi.org/10.1097/AOG.0000000000002964.
64. https://aidsinfo.nih.gov/guidelines. Accessed 15 Oct 2018.

15 Gynecologic Malignancies

Christine A. Prifti, Deborah Kwolek,
Whitfield Board Growdon, and Kerri Palamara

Learning Objectives

1. Review the epidemiology, risk factors, and prevention of uterine, ovarian, cervical, vulvar, and vaginal cancers.
2. Discuss screening, presenting symptoms, and early diagnosis of uterine, ovarian, cervical, vulvar, and vaginal cancers.
3. Describe the evaluation and staging of uterine, ovarian, cervical, vulvar, and vaginal cancers.
4. Explain the prognosis and typical treatment plans for uterine, ovarian, cervical, vulvar, and vaginal cancers.
5. Describe the survivorship issues in women with gynecologic malignancies including the potential sequelae from therapeutic chemoradiation and surgery.

Gynecologic Malignancies: An Overview

Gynecologic cancers include uterine, ovarian, cervical, vulvar, and vaginal cancers. Annually, approximately 107,000 women in the United States and nearly 1 million women globally are diagnosed [1, 2]. Major risk factors include high-risk HPV (hrHPV), estrogen excess, smoking, immunodeficiency, diethylstilbestrol (DES) exposure, and genetics. Except for the Pap test and HPV testing, which are used to screen for cervical cancer, there are no approved screening tests to detect gynecologic cancers in asymptomatic women of average risk. Primary care providers assess risk, discuss prevention strategies, and recognize and evaluate early symptoms. The primary symptoms in gynecologic malignancies are bleeding abnormalities, abdominal or pelvic pain or discomfort, bowel or urinary complaints, unexplained vulvar pruritus, and masses or lesions.

The prognoses of gynecologic malignancies vary by cancer type and stage at diagnosis. Uterine cancer tends to be associated with postmenopausal bleeding, is often diagnosed early, and typically has a favorable prognosis. Ovarian cancer is often diagnosed in late stages and thus can have a relatively poor prognosis. Cervical cancer is caused by persistent HPV infection and is detected through routine screening where resources are available. Vulvar cancers may be preceded by dermatologic etiologies, such as lichen planus, and typically present with pruritus or lesions noted on routine pelvic exam. Vaginal cancer is rare and primarily related to hrHPV infection.

Several genetic syndromes, such as Lynch, Cowden, and BRCA 1 and 2 mutations, greatly increase the risk of gynecologic malignancies. Such patients require increased surveillance and should consider prophylactic surgery. Patients should be screened during preventive visits for a family history of cancer or genetic mutations, and appropriate patients should undergo genetic counseling and testing (see Chap. 17 on "The Primary Prevention of Breast Cancer" for a discussion of genetic syndromes and screening).

C. A. Prifti (✉)
Boston University Medical Center, Department of Medicine, Women's Health Unit, Boston, MA, USA
e-mail: christine.prifti@bmc.org

D. Kwolek
Harvard Medical School, Massachusetts General Hospital, Department of Medicine, Boston, MA, USA

W. B. Growdon
Massachusetts General Hospital, Department of Obstetrics, Gynecology and Reproductive Medicine, Division of Gynecologic Oncology, Boston, MA, USA

K. Palamara
Center for Physician Well-Being, Massachusetts General Hospital, Department of Medicine, Boston, MA, USA

S. A. Tilstra et al. (eds.), *Sex- and Gender-Based Women's Health*, https://doi.org/10.1007/978-3-030-50695-7_15

Table 15.1 Overview of gynecologic malignancies [3, 4]

	Uterine cancer [5]	Ovarian cancer [6]	Cervical cancer [7]	Vulvar cancer [8]	Vaginal cancer [9]
Projected new cases: annual US 2019 [4]	61,880	22,530	13,170	6070	5350
Deaths: annual US 2015 [4]	12,160	13,980	4250	1280	1430
Average age at diagnosis	62	63	50	68	60
Mean 5-year survival: US 2008–2014	81.1%	47.4%	66.2%	71% (13% for vulvar melanomas)	55–60% (13% for vaginal melanomas)
Major risk factors	Estrogen excess; obesity; genetics (Lynch, Cowden syndromes)	Uninterrupted ovulation; genetics (BRCA 1 and 2, Lynch syndrome)	hrHPV; immunosuppression; DES[a]	hrHPV; immunosuppression; lichen sclerosis	hrHPV; immunosuppression; DES[a]
Screening test	None	None	HPV and Pap testing	None	None
Early detection	Evaluation of postmenopausal bleeding or AUB; evaluation of incidental abnormal glandular, atypical endometrial, or abnormal squamous cells on Pap; genetic testing in certain populations[a]	Evaluation of abdominal/GI/ pelvic symptoms; genetic testing in certain populations[b]; incidental cancer cells on Pap (rarely)	Routine Pap; workup of vaginal bleeding (classically postcoital) or discharge	Biopsy of unexplained vulvar pruritis or lesions; routine follow-up of lichen sclerosis	Workup of vaginal bleeding or discharge; biopsy of suspicious lesions; incidental finding on Pap

[a]Populations at risk are discussed in the sections on uterine and ovarian cancer
[b]DES exposure may impact women born prior to 1971

The treatment for gynecologic malignancies may include surgery, radiation, and/or chemotherapy and should be managed by a gynecologic oncologist. Where clinically appropriate, clinicians may attempt fertility preservation for younger women and consider definitive surgical approaches such as hysterectomy for women who have completed childbearing. Survivorship care is important for women who may have postsurgical and/or chemoradiation sequelae resulting in gastroenterological, urological, neurological, psychological, and sexual issues posttreatment. Women may or may not be able to take estrogen therapy for treatment-induced menopause, depending upon the type of malignancy.

The prevention and early detection of gynecologic cancers relies on excellent comprehensive preventive care for women. In particular, educating women about how to recognize symptoms that are warning signs for malignancy and the conditions which require careful follow-up can prevent mortality. Access to care, lack of resources, fear, shame, social stigma, religious traditions, limited education, or cultural beliefs may be barriers to care for patients. Healthcare providers can help patients navigate these obstacles with routine health education that empowers patients and contributes to early cancer detection (Table 15.1).

Uterine Cancer

Keesha is a 65-year-old woman with a past medical history of obesity (BMI 40) and non-insulin-dependent diabetes mellitus who presents with 1 month of intermittent vaginal bleeding. She had severe vasomotor symptoms when she went through menopause 15 years ago and was treated with 12 months of combined estrogen and progestin therapy by her previous physician. She wants to know if she should be concerned about the bleeding.

Overview

Uterine cancer is the most common gynecologic malignancy in the United States [1]. The majority of uterine cancers are type I endometrial cancers. These tumors are associated with estrogen excess, have a classic presentation of abnormal bleeding, and are typically diagnosed early, leading to an overall favorable prognosis. Despite this, the incidence and mortality of endometrial cancer is increasing in the United States, which is thought to be related to rising rates of obe-

Table 15.2 Classification of uterine cancers [13, 14]

	Endometrial type I	Endometrial type II	Sarcoma
Percentage of uterine cancers	80%	10–15%	5%
Major risk factors	Estrogen excess	BRCA 1 and 2 for serous carcinoma	Genetics, history of radiation
Examples	Endometrial adenocarcinoma (grade 1 or 2)	Poorly differentiated endometrial adenocarcinoma (grade 3), clear cell and uterine serous carcinomas, and carcinosarcomas	Leiomyosarcomas, endometrial stromal tumors, and adenosarcomas
Prognosis	Good	Poor	Poor

sity [10]. Fat tissue converts androgen precursors to estrogen, and the consequent estrogen excess out of proportion to progesterone levels is a major risk factor for type I endometrial carcinoma. Although endometrial cancer is twice as common in Caucasian women as in Black women, Black women have a less favorable prognosis regardless of stage at diagnosis [10]. Black women are more commonly diagnosed with the more aggressive type II subtype for reasons that are not well understood, and rates of endometrial carcinoma are increasing faster in Blacks as compared to White women [11]. There are no currently available routine screening tests for uterine cancer, although some cases can be detected incidentally on Pap test, or during the evaluation of abnormal uterine bleeding. Most cases of uterine cancer are diagnosed in the workup of postmenopausal bleeding and are still curable when discovered.

Keesha had a Pap test 1 year ago which was HPV+ with AGC-US cytology results. She was sent a letter suggesting she come in for follow-up, but she does not remember getting the letter. Her mother died of "female cancer"; the details are unknown.

Epidemiology

Uterine cancer is the fourth most common cancer in women in the United States, after lung, breast, and colorectal cancers [1]. Worldwide, uterine cancer is the sixth most common malignancy in women [1, 12]. Endometrial cancer accounts for 95% of uterine cancers, while the remaining 5% are sarcomas [13]. Endometrial cancer most commonly presents in women over 55-years-old, has a mean age at diagnosis of 62 years, and is uncommon in women under 45 years of age [1, 5]. Endometrial cancer is subdivided into two types, which reflect grading and histology:

- *Type I* tumors are estrogen-dependent, low- to moderate-grade malignancies exclusively of endometrioid histology. They comprise 85% of endometrial cancers and have an excellent prognosis.
- *Type II tumors* are less associated with estrogen excess, are more aggressive, and have a less favorable prognosis. Type II endometrial cancer includes poorly differentiated (grade 3) endometroid tumors, papillary serous carcinomas, clear cell carcinomas, carcinosarcomas, and choriosarcomas.

Uterine sarcomas make up about 5% of uterine cancers. The most common subtypes are endometrial stromal sarcoma, leiomyosarcoma, and undifferentiated uterine sarcoma. The mean age at diagnosis is 60 years, and presenting complaints of abnormal vaginal bleeding and abdominal fullness are similar to endometrial cancer (see Table 15.2).

Pathophysiology and Risk Factors

Type I Endometrial Carcinoma Most cases of endometrial adenocarcinoma arise from prolonged estrogenic stimulation of the endometrium, leading to endometrial hyperplasia and atypical hyperplasia (also known as endometrial intraepithelial neoplasia; see discussion below on classification of noncancerous and precancerous endometrial lesions). Nonhormonal risk factors for endometrial adenocarcinoma include increased age, genetic predisposition, and diabetes.

Estrogen excess unopposed by progesterone is the most important risk factor for endometrial adenocarcinoma. Obesity, anovulation, estrogen-producing tumors, tamoxifen, hormone replacement therapy with unopposed estrogen, nulliparity, and early menarche or late menopause all increase estrogen exposure in the endometrium and therefore increase the risk of endometrial adenocarcinoma.

Obesity increases estrogen exposure because adipose cells convert androstenedione into estrone. As such, women with BMIs greater than 30 have a two- to sevenfold increased risk of endometrial cancer (odds ratio 1.5 for BMI 25 to <30; 2.5 for BMI 30 to <35; 4.5 for BMI 35 to <40; 7.1 for BMI ≥ 40) [15, 16].

Anovulation results in continuous unopposed estrogenic stimulation as without ovulation there is no corpus luteum to produce progesterone. The corpus luteum, which develops in the ovary after ovulation, produces progesterone until it dissolves in concert with the regular shedding of the endometrium in the absence of implantation. Use of *oral contraceptive pills*, which regulates this hormonal milieu, is associated with decreased endometrial cancer risk [16].

Tamoxifen is a selective estrogen receptor modulator that acts as an estrogen antagonist in breast tissue and an agonist in the endometrium. Women on tamoxifen therapy for breast cancer treatment or prevention have a 2- to 2.7-fold increased risk of endometrial cancer and should routinely be asked about symptoms of abnormal bleeding [17]. However, routine surveillance of asymptomatic women being treated with tamoxifen either with transvaginal ultrasound or endometrial biopsy is not recommended due to low specificity and low positive predictive value in this population [18–20].

Age is a significant risk factor for endometrial carcinoma. Ninety percent of cases occur in women aged greater than 50 years [21]. Only 20 percent are diagnosed in premenopausal women. Women with predisposing genetic cancer syndromes have a higher incidence of premenopausal uterine cancer than the sporadic cases that occur among other premenopausal women [22].

Diabetes is associated with an increased risk of endometrial cancer, though this is likely due to inflammatory factors and comorbid obesity [23].

Genetics, specifically *Lynch syndrome*, known as *hereditary nonpolyposis colorectal cancer or (HNPCC)*, is an uncommon autosomal dominant disorder which affects less than 1% of women and increases the risk of colon, endometrial, ovarian, brain, and other GI cancers. HNPCC patients have a lifetime risk of 40–60% of developing endometrial cancer, which tends to develop 10–20 years earlier than endometrial cancers caused by sporadic mutations [22, 24]. Patients with Lynch syndrome require intensive screening for a variety of cancers, starting in their 20s, including yearly endometrial biopsy (EMB). Patients should be referred to gynecology for annual screening and consideration of prophylactic hysterectomy with bilateral salpingo-oophorectomy after childbearing is complete [22]. There is also an increased risk in patients with *Cowden syndrome*, *BRCA 1* and 2, and other genetic defects. Clinicians should consider genetic counseling for patients diagnosed with endometrial cancer at age <50 years or who have a strong family history of colon and endometrial cancer [22, 25, 26]. Positive genetic testing impacts both screening and therapeutic options. When endometrial cancer does arise in the setting of Lynch syndrome, these tumors tend to present with a high mutational burden due to DNA mismatch repair deficiencies that translate into a heightened response to immunotherapy [27].

Although it is a risk factor for many types of cancer, *smoking* is associated with decreased endometrial cancer risk [16].

Table 15.3 Risk factors for endometrial cancer [15, 16]

	Type	Risk factors	Relative risk
Estrogen-associated uterine cancers	Type I only	Obesity, BMI > 35–40	OR 1.5 for BMI 25 to <30; 2.5 for BMI 30 to <35; 4.5 for BMI 35 to <40; 7.1 for BMI ≥40
		Tamoxifen use	2–2.7
		Chronic anovulation (e.g., PCOS)	3
		Unopposed estrogen use (i.e., inappropriately dosed menopausal hormone therapy)	2–10
		Estrogen-producing tumors	Unknown
		Nulliparity	2
		Early menarche	Unknown
		Late menopause	2
Non-estrogen-associated uterine cancers	Type I or type II	Increased age (50–70)	Incidence rises with age
		Pelvic irradiation	Unknown
		Genetic syndromes: Lynch syndrome Cowden syndrome BRCA	13–50% lifetime risk

Type II endometrial cancers do not have a clear precursor lesion, are not associated with estrogen excess, are more likely to be stage III or IV at diagnosis, and are more common in Black women. For example, papillary uterine serous carcinoma (USC) is a very aggressive tumor much like ovarian serous carcinoma. USC represents less than 10 percent of endometrial cancer cases, but accounts for 40 percent of deaths from endometrial carcinoma. Risk factors for these tumors are described in Table 15.3.

Risk factors for *uterine sarcomas* include Black race (for leiomyosarcoma), long-term tamoxifen use, and history of pelvic irradiation. Hereditary leiomyomatosis, renal cell carcinoma syndrome, and hereditary childhood retinoblastoma are genetic syndromes associated with uterine sarcoma.

Screening

There are currently no recommended routine screening tests to detect uterine cancer in asymptomatic patients. Routine Pap tests performed for cervical cancer may incidentally detect uterine cancers based upon the presence of abnormal cells, such as *atypical glandular cells* after further investigation is performed [28]. Patients at increased risk, including those on tamoxifen, should not receive surveillance ultrasonography or endometrial biopsy, except those with genetic syndromes. Imaging and EMB are invasive and expensive, cause discomfort, and have not been shown to save lives [29, 30]. Clinicians should "screen" for gynecologic cancer by asking about abnormal vaginal bleeding, pain, bloating, or masses on review of systems.

Clinical Presentation

Postmenopausal bleeding is the classical presentation of uterine cancer, though premenopausal women may present with *abnormal uterine bleeding (AUB)***.** Nearly 70 percent of cases are confined to the uterus at time of diagnosis with a 5-year survival rate of greater than 90 percent [5]. Women should be educated regarding symptoms of pain, bleeding, or fullness which might indicate the presence of a gynecologic abnormality or cancer and be asked to report such symptoms to their care providers.

Keesha reports that her bleeding is very light; she uses a panty liner a few times a week. A pelvic exam reveals a normal-sized uterus, no blood in the vaginal vault, and no abnormal lesions of the cervix, vagina, or vulvae. Bimanual exam is normal. There is no cervical motion tenderness, and testing for sexually transmitted infections and a stool guaiac are negative.

Evaluation and Diagnosis

Endometrial cancer most commonly presents as *postmenopausal bleeding***,** or as an *incidental Pap test abnormality* in women over age 55. In premenopausal women, especially those over age 45 or with BMI > 30, *abnormal uterine bleeding (AUB)*, defined as heavy menstrual bleeding or intermenstrual bleeding, may herald malignancy although a broad differential diagnosis exists (see Chap. 7 on "Abnormal Uterine Bleeding"). In *postmenopausal women*, all vaginal bleeding requires an evaluation to exclude malignancy. Similarly, all patients with *abnormal glandular cells* or *atypical endometrial cells* found incidentally on Pap test need an evaluation by gynecology. Further workup should include endometrial and endocervical sampling and/or colposcopy in addition to possible ultrasound or other tests to determine the source of the abnormal cells. In addition, any endometrial cells seen on a Pap in women who are postmenopausal should prompt further evaluation.

Given the impact of menopausal status on the physiology of vaginal bleeding and the increasing incidence of endometrial cancer with age, the evaluation of abnormal bleeding varies by the age of the patient. Seventy-seven percent of endometrial malignancies occur in women over 55, 16% in women 45–54 years of age, and only 7% in women under 44 years of age [5]. For postmenopausal women, a transvaginal ultrasound (TVUS) will usually exclude malignancy if the endometrial stripe is less than 4 mm [31]. A thicker stripe requires EMB, as does persistent bleeding (>3–6 months) with prior negative workup. In premenopausal women over 45, an EMB is needed after the exclusion of pregnancy. TVUS may be ordered to exclude structural lesions, but the endometrial stripe thicknesses on transvaginal ultrasound are nondiagnostic in premenopausal women and tissue sampling is needed. In women younger than 45-years-old with risk factors (see Table 15.3), evaluation with EMB should be performed after the exclusion of pregnancy [32] (see Chap. 7 on "Abnormal Uterine Bleeding").

Keesha is told that postmenopausal bleeding is abnormal and that additional testing is needed. She is worried and asks how likely it is that she has cancer.

Postmenopausal bleeding has many causes. The most common cause is endometrial atrophy. Atrophic changes can cause bleeding from the lower pelvic organs as well as the endometrium. Other benign causes include hyperplasia of the endometrium, polyps, fibroids, or hormonal therapy. Her risk of endometrial cancer is 3–20% [33, 34]. For a complete discussion, please see Chap. 7 on "Abnormal Uterine Bleeding", section on postmenopausal bleeding.

Transvaginal ultrasound reveals an endometrial stripe of 7 mm. Keesha is informed of the results, and an urgent referral to gynecology is requested for EMB. She is quite anxious and wonders what to expect.

Endometrial Biopsy

An *endometrial biopsy* (EMB) is typically a quick and simple procedure that occurs in a physician's office much like a Pap test or IUD insertion. The most popular method in the United States utilizes the thin plastic Pipelle (registered trademark) suction curette or equivalent device. Internists, family practitioners, and NPs can perform EMB with minimal training though most women are referred to gynecologists when EMB is needed. Pregnancy is excluded prior to the procedure and a dose of oral NSAID is often given 20–30 min prior to the EMB to minimize cramping. The patient assumes the dorsal lithotomy position and a speculum is inserted. The cervix is visualized and cleaned, and then the thin soft plastic Pipelle is inserted through the cervical os. Several samples are taken in succession by aspirating a small amount of endometrial tissue into the Pipelle from four to six sites on the sides of the uterine cavity. Providers should counsel patients that this may cause cramping. The Pipelle tip is not withdrawn from the os between samples. When sampling is complete, the Pipelle is withdrawn, the tissue is placed in fixative, and the specimen is sent to pathology for diagnosis. Cramping and bleeding are usually mild and self-limited, clearing rapidly after the procedure [35].

Endometrial Hyperplasia and Precancerous Lesions

Women with excess estrogen stimulation often develop *endometrial hyperplasia* which is most commonly diagnosed by *endometrial biopsy (EMB)***.** The clinical presentation of hyperplasia is identical to that of endometrial cancer, and the diagnosis is made pathologically by EMB. Traditionally, there were four types of endometrial hyperplasia, which were categorized as simple vs complex in terms of cell architecture and with or without atypia [36]. In 2015, the WHO revised its classification system into two categories: *hyperplasia without atypia (nonneoplastic)* and *atypical hyperplasia (endometrial intraepithelial neoplasm)* [37]. The *endometrial intraepithelial neoplasia classification* system is an alternate organizational schema [38]. The discussion of the various classifications is beyond the scope of this chapter.

Atypical hyperplasia is precancerous and has a high incidence of concurrent carcinoma (~42%) in an area of the uterus not sampled by the biopsy [39]. *Hyperplasia without atypia* has a <5% risk of concurrent malignancy [40, 41]. Hyperplasia with or without atypia is comanaged with a gynecologist. Sources of excess estrogen are eliminated, and treatment options include progestin therapy or hysterectomy. The desire for future fertility and surgical risk will guide management options. For women with atypical hyperplasia who have completed childbearing, hysterectomy is the safest option.

Strategies to *reduce estrogen exposure include* discontinuing medications containing estrogen, encouraging weight loss, and treating PCOS or hyperprolactinemia that leads to increased estrogen exposure from ovulatory dysfunction. In women not initially treated with hysterectomy, multiple options for administering progestins are available, including oral, intrauterine device (IUD), intramuscular (IM), and intravaginal preparations. Progesterone implants (i.e., Nexplanon™) have not been studied and are therefore not recommended. Common regimens include cyclic medoxyprogesterone 10 mg daily for 14 days per month, continuous megestrol acetate 20–40 mg daily, or a progestin-releasing IUD [42]. If progestins are used, response may be monitored with serial biopsies at 3- to 12-month intervals. Women with hyperplasia who fail medical therapy may undergo hysteroscopy with directed dilation and curettage to further evaluate for cancer.

Table 15.4 FIGO grading of endometrial carcinoma by histopathology [43]

	Meaning	Percentage of cases (%)	Classification
Grade 1	Well differentiated	50	Type I
Grade 2	Moderately differentiated	35	Type I
Grade 3	Poorly differentiated	15	Type II

A gynecologist evaluates Keesha and performs an EMB. The pathology report returns as adenocarcinoma. Keesha is referred to a gynecologic oncologist for staging and treatment which starts with a total hysterectomy and bilateral salpingo-oophorectomy. Following the diagnosis, Keesha calls and asks if she should start shopping for wigs in preparation for chemotherapy.

Patients who are diagnosed with endometrial carcinoma are referred to gynecologic oncologists for initial management and treatment planning. For more advanced cancers, radiation oncologists may help create a treatment plan. For patients requiring chemotherapy, in some centers, medical oncologists specializing in gynecologic cancers will provide patient care related to chemotherapy; in other centers, both surgical and chemotherapy management are managed by gynecologic oncologists. Patients often have questions about their diagnosis or potential treatment strategies as they await specialty appointments. The content included in this section may help primary care providers to help patients formulate appropriate questions and anticipate common treatments during that time.

Endometrial carcinoma is classified by the International Federation of Gynecology and Obstetrics (FIGO) grading and staging systems (see Table 15.4). Grading is based upon histology of biopsy specimens, which are rated as Grade 1, 2, or 3, and staging is divided into four categories depending upon the extent and spread of the disease (see section on "Staging" below). Grades 1 and 2 are classified as type I endometrial cancer, and Grade 3 is type II.

Staging

Prior to deciding on the treatment course, uterine cancer must be staged. Tumors are classified as low or high risk based on histopathology and grading. Endometrial cancer is not staged with imaging, but rather surgically via the joint

2010 International Federation of Gynecology and Obstetrics (FIGO)/TNM classification system. Complete physical exam, pelvic exam, and CXR to exclude pulmonary metastases are performed. Imaging with MRI is primarily ordered for women who are not surgical candidates or for those who wish to preserve fertility.

Standard staging surgery is a total hysterectomy with bilateral salpingo-oophorectomy with or without pelvic and para-aortic lymph node dissection. The ovaries and cervix are removed because they may contain endometrial cancer cells ("total" hysterectomy indicates removal of the cervix). There is no consensus on which patients require lymph node staging, or what constitutes an adequate lymphadenectomy in regards to the number of nodes removed and extent of lymphadenectomy. Lymph node resection can lead to lymphedema, which is a troubling side effect for endometrial cancer survivors. Because of the risks associated with comprehensive lymphadectomy, investigators now commonly employ sentinel lymph node dissections with fluorescent dye and infrared cameras. This universal and targeted approach has been prospectively validated and is a part of the NCCN guidelines [44].

Treatment Strategies

Early-stage endometrial cancer is treated with curative-intent surgery. As the disease advances, radiation and/or chemotherapy may also become necessary.

Premenopausal women who wish to preserve fertility with stage I disease can sometimes be treated by hysterectomy with preservation of the ovaries. Conservative management of women with atypical endometrial hyperplasia or endometrial cancer to preserve future fertility is controversial given the risk of disease progression. There are reports of therapeutic success with progesterone therapy [45]. Such patients should be closely followed by gynecologic oncology. The acceptance and availability of frozen oocytes and ovarian tissue cryopreservation are promising technologies which further inform this type of decision [46].

The vast majority of women with endometrial cancer will undergo simple hysterectomy with or without removal of the ovaries and fallopian tubes. Rarely radical hysterectomies can be utilized if cervical involvement is suspected on preoperative exam, biopsy, or imaging to spare the patient the need for postoperative radiation, but this practice is uncommon and has not been widely validated [47]. The various types of hysterectomies that can be performed range from type I to type V and the surgical nuances are beyond the scope of this chapter. A type I hysterectomy is simple, and type III is radical (Table 15.5).

Table 15.5 Types of hysterectomy

Type of hysterectomy	Supracervical	Simple	Radical
Description	Removal of uterine body; cervix left in place	Uterus, cervix, fallopian tubes, and ovaries removed	Total hysterectomy and BSO, plus removal of parametrium[a] and upper 1/3 of vagina
Sample indications	Benign conditions	Endometrial cancer, early-stage cervical cancer, ovarian cancer	Stage IA2 to IIA cervical cancer

[a]Connective tissue surrounding the uterus

TAHBSO is commonly used to refer to total hysterectomy and bilateral salpingo-oophorectomy. Technically, this is incorrect as the "A" stands for abdominal and this method is used less today. In endometrial cancer, the use of laparoscopy has been shown to have equivalent oncologic outcomes with decreased surgical morbidity when compared to open surgery [48]. The newer terminology commonly used is TLH/BSO. The DaVinci™ Robotic platform is a commonly used tool to complete laparoscopic staging for endometrial cancer though outcomes appear to be similar to nonrobotic laparoscopy at a significantly higher cost [49].

At diagnosis, approximately 72% of endometrial cancers are stage I, 12% are stage II, 13% are stage III, and 3% are stage IV [50, 51]. Carcinoma in situ is a precancerous lesion and is not included in the FIGO staging system. The prognosis depends primarily on the stage of the tumor as well as histology and grade. Table 15.6 summarizes the FIGO staging for endometrial carcinoma, 5-year survival rate, and usual treatment.

Many stage I–III tumors require the use of radiation and chemotherapy. Radiation therapy may take the form of internal therapy with vaginal brachytherapy or external beam pelvic radiation. If external been radiation is used, and ovarian preservation is desired, the ovaries can be surgically moved out of the field of radiation. Radiation therapy often has the unwanted side effects of cystitis, proctitis, and vaginal changes.

For metastatic or recurrent disease, chemotherapeutic regimens containing a combination of cisplatin or carboplatin, doxorubicin, and/or paclitaxel are often recommended. These chemotherapy agents have numerous side effects including nausea and vomiting, hematologic suppression, and temporary hair loss. Renal toxicity and cardiotoxicity are feared complications. Women with stage IV disease for whom there is no curative intent may be treated with hormonal treatments including tamoxifen or aromatase inhibi-

Table 15.6 Endometrial cancer prognosis and treatment by stage [50, 51]

Stage	Proportion of women at this stage at time of diagnosis (%)	Description	5-year survival rate (%)	Usual treatment
I	72	Tumor limited to the body of the uterus (limited to endometrium or showing only superficial invasion of myometrium)	90	Hysterectomy/BSO +/− radiation if high-risk features on biopsy
II	12	Tumor has spread to the cervical stroma (involving the cervix or invading deeply into the myometrium)	69	Hysterectomy, possible radical hysterectomy[a] with or without postoperative radiation
III	13	Tumor extends beyond the confines of the uterus but not outside the pelvis	50	Hysterectomy/BSO with lymph node dissection, radiation, and/or chemotherapy
IV	3	Tumor extends outside the pelvis +/− distant metastases	15	No curative intent. Palliation includes primary chemotherapy, attempted debulking, hormonal therapy with progestins, tamoxifen or aromatase inhibitors

tors which are generally well tolerated. Further discussion of stage II–IV is beyond the scope of this chapter.

Keesha returns 6 months after her surgery with total hysterectomy and bilateral salpingo-oophorectomy. She was diagnosed with stage 1 endometrial adenocarcinoma with low-grade histology (type I). She has a follow-up appointment with her gynecologic oncologist later that week but wonders why she does not have to do any imaging or lab work beforehand "like my friend with breast cancer."

Survivorship Care

The greatest risk of recurrence in endometrial cancer patients is within the first 2 years after treatment. The most common site of recurrence for stage I disease is the vagina. Following therapy, patients should be seen every 3–4 months for 2 years by a gynecologic oncologist to assess for symptoms of recurrence and then every 6 months for the next 3 years. Physical exam includes speculum and bimanual pelvic exam. Most vaginal recurrences are treated with radiation therapy. Vaginal Pap tests are no longer recommended as the sensitivity is poor [52]. Cytology is affected by radiation which decreases the yield and sensitivity of Pap tests.

Surveillance imaging is obtained only if there are signs or symptoms of recurrence. Whole-body PET/CT scanning is the imaging modality of choice [53].

During treatment, women are typically comanaged by their primary care provider and oncologist. After treatment, depending on institutional resources, the primary care clinician may be responsible for monitoring women for symptoms of disease recurrence and assisting women in coping with the long-term sequelae of therapy: treatment-induced menopause, anxiety and depression, bowel and bladder issues, surgical adhesions, and issues with sex or intimacy. Women who have received radiation are more likely to have bowel or bladder symptoms, especially in the first 1–2 years. A full discussion is found in the section on survivor care at the end of the chapter.

Ovarian Cancer

Cindy, a 30-year-old G2P2, presents for an urgent care visit. Three weeks ago, her mother was diagnosed with advanced ovarian cancer at age 50. Her mother is an only child whose parents died in a car accident many years ago. Cindy is very upset and wants to learn more about her risk of ovarian cancer.

Overview

Ovarian cancer has the highest fatality rate of the gynecologic malignancies [6]. This is because ovarian cancer may be asymptomatic or present with vague abdominal symptoms, delaying diagnosis until it is at an advanced stage. There is no validated method for screening asymptomatic women of average risk although several, including transvaginal ultrasound (TVUS) and serum CA 125 levels, alone and in combination, have been studied [54–56]. Multiple large prospective trials have studied routine transvaginal ultrasound with or without CA-125 as possible screening modalities. Though some stage shift has been described (i.e., cancer diagnosis at early stages), no trial has demonstrated a survival benefit. Routine screening in an asymptomatic, low-risk population is therefore not recommended. Suspected ovarian cancer cannot be biopsied given the risk of seeding the peritoneum; the mass must be removed en bloc. Any proposed screening strategy must therefore have high specificity since any positive test requires confirmatory surgery. The best current defenses against ovarian cancer include screening for genetic susceptibilities and maintaining a high index of suspicion when patients present with vague symptoms.

Epidemiology

Ovarian cancer is the leading cause of death from a gynecologic malignancy and has surpassed cervical cancer as the second most common type of gynecologic cancer in the United States, likely due to improved cervical cancer screening [6, 7] (see Table 15.1). Despite overall advances in ovarian cancer treatment, mortality is essentially unchanged over the past three decades [57]. The average age at diagnosis is 63 years old, with a 1.3% lifetime risk of developing the disease in women of average risk [6]. When caught early, survival rates improve markedly; however, screening is ineffective, and most patients are not diagnosed until metastatic symptoms appear. If ovarian cancer is found incidentally and treated in stage 1, the 5-year survival rate is approximately 90%. Unfortunately, only 15% of ovarian cancers are diagnosed at this stage [6]. In contrast, stage IV patients with distant metastasis at diagnosis have a 25% survival rate at 5 years [6].

Pathophysiology

Ninety-five percent of ovarian tumors originate from the epithelial ovarian cells and are referred to as epithelial ovarian carcinoma [58]. The most common type of epithelial ovarian cancer is *high-grade serous carcinoma*. High-grade serous carcinomas of the ovary, fallopian tube, and peritoneum have identical pathologic characteristics and clinical behavior and therefore are treated in the same manner both in clinical practice and trials [59]. Recent data from women undergoing prophylactic bilateral salpingo-oophorectomy for BRCA gene mutations has revealed precursor neoplastic lesions in the fallopian tubes leading some investigators to assert that the fallopian tube may be the organ of origin for a significant subset of ovarian and peritoneal cancers [59, 60]. The remainder of nonepithelial ovarian cancers arise from the germ and stromal cells in the ovary. While sex cord stromal tumors affect women of all ages, germ cell tumors are more common in adolescents (see Table 15.7).

Cindy asks if she is at increased risk for ovarian cancer and whether she should go for genetic testing. She is asymptomatic and G2P2 and has never taken OCPs. Family history reveals that aside from her mother, no one else in the family has had ovarian cancer; neither she nor her mother has siblings. A paternal great aunt had breast cancer in her 70s, and there is no other family history of breast cancer or other cancers in men or women. Her ethnic background is Pakistani, with no Ashkenazi Jewish grandparents.

Risk Factors

Ovarian cancer risk is increased primarily through genetic factors, inflammation, and uninterrupted ovulation. *BRCA mutations*, *Lynch syndrome*, and *Ashkenazi Jewish heritage* have all been linked to ovarian cancer. *BRCA1* mutation carriers have a 44% lifetime risk of ovarian cancer, and *BRCA 2* mutation carriers have a 17% lifetime risk [61]. Patients who test positive for BRCA 1 or 2 or Lynch syndrome should be referred to specialty care to consider a prophylactic bilateral salpingo-oophorectomy (see Chap. 17 on "The Primary Prevention of Breast Cancer"). Prophylactic surgery is preferably performed prior to 35–40 years of age, but after a woman has completed her desired childbearing. *Endometriosis*, *cigarette smoking*, and *PCOS* lead to increased ovarian cancer risk, likely related to chronic inflammation leading to cellular damage and the need for repair [62]. Errors in copying the genetic code in the DNA repair process are thought to lead to increased cancer risk [62, 63].

Ovarian rest, or time spent without ovulation events, decreases the risk of ovarian cancer. When cells do not divide in the ovulation process, there is less risk of introducing error when copying the genetic code. *Parity* and *breastfeeding* both increase ovarian rest and are associated with decreased risk. Notably, *combined oral contraceptives* which inhibit

Table 15.7 Malignant ovarian tumors

Tumor type	Cells of origin	Epidemiology	Malignant subtypes
Epithelial tumors (epithelial ovarian carcinoma)	Epithelial ovarian cells	95% of malignant ovarian tumors are epithelial ovarian carcinoma	Serous (most common), clear cell, mucinoid, and endometrioid epithelial carcinomas
Germ cell tumors	Ova	2% of malignant ovarian tumors. Typically impact young women and girls. Best prognosis	Immature teratomas, dysgerminomas, choriocarcinomas, and endodermal sinus (yolk sac) tumors
Sex cord stromal tumors	Ovarian stroma (granulosa, theca, Sertoli, and Leydig cells; fibroblasts)	1% of malignant ovarian tumors. More common in postmenopausal women. Some produce estrogen or androgens	Granulosa cell (most common), Sertoli-Leydig

ovulation decrease risk by 50% when used for at least 10 years [64]. Tubal ligation and salpingo-oophorectomy also reduce risk. Tubal ligation may be a proxy for multiparty. IUDs likely "increase" risk because ovulation does not cease with IUD use as it does with oral contraceptive pills (see Table 15.8).

Patients with a strong family history of breast and ovarian cancer should be referred for *genetic counseling* and possible testing. Notably, *genetic evaluation and possible testing are recommended for anyone with a personal history of ovarian cancer*, as well as anyone with a close relative with ovarian cancer when testing the affected family member is not possible. A close relative is a first-, second-, or third-degree relation. Multiple organizations have issued guidelines, including the American Cancer Society (ACS), the United States Preventive Services Task Force (USPSTF), and the National Comprehensive Cancer Network (NCCN).

The decision of whom to refer for genetic counseling and testing ultimately resides with the physician and patient on an individualized basis. Of note, genetic testing is now increasingly available to patients with home kits and send away DNA tests such as 23andMe™ which may bypass the initial consultation by the genetic counselor. Patients may be referred to genetic counselors, or to gynecologic oncology, to discuss the implications of DNA tests obtained through outside sources. It should be noted that commercial DNA tests are not validated and are not a substitute for the testing ordered by a certified genetic counselor. The results may not be accurate or may only cover a few mutations or genetic variations for a given syndrome (see Chap. 17 on "The Primary Prevention of Breast Cancer" for further information on genetic syndromes and genetic screening).

Table 15.8 Risk factors and protective factors in ovarian cancer [65–72]

Factors associated with increased risk of ovarian cancer	Factors associated with decreased risk of ovarian cancer
Increasing age Nulliparity Infertility Endometriosis PCOS Smoking Use of an intrauterine device Cigarette smoking (mucinous carcinomas) Lynch syndrome BRCA1 and 2 Ashkenazi Jewish heritage	Previous pregnancy History of breastfeeding Oral contraceptives Tubal ligation Salpingo-oophorectomy

Cindy is informed that she and her mother should be referred to a genetic counselor and that ovarian cancer screening with ultrasound, CA125, or other testing is not recommended, even for women at "increased" risk. If she is found to have a BRCA or a Lynch syndrome mutation, she would be considered "high" risk, and prophylactic salpingo-oophorectomy or other surgery should be considered. She wonders what symptoms she should "watch out for" and what the downside would be to a transvaginal ultrasound, which was how her mother's mass was found.

Screening

At present, there is no effective screening test for ovarian cancer. CA-125 levels and TVUS have been studied both together and separately, but are not sufficiently specific to justify routine screening. A persistent challenge in identifying an appropriate screening test is that, with current diagnostic methods, any positive screening test would then likely necessitate a laparoscopy or laparotomy for further investigation. A suspected ovarian cancer cannot be biopsied; it must be removed intact to avoid seeding the peritoneal cavity. Although ovarian cancer carries a high mortality, given that these procedures are associated with morbidity and the overall prevalence of ovarian cancer is low, the risks outweigh the benefits for available screening methods [55]. Several large, prospective randomized trials have examined the role of CA-125 and TVUS for ovarian cancer screening in asymptomatic women and all failed to lead to statistically significant mortality reduction and therefore did not reach their end points [73]. A test that looks for shed ovarian and endometrial tumor cells in endocervical brushings is currently being investigated, but will face the same challenges [74].

The UK Collaborative Trial of Ovarian Screening is the largest randomized trial of both CA125 and TVUS methods to date and showed a nonsignificant 15% reduction in mortality from ovarian cancer with multimodal CA-125 screening (95% CI −3 to 30 p = 0.10) [75]. The trial randomized approximately 200,000 women of average ovarian cancer risk into three groups: annual CA-125 screening, annual transvaginal ultrasound, and no screening. Women in the first group were further stratified into normal CA-125 levels, indeterminate CA-125 levels, and elevated CA-125 levels. Women with indeterminate CA-125 levels had a repeat CA-125 drawn in 3 months, and women with elevated CA-125 levels were evaluated with transvaginal ultrasound. Findings from the trial suggest that one ovarian cancer death may be prevented by screening 641 women with CA-125 levels on an annual basis for 14 years. The investigators observed that there were more stage I and II cancers observed in the experimental arm suggesting a promising stage migration signal, though this did not translate into a survival benefit. The long term follow-up phase is in process.

Pelvic exam is not sensitive or specific enough to be a reliable method of screening for ovarian cancer, as it does not reliably correlate with ultrasound or surgical findings, even among experienced providers [76–78].

High-risk women with known genetic predispositions may benefit from screening in selected circumstances. A women with BRCA 1 or 2, or Lynch syndrome, who has rejected or wishes to postpone surgery, may be screened with serial TVUS and/or CA-125 in coordination with a gynecologic oncologist [79].

Clinical Presentation

Traditionally, ovarian cancer has been considered to be asymptomatic until the late stages. However, a sizable number of women may have symptoms in early disease that are missed. Ovarian cancer patients present with abdominal and gastrointestinal symptoms such as bloating in over 70% of cases, pain in 58% of cases, constitutional symptoms in 50% of cases, urinary symptoms in 34% of cases, and pelvic symptoms in 26% of cases [80]. A symptom index has been developed to determine which women should be evaluated for ovarian cancer. Any of the following symptoms present more than 12 times per month for less than 1 year is considered a positive screen: abdominal or pelvic symptoms of pain, bloating, increased abdominal size, and changes in appetite or early satiety [80].

Evaluation and Diagnosis

Physical examination should include an abdominal exam (attention to masses in the lower abdomen), breast exam, pelvic exam, rectal exam with stool guaiac, and lymph node exam (attention to inguinal and supraclavicular nodes). Imaging of patients with pelvic or lower abdominal symptoms begins with a TVUS which visualizes the ovaries and pelvic structures. If the TVUS is negative, and no other explanation is found, patients should undergo an abdominal/pelvic CT and possible colonoscopy or urinary tract evaluation to evaluate all possible sources of the symptoms. Ovarian cancer can present as peritoneal carcinoma alone or as an incidental finding on imaging done for another purpose. A CA-125 should not be checked until concern for ovarian cancer is established by imaging. If a suspicious lesion is identified on exam or imaging, the patient is referred to a gynecologic oncologist for urgent evaluation and surgical staging.

Ovarian cancer is a histologic diagnosis that is made via a laparoscopy or laparotomy with surgical removal of the ovary and fallopian tube, peritoneal lymph node biopsies, and/or pelvic washings. Masses suspicious for ovarian cancer must be removed intact – puncturing an ovarian mass for a biopsy could lead to seeding throughout the peritoneal cavity and therefore a worse prognosis. Preoperatively, abdominal and pelvic imaging with CT or MRI may be used for surgical planning. A CXR is obtained to exclude metastasis.

Staging and Treatment Strategies

Ovarian cancer staging is based on operative findings (see Table 15.9). For more advanced cases, surgery is used for cytoreduction prior to beginning platinum-based chemotherapy. The administration of chemotherapy prior to cytoreductive surgery (neoadjuvant) has been shown to have noninferior survival outcomes compared to surgery followed by chemotherapy allowing the clinician discretion based on patient factors to decide how to best sequence care [81]. Regardless of stage or the interval nature of chemotherapy, patients who have high-quality, "optimal" debulking surgeries that remove as much tumor as possible have increased survival rates.

Chemotherapy regimens typically include paclitaxel plus carboplatin and may be given intrapertonially and/or intravenously. *Intraperitonal chemotherapy* is introduced through an abdominal catheter and allows for higher doses of chemotherapeutic agents with lesser effects on healthy tissue. Side effects are related to the chemotherapy drugs (neuropathy and nephrotoxicity being most common), the port (catheter malfunction), or the mechanism of infusion (abdominal pain from instilling a large amount of fluid).

Survivorship Care

Following the completion of treatment, patients should be seen in the office for a history, general physical, and pelvic exam to monitor for recurrence. A pelvic exam should be performed every 2–4 months for 2 years, then every 3–6 months for 3 years, and then annually after 5 years. CA-125 levels, if they were elevated during the time of active disease, are typically checked at these visits following discussions between women and their clinicians on both the pros and cons of these measurements. A rise in CA-125 often but does not always signal recurrence, and following these levels has not been found to impact survival [84]. Other laboratory testing and imaging are obtained only as clinically indicated, such as to investigate a concerning symptom, exam findings, or rising CA-125 level. If not already completed, survivors should be referred for genetic counseling and undergo prophylactic mastectomy if appropriate. If the cervix was removed during surgery, Pap tests are no longer required.

Many survivors have ongoing sequelae from treatment. Neurotoxicity from platinum-based chemotherapy, gastroin-

Table 15.9 Ovarian cancer staging, 5-year survival, and treatment [82]

FIGO stage	Stage description[a]	5-year survival (%) [83]	Treatment
IA IB IC1,2,3	The cancer is only in the ovary (or ovaries) or fallopian tube(s) IA – Confined to one ovary, no surface involvement, no rupture upon removal IB – Both ovaries, no surface involvement, no rupture upon removal IC1 – Confined to one or both ovaries, surgical spill IC2 – Confined to one or both ovaries, capsule rupture prior to surgery, surface involvement IC3 – malignant cells in pelvic wash	78–93	If completely resected, observation. If high-risk features, treated with three to six cycles of platinum-based chemotherapy
IIA IIB	The cancer is in one or both ovaries or fallopian tubes and has spread to other organs within the pelvis (such as the uterus, bladder, sigmoid colon, or rectum) IIA – Extension or implant into uterus or fallopian tubes IIB – Extension or implant into other pelvic organs	61–82	If completely resected, adjuvant chemotherapy, typically paclitaxel plus carboplatin, for six cycles
IIIA IIIB IIIC	No longer confined to the pelvis; has spread into the abdomen IIIA1 – Cancer spread to pelvic and/or para-aortic lymph nodes IIIA2 – Microscopic tumor involvement in upper abdominal tissues or organs IIIB – Macroscopic tumor <2 cm in size involving upper abdominal tissues or organs IIIC – Macroscopic tumor >2 cm in size involving upper abdominal tissues or organs	28–63	Surgical cytoreduction, intravenous or intraperitoneal adjuvant platinum-based chemotherapy, consideration of maintenance therapy with poly ADP-ribose polymerase inhibitors (PARPi) or bevacizumab
IVA IVB	The cancer has spread to the inside of the spleen or liver, or outside the abdomen IVA – Malignant pleural effusion IVB – Parenchymal liver or spleen metastasis, distant metastasis	19	Platinum-based chemotherapy before or after surgical cytoreduction, consideration of maintenance therapy with PARPi or bevacizumab

testinal symptoms from surgery, abrupt menopause from ovarian removal, and sexual dysfunction are among the many common symptoms. For a full discussion, please see the section on survivorship care at the end of the chapter.

Cervical Cancer

Cindy is a 44-year-old G4P4 woman with a history of obesity and AUB. She had her last child at age 34 and presents to the office to establish care because "I haven't had a physical since my gynecologist put that copper IUD in 10 years ago. I think it's time to take it out." In the past she was HPV positive on screening, but was lost to follow-up. She has always had heavy periods, but now she notices that she is having bleeding after intercourse.

Overview

Cervical cancer is the only gynecologic cancer with a screening test, and all women should be screened with Pap and/or HPV testing using evidence-based guidelines (see Chap. 14 on "Cervical Cancer and Human Papillomavirus"). Most precancerous cervical abnormalities are diagnosed by screening, and thus, invasive cervical cancer is relatively uncommon in developed countries. For those who do not undergo screening, are lost to follow-up, or who live in low- and middle-income countries, cervical cancer is still a significant cause of mortality. Cervical cancer classically presents with postcoital bleeding.

Epidemiology

Worldwide, over 500,000 women are diagnosed with cervical cancer each year; of those, over half will die of the disease [85, 86]. The majority of cases (>85%) occur in low- and middle-income countries where cervical cancer is the second most common cancer in women, compared to being the 16th most common cancer in US women [4]. Cervical cancer incidence peaks between the ages of 48 and 55, and the peak incidence of carcinoma in situ is between the ages of 25 and 40. It is estimated that 50% of invasive cervical cancer is diagnosed in women who have never had a Pap test, who have not received cervical cancer screening for 5–10 years, or who have been lost to follow-up after an abnormal Pap [87].

Pathophysiology and Risk Factors

High-risk HPV (hrHPV) is the underlying cause of 99% of cervical cancers, including squamous, adenosquamous, and adenocarcinomas [85, 88]. When a woman's immune system does not clear HPV from her body, the persistent viral infection leads to cellular atypia and slowly occurring premalignant cellular changes in the basal layer in the cervical epithelium over time [88]. The length of time of hrHPV infection, age, immunosuppressive conditions, multiparity, multiple partners, long-term oral contraceptive use, coinfection with other sexually transmitted infections, and smoking increase the risk of progression to cervical intraepithelial neoplasia 3 (CIN3) [86, 89]. HPV-16 infections have the lowest 18-month clearance rates and carry the highest likelihood of progression to CIN3 or cervical cancer compared to other hrHPV infections [89] (see Chap. 14 on "Cervical Cancer and Human Papillomavirus").

Diethylstilbestrol (*DES*) exposure also increases cervical cancer risk and may impact women born prior to 1971. DES was a "synthetic estrogen" prescribed to pregnant women from 1938 to 1971 when it was thought to prevent miscarriage and preterm birth. Women exposed to DES in utero should follow a specialized screening protocol.

Screening

Cervical cancer is the only gynecologic cancer with a routine screening test for average-risk women. Pap testing detects the vast majority of cervical cancers and precursor lesions, where resources are available.

Clinical Presentation

Women who are screened regularly for cervical cancer rarely present with clinical signs and symptoms. Women who have not been screened adequately, and develop invasive cervical cancer, may present with postcoital bleeding, pain, unprovoked vaginal bleeding, or foul-smelling discharge.

A Pap test and HPV co-test are obtained, as well as a cervical culture. Cindy's Pap result returns suspicious for invasive cervical cancer, + HPV 16. She is devastated and wonders how this could happen to her and whether she is going to die from this. She asks what to do next.

Evaluation and Diagnosis

In high-income countries, abnormal Pap tests that are positive for *hrHPV* are typically referred to a gynecologist for colposcopy and biopsy of suspicious lesions. It is important that women return for follow-up and complete treatments in a timely manner. High-grade biopsy results or carcinomatous findings are referred to gynecologic oncologists for evaluation and treatment.

In low-resource settings where the Pap test is not available, women may be screened by "visual inspection with acetic acid" (VIA) in which the cervix is inspected for acetowhite lesions indicative of HPV infection or premalignant or malignant lesions. The "see and treat" approach further treats visible lesions with cryotherapy without cervical biopsy or pathology [88]. These approaches lack sensitivity and specificity and have disadvantages, but lives are saved with these programs when screening with Pap, colposcopy, and biopsy are not available.

Staging

The clinical staging of cervical cancer is accomplished by pelvic exam, biopsy, and imaging. Imaging to assess for metastases and lymph node involvement is most often PET-CT or PET-MRI [90]. Staging follows the FIGO system [91]. The prognosis worsens with advanced stages and metastases – early-stage localized disease has a 91% 5-year survival rate, whereas locally advanced and metastatic cervical cancer 5-year survival rates are far lower (57% and 16%, respectively), with a median survival of 8–13 months [85, 90] (see Table 15.10). Cervical cancer metastasizes in two ways: hematogenous metastases and lymphatic metastasis. Hematogenous metastases carry a worse prognosis.

Cindy is referred for colposcopy and biopsy, which confirm invasive cervical cancer with extension to the margins. A pelvic MRI reveals no extension of disease beyond the cervix. She is referred to a gynecologic oncologist, who recommends total hysterectomy.

Treatment Strategies

The treatment of cervical cancer depends upon the stage. Preinvasive disease (CIN3 and CIS) is treated with LEEP or conization. In a LEEP (loop endocervical excision procedure), the speculum is inserted, a paracervical block is applied, and acetic acid is placed on the cervix to highlight abnormal tissue. A small metal loop heated with an electric current then slices an ovoid tissue specimen containing abnormal cells, much like a wire cheese cutter takes a slice from a block of cheese. A second swipe deeper into the endocervical canal can then effectively replicate a conization procedure, removing the transformation zone. A LEEP is an outpatient office procedure that removes less tissue than a cold-knife conization, which is typically performed in an ambulatory

Table 15.10 Cervical cancer staging, prognosis, and treatment [7, 92, 93]

Stage	Description	5-year survival (%)	Treatment[a]
I	The cancer has not grown beyond the cervix	80–93	Dependent on disease extension and desire for future fertility. Options: conization, simple hysterectomy, radical trachelectomy, radical hysterectomy, radiotherapy, chemoradiation
II	The cancer has grown beyond the cervix but has not spread to the walls of the pelvis or lower part of the vagina	58–63	Radical hysterectomy for a subset of stage II patients; radiosensitizing chemotherapy with concurrent radiation therapy
III	The carcinoma involves the lower third of the vagina and/or extends to the pelvic wall and/or causes hydronephrosis or nonfunctioning kidney and/or involves pelvic and/or para-aortic lymph nodes	32–35	Radiosensitizing chemotherapy and volume-directed concurrent radiation
IV	The carcinoma has extended beyond the true pelvis or has involved the mucosa of the bladder or rectum (biopsy proven)	15–16	Platinum-based systemic chemotherapy with antiangiogenic agents, palliative radiation, immune checkpoint inhibitors

surgery suite. Conization uses a scapel or laser to remove a "cone" of tissue at the os. Hysterectomy may be considered in women for whom future childbearing is not a concern.

The treatment of invasive cervical cancer depends upon the degree of lymphovascular invasion and the patient's desire for future fertility. Fertility-sparing treatments may be safely performed in patients with early disease, but are not recommended in patients with locally advanced or metastatic cancer [85]. In early-stage cancers, conization +/− lymph node sampling or trachelectomy (a surgery that removes the cervix, upper portion of the vagina, and pelvic lymph nodes) may be possible for women who desire future fertility. Women who have finished childbearing and have pelvic confined disease (stage < IIB) can undergo simple or radical hysterectomy or definitive radiation with curative intent. Treatment of metastases is based on location and may involve surgery, chemoradiotherapy, radiation, or chemotherapy. The multitude of treatment modalities highlight the importance of referring women to experienced gynecologic oncologists for optimal care [85, 90, 92].

During treatment, the patient is managed by a gynecologic oncologist. The role of the primary care clinician during active treatment is primarily supportive: assisting in the management of complications and treating other medical conditions.

Cindy undergoes total hysterectomy with close follow-up by her gynecologic oncologist. She is doing well and wants to discuss long-term plans and side effects of treatment.

Survivorship Care

Patients with cervical cancer are monitored by gynecologic oncologists for at least 5 years following treatment. Recurrence, if and when it occurs, is typically local or regional. Patients should be reassured that the prognosis is typically favorable, even with locally advanced disease, and that cervical cancer is not inheritable. It is important to set a clear follow-up plan, especially when care is returned to the primary care provider. The cancer survivor plan should be made in conjunction with the gynecologic oncologist and include specifications for the frequency of Pap testing, when it is safe to space out Pap tests beyond 1 year, and when to eventually stop. There are no set guidelines, but many gynecologic oncologists continue annual Pap tests until age 65, followed by every other year Pap tests as long as there is an expected life expectancy of 5 years or more [94].

Approximately 30–50% of patients will have treatment failure or recurrence, which is more common with large tumors and with involved pelvic and para-aortic lymph nodes [95]. If recurrence is suspected, PET-CT is the recommended imaging modality. When recurrence is limited to the cervix or vagina, curative intent surgery and radiation are the treatments of choice. Surgery is often chosen in patients who had prior radiation therapy. Radiation is the treatment of choice in patients without prior radiation, or who are not surgical candidates. Metastatic disease that is not amendable to surgery or radiation is treated with cisplatin, paclitaxel, and bevacizumab.

Most cervical cancer patients have a good prognosis and may return to primary care with long-term quality of life issues that are sequelae of therapy. Cervical cancer survivors are able to take estrogen treatment, if needed, since cervical cancer is not related to estrogen exposure (see section below on care of the cancer survivor). If and when it appears likely that the patient will survive for at least another 5–10 years, then routine screening for other malignancies should resume.

Studies are underway on the utility of using therapeutic HPV vaccination in cervical cancer patients as a treatment modality. These studies use formulations of HPV vaccinations (not those in current use) which stimulate cellular immunity [96].

Vulvar and Vaginal Cancers

Aditi is a 62-year-old woman who presents for her annual physical exam. She is due for a Pap test. On pelvic exam, a 5-mm white plaque is seen on her vulva. The lesion was not previously noted in the record and Aditi was not aware of it.

Overview

Vulvar and vaginal cancers, the least common of the gynecologic cancers, typically present as asymptomatic lesions, or with pruritus, pain, or vaginal bleeding. Because the morphology of malignant lesions is variable, *any lesion of the vulva or vagina that is not obviously benign must be biopsied for definitive diagnosis.* Most vulvar and vaginal malignancies are squamous cell cancers related to *hrHPV* or *lichen sclerosis* of the vulva.

Epidemiology

Vulvar cancer is the fourth most common gynecologic malignancy (after uterine, ovarian, and cervical). US women have a 0.3% lifetime risk of being diagnosed with vulvar cancer, and the average age at diagnosis is 68 years [8]. Nearly 60% of vulvar cancers are confined to the primary site at diagnosis, 30% show regional spread, and 6% have distant metastasis. Survival for women in the United States with vulvar cancer is 72.1% at 5 years. Seventy-five percent are squamous cell carcinomas; other types include melanoma, basal cell carcinoma, clear cell carcinoma, Bartholin gland adenocarcinoma, sarcoma, and Paget's disease [97].

Vaginal cancer is the least common gynecologic malignancy. Metastatic disease to the vagina is more common than primary cancers of the vagina. The mean age at diagnosis for primary vaginal carcinoma is 60 years. Most lesions (83%) are squamous cell carcinoma [98]. In utero *DES* exposure and *hrHPV* are known risk factors. Other subtypes include adenocarcinoma, sarcoma, clear cell carcinoma, and melanoma.

Pathophysiology and Risk Factors

hrHPV is a major risk factor for vulvar and vaginal cancers. Persistent HPV infection may lead to precancerous changes in the vulva and vagina similar to precancerous abnormalities in the cervix with atypia, intraepithelial neoplasia, and carcinoma in situ (see tables below). The cervix, vagina, vulva, anus, and rectum to the dentate line are all derived from the same embryonic tissue which matures into squamous epithelia. These tissues are susceptible to persistent HPV infection which can cause neoplastic changes. The metabolically active transformation zone of the cervix is more vulnerable to neoplastic changes due to HPV than the vulva or vagina, which are covered by stable, mature squamous tissue – leading to high rates of cervical cancer compared to vaginal and vulvar cancer. Cigarette smoking, HIV infection, and immunosuppression are cofactors which increase the risk of HPV-related cancer.

Women with in situ *DES* exposure can have metaplastic tissue in the vagina and are at increased risk of vaginal cancers, including clear cell carcinoma.

Chronic inflammatory processes such as *lichen sclerosis* elevate the risk of vulvar malignancy due to increased cell turnover, which leads to greater chances for errors in DNA replication. Although hrHPV is responsible for the majority of vulvar intraepithelial changes on biopsy, tissues with lichen sclerosis give rise to the majority of malignancies. Lichen sclerosis should be treated to reduce risk of progression to malignancy, and all women found to have premalignant or malignant lesions should be counseled to stop smoking (see Chap. 12 on "Vaginitis and Vulvar Conditions").

Screening

There is no validated screening test for vulvar or vaginal cancer. Women should be encouraged to report any abnormalities which develop in the perineal region or vagina. All vulvar and vaginal complaints need evaluation with inspection, palpation, and diagnostic testing.

As noted above, women with a history of *DES* exposure should have annual vaginal cytology. Women with *lichen sclerosis* should be followed by a gynecologist or dermatologist who specializes in this area for annual exams given the risk of progression to squamous cell carcinoma in lichen sclerosis.

Acetic acid is applied to the vulvar lesion and it turns white. Aditi consents to take a secure photo of the lesion for her medical chart. Aditi is told that she will need a referral and probable biopsy to determine the cause of the lesion. She is agreeable, and arrangements are made for her to see a gynecologist next week. Aditi is understandably anxious and asks what to expect.

Clinical Presentation, Evaluation, and Diagnosis

Vulvar cancer is often asymptomatic, but may present with pruritus or palpable lesions. Vulvar cancer should also be suspected in women with persistent vaginal itching refractory to treatment. *Vaginal cancer* typically presents with vaginal bleeding or discharge, but may be asymptomatic [99]. Bleeding is usually scant spotting or postcoital.

Review of systems at annual visits should contain questions regarding vulvar, vaginal, or pelvic pain, lesions, pruritus, discharge, and bleeding (see Chap. 3 on "Sex and Gender Specific History and Examination"). Exams should include inspection of the vulva, as with the rest of the skin, even when internal pelvic examinations are not performed. Since many dermatologists do not include the vulva in their complete skin exam, the primary care clinician should be sure women are monitored for lesions or abnormalities.

During pelvic exams, the vaginal walls are palpated for masses or induration and can be inspected for lesions or irregularities during removal of the speculum. The most common site for vaginal tumors is the posterior wall of the upper one-third of the vagina, an area that can be visualized with a careful speculum exam. Any abnormality should be referred to gynecology for evaluation and possible biopsy. Up to 20% of vaginal cancers are detected incidentally on routine Pap testing [99].

The morphology of vulvar and vaginal lesions varies greatly, and expertise is required for proper evaluation. Cancerous lesions may present as patches, plaques, nodules, or papules with red-, brown-, black-, white-, pink-, or flesh-colored pigment. *Any vulvar or vaginal lesion that cannot be easily explained should be biopsied for definitive diagnosis.* The differential diagnosis for vaginal or vulvar carcinoma includes physiologic or post-inflammatory hyperpigmentation, warts, lichen planus, acanthosis nigrans, vulvar or vaginal interepithelial neoplasia, melanocytic nevus, angiokeratoma, and seborrheic keratosis (see Chap. 12 on "Vaginitis and Vulvar Conditions").

Basal cell carcinoma and melanomas occur on the vulva and vagina. Vulvar and vaginal melanomas are more common in Caucasian women and may present as a blue-black mass, a black-brown mass, a nonpigmented plaque, or an ulceration. Vaginal melanomas occur most frequently on the distal one-third of the anterior vaginal wall. Sarcomas are more common in children, classically present as a "bunch of grapes" protruding from the vagina, and can arise from any structure in the lower genital tract.

Vulvar and vaginal cancers are diagnosed by biopsy of suspicious lesions, which is usually performed by a gynecologist. Most primary care offices do not have the expertise or equipment to evaluate these lesions without a consultation. However, if desired, the clinician may obtain consent to document the lesion with a photo in the medical record prior to referral for biopsy.

Vulvar and vaginal colposcopy are performed to look for lesions that may not be visible to the naked eye. Indications include unexplained symptoms, or abnormal cytology without corresponding lesions. Additionally, vulvar intraepithelial neoplasia (VIN) and vaginal intraepithelial neoplasia (VaIN) often coexist with cervical intraepithelial neoplasia or cancer. The application of acetic acid turns HPV-infected areas white, although this is not specific. A magnifying glass can be used for the examination if colposcopy is not available. Abnormal areas are biopsied.

Categories of vulvar and vaginal intraepithelial neoplasia – histology and treatment options – are outlined in Tables 15.11 and 15.12.

VIN lesions fall into three categories:

- LSIL is benign, usually regresses, and does not require treatment.
- HSIL is caused by *HPV*, is usually treated, and may progress to cancer.
- Differentiated VIN is associated with *Lichen sclerosis* and is most likely to be associated with malignancy.

Vaginal biopsies may also reveal vaginal intraepithelial neoplasia (VaIN). Invasive disease is excluded with vaginal

Table 15.11 Vulvar intraepithelial neoplasia (VIN) [100, 101]

Name	Description	Therapy
Vulvar LSIL (low-grade squamous intraepithelial lesion)	*Not* precancerous. Flat condyloma or HPV-related inflammatory changes	Monitor. Most will regress. Stop smoking. Treat if symptomatic
Vulvar HSIL (high-grade squamous intraepithelial lesion)	HPV related. May be associated with or progress to squamous cell carcinoma	Excision, or, less commonly, topical therapy with imiquimod
Differentiated VIN (vulvar intraepithelial neoplasia)	Not associated with HPV Typically associated with lichen sclerosis. Less common than HSIL. *Most likely to be associated with, or progress to, cancer*	Excision

Table 15.12 Vaginal intraepithelial neoplasia (VaIN)

Name	Description	Therapy
VaIN 1 LSIL (low-grade squamous intraepithelial lesion)	Pathology involves lower 1/3 of the epithelium	Close surveillance only
VaIN 2 HSIL (high-grade squamous intraepithelial lesion)	Pathology involves lower 2/3 of the epithelium	Treatment options include surgical excision, laser ablation, intracavitary radiation, and topical therapy with imiquimod
VaIN 3 (includes CIS[a]) HSIL	Pathology involves >2/3 of the epithelium	

[a]carcinoma in situ

colposcopy and biopsy. Less than 10% of VaIN progresses to invasive vaginal carcinoma [102].

Following treatment for precancerous conditions, women should be seen every 6 months for an exam, vaginal cytology, and HPV testing for 2 years, after which they can be followed annually by exam, vaginal cytology, and HPV co-testing [103]. There is no consensus on when to stop annual screening in this population although some clinicians stop after age 65 if the previous five screens were normal.

Staging

Vulvar cancer is staged via physical exam. Assessment includes pelvic and rectal exam and inspection of the perineum, anus, vagina, and urethra. The vulva, vagina, and cervix are evaluated with colposcopy as multicentric lesions may occur. Imaging with pelvic and abdominal MRI or PET scan may be obtained to evaluate for concurrent pathology, metastatic disease, or surgical planning, especially when symptoms are suggestive of possible metastatic disease, such as bowel or bladder dysfunction, a tumor ≥4 cm, or if there are palpable inguinal femoral notes (see Table 15.13).

Vaginal cancer is clinically (not surgically) staged via the International Federation of Gynecology and Obstetrics (FIGO) and Tumor, Node, Metastasis (TNM) system. Staging workup includes a physical examination and chest and skeletal radiography. Cystoscopy and anoscopy or proctoscopy are preformed when indicated by history, physical exam, or sexual practices, and a CT or MRI may be done for surgical planning (see Table 15.14).

Aditi's biopsy comes back as positive for squamous cell carcinoma. It is HPV positive and she is referred to a gynecologic oncologist.

Table 15.13 Vulvar cancer staging, prognosis, and treatment [8, 104, 105]

Stage	Description	5-year survival	Treatment
IA, IB	Tumor confined to the vulva IA: < 2 cm, < 1-mm invasion IB: > 2 cm, > 1-mm invasion	86%	Vulvectomy +/− inguinal node sampling, with or without postoperative chemotherapy and radiation
II	Tumor of any size with extension to adjacent perineal structures (lower third of urethra, lower third of vagina, anus) with negative lymph nodes		
III	Tumor of any size with or without extension to adjacent perineal structures (lower third of urethra, lower third of vagina, anus) with positive inguinofemoral nodes	54%	
IV	Tumor invades other regional (upper 2/3 urethra, upper 2/3 vagina) or distant structures	54% 18% if spread to distant organs or tissues	

Treatment Strategies

Vulvar and vaginal cancers are managed by gynecologic oncologists. Treatment for vaginal cancer is determined by expert opinion and is extrapolated from the care of cervical and anal cancers. There are no randomized clinical trials for vaginal cancer as it is rare. Vulvar cancer is better studied. For both cancers, surgical options, as well as radiation and chemotherapy, depend on the size and location of the cancer. Low-risk disease is confined to the vagina and may be treated with surgery alone. High-risk disease has spread to the pelvic wall, lymph nodes, or other structures. High-risk disease is treated with radiation +/− chemotherapy or surgery. Radiation may involve brachytherapy, in which a probe is inserted into the vagina to deliver therapy. Treatment alters the structure of the vagina and vulva, which may impact patient well-being.

Survivorship Care

Patients with a history of low-risk disease should be seen every 6 months for the first 2 years after diagnosis and then

Table 15.14 Vaginal cancer staging, prognosis, and treatment[a] [106]

Stage	Description	5-year survival (%)	Treatment
I	Cancer is confined to the vagina	75–95	Surgery +/− radiation
II	Cancer has grown through the vaginal wall, but does not extend to the pelvic wall or nearby lymph nodes	50–80	Radiation +/− chemotherapy or surgery
III	Cancer is growing into the pelvic wall and has spread to nearby lymph nodes but not distant sites	30–60	Radiation +/− chemotherapy
IV	Cancer has spread to distant organs	15—50%	

[a]Survival rates given as ranges given relative rarity of this cancer [107]

annually. Women with a history of high-risk disease should be seen every 3 months for the first 2 years, every 6 months years 3 through 5, and then annually. All patients with a history of vaginal or vulvar cancer should have cervical or vaginal Pap tests annually with HPV co-testing. If recurrence is suspected, PET CT is recommended [108].

> *Aditi is treated with local resection and returns to your clinic for follow-up. Since her surgery, she has found sex less pleasurable.*

Care of the Gynecologic Cancer Survivor in Primary Care

Care of the cancer survivor begins when the patient is diagnosed and continues throughout her life. The primary care provider (PCP) plays a critical role in this care and should be well versed in the issues which arise in cancer survivors. The management of common sequelae is covered in detail in other chapters of this volume and will not be repeated here, except those that are unique to gynecologic cancer survivors (see Chaps. 8, 9, 20, 23, 27, 30, 31, and 33 on "Menopause, Female Sexual Function and Dysfunction", "Care of the Breast Cancer Survivor", "Urinary Incontinence", "Irritable Bowel Syndrome", "Interstitial Cystitis", "Chronic Pelvic Pain", and "Depressive and Anxiety Disorders" for in-depth discussions).

During active treatment, side effects are managed by the oncology team. Once treatment is complete, the gynecologic malignancy survivor may experience treatment-induced menopause; urinary, gastrointestinal, pelvic, and psychologic symptoms; infertility; neuropathy; and intimacy or sexual health concerns. Patients who undergo radiation therapy and radical hysterectomies have the highest burden of side effects and the lowest posttreatment quality of life [109, 110]. Primary care providers should address long-term quality of life issues, assess the burden of treatment-induced sequelae, and discuss options to treat identified problems (see Chap. 20 on the "Care of the Breast Cancer Survivor") [11]. Symptoms and sequelae which are specific to surgery or radiation, or that are worrisome for recurrent malignancy, should be referred back to the gynecologic oncologist for evaluation and treatment (Fig. 15.1).

Long-Term Complications in Survivors of Gynecologic Cancers

Gastroenterological Complications

Pelvic surgery and radiation therapy to the pelvis, both common treatments for gynecologic malignancies, can have an adverse impact on bowel and bladder function. Bowel dysfunction may be the result of tissue damage from radiation, or postsurgical mechanical (related to adhesions) or neuropathic (related to disruption of sympathetic and parasympathetic nerve fibers) changes. For some survivors, particularly

Fig. 15.1 Common side effects and sequelae in the gynecologic cancer survivor

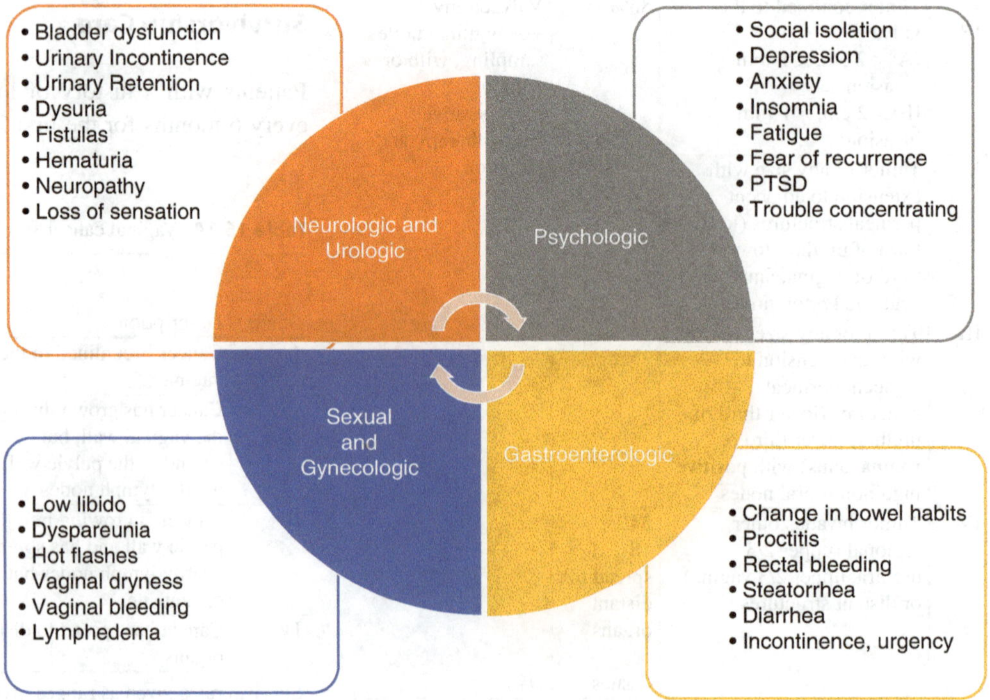

in the case of ovarian cancer, initial cancer symptoms may have been perceived as vague gastrointestinal distress. Gastrointestinal symptoms may therefore be particularly distressing in ovarian cancer survivors who fear that the symptoms signal recurrence.

As with any patient, the etiology of the presenting complaint should be identified, and recurrent malignancy should be excluded, when appropriate. Most therapy is supportive. Constipation, loose stools, urgency, and fecal incontinence may be complications of treatment and are managed with increasing the intake of high-fiber foods or with the addition of stool bulking agents like psyllium. Constipation is managed with polyethylene glycol and Senna, a plant-derived stimulant laxative, as necessary (for further discussion, see Chap. 27 on "Irritable Bowel Syndrome").

Radiation proctitis typically resolves on its own and is managed in the short term with hydration and antidiarrheal agents as needed. Severe symptoms of proctitis may require steroid enemas [111].

Urologic and Neurologic Complications

Chemotherapy, radiation, and surgery can all impact urologic function. Radiation therapy is associated with the highest likelihood of urologic complications. Symptoms include incontinence, pain, frequency, urgency, and hematuria. Infection should be excluded and management should be tailored to symptoms. Many of the urologic symptoms associated with radiation therapy will be treated similarly to other causes of the same symptoms (see Chaps. 23 and 30 on "Urinary Incontinence and Interstitial Cystitis"). These patients should be referred back to gynecology or to an urologist or urogynecologist for evaluation and treatment.

Neurologic complications are common in gynecologic cancer survivors. Peripheral neuropathy often results from platinum-based chemotherapy and several other agents that are mainstays of chemotherapy for gynecologic cancers. Some women may only have troublesome symptoms when exposed to hot or cold temperatures, or tight clothing, and should be encouraged to avoid triggers and/or wear gloves and socks to reduce symptoms. Duloxetine is the suggested pharmacotherapy agent for refractory symptoms. For further discussion, see Chaps. 26 and 31 on the "General Approach to Chronic Pain" and "Chronic Pelvic Pain".

Sexual and Gynecologic Complications

Sexual dysfunction following treatment for gynecologic cancer is common. Primary care providers should proactively inquire in a sensitive and skilled manner about sexual health as many women will not bring up this subject without prompting. In gynecologic cancer survivors, the NCCN (National Comprehensive Cancer Network) recommends asking directly if the patient is sexually active and whether they are having intercourse, if they are satisfied with their sex life, and if not, for how long? Providers should identify whether the problem is with pain, dryness/lubrication, fear, lack of interest, decreased sensation, or orgasm [112]. A full discussion of the assessment and management is outlined in Chap. 9 on "Female Sexual Function and Dysfunction". Women sometimes deny problems initially but may be willing to discuss issues in the future, once the provider has shown an openness to discuss sexuality concerns.

Women who have been treated for a gynecologic malignancy may have significant anatomic changes following surgery and/or skin changes from radiation. Further, women may be misinformed or have misconceptions about their posttreatment anatomy and ability to be sexually active. For example, a radical hysterectomy can make the vagina shorter and vaginal stenosis may occur. Women may experience difficulty with body image after treatment, and alopecia of the pubic hair may occur. Removal of the pelvic lymph nodes may also lead to lymphedema of the genital tissues, which can be painful and have a significant negative impact on quality of life [109, 110]. Dryness and dysthesia are also common issues after treatment. Vaginal infection, or bowel or bladder incontinence, can also negatively impact sexual health and should be addressed and treated appropriately. Treatment of sexual dysfunction should be targeted to the specific complaint.

A pelvic exam can assess for areas of scarring, atrophy, or stenosis that may be causing symptoms, and if needed, reevaluation should be performed by the treating gynecologic oncologist. Vaginal dryness can initially be managed with a trial of moisturizers and lubricants (see Chap. 8 on "Menopause", section on vaginal atrophy). For patients who have experienced the vaginal shortening of a radical hysterectomy, advice can be given for some couples to adjust to this change by using a penile ring to shorten the depth of penetration or by cupping a hand around the base of the penis during sex. Vaginal stenosis can be treated with dilators. Pelvic floor physical therapy may be helpful for many of these symptoms and can also help with urinary incontinence.

Referrals to certified sex therapists who are experienced in sexual issues after cancer treatment can provide specialized cognitive behavioral therapy and practical approaches to sexual dysfunction. Certified therapists can be found at https://www.aasect.org/, and some cancer centers have special clinics for this purpose [113] (for a full discussion, see Chap. 9 on "Female Sexual Function and Dysfunction"). Radiation can also cause rectovaginal or vesicovaginal fistulas, radiation cystitis or proctitis, and/or rectal strictures. Women with these complaints should be referred to urology or surgery for definitive treatment.

Chronic pelvic pain is another possible sequelae of therapy and may be related to the issues described above. Treatment is targeted to the etiology, and patients should be comanaged with gynecology.

May gynecologic cancers cannot be safely treated with fertility-preserving methods. Ideally, treatment's impact on reproductive potential is discussed prior to initiation of therapy as part of informed consent and shared decision making. Women in need of support adjusting to this "new normal" should be referred to counseling.

Surgical and Treatment-Induced Menopause

Many women who are survivors of gynecologic malignancies will experience treatment-induced menopause. The symptoms of surgical menopause are similar to those experienced in natural menopause except that symptoms can be more severe and can come on suddenly. A full discussion of the treatment of surgical menopausal symptoms is found in Chap. 8 on "Menopause:, and Chap. 20 on the "Care of the Breast Cancer Survivor". Survivors of cervical, vaginal, or vulvar malignancy are candidates for hormone therapy and have no restrictions for menopausal treatment options.

Ovarian and uterine cancer survivors have traditionally not been treated with hormonal therapy, as it is not safe for patients with certain types of tumors, or advanced malignancies. Recent data, however has shown that epithelial ovarian cancer and early (stage I) endometrial cancer survivors may be appropriate candidates for hormone therapy; treatment should only be initiated in consultation with a patient's treating gynecologic oncologist [114–116].

Psychologic Complications

Many cancer survivors experience anxiety, depression, PTSD, and fear of recurrence. Fatigue, trouble concentrating, and insomnia are also common. The primary care clinician should actively monitor for these conditions and provide treatment. Anxiety and depression should be assessed with validated tools and shared decision-making used to develop a treatment plan, which typically involves SSRIs and talk therapy (for a full discussion, please see Chaps. 20 and 33 on "Care of the Breast Cancer Survivor", and "Depressive and Anxiety Disorders").

Providers can educate their patients on the cancer surveillance plan, symptoms needing evaluation, and how to communicate concerns. Helping women identify peer support groups and ensuring regular check-ins on their well-being are also essential. A compassionate and patient-centered approach, which is evidence based and integrates the expertise of a multidisciplinary team of providers, will insure that survivors of gynecologic malignancies will experience the best possible quality of life. The primary care provider is uniquely positioned to help patients identify issues and manage symptoms, provide expert referral, and coordinate care.

Summary Points

1. Review the epidemiology, risk factors, and prevention of uterine, ovarian, cervical, vulvar, and vaginal cancers.
   (a) In the United States, uterine cancer is the most common gynecologic cancer and the 4th most common cancer overall in women. Rates of uterine cancer are increasing, likely due to rising rates of obesity. Ovarian cancer is less common, followed by cervical, vulvar, and vaginal cancers (see Table 15.1).
   (b) Major risk factors for gynecologic malignancies include unopposed estrogen exposure, hrHPV infection, in utero DES exposure, lichen planus, and certain genetic syndromes: BRCA 1 and 2, Lynch, and Cowden syndromes.
   (c) Options for risk reduction are limited and include maintaining a healthy weight, routine Pap and pelvic exams, oral contraceptives, and proper referral for patients at high genetic risk.
2. Discuss screening, presenting symptoms, and early diagnosis of uterine, ovarian, cervical, vulvar, and vaginal cancers.
   (a) Cervical cancer is the only gynecologic cancer with a recommended screening protocol for average-risk women.
   (b) The primary symptoms in gynecologic malignancies are bleeding abnormalities, abdominal or pelvic pain or discomfort, bowel or urinary complaints, unexplained vulvar pruritus, and masses or lesions.
   (c) Early diagnosis of uterine, ovarian, vulvar, and vaginal cancer is typically made based on clinical suspicion prompting further evaluation, or by abnormal cells found on routine Pap test.
   (d) Patients with in utero DES exposure lichen planus, BRCA 1 and 2, Lynch, or Cowden syndrome may be candidates for specialized screening protocols or preventative surgery. Such patients should be referred to specialty care.
3. Describe the evaluation and staging of uterine, ovarian, cervical, vulvar, and vaginal cancers.
   (a) Gynecologic cancers are staged by the FIGO system.
   (b) Formal evaluation and staging of gynecologic cancers should be completed by a gynecologic oncologist
4. Explain the prognosis and typical treatment plans for uterine, ovarian, cervical, vulvar, and vaginal cancers.

(a) Gynecologic cancer should always be managed in conjunction with a gynecologic oncologist and preferably in a specialized treatment center with up-to-date protocols and multispecialty support for women undergoing treatment.
(b) Uterine cancer has the best prognosis of all the gynecologic cancers because it has a classic presentation of abnormal uterine bleeding and is typically detected at an early stage. Ovarian cancer classically has the worst prognosis because the symptoms are often nonspecific and is diagnosed at late stages.
(c) Treatment varies by type of cancer and stage at diagnosis, but may include surgery, radiation, and/or chemotherapy.

5. Describe the survivorship issues in women with gynecologic malignancies including the potential sequelae from therapeutic chemoradiation and surgery.
   (a) Posttherapy sequelae may include treatment-induced menopause; gastrointestinal, urologic, psychologic, or neuropathic symptoms' mental health issues; or sexual health concerns.

Review Questions

1. A 58-year-old postmenopausal woman presents with vaginal spotting which has been present for 1 month. She had a normal Pap test last year. What is the next step in her management?
   A. Watchful waiting. Reevaluate if spotting persists more than 6 months.
   B. Genetic testing to screen for high-risk mutations.
   C. Transvaginal ultrasound.
   D. Repeat Pap test with HPV testing.

   The correct answer is C. A postmenopausal woman with vaginal spotting or bleeding (PMB) requires evaluation to exclude endometrial malignancy. Pap tests are used to screen for cervical cancer, but are not reliable to rule out endometrial cancer. Transvaginal ultrasound with measurement of the endometrial stripe is the first test used to evaluate a woman with postmenopausal bleeding. An endometrial stripe thickness over 4 mm is an indication for endometrial biopsy to exclude malignancy when postmenopausal bleeding is present, although many gynecologists would perform an EMB first in cases of PMB. Watchful waiting or repeat Pap test is not indicated, as all postmenopausal bleeding requires evaluation. Genetic testing is indicated in patients with a family history or personal history suspicious for inherited genetic syndromes associated with malignancy and would not help to define the diagnosis in this case [31, 33, 34].
2. A 48-year-old woman of Ashkenazi Jewish descent presents for her annual exam. Her last Pap co-testing was normal 3 years ago. She has no symptoms, but wants to be screened for ovarian cancer because her sister was diagnosed with metastatic ovarian cancer at age 50. She and her sister were adopted, and she does not know her family history. She read that an ultrasound and CA-125 level were the best screening procedures. What would be the next step in her evaluation?
   A. Pap co-testing
   B. Referral for genetic counseling and testing
   C. Transvaginal ultrasound and CA-125 level
   D. Pelvic MRI
   E. PET scan

   The correct answer is B. Ovarian cancer has a high mortality because most patients are asymptomatic until the cancer has spread. Unfortunately, there is no reliable screening test for asymptomatic women, even for those with a family history. A large study in the United Kingdom recently showed that the harm of screening outweighed the benefits because of the high incidence of false-positive findings which lead to unnecessary surgery. This woman is at risk for the BRCA 1 or 2 genetic mutation based on her Ashkenazi Jewish descent and family history of ovarian cancer in a close relative. She should be referred for genetic counseling and testing. If she is found to have a genetic syndrome which predisposes to ovarian cancer, then gynecologic referral is indicated, and prophylactic bilateral salpingo-oophorectomy should be considered to prevent ovarian cancer [75, 117].
3. A 65-year-old woman presents with vaginal spotting for 2 months. She has no history of malignancy and is not sexually active. Her last Pap co-test was 2 years ago. The physical exam is significant for the absence of visible lesions of the vulva, vagina, or cervix, and there are no adnexal masses or tenderness. Vaginal atrophy is noted. Transvaginal ultrasound reveals an endometrial stripe thickness of 2 mm. The most likely cause of her spotting is:
   A. Endometrial atrophy
   B. Vaginal intraepithelial neoplasia (VIN)
   C. Ovarian cancer
   D. Uterine cancer
   E. Cervical cancer

   The correct answer is A. The most common cause of postmenopausal bleeding (PMB) is endometrial atrophy. VIN is a very rare cause of vaginal bleeding, is typically caused by human papillomavirus (HPV). She tested negative for HPV 2 years ago, which makes VIN less likely. Ovarian cancer is not a common cause of PMB. Uterine cancer is of concern and must be excluded, but atrophy is more common than cancer as a source of PMB. Cervical cancer can present with PMB, but given her normal co-testing 2 years ago, this is not a likely diagnosis [33, 118].

4. A 75-year-old woman who is in excellent health presents to establish care. She has not had a pelvic exam for 10 years, as her previous primary care physician told her that gynecologic exams were not necessary after the age of 65. On review of systems, she notes that she has itching of the vulva off and on for years. On inspection of her perineum, there are marked atrophic changes and an indurated 1-cm excoriated lesion on the left labia. What is the next step in her management?
   A. HPV testing
   B. Referral to gynecology for evaluation and biopsy
   C. Treatment with topical steroids
   D. Pelvic exam followed by pelvic MRI

   The correct answer is B. Pap tests and routine bimanual examinations are not recommended for women over 65 who have no history of malignancy and have had regular screening prior to age 65; however, women should continue to be monitored for gynecological symptoms: dyspareunia, bleeding, pruritis, discharge, and vulvar lesions. Vulvar cancer is uncommon and can be caused by HPV or be associated with other etiologies such as lichen sclerosis or melanoma. Referral to a gynecologist for evaluation and possible biopsy is the correct answer. HPV testing would not change the need for referral. The gynecologist might offer topical steroids depending on the etiology of the lesion. Pelvic MRI would only be ordered if there were a concern about cancer staging in selected cases [108].

5. A 40-year-old woman had a radical hysterectomy 5 years ago for endometrial cancer. She underwent a course of radiation therapy, but no chemotherapy at that time. She presents for her annual general medical exam. She denies gynecologic symptoms of pain or bleeding, but she and her husband have not resumed intercourse after her surgery due to discomfort with penetration. Which treatment is the next best step?
   A. Prescribe topical estrogen and dilators, follow-up in 3 months.
   B. Screen the patient for PTSD and depression.
   C. Refer back to her gynecologist or gynecologic oncology physician for evaluation.
   D. Discuss vibrators and erotic movies with patient.

   The correct answer is C. Her gynecologist should be able to address these issues or send her to a specialized sex therapist if needed. There are many factors that may impact the couple's lack of sexual activity, and the issues will need evaluation and treatment. The pain she experiences with penetration could be atrophy, and/or radiation changes. After radical hysterectomy, the vagina is shortened. She may have PTSD or depression, but treatment for mental health issues alone does not address the physical issues which may be impeding their sexual activity. Estrogen may be contraindicated in patients with endometrial cancer and should be prescribed in consultation with the gynecologic oncologist [119, 120].

References

1. Siegel RL, Miller KD, Jemal A. Cancer statistics, 2017. 2017. Contract No.: 1.
2. Sankaranarayanan R, Ferlay J. Worldwide burden of gynaecological cancer: the size of the problem. Best Practice Res Clin Obstet Gynaecol. 2006;20(2):207–25.
3. Society TAC. Global burden of cancer in women: current status, trends, and interventions. The American Cancer Society; 2012. Contract No.: 10/25/2018.
4. Society AC. Cancer facts & figures: 2019. 2019.
5. Program NCIS. Cancer stat facts: uterine cancer 2018. Available from: https://seer.cancer.gov/statfacts/html/corp.html
6. Program NCIS. Cancer stat facts: ovarian cancer 2018. Available from: https://seer.cancer.gov/statfacts/html/ovary.html.
7. Program NCIS. Cancer stat facts: cervical cancer 2018. Available from: https://seer.cancer.gov/statfacts/html/cervix.html
8. Program NCIS. Cancer stat facts: vulvar cancer 2018. Available from: https://seer.cancer.gov/statfacts/html/vulva.html.
9. Society AC. Special section: rare cancers in adults. 2017.
10. Sorosky JI. Endometrial cancer. Obstet Gynecol. 2012;120(2 Pt 1):383–97.
11. Cote ML, Ruterbusch JJ, Olson SH, Lu K, Ali-Fehmi R. The growing burden of endometrial cancer: a major racial disparity affecting black women. Cancer Epidemiol Biomark Prev. 2015;24(9):1407–15.
12. Ferlay J, Soerjomataram I, Dikshit R, Eser S, Mathers C, Rebelo M, et al. Cancer incidence and mortality worldwide: sources, methods and major patterns in GLOBOCAN 2012. Int J Cancer. 2015;136(5):E359–E86.
13. Trope CG, Abeler VM, Kristensen GB. Diagnosis and treatment of sarcoma of the uterus. A review. Acta oncol (Stockholm, Sweden). 2012;51(6):694–705.
14. Felix AS, Weissfeld JL, Stone RA, Bowser R, Chivukula M, Edwards RP, et al. Factors associated with type I and type II endometrial cancer. Cancer Causes Control. 2010;21(11):1851–6.
15. Smith RA, von Eschenbach AC, Wender R, Levin B, Byers T, Rothenberger D, et al. American Cancer Society guidelines for the early detection of cancer: update of early detection guidelines for prostate, colorectal, and endometrial cancers. Also: update 2001--testing for early lung cancer detection. CA Cancer J Clin. 2001;51(1):38–75; quiz 7–80.
16. Setiawan VW, Yang HP, Pike MC, McCann SE, Yu H, Xiang YB, et al. Type I and II endometrial cancers: have they different risk factors? J Clin Oncol. 2013;31(20):2607–18.
17. Braithwaite RS, Chlebowski RT, Lau J, George S, Hess R, Col NF. Meta-analysis of vascular and neoplastic events associated with tamoxifen. J Gen Int Med. 2003;18(11):937–47.
18. Tamoxifen and Uterine Cancer - ACOG 2018. Available from: https://www.acog.org/Clinical-Guidance-and-Publications/Committee-Opinions/Committee-on-Gynecologic-Practice/Tamoxifen-and-Uterine-Cancer?IsMobileSet=false
19. Fung MF, Reid A, Faught W, Le T, Chenier C, Verma S, et al. Prospective longitudinal study of ultrasound screening for endometrial abnormalities in women with breast cancer receiving tamoxifen. Gynecol Oncol. 2003;91(1):154–9.
20. Bertelli G, Venturini M, Del Mastro L, Garrone O, Cosso M, Gustavino C, et al. Tamoxifen and the endometrium: findings

of pelvic ultrasound examination and endometrial biopsy in asymptomatic breast cancer patients. Breast Cancer Res Treat. 1998;47(1):41–6.

21. Braun MM, Overbeek-Wager EA, Grumbo RJ. Diagnosis and Management of Endometrial Cancer. Am Fam Physician. 2016;93(6):468–74.
22. Meyer LA, Broaddus RR, Lu KH. Endometrial cancer and lynch syndrome: clinical and pathologic considerations. Cancer Control. 2009;16(1):14–22.
23. Luo J, Beresford S, Chen C, Chlebowski R, Garcia L, Kuller L, et al. Association between diabetes, diabetes treatment and risk of developing endometrial cancer. Br J Cancer. 2014;111(7): 1432–9.
24. Resnick KE, Hampel H, Fishel R, Cohn DE. Current and emerging trends in lynch syndrome identification in women with endometrial cancer. Gynecol Oncol. 2009;114(1):128–34.
25. Lancaster JM, Powell CB, Kauff ND, Cass I, Chen LM, Lu KH, et al. Society of Gynecologic Oncologists Education Committee statement on risk assessment for inherited gynecologic cancer predispositions. Gynecol Oncol. 2007;107(2):159–62.
26. Bonnet D, Selves J, Toulas C, Danjoux M, Duffas JP, Portier G, et al. Simplified identification of Lynch syndrome: a prospective, multicenter study. Digest Liver Dis. 2012;44(6): 515–22.
27. Le DT, Uram JN, Wang H, Bartlett BR, Kemberling H, Eyring AD, et al. PD-1 blockade in tumors with mismatch-repair deficiency. N Engl J Med. 2015;372(26):2509–20.
28. Schorge JO, Hossein Saboorian M, Hynan L, Ashfaq R. ThinPrep detection of cervical and endometrial adenocarcinoma: a retrospective cohort study. Cancer. 2002;96(6):338–43.
29. Seoud M, Shamseddine A, Khalil A, Salem Z, Saghir N, Bikhazi K, et al. Tamoxifen and endometrial pathologies: a prospective study. Gynecol Oncol. 1999;75(1):15–9.
30. Love CD, Muir BB, Scrimgeour JB, Leonard RC, Dillon P, Dixon JM. Investigation of endometrial abnormalities in asymptomatic women treated with tamoxifen and an evaluation of the role of endometrial screening. J Clin Oncol. 1999;17(7):2050–4.
31. Karlsson B, Granberg S, Wikland M, Ylostalo P, Torvid K, Marsal K, et al. Transvaginal ultrasonography of the endometrium in women with postmenopausal bleeding--a Nordic multicenter study. Am J Obstet Gynecol. 1995;172(5):1488–94.
32. ACOG committee opinion no. 557: management of acute abnormal uterine bleeding in nonpregnant reproductive-aged women. Obstet Gynecol. 2013;121(4):891–6.
33. Clarke MA, Long BJ, Del Mar Morillo A, Arbyn M, Bakkum-Gamez JN, Wentzensen N. Association of Endometrial Cancer Risk with postmenopausal bleeding in women: a systematic review and meta-analysis. JAMA Int Med. 2018;178(9):1210–22.
34. Burbos N, Musonda P, Giarenis I, Shiner AM, Giamougiannis P, Morris E, et al. Age-related differential diagnosis of vaginal bleeding in postmenopausal women: a series of 3047 symptomatic postmenopausal women. Menopause Int. 2010;16(1):5–8.
35. Zuber TJ. Endometrial biopsy. Am Fam Physician. 2001;63(6):1131–5, 7–41.
36. Scully RE, Bonfiglio TA, Kurman RJ, Silverberg SG, Wilkinson EJ. Histological typing of female genital tract tumours. New York: Springer; 2018.
37. Emons G, Beckmann MW, Schmidt D, Mallmann P. New WHO classification of endometrial hyperplasias. Geburtshilfe Frauenheilkd. 2015;75(2):135–6.
38. Mutter GL. Endometrial intraepithelial neoplasia (EIN): will it bring order to chaos? The Endometrial Collaborative Group. Gynecol Oncol. 2000;76(3):287–90.
39. Trimble CL, Kauderer J, Zaino R, Silverberg S, Lim PC, Burke JJ 2nd, et al. Concurrent endometrial carcinoma in women with a biopsy diagnosis of atypical endometrial hyperplasia: a Gynecologic Oncology Group study. Cancer. 2006;106(4): 812–9.
40. Byun JM, Jeong DH, Kim YN, Cho EB, Cha JE, Sung MS, et al. Endometrial cancer arising from atypical complex hyperplasia: the significance in an endometrial biopsy and a diagnostic challenge. Obstet Gynecol Sci. 2015;58(6):468–74.
41. Trimble CL, Method M, Leitao M, Lu K, Ioffe O, Hampton M, et al. Management of endometrial precancers. Obstet Gynecol. 2012;120(5):1160–75.
42. Gynecologists ACoOa. Endometrial intraepithelial neoplasia. ACOG Committee Opinion 2015.
43. Lewin SN. Revised FIGO staging system for endometrial cancer. Clin Obstet Gynecol. 2011;54(2):215–8.
44. Rossi EC, Kowalski LD, Scalici J, Cantrell L, Schuler K, Hanna RK, et al. A comparison of sentinel lymph node biopsy to lymphadenectomy for endometrial cancer staging (FIRES trial): a multicentre, prospective, cohort study. Lancet Oncol. 2017;18(3):384–92.
45. Kim JJ, Chapman-Davis E. Role of progesterone in endometrial cancer. Sem Reprod Med. 2010;28(1):81–90.
46. Carneiro MM, Lamaita RM, Ferreira MC, Silva-Filho AL. Fertility-preservation in endometrial cancer: is it safe? Review of the literature. JBRA Assist Reprod. 2016;20(4):232–9.
47. Mariani A, Webb MJ, Keeney GL, Calori G, Podratz KC. Role of wide/radical hysterectomy and pelvic lymph node dissection in endometrial cancer with cervical involvement. Gynecol Oncol. 2001;83(1):72–80.
48. Walker JL, Piedmonte MR, Spirtos NM, Eisenkop SM, Schlaerth JB, Mannel RS, et al. Recurrence and survival after random assignment to laparoscopy versus laparotomy for comprehensive surgical staging of uterine cancer: Gynecologic Oncology Group LAP2 Study. J Clin Oncol. 2012;30(7):695–700.
49. Wright JD, Burke WM, Wilde ET, Lewin SN, Charles AS, Kim JH, et al. Comparative effectiveness of robotic versus laparoscopic hysterectomy for endometrial cancer. J Clin Oncol. 2012;30(8):783–91.
50. Pelikan HM, Trum JW, Bakers FC, Beets-Tan RG, Smits LJ, Kruitwagen RF. Diagnostic accuracy of preoperative tests for lymph node status in endometrial cancer: a systematic review. Cancer Imaging. 2013;13(3):314–22.
51. Amin MB, Greene FL, Edge SB, Compton CC, Gershenwald JE, Brookland RK, et al. The Eighth Edition AJCC Cancer Staging Manual: continuing to build a bridge from a population-based to a more "personalized" approach to cancer staging. CA Cancer J Clin. 2017;67(2):93–9.
52. Salani R, Backes FJ, Fung MF, Holschneider CH, Parker LP, Bristow RE, et al. Posttreatment surveillance and diagnosis of recurrence in women with gynecologic malignancies: Society of Gynecologic Oncologists recommendations. Am J Obstet Gynecol. 2011;204(6):466–78.
53. Atri M, Zhang Z, Dehdashti F, Lee SI, Marques H, Ali S, et al. Utility of PET/CT to evaluate retroperitoneal lymph node metastasis in high-risk endometrial cancer: results of ACRIN 6671/GOG 0233 trial. Radiology. 2017;283(2):450–9.
54. Menon U, Skates SJ, Lewis S, Rosenthal AN, Rufford B, Sibley K, et al. Prospective study using the risk of ovarian cancer algorithm to screen for ovarian cancer. J Clin Oncol. 2005;23(31): 7919–26.
55. Buys SS, Partridge E, Greene MH, Prorok PC, Reding D, Riley TL, et al. Ovarian cancer screening in the Prostate, Lung, Colorectal and Ovarian (PLCO) cancer screening trial: findings from the initial screen of a randomized trial. Am J Obstet Gynecol. 2005;193(5):1630–9.
56. Partridge E, Kreimer AR, Greenlee RT, Williams C, Xu JL, Church TR, et al. Results from four rounds of ovarian cancer screening in a randomized trial. Obstet Gynecol. 2009;113(4):775–82.

57. Barnholtz-Sloan JS, Schwartz AG, Qureshi F, Jacques S, Malone J, Munkarah AR. Ovarian cancer: changes in patterns at diagnosis and relative survival over the last three decades. Am J Obstet Gynecol. 2003;189(4):1120–7.
58. Desai A, Xu J, Aysola K, Qin Y, Okoli C, Hariprasad R, et al. Epithelial ovarian cancer: an overview. World J Transl Med. 2014;3(1):1–8.
59. Tone AA, Salvador S, Finlayson SJ, Tinker AV, Kwon JS, Lee CH, et al. The role of the fallopian tube in ovarian cancer. Clin Adv Hematol Oncol. 2012;10(5):296–306.
60. Karst AM, Levanon K, Drapkin R. Modeling high-grade serous ovarian carcinogenesis from the fallopian tube. Proc Nat Acad Sci U S A. 2011;108(18):7547–52.
61. Kuchenbaecker KB, Hopper JL, Barnes DR, Phillips KA, Mooij TM, Roos-Blom MJ, et al. Risks of breast, ovarian, and contralateral breast cancer for BRCA1 and BRCA2 mutation carriers. JAMA. 2017;317(23):2402–16.
62. Maccio A, Madeddu C. Inflammation and ovarian cancer. Cytokine. 2012;58(2):133–47.
63. Savant SS, Sriramkumar S, O'Hagan HM. The role of inflammation and inflammatory mediators in the development, progression, metastasis, and chemoresistance of epithelial ovarian cancer. Cancers. 2018;10(8):251.
64. Havrilesky LJ, Moorman PG, Lowery WJ, Gierisch JM, Coeytaux RR, Urrutia RP, et al. Oral contraceptive pills as primary prevention for ovarian cancer: a systematic review and meta-analysis. Obstet Gynecol. 2013;122(1):139–47.
65. Ness RB, Cramer DW, Goodman MT, Kjaer SK, Mallin K, Mosgaard BJ, et al. Infertility, fertility drugs, and ovarian cancer: a pooled analysis of case-control studies. Am J Epidemiol. 2002;155(3):217–24.
66. Chittenden BG, Fullerton G, Maheshwari A, Bhattacharya S. Polycystic ovary syndrome and the risk of gynaecological cancer: a systematic review. Reprod Biomed Online. 2009;19(3):398–405.
67. Pearce CL, Templeman C, Rossing MA, Lee A, Near AM, Webb PM, et al. Association between endometriosis and risk of histological subtypes of ovarian cancer: a pooled analysis of case-control studies. Lancet Oncol. 2012;13(4):385–94.
68. Jordan SJ, Whiteman DC, Purdie DM, Green AC, Webb PM. Does smoking increase risk of ovarian cancer? A systematic review. Gynecol Oncol. 2006;103(3):1122–9.
69. Tworoger SS, Fairfield KM, Colditz GA, Rosner BA, Hankinson SE. Association of oral contraceptive use, other contraceptive methods, and infertility with ovarian cancer risk. Am J Epidemiol. 2007;166(8):894–901.
70. Beral V, Doll R, Hermon C, Peto R, Reeves G. Ovarian cancer and oral contraceptives: collaborative reanalysis of data from 45 epidemiological studies including 23,257 women with ovarian cancer and 87,303 controls. Lancet (London, England). 2008;371(9609):303–14.
71. Cibula D, Widschwendter M, Majek O, Dusek L. Tubal ligation and the risk of ovarian cancer: review and meta-analysis. Hum Reprod Update. 2011;17(1):55–67.
72. Ip S, Chung M, Raman G, Trikalinos TA, Lau J. A summary of the Agency for Healthcare Research and Quality's evidence report on breastfeeding in developed countries. Breastfeed Med. 2009;4 Suppl 1:S17–30.
73. Buys SS, Partridge E, Black A, Johnson CC, Lamerato L, Isaacs C, et al. Effect of screening on ovarian cancer mortality: the Prostate, Lung, Colorectal and Ovarian (PLCO) Cancer Screening Randomized Controlled Trial. JAMA. 2011;305(22): 2295–303.
74. Wang Y, Li L, Douville C, Cohen JD, Yen T-T, Kinde I, et al. Evaluation of liquid from the Papanicolaou test and other liquid biopsies for the detection of endometrial and ovarian cancers. Sci Transl Med. 2018;10(433):eaap8793.
75. Jacobs IJ, Menon U, Ryan A, Gentry-Maharaj A, Burnell M, Kalsi JK, et al. Ovarian cancer screening and mortality in the UK Collaborative Trial of Ovarian Cancer Screening (UKCTOCS): a randomised controlled trial. Lancet. 2016;387(10022):945–56.
76. Guirguis-Blake JM, Henderson JT, Perdue LA. Periodic screening pelvic examination: evidence report and systematic review for the US preventive services task force. JAMA. 2017;317(9): 954–66.
77. Padilla LA, Radosevich DM, Milad MP. Accuracy of the pelvic examination in detecting adnexal masses. Obstet Gynecol. 2000;96(4):593–8.
78. Padilla LA, Radosevich DM, Milad MP. Limitations of the pelvic examination for evaluation of the female pelvic organs. Int J Gynaecol Obstet. 2005;88(1):84–8.
79. NCCN. Genetic/familial high-risk assessment: breast and ovarian. Version 2.2019. www.nccn.org
80. Goff BA, Mandel LS, Drescher CW, Urban N, Gough S, Schurman KM, et al. Development of an ovarian cancer symptom index: possibilities for earlier detection. Cancer. 2007;109(2):221–7.
81. Vergote I, Trope CG, Amant F, Kristensen GB, Ehlen T, Johnson N, et al. Neoadjuvant chemotherapy or primary surgery in stage IIIC or IV ovarian cancer. N Engl J Med. 2010;363(10): 943–53.
82. Mutch DG, Prat J. 2014 FIGO staging for ovarian, fallopian tube and peritoneal cancer. Gynecol Oncol. 2014;133(3):401–4.
83. Society AC. Survival Rates for ovarian cancer, by stage 2018. Available from: https://www.cancer.org/cancer/ovarian-cancer/detection-diagnosis-staging/survival-rates.html.
84. Rustin GJ. Follow-up with CA125 after primary therapy of advanced ovarian cancer has major implications for treatment outcome and trial performances and should not be routinely performed. Ann Oncol. 2011;22 Suppl 8:viii45–viii8.
85. Koh WJ, Greer BE, Abu-Rustum NR, Apte SM, Campos SM, Cho KR, et al. Cervical cancer, version 2.2015. J Natl Compr Cancer Netw. 2015;13(4):395–404; quiz.
86. Hillemanns P, Soergel P, Hertel H, Jentschke M. Epidemiology and early detection of cervical cancer. Oncol Res Treat. 2016;39(9):501–6.
87. Brown RK, Barker WH Jr. Pap smear screening and invasive cervical cancer. J Fam Pract. 1982;15(5):875–9.
88. Goodman A. HPV testing as a screen for cervical cancer. BMJ (Clinical research ed). 2015;350:h2372.
89. Chelimo C, Wouldes TA, Cameron LD, Elwood JM. Risk factors for and prevention of human papillomaviruses (HPV), genital warts and cervical cancer. J Infect. 2013;66(3):207–17.
90. Li H, Wu X, Cheng X. Advances in diagnosis and treatment of metastatic cervical cancer. J Gynecol Oncol. 2016;27(4):e43.
91. Bhatla N, Aoki D, Sharma DN, Sankaranarayanan R. Cancer of the cervix uteri. Int J Gynaecol Obstet. 2018;143 Suppl 2:22–36.
92. Eskander RN, Tewari KS. Immunotherapy: an evolving paradigm in the treatment of advanced cervical cancer. Clin Therap. 2015;37(1):20–38.
93. Bhatla N, Aoki D, Sharma DN, Sankaranarayanan R. Cancer of the cervix uteri. Int J Gynaecol Obstet. 2018;143(S2):22–36.
94. Salani R, Khanna N, Frimer M, Bristow RE, Chen LM. An update on post-treatment surveillance and diagnosis of recurrence in women with gynecologic malignancies: Society of Gynecologic Oncology (SGO) recommendations. Gynecol Oncol. 2017;146(1):3–10.
95. Kumar L, Harish P, Malik PS, Khurana S. Chemotherapy and targeted therapy in the management of cervical cancer. Curr Prob Cancer. 2018;42(2):120–8.
96. Bogani G, Leone Roberti Maggiore U, Signorelli M, Martinelli F, Ditto A, Sabatucci I, et al. The role of human papillomavirus vaccines in cervical cancer: prevention and treatment. Crit Rev Oncol Hematol. 2018;122:92–7.

97. Saraiya M, Watson M, Wu X, King JB, Chen VW, Smith JS, et al. Incidence of in situ and invasive vulvar cancer in the US, 1998-2003. Cancer. 2008;113(10 Suppl):2865–72.
98. Yagi A, Ueda Y, Kakuda M, Tanaka Y, Egawa-Takata T, Morimoto A, et al. Descriptive epidemiological study of vaginal cancer using data from the Osaka Japan population-based cancer registry: Long-term analysis from a clinical viewpoint. Medicine. 2017;96(32):e7751.
99. Underwood PB Jr, Smith RT. Carcinoma of the vagina. JAMA. 1971;217(1):46–52.
100. Oluwatosin G. Management of vulvar intraepithelial neoplasia - ACOG 2019. Available from: https://www.acog.org/Clinical-Guidance-and-Publications/Committee-Opinions/Committee-on-Gynecologic-Practice/Management-of-Vulvar-Intraepithelial-Neoplasia
101. van de Nieuwenhof HP, Bulten J, Hollema H, Dommerholt RG, Massuger LF, van der Zee AG, et al. Differentiated vulvar intraepithelial neoplasia is often found in lesions, previously diagnosed as lichen sclerosus, which have progressed to vulvar squamous cell carcinoma. Mod Pathol. 2011;24(2):297–305.
102. Jentschke M, Hoffmeister V, Soergel P, Hillemanns P. Clinical presentation, treatment and outcome of vaginal intraepithelial neoplasia. Arch Gynecol Obstet. 2016;293(2):415–9.
103. Frega A, French D, Piazze J, Cerekja A, Vetrano G, Moscarini M. Prediction of persistent vaginal intraepithelial neoplasia in previously hysterectomized women by high-risk HPV DNA detection. Cancer Lett. 2007;249(2):235–41.
104. FIGO staging for carcinoma of the vulva, cervix, and corpus uteri. Int J Gynaecol Obstet. 2014;125(2):97–8.
105. Rogers LJ, Cuello MA. Cancer of the vulva. Int J Gynaecol Obstet. 2018;143 Suppl 2:4–13.
106. Rajaram S, Maheshwari A, Srivastava A. Staging for vaginal cancer. Best Pract Res Clin Obstet Gynaecol. 2015;29(6):822–32.
107. Hacker NF. Vaginal cancer. Berek JS, Hacker NF. Berek and Hacker's gynecologic oncology. Lippincott Williams & Wilkins Philadelphia; 2010; pp. 576–92.
108. Koh WJ, Greer BE, Abu-Rustum NR, Campos SM, Cho KR, Chon HS, et al. Vulvar Cancer, version 1.2017, NCCN clinical practice guidelines in oncology. J Nat Compreh Cancer Network. 2017;15(1):92–120.
109. Pfaendler KS, Wenzel L, Mechanic MB, Penner KR. Cervical cancer survivorship: long-term quality of life and social support. Clin Therap. 2015;37(1):39–48.
110. Ye S, Yang J, Cao D, Lang J, Shen K. A systematic review of quality of life and sexual function of patients with cervical cancer after treatment. Int J Gynecol Cancer. 2014;24(7):1146–57.
111. Bansal N, Soni A, Kaur P, Chauhan AK, Kaushal V. Exploring the management of radiation proctitis in current clinical practice. J Clin Diag Res. 2016;10(6):XE01–6.
112. Hatzichristou D, Rosen RC, Derogatis LR, Low WY, Meuleman EJ, Sadovsky R, et al. Recommendations for the clinical evaluation of men and women with sexual dysfunction. J Sexual Med. 2010;7(1 Pt 2):337–48.
113. AASECT: American Association of Sexuality Educators, Counselors and Therapists. 2019 [cited 2018 12/10]. Available from: https://www.aasect.org/
114. Li D, Ding C-Y, Qiu L-H. Postoperative hormone replacement therapy for epithelial ovarian cancer patients: a systematic review and meta-analysis. Gynecol Oncol. 2015;139(2):355–62.
115. Del Carmen MG, Rice LW. Management of menopausal symptoms in women with gynecologic cancers. Gynecol Oncol. 2017;146(2):427–35.
116. Suriano KA, McHale M, McLaren CE, Li KT, Re A, DiSaia PJ. Estrogen replacement therapy in endometrial cancer patients: a matched control study. Obstet Gynecol. 2001;97(4):555–60.
117. Network NCC. NCCN clinical practice guidelines in oncology: genetic/familial high-risk assessment: breast and ovarian, version 1.2018. NCCN; 2017.
118. Ferenczy A. Pathophysiology of endometrial bleeding. Maturitas. 2003;45(1):1–14.
119. DeSimone M, Spriggs E, Gass JS, Carson SA, Krychman ML, Dizon DS. Sexual dysfunction in female cancer survivors. Am J Clin Oncol. 2014;37(1):101–6.
120. Krychman ML, Pereira L, Carter J, Amsterdam A. Sexual oncology: sexual health issues in women with cancer. Oncology. 2006;71(1–2):18–25.

Part III

Breast Health and Disease

Benign Breast Conditions

16

Brielle M. Spataro and Amy Fitzpatrick

Learning Objectives

1. Evaluate a patient with a palpable breast mass by performing an appropriate history, physical examination, and evaluation.
2. Formulate evaluation and treatment plans for benign breast masses based on BI-RADS classifications and biopsy results.
3. Identify which classes and types of benign breast masses increase the risk for breast cancer.
4. Compare the presentation of different types of breast inflammation and infection, and discuss appropriate treatment strategies.
5. Develop a differential diagnosis, evaluation, and treatment plan for patients presenting with different types of breast pain: cyclic, noncyclic, and extramammary.
6. Assess a patient presenting with nipple discharge including diagnostic testing as indicated.

Benign breast conditions include a wide variety of presentations: asymptomatic incidental findings on mammography, palpated masses, breast infections, abnormal nipple discharge, and breast pain. The incidence of benign breast conditions peaks in the fourth and fifth decade of life, whereas breast cancer peaks at age 70. Benign breast conditions are much more common than breast cancer and are estimated to effect up to 90% of women at some time in their lives [1]. The goal in the initial evaluation and management of breast complaints is first to exclude malignancy and then to manage the condition. In addition to evaluating and treating benign breast conditions, patient education regarding breast health, benign breast conditions, future cancer risk, and cancer prevention is paramount. This chapter discusses the broad range of benign breast conditions which present for evaluation to the primary care provider.

Normal Breast Anatomy

Breasts are composed of milk-producing glands and surrounding fat. They rest on the pectoralis major but the breasts themselves have no muscle tissue. Breast tissue is responsive to three main hormones: estrogen, progesterone, and prolactin. These hormones drive normal breast development, enlargement, and milk production. Each breast contains about 15–20 lobes arranged in a circular fashion. Each lobe is, in turn, made up of many lobules. At the end of the lobes are tiny bulblike glands where milk is produced. Ducts connect the lobes, lobules, and glands and deliver milk to openings in the nipple. The areola is the darker pigmented area around the nipple. Breast tissue is drained by lymphatic vessels that drain into the axillary lymph nodes [2] (Fig. 16.1).

Janet is a 35-year-old woman who presents with a palpable breast mass in her right breast. She first noticed the mass 6 weeks ago and has noticed no changes since that time. She has no pain, no family history of breast cancer, no history of prior breast biopsies, or history of chest irradiation. On clinical breast exam, a 1-cm, mobile, pea-sized mass, at 9:00, 5 cm from the nipple, is appreciated.

Every patient with a palpable breast mass should be evaluated and followed until there is a satisfactory diagnosis, and malignancy is excluded. The physician must take a thorough

B. M. Spataro
University of Pittsburgh Medical Center, Department of Internal Medicine, Pittsburgh, PA, USA

A. Fitzpatrick (✉)
Boston Medical Center/Boston University School of Medicine, Department of Internal Medicine, Boston, MA, USA
e-mail: amy.fitzpatrick@bmc.org

S. A. Tilstra et al. (eds.), *Sex- and Gender-Based Women's Health*, https://doi.org/10.1007/978-3-030-50695-7_16

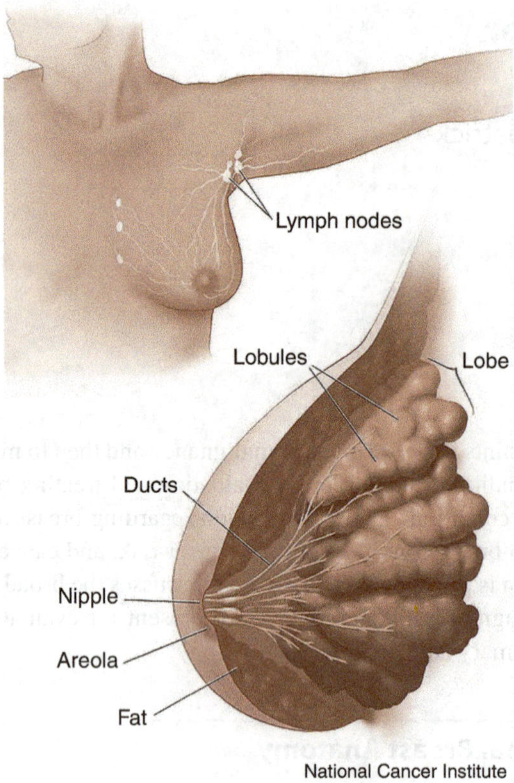

Fig. 16.1 Normal breast anatomy [3]. (Reprinted from NIH. The National Cancer Institute [3])

patient history, perform a careful and systematic breast examination, and order appropriate diagnostic imaging. An overview of this process is outlined below.

The Comprehensive Evaluation of the Breast

The following items should be included when evaluating a patient with breast concern [4, 5]:

- Chief concern involving the breast(s)
- History of present illness:
  - Elaboration of concern: presence of mass(es), pain, skin changes, nipple discharge, axillary symptoms, swelling, erythema, or fever
  - Timing: duration of symptoms, change over time, change with menstrual cycle
  - Current reproductive status: last menstrual period, pregnancy status, breastfeeding status
- Past medical, social, and family history:
  - History of chest irradiation, any cancer, polycystic ovary syndrome (PCOS), and/or obesity
  - Medications (past and present): hormonal therapy, dopamine antagonists, selective serotonin reuptake inhibitors
  - Reproductive and gynecologic history: age of menarche, pregnancies and births including age of first delivery, contraceptive use, age of menopause
  - Breast history: prior history of breast cancer, breast masses, breast trauma, breast abnormalities or symptoms, prior imaging including breast density or abnormalities, prior biopsy and results, history of breast cancer and any surgery, radiation, chemoprophylaxis or chemotherapy
  - Family history: breast or ovarian cancer in family including age of diagnosis, other cancer history, or known genetic testing
  - Habits: smoking, alcohol, diet, physical activity, living situation, and occupation

The Clinical Breast Exam

The clinical breast exam (CBE) is a systematic and thorough exam which is essential for evaluating all breast concerns. A careful CBE can take up to 6 min. During the exam, additional history may be obtained, and general breast health education can be discussed. The patient should be gowned with the opening of the gown in the front of the patient. Inspection of breast should take place while the patient is sitting or standing upright. Asymmetry, skin changes, puckering, nipple inversion, retraction, or discharge are noted, and supraclavicular and axillary lymph nodes are palpated. The patient assumes the supine position, and each breast examined, with the ipsilateral arm raised above the head, from the clavicle to the sixth rib and from the sternum to the midaxillary line. A systematic method, such as vertical lines, is used to ensure that no tissue is missed. Using the pads of the index, middle, and ring fingers of one hand, the breast tissue is palpated in three planes – superficial, medium, and deep – applying increasing pressure in a circular motion (see Chap. 18 on "Breast Cancer Screening" for a detailed discussion and description of the CBE).

Any mass or thickening appreciated should be examined closely. The approximate size, mobility, shape, texture, tenderness, and location should be described and documented. Standard descriptions of location include laterality, position in the breast using a clockface nomenclature, distance in centimeters from the edge of the mass to the nipple, and subareolar position or quadrant, such as upper versus lower and medial (inner) versus lateral (outer). When ordering breast imaging or consultations, location needs to be described accurately [4, 5] (Fig. 16.2).

Breast Imaging

In patients over 30 years old with a palpable breast mass, focal pain, or pathologic nipple discharge, diagnostic mammography and ultrasound are recommended. In patients

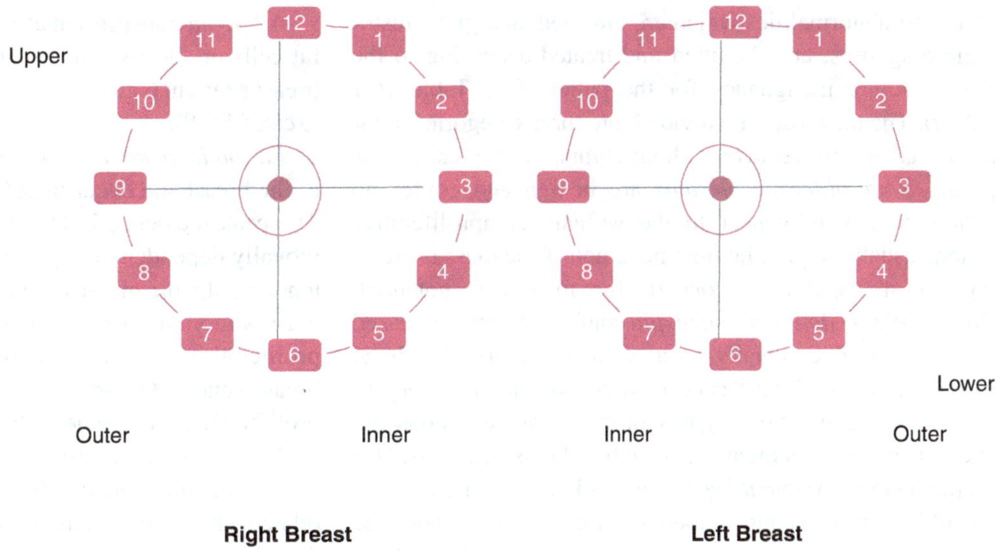

Fig. 16.2 Breast diagram with superimposed clockface and quadrants

under 30 years old, an ultrasound is recommended without mammography. For the woman under 30 years old, observation over one or two menstrual cycles is an acceptable alternative to imaging, for low clinical suspicion abnormalities. If the mass persists longer than 2 cycles, the mass should be imaged. In high-risk or suspicious cases, however, consultation with a breast specialist is required, and MRI or mammography may be recommended [6, 7].

In patients with an average cancer risk and a lesion of low suspicion, the negative predictive value of diagnostic mammography with ultrasound ranges from 97.4% to 100% [6]. In general, women are average risk if there is no family history of breast or ovarian cancer, no history of prior breast problems or breast biopsy, and no history of radiation to the chest prior to age 30 (please see Chap. 17 on "The Primary Prevention of Breast Cancer" and Chap. 18 on "Breast Cancer Screening" for a full discussion of assessing breast cancer risk). In higher-risk women or if clinical suspicion is high, consultation with a breast specialist and possible MRI or core needle biopsy should be considered, even in the setting of negative imaging. An MRI should be performed, if needed, prior to biopsy, as a biopsy can affect images. If biopsy is not performed after consultation, then the patient needs close follow-up every 6 months with CBE and imaging, usually ultrasound, to ensure stability, for 2 years. In addition, the patient should perform breast self-examination and practice breast awareness (see Chap. 18 on "Breast Cancer Screening") and report any changes in her symptoms urgently. Masses should be followed until there is a successful resolution. As a risk management point, failure to diagnose breast cancer is one of the most common malpractice complaints. Careful documentation, open communication with the patient, and continued evaluation of patient concerns will help ensure that the patient is properly treated and satisfied with care rendered.

A diagnostic mammography and ultrasound are ordered, and the results read BI-RADS 3, likely fibroadenoma. The patient wants to discuss the results.

The patient's palpable mass is most likely a fibroadenoma based on mammography and ultrasound. A BI-RADS 3 interpretation describes lesions that are most likely benign, but given their radiologic appearance, there is a less than 2% chance of malignancy (see Chap. 18 on "Breast Cancer Screening" for table on BI-RADS categories and follow-up). BI-RADS 3 lesions must be monitored with short-interval follow-up. Diagnostic mammography and ultrasound are performed at 6, 12, and 24 months to ensure stability. If the patient has other risk factors that increase the provider's suspicion for underlying carcinoma, then core needle biopsy should be performed [7].

Differential Diagnosis of Benign Breast Lesions

Breast concerns are common, as are incidental findings on breast imaging. Most benign breast lesions, physiologic nipple discharge, and breast pain collectively are blamed on fibrocystic changes (FCC), or fibrocystic breast disease, which is a broad clinical diagnosis encompassing many benign breast changes. FCC occurs most commonly in premenopausal women and appears to be hormone related. The definition of FCC is not standardized and may include all benign breast lesions or nonproliferative breast lesions only. FCC has also been referred to as chronic cystic mastitis and mammary dysplasia. More specific diagnoses than the broad term FCC help in determining the treatment needed and the cancer risk for individual women.

Breast abnormalities which are biopsied, and given histologic diagnoses, are classified and treated according to the risk of future malignancy for the patient (see Table 16.1 below). The diagnoses are divided into three categories: nonproliferative, proliferative without atypia, or atypical hyperplasia. *Nonproliferative lesions* are benign and confer no additional risk of cancer to the woman. Nonproliferative lesions usually require no treatment, unless the mass is growing, or if there is a concern for malignant potential. *Proliferative lesions without atypia* confer a slightly increased risk of cancer, especially in a woman who is already at increased risk of breast cancer based on family history or other risk factors. Some types of proliferative lesions are excised, and management is guided by a breast specialist (see section below). *Atypical hyperplasia* is known to increase the risk of breast cancer and women with this diagnosis should be offered chemoprevention which can decrease the risk of developing breast cancer by approximately 50%. These patients should undergo risk assessment with the GAIL or IBIS model to determine whether yearly MRI, in addition to routine mammography and increased surveillance, should be performed (see Chap. 17 on "The Primary Prevention of Breast Cancer" and Chap. 18 on "Breast Cancer Screening").

Nonproliferative Benign Lesions

Nonproliferative lesions are not associated with any increased risk of future breast cancer. *Cysts*, the most common type of benign breast disease, are fluid-filled round or ovoid structures. They are found in up to one-third of women aged 35–50. Cysts are classified as simple or complex based on ultrasound findings. Simple cysts are benign and do not require treatment. If the cyst is bothersome, then a fine needle aspiration (FNA) with drainage can be both curative and reassuring to the patient. Follow-up of simple cysts is not needed. *Complex cysts*, also called complicated or atypical cysts, are diagnosed based on ultrasound findings of internal echos, thin septations, thickened or irregular walls, or absent posterior enhancement. Complex cysts are managed with follow-up imaging to document stability or resolution. Intracystic masses, when present, are managed as other solid masses with biopsy, either excisional or core as indicated, to ensure appropriate tissue diagnosis. The risk of malignancy for complex cysts is approximately 0.3% [8, 9].

Fat necrosis may present as a mass or as an oil cyst and may be the result of breast trauma or surgery. Fat necrosis may require biopsy, but once diagnosis is confirmed, no further treatment is necessary.

A *galactocele* is a cystic collection of fluid caused by an obstructed milk duct. The diagnosis is confirmed with aspiration of milky fluid from the cyst. No further management is necessary.

A *lipoma* may present as a breast mass and reveals mature fat cells on biopsy. The recommended follow-up is clinical breast exam in 6 months; if lesion grows rapidly, it should be excised [1, 8].

Fibroadenomas are the most common benign neoplasm of the breast and occur in 25% of asymptomatic women [1]. The peak incidence is 15–35 years of age. Lesions are hormonally dependent and present as highly mobile, firm, nontender, palpable masses. Fibroadenomas are common breast masses in young women, half of which are simple, or nonproliferative, and are not associated with an increased risk of breast cancer. One-half of fibroadenomas are complex, or proliferative, and are described below [1, 8].

The other nonproliferative breast conditions listed in Table 16.1 include papillary apocrine change, epithelial-related calcifications, mild hyperplasia of the usual type, ductal ectasia, nonsclerosing adenosis, and periductal fibro-

Table 16.1 Benign breast lesions and the relative risk of future breast cancer [8, 9]

Diagnosis based on clinical evaluation including imaging and biopsy	Relative risk of future breast cancer	
Nonproliferative lesions: Simple cysts[a] Papillary apocrine change Epithelial-related calcifications Mild epithelial hyperplasia Ductal ectasia Nonsclerosing adenosis Periductal fibrosis Simple fibroadenoma Fat necrosis Galactocele Lipoma	*No increased risk*	
Proliferative lesions without atypia:	*Slightly increased risk*	
Epithelial hyperplasia (ductal or lobular) Sclerosing adenosis Radial scar Intraductal papilloma Papillomatosis Complex fibroadenoma Hamartoma	No family history of breast cancer RR 1.3–1.9	Family history of breast cancer RR 2.4–2.7
Proliferative lesions with atypia:	*Increased risk of breast cancer*	
Atypical ductal hyperplasia (ADH) Atypical lobular hyperplasia (ALH)	No family history RR 4.1–4.3	Family history RR 4.7–22
Lobular carcinoma in situ (LCIS)	RR 10.0	
Ductal carcinoma in situ (DCIS)	RR 17.3 after biopsy without treatment[b]	

[a]Simple cysts may be diagnosed without biopsy, although fine needle aspiration (FNA) with drainage may be curative. Complex cysts require additional evaluation to exclude malignancy

[b]DCIS is a noninvasive malignancy with a variable history. RR of invasive cancer is high without treatment [10, 11]

sis. These changes are benign and do not require additional evaluation or treatment.

Proliferative Lesions Without Atypia

Proliferative lesions without atypia are associated with an increased risk of subsequent breast cancer. The relative risk (RR) of future breast cancer is 1.3–1.9 if there is no family history of breast cancer and increases to 2.4–2.7 if there is a family history of breast cancer [8, 9].

Complex Fibroadenoma. Approximately half of fibroadenomas are complex meaning they have proliferative changes: sclerosing adenosis, adenosis, or duct epithelial hyperplasia. Complex fibroadenomas confer a slightly higher risk for subsequent cancer [9]. The management of proliferative lesions varies and is often based on size. The majority are monitored closely with imaging every 6 months for 2 years to ensure stability. Biopsy is indicated for lesions with suspicious findings on imaging, growth during the surveillance period, or increased clinical concern. Biopsy-proven fibroadenomas greater than 4 cm in size are removed surgically or treated with office-based, ultrasound-guided cryoablation [8, 12].

Epithelial hyperplasia is the most common form of proliferative breast disease and refers to any increase in the number of cells in the ductal space. Hyperplasia may involve cells of ductal or lobular origin. Hyperplasia is stratified into three categories: mild, moderate, and florid. Mild hyperplasia consists of three to four cell layers of epithelial cells, moderate hyperplasia is greater than four cells in depth, and florid hyperplasia fills the ductal lumen, which may become obliterated and distended [9]. Mild hyperplasia occurs normally as breast tissue responds to hormonal influences and is not pathologic. Hyperplasia without atypia does not require specific treatment, regardless of severity.

Adenosis of the breast is a proliferative lesion that consists of an increased number of glandular components. *Sclerosing adenosis* is a lobulocentric lesion of disordered acinar, myoepithelial, and connective tissue. Sclerosing adenosis can mimic infiltrative carcinoma histologically and therefore can be diagnostically challenging for pathologists. *Microglandular adenosis* is a proliferation of round, small glands distributed irregularly in dense fibrous or adipose tissue that recurs if not completely excised [8]. These lesions may or may not be excised, and no further treatment is needed.

A radial scar is a fibroelastic core with entrapped ducts surrounded by radiating ducts and lobules which can mimic carcinoma on mammography. The lesion often has the appearance of a scar, thus its name, although it is often not a true scar. It is recommended that radial scars be completely excised when found on biopsy. Radial scars require careful management as they may be premalignant markers or coexist with lesions of atypical hyperplasia, lobular carcinoma in situ (LCIS), ductal carcinoma in situ (DCIS), or invasive breast carcinoma [8].

An *intraductal papilloma* is a tumor of the epithelium of mammary ducts that usually presents with serous or serosanguinous nipple discharge (see section "Nipple Discharge"). While central, single papillomas are not considered to be premalignant or carry an increased risk of breast cancer, there is a correlation between papillomas and atypical ductal hyperplasia. Excisional biopsy is recommended with no further treatment needed, assuming benign pathology. *Papillomatosis* describes a minimum of five separate papillomas. It is more likely to occur bilaterally and to have an associated in situ or invasive carcinoma than central papillomas. It may indicate a slightly increased risk of breast cancer. Surgical excision of papillomatosis is recommended [8]. A small number of papillary tumors will be found upon excision to contain invasive carcinoma and should be treated accordingly.

Phyllodes tumor is a benign fibroepithelial tumor of the breast which arises from the connective tissue and may display a spectrum of cellular changes like fibroadenomas. Women with Li-Fraumeni syndrome are at increased risk of phyllodes tumors. Tumors with recurrent or malignant behavior are identified by hypercellular stroma with atypia, increased mitoses, and infiltrative margins. Phyllodes tumors need to be surgically excised with clear margins, and recurrence is often treated with mastectomy [8]. Malignant phyllodes tumors, those with distant metastases, are technically sarcomas and may be resistant to therapy. Malignant tumors are treated with surgical excision and may often require radiation and sometimes chemotherapy.

Adenomas are pure epithelial neoplasms that are further classified as tubular, lactating, apocrine, ductal, or pleomorphic. Adenomas usually present as a solitary palpable mass, do not recur, have no malignant potential, but may require excision due to mass effect [2, 8].

A *hamartoma* is an uncommon tumor and is composed of glandular, adipose, and fibrous tissue. Coincidental malignancy can exist, and therefore, surgical excision is recommended [1, 8].

Janet returns 6 months later for follow-up with a clinical breast exam and repeat imaging. She is doing well and believes the mass has gotten smaller. On clinical exam, it is unclear whether the mass has changed in size. Repeat imaging shows a stable mass, likely fibroadenoma. She is followed with imaging every 6 months for 2 years to ensure stability, at which point her mammography changes to BI-RADS 2.

Norah is a healthy 46-year-old woman who had a screening mammogram. It is read as having suspicious calcifications and is classified as BI-RADS 4. Norah is referred for biopsy.

A core needle biopsy is recommended in cases where initial imaging is read as BI-RADS 4 or 5 or if there is a high clinical suspicion for invasive carcinoma, even if there is no palpable mass [7]. A reading of BI-RADS 4 is "suspicious" and the risk of malignancy ranges from low (2–9%) for 4A, moderate (10–49%) for 4B to high (50–94%) for 4C. BI-RADS 5 is "highly suggestive of malignancy" and carries a risk of 95–100% for malignancy.

If the results of a core needle biopsy are benign and concordant with imaging, these patients may return to routine screening or continue short interval follow-up with CBE and mammography every 6–12 months for a year. If there is a significant increase in size in the lesion or high clinical suspicion for carcinoma, then surgical excision is performed [8].

Surgical excision is indicated for lesions that are indeterminate on core needle biopsy, benign, and image discordant or show atypical ductal hyperplasia, mucin-producing lesions, phyllodes tumor, or other histology of concern to the pathologist. Some patients with flat epithelial atypia, papillomas, fibroepithelial lesions, or radial scars, in consultation with a breast specialist, may be candidates for close monitoring rather than excision. Treatment decisions are agreed upon by the patient and breast specialist through shared decision-making [8].

Norah undergoes biopsy, and the pathology report shows atypical ductal hyperplasia. She is seen by a breast surgeon and has a subsequent surgical excision. Final pathology is consistent with "atypical ductal hyperplasia, no invasive or in situ carcinoma seen." The patient understands that her risk of breast cancer is increased and agrees to chemoprevention. She is premenopausal and is prescribed tamoxifen (see Chap. 17 on "The Primary Prevention of Breast Cancer").

Proliferative Lesions with Atypia

Proliferative lesions with atypia are associated with an increased risk of breast cancer. Atypical lesions are classified as lobular or ductal. Women with a history of atypical lobular hyperplasia or atypical ductal hyperplasia should avoid exogenous hormones like hormonal contraceptives or hormone replacement therapy and should be offered chemoprevention: with tamoxifen if she is premenopausal, and raloxifene or aromatase inhibitor therapy if she is postmenopausal. The choice of hormonal therapy agents and duration of therapy are discussed separately (see Chap. 17 on "The Primary Prevention of Breast Cancer" for a full discussion).

Lobular neoplasia is a term which includes *atypical lobular hyperplasia (ALH)* and *lobular carcinoma in situ (LCIS)*. Lobular neoplasia is nonmalignant and primarily affects premenopausal women. It is often multifocal and is bilateral in a third of cases. Lobular neoplasia is usually an incidental finding on mammography or biopsy and traditionally has not been considered premalignant. Lobular abnormalities resemble adipose cells in terms of density, can grow in a weblike pattern, are usually without calcifications, and can be invisible on mammography, even if malignant. If lesions with the pathologic diagnosis of atypical lobular hyperplasia (ALH), or lobular carcinoma in situ (LCIS), are nonconcordant with imaging, or if the biopsy reveals pleomorphic LCIS, then surgical excision is recommended. However, if ALH or LCIS are concordant with imaging and are not pleomorphic, then observation with physical exam and breast imaging every 6–12 months for a year may be considered [7].

The relative risk of subsequent breast cancer is increased 4 times in women with ALH and is increased 10 times in patients with LCIS compared to women without these lesions. Patients with ALH or LCIS should be offered chemoprophylaxis and increased surveillance (exam every 6–12 months and yearly mammography for the remainder of her life) to decrease the risk of breast cancer (see Chap. 17 on "The Primary Prevention of Breast Cancer"). Recent studies have called into question the idea that ALH and LCIS have a more benign natural history than atypical ductal hyperplasia [7, 13].

Atypical ductal hyperplasia (ADH) is morphologically similar to DCIS and is more likely to manifest as calcifications on mammography then as a palpable mass. ADH is a high-risk, premalignant lesion and is a direct precursor to invasive ductal carcinoma. The associated risk of breast cancer is highest in the 5–15 years following the diagnosis of ADH and may occur in the ipsilateral or contralateral breast. Surgical excision is the standard recommendation for ADH lesions, as a significant percentage of lesions are upgraded to DCIS or invasive carcinoma on surgical pathology [7]. Chemoprophylaxis with selective estrogen receptor modulators (SERMs) or aromatase inhibitors (AIs) is recommended for women with ADH. It should be noted that prophylactic treatment is currently greatly underutilized by patients and primary care providers despite the safety and efficacy of chemopreventive agents (see Chap. 17 on "The Primary Prevention of Breast Cancer") [13, 14]. DCIS is a noninvasive malignancy and is discussed elsewhere (see Chap. 19 on "Breast Cancer Diagnosis and Management").

All women with a history of LCIS, ADH, or ALH are considered high risk for breast cancer. From the time of diagnosis, patients should have a breast risk assessment clinical encounter every 6–12 months. During this encounter, updated medical and family history should be reviewed to update risk assessment. The patient should have risk reduction counseling and a clinical breast exam. Annual screening mammography is recommended to begin at the diagnosis of ADH/ALH or LCIS but not prior to age 30. Annual breast MRI is recommended in high-risk women over the age of 25 who have an estimated lifetime risk of breast cancer greater than 20–25 percent (see Chap.18 on "Breast Cancer Screening"). Chemoprevention with a SERM or AI should be offered to all patients with ALH, ADH, or LCIS [5, 9] (see Chap. 17 on "The Primary Prevention of Breast Cancer").

For chemoprevention, premenopausal women should be offered tamoxifen, 20 mg per day for 5 years, which has been shown to decrease the risk of breast cancer by up to 49% in women with ALH or LCIS. In premenopausal women with ADH, the benefit is greater, and tamoxifen use has been associated with an 86% reduction in breast cancer risk. In postmenopausal women, the preferred treatment is raloxifene 60 mg per day for 5 years. Raloxifene is as effective as tamoxifen in decreasing the risk of invasive breast cancers but may be slightly less efficacious in preventing DCIS. For women with a uterus, this difference is offset by the fact that raloxifene does not increase the risk of uterine cancer.

Both tamoxifen and raloxifene increase bone mass, and raloxifene is approved in both the prevention and treatment of osteoporosis. The risk of venous thrombotic events is 1–3/1000 for patients taking tamoxifen or raloxifene. Contraindications to the use of tamoxifen and raloxifene include prior deep vein thrombosis, pulmonary embolus, thrombotic stroke, transient ischemic attack, or clotting disorder. Major side effects include menopausal symptoms. Vaginal bleeding on tamoxifen must be further evaluated as it is associated with an increased risk of endometrial cancer (see Chap. 15 on "Gynecologic Malignancies"). Ongoing trials evaluating lower doses of tamoxifen for chemoprophylaxis suggest comparable efficacy and lower complication rates to the traditional dose of tamoxifen 20 mg per day. Further study is needed to define optimal chemoprevention strategies and increase the acceptance of chemoprevention among patients and PCPs.

Aromatase inhibitors (AIs), including exemestane and anastrozole, are prescribed to postmenopausal women who cannot tolerate selective estrogen receptor modulators (SERMS). Exemestane, 25 mg daily, reduces breast cancer incidence by 65% at 3 years. Anastrozole, 1 mg daily, reduces the relative incidence of breast cancer by 53% at 5 years [9].

The major disadvantage of AIs is the increased risk of osteoporosis associated with antiestrogen therapy. Baseline bone density should be evaluated in all postmenopausal women prior to starting treatment with SERMs or AIs and monitored every 2 years, especially when aromatase inhibitors are used. Major side effects of all antiestrogen treatments include hot flashes, vaginal atrophy, and menopausal symptoms. AIs can be associated with fatigue and muscle and joint aches; however, the side effects associated with placebo use are nearly equivalent to AI use [9]. Some AIs may increase risk of thromboembolic events to a similar degree as SERMs. A full discussion or AI and SERM use is beyond the scope of this chapter.

Mastitis and Breast Abscess

Adriana is a 42-year-old woman who reports severe breast pain on the left for the past 8 h. She is breastfeeding her third child. She is advised by the nurse to keep breastfeeding, get rest, apply warm and cold compresses, and use nonsteroidal anti-inflammatory agents (NSAIDS). She will come in to clinic tomorrow morning to be seen if her symptoms do not improve by then.

Puerperal Mastitis

The most common type of breast infection is lactational or puerperal mastitis. The incidence ranges from 2% to 11% of all breastfeeding women, although some studies have estimated the incidence to be as high as 27% [14, 15]. It most commonly occurs in the first 12 weeks of breastfeeding and often presents as a swollen, painful, and red breast. Women may develop a low-grade fever and generalized malaise 12–24 h after symptoms appear. Breast engorgement initially occurs due to poor milk drainage which can be caused by a number of factors, including interrupted or erratic feeding patterns, a sudden change in the number of feeds, skipped feedings, nipple trauma, poor positioning and latch-on, a short frenulum in the infant, mother or infant illness, and separation of mother and infant with reduced frequency of breastfeeding [16].

If symptoms persist beyond 12–24 h, the condition is considered to be infective lactational mastitis and bacteria are found in both the milk and within the mother's skin. Lactational infections are frequently located peripherally. Lactational infections are readily recognized and treated by primary care or obstetric providers and therefore account for <15% of infections seen in breast clinics [17].

Adriana comes in to clinic the next day with increasing pain. Any movement of the breast is excruciatingly painful, and there is a mass in the center of the painful area. She does not have a fever, but reports she has been experiencing shaking chills for the past 30 min.

When the treatment of lactational mastitis is delayed or inadequate, a lactational abscess may develop [14–16]. A palpable mass may be present and may represent a preexisting breast mass, a blocked duct, or an abscess. If a palpable mass is present, an ultrasound will differentiate the etiology, i.e., whether edema, a mass, or an abscess is present. Women can become toxic with high fevers and experience extreme pain, requiring intravenous antibiotics, intravenous fluids, analgesia, and ultrasound drainage of any fluid collection.

Fungal mastitis is a less common entity that presents with pain out of proportion to physical findings. Fungal mastitis occurs in the setting of thrush in the infant and is treated with topical or oral antifungals for mother and infant.

Treatment of Lactational Mastitis and Abscess

Lactational mastitis generally does not require diagnostic imaging. Symptomatic treatment with NSAIDS, cold or warm compresses, and complete emptying of the breast by breastfeeding or pumping are recommended during the first 12–24 h. If symptoms persist for more than 12–24 h, then antibiotics are recommended in addition to symptomatic treatment [14, 15].

In infective lactational mastitis or abscess, the most common causative organism is *Staphylococcus aureus*. Empiric antibiotic therapy for lactational mastitis depends upon *methicillin-resistant Staphylococcus aureus* (MRSA) risk and age of the newborn. Risk factors for MRSA include recent hospitalizations, residence in a long-term care facility, hemodialysis, a history of intravenous drug use (IVDU), a history of incarceration, and being a health-care worker. In many communities, MRSA has become common without significant risk factors.

Choices of antibiotics for empiric therapy include:

- No MRSA risk factors:
  - Dicloxacillin 500 mg four times daily or
  - Cephalexin 500 mg four times daily or
  - Clindamycin 300 or 450 mg three times daily (indicated if beta-lactam hypersensitivity present)
- MRSA risk factors:
  - Trimethoprim-sulfamethoxazole 1 double-strength tablet twice daily (only if infant is >2 months old, or beyond the newborn period) or
  - Clindamycin 300 or 450 mg three times daily

Treatment should be given for 10–14 days. Trimethoprim-sulfamethoxazole should not be used in mothers nursing newborns or in immunocompromised infants due to the increased risk of kernicterus. Lactational mastitis does not usually recur, but women should be counseled about the prevention and management of blocked ducts with adequate fluid intake, rest, frequent breastfeeding, warm compresses and gentle massage, and expulsion of duct plugs when possible.

Bridgette is a 40-year-old African American woman who presents to clinic with a painful, warm, and erythematous right breast. She reports that she developed pain and redness around the areola which progressed into ulceration and drainage 2 days ago. Bridgette reports the pain is so severe, that she is unable to wear a bra and has not been able to sleep. She denies fevers but reports that she has pain when she bumps or jostles her right breast. She is not pregnant or breastfeeding, and her youngest child is 22-year-old.

Nonpuerperal Mastitis

Nonpuerperal, or nonlactational, mastitis is an uncommon disorder and describes all the causes of inflammatory changes in the breast not related to lactation. Nonpuerperal mastitis may occur due to a ruptured cyst and may be self-limited; however, malignancy should be excluded.

Mammary duct ectasia, also referred to as *periductal mastitis*, is a benign condition that becomes more common as women approach menopause. The lactiferous ducts become shorter and wider and may become clogged. Initially, squamous metaplasia of the cuboidal epithelium of the ducts leads to increased keratin formation and obstruction of the duct lumen. Blockage of ducts with cellular debris results in dilatation and, ultimately, the formation of a foreign body inflammatory reaction around the extruded keratin. A greenish discharge may be noted from the nipple. Secondary infection may occur due to stagnation of the intraductal fluid, which predisposes to abscess formation and cutaneous fistulas [17, 18].

Nonpuerperal abscesses have been characterized into two types and are differentiated by location. Peripheral nonpuerperal abscesses are uncommon compared to central or periareolar abscesses. Risk factors for the development of nonpuerperal abscesses are Black race, obesity, and smoking [18]. It is thought that nonpuerperal abscesses form as a complication of mammary duct ectasia.

Peripheral nonpuerperal abscesses are generally associated with trauma, acne, epidermal cysts, and chronic conditions such as diabetes and rheumatoid arthritis [17]. *Central or subareolar abscesses* affect women in a wide age range, from teens to the eighth decade, with peak incidence in mid- to late forties [17]. Subareolar abscesses may present unilaterally or bilaterally and symptoms vary depending on the age of the patient. Younger patients often report more breast pain than older patients. Palpable masses associated with this type of breast infection are common and are generally associated with overlying erythema. Approximately 15–20% of women with subareolar abscesses report discharge or drainage, and infections often involve anaerobic bacteria. Nonpuerperal abscesses frequently recur (>50%) and often require multiple drainage or surgical procedures. Fistulas form in up to one-third of recurrent cases and are associated with mixed aerobic and anaerobic infections [17].

Bridgette reports that she is nervous about having any sort of procedure and would like to avoid "needles" if possible. Her clinical breast exam is notable for swelling and erythema of the right areola extending into the surrounding skin laterally, at 9 o'clock. There is a small open area that is draining purulent material.

The treatment of nonpuerperal abscesses includes ultrasound-guided aspiration and drainage and antibiotic therapy. Abscesses that are not amenable to ultrasound-guided drainage are treated with antibiotics and warm compresses. The most common organisms are *Staphylococci, Enterococci, anaerobic Streptococci, Bacteroides,* and *Proteus.*

Empiric antibiotic therapy for nonpuerperal abscess [17, 18] include the following:

- No MRSA risk factors:
  - Amoxicillin-clavulanate 875–125 mg twice daily or
  - Dicloxacillin 500 mg four times daily or
  - Cephalexin 500 mg four times daily
- If anaerobes are suspected (especially subareolar infections):
  - Clindamycin 300 or 450 mg three times daily PLUS metronidazole 500 mg three times daily or
  - Amoxicillin-clavulanate 875–125 mg twice daily or
  - Clarithromycin 500 mg PO BID, *plus* metronidazole 500 mg PO TID [19]
- MRSA risk factors:
  - Trimethoprim-sulfamethoxazole one double-strength tablet twice daily or
  - Doxycycline 100 mg twice daily or
  - Clindamycin 300 or 450 mg three times daily

Cases that are refractory to medical management are referred for surgical intervention [17]. The optimal duration of antibiotics is not known. Mild to moderate cases can be treated with 7 days of antibiotics, with more severe cases requiring 10–14 days of antibiotics [17, 18].

Bridgette's breast ultrasound revealed a large subareolar fluid collection which was amenable to drainage. The patient was screened for MRSA risk factors and found to have none. She was prescribed cephalexin 500 mg four times daily for 7 days. During her follow-up visit 2 weeks later, the patient was doing well with resolution of her right breast abscess. Now, 3 months later, Bridgette returns with the same symptoms.

Recurrences of subareolar abscesses are common and occur in more than 50% of cases. Several risk factors are associated with higher rates of recurrence and delayed recovery, including cigarette smoking, the presence of mixed flora infections, anaerobic infections, and *Proteus* organisms [17]. The relative risk of subareolar abscess recurring is directly related to the intensity of cigarette smoking, with heavier smokers more likely to experience recurrence [16]. The exact mechanism by which smoking increases the risk of abscess is not known; however, one theory is that squamous metaplasia occurs in a similar fashion to the smoking-related squamous metaplasia of bronchial mucosa, which is related to the level of smoking intensity. Nicotine and its metabolite cotinine can be detected in breast milk within 30 min of smoking. Another theory suggests that smoking decreases the bioavailability of estrogen which negatively affects ductal integrity [16].

Bridgette again underwent ultrasound-guided drainage of her right breast abscess and was started back on cephalexin. She admitted to smoking ½ pack per day for more than 20 years and reported that she would try to cut back. On follow-up 2 weeks later, she had resolution of her abscess. Now, 2 months later, she presents with a third recurrence. On clinical exam, she has no drainage or discharge, but has more significant skin thickening, a 1-cm palpable mass, and a slight retraction of her right nipple on exam.

In patients who present with signs of skin thickening, subareolar mass, and retraction of the nipple, there is often concern for a malignancy, such as inflammatory breast cancer. Mammographic findings in inflammatory breast cancer and those found with subareolar abscess or infection often overlap and can include skin thickening, trabecular prominence or edema, and asymmetric density [17]. Frequently, masses associated with inflammatory breast cancer are solid masses, whereas those associated with abscess or infections are cystic or mixed [17]. If imaging with breast mammogram and ultrasound are not diagnostic, a biopsy will confirm the diagnosis. In addition to inflammatory breast cancer, the differential diagnosis includes granulomatous mastitis, Mondor's disease (superficial thrombophlebitis of a vein in the anterolateral thoracoabdominal wall), and sarcoidosis of the breast, or more rarely, cat scratch disease and tuberculosis of the breast. Further management depends upon biopsy and culture results, in consultation with a breast specialist.

Granulomatous mastitis presents similarly to breast abscesses and patients are generally referred to a breast clinic after multiple unsuccessful antibiotic courses and drainage attempts. Core needle biopsy provides a definitive diagnosis with the presence of nonnecrotizing granulomas that are negative for microorganisms in the setting of no other systemic granulomatous disease. The treatment for persistent or severe granulomatous mastitis includes corticosteroid therapy or methotrexate [20].

Bridgette has a diagnostic mammogram and repeat ultrasound performed, which shows an irregularly shaped subareolar mass that is cystic with some internal debris and small associated fluid collection (BI-RADS 4). A core needle biopsy is performed which demonstrates inflammation but no granulomatous disease or malignancy. The patient is referred to a breast surgeon for further evaluation.

Patients who fail medical management with ultrasound-guided drainage and antibiotics should be referred to breast surgeon for possible surgical excision of the abscess and involved ducts. There have been several studies suggesting that surgical excision of the abscess, affected ducts, and fistulae should be done early, on initial presentation, resulting in lower recurrence rates. One study showed the recurrence rate after excision was 28% versus 79% after management without surgical excision [21].

Breast Pain

Tatiana is a 27-year-old Columbian woman who presents to clinic complaining of cyclic breast pain for 4 months. She reports pain for 1–2 weeks at a time before the pain resolves. The pain seems worse in the weeks prior to menses. She reports she has more pain on the left side than the right. When asked where the pain is located, Tatiana indicates the entire breast is painful. She reports regular menses and denies the use of contraceptives. On clinical breast exam, the patient has diffuse tenderness to palpation without a discrete or dominant mass.

Mastalgia or breast pain is a common complaint of women and the most frequent reason for breast-related office visits [22, 23]. One large population study showed that approximately 50% of women experience breast pain with 41% reporting a negative impact on their sex life and 35% reporting a negative impact on sleep [22]. Other studies estimate the prevalence as high as 70% [24]. Although some women visit the doctor for breast pain out of fear for breast cancer, the prevalence of breast pain is likely underreported because many women do not go to the doctor for this problem.

The history in the breast pain patient includes (1) the quality, location, duration, and radiation of the breast pain as well as triggering and alleviating factors; (2) breast symptoms such as a breast mass, nipple discharge, or skin changes; and (3) hormonal influences such as relation to menses, pregnancy, contraceptive use, and, in postmenopausal women, hormonal therapies [25]. Medications are reviewed, because some medications can be associated with breast pain (see below). Risk assessment for breast cancer includes a detailed reproductive, family, and medical history. The medical history sometimes provides clues to extramammary etiologies. For example, hidradenitis suppurativa, neck or back arthritis, fibromyalgia, depression, or anxiety may provide clues to underlying causes of the report of breast pain. Finally, a thorough CBE should be performed.

There are three broad classifications of breast pain including *cyclical, noncyclical*, and *extramammary* breast pain. *Cyclical breast pain* by definition occurs in premenopausal women and fluctuates in intensity throughout the menstrual cycle. Cyclical breast pain is generally diffuse and bilateral although it may be worse in one breast and often occurs in the upper outer quadrants, radiating to the axilla. Cyclical breast pain starts during the luteal phase of the menstrual cycle, increasing in intensity until the onset of menses. Some women report pain during the entire cycle, with intensification of pain during luteal phase prior to the onset of menses. Breast pain may increase in the luteal phase because luteal hormones increase water content in the breast stroma [25]. Psychological factors may also play a role, as several studies have shown higher rates of anxiety and depression in women with breast pain compared to asymptomatic women, and mood may worsen in the premenstrual weeks [26]. Cyclical breast pain resolves spontaneously in 20–30% of women, but recurs in 60% of women [24]. Remission of cyclical mastalgia can occur after hormonal events such as pregnancy or menopause [25].

Noncyclical breast pain is intermittent or constant breast pain that is not related to the menstrual cycle. It is less common than cyclical mastalgia and tends to be unilateral and is often localized to a quadrant of the breast. There is a spectrum, however, and some women present with diffuse breast pain that radiates to the axilla. Noncyclical breast pain tends to present later in life and affects women in the fourth and fifth decades, although many of the women are postmenopausal at the onset of symptoms [25]. In the majority of cases, there is no identified cause for noncyclical breast pain; however, some identified causes include trauma, mastitis, cysts, benign tumors, or cancer. The cause of noncyclical breast pain is thought to be more anatomical than hormonal [25]. Large pendulous breasts may cause ligamentous pain and may be improved with the use of a well-fitting support bra [27].

There has been some association between medications and noncyclical breast pain, especially with hormonal medications such as estrogen, progestin, and menopausal hormonal therapy. Other medications associated with breast pain include some antidepressants (specifically selective serotonin reuptake inhibitors, SSRIs), antipsychotics, antifungals, and methadone [25]. These medications are suspected to cause breast pain through several pathways: antipsychotics and methadone (opiates) are thought to contribute to breast pain by their antagonism of dopamine receptors in the CNS, which causes an increase in prolactin by the pituitary gland. Antifungals are known to inhibit androgen synthesis which increases breast tissue growth.

There is also a high incidence of breast pain after breast surgery, including mastectomy, augmentation, reduction, lumpectomy, and excision [25]. Noncyclical breast pain responds poorly to treatment but tends to resolve spontaneously in half of women [24].

Extramammary pain presents as breast pain but has many other etiologies. The most frequent extramammary cause of breast pain is costochondritis or other chest wall conditions including Tietze syndrome (swelling and pain of the 1st two costo-sternal joints), slipping and clicking ribs, bruised or fractured ribs, and cervical arthritis [25]. Other extramammary causes include fibromyalgia, back or shoulder pain, pericarditis, gastroesophageal reflux, cholelithiasis, or angina [25]. Extramammary causes can usually be identified on history and clinical breast exam; however, in the cases of diffuse pain syndromes or patients who are unable to give an accurate history, additional investigation may be required. Musculoskeletal causes of pain are treated with heat, nonsteroidal anti-inflammatory medication, and physical therapy as indicated.

Treatment of Breast Pain

The majority of women who present with mastalgia are reassured after normal findings on evaluation (either clinical breast exam or imaging) and decline other interventions [25]. Many nonpharmacological interventions are used to treat cyclical or noncyclical breast pain; however, there are very few studies to support their efficacy. These interventions include recommending a properly fitted and supportive bra, physical exercise, relaxation training, dietary changes such as reducing dietary fat and reducing or eliminating caffeine, and warm or cold compresses. Vitamin E and evening primrose oil (EPO) are sometimes recommended although a recent systematic review found that the effectiveness of vitamin E was unknown and that evening primrose oil (EPO) lacked efficacy [24]. Despite mixed reviews, EPO is recommended by many breast specialists as a benign remedy which may help some patients with breast pain. NSAIDs such as diclofenac gel have been found to be effective in relieving breast pain and should be considered as a first-line agent, as benefits outweigh the risks for most women [24]. Women with large painful breasts who also experience neck or back pain may be candidates for breast reduction surgery.

Many women with *cyclical breast pain* experience relief with hormonal contraceptives which prevent the monthly hormonal fluctuations associated with ovulation; however, there have been no high-quality randomized controlled studies to evaluate efficacy [25]. In contrast, some women, especially young women and teenagers, experience breast swelling and tenderness when using oral contraceptives. Other hormonally active medications used to treat severe breast pain, including danazol and tamoxifen, are effective at reducing breast pain; however, they are associated with a number of adverse effects and are not frequently used for this purpose. Danazol is the only FDA-approved medication for the treatment of mastalgia and it works by suppressing gonadotropin secretion, preventing the luteinizing hormone surge, and inhibiting ovarian steroid formation. Its adverse effects include weight gain, deepening of the voice, menorrhagia, and muscle cramps [24, 25]. Tamoxifen is a selective estrogen receptor modulator and is effective in reducing both cyclic and noncyclic mastalgia in clinical trials [25]. Tamoxifen increases the risk of potentially fatal events such as blood clots, stroke, and endometrial cancer, and its adverse effects include hot flashes, mood swings, and gastrointestinal symptoms [24]. Tamoxifen has the benefit of reducing breast cancer risk and is discussed in Chap. 17 on "The Primary Prevention of Breast Cancer". Bromocriptine, a dopamine agonist, has been shown to reduce breast pain; however, it is no longer licensed for this indication in the USA due to the intolerable adverse effects of nausea, postural hypotension, and constipation [25].

Tatiana reports that she had some improvement in pain after eliminating caffeine and buying a new, more supportive bra. However, she reports she is now having more pain in her left breast on the lateral side. Her clinical breast exam is notable for focal tenderness in the left breast, laterally, at 2 o'clock, 6 centimeters from the nipple.

Women with nonfocal breast pain can be provided reassurance and do not need diagnostic imaging. Nonfocal mastalgia can be managed with both pharmacological and nonpharmacological treatments.

Women with focal breast pain should be evaluated with diagnostic imaging according to National Comprehensive Cancer Network (NCCN) guidelines. Women under the age of 30 are evaluated with a diagnostic breast ultrasound of the painful area. Women aged 30 and over are evaluated with a diagnostic bilateral mammogram and diagnostic breast ultrasound [7, 27].

The left breast ultrasound shows normal breast tissue and the patient is relieved. She is offered a trial of diclofenac gel to the affected area; however, she does not want to take medication and will continue with lifestyle and dietary changes.

Nipple Discharge

Claudette is a 38-year-old woman presenting with bilateral nipple discharge. She states that when she squeezes her nipples, a small amount of milky fluid appears. She denies that the discharge is ever spontaneous or bloody.

Nipple discharge is a chief concern for approximately 5% of women who are presenting to a health-care provider with breast-related concerns [28]. Nipple discharge can be a symptom of breast cancer, and therefore, it causes a significant amount of anxiety for women. Nipple discharge is associated with benign conditions in 97% of cases [28]. In the evaluation and management of nipple discharge, the most important factor is to determine whether the discharge is physiologic or pathologic. A thorough history and physical exam should be done to characterize the discharge including color, unilateral versus bilateral, spontaneous or only with manual expression, the number of ducts involved, and whether it is associated with a mass or skin change. During the clinical breast exam, the provider should attempt to elicit the nipple discharge and, if possible, to identify the number of ducts involved. The discharge should be tested for blood with a Hemoccult, or similar, test. Cytologic examination of the discharge is no longer recommended because of the low sensitivity for detection of cancer and because the absence of malignant cells does not exclude cancer [27, 28].

The clinical breast exam reveals no breast masses and the patient demonstrates manual expression which produces a drop of milky fluid bilaterally. The discharge tests negative for blood on Hemoccult. Serum prolactin and TSH are normal.

Physiologic discharge often is bilateral, involves multiple ducts, tests negative for blood, and is associated with nipple stimulation or breast compression [29]. *Galactorrhea* is a bilateral milky white discharge that is normal in women who are pregnant or breastfeeding. After pregnancy, it is normal to have discharge for up to 1 year after cessation of breastfeeding. Galactorrhea in nonpregnant, nonbreastfeeding women may be caused by hyperprolactinemia. Women presenting with galactorrhea should have a pregnancy test and prolactin level and thyroid-stimulating hormone tests completed to rule out pregnancy or endocrinopathy [29]. Medications, especially psychoactive medications which inhibit dopamine, can raise prolactin levels and cause galactorrhea, which is why it is important to review the medication history of a woman with nipple discharge. Medications associated with galactorrhea include phenothiazines, metoclopramide, risperidone, SSRIs, estrogen, and verapamil. Prolactin levels can be quite high, as high as 200–300 ng/mL in women taking risperidone, a potent dopamine antagonist which can lead to galactorrhea and menstrual irregularities. Pituitary imaging is indicated in cases of high prolactin levels, especially when levels are over 100 ng/mL, in the absence of dopamine inhibitor use, or when headaches or visual symptoms are present. The evaluation and treatment of pituitary tumors is beyond the scope of this book.

If the history and physical examination indicate that the discharge is physiologic, and breast cancer screening is up to date, then no breast imaging is required. Women who are expressing discharge should be counseled to avoid nipple stimulation [27].

Claudette returns to clinic 3 years later (age 41), with a chief concern of unilateral, spontaneous left nipple discharge. Her clinical breast exam shows no breast masses. There is spontaneous discharge from her left nipple that is dark brown and guaiac positive.

Pathologic nipple discharge is often spontaneous, unilateral, bloody, serous, or associated with a mass [27, 29] (see Table 16.2 below).

Table 16.2 Nipple discharge [8]

	Characteristics	Evaluation	Management
Pathologic discharge	Spontaneous, unilateral, single duct, serous, sanguineous, or serosanguinous	< 30-year-old: ultrasound and consider diagnostic mammogram ≥30-year-old: diagnostic mammogram and ultrasound If mammogram is BI-RADS 1–3, consider adding breast MRI	Follow imaging recommendations (i.e., serial imaging versus biopsy). May require excision if mass present Refer to breast surgeon for evaluation
Physiologic discharge	Nonspontaneous: elicited with squeezing or pinching Multiductal expression Color can be white, clear, yellow, green, gray, or brown	If <40-year-old, observation If >40-year-old, recommend mammogram and, if negative, observation	Educate patient to stop manual compression of breast and nipple stimulation Optional to have a 3- to 6-month follow-up to reassess Return to clinic if discharge becomes pathologic, or if exam changes

The most common causes of pathologic nipple discharge are intraductal papilloma, duct ectasia, infection, and carcinoma [27, 29]. *Intraductal papilloma,* discussed above, is the most common cause of nipple discharge and has been reported in up to 57% of cases of pathologic nipple discharge [26, 27, 29]. *Duct ectasia* is another common cause of nipple discharge and has been identified in up to 33% of cases of pathologic nipple discharge. Malignancy is associated with pathologic nipple discharge in 5–15% of cases [29]. Pathologic nipple discharge always requires further investigation. NCCN guidelines recommend breast ultrasound, and sometimes a diagnostic mammogram (at the discretion of radiologist), in women under the age of 30 and both diagnostic mammogram and ultrasound in women 30-year-old and older. If imaging is abnormal, the patient will proceed to tissue biopsy. If the imaging is normal, the provider should consider further evaluation with breast MRI or ductogram in consultation with a breast specialist [7, 27, 29].

Summary Points

1. Patients presenting with a palpable breast mass should be evaluated with a thorough history, review of risk factors for breast cancer, and a clinical breast exam [4]. Diagnostic mammography and ultrasound should be performed on women over 30-year-old; those under 30-year-old should have an ultrasound of the mass [5, 6].
2. Further evaluation and treatment of breast masses is based on the results of imaging and clinical suspicion. Some lesions require biopsy, while others are diagnosed on radiologic findings alone. Treatment varies from close interval follow-up to surgical excision [1–7]. Persistent palpable masses with negative imaging should be referred to a breast specialist for further evaluation and possible biopsy.
3. Breast masses are cystic or solid. Cystic masses can be simple or complicated. Solid masses can be classified by pathologic diagnosis as nonproliferative, proliferative without atypia, atypical hyperplasia, ductal carcinoma in situ, lobular carcinoma in situ, or invasive carcinoma. Simple cysts and nonproliferative lesions do not increase the risk of subsequent breast cancer, but all other diagnoses potentially increase breast cancer risk.
4. Lactational mastitis is common and antibiotics that are effective against *S. aureus* are recommended for women with symptoms that persist beyond 12–24 h. Women with risk factors for methicillin-resistant *Staphylococcus aureus* (MRSA) should be treated with antibiotics that cover MRSA. Nonpuerperal breast abscesses are less common but are treated similarly to lactational mastitis with antibiotics and possible drainage. Underlying malignancy should be excluded.
5. Cyclic (diffuse, bilateral) breast pain is physiologic pain that can be managed with lifestyle and dietary changes or medications such as acetaminophen, oral NSAIDs, or topical diclofenac gel. Noncyclic or focal breast pain warrants diagnostic imaging to rule out underlying pathology.
6. Physiologic nipple discharge is nonbloody, often bilateral, and associated with nipple stimulation or breast compression. Women ≥40-year-old should have a mammogram and women <40-year-old should undergo education and clinical observation. Pathologic nipple discharge is spontaneous, unilateral, or bloody and always warrants a diagnostic workup. For women ≥30-year-old, workup includes a mammogram and breast ultrasound. In women <30-year-old, a breast ultrasound is recommended.

Review Questions

1. A 25-year-old woman presents with a palpable mass in her left breast for the last 2 months. She denies any changes in the mass with her menstrual cycle and denies any breast pain. She is otherwise healthy, has never been pregnant, and has a mother who was recently diagnosed

with breast cancer at age 55. She has no other risk factors for breast cancer. On breast exam, there is a nontender, soft, round, mobile mass on the left. What is the next step in the evaluation of this patient?

A. Diagnostic mammography of the left breast
B. Left breast ultrasound
C. Bilateral breast ultrasound
D. Breast MRI

The correct answer is B. NCCN and American College of Radiology (ACR) guidelines recommend ultrasound imaging for palpable breast masses in patients under the age of 30 [6, 7]. Diagnostic mammography followed by ultrasound would be the first step in the workup of a patient over the age of 30; however, this patient is 25-year-old. Bilateral breast ultrasound is not indicated, as there are no palpable lesions on the right breast. There is no indication for right breast imaging. Breast MRI would be inappropriate to order in this patient as an initial screening test [6].

2. A 40-year-old woman presents for follow-up after screening mammography. The mammography was read as BI-RADS 3, with a small mass seen in her right breast, likely a fibroadenoma. An ultrasound to the area in question was consistent with a fibroadenoma. The patient is a healthy, nonsmoker with no history of prior breast biopsy; she had her first child at age 18 and is not taking any chronic medications. She has no family history of breast cancer. What is the next step in the management of this patient?

   A. Refer her to breast surgery for evaluation and possible surgical excision.
   B. Discuss the use of tamoxifen to reduce her risk of developing breast cancer.
   C. Order a short interval follow-up with breast MRI in 6 months.
   D. Order a short interval follow-up with diagnostic breast mammography and ultrasound in 6 months.

   The correct answer is D. Follow-up imaging with diagnostic mammography and ultrasound is recommended for BI-RADS 3, likely benign imaging, every 6 months for 2 years [7]. Most likely this recommendation would have been made on the mammography report. There is no indication for surgical excision at this time given the low clinical suspicion of malignancy and the likely benign reading on imaging. Tamoxifen is only indicated as chemoprophylaxis in patients with a greater than 1.7% chance of developing a diagnosis of breast cancer in the next 5 years and patients with ADH, ALH, and LCIS, or with certain genetic conditions [14].

   While short-interval follow-up is indicated is patients with BI-RADS 3 imaging, there is no indication for MRI in this patient. MRI is indicated as a screening tool in patients with a lifetime risk for breast cancer of >20% [6, 7].

3. A 34-year-old nurse, who is 6 weeks postpartum and breastfeeding, reports pain, swelling, and redness of her right breast for the last 24 h with a low-grade temperature (100.1F). She is diagnosed with lactational mastitis. The most appropriate management is:

   A. Nonsteroidal anti-inflammatory agents, compresses, and expression of milk by feeding or pumping
   B. Dicloxacillin 500 mg four times daily
   C. Cephalexin 500 mg four times daily
   D. Clindamycin 300 mg four times daily

   The correct answer is D. Clindamycin is an appropriate choice for mastitis in a woman with risk factors for MRSA, such as a nurse. Trimethoprim/sulfamethoxazole DS (TMP/SMX) also covers MRSA but is contraindicated in women who are breastfeeding newborn infants, younger than 2 months of age, due to the increased risk of kernicterus [15, 16]. Symptomatic treatment is generally effective for women with mild cases of inflammation who have been symptomatic for less than 24 h. If symptoms persist for more than 12–24 h, then antibiotics are indicated [15, 16]. Dicloxacillin and cephalexin are appropriate antibiotic treatment choices for lactational mastitis in women who do *not* have risk factors for methicillin-resistant *Staphylococcus aureus* (MRSA). This patient is a health-care provider (a nurse) who works in a hospital, and therefore, MRSA should be covered [15, 16].

4. A 36-year-old woman presents with bilateral breast pain that generally starts 2 weeks prior to her menses and sometimes lasts 1 week after her menses. She reports the pain is "everywhere." Clinical breast exam is significant for diffuse, bilateral tenderness without palpable masses or focal tenderness. Appropriate treatment would include:

   A. Counseling on dietary and lifestyle modifications such as cutting down on caffeine, exercising several days per week, and recommending a professionally fitted bra.
   B. Recommending tamoxifen 10 mg daily for 3 months.
   C. Ordering a diagnostic bilateral mammogram for further evaluation
   D. Ordering bilateral breast MRI to rule out dense breasts.

   The correct answer is A. Dietary changes such as low-fat, high-carbohydrate diets have shown some positive effects in observational studies. Eliminating caffeine has also been shown to be effective in small studies. Some women find relief with a well-fitted bra that provides support, or from compression with a sports bra. Tamoxifen can be used for severe breast pain; however, given the potential adverse events associated with it, other options should be tried and fail first. There is no indication for imaging given the cyclical, diffuse nature of the pain and the fact that the patient is only 36-year-old which is below the recommended age to start mammography in women at average risk for breast cancer [7, 21, 22].

5. A 40-year-old woman presents with spontaneous left-sided nipple discharge. She denies any blood in the discharge. On clinical breast exam, the patient has no masses and has a yellow discharge from her left nipple with palpation of the left breast. The discharge is guaiac negative. What is the next appropriate treatment for the patient?
   A. Provide reassurance as the patient is having non-bloody nipple discharge that is not associated with any palpable mass.
   B. Tell the patient to monitor the discharge for the development of blood and begin her screening mammograms at age 50 as recommended by the USPSTF.
   C. Order a diagnostic bilateral mammogram and a left breast ultrasound because the patient has pathologic nipple discharge.
   D. Order a left breast ultrasound to assess for subareolar dilated ducts.

   The correct answer is C. Pathologic nipple discharges are unilateral and spontaneous. The patient has a suspicious or pathologic discharge and needs diagnostic imaging. Although a left breast ultrasound may show dilated ducts, imaging needs to include a diagnostic mammogram in women over 30-year-old. Ultrasound is appropriate for pathologic discharge for women who are under the age of 30. Because the patient is over 30-year-old, a diagnostic bilateral mammogram and a left breast ultrasound would be the appropriate imaging. If the patient were having physiologic bilateral nipple discharge and was under the age of 40, observation would be appropriate. For women having physiologic discharge who are age 40 and above, a screening mammogram is recommended [7, 20].

References

1. Rungruang B, Kelley JL. Benign breast diseases: epidemiology, evaluation and management. Clin Obstet Gynecol. 2011;54(1):110–24.
2. The National Cancer Institute. SEER training module: breast cancer. https://training.seer.cancer.gov/breast/. Accessed 05 Oct 2018.
3. NIH. The National Cancer Institute. Visuals Online. Breast and Adjacent Lymph Nodes. Don Bliss, Illustrator. https://visualsonline.cancer.gov/details.cfm?imageid=4347. Accessed 19 Jan 2019.
4. Klein S. Evaluation of palpable breast masses. Am Fam Physician. 2005;71(9):1731–8.
5. Stein L, Chellman-Jeffers M. The radiologic workup of a palpable breast mass. Cleve Clin J Med. 2009;76(3):175–80.
6. Harvey JA, Mahoney MC, Newell MS, et al. ACR appropriateness criteria palpable breast masses. J Am Coll Radiol. 2013;10:742–9.
7. National Comprehensive Cancer Network Clinical Practice Guidelines in Oncology (NCCN Guidelines). Breast cancer screening and diagnosis. Version 1.2017. June 2, 2017.
8. Guray M, Sahin AA. Benign breast diseases: classification, diagnosis and management. Oncologist. 2006;11(5):435–49.
9. Schnitt SJ. Benign breast disease and breast cancer risk morphology and beyond. Am J Surg Pathol. 2003;27(6):836–41.
10. Miller ME, Muhsen S, Olcese C, Patil S, Morrow M, Van Zee KJ. Contralateral breast cancer risk in women with ductal carcinoma in situ: is it high enough to justify bilateral mastectomy? Ann Surg Oncol. 2017;24(10):2889–97. https://doi.org/10.1245/s10434-017-5931-2.
11. Collins LC. Precursor lesions of the low-grade breast neoplasia pathway. Surg Pathol Clin. 2018;11(1):177–97.
12. The American Society of Breast Surgeons. Management of fibroadenomas of the breast. 2008.
13. Hartmann LC, Radisky DC, Frost MH, et al. Understanding the premalignant potential of atypical hyperplasia through its natural history: a longitudinal cohort study. Cancer Prev Res (Phila). 2014;7(2):211–7.
14. National Comprehensive Cancer Network (NCCN) Clinical Practice Guidelines in Oncology. Breast cancer risk reduction. Version 1.2018. February 2, 2018.
15. Dixon JM, Khan LR. Treatment of breast infection. BMJ. 2011;342:d396.
16. Spencer JP. Management of mastitis in breastfeeding women. Am Fam Physician. 2008;78:727.
17. Kasales C, Han B, Smith JS, et al. Nonpuerperal mastitis and subareolar abscess of the breast. Am J Roentgenol. 2014;202(2):W133–9.
18. Trop I, Dugas A, David J, et al. Breast abscesses: evidence-based algorithms for diagnosis, management, and follow-up. Radiographics. 2011;31:1683–99.
19. Jahanfar S, Ng CJ, Teng CL. Antibiotics for mastitis in breastfeeding women. Cochrane Database Syst Rev. 2013;2:CD005458.
20. Patel BK, Falcon S, Drukteinis J. Management of nipple discharge and the associated imaging findings. Am J Med. 2015;128(4):353–60.
21. Smith RL, Pruthi S, Fitzpatrick LA. Evaluation and management of breast pain. Mayo Clin Proc. 2004;79:353–72.
22. Goyal A. Breast pain. BMJ Clin Evid. 2011;2011:pii: 0812.
23. Fetherston C. Characteristics of lactation mastitis in a Western Australian cohort. Breastfeed Rev. 1997;5(2):5–11.
24. Committee on Health Care for Underserved Women, American College of Obstetricians and Gynecologist. ACOG committee opinion no. 361: breastfeeding: maternal and infant aspects. Obstet Gynecol. 2007;109:479.
25. Marchant DJ. Inflammation of the breast. Obstet Gynecol Clin N Am. 2002;29(1):89–102. Review
26. Scurr J, Hedger W, Morris P, Brown N. The prevalence, severity, and impact of breast pain in the general population. Breast J. 2014;20(5):508–13.
27. Barton MD, Elmore JG, Fletcher SW. Breast symptoms among women enrolled in a health maintenance organization: frequency, evaluation, and outcome. Ann Intern Med. 1999;130:651–7.
28. Salzman B, Fleegle S, Tully AS. Common breast problems. Am Fam Physician. 2012;86(4):343–9.
29. Ramirez AJ, Jarrett SR, Hamed H, Smith P, Fentiman IS. Psychosocial adjustment of with mastalgia. Breast. 1995;4:48–51.

17 The Primary Prevention of Breast Cancer: Risk Assessment, Genetic Screening, Chemoprevention, and Modifiable Risk Factors

Jennifer Rusiecki and Deborah Kwolek

Learning Objectives

1. Describe how lifestyle, genetic, reproductive, and hormonal factors affect breast cancer risk.
2. Assess all women starting at age 18 for breast cancer risk, and teach breast awareness as part of routine preventive care throughout the life span.
3. Using three basic questions, triage to determine which women will benefit from a detailed breast cancer risk evaluation, and formulate a personalized prevention plan.
4. Appropriately identify women who would benefit from genetic testing.
5. Identify women with high-risk breast lesions and counsel appropriate patients on the use of screening breast MRI and chemoprevention.
6. Co-manage prevention and screening for women at highest risk with specialists.

Jeanne is a 35-year-old white woman who presents to establish primary care. She has no significant past medical or surgical history. Her reproductive history is significant for menarche at age 10, G1P1, and first birth at age 30. She breastfed her infant for more than 1 year and took birth control pills for 5 years prior to her pregnancy. Her BMI is 30 and she does not exercise regularly. She drinks a glass of wine every night.

J. Rusiecki (✉)
University of Chicago, Department of General Internal Medicine, Chicago, IL, USA
e-mail: jrusiecki@medicine.bsd.uchicago.edu

D. Kwolek
Harvard Medical School, Massachusetts General Hospital, Department of Medicine, Boston, MA, USA

Introduction

Breast cancer is the most common cancer in women and will affect 1 in 8 women in their lifetime. While breast cancer risk increases as women age, peaking in the 70s, it remains a leading cause of death for women in their 40s [1, 2]. Primary care providers (PCPs) regularly recommend mammography screening for women according to current guidelines, yet more can be done to address the risk of cancer in individual patients. Approximately 10% of breast cancer cases are due to genetic factors, 40% are caused by known hormonal or reproductive factors, and 40% are attributed to modifiable risk factors [3]. With prudent lifestyle changes and judicious use of chemoprevention, more than half of all breast cancers could be prevented, representing 150,000 fewer breast cancer diagnoses and 20,000 fewer breast cancer deaths annually in the USA [4].

Primary care providers (PCPs) are in the position, through the provision of routine preventive care, to reduce breast cancer morbidity and mortality substantially. The United States Preventive Services Task Force (USPTF) recommends that breast cancer education and family history screening be provided to all women starting at age 18, analogous to the way that adult patients are screened for cardiovascular risk factors [5]. After risk assessment, PCPs can recommend appropriate prevention.

Although proven prevention strategies are available, studies suggest that screening mammography for all populations at risk and targeted interventions (Table 17.1) including genetic screening, MRI imaging for women at high risk of breast cancer, prophylactic mastectomy in extremely high-risk patients, and the use of chemoprevention medications are grossly underutilized [6–8]. This inequity is largely due to the fragmented care that women receive and the lack of breast cancer prevention training for PCPs (see Chap. 1 on "Women's Health and Sex and Gender Based Medicine"). The purpose of this chapter is to simplify breast cancer risk assessment and prevention with the goal that primary care

S. A. Tilstra et al. (eds.), *Sex- and Gender-Based Women's Health*, https://doi.org/10.1007/978-3-030-50695-7_17

providers will be equipped to address breast cancer prevention with all their women patients.

Breast Cancer Risk Assessments in Primary Care

Risk Factors for Breast Cancer

Risk factors for breast cancer fall into four major categories, as seen in Box 17.1.

The degree of risk associated with each factor varies substantially. Table 17.1 presents a list of known risk factors grouped from strongest to weakest risk conferred. Protective factors and factors for which there is currently not sufficient proof of effect are also included.

Patient Evaluation and Documentation at Preventive Visits

The authors recommend that "breast cancer risk" be a permanent entry in the problem list of each woman and that the information be reviewed and updated at annual preventive visits. At these visits, primary care providers should also screen for current breast or gynecologic concerns. Past medical history should record breast and gynecologic histories, such as age of menarche, parity, age of first live birth, age of menopause and hormonal therapies, as these details are used in breast cancer risk calculators. A breast history includes any history of breast biopsies with results, breast imaging including density, and treatments given for any abnormalities. Family history, social history, and lifestyle habits should be obtained with attention to factors which affect breast cancer risk (see Chap. 3 on "Sex and Gender Specific History

Box 17.1 Categories of Risk Factors for Breast Cancer

Breast cancer risk factors can be divided into major categories:

- *Patient characteristics* including sex, age, race, body mass index (BMI), and lifestyle habits.
- *Genetic factors* as manifest through family history or genetic testing.
- *Breast factors* including history of chest radiation, breast density, and history of breast biopsy.
- *Reproductive and hormonal factors* including menstrual and obstetric histories.

Table 17.1 Risk factors for breast cancer [9–16]

Relative risk (RR)	Risk factor
Highest risk RR > 4.0	Chest radiation as child to age 30
	Genetic factors: Personal or family history of known genetic mutation Hereditary breast and ovarian cancer syndromes: BRCA 1 and BRCA2, PALB2, Peutz-Jeghers syndrome Li-Fraumeni syndrome – TP53 PTEN hamartoma tumor, Cowden, RBBS Hereditary diffuse gastric cancer syndrome Neurofibromatosis 1 Strong family history of breast cancer – 1st or 2nd degree relative with: 2 + family members with breast cancer Bilateral breast cancer Premenopausal breast cancer Ovarian cancer Male breast cancer Personal history of ovarian cancer
	Breast factors: Personal history of breast cancer Ductal carcinoma in situ (DCIS) Lobular carcinoma in situ (LCIS) Atypical ductal or lobular hyperplasia
Moderate risk RR 2.1–4.0	Genetic factors: CHEK2 mutation carrier (checkpoint kinase 2) Lynch syndrome Ataxia telangiectasia One first-degree relative with postmenopausal breast cancer
	Breast factors: Extremely or heterogeneously dense breast tissue
Modest RR 1.1–2.0	Genetic factors: History of melanoma or thyroid cancer Personal history of endometrial cancer
	Breast factors: History of one or more breast biopsies Proliferative breast lesions without atypia
	Hormonal/reproductive factors: Early menarche (<12 years) Age of first live birth at 30 years or older, or nulliparity Never breastfed an infant Late menopause (>55 years) Recent OC use (within past 10 years) Recent use of HT (within past 5 years) DES use during pregnancy or in utero DES exposure PCOS High circulating estrogens, androgens, IGF-1, and IGFBP-3
	Lifestyle factors: Postmenopausal obesity or inactivity Alcohol consumption Current smoking

Table 17.1 (continued)

Relative risk (RR)	Risk factor
Protective RR <1.0	Giving birth (compared to nulliparity) Four pregnancies or more (compared to one or less) Age at first birth <25 years (compared to >29 years) History of breastfeeding Use of tamoxifen or raloxifene Physical activity
Inconclusive data	Diet: Soy intake Fruits and vegetable intake, olive oil, fish Fat intake in diet, red meat Vitamins A, E, C, D, beta carotene Other factors: In vitro fertilization Less than 3 years HT Aspirin or other NSAIDs Bisphosphonate use
No known effect	Abortion or pregnancy termination Second-hand smoke Silicone implants Caffeine Stress Underarm deodorant or antiperspirant Wearing a bra or a particular type of bra Environmental pollutants Hair dye Electric blankets

DCIS ductal carcinoma in situ, *LCIS* lobular carcinoma in situ, *OC* oral contraception, *HT* hormone therapy, *DES* diethylstilbestrol, *PCOS* polycystic ovarian syndrome, *NSAID* nonsteroidal anti-inflammatory drug, *BRRS* Bannayan-Riley-Ruvalcaba syndrome

and Examination"). Details from the history predict risk and direct which risk calculator to use when a more specific risk percentage is needed to guide management (see discussion below on risk calculators).

Based on the results of the risk assessment, preventative strategies should be discussed for all women based on their level of risk. An overview of preventative interventions is outlined in Table 17.2.

Breast Risk Triage: Three Questions

If a woman has no current breast concerns, then an expedited risk assessment can begin with three questions. If the answer to all three questions is "no," then no further assessment is required beyond routine lifestyle counseling and age-based mammographic screening [17]. *See* Box 17.2.

Patients who answer "yes" to one or more of the three triage questions have a potentially increased risk and require further evaluation; if time does not permit the PCP to fully

Table 17.2 Breast cancer preventive interventions

Preventive interventions which apply to all patients include:
Lifestyle, hormonal, and reproductive review and counsel.
Breast awareness instruction.
Age-based mammography screening.
Advanced interventions offered to selected patients with higher than average risk include:
Clinical breast exams.
Imaging with early mammography or MRI.
Genetic counsel and screening.
Chemoprevention medication prescriptions.
Specialty referral to develop a comprehensive management plan.
Prophylactic surgery.

access risk and discuss recommended interventions during the annual exam, a separate office visit should be scheduled. An algorithm for expedited risk assessment is found in Fig. 17.1. The results of the risk assessment and recommendations can be formulated into a personalized prevention plan for each woman [17].

Jeanne has never had radiation to her chest. Her family history is significant for breast cancer in her mother at age 55, breast cancer in her sister at age 42, and ovarian cancer in her maternal grandmother at approximately age 60. Her breast history is significant for a breast biopsy 3 years ago with atypical ductal hyperplasia.

Evaluation and Management Based on Triage Question Answers

Next steps, depending on the answers to the triage questions, are discussed below.

Box 17.2 Three Questions to Triage for Increased Breast Cancer Risk

Three questions to start breast cancer risk assessment:

1. *Have you ever had radiation treatment to the chest for cancer or other conditions?*
2. *Do you or your family members have a history of cancer, or a genetic mutation associated with increased breast cancer risk?*
3. *Have you ever had a breast biopsy or a diagnosis of dense breasts on mammogram?*

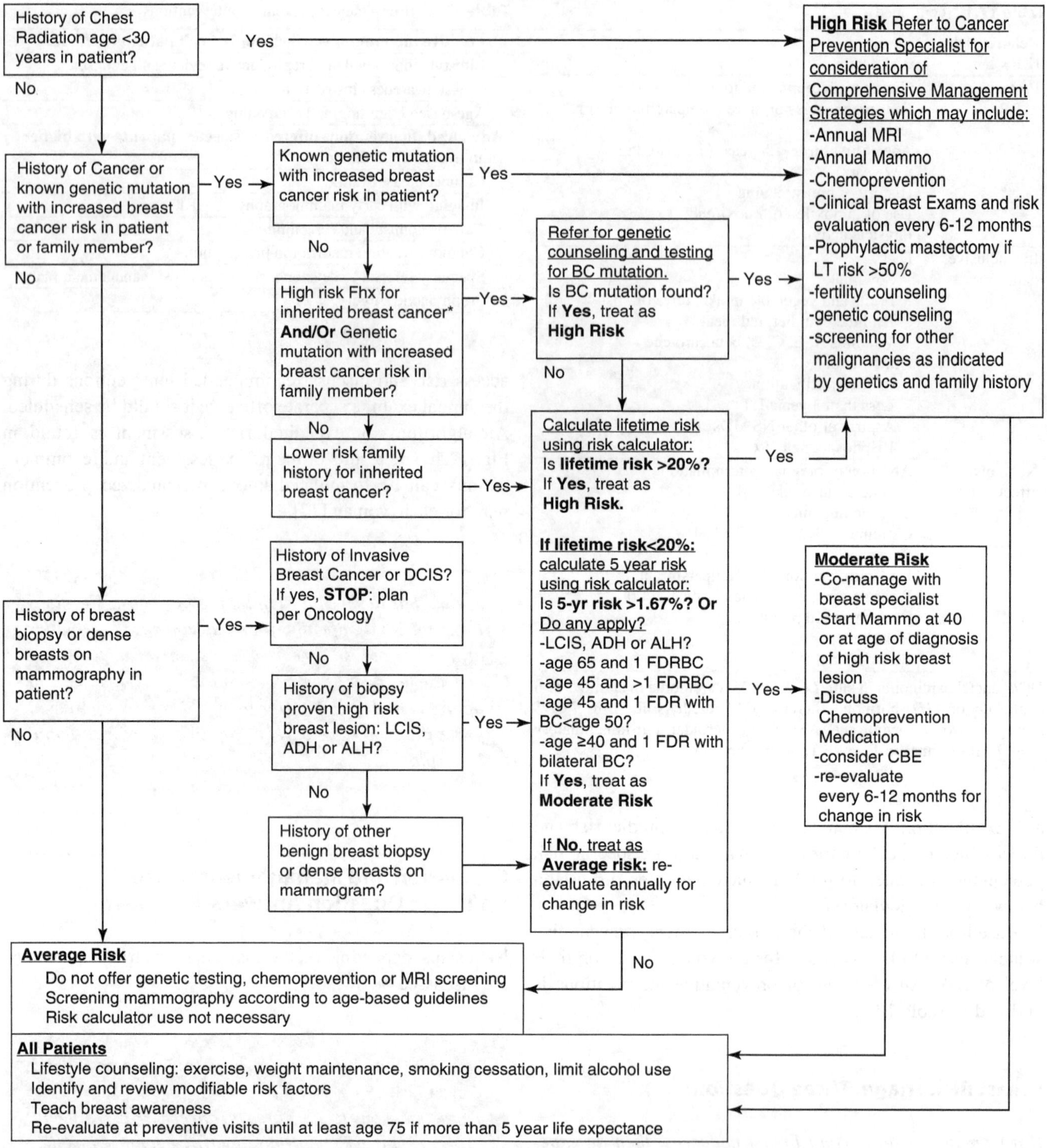

Abbreviations: LCIS= lobular carcinoma in situ, ADH= atypical ductal hyperplasis, ALH= atypical lobular hyperplasia, DCIS= ductal carcinoma in situ, FDRBC= first degree relative with breast cancer, FDR= first degree relative, BC= breast cancer, MRI= magnetic resonance imaging, Mammo= mammogram, CBE= clinical breast exam Fhx= family history HR= High Risk MR= Moderate Risk

*Per NCCN screening (Table 5) a high risk or suspicious family history includes 1) breast cancer in 2 or more family members on the same side of the family (maternal or paternal); 2) a family history of premenopausal, bilateral, or male breast cancer, or 3) a family history of ovarian cancer, or 4) colon, thyroid, peritoneal, endometrial, uterine or other cancers in multiple family members. Ashkenazi Jewish descent increases the risk of BRCA mutation.

Figure is original to author Kwolek

References:5, 6, 9, 13, 14

When the Answer Is "No" to All Three Questions: No Radiation, No Genetic or Family History, and No Breast History

Women who answer no to all three questions have an average risk for breast cancer and do not need further risk evaluation with a risk calculator or advanced interventions at this time.

The majority of women seen in primary care are in the average risk category and should be counseled on lifestyle prevention strategies, be taught breast awareness, and be screened according to age-based mammography screening guidelines [18]. Reproductive and hormonal factors affect risk, but are not of sufficient strength, in the absence of family history, genetic, or breast history factors, to alter age-based screening guidelines. Although the majority of cases of breast cancer occur in this group, these women do not require a detailed risk factor calculation and should not be offered MRI screening, genetic testing, or chemoprevention [4, 19, 20]. Women should be reassessed periodically for changes in risk status by readdressing family history and breast history at routine preventive visits (see Chap. 18 on "Breast Cancer Screening").

When the Answer to Question One Is "Yes": History of Chest Radiation

Patients with a history of childhood chest radiation require referral to develop a comprehensive management plan.

A history of childhood or young adulthood (10- to 30-year-old) radiation to the chest, although uncommon, confers at 40% lifetime risk of breast cancer. These patients are primarily those who were treated for Hodgkin's or non-Hodgkin's lymphoma as teens or young adults. Screening and prevention recommendations for high-risk patients are outlined in Table 17.3. These patients should be seen at least annually in primary care clinic to review family history, perform a clinical breast exam, and advise patients with risk-reduction counseling including consideration of chemoprevention. Patients with this risk factor begin breast cancer screening with clinical breast exams 8–10 years after the radiation therapy was given up to age 25. For patients over 25-year-old, mammography and MRI screening can be initiated [5, 20]. Patients are best managed in conjunction with a breast cancer prevention specialist.

When the Answer to Question Two Is "Yes": Personal or Family History of Cancer or Genetic Mutations

All patients who have a family history of cancer, or a suspected genetic syndrome which increases cancer risk, require further evaluation. Patients are triaged to determine whether referral for genetic counseling and testing is indicated. Advanced preventive interventions should be considered for most patients (see Fig. 17.1).

Patients with a positive screen for family history or genetics are further classified according to risk status: (1) known genetic mutation, (2) family member with a known genetic mutation, (3) history suspicious for mutation, (4) strong family history with negative genetic testing, or (5) one first-degree relative with postmenopausal breast cancer.

- *Patient with a known genetic mutation*

Patients with a BRCA mutation or other known genetic mutation associated with an increased risk of breast cancer will need comprehensive management strategies and should be co-managed with a breast cancer prevention specialist.

Table 17.4 lists the major known mutations associated with increased breast cancer risk, associated conditions, and recommended prevention strategies.

- *Family member with a known genetic mutation*

Patients, who have a first-degree relative with a BRCA genetic mutation, or other genetic mutation associated with breast cancer, should be referred for genetic counseling and evaluation by a breast cancer prevention specialist.

If genetic testing of the patient is negative, follow recommendations for *strong family history with negative genetic testing*. If the genetic testing of the patient is positive, refer to the specific mutation for recommended screening and co-manage with specialist. See Table 17.4.

Fig. 17.1 Breast cancer risk triage: three questions for asymptomatic women [5, 6, 9, 13, 14]. Abbreviations: LCIS lobular carcinoma in situ, ADH atypical ductal hyperplasia, ALH atypical lobular hyperplasia, DCIS ductal carcinoma in situ, FDRBC first-degree relative with breast cancer, BC breast cancer, MRI magnetic resonance imaging, Mammo mammogram, CBE clinical breast exam, Fhx family history, HR high risk, MR moderate risk. *Per NCCN screening (Table 17.5) a suspicious family history includes (1) breast cancer in 2 or more family members on the same side of the family (maternal or paternal); (2) a family history of premenopausal, bilateral, or male breast cancer; or (3) a family history of ovarian cancer, or (4) Colon, thyroid, peritoneal, endometrial, uterine or other cancers in multiple family members. Ashkenazi Jewish descent increases the risk of BRCA mutation

Table 17.3 Breast cancer prevention using comprehensive management strategies for high-risk women [13, 14, 20, 21, 25–27]

High-risk type	Screening breast imaging	Counseling and clinical exam, including recommended visit intervals	Management of breast cancer risk
History of chest radiation between age 10 and 30 years	Annual screening mammogram with or without tomography *and* MRI starting 8–10 years after radiation treatment, but not before age 25	Age 18–25 clinical breast exam starting 10 years after radiation therapy every 6–12 months Discuss breast awareness	Co-manage with specialist Consider chemoprevention Consider prophylactic mastectomy
Known genetic mutation: BRCA 1, BRCA 2, or other high-risk genetic mutation (see Tables 17.1 and 17.4)	Age 25–29 annual breast MRI[a] Age 30–75 annual mammogram with or without tomography *and* breast MRI Age > 75, individualized discussion	Clinical breast exam every 6–12 months starting at age 18 Discuss breast awareness	Co-manage with specialist Consider chemoprevention Consider prophylactic mastectomy
Family history of breast cancer without identified mutation *and* lifetime risk >20% according to IBIS or other risk assessment model	Begin annual mammogram with or without tomography 10 years younger than when youngest family member developed breast cancer, but not before age 30 Start annual breast MRI 10 years younger than when youngest family member developed breast cancer, but not before age 25	Discuss breast awareness Optional annual clinical breast exam, but continue annual preventive reevaluation	Co-manage with specialist Consider chemoprevention
History of high-risk breast lesion: LCIS, ADH, or ALH	Annual screening mammogram with or without tomography to begin at time of lesion diagnosis, but not before age 30 Consider annual MRI starting at time of diagnosis, but not before age 25	Clinical breast exam every 6–12 months Discuss breast awareness	Co-manage with specialist Consider chemoprevention
Lifetime risk >20% according to risk assessment tools based on a combination of factors	Annual screening mammogram with or without tomography to begin at time of risk exceeding 20% Consider annual MRI at time of risk exceeding 20%. Stop when risk decreases below 20%	Optional annual clinical breast exam Discuss breast awareness	Co-manage with specialist Consider chemoprevention

MRI magnetic resonance imaging, *LCIS* lobular carcinoma in situ, *ADH* atypical ductal hyperplasia, *ALH* atypical lobular hyperplasia, *BCSC* Breast Cancer Surveillance Consortium, *IBIS* International Breast Cancer Intervention Study, *BRCA* BReast CAncer tumor suppressor gene mutation

[a]Breast MRI should be performed with contrast, during days 7–14 of menstrual cycle. For women <30 years, perform mammogram with or without tomography if MRI is not available

- *Family history suspicious for a genetic mutation*

A detailed cancer history will determine whether genetic referral for counseling and testing is indicated.

A detailed family history is conducted to review any cancer diagnosis in first-, second-, and third-degree relatives. For each cancer, the age of onset is noted. A suspicious family history includes (1) breast cancer in two or more family members on the same side of the family (maternal or paternal); (2) a family history of premenopausal, bilateral, or male breast cancer; or (3) a family history of ovarian cancer, or (4) colon, thyroid, peritoneal, endometrial, uterine, or other cancers in multiple family members. Ashkenazi Jewish descent increases the risk of BRCA mutation. The National Comprehensive Cancer Network (NCCN) guidelines [13] for referral for genetic counseling are outlined in Table 17.5. Table 17.5 is not a complete list of patients who should be considered for genetic counseling. Clinical decision making as well as patient preference should be included in the discussion of genetic counseling referral. With advances in genetic testing and the availability of home-based testing for a low cost, many patients will present with results obtained privately and will need counseling and confirmation of results.

- *Strong family history for breast cancer with negative genetic testing or without genetic testing in the patient*

For patients with a strong family history of breast cancer, but in whom a specific genetic syndrome is not found, preventive strategies, including MRI imaging and chemoprevention, may be indicated.

A "strong family history" is defined as either (1) one or more first-, second-, or third-degree relative(s) with pre-

Table 17.4 Selected genetic mutations and recommended comprehensive management strategies [13, 28–32]

Genetic syndrome	Gene	Prevalence (approximate)	Breast cancer risk	Ovarian cancer risk	Approximate age to begin mammography (Mammo) and/or MRI screening[a]	Other cancers associated with syndrome or mutation	Other prevention considerations
PTEN Hamartoma Tumor syndrome Cowden syndrome Bannayan-Riley-Ruvalcaba syndrome	*PTEN*	*1/200,000*	77% lifetime	No increase in risk	Age 30–35 Mammo Age 30–35 MRI *or* 5–10 years before the age of the youngest breast cancer case in the family (whichever comes first)	Endometrial, follicular, or papillary thyroid, colon polyps, renal cell carcinoma	Consider prophylactic mastectomy, hysterectomy, and colectomy Screen for uterine cancer age 30–35 annually Annual thyroid ultrasound Renal ultrasound every other year starting at age 40 Colonoscopy starting at age 35 or earlier and repeat every 5 years
Hereditary breast and ovarian cancer syndrome	*BRCA1*	*1/500* *1/40 Jewish*	57% at age 70 (often triple negative breast cancer)	40% at age 70	Age 30 Mammo Age 25 MRI	Prostate	Consider prophylactic mastectomy and salpingo-oophorectomy
Hereditary breast and ovarian cancer syndrome	*BRCA2*	*1/500* *1/40 Jewish*	49% at age 70	18% at age 70	Age 30 Mammo Age 25 MRI	Prostate, pancreas, and melanoma	Consider prophylactic mastectomy and salpingo-oophorectomy
Li-Fraumeni Syndrome[b]	*TP53*	*1/500*	54% at age 70	No increase in risk	Age 30 Mammo Age 20 MRI	Soft tissue sarcoma, osteosarcoma, central nervous system tumors, adrenocortical malignancies	Consider prophylactic mastectomy
Hereditary diffuse gastric cancer syndrome	*CDH1*	*Unknown*	52% at age 75 (often lobular)	No increase in risk	Age 30 Mammo Consider adding MRI at 30	Gastric cancers	Consider prophylactic mastectomy and gastrectomy
Hereditary breast and ovarian cancer syndrome	*PALB2* (BRCA 2 interacting protein)	*Unknown*	35% at age 75 (can occur in males)	Unclear association	Age 30 Mammo Age 25–30 MRI	Pancreatic cancer	Consider prophylactic surgery
Peutz-Jeghers syndrome	*STK11*	*1/8000–1/200,000*	45% at age 70	18% at age 70[d]	Age 25 Mammo Age 25 MRI	Colon cancer and polyps	Colonoscopy and upper endoscopy every 2–3 years starting in late teen years
Neurofibromatosis type 1 (NF1)	*NF1*	*1/3000*	8.4% at age 50	No increased risk	Age 30 Mammo Consider adding MRI ages 30–50	Peripheral nerve sheath tumors, central nervous system tumors and gastro-intestinal stromal tumors	Consider mastectomy, based on family history

(continued)

Table 17.4 (continued)

Genetic syndrome	Gene	Prevalence (approximate)	Breast cancer risk	Ovarian cancer risk	Approximate age to begin mammography (Mammo) and/or MRI screening[a]	Other cancers associated with syndrome or mutation	Other prevention considerations
CHEK 2	CHEK2	*Not available*	28% lifetime	No increased risk	Age 40 Mammo Consider adding MRI at 40	Colon cancer	Consider mastectomy based on family history Colonoscopy every 5 years starting at age 40
Lynch syndrome	*MLH1*[a]	*1/2000*	18% at age 70	24% lifetime risk	Age 40 Mammo MRI based on other risk factors[c]	Colon and endo-metrial cancer	Consider prophylactic salpingo-oophorectomy Colonoscopy age 20 every 2–5 years
Ataxia Telangiectasia	*ATM*	*Not available*	38% lifetime	No increased risk	Age 40 Mammo Consider adding MRI at 40		Consider mastectomy, based on family history

[a]Varies by family history and age of family member when diagnosed with breast cancer
[b]Radiation sensitivity refers to the vulnerability of tissues exposed to radiation to develop secondary malignancies. Breasts in women less than 30 years of age are considered to be sensitive to radiation. Patients with Li-Fraumeni and NF1 are especially prone to radiosensitivity
[c]only gene with increased risk of breast cancer in Lynch syndrome
[d]Includes risk of ovarian, uterine, and cervical cancer

Table 17.5 National Comprehensive Cancer Network NCCN Guidelines for referral to genetic counselor [13]

First- or second-degree relative[a] with any of the following	A known mutation ≥2 breast cancer primaries in a single individual Ovarian cancer Metastatic prostate cancer Pancreatic cancer Male breast cancer
Anyone of Ashkenazi Jewish decent with a personal history of breast or high-grade prostate cancer diagnosed at any age Anyone with a personal history of ovarian or pancreatic cancer diagnosed at any age	
Family history of three or more of these cancers in any combination	Breast, pancreatic or prostate cancer Melanoma, sarcoma, adrenocortical carcinoma Brain tumor or leukemia Diffuse gastric, colon, endometrial, thyroid, or kidney cancer Macrocephaly (large head) or hamartomatous polyps of the gastrointestinal tract

Adapted with permission from the NCCN Guidelines® for Genetic/Familial High-Risk Assessment: Breast and Ovarian V.3.2019.
[a]When possible, genetic testing should be performed on an affected family member

menopausal breast cancer (prior to age 45), bilateral disease, ovarian cancer, or (2) at least two family members with postmenopausal breast cancer (over age 50) [6]. The lifetime and 5-year breast cancer risk is calculated for women in this group using the International Breast Cancer Intervention Study (IBIS) risk calculator [24] to determine the appropriateness of MRI screening or chemoprevention (see Box 17.3).

- *One first-degree relative with postmenopausal breast cancer*

For women who have only one first-degree relative with postmenopausal breast cancer, usually the mother, risk assessment with the Gail model is used to determine if the patient should be offered MRI screening or chemoprevention medication.

Having a mother or sister with postmenopausal breast cancer is concerning to patients and is a moderate risk factor for breast cancer (see Table 17.1). The Gail model calculator [22] is used to quickly determine if women would benefit from chemoprevention or MRI based on 5-year and lifetime risk percentages, respectively. If the patient also has dense breasts, the BCSC calculator [23] may be used as another measure. Starting annual mammograms at age 40 can be considered for these women after a shared decision-making discussion of risks and benefits [14, 21, 25–27].

When the Answer to Question 3 Is "Yes": History of Breast Biopsy or Dense Breasts

Clinical or mammographic breast abnormalities may prompt a breast biopsy, which is often benign. Even when noncancerous, biopsy results contribute to breast cancer risk assessment. The pathologic report should be obtained to confirm results, if not clear.

- *History of DCIS or invasive breast cancer*

The records of patients with a history of DCIS or invasive cancer are reviewed, when possible, to be sure that all recommended treatments have been completed. Many women will have been given tamoxifen to prevent future breast cancer, but those who declined may want to reconsider, and this is decided together with a breast oncologist. The prevention of breast cancer in survivors involves attention to both new cancers and to the early detection of recurrence (see Chap. 19 on "Breast Cancer Diagnosis and Management"). Patients continue yearly mammography, breast exam, and management according to a survivorship care plan prescribed by the oncologist (see Chap. 20 on "Care of the Breast Cancer Survivor"). Of note, women with DCIS or a history of invasive breast cancer are excluded from risk prediction calculators.

Jeanne declined chemoprevention with tamoxifen at the time of her atypical hyperplasia diagnosis and has not received follow-up care for this condition.

- *History of atypical hyperplasia or lobular carcinoma in situ (LCIS)*

Patients with a history of biopsy-proven high-risk breast lesions, namely, atypical hyperplasia or LCIS, should be evaluated for MRI screening schedules and chemoprevention strategies and be co-managed with a breast specialist [5] (see Tables 17.3 and 17.6).

In general, high-risk breast lesions should be removed, and women who have not had an excisional biopsy should be referred to a breast surgeon for possible excision. It is common to find women who refused tamoxifen prophylaxis after treatment for LCIS or atypical ductal hyperplasia (ADH) or atypical lobular hyperplasia (ALH) many years ago. A woman's risk changes as she ages, as additional family members are diagnosed with cancer, and as her personal breast history evolves. The issue of chemoprevention should be periodically reexplored in the context of the patient's changing risk status, current data, and perhaps a changed patient perspective on the importance of preventive strategies.

- *History of a proliferative breast lesion*

Proliferative breast lesions increase the risk of breast cancer, especially in a woman with a positive family history for breast cancer (see Chap. 16 on "Benign Breast Conditions"). The Gail or IBIS (in cases with a strong family history) risk calculators [22, 24] are used to help determine whether the patient should be offered chemoprevention medication or MRI screening.

Table 17.6 Chemoprevention: patient selection, medication choice and precautions. High-risk conditions including childhood chest radiation, known genetic mutations, and a history of high-risk breast biopsy benefit from specialty consultation in planning prevention strategies

Diagnosis or indication any one of the following:	Medication options	Contraindications and precautions	Adverse effects
Chest radiation before age 30[a] *Known genetic mutations increasing breast cancer risk*[a] *Lobular carcinoma* in situ *Atypical hyperplasia, ductal or lobular* *Any combination of risk factors with:* *>1.67% per NCCN (>3% per USPSTF) 5-year risk of breast cancer and >10-year life expectance* *>65 years with one first-degree relative with breast cancer* *>45 years with more than one first-degree relative OR one relative with bilateral breast cancer OR one first-degree relative with breast cancer under age 50* *>40 years with one first degree relative with bilateral breast cancer*	*Premenopausal* Tamoxifen 20 mg daily *Postmenopausal* Tamoxifen 20 mg daily Raloxifene 60 mg daily Anastrozole 1 mg daily Exemestane 25 mg daily *Suggested duration*: 5 years	*Hormonal and Reproductive* Pregnancy and lactation Undiagnosed uterine bleeding Estrogen use *Cardiovascular Risk* Active or past history of venous thromboembolism (VTE), including deep vein thrombosis, pulmonary embolism, and retinal vein thrombosis Clotting disorder Stroke or transient ischemic attack Ischemic cardiac disease Congestive heart failure Increased cardiovascular risk: smoking, diabetes, hypertension	*All agents* Venous thromboembolism Hot flashes Fatigue Joint and muscle aches *Tamoxifen* Endometrial hyperplasia and cancer Avoid paroxetine, bupropion, and fluoxetine during use *Anastrozole and exemestane* Decreased bone mass and Osteoporosis

Table adapted from data in the American Cancer Society, United States Preventative Services Task Force (USPSTF) 2019, and National Comprehensive Cancer Network [5, 14, 25]

[a]There is limited data on chemoprevention in these patients. Consultation with a breast cancer prevention specialist is advised

- *History of a nonproliferative breast lesion*

Nonproliferative breast lesions are not associated with an increased breast cancer risk; however, the Gail model includes a history of breast biopsy as one of the factors used in risk calculations. Women undergo calculation of risk with the Gail model to determine whether chemoprevention medication or MRI screening might be of benefit.

- *Dense breasts on mammography*

Breast density is a finding on mammography related to the ratio of glandular breast tissue to fat as interpreted by the radiologist. Density is primarily determined by genetics, but estrogen use and premenopausal status can lead to slight increases in density. Breasts that fall into "extremely dense" and "heterogeneously dense" classifications are often reported as "dense" in the literature or in reports (about 40% prevalence). Increased breast density increases the risk of cancer by both decreasing the sensitivity of mammography and as an independent risk factor. The risk associated with dense breasts also varies by the age of the patient. Dense breasts are more significant as a risk factor in postmenopausal women than in premenopausal women. The Breast Cancer Surveillance Consortium (BCSC) or International Breast Cancer Intervention Study (IBIS) calculators [23, 24] are used to determine whether these women would benefit from chemoprevention or MRI screening (see Chap. 18 on "Breast Cancer Screening").

Jeanne is found to be at high risk on the basis of both her family history and breast biopsy results. Her risk of breast cancer over the next 5 years and lifetime risk were calculated using the IBIS risk calculator. The results were: 5-year risk 3.5%, lifetime risk 44%.

Box 17.3 Calculators for Breast Cancer Risk in Women Without a History of Breast Cancer or DCIS

Risk calculators:

- Gail model or NIH Breast Cancer Risk Assessment Tool (BCRAT) www.mdcalc.com/gail-model-breast-cancer-risk. Accessed 3/8/19 [22]
- Breast Cancer Surveillance Consortium (BCSC) www.tools.bcsc-scc.org/BC5yearRisk. Accessed 3/8/19 [23]
- International Breast Cancer Intervention Study (IBIS) or Tyrer-Cuzick model www.ems-trials.org/riskevaluator. Accessed 3/8/19 [24]

Box 17.4 Use of 5-Year and Lifetime Risk Percentages [5, 14, 25, 27]

The *5-year risk* is used to determine whether a woman should be offered *chemoprevention.*

- <1.67% average 5-year risk – do not offer chemoprevention
- 1.68–3% moderate 5-year risk – may benefit from chemoprevention
- >3% high 5-year risk – most likely to benefit from chemoprevention

The *lifetime risk* is updated yearly to guide ongoing screening with *MRI.*

- <15% average lifetime risk – do not offer MRI screening
- 15–20% moderate lifetime risk – do not offer MRI screening
- >20% high lifetime risk – offer annual MRI in addition to mammography.

Risk Calculators

Risk calculators are used to determine a patient's 5-year and lifetime risk of breast cancer (see Box 17.3).

The Gail model, also known as the *Breast Cancer Risk Assessment Tool (BCRAT),* is the most widely used and most easily available risk calculator. The Gail model cannot be used in patients with LCIS, increased breast density, or an extensive family history. The Gail model uses reproductive factors, a history of breast biopsy and results, and history of breast cancer in first-degree relatives in the calculations. The model calculates 5-year and lifetime risk percentage estimates in women over 35 years.

The Breast Cancer Surveillance Consortium (BCSC) Risk Calculator incorporates breast density into calculations, but does not use reproductive data. The BCSC calculates 5-year and 10-year risk in women over 35 years.

The International Breast Cancer Intervention Study (IBIS) or Tyrer-Cuzick calculator is used for patients with: more than two relatives with cancer, LCIS, dense breasts, Ashkenazi Jewish heritage (due to increased risk of BRCA in that population), male breast cancer in the family, ovarian cancer in the family, or cancer in second- and third-degree relatives. The 5-year risk, 10-year risk, and lifetime risk estimates are calculated (see Box 17.4).

Developing a Personalized Prevention Plan

A personalized prevention plan (PPP) includes a discussion of lifestyle and behavioral modifications to reduce risk with specific, actionable goals for the patient to follow. A copy of the prevention plan can be provided to the patient, included in her medical record, and reviewed for progress at subsequent visits. The prevention plan is revised periodically and updated when there is a change in the patient's health status, family history, or risk factors. To aid clinical documentation, a standardized form outlines risk and a PPP (see Fig. 17.2).

Jeanne asks if she should have a mammogram. A thorough breast cancer risk evaluation and a personalized prevention plan are discussed with the patient, using a standard form.

Jeanne's risk factor assessment:

Genetics: Positive family history for breast and ovarian cancer (major risk factor)

Breast: Positive history of biopsy with atypical hyperplasia (major risk factor)

Reproductive and hormonal: Age of menarche, age of first birth increase risk

Protective factor: History of breastfeeding

Lifestyle: Elevated BMI, lack of exercise, and alcohol use

Jean's completed form, with assessment and plan, is in Fig. *17.3. Jeanne has questions about self-breast exams and use of alcohol.*

Preventive Interventions

Principles of Counseling and Explaining Risk to Patients

Providers present a balanced perspective when counseling women about breast cancer risk, recognizing that these discussions have the potential to invoke fear or stress. Providers relay basic risk data and interpret the information using terms like "average risk" or "increased risk" [33]. Conversations focus on the provider and patient working together as a team, utilizing shared decision making with the goal of decreasing cancer risk.

When explaining risks to patients, both the absolute and relative risks (RR) are explained as necessary. For example, a chemoprevention medication may lower the relative risk (RR) of breast cancer by 50%, but if the absolute risk of the cancer is low, then the benefit will be small. In the Breast Cancer Prevention Trial, tamoxifen use in women at high risk of breast cancer was associated with a RR of 0.51, which translates to a 49% reduction in the development of invasive breast cancer compared to placebo. In terms of absolute risk, 1.3% of women in the tamoxifen arm developed breast cancer compared to 2.7% of women in the placebo arm, for an absolute risk reduction of 1.4% [34].

To help patients understand risk factors, many factors can be described as conferring a high, moderate, or modest increase in breast cancer risk. Other factors have mildly protective effects or no known effect on breast cancer risk (see Table 17.1). Relative risk (RR) involves a comparison to what is considered as the "standard level of risk." For many risk factors, the "standard level of risk" can differ based on the author's interpretation. Using the example of breast density, if fatty breasts (category A) are the "standard level of risk," the RR for extremely dense breasts (category D) is 4.5, placing breast density in the "high-risk" group of factors. When the "standard level of risk" is scattered areas of fibroglandular density (category B), the RR for extremely dense breasts (category D) is 1.3, conferring only a "modest" increase in risk [15]. Statistical concepts may be confusing to patients, and it is the responsibility of the PCP to put each diagnosis and risk factor into perspective for the patient.

Lifestyle Counseling

Physical Activity

The 2018 World Cancer Research Fund (WCRF) report on global cancer perspectives acknowledges that physical activity and achieving a normal weight is protective against postmenopausal breast cancer (this resource is continuously updated; see this link for updated review: https://www.wcrf.

Fig. 17.2 Use this standard form to uniformly collect information on risk factors, to aid in breast cancer risk assessment, and to track a personalized prevention plan. This form is intended to print and fill in blanks and circle yes or no; alternatively, a smart form or phrase could be customized to an electronic health record. A nurse could be trained to complete the history part of this form with the patient, to be confirmed by the primary care provider. *Abbreviations: BMI body mass index, ALH atypical lobular hyperplasia, ADH atypical ductal hyperplasia, LCIS lobular carcinoma in situ, DCIS ductal carcinoma in situ, RT radiation therapy, SERM selective estrogen receptor modulators, HT hormonal therapy. Make note of Ashkenazi, Hispanic from southwest USA, or other race designation with increased incidence of BRCA or increased risk of breast cancer

Breast Cancer Risk Assessment/ Personalized Prevention Plan

Age ____HT_____WT______BMI _____ Race*____________________________

1. History of chest radiation age <30: Yes No

2. Family history and genetics: Known genetic mutation: Yes-patient Yes-family No

Prior genetic testing? Yes No __________ BRCA 1/ 2/ other mutation__________

Strong family history breast cancer risk: 2+ relatives/ male/ bilateral/premenopausal

Family history other cancers: ovarian/ colon/ other (list)______________

Postmenopausal breast cancer in one first degree relative only Yes No

3. Breast history: History of biopsy(s): Yes No Number of biopsies? ________

Diagnosis: unknown/ non-proliferative/ proliferative/ ALH/ ADH/ LCIS/ DCIS/ cancer

Treatment: excision/ chemoprevention/ mastectomy/ radiation therapy/ Chemotherapy

Completed treatment Yes/ No Declined Chemoprevention Yes/No

Mammogram or breast imaging (type, date, results): ____________________

Breast Density:_______Extremely Dense: Yes No

4. Reproductive and hormonal history:

Age of menarche:____ Parity G__ P __ Age at first birth:______________

Age of menopause:___Breastfed infant? Yes/ No Duration (months)__________

H/o Hormonal contraceptive /HT / SERM/ AI use_____________________

5. Lifestyle habits: Exercise:______________________________________

Alcohol: Yes No How much:____________________________________

Smoking/ Nicotine/ Other substance: Yes No_________________________

6. Risk Calculations: If #1-3 are negative, and breast cancer risk appears low, risk calculation is not necessary; follow plan for average risk below.

Risk Calculation using Gail/ BCSC/ IBIS/ other: 5-year_______% lifetime______%

Low/ Moderate/ High (and Highest) risk as follows:

5-year <1.67%/ 1.68-3%/ >3% lifetime <15%/ 15-20%/ 20-49%/ (>50%)

7. Assessment and Plan: Risk-Average/ Moderate or unknown/ High Risk/ Highest Risk

Genetic Screen referral: Yes No ____________________________________

Imaging early (mammogram less than 45 years) or MRI: Yes No________________

Chemoprophylaxis: Yes No ____

Specialty referral for Comprehensive Management Strategies: Yes No____________

Consider Prophylactic Surgery Yes No_________________________________

Risk reduction goals: increase exercise/ decrease alcohol/quit smoking/ limit hormone Rx

Clinical Breast Exams: Yes No_____ Teach breast awareness / Other__________

Referrals: Genetics/ Cancer Prevention/ Breast Surgeon/Medical Oncology/ other_________

Follow-up____

* make note of Ashkenazi, hispanic from southwest US, or other race designation with increased incidence of BRCA or increased risk of breast cancer. {abbreviations: BMI= body mass index, ALH= atypical lobular hyperplasia, ADH= atypical ductal hyperplasia,
LCIS= lobular carcinoma in-situ, DCIS= ductal carcinoma in-situ, RT=radiation therapy,
SERM= selective estrogen receptor
modulators, HT=hormonal therapy}
Figure original made by authors Kwolek, Rusiecki

Fig. 17.3 Case patient: personalized prevention plan worksheet

Breast Cancer Risk Assessment/ Personalized Prevention Plan

Age _35___HT_____WT______BMI___30__ Race*__White, non-Hispanic

1. **History of chest radiation age <30**: Yes/ (No)
2. **Family history and genetics**: Known genetic mutation: Yes-patient Yes-family (No)
   Prior genetic testing? Yes (No)________ BRCA 1/ 2/ other mutation__________
   Strong family history breast cancer risk: (2+ relatives)/ male/ bilateral/ (premenopausal)
   Mom (50) & sister (42) breast ca, MGM ovarian ca
   Family history other cancers: (ovarian)/ colon/ other (list)____________________
   Postmenopausal breast cancer in one first degree relative only Yes No
3. **Breast history:** History of biopsy(s): (Yes) No Number of biopsies? _____/___
   Diagnosis: unknown/ non-proliferative/ proliferative/ ALH/ (ADH)/ LCIS/ DCIS/ cancer
   Treatment: excision/ chemoprevention/ mastectomy/ radiation therapy/ Chemotherapy/ (none)
   Completed treatment Yes/ No Declined Chemoprevention (Yes)/ No
   Mammogram or breast imaging (type, date, results): *none*
   Breast Density:_______Extremely Dense: Yes No
4. **Reproductive and hormonal history:**
   Age of menarche:__*10*__ Parity G_*1*_ P _*1*_ Age at first birth:_________*30*____________
   Age of menopause: ___Breastfed infant? (Yes)/ No Duration (months)____*12 months*_________
   H/o Hormonal contraceptive /HT / SERM/ AI use *OCP for 5 yrs, not current*
5. **Lifestyle habits:** Exercise: *not regularly*
   Alcohol: (Yes) No How much: *1 glass of wine per night*
   Smoking/ Nicotine/ Other substance: Yes (No)
6. **Risk Calculations:** If #1-3 are negative, and breast cancer risk appears low, risk calculation is not necessary; follow plan for average risk below.
   Risk Calculation using Gail/ BCSC/ (IBIS)/ other: 5-year__3.5_____% lifetime__44____%
   Low/ Moderate/ High (and Highest) risk as follows:
   5-year <1.67%/ 1.68-3%/ (>3%) lifetime <15%/ 15-20%/ (20-49%)/ (>50%)
7. **Assessment and Plan:** Risk-Average/ Moderate or unknown/ (High Risk)/ Highest Risk
   Genetic Screen referral: (Yes) No __request genetic testing results on other family members_____
   Mammogram or MRI: (Yes) No *start yearly mammogram, alternate with yearly MRI*
   Chemoprophylaxis: Yes No __*discussed tamoxifen with patient, will consider*
   Specialty referral for Comprehensive Management Strategies: Yes No ____ refer breast center ___
   Consider Prophylactic Surgery Yes No _______ *await genetic testing results* ______________
   Risk reduction goals: (increase exercise)/ (decrease alcohol)/ quit smoking/ limit hormone Rx_____
   Clinical Breast Exams: (Yes) No_____ (Teach breast awareness)/ Other_______________
   Referrals: Genetics/ Cancer Prevention/ Breast Surgeon/Medical Oncology/ other__________
   Follow-up________*3-6 months to follow-up on above plan*

org/dietandcancer/breast-cancer) [16]. Physical activity may be protective against premenopausal breast cancers as well; however, the report concluded the evidence was inconclusive. From a primary care perspective, it is still worthwhile to discuss weight loss with premenopausal women to avoid obesity-related health complications as well as postmenopausal obesity. In postmenopausal women, any level of physical activity appears protective, though a statistically significant 20% reduction in breast cancer risk was seen in women of all weights who performed more than 6.7 metabolic equivalents (MET)-hr/week of physical activity (odds ratio [OR] 0.82; confidence interval [CI] 0.7–0.92) [35]. This MET-hr/week is equal to briskly walking for 30 min 4 times a week or 1 h of singles tennis a week.

Postmenopausal Obesity

Maintaining or achieving a normal postmenopausal weight is an important reduction of breast cancer risk. A meta-analysis of 17 studies evaluating postmenopausal breast cancer risk demonstrated an increased risk of 1.03 (95% CI 1.01–1.04) per 2 kg/m^2 point increase in body mass index (BMI). For example, in a woman with a height of 5 foot, 4 inches, increasing weight from 130 pounds to 142 pounds represents a BMI increase of 2 and an increased risk of 3%. Women with postmenopausal weight gain can decrease risk of breast cancer by 8% for each 5 kg/m^2 reduction in BMI [36]. The Nurses' Health Study of postmenopausal women not using hormone therapy found that the women who maintained a weight reduction of at least 10 kg (22 pounds) had a 50% reduction in the risk of breast cancer [37]. Physicians often counsel patients on the connection of physical activity and obesity to cardiovascular and diabetes risk, but the importance of these factors in breast cancer risk is also important.

Alcohol Use

Limiting alcohol use reduces the risk of breast cancer in both pre- and postmenopausal women. There appears to be a dose-dependent relationship, yet the 2018 WCRF report did not identify a threshold level of excessive alcohol consumption, instead stating that the safest level is no alcohol [16]. The Nurses' Health Study found an increased breast cancer risk (RR 1.15; 95% CI 1.06–1.24) for women who had 3–6 drinks per week [38]. A suggested limit to discuss with patients is no more than 1 drink a day and to have 2–3 alcohol-free days a week to reduce their breast cancer risk. Of note, current guidelines *do not* recommend that people who do not drink alcohol start drinking for any reason [39].

Smoking

Cohort studies suggest that long-term cigarette smoking leads to breast cancer development, as well as increased progression of existing breast cancer. Some components of tobacco smoke have a carcinogenic effect on many cells lines and have been shown to have a toxic effect on normal mammary epithelial cells [40]. All smokers are counseled to quit in order to reduce the risk of cancer, including breast cancer, and the risk of cardiopulmonary diseases.

Reproductive and Hormonal Factor Counseling

Pregnancy

Past pregnancy is not a modifiable risk factor for women, the timing of pregnancy may not be possible, and the decision to plan a pregnancy has a myriad of considerations outside of the discussion of breast cancer risk. Pregnancy increases the short-term risk and then lowers the long-term risk of breast cancer. Nulliparous women have a 2.0 relative risk of breast cancer compared to women who have given birth to children, and early pregnancy is protective against breast cancer in the long run [35]. Women who have their first child at or after age 30 are at an increased risk for breast cancer. Women with known genetic syndromes or elevated breast cancer risk who wish to be become pregnant in the future may plan for pregnancy at a younger age to help lower risk and to allow for earlier prophylactic surgery when indicated.

Breastfeeding

Women who have breastfed have a lower incidence of breast cancer compared to women who have not. It is proposed that women who breastfeed are exposed to lower levels of endogenous sex hormones during the amenorrhea that accompanies lactation. A pooled analysis by the World Cancer Research Fund (WCRF) including 140,000 women from 30 countries demonstrated a statistically significant 4.3% decreased relative risk of breast cancer for every 12 months of nursing compared to women who never breastfeed, which persists through menopause. There is a dose-response effect in which a longer duration of breastfeeding produces further risk reduction, though a benefit is seen with as few as 5 months of nursing [35]. While this is not always a modifiable risk factor, reproductive aged women who plan to bear children are counseled on the benefits of lactation, including the lifelong breast cancer risk reduction.

Hormonal Contraceptive Use

Studies have shown an increased risk of breast cancer in current users of oral contraceptives (OCs), which increases with prolonged use, increased age, and triphasic formulations. A recent study from Denmark including 1.8 million women over 10 years found that all forms of hormonal contraception mildly increase the risk of breast cancer: for OCs, RR 1.20 (CI 1.14–1.26) and for progesterone IUDs, RR 1.21 (CI 1.11–1.33) [41]. Women who are concerned for breast cancer risk are counseled to limit OC use to a duration of less than 5–10 years and to consider a different form of contraception after age 40 [42]. Of note, OC use is associated with a decreased risk of ovarian cancer, and thus recommendations are individualized for each patient.

Postmenopausal Hormone Therapy

Hormone therapy (HT) for the treatment of menopausal vasomotor symptoms has fallen in and out of favor over the last 50 years. One of the major concerns that many women and providers have with the use of hormones is the risk of breast cancer. The Women's Health Initiative (WHI) was a 16,000-women randomized controlled trial studying the use of HT. The study was stopped early, partially due to an increased risk of breast cancer in the treatment arm. This risk was seen only in the group of women receiving combined estrogen and progesterone therapy, while the use of estrogen alone appeared to be protective (hazard ratio [HR] 1.25 for estrogen+progesterone [E + P]; HR 0.77 for estrogen only) [43, 44]. There are important caveats to these data. First, the patients in the WHI were an older population (average age 63). Second, the long-term WHI study did not show a significant difference in cancer mortality at 18-year follow-up for combined E + P, although the trend was towards increased risk (HR 1.44, 95% CI 0.97–2.15). The estrogen only arm, however, continued to show a decreased risk (HR 0.55, 95% CI 0.33–0.92).

The Nurse's Health Study, although a cohort study, may be a better predictor of breast cancer risk with current HT prescribing practices, since it was a younger patient group (average age 56) and the majority of women who used hormone therapy did so for only 5 years in the perimenopausal and early menopausal stages, in concordance with current guidelines. For all women using HT (E only and E + P), breast cancer mortality in past and current HT users was not increased: current users (RR 0.76, CI 0.56–1.02) and past users (RR 0.83, CI 0.63–1.09) [45]. Women using only estrogen were stratified by duration of hormone use: an increase in breast cancer risk was not seen until after 5 years of estrogen and did not reach statistical significance until after 15 years of use [46]. Of note, the level of risk seen with 15 years of use is equal to that of 1 alcohol drink a day (RR 1.1).

Hormone therapy has risks and benefits beyond breast cancer risk (see Chap. 8 on "Menopause"). Women can be counseled that the risk of breast cancer from HT use is small if used according to current guidelines.

Breast Awareness

Teach Breast Awareness to All Patients

While we no longer recommend routine self-breast exams for women, breast awareness is discussed with patients, including a discussion of the symptoms of breast cancer. Breast awareness empowers women to know the look and feel of their breast so as to present to a health-care provider if changes occur [13]. Specifically, women should pay attention to their breasts when they dress or bathe and watch for lumps, focal pain, discharge, or any other changes. Breast changes, and any changes in family history of cancer, should be brought to the attention of the PCP.

Jeanne asks about lifestyle changes to reduce her risk of breast cancer. She is advised to increase her exercise to at least 30 min, 3 times per week. She is advised to lower her BMI from 30 to 25 with healthy eating for a general health benefit. She is informed that alcohol use increases the risk of breast cancer, and she should reduce intake to a few days per week or less. Breast awareness is explained to Jeanne so that she will notify her physician of any changes in her breast, or changes in her family history for cancer.

Age-Based Mammography Screening

In average-risk patients, breast cancer screening is age-based. Screening mammography begins at age 45 or 50, but no later than 50 (see Chap. 18 on "Breast Cancer Screening").

Advanced Interventions Offered to Selected Patients

Clinical Breast Exams

Clinical breast exams are essential for the evaluation of breast complaints and are an important part of the follow-up of high-risk patients and patients with a history of cancer or DCIS (see Chap. 18 on "Breast Cancer Screening").

Referral for Genetic Counseling

The primary care provider is well positioned to perform a detailed family history to assess genetic risk. The family history includes a review of cancers in first-, second-, and third-degree relatives with attention to the age at which each family member was diagnosed. To assist in determining who needs a referral, the USPSTF recommends a brief patient questionnaire such as the Ontario Family History Assessment Tool, Manchester Scoring System, Referral Screening Tool, Pedigree Assessment Tool, or Family History Screen (FHS-7), which are available on the USPSTF website [28]. Family history factors associated with increased likelihood of potentially harmful BRCA mutations include breast cancer diagnosis before age 50 years, bilateral breast cancer, presence of breast and ovarian cancer, one or more male family members with breast cancer, multiple cases of breast cancer in the family, one or more family members with two primary types of BRCA-related cancer, and Ashkenazi Jewish ethnicity [28]. The National Comprehensive Cancer Network (NCCN) guidelines to determine who should be referred for genetic counseling are outlined in Table 17.5. Current guidelines recommend patients of Ashkenazi Jewish decent be tested for BRCA mutations, due to increased risk. Hispanic Americans in the southwestern United States also have a high risk, and providers must maintain a high degree of clinical suspicion in these populations [47].

The most recent drafted guidelines from the United States Preventative Services Task Force (USPSTF) suggest that PCPs who have received training in genetic counseling can order genetic tests and provide counseling. It is suggested, however, that primary care providers not order BRCA or other genetic testing without the availability of genetic counseling [28]. Patients benefit from a certified genetic counselor to fully understand the risk, benefits, and implications of genetic testing. As genetic testing and DNA sequencing becomes more widespread and affordable, many patients will obtain testing through mail-in tests and present for advice; therefore, PCPs should be prepared to discuss these results.

A challenge with genetic testing is to interpret the result in the context of the individual patient and the risk of breast cancer associated with each mutation (see Table 17.4). Genetic counseling will continue to be important as the list of mutations associated with cancer expands. Patients who test at home will need to be advised on preventive strategies if genetic risk is identified. Currently, home testing panels vary greatly as to which mutations are included, and therefore, a negative test result is approached with caution in patients with a significant family history. Patients who qualify for genetic testing (Table 17.5) are referred to a genetic counselor even if they had a negative home test. The patient is advised to bring the home test results to their appointment with the counselor to determine if additional testing is needed.

Preventive Care of Patients with BRCA and Other High-Risk Genetic Mutations

Hereditary breast and ovarian cancer syndromes (HBOCs), the most common of which are BRCA1 and BRCA2 germline mutations, are responsible for 30% of inherited breast cancers [28]. BRCA genes are inherited in an autosomal dominant pattern and are mutations in a tumor suppressor gene.

If a BRCA1 or BRCA2 mutation is detected, breast cancer screening is adjusted as outlined in Table 17.3. The NCCN guidelines state that BRCA1- and BRCA2-positive women who have completed childbearing should undergo risk-reducing bilateral mastectomy and salpingo-oophorectomy [13]. Risk-reducing mastectomy has been shown to decrease the risk of developing breast cancer in patients with BRCA mutations by 95% (CI 41.4–100%) [48]. For younger patients who are hesitant to undergo mastectomy and salpingo-oophorectomy, there are currently trials underway investigating salpingectomy with delayed oophorectomy since much of ovarian cancer is thought to originate in the fallopian tubes [29]. This is not part of the NCCN guidelines at this time. The care of these patients is best performed in partnership with a comprehensive breast cancer management program and primary care provider.

Breast cancer screening recommendations for patients positive for BRCA and other genetic mutations are outlined in Table 17.4. Prior to age 30, mammography is avoided, and screening with an MRI or ultrasound is recommended. After age 30, yearly clinical exam, mammography, and MRI are recommended.

Prophylactic mastectomy should be considered for patients with PTEN mutation, Li-Fraumeni syndrome, hereditary diffuse gastric cancer syndrome, PALB2 mutations, or any other mutation which is associated with a greater than 50% lifetime risk of breast cancer [13]. Patients with Peutz-Jeghers syndrome and Lynch syndrome need aggressive colorectal cancer screening [30]. Depending on the mutation and vulnerabilities of patients with genetic mutations, screening for colon cancer, ovarian, thyroid, or other cancers might also be recommended. Chemoprevention is recommended in many cases of genetic mutations if prophylactic mastectomy is not performed. Given the complexity of genetically susceptible patients, co-management with specialists utilizing comprehensive management strategies is recommended (see Table 17.4).

Imaging with MRI and Early Mammography

The decision as to when to start mammography, and whether to order MRI screening, depends on the overall risk of breast cancer. In general, early mammogram and MRI are recommended for patients with a history of prior chest radiation, known genetic syndrome, high-risk breast lesions, and those with a > 20% lifetime risk of breast cancer. Despite the known benefit of supplemental MRI screening for high-risk patients, it remains underutilized. A recent study found that, despite recommendations, only 6% of high-risk women are currently being screened by breast MRI [49] (for details, see Box 17.4).

Jeanne engages in a discussion about chemoprevention with tamoxifen to reduce her risk of breast cancer. The potential risks of thromboembolism and vaginal bleeding with this medication are discussed, and the patient is counseled about the warning signs of blood clots and possible uterine bleeding abnormalities. She is educated about the potential for menopausal symptoms such as hot flashes and vaginal dryness. She agrees to start the medication.

Chemoprevention: Effectiveness and Selecting an Agent

Evidence of Impact

Selective estrogen receptor modulators (SERM) and aromatase inhibitors (AI) are the most common agents for primary chemoprevention; they are also used to prevent recurrence of breast cancer. When used in select women, these medications can reduce the risk of estrogen-receptor-positive (ER+) breast cancer by 50% [34]. For women with atypical hyperplasia, this can help reduce risk as much as by 86% [34]. Despite being one of the most effective prevention options, chemoprophylaxis remains underutilized with only 1% of eligible women taking the medications [50]. Some of the proposed barriers include limited knowledge of PCPs about chemoprevention, lack of prevention focus by oncologists, time constraints, and perceptions that fail to see breast cancer as a preventable disease [50, 51]. Patients may be concerned about adverse effects and, while this is an important concern, these medications are generally well tolerated. Primary care providers can help to move breast cancer from a treatment-focused disease to a potentially preventable disease with the use of chemoprevention.

Candidates for Chemoprevention

While there is some variation in patient qualifications between guidelines, all are founded on identifying women at an increased risk of breast cancer, either by identification of certain high-risk factors or by estimation of the 5-year risk of breast cancer. Current recommendations for women over age 35 are summarized in Table 17.6 [5, 14, 25]. The choice of calculator affects risk estimation (see Box 17.4). All of the guidelines support the use of the Breast Cancer Risk Assessment Tool (or Gail model), but to determine 5-year breast cancer risk, other calculators may be more appropriate. Women with dense breasts may be assessed using the BCSC tool. The IBIS model also incorporates breast density, a diagnosis of LCIS, Ashkenazi Jewish decent, family history of breast or ovarian cancer in second-degree relatives, a family history of male breast cancer, genetic findings of BRCA 1 and 2, and other factors into its calculations.

The American Cancer Society (ACS) and NCCN advise chemoprevention in women with a greater than 1.66% 5-year risk and at least a 10-year life expectancy [14, 25]. The USPFTS guidelines state that 1.66% 5-year risk treatment cutoff may overestimate the benefit from risk-reduction medications and recommend 3% as the level of risk in which patients may have a greater benefit from these interventions [5]. All guidelines support the use of these risk-reduction agents for 5 years to reduce the risk of future estrogen-receptor-positive cancers.

Based on the 2019 USPSTF drafted guideline on chemoprophylaxis, clinicians can also use a combination of risk factors to determine if a patient would benefit from these medications [5]. This includes the following:

- Patients 65-year-old or older with one first-degree relative with breast cancer
- Patients 45-year-old or older with more than one first-degree relative with breast cancer or one first-degree relative who developed breast cancer prior to age 50
- Patients 40-year-old or older with a first-degree relative with bilateral breast cancer

The USPSTF also has a "D" (evidence of harm) recommendation for using chemoprevention medications in women who are not at increased risk of breast cancer. "Women who are younger than 60 years and with no additional breast cancer risk factors or women with a low 5-year risk should not routinely be offered this medication as the harms of the medication outweigh the benefit in this population" [5]. Women over 60 years of age might qualify for chemoprevention with no family history or high-risk breast lesion, but the increased risk of vascular events in older women must be considered in the shared decision-making process.

Providers who would like to gain more experience in managing chemoprevention medications are encouraged to start by offering chemoprevention to women with known atypical ductal hyperplasias and lobular carcinoma in situ. PCPs are encouraged to identify and discuss risks and benefits with women who have a new diagnosis and with those who may have refused or deferred chemoprevention in the past.

Selective Estrogen Receptor Modulators (SERMs)

SERMs block some estrogen receptors and stimulate others. These effects differ by each drug within this class of medication. The two SERMs currently approved for breast cancer prevention are tamoxifen and raloxifene. Tamoxifen blocks estrogen effects in the breast but has an estrogenic effect on the uterus and bones. Tamoxifen increases the risk of endometrial dysplasia and uterine cancer and thus is typically reserved for premenopausal women and those who have undergone a hysterectomy. In a review of placebo-controlled trials, tamoxifen (RR 0.70 [95% CI, 0.59–0.82] or 7 cases in 1000 women) and raloxifene (RR 0.44 [95% CI, 0.27–0.71] or 9 cases in 1000 women) both demonstrated decrease in breast cancer among women who used these therapies [52].

Raloxifene has a similar profile to tamoxifen with agonist activity in the bone and lipids and an antagonist effect on the breast and uterus. Raloxifene is approved for chemoprevention in postmenopausal women only and is approved for both the prevention and treatment of postmenopausal osteoporosis. Both agents improve bone density which is important since these medications are often given after peak bone mass has been established (see Chap. 25 on "Osteoporosis").

Contraindications to SERM Use

SERMs should not be used in women who have a history of venous thrombosis or pulmonary embolism, a history of stroke, a condition increasing the risk of clotting such as prolonged immobilization and pregnancy, or lactation. When these medications are used in reproductive-aged women, it is important to discuss contraceptive options, focusing on non-estrogen options since estrogen will interact with the SERM. While both SERMs carry the risk of thromboembolism, the risk appears to be more pronounced with tamoxifen (RR 1.93 [95% CI, 1.41–2.64]) [52]. The most commonly reported adverse effects with both agents are vasomotor symptoms and vaginal dryness.

In a direct comparison of tamoxifen and raloxifene in the STAR trial, there were more invasive breast cancers with raloxifene (RR 1.24, 95% CI, 1.05–1.47), suggesting a superiority of tamoxifen for chemoprevention; however, there were fewer adverse events with raloxifene, including invasive uterine cancer (RR 0.55, $p = 0.003$) and thrombosis (RR 0.75, $p = 0.007$). The absolute increased risk of thrombosis with tamoxifen was 0.83 events per 1000 women (3.30 per 1000 with tamoxifen vs 2.47 with raloxifene) [53]. It is important to note that the effects of these medications on overall survival are unknown because the length of follow-up is limited (longest study has a 13-year follow-up interval).

Clinically, tamoxifen is used for chemoprophylaxis primarily in premenopausal women and in postmenopausal women who have had a hysterectomy; raloxifene or AIs are used in postmenopausal women. Patients should plan to take the medication for 5 years, but women are free to stop the medication at any time if they experience side effects. The use of tamoxifen and AIs for secondary prevention in patients with DCIS and breast cancer is discussed in Chap. 19 on "Breast Cancer Diagnosis and Management".

Aromatase Inhibitors (AIs)

AIs are used as adjuvant treatment in breast cancer (see Chap. 19 on "Breast Cancer Diagnosis and Management") and can be used for chemoprevention. AIs block the conversion of androgens to estrogen by aromatase thereby decreasing the amount of circulating estrogen. Conversion of androgens is the main method of estrogen production after menopause, and therefore, this method is reserved for postmenopausal women.

Two AIs have been studied for chemoprevention. Anastrazole, when compared to placebo, demonstrated a lower incidence of breast cancer (HR 0.47, 95% CI 0.32–0.68) [54]. Of note, there was a slightly higher incidence of fracture in the anastrazole group, though this was not statistically significant. Exemestane, when compared to placebo, also demonstrated a lower incidence of breast cancer (HR 0.47, 95% CI 0.27–0.79). There was not a significant change in fracture risk between placebo and exemestane [25]. In addition to bone effects, other common adverse effects of AIs are worsening of vasomotor symptoms, vaginal dryness, and joint pain. AIs should be used with caution for women with a history of osteoporosis.

Jeanne returns to clinic 3 months later complaining of severe hot flashes 3–4 times a day, including nocturnal symptoms. She notes feeling tired in the morning due to poor sleep. She is still having regular periods. She would like to know if she should take hormones like her friend did when going through menopause, or if there are other options. The patient is counseled that her hot flashes are an expected side effect of tamoxifen and that estrogen therapy is not appropriate. Nonhormonal options for treating the vasomotor symptoms of SERMs including SSRIs, SNRIs, and gabapentin are discussed. She would like to try venlafaxine.

Managing the Adverse Effects of Chemoprevention

Vasomotor symptoms can be bothersome to patients taking either SERMs or AIs. Menopausal hormone therapy is not appropriate for the treatment of vasomotor symptoms in women on these medications. Hot flashes are caused by a complicated system of neurotransmitter changes due to low estrogen levels, increased levels of FSH, and possible LH surges. Thermoregulatory control is destabilized as norepinephrine, serotonin, GABA, and other neurotransmitters are affected. This provides the mechanisms for pharmacologic treatment when estrogen treatment is contraindicated (for further discussion see Chap. 8 on "Menopause"). Venlafaxine and serotonin reuptake inhibitors (SSRIs) have been shown to ameliorate hot flashes in women with a history of breast cancer [55]. Venlafaxine decreases the hot flash frequency by as much as 50% in breast cancer survivors and men with prostate cancer taking androgen deprivation therapy. While a dose response was present, there was no additional improvement seen in venlafaxine doses above 75 mg daily [56]. Gabapentin has also been shown to decrease frequency of hot flashes at doses of 900 mg daily when compared to placebo [56].

Venlafaxine is the drug of choice for treating hot flashes in women on tamoxifen. Paroxetine, bupropion, and fluoxetine should be used with caution in women taking tamoxifen since they are strong inhibitors of the CYP2D6 enzyme. This enzyme converts tamoxifen to its active metabolite; inhibitors of this enzyme can decrease the effectiveness of tamoxifen. A Canadian cohort study estimates use of paroxetine results in 1 additional death for every 19 breast cancer patients taking tamoxifen for breast cancer treatment. This effect has not been demonstrated with other SSRIs [57].

Venlafaxine minimally blocks the activity of the CYP2D6 enzyme and is considered the preferred agent to use with tamoxifen [58].

Vaginal dryness and dyspareunia are also commonly reported by women taking both SERMs and AIs. The first-line treatments include water-based (KY and Astroglide) lubricants; olive and coconut oil can also be used for lubrication. Vaginal moisturizers such as Replens can be helpful for women who have symptoms outside of intercourse. These options will not reverse vaginal atrophy which requires estrogen to treat. The use of topical estrogens in women at high risk of breast cancer and in breast cancer survivors is controversial; see Chap. 8 on "Menopause" for a discussion on the genitourinary syndrome of the menopause.

Bone health is an important consideration in all postmenopausal women but particularly in those taking AIs. Given the risk of osteoporosis with AIs, raloxifene is recommended as the first-line chemoprevention agent for postmenopausal women. There are no clear guidelines for bone health in women using AIs for chemoprevention, but recommendations for breast cancer survivors who are taking AIs may be applicable to this population. The American Cancer Society (ACS) and the American society of Clinical Oncology (ASCO) recommend a baseline DEXA scan for all women when starting AIs and again every 2 years [59]. In addition to counseling on weight-bearing exercise, limiting alcohol, and avoiding tobacco, the ACS/ASCO recommends all women taking AIs also consider supplemental calcium (1200 mg/day) and vitamin D3 (600–1000 U/day) [59]. For women taking AIs found to have osteoporosis, bisphosphonates are the first-line treatment option (see Chap. 25 on "Osteoporosis").

Vaginal bleeding occurs in one-quarter of women taking tamoxifen, due to the agonistic activity of tamoxifen on the endometrium. This same mechanism is the cause of increased risk of endometrial hyperplasia, polyps, and cancer. Postmenopausal and premenopausal women with irregular vaginal bleeding or a change in menstrual bleeding should be biopsied and referred to a gynecologist as necessary (see Chaps. 7 and 15 on "Abnormal Uterine Bleeding" and "Gynecologic Malignancies, Section on Uterine Cancer").

Jeanne starts venlafaxine 37.5 mg daily and titrates up to 75 mg; her hot flash symptoms improve. She is now having only 1–2 hot flashes a day, with nocturnal symptoms about once a week, and finds this tolerable. Vaginal dryness has not been a problem. The plan is to continue the tamoxifen for a total of 5 years with venlafaxine 75 mg daily.

Future Directions for Chemoprophylaxis

With advances in breast cancer risk assessment, genetic counseling, and chemoprophylaxis, the goal is that many breast cancers will be prevented. Just as PCPs evaluate all patients for cardiovascular risk, breast cancer risk should be evaluated in all women. The use of chemoprevention is a powerful tool to reduce breast cancer risk in women over age 35. Its clinical usefulness is currently limited by difficulty in tolerating adverse effects such as vasomotor symptoms. Currently, a phase III clinical trial is underway to determine if tamoxifen can be used at a 5-mg dose for secondary prophylaxis in breast cancer with the hope that this would reduce the risk of adverse side effects [60]. If this is successful, these data may be able to be extrapolated to a chemoprophylaxis application.

Prophylactic Mastectomy

Prophylactic mastectomy is generally offered to women with a lifetime breast cancer risk of over 50% after the completion of childbearing. Very-high-risk women could undergo mastectomy before the completion of childbearing if needed.

Comprehensive Management Strategies

Women at very high risk of breast cancer are generally women with history of chest radiation, genetic syndromes, lifetime risk >20%, or high-risk abnormal breast biopsies (such as DCIS, LCIS, and atypical hyperplasia). These women should be followed using comprehensive management strategies in conjunction with specialists who may include breast oncologists or surgeons, gynecologists, genetic counselors, and radiologists. This team can devise a plan to address screening, genetic counseling, general preventive strategies, chemoprevention, and prophylactic surgery if indicated.

Summary Points

1. Breast cancer risk can be modified through lifestyle modifications including weight loss, regular exercise, breastfeeding, and decreasing alcohol intake.
2. All women should undergo a breast cancer risk assessment by their primary care provider starting at age 18. Patients should be educated on breast health and breast awareness, risk factors, and prevention strategies.
3. Women can be triaged with three questions about history of chest radiation, family and genetic risk, and history of

breast biopsy to determine if further risk calculations will be helpful. A personalized prevention plan addresses modifiable risk factors, as well as screening and prevention strategies appropriate for each woman.

4. High-risk women, including those with known genetic syndrome, a history of chest irradiation, or a history of cancer, DCIS, LCIS, ADH or ALH, or lifetime risk of >20%, should be referred and co-managed with specialists.
5. Patients with (1) a family history of ovarian cancer, (2) a family history of male breast cancer, (3) breast cancer in 2 or more family members on the same side of the family, or (4) a family member diagnosed with breast cancer at a young age (<45-year-old) should be referred to a genetic counselor. Women at high risk may benefit from chemoprevention or adding MRI to mammogram screening.
6. Use of SERMS and AIs in high-risk women (>1.66% 5-year risk) over age 35 can decrease breast cancer risk by approximately 50%. PCPs can become comfortable in prescribing SERMs for the primary prevention of breast cancer in selected patients.

Acknowledgments The authors would like to acknowledge Diane Altkorn for her assistance in reviewing this chapter and Jacqueline Falk for her patient and skilled assistance in the graphic design of Fig. 17.1.

Review Questions

1. A 37-year-old G1P1 female presents for a new patient appointment. Her family history is significant in that her maternal grandmother had breast cancer and her maternal aunt died of breast cancer at age 44. Her mother and sister have not had any breast disease. Her Gail 5-year risk score is 1.4% and lifetime risk is 10%. In addition to a complete history and physical, what is the next step for her in regards to breast cancer screening and prevention?
   A. Start mammograms when she turns 40 and screen annually
   B. Order mammogram now and refer for genetic counseling
   C. Refer her for genetic counseling
   D. Start mammograms with supplemental breast MRIs annually when she turns 40

   The correct answer is C. This woman should be referred now for genetic counseling given the age of her aunt at time of her breast cancer diagnosis. Per the NCCN guidelines, any first-, second-, or third-degree relative with breast cancer diagnosed at age 45 or younger qualifies for a genetic counseling referral to evaluate for high-penetration genetic mutations [13]. This is the *next* step because the results of her genetic testing will determine an appropriate screening regimen. Only patients with a greater than 20% lifetime risk require MRI or screening mammograms before age 40.
2. A 50-year-old premenopausal female presents to discuss breast cancer risk. She is very upset that her best friend was recently diagnosed with breast cancer. Her BMI is 35 and she regularly attends a yoga class on the weekends. She has 5–7 alcoholic drinks a week. There is no family history of breast or ovarian cancer. Mammogram earlier this year was normal with density "almost entirely fat." Her 5-year breast cancer risk by Gail model is 0.8% and lifetime risk 9.5%. She would like to know what she can do to reduce her risk of breast cancer. Which of the following interventions would decrease her risk of breast cancer?
   A. Encourage her to decrease her alcohol consumption to less than 4 drinks per week and to work towards weight loss
   B. Advise her to avoid soy in her diet as this has weak estrogen-like properties.
   C. Advise her to start taking tamoxifen daily for the next 5 years
   D. Encourage her to limit caffeine to less than 200 mg daily

   The correct answer is A. Reducing her alcohol consumption and losing weight have both been shown to reduce breast cancer risk. She should also increase her physical activity. While taking a chemoprevention agent like tamoxifen may reduce her risk of breast cancer, it is not indicated in women with a 5-year risk of <1.67% by Gail or IBIS [14, 22, 23, 25]. Soy and caffeine do not affect breast cancer risk.
3. Which of the following is a known adverse effect of raloxifene?
   A. Raloxifene, like other SERMS, can increase the risk of osteoporosis
   B. Raloxifene can increase the risk for deep venous thrombosis and pulmonary embolism
   C. Raloxifene can increase the risk of ovarian cancer
   D. Raloxifene can increase the risk of uterine cancer

   The correct answer is B. Raloxifene is a SERM which has estrogenic effects on the bones, but antiestrogen effects on breast and uterine tissue. Raloxifene increases the risk of thrombosis. Raloxifene does not increase the risk of ovarian cancer or uterine cancer. Raloxifene is approved for the prevention and treatment of osteoporosis. Raloxifene is only approved for use in postmenopausal women [51–53].
4. A 31-year-old female with a history of Hodgkin's lymphoma at age 11 had treatment with chemotherapy and radiation therapy to her chest. She was not aware of her increased risk of breast cancer. What is the recommended prevention plan for women with her history?

A. Start mammograms with possible tomosynthesis at age 40 and continue annually
B. Start mammograms now with possible tomosynthesis and supplemental breast MRI
C. Start mammograms now with supplemental whole breast ultrasound
D. Start annual whole breast ultrasound and add mammogram with possible tomosynthesis at age 40

The correct answer is B. Women with a history of childhood chest radiation are at a significantly increased risk of developing breast cancer. These patients should be referred to a high-risk breast specialist for co-management with primary care. Per the NCCN guidelines, these patients should start annual screening mammograms with possible tomosynthesis and supplemental breast MRI at age 25 [21]. There are currently no guidelines recommending screening whole breast ultrasound for high-risk women. Chemoprevention should also be considered in high-risk patients.

5. A 60-year-old postmenopausal female recently received breast biopsy results significant for atypical ductal hyperplasia. You have counseled the patient on these results, need for surgical excision, and options for prevention including chemoprevention. She developed a rash with raloxifene and had to stop taking it. She saw the breast surgeon who recommended an aromatase inhibitor for chemoprevention. She is concerned about the risk of osteoporosis because her mother suffered a hip fracture in her 70s. What would be the appropriate timing of DXA use in this patient for osteoporosis screening?
A. Obtain a baseline DXA now and repeat every 2 years during treatment
B. Start DXA screening at age 65 per the USPSTF guideline
C. Obtain a baseline DXA now and repeat at age 65
D. Check a vitamin D level now and order DXA if the vitamin D level is <25 ng/mL

The correct answer is A. Aromatase inhibitors (AI) like anastrozole can be used for chemoprevention in postmenopausal women. The major concern with AIs is the increased risk of osteoporosis, as well as risk of thrombosis. Therefore, the American Cancer Society and American Society of Clinical Oncology recommend obtaining a baseline DXA at time of starting AI therapy and repeating at least every 2 years during treatment. While the ACS and ASCO recommend calcium and vitamin D supplements for all women taking AIs, the recommendations for DXA testing are independent of vitamin D levels. If osteoporosis is detected, this should be treated aggressively with consideration of stopping the AI [58].

References

1. Centers for Disease Control. United States cancer statistics: data visualization. https://gis.cdc.gov/Cancer/USCS/DataViz.html. Accessed 6 Nov 2018.
2. Anders CK, Johnson R, Litton J, et al. Breast cancer before age 40 years. Sem Oncol. 2009;36(3):237–49.
3. Sprague B, Trentham-Dietz A, Egan K, et al. Proportion of invasive breast cancer attributable to risk factors modifiable after menopause. Am J Epidemiol. 2008;168(4):404–11.
4. Colditz GA, Bohlke K. Priorities for the primary prevention of breast cancer. CA Cancer J Clin. 2014;64(3):186–94. https://doi.org/10.3322/caac.21225.
5. United States Preventative Services Task Force. Medication use to reduce risk of breast cancer USPSTF recommendation statement. JAMA. 2019;322(9):857–67.
6. Moyer V. Risk assessment, genetic counseling, and genetic testing for BRCA-related cancer in women: US Preventive Services Task Force recommendation statement. Ann Int Med. 2014;160(4):271–81.
7. Peek M, Han J. Disparities in screening mammography current status, interventions, and implications. J Gen Intern Med. 2004;19(2):184–94.
8. Nelson HD, Smith MB, Griffin JC, Fu R. Use of medications to reduce risk for primary breast cancer: a systematic review for the US Preventive Services Task Force. Ann Intern Med. 2013;158(8):604–14.
9. National Breast and Ovarian Cancer Centre. Breast cancer risk factors: a review of the evidence. National Breast and Ovarian Cancer Centre, Surry Hills, NSW; 2009. https://canceraustralia.gov.au/system/tdf/publications/breast-cancer-risk-factors-review-evidence/pdf/rfrw-breast-cancer-risk-factors-a-review-of-the-evidence_1.15.pdf?file=1&type=node&id=3074. Accessed 28 Nov 2018.
10. Hulka B, Moorman P. Reprint of breast cancer: hormones and other risk factors. Maturitas. 2008;61(1–2):203–13.
11. Hartmann L, Sellers T, Frost M, et al. Benign breast disease and the risk of breast cancer. N Engl J Med. 2005;353(3):229–37.
12. Nelson H, Zakher B, Cantor A, et al. Risk factors for breast cancer for women age 40 to 49 years: a systematic review and meta-analysis. Ann Intern Med. 2012;156(9):635–48.
13. National Comprehensive Cancer Network. NCCN clinical practice guidelines in oncology: genetic/familial high-risk assessment: breast and ovarian, version 3.2019; January 2019. https://www.nccn.org/professionals/physician_gls/pdf/genetics_screening.pdf. Accessed 12 Oct 2019.
14. National Comprehensive Cancer Network. NCCN clinical practice guideline in oncology: breast cancer risk reduction. Version 2.2018; 2018. https://www.nccn.org/professionals/physician_gls/PDF/breast_risk.pdf. Accessed 13 Aug 2018.
15. Nattinger AB, Mitchell JL. Breast cancer screening and prevention. Ann Intern Med. 2016;164(11):ITC81–96. https://doi.org/10.7326/AITC201606070.
16. World Cancer Research Fund/American Institute for Cancer Research. Diet, nutrition, physical activity and breast cancer. Continuous update project expert report 2018. Available at dietandcancerreport.org. Accessed 25 Feb 2019.
17. Kwolek D. Three questions to triage breast cancer risk and the personalized prevention plan. Oral presentation in workshop; Benign breast diseases. Presented at the annual meeting of the Society of General Internal Medicine, Washington DC; 2019, May.
18. Oeffinger K, Fontham E, Etzioni R, et al. Breast cancer screening for women at average risk: 2015 guideline update from the American Cancer Society. JAMA. 2015;314(15):1599–614.
19. DeSantis C, Ma J, Bryan L, Jemal A. Breast cancer statistics, 2013. CA Cancer J Clin. 2014;64(1):52–62. https://doi.org/10.3322/caac.21203.

20. US Preventive Services Task Force. Screening for breast cancer: US Preventative Services Task Force recommendation statement. Ann Intern Med. 2016;164(4):279–96.
21. NCCN Clinical Practice Guideline in Oncology. Breast cancer screening and diagnosis. Version 3.2019; 2019. https://www.nccn.org/professionals/physician_gls/pdf/genetic_screening.pdf. Accessed 10 Sept 2019.
22. www.mdcalc.com/gail-model-breast-cancer-risk. Accessed 8 Mar 2019.
23. www.tools.bcsc-scc.org/BC5yearRisk. Accessed 8 Mar 2019.
24. www.ems-trials.org/riskevaluator. Accessed 8 Mar 2019.
25. Visvanathan K, Hurley P, Bantug E, et al. Use of pharmacologic interventions for breast cancer risk reduction: American Society of Clinical Oncology clinical practice guideline. J Clin Oncol. 2013;31(23):2942–62.
26. Moyer V. Medications to decrease the risk for breast cancer in women: recommendations from the US Preventive Services Task Force recommendation statement. Ann Intern Med. 2013;159(10):698–708.
27. Saslow D, Boetes C, Burke W, et al. American Cancer Society guidelines for breast cancer screening with MRI as an adjunct to mammography. CA Cancer J Clin. 2007;57(2):75–89.
28. United States Preventative Service Task Force. Risk assessment, genetic counseling, and genetic testing for BRCA-related cancer: US Preventive Services Task Force Recommendation Statement. JAMA. 2019;322(7):652–65.
29. Kwon J, Tinker A, Pansegrau G. Prophylactic salpingectomy and delayed oophorectomy as an alternative for BRCA mutation carriers. Obstet Gynecol. 2013;121(1):14–24.
30. National Comprehensive Cancer Network. NCCN clinical practice guidelines in oncology: genetic/familial high-risk assessment: colorectal. Version 1.2018. July 2018. https://www.nccn.org/professionals/physician_gls/pdf/genetics_colon.pdf. Accessed 27 Nov 2018.
31. Valencia OM, Samuel SE, Viscusi RK, Riall TS, Neumayer LA, Aziz H. The role of genetic testing in patients with breast cancer: a review. JAMA Surg. 2017;152(6):589–94.
32. Easton DF, Pharoah PD, Antoniou AC, et al. Gene-panel sequencing and the prediction of breast-cancer risk. N Engl J Med. 2015;372(23):2243–57.
33. Paling J. Strategies to help patients understand risks. BMJ. 2003;327(7417):745–8.
34. Fisher B, Costantino J, Wickerham D, et al. Tamoxifen for prevention of breast cancer: report of the National Surgical Adjuvant Breast and Bowel Project P-1 Study. JNCI. 1998;90(18):1371–88.
35. Marmot M, Atinmo T, Byers T; World Cancer Research Fund / American Institute for Cancer Research, et al. Food, nutrition, physical activity, and the prevention of cancer: a global perspective. Washington, DC: AICR; 2007.
36. Bernstein L, Patel AV, Ursin G, et al. Lifetime recreational exercise activity and breast cancer risk among black women and white women. J Natl Cancer Inst. 2005;97(22):1671–9.
37. Eliassen AH, Colditz GA, Rosner B, Willett WC, Hankinson SE. Adult weight change and risk of postmenopausal breast cancer. JAMA. 2006;296(2):193–201.
38. Chen WY, Rosner B, Hankinson SE, Colditz GA, Willett WC. Moderate alcohol consumption during adult life, drinking patterns, and breast cancer risk. JAMA. 2011;306(17):1884–90.
39. US Department of Health and Human Services and US Department of Agriculture. 2015–2020 dietary guidelines for Americans. 8th ed. https://health.gov/dietaryguidelines/2015/. Accessed 6 Nov 2018.
40. Kispert S, McHowat J. Recent insights into cigarette smoking as a lifestyle risk factor for breast cancer. Breast Cancer (Dove Med Press). 2017;9:127–32.
41. Morch L, Skovlund C, Hannaford P, et al. Contemporary hormonal contraception and the risk of breast cancer. N Engl J Med. 2017;377:2228–39.
42. Marchbanks P, McDonald J, Wilson H, et al. Oral contraceptives and the risk of breast cancer. N Engl J Med. 2002;346(26):2025–32.
43. Chlebowski RT, Anderson GL, Gass M, et al. Estrogen plus progestin and breast cancer incidence and mortality in postmenopausal women. JAMA. 2010;304(15):1684–92.
44. Anderson GL, Chlebowski RT, Aragaki AK, et al. Conjugated equine oestrogen and breast cancer incidence and mortality in postmenopausal women with hysterectomy: extended follow-up of the Women's Health Initiative randomized placebo-controlled trial. Lancet Oncol. 2012;13(5):476–86.
45. Manson JE, Aragaki AK, Rossouw JE, et al. Menopausal hormone therapy and long-term all-cause and cause-specific mortality: the Women's Health Initiative randomized trials. JAMA. 2017;318(10):927–38.
46. Chen WY, Manson JE, Hankinson SE, et al. Unopposed estrogen therapy and the risk of invasive breast cancer. Arch Intern Med. 2006;166(9):1027–32.
47. Weitzel JN, Clague J, Martir-Negron A, et al. Prevalence and type of BRCA mutations in Hispanics undergoing genetic cancer risk assessment in the southwestern United States: a report from the Clinical Cancer Genetics Community Research Network. J Clin Oncol. 2012;31(2):210–6.
48. Hartmann LC, Sellers TA, Schaid DJ, et al. Efficacy of bilateral prophylactic mastectomy in BRCA1 and BRCA2 gene mutation carriers. J Natl Cancer Inst. 2001;93(21):1633–7.
49. Miles R, Wan F, Onega T, et al. Underutilization of supplemental magnetic resonance imaging screening among patients at high breast cancer risk. J Womens Health (Larchmt). 2018;27(6):748–54.
50. Peres J. Why is breast cancer chemoprevention such a hard sell? JNCI. 2014;106(5):4–6.
51. Armstrong K, Quistberg A, Micco E, et al. Perscription of Tamoxifen for breast cancer prevention by primary care physicians. JAMA. 2006;166(20):2260–5.
52. Vogel VG, Costantino JP, Wickerham DL, et al. Update of the national surgical adjuvant breast and bowel project study of tamoxifen and raloxifene (STAR) P-2 trial: preventing breast cancer. Cancer Prev Res (Phila Pa). 2010;3(6):696–706.
53. Freedman AN, Yu B, Gail MH, et al. Benefit/risk assessment for breast cancer chemoprevention with raloxifene or tamoxifen for women age 50 years or older. J Clin Oncol. 2011;29(17):2327.
54. Cuzick J, Sestak I, Forbes JF, et al. Anastrozole for prevention of breast cancer in high-risk postmenopausal women (IBIS-II): an international, double-blind, randomised placebo-controlled trial. Lancet. 2014;383(9922):1041–8.
55. Cella D, Fallowfield LJ. Recognition and management of treatment-related side effects for breast cancer patients receiving adjuvant endocrine therapy. Breast Cancer Res Treat. 2008;107(2):167–80.
56. Pachman DR, Jones JM, Loprinzi CL. Management of menopause-associated vasomotor symptoms: current treatment options, challenges and future directions. Int J Women's Health. 2010;2:123.
57. Kelly CM, Juurlink DN, Gomes T, et al. Selective serotonin reuptake inhibitors and breast cancer mortality in women receiving tamoxifen: a population based cohort study. BMJ. 2010;340:c693.
58. Desmarais JE, Looper KJ. Interactions between tamoxifen and antidepressants via cytochrome P450 2D6. J Clin Psychiatry. 2009;70(12):1688–97.
59. Runowicz CD, Leach CR, Henry NL, et al. American cancer society/American society of clinical oncology breast cancer survivorship care guideline. CA Cancer J Clin. 2016;66(1):43–73.
60. DeCensi A, Puntoni M, Guerrieri Gonzaga A, et al. Abstract GS3–01: A randomized placebo controlled phase III trial of low dose tamoxifen for the prevention of recurrence in women with operated hormone sensitive breast ductal or lobular carcinoma in situ. Published 2019: Presented at the 2018 San Antonio Breast Cancer Symposium, December 4–8, 2018.

18 Breast Cancer Screening

Anna Golob, Traci A. Takahashi, and Kay M. Johnson

Learning Objectives

1. Assess breast cancer risk to determine whether women are of average, moderate, or high risk for breast cancer over the next 5 years and in their lifetimes.
2. Discuss screening and diagnostic imaging tools including mammography types (2D conventional vs 3D tomosynthesis), MRI, and ultrasound, including the risks and benefits for patients.
3. Discuss the recommended ages and screening intervals for mammography for average-risk women according to the US Preventive Services Task Force (USPSTF) and American Cancer Society (ACS) guidelines.
4. Describe the categories of mammographic breast density, the implications for breast cancer risk, and imaging options for dense breasts.
5. Identify women at increased risk for breast cancer who may benefit from earlier initiation of mammography screening, MRI imaging, referral for genetic testing, and referral to a breast specialist for prophylactic treatment recommendations.
6. Perform a clinical breast exam when indicated and list clinical scenarios in which it is most likely to add benefit.
7. Interpret mammography results and initiate appropriate follow-up.
8. Describe initial patient counseling issues in women with suspected breast cancer who are being referred for further evaluation and treatment by breast oncologists.

LuAnn is a 44-year-old African American woman who presents to her primary care provider for a routine health care visit. She has several questions about breast cancer screening. She is worried because her mother was recently diagnosed with breast cancer at the age of 68. Also, LuAnn had a mammogram at age 40 and received a letter stating that her mammogram was normal but that she had "heterogeneously dense breasts." The letter advised that she discuss further screening options with her primary care provider. She underwent menarche at age 10, is nulliparous and is still menstruating. Today she asks whether she needs a breast MRI and whether she should get a genetic test, because of her dense breasts, and because of her mother's recent breast cancer diagnosis.

Introduction

Breast cancer is the most common invasive cancer in women worldwide and is responsible for more deaths than any other cancer in women. In the USA, cancers are the leading cause of death in women aged 35–65 [1]. Over their lifetime, one out of eight women in the USA will be diagnosed with breast cancer [2]. Although breast cancer incidence has increased in the USA since the 1970s, breast cancer mortality has steadily decreased at a rate of approximately 2.2% per year since the 1990s. This decrease in mortality is attributed to improvements in breast cancer treatment in addition to earlier detection with more widespread screening with mammography.

While there is good evidence that mammography reduces mortality from breast cancer in women at average-risk ages 50–69, optimal screening protocols for younger women and women at intermediate risk are debated among professional organizations. Values placed by patients and physicians upon

A. Golob (✉) · T. A. Takahashi · K. M. Johnson
Department of Medicine, University of Washington and VA Puget Sound Healthcare System, Seattle, WA, USA
e-mail: anna.golob@va.gov

S. A. Tilstra et al. (eds.), *Sex- and Gender-Based Women's Health*, https://doi.org/10.1007/978-3-030-50695-7_18

early detection versus the burden of false-positive findings, with the resulting unnecessary diagnostic and treatment modalities, inform shared decision-making in such cases. Newer imaging technologies, such as 3D breast tomosynthesis, may augment conventional 2D mammography for breast cancer screening, particularly for women with dense breasts. Women at moderate and high risk (referred to in the literature as "increased risk") should be identified and referred for appropriate genetic testing and discussion of prophylactic treatments. Breast MRI in addition to mammography has become a standard screening modality for women at high risk for breast cancer. This chapter will address breast cancer risk assessment, screening recommendations, shared decision-making, and patient counseling issues in women with suspected breast cancer who are being referred for further evaluation and treatment by breast specialists.

Breast Cancer Risk Factors and Risk Assessment

Breast cancer screening guidelines depend foremost on breast cancer risk category. Current screening guidelines for mammography are applicable to the majority of women patients who are at average or moderate risk for the development of breast cancer. Women who are at high risk of breast cancer are screened according to separate protocols utilizing MRI in addition to mammography beginning in the third and fourth decades of life.

Risk Factors

Breast cancer risk assessment should be part of the health care maintenance of all adult women, starting at age 18. (See Chap. 17 on The Primary Prevention of Breast Cancer.) Risk factors are identified through history-taking and by reviewing diagnostic imaging and testing, if any, related to the breast.

The major risk factor categories for breast cancer risk include:

1. History of chest radiation prior to age 30 (usually for Hodgkin's disease)
2. Genetics: family history of cancer or known genetic syndrome, race
3. Personal breast characteristics: lumps, pain, discharge, prior biopsies and result, density
4. Reproductive and hormonal factors: age of menarche, parity, age of first birth, menstrual status, age at menopause (if postmenopausal), history of breastfeeding, past or current exogenous hormone use

Breast Cancer Risk Assessment

The identification of risk factors for individual patients allows for risk assessments which categorize women into average-, moderate-, and high-risk categories. The risk assessments inform several decision points (see Table 18.1):

1. Which imaging modalities should be employed, starting at what age and how often?
2. Which women should be offered chemoprophylaxis or prophylactic mastectomy?
3. Which women should be referred for genetic counseling and possible genetic testing?

Some women are easily identified to be at average risk due to the absence of risk factors, and others are clearly at high risk based on the presence of strong predisposing factors: chest radiation and known genetic mutation. Women with one or more risk factors or a positive family history for cancer, however, may require more detailed risk assessment and calculation to determine risk category. Risk assessment tools are useful to determine 5- or 10-year risk and lifetime risk of developing invasive breast cancer in individual patients. These tools are widely available to the public and to clinicians on the Internet. A woman is at *average risk* if her lifetime risk of developing breast cancer is 15% or less, at *moderate risk* if her lifetime risk is 15–20%, and at *high risk* if her lifetime risk exceeds 20–25% [5]. Women at moderate risk are screened according to the same guidelines as average risk women. All women should be assessed annually to determine if new information places the patient into a higher risk category.

Table 18.1 Breast cancer risk categories for screening

Risk category	Lifetime risk of developing breast cancer	Screening recommendations
Average	<15%	Offer routine mammography per average risk screening guidelines by the ACS or USPSTF (see Table 18.3)
Moderate	15–20%	Offer routine mammography per average risk screening guidelines by the ACS or USPSTF (see Table 18.3) Consider 3D tomosynthesis rather than conventional 2D mammography when available for women with dense breasts
High	>20%	Offer annual mammography and breast MRI starting at age 30 or as recommended by breast specialist Consider annual breast exam (recommended by NCCN but not ACS)

ACS American Cancer Society, *USPSTF* US Preventative Services Task Force, *NCCN* National Comprehensive Cancer Network

Average Risk

Women with an average risk of breast cancer have a <15% lifetime risk of developing invasive breast cancer and are screened per USPTF guidelines. Per American Cancer Society guidelines, a woman may be presumed to be of average risk for screening purposes if she has *none* of the following risk factors:

- Personal history of breast cancer or abnormal breast biopsy
- Strong family history of breast cancer or a genetic mutation known to increase the risk of breast cancer (such as a *BRCA* gene mutation)
- Chest radiation therapy before the age of 30 [6]

Most women who develop breast cancer are considered average risk, with no additional strong risk factors beyond age and sex.

High Risk

Some women are known to be high risk without the use of risk assessment tools and should be referred to a breast health specialist for evaluation and counseling. These include women with:

- Known BRCA1 or 2 mutation carriers or known genetic mutation with increased risk
- Untested first-degree relatives of a known BRCA mutation carrier
- History of chest irradiation between 10 and 30 years of age
- >20% lifetime risk of cancer based on a risk assessment tool

These patients often begin screening with annual mammography and MRI prior to age 40, and options of prophylactic mastectomy, oophorectomy, or chemoprophylaxis should be discussed with the patient. (See Chap. 17 on Primary Prevention of Breast Cancer.)

Breast cancer risk assessment is highly dependent on an accurate and up-to-date family history. The USPSTF recommends that all women be screened at 18, and then periodically every 3–5 years as family history changes, to determine who should be tested for inheritable cancer genes. Women with a family history of premenopausal breast cancer, male breast cancer or ovarian cancer in first-degree relatives, or multiple cases of cancers in the immediate or extended family should be considered for genetic counseling and testing. (See Chap. 17 on Primary Prevention of Breast Cancer.)

Women with a personal history of dense breasts or abnormal breast biopsies need closer evaluation. Patients with a history of *ductal carcinoma in situ* (*DCIS*) or a *previous history of breast cancer* are excluded from most risk assessment tools and should be managed in consultation with a breast specialist. Women with biopsy-proven *atypical lobular* (*ALH*) and *atypical ductal hyperplasia* (*ADH*) *or lobular carcinoma in situ* (*LCIS*) should be offered chemoprevention and be evaluated for lifetime breast cancer risk. Patients with dense breasts should be evaluated for risk in conjunction with other risk factors. Consultations from breast health specialists will assist in decisions regarding appropriate genetic testing, prophylactic therapies, and screening regimens for women at higher than average or unclear risk status. (See Chap. 17 on Primary Prevention of Breast Cancer.)

Use of Risk Assessment Tools in Women at Possible Increased Risk

Risk assessments may be performed using one of several risk assessment tools. For breast cancer screening purposes, the goal is to identify women with a greater than 20% lifetime risk who should be offered annual MRI screening in addition to mammography. The most commonly used tool is the National Cancer Institute's "Breast Cancer Risk Assessment Tool (BCRAT)" also called the *Gail Model* that is available on the National Cancer Institute website: https://bcrisktool.cancer.gov/ [7, 8].

The Gail Model is valid for use in women aged 35–85, with no history of breast cancer, DCIS, or LCIS. Other tools should be used for women with known mutations in BRCA1, BRACA2, and other hereditary syndromes associated with breast cancer and in patients with a strong family history of breast or ovarian cancer.

The Gail Model calculator can be used for 35- to 85-year-old women, and asks for:

- Age
- Age of menarche
- Age at first live birth (or nulliparity)
- Number of first-degree female relatives with breast cancer (mother, sisters, and daughters only)
- Number of previous breast biopsies and results (with or without atypical hyperplasia)
- Race/ethnicity (White, Hispanic, Asian American (with subcategories), or American-Indian/Alaskan Native

Five-year and lifetime risks of developing invasive breast cancer are then calculated. According to the Gail Model, a

5-year risk >1.7% is interpreted as increased risk (including both moderate- and high-risk women). Women in this risk category are candidates for chemoprevention with selective estrogen receptor modulators or aromatase inhibitors or consideration of surgical prophylactic options. (See Chap. 17 on Primary Prevention of Breast Cancer.) Patients with a lifetime risk over 20% are offered screening MRI in addition to mammography.

The Gail Model's strengths include validation in three large population databases [9] and ease of use during an office visit. Limitations of the Gail Model include (1) a relatively low sensitivity (28–44%) and moderate specificity (66–88%) for predicting breast cancer diagnosis in all women and (2) worsened performance characteristics in women with a strong family history of breast cancer (e.g., more than one first-degree relative or multiple non-first-degree relatives or male relatives) or family history of other cancers such as ovarian cancer [9–11]. The Gail Model is not well validated among women of Hispanic or Asian descent and may underestimate breast cancer risk in women of some races and ethnic backgrounds including African American and Jewish women. Many women are of mixed racial decent, so while the Gail Model makes an attempt to incorporate data on race, these are significant limitations which the creators acknowledge. Lastly, breast density is not included in the Gail Model calculation.

For women in whom an inherited breast cancer syndrome is suspected based on strong family history of breast, ovarian, tubal, or peritoneal cancer, the USPSTF recommends the use of other clinical risk prediction tools with better predictive accuracy than the Gail Model to determine which patients should be referred for genetic counseling/testing or undergo other preventive strategies [11]. (See Chap. 17 on Primary Prevention of Breast Cancer.)

The Tyrer-Cuzick or International Breast Cancer Intervention Study (IBIS) Model

The Tyrer-Cuzick or International Breast Cancer Intervention Study (IBIS model) is considered superior to other online screening tools, in that it does not underestimate risk, considers both clinical and family history data in depth, and includes breast density in risk calculations. The calculator estimates probability of BRCA1 and 2 mutations, lifetime risk of breast cancer, and 5- or 10-year risk.

The International Breast Cancer Intervention Study (IBIS: version 8 released Sept 2017) calculator asks for [12]:

- Age of patient
- Age at menarche
- Age at first live birth (or nulliparity)
- Number of first-degree female relatives with breast cancer
- Number of previous breast biopsies and results (with or without atypical hyperplasia)
- Height and weight
- Hormone therapy use
- Breast density category
- Ashkenazi grandparent
- BRCA or another genetic syndrome
- History of LCIS
- Family history that includes breast and ovarian cancer in first- and second-degree relatives on both sides of the family including age of diagnosis
- Male breast cancer in first-degree relative
- Bilateral breast cancer
- Breast cancer in half-sisters, female cousins, and nieces is also considered

The IBIS calculator can be downloaded without charge from http://www.ems-trials.org/riskevaluator/ [12].

There are numerous other risk calculators that are not as widely known, the discussion of which is beyond the scope of this chapter. These tools may be used by breast health specialists, researchers, or genetic counselors and can give more detailed risk information for risk of 5- or 10-year and lifetime breast cancer risk.

Case Resolution

Per the Gail Model (BCRAT), LuAnn has a 5-year risk of 1.9% and a 14.5% lifetime risk of breast cancer. The 5-year risk is such that she should consider chemoprevention and would warrant referral to a breast specialist. Her lifetime risk, however, is in the average-risk category (<15% lifetime risk).

Knowing that the Gail Model underestimates risk in African American women and does not account for breast density, a second risk calculation was performed for LuAnn. Per the Tyrer-Cuzick (IBIS) tool, she has a 26% lifetime risk of breast cancer which puts her into the high-risk category (>20–25% lifetime risk). Given this risk prediction from a more appropriate tool, she should be referred to a breast health specialist for consideration of genetic testing, begin annual imaging with breast MRI in addition to annual screening mammography, and also consider preventive strategies such as chemoprevention to reduce her risk of future breast cancer.

Breast Cancer Screening Modalities

Mammography

Conventional digital mammography has essentially replaced film mammography in the US. Digital breast tomosynthesis (DBT), sometimes referred to as "3D mammography", is a newer technology that has been approved by the FDA as an adjunct to conventional digital mammography, and is now routinely built into newer-generation mammography units [13]. Using the same breast compression required for standard 2D digital mammography, DBT images are obtained using a moving x-ray source that arcs over the breast (See Fig. 18.1). These images from multiple angles are then processed into thin "slices." The radiologist can scroll through the different projections slice by slice, as in other cross-sectional imaging examinations, comparing them to the standard 2D images. The main advantage of DBT is that it can mitigate the problem of focal asymmetry due to overlapping breast tissue. On standard digital projections, overlapping tissue can create the appearance of a tumor that isn't there or can make it hard to see small cancers that are present.

Potential benefits of using tomosynthesis with conventional digital mammography compared to conventional digital mammography alone include increased cancer detection (better sensitivity) and decreased rates of false positives (better specificity). Though no randomized trials have been done, prospective studies evaluating this technology have confirmed increased cancer detection rates with the addition of tomosynthesis but have conflicting results regarding its effect on false positives. One large prospective trial of 12,631 exams interpreted either with conventional digital mammography alone or with tomosynthesis combined with conventional mammography found cancer (invasive and in situ) in 6.1 per 1000 exams with conventional mammography alone vs 8.0 per 1000 exams with added 3D tomosynthesis, resulting in a 27% increased detection rate with the addition of tomosynthesis. There were 15% fewer false positives with the addition of tomosynthesis: 61.1 per 1000 exams with mammography alone vs 53.1 per 1000 exams with added tomosynthesis [15]. In another prospective study of 9672 exams using conventional digital mammography alone vs tomosynthesis combined with conventional digital mammography, there was a similar increase in cancer detection rate but also an increased rate of false positives with tomosynthesis views (4.0–4.5%) vs conventional mammography alone (3.4%) [16]. In this study, the increased cancer detection rate was particularly notable in women with dense breasts.

The downsides of 3D tomosynthesis include increased radiation exposure, longer duration of exam, and increased radiologist reading time, in addition to higher costs of these studies. Newer tomosynthesis technology that allows reconstruction of standard 2D images from the tomosynthesis data aims to reduce radiation exposure and duration of exam.

There are not yet clear consensus guidelines regarding the appropriate use of 3D tomosynthesis as a primary screening modality. The USPSTF 2016 guidelines give it an "I" grade: insufficient evidence to assess harms and benefits for tomosynthesis as a primary screening modality [17].

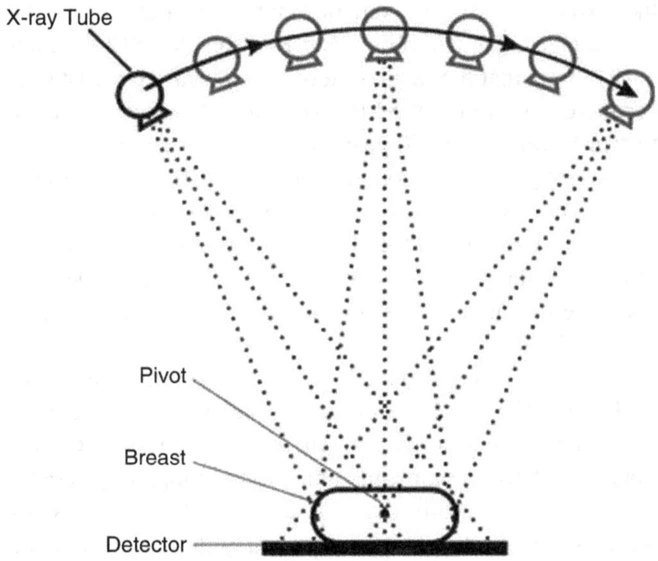

Fig. 18.1 Schematic representation of image acquisition in breast tomosynthesis [14]. (Reprinted from Yaffe MJ. Measurement of mammographic density. Breast Cancer Res. 2008;10:209)

Breast MRI

Women at high risk for breast cancer should be offered gadolinium contrast-enhanced breast MRI in combination with mammography to screen for breast cancer (See Table 18.1). While breast MRI has not yet been shown to reduce breast cancer mortality, it has been shown to detect smaller breast cancers and cancers at an earlier stage in high-risk women. Since half of all abnormal breast lesions seen on MRI are not seen on other imaging modalities, facilities performing breast MRIs should be capable of performing MRI-guided breast biopsies. Breast MRIs have a significantly lower specificity compared to mammography, resulting in higher call back rates and biopsies. Glandular enhancement by gadolinium can occur in the lactating breast and during certain days of the menstrual cycle [18]. Despite the clear benefits of breast MRI as an adjunct to mammography to screen high-risk women, it remains greatly underutilized in the high-risk population [19].

Benefits of Screening Mammography

The goal of screening mammography (whether 2D or 3D) is early detection of clinically important breast cancer to allow earlier treatment and therefore decrease breast cancer mortality. Though the effectiveness of mammography in detecting only clinically important breast cancer is still debated, the evidence supports that screening mammography programs do decrease breast cancer mortality by 12–33% [5, 17]. Not surprisingly, since breast cancer risk increases with age, the benefit of screening also increases with age. A 2016 meta-analysis of mammography breast cancer screening trials found that for every 10,000 women screened with repeat mammography for 10 years, 3 deaths were avoided in women aged 39–49 years, 8 deaths were avoided in women aged 50–59 years, 21 deaths were avoided in women aged 60–69 years, and 13 deaths were avoided in women aged 70–74 years [20].

Harms of Screening Mammography

Identified harms of screening mammography include (1) false-positive results that lead to unnecessary further testing, including diagnostic imaging and biopsies, and (2) overdiagnosis and overtreatment of breast cancer, defined as the detection or treatment of a cancer that would never have been detected or threatened health in the absence of screening. For example, a small DCIS lesion that might never have progressed to invasive breast cancer would currently be treated similarly to invasive cancer. The natural history of DCIS is not fully understood, and it is possible that this treatment will not benefit the patient as compared to no treatment.

Risk of False Positives and Biopsy Recommendations

False-positive mammograms are extremely common. Based on observational study data from the Breast Cancer Surveillance Consortium (BCSC), a large population-based database of mammogram and tumor registries in the USA, if a woman starts annual screening at age 40, her risk of having a false positive in the first decade is 61%; if she has biennial screening starting at 40, her risk over the first decade is 42% [21]. The rates of false positives were similar in women who began screening at age 50 compared to women who began at age 40.

A significant number of false-positive mammograms lead to breast biopsy. Among women who start screening at age 40 years, 7% of those with annual screening and 5% of those with biennial screening will have a false-positive screening mammogram leading to a biopsy recommendation. Similarly, among women who start screening at age 50 years, 9% of women with annual screening and 6% of women with biennial screening will have a false-positive mammogram and biopsy recommendation [22].

Risk of Overdiagnosis and Overtreatment

It is not currently possible to determine the exact proportion of mammogram-detected breast cancer that represents overdiagnosis since available diagnostic studies cannot differentiate clinically important from clinically unimportant cancers. However, estimates from randomized controlled trials (RCTs) suggest an overdiagnosis rate of 1 in 5 women who are diagnosed with breast cancer via mammography over a 10-year period [23]. A 2016 USPSTF-commissioned modeling study found a median overdiagnosis risk of 1 in 8 women who are diagnosed with breast cancer with biennial screening from ages 50–75 [24]. The task force concludes that with this conservative estimate of breast cancer overdiagnosis risk of 1 in 8, two to three women will be treated unnecessarily for every breast cancer death avoided.

Breast Cancer Screening Guidelines in Average-Risk Women

Increasing age is the most important risk factor for most women, which is why screening guidelines, including the USPSTF, publish recommendations which are based upon the age of the patient. A woman in her 70s has a relative risk of 18 compared to a woman in her 30s [25]. Similarly, the 2017 US cancer statistics summary data from the Surveillance, Epidemiology, and End Results (SEER) database reports that the odds of developing invasive breast cancer increases from 1 in 52 for women under 50 years of age to 1 in 15 for women 70 years of age and over [26].

Several professional organizations, societies, and national health care systems have created breast cancer screening guidelines based upon their own interpretations of the literature, particularly their assessment of the balance of benefits and potential harms of mammography. These are summarized in Table 18.2.

To highlight key differences, the US Preventive Services Task Force (USPSTF) recommends biennial mammography screening starting at age 50, whereas the American Cancer Society (ACS) recommends annual mammography screening starting at 45 with transition to biennial screening starting at age 55. Both guidelines generally do not recommend screening younger average-risk women (40–49 for USPSTF and 40–44 for ACS) but rather that providers use individual shared decision-making regarding screening in these age groups.

Table 18.2 Comparison of breast cancer screening guidelines for average-risk women from multiple organizations [5, 14, 27–31]

Organization	Year	Start screening mammography	Frequency/duration of screening mammography
US Preventative Services Task Force (USPSTF) [14]	2016	Start routine screening at age 50 Women may choose to start screening between ages 40 and 49	Biennial Insufficient evidence to recommend for or against screening >75 years old
American Cancer Society (ACS) [5]	2015	Start routine screening at age 45 Women may choose to start at age 40	Annual for women ages 45–54 Biennial for women aged ≥55 (Women may choose to continue annual screening after age 54) Continue screening if overall good health and life expectancy ≥10 years
American College of Obstetrics and Gynecology (ACOG) [27]	2017	Offer starting at age 40 Initiate no later than age 50	Annual or biennial Continue until age 75; women may choose to continue longer
American Academy of Family Physicians (AAFP) [28]	2013	Start at age 50 Women may choose to start screening between ages 40 and 49	Annual or biennial Continue until age 75; consider longer with shared decision-making
American College of Radiology (ACR) [29]	2017	Start at age 40	Screen annually Consider stopping when life expectancy is <5–7 years
Canadian Task Force [30]	2011	Start at age 50	Screen every 2–3 years for women ages 50–74
National Health Service (UK) [31]	2010	Start at age 50	Screen every 3 years from ages 50–70

The USPSTF acknowledges that the evidence suggests women aged 40–49 do have a net benefit from screening mammography, but this is small (3 deaths avoided per 10,000 women screened for 10 years, compared to 8–21 deaths avoided for women aged 50–75) and may not be acceptable to some women when potential harms are considered.

The ACS argues that women aged 45–49 are more similar in risk of breast cancer, with a 5-year absolute breast cancer risk of 0.9%, compared to women aged 50–54, whose 5-year absolute risk is 1.1% than they are to women aged 40–44 who have a 5-year risk of 0.6%. The risk of false positives is similar whether screening begins at 40 or 50, hence their recommendation to start screening at 45 [5]. Regarding their recommendation to screen women annually from 45 to 54, the ACS acknowledges that direct evidence comparing breast cancer mortality by screening interval is limited. However, they cite observational data, meta-analyses, and modeling studies that show greater mortality benefit for annual screening in younger women as compared to older women, likely due to a combination of more aggressive tumor characteristics and decreased sensitivity of mammography in younger premenopausal women. The ACS does note that annual screening also increases risks of false positives [5].

The above discordance in guideline recommendations highlights the need for individual shared decision-making between clinicians and patients. In summary, all women at average risk for breast cancer are recommended to begin screening no later than age 50. Clinicians should discuss screening with average-risk women starting in their 40s. Women who are strongly interested in screening mammography between 40 and 50 years of age and who are willing to accept an increased risk of false positives should be offered earlier screening after a risk versus benefit discussion. By contrast, other women may prefer to start later and screen every other year.

Breast Cancer Screening for Women with Dense Breasts

Breasts with a high proportion of glandular and fibrous connective tissue compared to fat appear dense on mammography. The American College of Radiology's Breast Imaging Reporting and Data System (BI-RADS) classification of breast density is shown in Table 18.3.

"Dense breasts" (BI-RADS C or D) are common, occurring in approximately 43% of women aged 40–74 years. A woman's BI-RADS density category may vary from one year to the next, due to both biological reasons (primarily body weight and hormonal status) and variation in readings by radiologists [32].

Dense breasts are at an increased risk of developing breast cancer, estimated to be about 20–30% higher risk than women with normal breast density [17, 33] and may obscure breast tumors on mammography. The sensitivity of mammography to detect breast cancer ranges from 87% in women with BI-RADS A to 63% in women with BI-RADS D density [34]. This raises the question of whether supplemental screening (with ultrasound, MRI, or other modality) should be done when a mammogram is negative in women with dense breasts. There are no published randomized trials to answer this question. The USPSTF funded a systematic review of the literature and concluded in its 2016 Breast Cancer Screening guidelines that there is insufficient evi-

Table 18.3 Breast density classification [3] and prevalence of each category among US women age 40–74 [4]

Breast composition category	Description of breast tissue appearance	Prevalence (%)
A	Almost entirely fat	13.3
B	Scattered areas of fibroglandular density	43.4
C	Heterogeneously dense, which may obscure small masses	35.9
D	Extremely dense, which lowers the sensitivity of mammography	7.4

dence to assess the balance of benefits and harms of adjunctive screening using digital breast tomosynthesis, breast ultrasound, MRI, or other methods in women identified to have dense breasts on an otherwise negative mammogram [17]. Digital 3D breast tomosynthesis may increase sensitivity and decrease recalls in patients with dense breasts; however randomized trials are lacking to confirm this with direct evidence. Ultrasound is limited by a very high rate of false positives. MRI is limited by cost, lack of widespread availability, and potential for adverse events related to the use of gadolinium contrast, especially if used annually for decades.

No major guidelines recommend supplemental screening for women with dense breasts; however, due to grassroots efforts, more than half of US states require mammography result letters to include information on breast density. Mammography result letters are required to include the woman's breast density in the report or to include a comment stating that breast density decreases the sensitivity of mammography screening. Some statements encourage women to discuss supplemental screening with ultrasound or MRI with their health care provider. This can cause stress and confusion for patients whose providers may not always agree and whose insurance may not pay for supplemental screening. Providers should be prepared to assess a woman's overall risk.

For women with dense breasts and a high risk of breast cancer, the clinician should discuss the potential risks and benefits of additional screening with MRI or referral to a breast specialist. As mentioned above, the IBIS tool does include breast density in its risk assessment. At this time, decisions for supplemental screening with MRI are based on estimates of breast cancer risk as described in the section above and are only recommended for women with high risk. Women should be reassured that they will be followed clinically, and their risk will be assessed annually. As emerging technologies and future studies improve screening modalities and inform care, providers will notify patients and advise them accordingly.

Breast Cancer Screening in Women at Increased Risk for Breast Cancer: Moderate and High Risk

Moderate Risk

For women at moderately increased risk for breast cancer (15–20% lifetime risk) but no identified genetic mutation, there is currently no data from randomized trials to show that early mammography prior to age 50 or adjunctive imaging studies including breast ultrasound or MRI reduce mortality. This group includes many women in the 40–49 age group with one first-degree relative with postmenopausal breast cancer, but no other risk factors. The ACS and USPSTF guidelines state that the current evidence is insufficient to recommend for or against adjunctive MRI in women at moderate risk [35]. Clinicians may discuss uncertain benefits with individual patients in this moderate-risk category and consider individual risks/benefits/preferences, availability, cost, and insurance coverage factors when deciding about adjunctive imaging. Alternately, primary care clinicians may consider referral to a breast health specialist for advice regarding appropriate screening.

High Risk

Women who are assessed as having high risk to develop breast cancer, defined as a lifetime risk >20–25% based on a risk prediction tool such as the Gail Model (BCRAT) or Tyrer-Cuzick (IBIS) model, known BRCA carrier state, untested first-degree relative of BRCA carrier, history of chest radiation between 10 and 30 years of age, or another high-risk genetic syndrome, should be referred to a breast health specialist as soon as possible for evaluation and counseling. The breast health specialist will make recommendations regarding appropriate genetic testing, prophylactic therapies, and screening regimens. (See Chap. 17 on The Primary Prevention of Breast Cancer.) *In general, for women at high risk of developing breast cancer* (*see* Table 18.4), *the American Cancer Society recommends adjunct annual MRI screening in addition to annual mammography starting at age 30;* however, they note that this recommendation is based on data from nonrandomized screening trials, observational studies, and expert opinion [35]. The MRI and the mammogram should be scheduled approximately 6 months apart to effectively screen twice yearly.

Ultrasounds should be considered in lieu of MRI in women who are unable to undergo MRI examinations. The age to start screening should be individualized, with consideration of patient-specific risk factors and the age of diagno-

Table 18.4 American Cancer Society recommendations for or against adjunctive breast MRI for breast cancer screening in women [35]. (Adapted with permission from Saslow D, Boetes C, Burke W, Harms S, Leach MO, Lehman CD, et al. American Cancer Society guidelines for breast screening with MRI as an adjunct to mammography. CA Cancer J Clin. 2007;57(2):75–89)

Recommend annual MRI screening	Insufficient evidence to recommend for or against MRI screening	Recommend against MRI screening
Women at high risk: Lifetime risk >20–25% based on risk prediction model	*Women at moderate risk:* Lifetime risk 15–20% based on risk prediction models	*Women at average risk:* Women <15% lifetime risk
BRCA1 or BRCA2 mutation	Lobular carcinoma in situ (LCIS) or atypical lobular hyperplasia (ALH)	
Untested first-degree relative of BRCA carrier	Atypical ductal hyperplasia (ADH)	
Radiation to chest between 10 and 30 years of age	Heterogeneously or extremely dense breast on mammography (BIRADS C and D)	
Li-Fraumeni, Cowden, or PTEN hamartoma tumor syndromes and first-degree relatives	Women with a personal history of breast cancer including ductal carcinoma in situ (DCIS)	

sis of affected relatives. (The use of ultrasounds in women with breast complaints, mammographic abnormalities, or palpable masses is discussed separately in Chap. 16 on Benign Breast Conditions.)

Mammography Interpretation and Appropriate Follow-Up

The American College of Radiology has developed standardized guidelines by which the FDA mandates all mammograms, breast ultrasounds, and breast MRIs be interpreted. These are called the "Breast Imaging Reporting and Data System," referred to as "BI-RADS" [36]. The BI-RADS manual specifies that mammogram reports must include an indication, an assessment of breast density, a description of abnormalities, and a summary that includes the most important findings and specification of a final BI-RADS assessment category, of which there are seven (see Table 18.5).

The Clinical Breast Exam

The clinical breast exam (CBE) described in this chapter is a physical exam which is performed by a clinician, in contrast to a self-breast exam (SBE), which is done by the patient

Table 18.5 BI-RADS mammography categories and management recommendations. (Reprinted by permission of the American College of Radiology. ACR BIRADS Atlas Mammography; Table 6: https://www.acr.org/-/media/ACR/Files/RADS/BIRADS/Mammography-Reporting.pdf. All rights reserved. The most current version of the ACR BI-RADS® Atlas can be found at http://www.acr.org/Quality-Safety/Resources/BIRADS [36])

BIRADS category	Appropriate management
0: Incomplete assessment – need additional imaging evaluation and/or prior mammograms for comparison	Recall for additional imaging and/or comparison with prior examination(s)
1: Negative	Return to routine mammography screening
2: Benign	Return to routine mammography screening
3: Probably benign	Short interval (every 6 months) follow-up with diagnostic mammogram and/or ultrasound × 1–2 years; return to routine screen when determined benign
4: Suspicious 4A: Low suspicion for malignancy 4B: Moderate suspicion for malignancy 4C: High suspicion for malignancy	Refer for tissue diagnosis
5: Highly suggestive of malignancy (95–100%)	Refer for tissue diagnosis
6: Known biopsy-proven malignancy	Oncology referral for comprehensive cancer treatment evaluation

herself. CBEs are essential when evaluating and following a woman with a breast mass, pain, or discharge (see Chap. 16 on Benign Breast Conditions) and for evaluating and following women at high risk of breast cancer. The CBE is also used by breast specialists for patients in the evaluation of known breast abnormalities, increased breast risk, and malignancies. The CBE is also used by many clinicians to screen for breast cancer, both in the US and worldwide. Like mammography, CBEs can help with the early detection of breast cancer but also can result in harms associated with false-positive results. It is not known whether screening CBEs decrease breast cancer mortality either in addition to imaging or as the only screening modality. An ongoing randomized trial comparing CBE to no screening in India should answer part of this question in the next several years [37]. The Canadian National Breast Screening Study-2 provides some evidence for the effectiveness of CBE [38]. All the women in the study received CBE, and half the women were also screened by mammography. The mammography group had no reduction in breast cancer mortality compared to CBE alone. CBE detected most of the invasive breast cancers but did not detect cancer as early as mammography;

however, the percent of women whose cancer was diagnosed prior to lymph node spread was the same whether detected by mammography or CBE. The sensitivity of CBE to detect breast cancer appears to be 40–69% and specificity 88–99% [39].

There are no randomized trials evaluating the effectiveness of adding CBE to the assessment of average-risk women already being screened by mammography. The USPSTF last addressed CBE in its 2009 guidelines, stating that the current evidence is insufficient to assess the additional benefits and harms of clinical breast exam (CBE) beyond screening mammography in women 40 years or older. The latest ACS Breast Cancer Screening Guidelines do not recommend CBE for average-risk, asymptomatic women given lack of demonstrated benefit and an increase in false positives [5]. Based on consensus and expert opinion, ACOG's view is that screening CBE may be offered "in the context of an informed, shared decision-making approach that recognizes the uncertainty of additional benefits and the possibility of adverse consequences of clinical breast examination beyond screening mammography. If performed for screening, intervals of every 1–3 years for women aged 25–39 years and annually for women aged 40 years and older are reasonable" [27]. Reflecting the diversity of opinion in the medical community, some authors of this textbook do not routinely offer CBE to asymptomatic women who are getting regular screening via mammography, but others feel strongly that a CBE (albeit shortened) should be offered to all women as part of an annual complete physical exam and breast health education.

There are multiple scenarios in which a CBE is especially useful in clinical practice. A thorough and skilled breast exam is essential for patients who present to clinic with breast lumps and other breast complaints. When ordering diagnostic mammograms or other imaging, clinicians must locate and confirm a breast mass and perform a lymph node exam (see Chap. 16 on Benign Breast Conditions). Mammography, in addition, misses 13–15% of breast cancers that are palpable on exam and is less sensitive in women with dense breasts. Although uncommon, a breast cancer can present first as an axillary node with no detectable primary tumor in the breast. Some women may not mention a breast or axillary mass to their clinician due to high anxiety or denial, leading to a delay in medical attention if a routine exam is not performed. Not all women want mammograms; some of them may accept a CBE for screening, and this may be beneficial in age groups at highest risk for breast cancer (e.g., ages 50–75). Some elderly women forego mammography, but the detection and treatment of palpable cancers may reduce morbidity and mortality. As mentioned previously, CBE may detect a substantial proportion of cases of cancer if it is the only screening test available [40].

One limitation of the CBE is that it has not been fully standardized. When a clinician performs a CBE, the exam should be careful and systematic [18, 41], particularly when assessing a breast complaint, evaluating a woman at increased risk, or when examining a woman who is not receiving screening mammography. Gloves should not be used. Inspection of breast contour (looking for puckering, dimpling, nipple retraction, or asymmetry) and palpation of axillary and supraclavicular lymph nodes is done while the patient is sitting up or standing. Though there are no adequate data to support specific positioning of the patient for inspection [41], some clinicians inspect while the woman raises her arms above her head, as she puts her hands on her hips and contracts her pectoralis muscles or leans slightly forward. After the patient is supine, breast palpation should be performed with the pads of the fingers using circular motions (not "walking" of the finger tips). Each area should be palpated using three different pressures (light, medium, and deep) to detect a mass at any of these levels. The best coverage of breast tissue is accomplished by examining tissue in vertical strips beginning at the axilla and extending down the midaxillary line to the bra line, then back up to the clavicle, moving medially in rows to the center of the chest. This is sometimes referred to as the lawnmower method and is more thorough than a circular or wheel-and-spoke method [41, 42]. The nipples should be inspected for skin changes, discharge, or asymmetry. It has been suggested by some authors that truly careful palpation should take about 3 minutes per breast.

The Self-Breast Examination and Breast Awareness

Clinicians in the USA used to routinely teach SBE to patients, but after a randomized trial in Shanghai showed no benefit and increased harms (false positives, extra biopsies, complications of treatment) [43], this practice has fallen out of favor. In 2003, the ACS stopped recommending SBE, and the USPSTF also recommends against teaching women how to perform SBE [40].

In lieu of teaching patients SBE, there is a newer concept of teaching patients breast self- awareness. Unlike breast self-examination, which entails women examining their breasts in a systematic way on a routine basis, breast self-awareness empowers a woman to notice a change or potential problem with her breasts and to take action. Women should be educated about the signs and symptoms of breast cancer and advised to notify their health care provider as soon as they notice a change such as pain, a mass, new onset of nipple discharge, or redness in their breasts [44]. Teaching points include the fact that most masses are found by women during normal activities such as bathing and dressing, the underlying structures of normal breast architecture, and the feel of normal glandular tissues. Given the strong public awareness, fear and attention given to the subject of breast cancer, and the perceived importance of SBE, it is critical that providers arm patients with accurate up-to-date information, to encourage appropriate screening and awareness and to educate women about the prevention and early detection of breast cancer.

The Palpable Breast Lump

It is critical that any patient who presents with a concerning breast lump on physical exam should have a full diagnostic workup with ultrasound, possible biopsy, and/or referral to a breast specialist even if initial mammography is normal (BI-RADS 1–3). Not all cancers are apparent on mammographic images, and the rate of false negatives for screening mammography is reported between 10% and 30% and is highest in women with very dense breast tissue [45]. Lobular cancer in particular may not show on mammogram as it can have a very low density and grow in a fishnet-type pattern rather than forming masses with calcifications [46]. From a risk management standpoint, all palpable lesions must be well documented and followed through to resolution. (See Chap. 16 on Benign Breast Conditions for a detailed discussion.)

Counseling Women with Suspected Breast Cancer

Over 90% of breast cancers in the USA are initially detected by mammography and the remainder by physical exam alone (i.e., a palpable lump) [47]. When a suspicious lesion has been identified, tissue should be obtained with a percutaneous needle biopsy, which has been shown to be as accurate as an open surgical biopsy [48]. A core needle biopsy can confirm malignancy and provide information of breast cancer histology. (See section on breast mass evaluation in Chap. 16 on Benign Breast Conditions.)

Malignant Findings on Breast Biopsy

Ductal carcinoma in situ (DCIS, stage 0 breast cancer) is a noninvasive carcinoma of the breast that is confined to the breast ducts and lobules and is a distinct entity from invasive breast cancer. The diagnosis of DCIS has increased significantly in the 1980s and 1990s as a result of increased breast cancer screening with mammography [2]. An estimated 20–25% of all breast cancers detected by mammography are proven to be DCIS upon biopsy [49]. In general, DCIS has a more favorable prognosis compared to invasive breast cancer, with an estimated overall breast cancer-specific mortality rate of 3.3% at 20 years [50]. Having DCIS increases the risk of developing a subsequent invasive breast cancer and thus, the goal of treating DCIS is to reduce the risk of invasive breast cancer and the associated increase in mortality. Lobular carcinoma in situ is commonly found incidentally in breast biopsy specimens and is discussed in Chaps. 16 and 17 on Benign Breast Conditions and The Primary Prevention of Breast Cancer respectively.

Invasive cancer, in contrast, shows infiltration of tumor cells through the ductal or lobar basement membrane on histology. (See Chap. 19 on Breast Cancer Diagnosis and Management.) There are several different histologic types of invasive breast cancer.

Ductal carcinoma is the most common histologic type, accounting for approximately 74% of invasive breast cancer. Lobular carcinoma and mixed lobular/ductal carcinomas comprise 8%, and 7% of invasive carcinomas. Lobular cancer may be invisible on mammogram and thus may present with a breast mass not seen on mammogram or at later stages with adenopathy in the neck, supraclavicular fossa, or axilla. Other rarer types of breast cancers comprise the remaining cases.

The Initial Evaluation of Newly Diagnosed Breast Cancer

Once a woman has biopsy-proven invasive breast cancer, the following important steps will be taken by the oncologist:

1. Staging or extent of disease (size, lymph node involvement, metastatic disease)
2. Hormone receptor and tumor marker analysis
3. Surgical staging and treatment planning
4. Genetic counseling +/− genetic testing if high risk for hereditary breast cancer

In general, the tumor size, lymph node involvement, and the presence of metastatic disease are all important prognostic determinants. The size of the tumor will be determined by imaging (mammography, ultrasound, or MRI) and clinical findings. Axillary lymph node involvement significantly impacts prognosis and removal of involved lymph nodes can reduce local recurrence. If patients have clinical evidence of lymph node involvement such as a palpable, enlarged node or evidence of nodal involvement on imaging, they will undergo an axillary lymph node dissection (ALND). Patients who have early-stage breast cancer without clinical evidence of lymph node involvement will undergo sentinel lymph node biopsy to confirm the presence or absence of lymph node involvement [51]. Women with symptoms or signs of metastatic disease will undergo appropriate imaging to define the extent of disease.

Tumor Biology and Receptor Testing

Invasive breast cancers are tested for hormone receptor status to determine the expression of estrogen receptors (ER) and progesterone receptors (PR). Approximately 80% of invasive breast cancers are ER and/or PR positive and tumors that express these hormone receptors generally have a more favorable prognosis [52]. The presence of estrogen receptors and progesterone receptors also predicts responsiveness to endocrine-based therapies [53]. Expression of human epidermal growth factor 2 (HER2) is measured in all invasive breast cancers at the time of diagnosis or recurrence. Approximately 20% of invasive breast cancers overexpress HER2 and in general, HER2 overexpression is associated with more aggressive tumors. Patients with HER2+ breast cancers may benefit from HER2-directed therapies. Breast cancers can be subtyped according to the presence or absence of ER, PR, and HER2. Approximately 13% of breast cancers are ER, PR, and HER2 negative, also known as triple-negative disease which tends to be more aggressive than ER+ tumors.

Staging

The formal staging of breast cancer has been standardized using the American Joint Committee on Cancer and the International Union for Cancer Control (AJCC-UICC) classification system for tumor, nodes, and metastases (TNM). Initially, patients are assigned a TNM stage clinically (cTNM) and then they are restaged after surgery (pTNM). Tumor stage is the most important prognostic factor for women with breast cancer. For women with nonmetastatic breast cancer, the number of axillary lymph nodes involved is the strongest predictor of recurrent, distant disease [54].

All patients diagnosed with invasive breast cancer should undergo a detailed family history to determine if they are at high risk for hereditary breast cancer and undergo genetic testing if indicated (see Chap. 17 on The Primary Prevention of Breast Cancer).

Treatment Planning for Breast Cancer

Ductal Carcinoma In Situ

DCIS accounts for approximately 20% of all breast cancer diagnoses. DCIS is not an invasive cancer but increases the risk of invasive breast cancer. DCIS lesions are treated by lumpectomy followed by whole breast radiation therapy, mastectomy, or lumpectomy with clinical observation. Whole breast radiation therapy has been shown to reduce local recurrence but does not improve breast cancer-specific survival. For low-risk DCIS, XRT may not provide a clinically significant benefit [55]. Debate currently exists about whether some women with low-grade DCIS can undergo close active surveillance in lieu of immediate surgical treatment. The results of the low-risk DCIS (LORIS) trial comparing surgery with active monitoring for low-risk DCIS in the UK will provide important information to help solve this question, and information can be found on the LORIS website: www.birmingham.ac.uk/research/activity/mds/trials/crctu/trials/loris/index.aspx [56].

Invasive Breast Cancer

The treatment of invasive breast cancer is broadly determined by type and size of tumor, lymph node involvement, specific hormone receptors and tumor markers, and the presence or absence of metastatic disease. Most women with early-stage invasive breast cancer (stage I or stage II) can be offered breast-conserving therapy (lumpectomy followed by whole breast radiation therapy) which has been shown to have equivalent survival rates to mastectomy [57]. Women with early-stage breast cancer who are at increased risk of recurrence may also be offered adjuvant systemic chemotherapy. Women with stage III breast cancer may be offered surgical resection with radiation therapy and adjuvant or neoadjuvant chemotherapy. Women with non-operable breast cancer are offered systemic chemotherapy with consideration of specific hormone receptor status and tumor markers [54]. A more detailed discussion of breast cancer and management can be found in Chap. 19 on Breast Cancer Diagnosis and Management.

Psychosocial Impact of Breast Cancer Diagnosis and Treatment

A diagnosis of breast cancer can have a negative impact on a woman's sense of well-being and mental health and can cause significant distress. Nearly half of women newly diagnosed with breast cancer screen positive for distress or a psychiatric disorder [58]. Younger women diagnosed with breast cancer have more distress compared to their older counterparts and both the diagnosis of cancer and the effects of surgical and medical treatment may negatively affect quality of life and self-image [59]. The National Comprehensive Cancer Network (NCCN) recommends screening all patients diagnosed with breast cancer for distress at the time of diagnosis and ideally at every subsequent visit. At a minimum, women should be screened at clinically appropriate intervals and particularly when there is a change in disease status. The NCCN Distress Thermometer Screening Tool may be used to determine severity of distress. Patients should also be screened for depression and anxiety, if indicated. A treatment plan should be developed to provide appropriate psychosocial support and care via the oncologic team, mental health professionals, social workers, and spiritual and/or chaplaincy care with periodic reassessments and modifications of the treatment plan as needed [60]. For further discussion, see Chap. 20 on Care of the Breast Cancer Survivor.

Summary Points

1. Breast cancer risk categories include average (lifetime risk of <15%), moderate (lifetime risk 15–20%), and high (lifetime risk >20%). Women with any of the following conditions are considered to have high risk for breast cancer: known BRCA1 or 2 mutations, untested first-degree relatives of a BRCA mutation carrier, a history of chest irradiation between 10 and 30 years of age, or another high-risk genetic syndrome. To assess risk in women who do not have high-risk conditions, we advise clinicians to use a risk assessment tool. The Gail Model (BCRAT) risk assessment tool is most appropriate for women without risk factors for a familial breast cancer syndrome and the Tyrer-Cuzick (IBIS) tool should be used for women with risk factors.
2. Tomosynthesis "3D" mammography has been approved by the FDA as an adjunct to conventional "2D" mammography. It has been shown to increase sensitivity of screening mammography, especially in women with dense breasts, but has an unclear impact on rates of false positives and breast cancer clinical outcomes.
3. The ACS recommends screening women at average risk annually from ages 45–54 and then biennially from age 55 until their life expectancy is <10 years. The ACS recommends using shared decision-making for women aged 40–44.
4. The American College of Radiology's Breast Imaging Reporting and Data System (BI-RADS) classifies breast density on mammography as ranging from A to D, where A is almost entirely fatty and D is extremely dense breast tissues. High breast density (BI-RADS C and D) increases the risk of developing breast cancer by about 20–30% and can also make it harder to see tumors on mammography.
5. At this time, additional imaging such as MRI is not recommended for women at moderate risk, but clinicians should consider referral to a breast health specialist for further evaluation and screening recommendations on an individual basis. Women in the high-risk category (>20–25% lifetime risk) should be referred to a breast specialist whenever possible and should have annual screening breast MRI in addition to annual screening mammography.
6. A careful and systematic breast exam should include palpation performed with the pads of the fingers using circular motions using the vertical strip (lawnmower) method for breast tissue coverage. CBE is essential when evaluating breast symptoms, such as a breast mass noticed by a patient. CBE is often used for breast cancer screening, though its additional benefit in women getting mammography is not known.

Review Questions

1. A 40-year-old woman who is at average risk for breast cancer presents for a routine visit. After a thorough discussion of the risks and benefits of screening mammography, she says that she truly has no preference about when to start screening. She wants to know your recommendation. Based on recent guidelines, which screening strategy is most appropriate?
   A. Biennial screening mammography starting at age 55
   B. Annual screening mammography starting at age 40
   C. Annual screening mammography from 45 to 54, then biennial screening, or biennial screening starting at age 50
   D. Annual screening with mammography and breast MRI starting at age 40

   The correct answer is C. Answer C describes the recommended screening strategy for average-risk women per ACS and USPSTF, respectively. Answer A is incorrect because no organizations advise waiting until 55 to start screening. Answer B is incorrect because most organizations (except for the American College of Radiology) do not advise starting screening at age 40 for average-risk women, although it is an option. Answer D is incorrect because MRI is not indicated for average-risk women [5, 17].
2. A 50-year-old patient with an average risk for breast cancer based on careful review of personal and family history had her screening mammogram two weeks ago. She received a letter stating that, though the mammogram was normal, she has extremely dense breasts. It further states women with dense breasts have a higher risk of breast cancer than average, and she should talk with her doctor about possible supplemental screening. What is recommended?
   A. Order a breast MRI.
   B. Order a breast ultrasound.
   C. Refer to a breast health specialist for genetic counseling and testing.
   D. Tell her it's unknown whether supplemental imaging improves survival in average-risk women with dense breasts and is not recommended.

The correct answer is D. Explanation: The USPSTF concluded in its 2016 Breast Cancer Screening guidelines that there is insufficient evidence to assess the balance of benefits and harms of adjunctive screening using digital breast tomosynthesis, breast ultrasound, MRI, or other methods in women identified to have dense breasts on an otherwise negative mammogram. The other answer choices are incorrect because she is at average risk otherwise and so is not recommended to have supplemental screening with ultrasound and MRI or see a breast specialist [17].

3. A 42-year-old woman presents to establish care. Her family history is notable for breast cancer diagnosed in her mother at age 50 and her older sister at age 46 and ovarian cancer in a maternal aunt at age 55. She has never had a mammogram or other breast cancer screenings. As far as she knows, her family members have not had genetic testing for their cancers. What is the most appropriate tool to estimate her breast cancer risk?
   A. Tyrer-Cuzick (IBIS) tool.
   B. Gail Model (BCRAT).
   C. Atherosclerotic cardiovascular disease (ASCVD risk calculator).
   D. No tool is needed; proceed with average-risk screening.

   The correct answer is A. Explanation: This patient is clearly at high risk for a familial breast cancer syndrome; hence, the IBIS tool should be used as this has better risk prediction in patients with inherited breast cancer risk factors. The Gail Model (BRCAT) is *not* recommended when a familial breast cancer syndrome is strongly suspected. The ASCVD tool is not relevant, and it would be inappropriate to proceed with average-risk screening given her concerning family history [11].
4. A 42-year-old patient has an estimated lifetime risk of breast cancer of over 20% using the IBIS calculator. What is the next step regarding breast cancer screening?
   A. Annual 3D tomosynthesis mammography starting now
   B. Annual breast MRI in addition to annual mammography, genetic risk evaluation, and referral to a breast health specialist for consideration of prophylactic therapies
   C. Referral to a surgeon for consideration of prophylactic mastectomy and oophorectomy
   D. Biennial mammography starting at age 50

   The correct answer is B. Explanation: A patient with a lifetime risk of cancer which is >20% should be referred to a breast specialist and be considered for: annual MRI in addition to mammography screening (staggered by 6-month intervals), evaluation of genetic risk, and consideration for prophylactic therapies. The other answer choices are incorrect because mammography alone is not sufficient to screen women at high risk for breast cancer; and referral directly to a surgeon without genetic testing and consultation with a breast specialist would be premature [35].
5. A 39-year-old woman presents to her primary care provider with concerns for a new dime-sized lump in her right breast that she discovered incidentally while showering. The lump is not painful. She denies associated redness, fevers, or nipple discharge; she is not breastfeeding. She has never had a mammogram; no family history of breast or other cancers. On exam, her provider palpates a firm nontender nodule in the upper outer quadrant of her right breast without associated skin changes, nipple discharge, or lymphadenopathy. She is referred for a diagnostic mammogram, which is normal (BIRADS-1). What is the next step?
   A. Reassure her based on the normal diagnostic mammogram; no other testing is indicated.
   B. Advise her that she should have a repeat diagnostic mammogram in 6 months.
   C. Refer her to a breast surgeon for prophylactic mastectomy.
   D. Despite a negative mammogram, she should also have a diagnostic ultrasound with consideration of image-guided biopsy and referral to a breast health specialist.

   The correct answer is D. Explanation: Not all cancers are apparent on mammographic images. The rate of false negatives for screening mammography is reported between 10% and 30% and is highest in women with very dense breast tissue [45]. Palpable lumps must be fully evaluated with diagnostic mammogram, diagnostic ultrasound, consideration of image-guided biopsy, and referral to a breast health specialist. Answer choices A and B are incorrect because she needs further evaluation with diagnostic US and consideration of biopsy. Answer choice C is incorrect because a tissue diagnosis must be obtained to guide treatment decisions.
6. A 52-year-old patient with an average risk of breast cancer reports having a mammogram 2 years ago which was negative. She shares that having the mammogram was extremely uncomfortable and despite a detailed discussion about the benefits of mammography to screen for breast cancer and potential options to lessen discomfort, she is adamant about avoiding another. What other option, if any, could be offered to her?

A. Breast MRI.
B. Breast ultrasound.
C. Clinical breast exam (CBE).
D. No other options should be offered.

The correct answer is C. Explanation: Currently, mammography is the only recommended breast cancer screening modality for average-risk women. Breast MRIs and ultrasounds are used as adjunctive imaging to mammography for diagnostic purposes and breast MRI is recommended for women at high risk for breast cancer screening. Patients can be offered a well-performed, systematic clinical breast exam (CBE) to assist with screening. While there is no evidence at this time that clinical breast exams reduce breast cancer mortality, a randomized trial comparing CBE to no screening in India will hopefully answer this question in the next several years [37]. There is some evidence that CBE can detect a substantial proportion of cases of cancer if it is the only screening test available [40].

References

1. Centers for Disease Control and Prevention. 2015 [cited 2018 Jun 14 2018]. Available from: https://www.cdc.gov/women/lcod/2015/all-females/index.htm.
2. DeSantis C, Ma J, Bryan L, Jemal A. Breast cancer statistics, 2013. CA Cancer J Clin. 2014;64(1):52–62.
3. D'Orsi CJSE, Mendelson EB, et al. ACR BI-RADS atlas, breast imaging reporting and data system. 5th ed. Reston: American College of Radiology; 2013.
4. Sprague BL, Gangnon RE, Burt V, Trentham-Dietz A, Hampton JM, Wellman RD, et al. Prevalence of mammographically dense breasts in the United States. J Natl Cancer Inst. 2014;106(10):dju255.
5. Oeffinger KC, Fontham ET, Etzioni R, Herzig A, Michaelson JS, Shih YC, et al. Breast cancer screening for women at average risk: 2015 guideline update from the American Cancer Society. JAMA. 2015;314(15):1599–614.
6. Society AC. American cancer society recommendations for the early detection of breast cancer 2017 updated Oct 9, 2017. Available from: https://www.cancer.org/cancer/breast-cancer/screening-tests-and-early-detection/american-cancer-society-recommendations-for-the-early-detection-of-breast-cancer.html#written_by.
7. Amir E, Freedman OC, Seruga B, Evans DG. Assessing women at high risk of breast cancer: a review of risk assessment models. J Natl Cancer Inst. 2010;102(10):680–91.
8. National Cancer Institute website: https://bcrisktool.cancer.gov/.
9. Rockhill B, Spiegelman D, Byrne C, Hunter DJ, Colditz GA. Validation of the Gail et al. model of breast cancer risk prediction and implications for chemoprevention. J Natl Cancer Inst. 2001;93(5):358–66.
10. Tice JA, Cummings SR, Smith-Bindman R, Ichikawa L, Barlow WE, Kerlikowske K. Using clinical factors and mammographic breast density to estimate breast cancer risk: development and validation of a new predictive model. Ann Intern Med. 2008;148(5):337–47.
11. Moyer VA, Force USPST. Risk assessment, genetic counseling, and genetic testing for BRCA-related cancer in women: U.S. Preventive Services Task Force recommendation statement. Ann Intern Med. 2014;160(4):271–81.
12. IBIS breast cancer risk evaluation tool. http://www.ems-trials.org/riskevaluator/.
13. Takahashi TA, Lee CI, Johnson KM. Breast cancer screening: does tomosynthesis augment mammography? Cleve Clin J Med. 2017;84(7):522–7.
14. Yaffe MJ. Measurement of mammographic density. Breast Cancer Res. 2008;10:209.
15. Skaane P, Bandos AI, Gullien R, Eben EB, Ekseth U, Haakenaasen U, et al. Comparison of digital mammography alone and digital mammography plus tomosynthesis in a population-based screening program. Radiology. 2013;267(1):47–56.
16. Bernardi D, Macaskill P, Pellegrini M, Valentini M, Fanto C, Ostillio L, et al. Breast cancer screening with tomosynthesis (3D mammography) with acquired or synthetic 2D mammography compared with 2D mammography alone (STORM-2): a population-based prospective study. Lancet Oncol. 2016;17(8):1105–13.
17. Siu AL, Force USPST. Screening for breast cancer: U.S. Preventive Services Task force recommendation statement. Ann Intern Med. 2016;164(4):279–96.
18. Saslow D, Hannan J, Osuch J, Alciati MH, Baines C, Barton M, et al. Clinical breast examination: practical recommendations for optimizing performance and reporting. CA Cancer J Clin. 2004;54(6):327–44.
19. Miles R, Wan F, Onega TL, Lenderink-Carpenter A, O'Meara ES, Zhu W, et al. Underutilization of supplemental magnetic resonance imaging screening among patients at high breast cancer risk. J Womens Health (Larchmt). 2018;27(6):748–54.
20. Nelson HD, Fu R, Cantor A, Pappas M, Daeges M, Humphrey L. Effectiveness of breast cancer screening: systematic review and meta-analysis to update the 2009 U.S. Preventive Services Task force recommendation. Ann Intern Med. 2016;164(4):244–55.
21. Hubbard RA, Kerlikowske K, Flowers CI, Yankaskas BC, Zhu W, Miglioretti DL. Cumulative probability of false-positive recall or biopsy recommendation after 10 years of screening mammography: a cohort study. Ann Intern Med. 2011;155(8):481–92.
22. Nelson HD, Pappas M, Cantor A, Griffin J, Daeges M, Humphrey L. Harms of breast cancer screening: systematic review to update the 2009 U.S. Preventive Services Task force recommendation. Ann Intern Med. 2016;164(4):256–67.
23. Marmot MG, Altman DG, Cameron DA, Dewar JA, Thompson SG, Wilcox M. The benefits and harms of breast cancer screening: an independent review. Br J Cancer. 2013;108(11):2205–40.
24. Mandelblatt JS, Stout NK, Schechter CB, van den Broek JJ, Miglioretti DL, Krapcho M, et al. Collaborative modeling of the benefits and harms associated with different U.S. breast cancer screening strategies. Ann Intern Med. 2016;164(4):215–25.
25. Clemons M, Goss P. Estrogen and the risk of breast cancer. N Engl J Med. 2001;344(4):276–85.
26. Siegel RL, Miller KD, Jemal A. Cancer statistics, 2017. CA Cancer J Clin. 2017;67(1):7–30.
27. Committee on Practice Bulletins—Gynecology. Practice bulletin number 179: breast cancer risk assessment and screening in average-risk women. Obstet Gynecol. 2017;130(1):e1–e16.
28. Tonelli M, Connor Gorber S, Joffres M, Dickinson J, Singh H, Lewin G, et al. Recommendations on screening for breast cancer in average-risk women aged 40–74 years. CMAJ. 2011;183(17):1991–2001.
29. Tria Tirona M. Breast cancer screening update. Am Fam Physician. 2013;87(4):274–8.
30. Radiology EPoBIAACBCSACo. 2017. Available from: https://acsearch.acr.org/docs/70910/Narrative/.
31. NHS Breast Cancer Screening. https://www.nhs.uk/conditions/breast-cancer-screening/.
32. Melnikow J, Fenton JJ, Whitlock EP, Miglioretti DL, Weyrich MS, Thompson JH, et al. Supplemental screening for breast cancer in women with dense breasts: a systematic review for the U.S. preventive services task force. Ann Intern Med. 2016;164(4):268–78.
33. Mandelblatt JS, Cronin K, deKoning H, Miglioretti DL, Schechter C, Stout N. Collaborative modeling of U.S. breast cancer screening strategies. Quality AfHRa, editor. Rockville; 2015.
34. Carney PA, Miglioretti DL, Yankaskas BC, Kerlikowske K, Rosenberg R, Rutter CM, et al. Individual and combined effects of age, breast density, and hormone replacement therapy use on the accuracy of screening mammography. Ann Intern Med. 2003;138(3):168–75.
35. Saslow D, Boetes C, Burke W, Harms S, Leach MO, Lehman CD, et al. American Cancer Society guidelines for breast screening

with MRI as an adjunct to mammography. CA Cancer J Clin. 2007;57(2):75–89.
36. Atlas-Mammography ACoRB. ACR BIRADS atlas mammography; Table 6: https://www.acr.org/-/media/ACR/Files/RADS/BIRADS/Mammography-Reporting.pdf. Available from: https://www.acr.org/Clinical-Resources/Reporting-and-Data-Systems/Bi-Rads. Accessed 29 Jan 2018.
37. Sankaranarayanan R, Ramadas K, Thara S, Muwonge R, Prabhakar J, Augustine P, et al. Clinical breast examination: preliminary results from a cluster randomized controlled trial in India. J Natl Cancer Inst. 2011;103(19):1476–80.
38. Miller AB, To T, Baines CJ, Wall C. Canadian National Breast Screening Study-2: 13-year results of a randomized trial in women aged 50–59 years. J Natl Cancer Inst. 2000;92(18):1490–9.
39. Humphrey LL, Helfand M, Chan BK, Woolf SH. Breast cancer screening: a summary of the evidence for the U.S. Preventive Services Task Force. Ann Intern Med. 2002;137(5 Part 1):347–60.
40. Force USPST. Screening for breast cancer: U.S. Preventive Services Task Force recommendation statement. Ann Intern Med. 2009;151(10):716–26, W-236.
41. Barton MB, Harris R, Fletcher SW. The rational clinical examination. Does this patient have breast cancer? The screening clinical breast examination: should it be done? How? JAMA. 1999;282(13):1270–80.
42. Saunders KJ, Pilgrim CA, Pennypacker HS. Increased proficiency of search in breast self-examination. Cancer. 1986;58(11):2531–7.
43. Thomas DB, Gao DL, Ray RM, Wang WW, Allison CJ, Chen FL, et al. Randomized trial of breast self-examination in Shanghai: final results. J Natl Cancer Inst. 2002;94(19):1445–57.
44. Committee on Practice Bulletins—Gynecology. Breast cancer risk assessment and screening in average-risk women. 2017.
45. Yankaskas BC, Klabunde CN, Ancelle-Park R, Renner G, Wang H, Fracheboud J, et al. International comparison of performance measures for screening mammography: can it be done? J Med Screen. 2004;11(4):187–93.
46. Porter AJ, Evans EB, Foxcroft LM, Simpson PT, Lakhani SR. Mammographic and ultrasound features of invasive lobular carcinoma of the breast. J Med Imaging Radiat Oncol. 2014;58(1):1–10.
47. Smart CR, Hartmann WH, Beahrs OH, Garfinkel L. Insights into breast cancer screening of younger women. Evidence from the 14-year follow-up of the Breast Cancer Detection Demonstration Project. Cancer. 1993;72(4 Suppl):1449–56.
48. Silverstein MJ, Recht A, Lagios MD, Bleiweiss IJ, Blumencranz PW, Gizienski T, et al. Special report: consensus conference III. Image-detected breast cancer: state-of-the-art diagnosis and treatment. J Am Coll Surg. 2009;209(4):504–20.
49. Ernster VL, Ballard-Barbash R, Barlow WE, Zheng Y, Weaver DL, Cutter G, et al. Detection of ductal carcinoma in situ in women undergoing screening mammography. J Natl Cancer Inst. 2002;94(20):1546–54.
50. Narod SA, Iqbal J, Giannakeas V, Sopik V, Sun P. Breast cancer mortality after a diagnosis of ductal carcinoma in situ. JAMA Oncol. 2015;1(7):888–96.
51. Lyman GH, Temin S, Edge SB, Newman LA, Turner RR, Weaver DL, et al. Sentinel lymph node biopsy for patients with early-stage breast cancer: American Society of Clinical Oncology clinical practice guideline update. J Clin Oncol. 2014;32(13):1365–83.
52. Parise CA, Bauer KR, Brown MM, Caggiano V. Breast cancer subtypes as defined by the estrogen receptor (ER), progesterone receptor (PR), and the human epidermal growth factor receptor 2 (HER2) among women with invasive breast cancer in California, 1999–2004. Breast J. 2009;15(6):593–602.
53. Harris L, Fritsche H, Mennel R, Norton L, Ravdin P, Taube S, et al. American Society of Clinical Oncology 2007 update of recommendations for the use of tumor markers in breast cancer. J Clin Oncol. 2007;25(33):5287–312.
54. Warner E. Clinical practice. Breast-cancer screening. N Engl J Med. 2011;365(11):1025–32.
55. Gradishar WJ, Anderson BO, Balassanian R, Blair SL, Burstein HJ, Cyr A, et al. NCCN guidelines insights: breast cancer, version 1.2017. J Natl Compr Cancer Netw. 2017;15(4):433–51.
56. Merrill AL, Esserman L, Morrow M. Clinical decisions. Ductal carcinoma in situ. N Engl J Med. 2016;374(4):390–2.
57. Early Breast Cancer Trialists' Collaborative Group, Darby S, McGale P, Correa C, Taylor C, Arriagada R, et al. Effect of radiotherapy after breast-conserving surgery on 10-year recurrence and 15-year breast cancer death: meta-analysis of individual patient data for 10,801 women in 17 randomised trials. Lancet. 2011;378(9804):1707–16.
58. Hegel MT, Moore CP, Collins ED, Kearing S, Gillock KL, Riggs RL, et al. Distress, psychiatric syndromes, and impairment of function in women with newly diagnosed breast cancer. Cancer. 2006;107(12):2924–31.
59. Baucom DH, Porter LS, Kirby JS, Gremore TM, Keefe FJ. Psychosocial issues confronting young women with breast cancer. Breast Dis. 2005;23:103–13.
60. Network NCC. NCCN clinical practice guidelines in oncology distress management 2017 September 7, 2017.

Breast Cancer Diagnosis and Management

19

Mita Sanghavi Goel and Aarati Didwania

Learning Objectives

1. Classify the stage of breast cancer based on data from imaging and biopsy in the preoperative setting.
2. Discuss how treatment modalities are chosen based on the preoperative classification of breast cancer.
3. Anticipate and counsel patient about adverse effects related to possible treatment modalities.
4. Prepare patients for the initial and subsequent meetings with the oncology team.
5. Describe clinical factors that influence the prognosis of patients with breast cancer.

Khadijah is a premenopausal 40-year-old woman with an abnormal screening mammogram (BI-RADS-5) showing a 3 cm area with calcifications in her left breast. She returns to discuss her results and wants to know what to expect going forward.

The Primary Care Provider in the Care of Patients with Breast Cancer

The primary care provider (PCP) has a variety of different roles to assume in caring for a patient with breast cancer, throughout the continuum of breast cancer care. Traditionally, PCPs bear responsibility for managing preventive health and screening exams in their patient population; however, most patients also see their PCPs while they are undergoing diagnostic testing for breast cancer [1]. During these visits, PCPs have opportunities to educate patients about the test findings to date and to advocate for timely follow-up of any remaining diagnostic testing. Furthermore, primary care providers may be involved in breast cancer treatment decisions. In a survey of women recently diagnosed with breast cancer, nearly one third reported involving their PCP, and higher levels of PCP engagement were associated with higher decision satisfaction [2]. These findings suggest that PCPs are able to draw upon an established relationship to prepare patients for their initial oncology visit and that they may also enhance communication between the patient and their oncology team.

When a patient has an abnormal mammogram requiring biopsy, the PCP is often notified and given the opportunity to let the patient know that a biopsy is recommended. The PCP can then inform the patient and make a referral. The primary care office should arrange timely consultation with a surgeon or breast specialist, ideally within 3–7 days, to evaluate the patient, perform a biopsy, review biopsy results, and begin the initial evaluation and treatment of any breast abnormality. If the diagnosis of cancer is confirmed, the primary care provider or the surgeon can refer to a medical oncologist and possibly a radiation oncologist to plan treatment.

Khadijah is referred to the breast clinic, and biopsy reveals infiltrating ductal carcinoma that is estrogen receptor negative (ER-), progesterone receptor negative (PR-), and HER-2/neu receptor negative. She comes to the office and wants to know what these results mean and what type of treatment will be recommended. She understands that her results are consistent with "triple-negative" breast cancer in a premenopausal patient, and she is very worried.

Recommending a course of treatment in a newly diagnosed breast cancer patient depends on a number of factors: tumor characteristics, tumor biology, and patient characteristics. Tumor characteristics and biology predict how aggressive the

M. S. Goel (✉) · A. Didwania
Northwestern University, Feinberg School of Medicine, Division of General Medicine & Geriatrics, Chicago, IL, USA
e-mail: m-goel@northwestern.edu; a-didwania@northwestern.edu

S. A. Tilstra et al. (eds.), *Sex- and Gender-Based Women's Health*, https://doi.org/10.1007/978-3-030-50695-7_19

cancer may be, how probable the cancer is to spread or recur, and how effective a treatment may be. Patient characteristics such as menopausal status, genetic mutations which confer a high risk of breast cancer, and comorbid conditions also influence the likelihood of recurrence and determine the risk-benefit ratio. Patient preferences may also influence treatment decisions, especially when considering surgical treatments such as mastectomy vs. lumpectomy and reconstruction.

Histopathology

Most cases of breast cancer arise from epithelial breast cells and are classified as carcinomas. Rarely, lymphomas, sarcomas, and melanomas occur in the breast.

The most common histopathologic types of carcinomas on biopsy are the following.

Lobular Carcinoma In Situ (LCIS)

LCIS is a unique entity which is not cancerous, but which increases the risk of breast cancer. LCIS consists of noncancerous, abnormal cells that are found in the lobules of breast tissue, where milk is produced. LCIS is often multicentric. Women with LCIS should be followed closely and offered chemoprevention (see Chaps. 16 and 17 on "Benign Breast Conditions", and "The Primary Prevention of Breast Cancer").

Ductal Carcinoma In Situ (DCIS)

DCIS is a noninvasive or preinvasive breast cancer. DCIS is diagnosed when abnormal cells replace the normal cells lining the breast ducts but have not extended beyond their original tissue layer. DCIS is most commonly identified on mammography as a cluster of microcalcifications and accounts for approximately 25% of cancers found on mammography. DCIS, by definition, does not spread to other organs; however, it is estimated that 20–30% of DCIS lesions progress to invasive cancer. Intermediate- and high-grade DCIS are generally treated with excision and XRT, and chemoprevention is offered to reduce the risk of the development of invasive breast cancer (see Chap. 17 on "The Primary Prevention of Breast Cancer"). The full discussion of DCIS treatment algorithms is beyond the scope of this chapter.

Debate currently exists about whether some women with low-grade DCIS can undergo close active surveillance in lieu of immediate surgical treatment. Whichever treatment is offered, it is critical that women with DCIS understand that continued close follow-up and monitoring are essential to prevent and detect invasive cancer. The low-risk DCIS (LORIS) trial comparing surgery with active monitoring for low-risk DCIS in the United Kingdom will provide important information to help solve this question: information can be found on the LORIS website www.birmingham.ac.uk/research/activity/mds/trials/crctu/trials/loris/index.aspx [3].

Invasive Ductal Carcinoma (IDC)

Invasive ductal carcinoma consists of cancerous cells that line breast ducts and have invaded beyond the original tissue layer. IDC represents 75% of invasive breast cancers and typically requires treatment with surgery. Chemotherapy or radiation therapy may also be recommended depending on the stage of the cancer.

Invasive Lobular Carcinoma (ILC) and Mixed Lobular/Ductal Carcinoma. Lobular carcinoma consists of invasive, cancerous cells that originate in the breast lobules, where milk is produced. Lobular cancer may be invisible on mammogram and thus present at later stages with axillary or supraclavicular adenopathy. ILC constitutes fewer than 15% of all breast cancers. Similar to IDC, treatment typically requires surgery and possibly chemotherapy and/or radiation therapy.

Rarer breast carcinomas include:

Mucinous or colloid carcinoma accounts for 2.3% of invasive carcinoma. It is more common in older women and is notable for producing mucus. These tumors can grow large and have a soft texture.

Tubular carcinoma (TC) is a subtype of IDC which tends to be small, full of tubules, and not aggressive. TC is often detected by mammography before there is a palpable mass.

Papillary carcinoma is usually small, ER/PR+ HER2- and has a good prognosis. Papillary tumors should be resected whole and sent to pathology to clarify whether or not invasive cancer is present.

Metaplastic carcinoma contains two or more cell types and is treated similarly to IDC.

Phyllodes tumors are rapidly growing tumors which arise in connective tissues, are classified as sarcomas, and occur in premenopausal women. Phyllodes tumors do not respond to hormone therapy and can be resistant to XRT and chemotherapies. Women with *Li-Fraumeni syndrome* are at increased risk of phyllodes tumors. Malignancy is seen in 10–25% of cases.

Mammary Paget's disease presents as changes in the nipple and areola, and DCIS or invasive cancer is often concomitantly present in the ipsilateral breast.

Inflammatory breast cancer (IBC), less than 5% of newly diagnosed breast cancers, is an extremely aggressive, locally advanced cancer. Most women develop diffuse erythema and edema of the breast itself, and many have distant, metastatic disease on presentation.

A full discussion of treatment strategies for each of these cancer types is beyond the scope of this volume.

Tumor Grade

Grading is a scoring system to describe how abnormal tumor cells appear, compared with normal cells. For breast cancer, grading is typically determined by reviewing tubule formation, the size and shape of the nucleus, and the mitotic rate and then assigning a score for each characteristic. Tumors are then categorized as grade 1 (low grade or well differentiated), grade 2 (intermediate grade or moderately differentiated), or grade 3 (high grade or poorly differentiated). Tumors that have higher grades are considered more aggressive and tend to grow faster and spread more rapidly than lower grades [4].

Tissue Markers and Molecular Profiling

Specific molecular profiles of breast carcinomas provide additional insight into a tumor's potential for metastasis and recurrence and help oncologists determine the appropriate, effective treatments for each patient. A full discussion of microarray and molecular profiling tests is beyond the scope of this chapter. Common current molecular profiles that strongly influence treatment choice include the following.

Estrogen Receptor and Progesterone Receptor (ER/PR) Status

Hormone receptor status describes whether, and how many, receptors for estrogen and progesterone are present on or in the tumor cells. The presence of these receptors is important to identify because when hormones attach to their receptors, they can fuel tumor growth. Approximately two-thirds of all breast cancers have at least one hormone receptor positive. Negative hormone status is conferred when less than 1% of cells tested have the receptor in question. Tumors that are ER-negative and PR-negative tend to grow more rapidly than hormone receptor positive tumors, are more likely to recur within the first few years of treatment, and are more common among premenopausal women [5].

Human Epidermal Growth Factor Type 2 Receptor (HER2/neu or Simply HER2)

The HER2 receptor allows for the binding of a growth-promoting protein; thus its presence indicates a more aggressive tumor type and one that may be less responsive to hormonal therapy. While all breast cancer cells have some HER2 receptors, those with an overexpression are considered positive. At times, initial testing is equivocal, requiring additional testing to conclusively determine HER2 receptor status.

Gene Profile Testing

Examining patterns of gene activity, also referred to as gene expression tests, genomic testing, or microarray testing, in breast cancer can help determine the risk of recurrence, thereby informing discussions regarding the benefits of treatment with chemotherapy. Additionally, specific genetic profiles can inform oncologists and patients when targeted therapies or clinical trials may be applicable to the individual patient based upon tumor biology.

Oncologists choose to order a gene profile test based on the patient characteristics, availability and familiarity of a certain test, and insurance coverage. Multiple assays should not be used on the same patient, because their results may be discordant. Some examples are as follows:

- The *recurrence score (Oncotype Dx®)* is a validated assay to assess the risk of recurrence in node-negative, ER+, and HER2- disease. The calculations assume that women would complete 5 years of hormonal therapy and thus estimate the additive benefit of adjuvant chemotherapy for an individual woman. Results are reported as recurrence scores ranging from 0 to 100 to indicate high (score > 30), intermediate (score 18–30), and low (score < 18) likelihood of recurrence. Chemotherapy is generally indicated for women at high risk of recurrence and may be of limited benefit in women with both low and intermediate scores [6, 7].
- *Amsterdam 70-gene profile (MammaPrint®)* also estimates risk of recurrence in ER+ and HER2- disease. Although it may be used in select patients with ER-/PR+ disease, it is not recommended in women with triple-negative disease or HER2+ tumors. Testing is designed to help determine which patients might benefit from adjuvant chemotherapy. Testing is indicated in women younger than 61 years old with:
  - Tumors 5 cm or smaller
  - No lymph node involvement (although some trials indicate benefit when up to three lymph nodes are involved)

Results are reported as "low risk" and "high risk" of distant recurrence, thereby indicating those who are more likely to benefit from chemotherapy.

Additional profile tests are presented at: https://www.asco.org/sites/new-www.asco.org/files/content-files/practice-and-guidelines/documents/2017-adjuvant-biomarkers-summary-table.pdf [8].

Staging

"Stage" is a summative method for describing the extent of cancer. There are two types of stages: clinical stage (assigned prior to surgery using clinical information such as physical exam, imaging, and biopsy results or when surgery is not an option) or anatomic or pathologic stage (using surgical specimens). Stage is often assigned using the American Joint Commission on Cancer (JCC) TNM System [9] that incorporates the following different data points.

Tumor Size (T)

Higher numbers following the T indicate a larger, more advanced tumor. Typical categories include:

- T1 – tumor is ≤20 mm across its widest point.
- T2 – tumor is >20 mm and ≤50 mm across.
- T3 – tumor is >50 mm across.
- T4 – tumor of any size growing into the chest wall or skin, including inflammatory breast cancer.
- Tx – unable to assess tumor.
- T0 – no evidence of primary tumor.
- Tis – ductal carcinoma in situ (DCIS) and Paget's disease of the breast, with no associated mass, that are not invasive cancers.

Nodal Involvement (N)

The N categories indicate how many and which lymph nodes are affected. With improving technology, smaller areas of nodal involvement can be detected; current cutoffs to change nodal status require at least 200 cancerous cells measuring at least 0.2 mm detected in a node. Categories include:

- N0 – no cancer in nearby lymph nodes
- N1 – cancer found in 1–3 lymph nodes in the axilla or cancer found in internal mammary lymph nodes on sentinel node examination
- N2 – cancer found in 4–9 axillary lymph nodes or internal mammary lymph nodes enlarged by imaging
- N3 – cancer involving 10 or more axillary lymph nodes or cancer found in both axillary lymph nodes and internal mammary nodes or cancer in the infra- or supraclavicular lymph nodes
- Nx – nodal status could not be determined

Metastases (M)

The M designation indicates whether the cancer has distant spread. Categories include:

- M0 – no distant spread
- M1 – distant spread present, most often to bone, brain, lung, or liver
- Mx – metastatic spread could not be assessed

The summative staging category is determined by the specific TNM results.

Table 19.1 Breast cancer staging, treatment options, and 5-year survival rates for primary care provider counseling purposes [10]

Stage	General treatments offered	5-year survival
Stage 0: DCIS *Stage 1*: Tumor ≤20 mm, no nodes, no metastatic lesions (mets)	Primary tumor resection Consider radiation therapy (RT) Consider hormonal chemoprevention therapy Less likely adjuvant chemotherapy	Nearly 100%
Stage 2A: Tumor >20 mm to ≤50 mm, no nodes, no mets *Stage 2B*: Tumor >20 mm to ≤50 mm, 1–3 nodes, *or* >50 mm, no nodes, no mets	Primary tumor resection Likely RT Likely adjuvant chemotherapy and/or hormonal therapy	93%
Stage 3A: Tumor of any size, with up to nine nodes, no mets *Stage 3B*: Tumor of any size with growth into chest wall or skin, including inflammatory cancer, with up to nine nodes, no mets *Stage 3C*: Any size tumor, more than ten nodes, no mets	Primary tumor resection Likely RT Likely chemotherapy and/or hormonal therapy	72%
Stage 4: Any T, any N, one met or more	Primary tumor resection Consider RT for local control or mets Curative intent unlikely Systemic therapies Hormonal therapy if ER+: SERM or AI Palliative and end-of-life care	22%

Adapted from Breast Cancer Survival Rates [10]

The classifications are described in detail on the American Joint Committee on Cancer (AJCC) website in their cancer staging manual [9]. Staging categories include early stage (IA, IB, IIA, IIB, IIIA) and advanced stage (IIIB, IIIC, and IV). These categories provide a method to allow comparison of average survivorship (Table 19.1). For example, 5-year survivorship for stage I breast cancer is 95.3% compared with 79.8% for stage IIB.

Hereditary Breast and Ovarian Cancer (HBOC) Syndromes and Gene Mutations in Breast Cancer Patients

Genetic Mutations

Certain genetic mutations, if present in the breast cancer patient, confer an increased risk of future breast cancer in the contralateral breast and an increased risk of other cancers. Patients with personal or family history characteristics suspicious for a genetic syndrome should be screened and managed accordingly. The presence of a genetic mutation has implications for surgical treatment, chemoprevention, and cancer screening with mammography, clinical breast exams, and annual breast MRI. A full discussion of testing for genetic syndromes in cancer patients is found in Chap. 20 on the "Care of the Breast Cancer Survivor". A discussion of genetic syndromes and the recommended screening schedules for affected patients is found in Chap. 17 on "The Primary Prevention of Breast Cancer".

BRCA 1/BRCA 2

Mutations in the *BRCA 1* and *2* genes are present in 2% of all women with breast cancer, with the prevalence increasing to 10% among women diagnosed with breast cancer younger than 40 years. Identifying patients with these mutations is important because it has implications for breast cancer screening, prophylaxis, and treatment, such as prophylactic mastectomy and salpingo-oophorectomy (see Chap. 17 on "The Primary Prevention of Breast Cancer"). Women with breast cancer who are positive for *BRCA 1* or *2* should consider contralateral prophylactic mastectomy, which reduces the future risk of breast cancer, through shared decision-making with the surgical oncologist. It is unclear whether prophylactic mastectomy reduces breast cancer associated mortality in women who already have breast cancer [11]. Similarly, risk-reducing salpingo-oophorectomy decreases risk of ovarian/peritoneal/fallopian cancers in patients with *BRCA* genes [12] (see Chap. 15 on "Gynecologic Malignancies").

Personal and family history factors, beyond age at diagnoses, that increase likelihood of a deleterious gene mutations include: a personal history of ovarian cancer, a history of bilateral breast cancer, breast cancer in a male relative, triple negative (i.e., ER/PR negative, HER2 negative) breast cancers diagnosed at younger than 60 years, and Ashkenazi or Sephardic Jewish heritage. Only 1 in 40 Ashkenazi Jews has a *BRCA* gene mutation compared to 1 in 300–500 individuals in the general US population. Though exact estimates vary, *BRCA 1* and *2* mutations confer a lifetime breast cancer risk of approximately 72% and 69%, respectively, and a lifetime ovarian cancer risk of 44% and 17%, respectively [13]. *BRCA* mutations also increase the risk of prostate and pancreatic cancers.

Risk models such as Breast and Ovarian Analysis of Disease Incidence and Carrier Estimation Algorithm (BOADICEA) and BRCAPRO help genetic counselors and oncologists identify women with breast cancer who may require genetic testing for *BRCA 1* and *2* gene mutations, although a recent study suggests that all breast cancer patients should be tested [14].

Other Genetic Mutations Which Increase Breast Cancer Risk

Other high-penetrance mutations that increase the risk of breast cancer include the following:

Li-Fraumeni syndrome (p53). This syndrome increases the risk of premenopausal breast cancer, and the breast *cancer risk in these patients* is 49% by age 60.

*PTEN Hamartoma Tumor Syndromes, Including Cowden Syndrome***.** The lifetime *breast cancer risk in these patients* is up to 50%. Diagnostic criteria can be found at: https://www.nature.com/articles/gim2014147/tables/4 [15].

Diffuse Gastric and Lobular Breast Cancer Syndrome. Pathogenic variations in the *CDH1* gene increase the risk of poorly differentiated invasive adenocarcinoma of the stomach and lobular breast cancer. The lifetime risk of breast cancer is 39% to over 50% in these patients.

Peutz-Jeghers Syndrome and *PALB2* also greatly increase the risk of breast cancer.

Lynch Syndrome Also known as *hereditary nonpolyposis colorectal cancer (HNPCC)*, this syndrome does not increase lifetime risk of breast cancer to the level that prophylactic mastectomy should be considered; the risk is approximately 18%, but has a high risk of right-sided colon cancer, endometrial cancer (second most common), and less commonly ovarian cancer [16, 17]. See Chap. 17 on "The Primary Prevention of Breast Cancer" for a full discussion of genetic syndromes with recommendations for screening and prevention in these patients.

Patient Characteristics

Patient characteristics influence the efficacy of recommended therapies and the choice of treatment therapies based on their side effects.

Menopausal status informs the choice of antiestrogen agents in women with ER/PR-positive tumors. Selective estrogen receptor modulators (SERMs) block estrogen receptors on breast tissue, and tamoxifen is first-line hormonal treatment in premenopausal women. Aromatase inhibitors (AIs) prevent the conversion of peripheral androgens into estrogen, are first line in postmenopausal women, and are generally not used in premenopausal women. Postmenopausal women generally benefit more from AIs than from SERMs in cancer treatment, which is different from how these agents are used for breast cancer prevention. (See Chap. 17 on "The Primary Prevention of Breast Cancer".)

Cardiovascular disease may impact the choice of chemotherapy: there is an increased risk of heart failure with anthracyclines, an increased risk of coronary artery disease with left-sided radiation therapy, and an increased risk of heart failure with trastuzumab for adjuvant therapy. The presence and severity of osteoporosis may limit use of treatment of aromatase inhibitors or dictate that bisphosphonate treatment be given concomitantly.

Lastly, numerous studies describe *disparities* in breast cancer stage at diagnosis, and mortality, by race/ethnicity, physical ability, and socioeconomic status [18–21]. For example, Black women have similar screening rates as White women, but they are more likely to be diagnosed with advanced cancers and have higher mortality [18]. Primary care clinicians are well positioned to promote equitable, high-quality care by identifying barriers affecting their individual patients, such as barriers to accessing recommended follow-up care and barriers to adhering to optimal therapy.

Treatment Options

Treatment for breast cancer consists of a range of options. Treatment for stages I–III breast cancer includes surgical excision, radiation therapy (RT), and often chemotherapy. Additional agents may be employed, depending on the status of molecular markers, such as ER/PR and HER2 receptors.

The American Society of Clinical Oncology recommends integrating palliative and end of-life care into standard oncology care for patients with advanced malignancies [22]. Advanced or metastatic breast cancer is incurable, although some patients will live many years after diagnosis. In women with ER+/PR+ tumors especially, hormonal therapies with AIs have extended life expectancy expectations, even in stage 4 cases. Palliative care specialists assist patients and families by addressing spiritual and emotional issues, assisting with decision-making, transitioning to end-of-life (hospice care), and providing grief counseling. Early referral in cases of metastatic breast cancer also decreases depression and improves survival [23].

Palliative care and hospice care are underutilized, as evidenced by the relatively short time between referral and death [24]. Primary care clinicians are well positioned to mitigate this gap by explaining to patients that the goal of palliative care is to reduce pain and discomfort and increase quality of life. PCPs may want to reinforce the message that the goal of palliative care is not to abandon treatment or hasten death, when providing referrals for patients.

Surgical Resection of the Primary Tumor

The mainstay of cancer treatment is removal of the primary tumor. Surgery is usually performed prior to chemotherapy; however, some women with large tumors benefit from neoadjuvant chemotherapy to reduce the size of the tumor prior to surgery. Depending on the size of the tumor, its location, and likely cosmetic outcome, breast conservation surgery may be an option. In breast-conserving surgery, only a portion of the breast is removed, and surgery is often followed by external beam radiation (XRT). Cancers that are multicentric or large may require a mastectomy, which removes all the breast tissue on the affected side(s) of the body. Shared decision-making is used in the selection of mastectomy over breast conservation therapy, since there is no difference in overall survival between these two treatments [25–27]. Support from the patient's PCP and oncologists for informed decision-making is critical and may reduce decisional conflict [28]. As a corollary, women undergoing mastectomy face myriad reconstruction options and demonstrate improved decisional satisfaction from the use of decision aids [28].

Radiation Therapy

Many women require additional treatment with radiation, based on the type of surgery, the involvement of lymph nodes, the size and location of the breast cancer, and the presence of metastatic lesions in the brain or bones. Radiation therapy is administered from an external source using external beam radiation (XRT) or via brachytherapy: implanting a radiation source into the affected area using seeds or pellets to deliver radiation locally.

Typical indications for radiation therapy to the breast include:

- Breast conservation surgery
- Removal of breast cancers that are 5 cm or larger (which may not have adequate margins)
- Breast cancers with positive lymph nodes (lymph nodes are then included in the radiation field)
- Metastatic disease to the brain or bones (targeted radiation is then directed to the metastatic lesions)

Chemotherapy

The need for chemotherapy is determined based on stage and tumor characteristics. Chemotherapy is administered as adjuvant chemotherapy after surgery or prior to surgery as neoadjuvant chemotherapy. Neoadjuvant chemotherapy is given prior to surgery in the hopes of reducing tumor size and thus reducing the extent of surgery needed.

Common chemotherapeutic agents used in locally advanced breast cancers include: anthracyclines, taxanes, 5-FU, cyclophosphamide, and carboplatin. The frequency and duration of chemotherapies vary greatly depending on the chemotherapy agents selected, patient comorbidities, and tolerability of the chemotherapy. Most recommended regimens include two or more drugs that act on cells during different phases of the cell cycle. Adverse effects of specific chemotherapeutic agents vary and are listed in the following section. The discussion of specific chemotherapeutic regimens is beyond the scope of this chapter.

Hormonal Therapies in ER-/PR-Positive Cancers

Hormonal therapies (HT) are active against breast cancer because they act as an antiestrogen in the breast tissue or by reducing levels of estrogen in the circulation. Hormonal therapies are recommended in the treatment of ER/PR-positive tumors, most commonly as a 5- to 10-year course of tamoxifen for premenopausal women or an aromatase inhibitor in postmenopausal women. These medications have been found to reduce both disease-free survival and breast cancer-related mortality [29]. Additional research is currently underway to determine the effects of transitioning between tamoxifen and aromatase inhibitors. Ovarian suppression or ablation may be considered for some women, especially those younger than 35 years at the time of diagnosis who also received chemotherapy [30]. Patients with *BRCA* mutations often undergo salpingo-oophorectomy for the additional benefit of preventing ovarian cancer.

Anti-HER2/neu Antibody

Numerous studies demonstrate the benefit of using the anti-HER2 antibody, trastuzumab, on disease-free survival and overall survival when given following chemotherapy with either anthracycline- or non-anthracycline-containing regimens, for patients who are HER2 positive [31, 32]. Trastuzumab is typically administered for 1 year in those with early-stage, HER2-positive breast cancer. Additional antibodies are currently being evaluated for their additive benefit to trastuzumab.

Bisphosphonates

Adjuvant bisphosphonates have many uses in breast cancer patients. Bisphosphonates are used in patients with osteoporosis and in those on AI therapy who are at increased risk of bone loss. In breast cancer patients with metastatic disease to the bone, bisphosphonates have long been used to prevent fractures, spinal cord compression, pain, and hypercalcemia. More recently, bisphosphonates have found an additional indication: to reduce bony recurrence and improve survival in postmenopausal patients with nonmetastatic breast cancer. Based on a review of the literature, ASCO guidelines recommend using bisphosphonates, particularly intravenous zoledronic acid or oral clodronate in patients with natural menopause or that are in menopause induced by ovarian suppression or ablation. The absolute benefit is greatest in those receiving systemic therapy and in those at higher risk of recurrence. The guidelines state:

"It is recommended that, if available, zoledronic acid or clodronate be considered as adjuvant therapy for postmenopausal patients with breast cancer who are deemed candidates for adjuvant systemic therapy. Further research comparing different bone-modifying agents, doses, dosing intervals, and durations is required. Risk factors for osteonecrosis of the jaw and renal impairment should be assessed, and any pending dental or oral health problems should be dealt with prior to starting treatment" [33].

A full discussion of bisphosphonates in breast cancer patients is beyond the scope of this chapter. Additional information may be found at www.asco.org/breast-cancer-adjuvant-bisphosphonatesguideline, www.asco.org/guidelineswiki, and https://www.cancercareontario.ca/guidelines-advice/types-of-cancer/breast [34–36].

Metastatic Disease Treatment

A diagnosis of metastatic disease was once considered untreatable, but currently, women diagnosed with metastatic breast cancer live a median of 2 years, with some living much longer. Given the advancements in the treatment of metastatic disease, particularly ER-positive cancers, some consider metastatic breast cancer to be a chronic illness that can be managed to support a good quality of life for many years. Thus, PCPs have a critical role in the care of breast cancer patients, even in those with advanced disease (see Chap. 20 on "Care of the Breast Cancer Survivor").

The treatment of metastatic disease is generally determined based on three different tumor characteristics: (a) ER-positive status, (b) HER2-positive status (regardless of ER status), and (c) triple-negative status. Of note, approximately 15% of metastatic tumors have discordant estrogen status compared with the primary tumor due to cell line mutations. For this reason, biopsy is recommended for recurrent, metastatic disease to confirm tumor characteristics, to see if they differ from the original tumor and inform treatment decisions.

Metastatic ER-positive tumors are treated primarily with antiestrogen hormonal therapy agents: tamoxifen or aromatase inhibitors. In stage 4 cancer, the primary tumor may or may not be resected, and XRT is given to control local growth and treat selected metastatic lesions to bone or brain. Recently, two additional classes of agents have been shown promise in treating ER-positive metastatic disease: CDK4/6 inhibitors, which include medications such as abemaciclib, palbociclib, and ribociclib, and mTOR inhibitors, such as everolimus. These medications increase progression-free survival, but have not yet demonstrated improvements in overall survival. In general, the CDK4/6 inhibitors seem better tolerated than mTOR inhibitors.

HER2-positive metastatic tumors in patients who are treatment naive are generally treated with a combination therapy of HER2-directed therapy with trastuzumab, and chemotherapy with a taxane. For select patients, additional targeted therapy has shown substantial increases in overall survival.

Triple-negative metastatic breast cancers are particularly aggressive and are typically treated with chemotherapy in either a sequential manner or in combination.

Novel and Emerging Therapies

Reviewing all trials examining breast cancer treatment is beyond the scope of this chapter; the following websites provide updated information on treatment advances:

- National Institutes of Health: https://www.cancer.gov/types/breast/hp/breast-treatment-pdq [37]
- Susan G. Komen: https://ww5.komen.org/BreastCancer/EmergingAreasInTreatment.html [38]

Khadija would like to discuss potential side effects from the various treatment options that she has researched. She wants to know, if she is given options for management by the oncologist, how much the treatment side effects should weigh into her decision. She has also been asked if she would like to enroll in a clinical trial and wants advice with this decision.

Participation in Clinical Trials

During the course of evaluation and treatment, patients may be offered participation in clinical trials. Patients may seek counsel from their PCPs about the risks and benefits of trial participation. Clinical trials test the safety and outcomes of evolving treatments, diagnostics methods, and screening tests. The goal of these trials is to determine whether a new therapy or test should be a part of standard treatment. While participation in these trials is voluntary, participation can make the patient feel like they are helping to advance medical care and potentially improve their outcomes by gaining exposure to experimental treatments. On the other hand, participation may introduce adverse effects and increase the amount of testing beyond that which is needed for standard of care. There are four phases of clinical trials, and patients will be offered enrollment based on whether they fit the enrollment criteria. It is important for primary care physicians to be cognizant of what the patient hopes to gain from participation before counseling them about their involvement. PCPs can refer patients to the following website to enhance their understanding of clinical trials: https://www.cancer.org/treatment/treatments-and-side-effects/clinical-trials/what-you-need-to-know.html [39].

Complications of Treatment

Treatment options for breast cancer depend on the underlying histology and extent of disease. The oncologist will also consider the patient's comorbidities and general health in terms of tolerance of treatment. All treatment options can be associated with immediate and late effects. For breast surgery and local radiation therapy, most complications are mild. Immediate side effects from XRT are dose and field dependent and may include fatigue and mucositis in addition to local pain and erythema. Patients do cite some degree of interference with their normal functioning or quality of life after surgery and radiation [40]. The greater the extent of surgery or the higher amount of radiation received increases the local effects. Table 19.2 lists commonly (>10% of patients) encountered local complications after treatment with surgery and/or radiation. Less than 10% of patients report developing cellulitis or pneumonitis from radiation therapy [41].

The surgical oncologist will likely refer the patient to a plastic surgeon to discuss breast reconstruction if mastectomy is performed. If reconstruction is undertaken, the optimal type of procedure will depend on the patient's preference and anatomy. Since these decisions have emotional components, PCPs with a good doctor-patient relationship are well positioned to assist in decision-making. There is no evidence suggesting that immediate or delayed reconstruction alters the long-term outcome of breast cancer or that it impedes or delays the detection of local or regional recurrence [42, 43]. Radiation therapy can contribute to complications and impair cosmetic results after reconstruction. According to Victor et al., the risk of cosmetic failure may be related to the higher percentage of

Table 19.2 Common local complications after surgery and/or radiation [41]

Complication[a]	Treatment-related risk factor
Pain or numbness in breast, chest wall, or axilla (15–75%)	Greater extent of surgery
Arm swelling or lymphedema (10–25%)	Greater extent of axillary surgery
Restricted arm motion or weakness (8–70%)	Greater extent of surgery, radiation therapy, recent surgery
Reoperation after breast implant or reconstruction (20–34%)	Radiation therapy

Adapted from Burstein and Winer [41]

[a]Percentage of patients reporting symptoms via patient survey or chart review

patients with advanced disease, those who received bolus application (a rubberlike disc placed on the skin to increase the dose of radiation to the tissue beneath), and those who received earlier delivery of radiation therapy after the cosmetic procedure in reconstructed breasts [44–46].

Lymphedema is one of the most concerning and well-known side effects for patients treated with lymph node dissection, surgery, and/or radiation. Symptoms can arise immediately after specific treatment type and persist. Most cases of lymphedema are mild and the cumulative incidence of breast cancer-related lymphedema within five years of surgery, as assessed in the Olmsted County Rochester Epidemiology Project Breast Cancer Cohort, was 9.1% [47]. The risk of lymphedema is directly related to the extent of axillary surgery and radiation treatment [48]. Sentinel lymph node biopsy requires less extensive axillary surgery than axillary dissection and is associated with a lower risk of lymphedema [49]. Additional risk factors for development of lymphedema include obesity, weight gain, and infection in the ipsilateral arm. Often patients will ask if there is anything they can do to minimize the risk of developing lymphedema. It is reasonable to protect the ipsilateral arm from infection, compression, venipuncture, and exposure to intense heat and abrasion. Although these measures can be suggested, the clinical effect of any or all of these measures has not been well studied [50]. Many comprehensive cancer centers have lymphedema clinics, volunteer networks, and gifts shops with experts to assist patients with these troubling issues. The full discussion of lymphedema is beyond the scope of this chapter.

Systemic Therapy

Most chemotherapeutic regimens are associated with toxic adverse effects. The common immediate side effects from these agents are listed in Table 19.3.

The likelihood of developing adverse effects is based on the duration and total dose of therapy, but also varies by the individual. Primary care physicians can discuss management and possible side effects with patients once their regimen has been determined by the oncologist.

Table 19.3 Immediate adverse effects from common chemotherapeutic agents in breast cancer

Medication or medication class (with examples)	Common adverse effects
Anthracyclines (doxorubicin or epirubicin)	Pancytopenia, nausea, vomiting and mucositis, complete alopecia
Taxanes (paclitaxel, docetaxel)	Pancytopenia, alopecia, arthralgias, peripheral neuropathy, nausea, vomiting, diarrhea, mucositis
5-Fluoruracil	Nausea, diarrhea, mucositis, decreased appetite, photophobia, taste changes, pancytopenia
Cyclophosphamide	Pancytopenia, hair thinning, nausea, vomiting, decreased appetite
Platinum-based agents (carboplatin or cisplatin)	Pancytopenia, nausea, vomiting, taste changes, alopecia, weakness
Vinorelbine	Nausea, vomiting, muscle weakness, constipation, peripheral neuropathy, diarrhea, alopecia, thrombocytopenia
Capecitabine	Neutropenia, anemia, hand-foot syndrome, diarrhea, elevated liver enzymes, fatigue, nausea, vomiting, rash, abdominal pain
Gemcitabine	Flu-like symptoms, fever, fatigue, hair thinning, nausea, vomiting, poor appetite, rash, pancytopenia
Ixabepilone	Peripheral neuropathy, weakness, muscle and joint pains, alopecia, nausea, vomiting, neutropenia
Eribulin	Pancytopenia, fatigue, alopecia, nausea, peripheral neuropathy

Alopecia

Anthracyclines and taxanes usually cause complete hair loss on the scalp within 2–3 weeks of the first chemotherapy treatment with possible loss of eyebrows, eyelashes, and pubic hair. Hair on the extremities and in the axilla tends to be spared. Cyclophosphamides and gemcitabine cause some degree of hair thinning of head hair for most patients over the course of treatment. The hair thinning is gradual over the course of treatment. Some patients will experience hair loss significant enough to warrant a wig or head covering. If the likelihood of hair loss is high, patients should prepare by determining how they would like to handle the loss. Patients often order wigs and shave their heads in advance to ease the transition. Women will find hair coverings besides wigs that are more comfortable for everyday use. Hair tends to grow back after treatment, and many women report thicker or curlier hair texture with the new growth. Options for mitigating the hair loss associated with chemotherapy are being developed. Scalp hypothermia during chemotherapy administration, either by an automated continuous cooling device or by cold packs designed for the scalp, is one such option. There are theoretical but not proven concerns with this option, for example, if the chemotherapy does not reach the scalp, and insurance generally does not cover these systems, which can be expensive. Nonetheless, in patients who value the avoidance of alopecia, a scalp hypothermia device may be considered. Most comprehensive cancer centers have volunteer networks and gifts shops with experts to assist patients with these troubling issues. The full discussion of hair loss is beyond the scope of this chapter.

Nausea and Vomiting

Nausea and vomiting are feared adverse effects for patients and often occur with chemotherapy and pain medications

[51]. Three classes of antiemetics are currently recommended for management of chemotherapy-induced nausea and vomiting because of their efficacy specifically in this setting: serotonin receptor antagonists, neurokinin-1 receptor antagonists, and corticosteroids. Alternatives are combination products or olanzapine when used with other antiemetics. Directing patients to resources [52] to understand adverse effects and management can be helpful for their discussion with the oncology team.

Antiestrogen and Anti-HER2 Therapies

Common adverse effects in patients taking tamoxifen include hot flashes, vaginal discharge, swelling, and loss of libido. Less commonly (<30%), patients can experience nausea, menstrual irregularities, vaginal bleeding, weight loss, thrombosis, and mood changes. Tamoxifen also increases the risk of uterine cancer.

Aromatase inhibitors are commonly associated with hot flashes, muscle and joint pain, and stomach upset. Less commonly, patients taking AIs experience decreased energy, mood disturbances, sore throat, high blood pressure, depression, nausea, and vomiting. AIs may increase the risk of osteoporosis. See Chap. 17 on "The Primary Prevention of Breast Cancer" for more discussion on managing adverse effects from tamoxifen and AIs.

Patients taking trastuzumab may experience chills and/or fever during the initial infusion [53]. Other common adverse effects include body pain, weakness, and nausea. Less commonly, patients may experience headache, diarrhea, abdominal pain, back pain, flu-like symptoms, vomiting, cough, shortness of breath, insomnia, rash, dizziness, or swelling.

Khadijah has a significant other that she has been with for some time and although they have discussed having children they are not ready to have children immediately. Khadijah wants to know how she can optimize her chances of having children after breast cancer therapy.

Infertility Risk in Breast Cancer Patients

Concerns for future childbearing potential are increasingly common among younger women with breast cancer. Systemic therapy for breast cancer is directly harmful to ovarian follicles and increases the risk of amenorrhea. Systemic therapy such as chemotherapy is the most well-defined risk factor for infertility in premenopausal cancer patients, followed by advanced maternal age [54]. A study of premenopausal women with breast cancer reports that the odds ratio of chemotherapy-induced amenorrhea is 10.1 in 35- to 39-year-olds and 39.5 in 40- to 44-year-olds compared with women younger than 35 years [55]. In premenopausal women, menstruation returned in 28% within 6 months after completion of systemic therapy, within 6–12 months for 14%, and after 1 year in 3% of patients. Fifty-five percent of women had amenorrhea at the end of 33 months of follow-up [55]. Breast cancer patients become menopausal at a younger age compared to the general population. One study found the median age of menopause to be 44 years after adjuvant therapy with cyclophosphamide/methotrexate/5-FU compared with the national average of 52 years [54].

Pre-chemotherapy anti-Mullerian hormone (AMH) and follicle-stimulating hormone (FSH) levels can predict the return of ovarian function and are used in prognostic scoring, along with age and body size, to estimate ovarian recovery. The assessment of ovarian reserve can help determine the probability of future pregnancies after the end of treatment. AMH and age can reliably estimate ovarian reserve and aid patients in fertility options prior to and after treatment. These discussions should be initiated by the oncologist [56, 57].

Gonadotoxic Chemotherapy Agents

In terms of specific chemotherapy agents, cyclophosphamide is gonadotoxic. Chemotherapy regimens with reduced lower cumulative dosing of cyclophosphamide have lower rates of amenorrhea. Studies of docetaxel, doxorubicin, and cyclophosphamide have found a greater than 80% risk of permanent amenorrhea in women 40 years and older and a less than 20% risk of permanent amenorrhea in women 30 years and younger [58, 59]. Data are limited with regard to taxanes, with mixed evidence as to whether adding a taxane to a regimen confers additional gonadotoxicity [60]. Selective estrogen receptor modulators, such as tamoxifen, have indirect effects on fertility and increase the risk of amenorrhea [58]. Pregnancy is contraindicated during treatment with endocrine therapy because of the risk of teratogenicity [61]. Trastuzumab has not been shown to definitely increase the likelihood of infertility [55].

Counseling Patients on Fertility Concerns

The responsibility for addressing fertility concerns falls on all providers caring for breast cancer patients. Often, it is the primary care physician who has a long-standing, therapeutic relationship with the patient and can address the issues early in the course of treatment. Counseling on fertility preservation includes discussion on risks and preservation strategies. Multiple guidelines state that preservation options should be discussed with all women of reproductive age, even if the threat of infertility is low, and the possibility of infertility should be discussed as part of patient education and informed consent, before initiating cancer therapy in patients of reproductive age [62]. Patients should be referred to reproductive specialists if they are interested or unsure about preservation, and referrals to psychosocial care providers should be offered if the possibility of infertility could cause distress [62].

Primary care physicians may assist the patient by introducing this important topic as some oncologists, although aware of these issues, lack knowledge of fertility preservation resources and are concerned about delaying treatment if a patient chooses to undergo preservation [63]. A survey of physicians in the United States found that fewer than half of all oncologists routinely refer cancer patients of childbearing age to fertility specialists [64]. Primary care physicians, through early intervention with counseling and referrals, can greatly improve patient anxiety and effect fertility outcomes. A patient who has an increased understanding of the management options for female infertility will be better able to participate in shared decision-making with their oncologist and fertility specialist.

Options for future motherhood include: preserving fertilized eggs, freezing ovarian tissue, egg or embryo donation, surrogacy, and adoption. Fertility preservation techniques include [65]:

- *Embryo cryopreservation*: Embryo cryopreservation occurs following in vitro fertilization. Hyperstimulation of the ovary may require a slight delay in initiating cancer treatment.
- *Oocyte cryopreservation*: Hormone-induced hyperstimulation can also be used in the absence of a sperm donor for oocyte cryopreservation. Improved technological processes have increased the egg survival rates after thaw to close to 90%.
- *Ovarian tissue cryopreservation*: An investigational technique, either an entire ovary or a portion of an ovary, is removed and cryopreserved.
- *Ovarian transposition*: The ovaries and fallopian tubes are surgically moved within the body out of the field of radiation exposure.
- *GnRH agonist treatment*: In investigational method, hormone agonists may prevent the iatrogenic loss of ovarian reserve but the precise mechanism of these drugs is unknown.

Education and resources are invaluable for the patient. Primary care physicians can refer patients to sites such as: http://www.breastcancer.org/treatment/side_effects/fertility_issues for further understanding of management options [66].

Khadijah appears distraught, but will not admit to anxiety or depression. Her primary care doctor, however, has developed a therapeutic relationship with her and recognizes the need to address her emotional needs.

The Psychological Impact of Breast Cancer Diagnosis and Treatment

The diagnosis and treatments of any cancer are life-changing events, having a significant psychological impact on patients, their extended families, and friends. Primary care providers have a therapeutic relationship with their patients and, therefore, the ability to detect emotional distress as it arises. During the first year after diagnosis and therapy, breast cancer patients may demonstrate intense psychosocial distress and problems with adjustment, which tends to improve over time [67]. In 2008, the Institute of Medicine report, "Cancer Care for the Whole Patient: Meeting Psychosocial Health Needs," described that the psychological needs of patients with cancer were not being addressed, posing a serious problem for the health care system [68].

The American Society of Clinical Oncology (ASCO) has adapted guidelines for the screening, assessment, and care of anxiety and depressive symptoms in adults with cancer. These guidelines recommend evaluating for depression and anxiety at periodic times, across the trajectory of care, via a validated, published measure and procedure [69]. Primary care physicians, who are familiar with patients at the time of their diagnosis, should perform screening for anxiety and depression. Validated screening measures, such as the PHQ-9 and GAD-7, for anxiety and depression, respectively, are not 100% sensitive and physicians should inquire about the patient's coping, anxiety, and depression throughout their treatment.

The diagnosis of cancer is a distressing, sometimes traumatic experience. Nearly half of newly diagnosed breast cancer patients experienced distress, depression, and anxiety, or post-traumatic stress disorder (PTSD) is common in this population [70, 71]. For a full discussion, please see Chap. 20 on "Care of the Breast Cancer Survivor" and Chap. 33 on "Depressive and Anxiety Disorders".

Khadijah would like to know when she should be seen next in the office and what specifics she should discuss with her oncologist at their visit.

The relationship between patient and primary care provider should not end or be put on hold at the time of diagnosis with breast cancer. Consistent attention to health maintenance needs and management of chronic disease processes should continue. The management of high blood pressure, diabetes, and hyperlipidemia throughout the treatment process can affect long-term morbidity and mortality unrelated to the cancer diagnosis. Patients often express concerns over the number of physician or health care-related appointments which are required during the time of active treatment. If management of their chronic diseases can be managed in conjunction with the oncology office, then lab work and adjustments to medications can be done at the time of their oncology visits. Open lines of communication, and the use of medical records, facilitate the flow of information between the patient, primary care physician, and oncologist.

The primary care clinician may further assist the breast cancer patient by helping her anticipate and frame questions that she would like answered when meeting with the oncologist. The oncology visit should readdress many of these concerns or questions. The authors suggest the following list of suggested questions that can be given to the patient to address with the oncologist:

- What is the stage of my cancer and the prognosis associated with this stage and histology?
- What are my treatment options and common immediate and late effects from this treatment?
- Can we address the diagnosis and treatment risk on my fertility?
- What else can I do to optimize my tolerance of the treatment and minimize side effects?

Khadijah has one final question before leaving the office. She knows that cancer has yet to be "cured" and wants to know her prognosis.

Breast Cancer Prognosis

Breast cancer prognosis is complicated and is best discussed with the oncologist. The stage of cancer and pathologic characteristics are needed to provide accurate prognostic information to patients. Principles of the cancer staging system, which requires information obtained by imaging and lymph node assessment, could be explained to the patient to help guide her understanding of prognosis. The PCP can reinforce and educate the patient in general terms and defer more detailed discussions to the oncologist. To help with a framework for discussion, the expected 5-year relative survival by stage at diagnosis is shown in Table 19.1.

The oncologist will provide the patient with the most current prognostic statistics based on the stage, pathology, and treatment regimen, but this information may need to be processed with the patient several times and with different providers. With the information in this chapter, PCPs can communicate in general terms about prognosis and treatment options, with the knowledge that the specific information regarding prognosis and treatment depends upon a number of specific clinical and tumor characteristics that are best addressed by an oncologist. Furthermore, given their longitudinal relationship with patients, PCPs are well positioned to promote their patient's adherence to recommended follow-up and adjuvant therapies and to help insure that patients are not lost to follow-up.

Conclusion

The care of breast cancer patients typically relies most heavily on surgical, medical, and radiation oncologists, but primary care providers are often well positioned to engage in discussions regarding diagnostic and treatment modalities, prepare patients for their initial oncology visits, and support patient adherence to recommended testing and treatment. In addition, understanding long-term implications of breast cancer and its treatment, especially as it relates to fertility, psychosocial adjustments, and prognosis, will position PCPs to provide longitudinal care for patients throughout the breast cancer care spectrum.

Summary Points

1. Breast cancer is staged based on results from imaging and biopsy. The four most commons types of histopathology are LCIS, DCIS, invasive lobular carcinoma, and invasive ductal carcinoma.
2. Treatment modalities for patients are chosen based on the classification of breast cancer and the extent of this disease process. Treatment modalities include surgical resection, chemotherapy, and radiation.
3. Primary care physicians should be familiar with adverse effects of the common treatment modalities so as to counsel patients on what to anticipate during the course of treatment and potentially aid patients in their decision-making process.
4. Primary care providers should prepare patients for the initial and subsequent meetings with the oncology team by reviewing common treatments, adverse effects of treatment, prognosis, and questions related to these categories.
5. Clinical factors that influence the prognosis of patients with breast cancer include: age of patient, existence of comorbid conditions, and presence of genetic markers.

Review Questions

1. A premenopausal 39-year-old woman with a normal clinical breast and axillary exam had an abnormal screening mammogram. Subsequent workup of the 3 cm area with calcifications in her left breast showed infiltrating ductal

carcinoma that was estrogen receptor negative, progesterone receptor negative, and HER-2 receptor negative. She calls to review her biopsy results and prepare for her upcoming appointment with a medical oncologist. What stage of breast cancer does she have?

A. She hasn't had surgery; therefore, she cannot be staged without pathology from her sentinel lymph node biopsy.
B. T1, cN0, pM0.
C. Clinical stage IIA.
D. Staging based on TNM classifications is no longer done, as it is not predictive of overall survival.

The correct answer is C. There are two types of stages: clinical stage which is assigned prior to surgery, or when surgery is not an option, and anatomic/pathologic stage which uses pathologic and surgical specimens. This patient has not yet had surgery, and her staging is considered clinical. Stage is assigned using the American Joint Commission on Cancer (JCC) TNM System that incorporates information on tumor size (T), involvement of lymph nodes (N), and presence of metastases (M). Her tumor is between 2 and 5 centimeters and is considered T2, and her nodal status is clinically negative given her normal axillary exam; however this may change after surgery is completed. While clinical stage may not provide as accurate overall survival predictions as surgical staging, it is still used to guide patient expectations of treatment prior to surgery [9].

2. Which statement regarding a 39-year-old premenopausal, stage II, triple-negative cancer patient is true?

A. Because of her age and triple negative status, she should undergo genetic counseling and possible testing for *BRCA* gene mutations.
B. She will require ovarian suppression treatment; therefore, she should discuss fertility preservation options.
C. She will probably require treatment with tamoxifen, which can lead to increased risk of endometrial cancer.
D. She should have a bilateral mastectomy regardless of *BRCA* status.

The correct answer is A. Her tumor is estrogen and progesterone receptor negative, and therefore hormonal therapies such as tamoxifen or ovarian suppression are unlikely to provide survival benefit. Given her triple-negative status and her age (<40) at diagnosis, she is at higher risk of having a *BRCA* gene mutation. Offering genetic counseling and testing is an important first step to identifying a mutation and is ideally completed before selecting a treatment course. Women with triple-negative breast cancers are typically treated with surgery and chemotherapy +/− XRT, but those who are found to have *BRCA* gene mutations may also elect prophylactic bilateral mastectomy and bilateral salpingo-oophorectomy [72, 73].

3. A 40-year-old premenopausal breast cancer patient is tested for the *BRCA* gene mutation and is found to be negative. She is interested in a future pregnancy and would like to undergo fertility preservation. After completion of fertility preservation with cryopreservation of oocytes, she undergoes neoadjuvant chemotherapy followed by a mastectomy. Lymph node sampling revealed two positive lymph nodes. She subsequently undergoes additional chemotherapy and XRT. Which statement is true regarding the likely adverse effects of her treatment regimen?
   A. She is not a candidate for immediate reconstruction with her mastectomy because of her need for XRT.
   B. As a result of axillary node dissection and radiation therapy, she is at risk of developing lymphedema.
   C. Radiation treatment is well tolerated and will not contribute to worsening fatigue.
   D. Given her young age at diagnosis, she is unlikely to develop amenorrhea during chemotherapy and does not need to be concerned about fertility preservation.

   The correct answer is B. The risk of lymphedema is directly related to the extent of axillary surgery and radiation treatment, and thus she is at risk for lymphedema. She would be eligible for immediate reconstruction, because there is no evidence that immediate or delayed reconstruction alters the long-term outcome of breast cancer or that it impedes or delays the detection of local or regional recurrence. Radiation is generally well tolerated, but fatigue is a common side effect. Lastly, all premenopausal women should consider the desire for fertility preservation into their treatment plans. A study of premenopausal women with breast cancer reports that the odds ratio of chemotherapy-induced amenorrhea is 10.1 in 35- to 39-year-olds and 39.5 in 40- to 44-year-olds compared with women younger than 35 years of age. This patient, at age 40, has a significant risk of amenorrhea after chemotherapy [42, 43, 48, 55].

4. Which of the following statements regarding a premenopausal triple-negative, *BRCA*-negative patient's breast cancer prognosis is most accurate?
   A. Her prognosis would depend upon the recurrence score as calculated by the Oncotype Dx.
   B. Her prognosis is better than if her HER-2 receptor status of her tumor was positive.
   C. Despite having no identified *BRCA* gene mutations, her risk of developing a contralateral breast cancer is still triple that of the average population.

D. Triple-negative breast cancer has about a 15% higher 5-year mortality than women with other forms of breast cancer.

The correct answer is D. The recurrence score (Oncotype Dx) can only be completed among women with estrogen receptor-positive tumors; therefore, the test would not be completed, nor impact treatment choice, in this patient. Having triple-negative breast cancer indicates a more aggressive cancer and has a higher mortality rate, about 15% higher at 5 years, than breast cancers with any of the other characteristics. Though having breast cancer increases risk of developing a contralateral breast cancer by about 50% over the average population, the overall risk of contralateral cancer remains low. In contrast, having a *BRCA* gene mutation may increase the risk of contralateral cancer from approximately 4% in under 10 years, up to 65% with certain mutations [13, 74].

5. A 63-year-old woman presents with a chronic cough, and chest x-ray demonstrates a pleural effusion with a suspicious, spiculated mass. Transthoracic biopsy demonstrates breast cancer that is ER+/PR+/HER2 negative. Which treatments, if any, may be options for this patient?
   A. Early referral to palliative care remains a cornerstone of therapy, as her overall prognosis is less than 6 months.
   B. A combination of trastuzumab and taxane therapy can increase her overall survival by as much as 12 months.
   C. Novel therapies such as palbociclib can be used to increase overall survival, even as a single agent.
   D. The use of aromatase inhibitors remains the mainstay of therapy for metastatic breast cancer that is estrogen receptor positive, but additional treatments are usually recommended.

The correct answer is D. The patient has stage 4 ER+/PR+/ HER2- breast cancer. While palliative care should be considered in symptomatic patients, median survival in those with metastatic breast cancer is 2 years, with some women surviving much longer. Combination therapy, directed at HER2, is not applicable to this patient, though it may increase survival in HER2+ patients. Palbociclib, a CDK 4/6 therapeutic agent, has shown promise in increasing the progression-free survival in women with estrogen-positive metastatic breast cancer, but data on increasing overall survival is not yet available, and it would not be used as sole therapy. For women with estrogen receptor-positive metastatic disease, hormonal therapy remains the primary treatment. This patient is over 60 years of age, can be considered postmenopausal, and would likely start on an aromatase inhibitor therapy combined with CDK 4/6 or mTOR novel therapies, given her initial presentation with metastatic disease. She may consider the risks and benefits of participating in a clinical trial if offered by her oncologist [75–77].

References

1. Jiang L, Lofters A, Moineddin R, et al. Primary care physician use across the breast cancer care continuum: CanIMPACT study using Canadian administrative data. Can Fam Physician. 2016;62(10):e589–98.
2. Wallner LP, Abrahamse P, Uppal JK, et al. Involvement of primary care physicians in the decision making and care of patients with breast cancer. J Clin Oncol. 2016;34(33):3969–75.
3. Society AC. The Low Risk DCIS (LORIS) trial comparing surgery with active monitoring for low risk DCIS in the United Kingdom. Info on LORIS website. Clinical trials: what you need to know; 2018. www.birmingham.ac.uk/research/activity/mds/trials/crctu/trials/loris/index.aspx
4. Institute NC. Tumor grade. 2013. https://www.cancer.gov/about-cancer/diagnosis-staging/prognosis/tumor-grade-fact-sheet.
5. Society TAC. Breast cancer hormone receptor status. 2017.
6. Paik S, Tang G, Shak S, et al. Gene expression and benefit of chemotherapy in women with node-negative, estrogen receptor-positive breast cancer. J Clin Oncol. 2006;24(23):3726–34.
7. Sparano JA, Gray RJ, Makower DF, et al. Adjuvant chemotherapy guided by a 21-gene expression assay in breast cancer. N Engl J Med. 2018;379(2):111–21.
8. Profile Tests. https://www.asco.org/sites/new-www.asco.org/files/content-files/practice-and-guidelines/documents/2017-adjuvant-biomarkers-summary-table.pdf
9. American Joint Committee on Cancer (AJCC). Cancer staging system. 2018. https://cancerstaging.org/references-tools/Pages/What-is-Cancer-Staging.aspx
10. Breast Cancer Survival Rates. 2013, December. Retrieved from https://www.cancer.org/cancer/breast-cancer/understanding-a-breast-cancer-diagnosis/breast-cancer-survival-rates.html
11. Lostumbo L, Carbine NE, Wallace J. Prophylactic mastectomy for the prevention of breast cancer. Cochrane Database Syst Rev. 2010;11:Cd002748.
12. Kauff ND, Satagopan JM, Robson ME, et al. Risk-reducing Salpingo-oophorectomy in women with a BRCA1 or BRCA2 mutation. N Engl J Med. 2002;346(21):1609–15.
13. Kuchenbaecker KB, Hopper JL, Barnes DR, et al. Risks of breast, ovarian, and contralateral breast cancer for BRCA1 and BRCA2 mutation carriers. JAMA. 2017;317(23):2402–16.
14. Beitsch PD, Whitworth PW, Hughes K, Patel R, Rosen B, Compagnoni G, et al. Underdiagnosis of hereditary breast cancer: are genetic testing guidelines a tool or an obstacle? J Clin Oncol. 2019;37(6):453–60. https://doi.org/10.1200/JCO.18.01631. Epub 2018 Dec 7.
15. Hampel H, Bennett RL, Buchanan A, Pearlman R, Wiesner GL. A practice guideline from the American College of Medical Genetics and Genomics and the National Society of Genetic Counselors: referral indications for cancer predisposition assessment. Genet Med. 2015;17:70–87.
16. Roberts ME, Jackson SA, Susswein LR, et al. MSH6 and PMS2 germ-line pathogenic variants implicated in Lynch syndrome are associated with breast cancer. Genet Med. 2018;20(10):1167–74.
17. Win AK, Lindor NM, Jenkins MA. Risk of breast cancer in Lynch syndrome: a systematic review. Breast Cancer Res. 2013;15(2):R27.
18. Bach PB, Schrag D, Brawley OW, Galaznik A, Yakren S, Begg CB. Survival of blacks and whites after a cancer diagnosis. JAMA. 2002;287(16):2106–13.

19. McCarthy EP, Ngo LH, Roetzheim RG, et al. Disparities in breast cancer treatment and survival for women with disabilities. Ann Intern Med. 2006;145(9):637–45.
20. Yu XQ. Socioeconomic disparities in breast cancer survival: relation to stage at diagnosis, treatment and race. BMC Cancer. 2009;9:364.
21. Li A, Burton G, Glass J. Breast cancer: a socioeconomic and racial comparison in northwest Louisiana. J La State Med Soc. 2001;153(8):420–5.
22. Smith TJ, Temin S, Alesi ER, et al. American Society of Clinical Oncology provisional clinical opinion: the integration of palliative care into standard oncology care. J Clin Oncol. 2012;30(8):880–7.
23. Rugno FC, Paiva BS, Paiva CE. Early integration of palliative care facilitates the discontinuation of anticancer treatment in women with advanced breast or gynecologic cancers. Gynecol Oncol. 2014;135(2):249–54.
24. Osta BE, Palmer JL, Paraskevopoulos T, et al. Interval between first palliative care consult and death in patients diagnosed with advanced cancer at a comprehensive cancer center. J Palliat Med. 2008;11(1):51–7.
25. Blichert-Toft M, Nielsen M, During M, et al. Long-term results of breast conserving surgery vs. mastectomy for early stage invasive breast cancer: 20-year follow-up of the Danish randomized DBCG-82TM protocol. Acta oncologica (Stockholm, Sweden). 2008;47(4):672–81.
26. Litiere S, Werutsky G, Fentiman IS, et al. Breast conserving therapy versus mastectomy for stage I-II breast cancer: 20 year follow-up of the EORTC 10801 phase 3 randomised trial. Lancet Oncol. 2012;13(4):412–9.
27. Veronesi U, Cascinelli N, Mariani L, et al. Twenty-year follow-up of a randomized study comparing breast-conserving surgery with radical mastectomy for early breast cancer. N Engl J Med. 2002;347(16):1227–32.
28. Waljee JF, Rogers MA, Alderman AK. Decision aids and breast cancer: do they influence choice for surgery and knowledge of treatment options? J Clin Oncol. 2007;25(9):1067–73.
29. Davies C, Pan H, Godwin J, et al. Long-term effects of continuing adjuvant tamoxifen to 10 years versus stopping at 5 years after diagnosis of oestrogen receptor-positive breast cancer: ATLAS, a randomised trial. Lancet. (London, England). 2013;381(9869):805–16.
30. Francis PA, Regan MM, Fleming GF, et al. Adjuvant ovarian suppression in premenopausal breast cancer. N Engl J Med. 2015;372(5):436–46.
31. Untch M, Rezai M, Loibl S, et al. Neoadjuvant treatment with trastuzumab in HER2-positive breast cancer: results from the GeparQuattro study. J Clin Oncol. 2010;28(12):2024–31.
32. Gianni L, Eiermann W, Semiglazov V, et al. Neoadjuvant chemotherapy with trastuzumab followed by adjuvant trastuzumab versus neoadjuvant chemotherapy alone, in patients with HER2-positive locally advanced breast cancer (the NOAH trial): a randomised controlled superiority trial with a parallel HER2-negative cohort. Lancet (London, England). 2010;375(9712):377–84. New from DK.
33. Dhesy-Thind S, Fletcher GG, Blanchette PS, Clemons MJ, Dillmon MS, Frank ES, et al. Use of adjuvant bisphosphonates and other bone-modifying agents in breast cancer: a Cancer Care Ontario and American Society of Clinical Oncology Clinical Practice Guideline. J Clin Oncol. 2017;35(18):2062–81. https://doi.org/10.1200/JCO.2016.70.7257.
34. Bisphosphonates in Breast Cancer Patients. www.asco.org/breast-cancer-adjuvant-bisphosphonatesguideline
35. Bisphosphonates in Breast Cancer Patients. www.asco.org/guidelineswiki
36. Bisphosphonates in Breast Cancer Patients. https://www.cancercareontario.ca/guidelines-advice/types-of-cancer/breast
37. National Institutes of Health. Breast cancer treatment – health professional version. 2018. https://www.cancer.gov/types/breast/hp/breast-treatment-pdq.
38. Susan G. Komen Foundation. Emerging areas in treatment. 2018. https://ww5.komen.org/BreastCancer/EmergingAreasInTreatment.html
39. Society AC. Clinical trials: what you need to know. 2018. https://www.cancer.org/treatment/treatments-and-side-effects/clinical-trials/what-you-need-to-know.html
40. Warmuth MA, Bowen G, Prosnitz LR, et al. Complications of axillary lymph node dissection for carcinoma of the breast: a report based on a patient survey. Cancer. 1998;83(7):1362–8.
41. Burstein HJ, Winer EP. Primary care for survivors of breast cancer. N Engl J Med. 2000;343(15):1086–94.
42. Johnson CH, van Heerden JA, Donohue JH, Martin JK Jr, Jackson IT, Ilstrup DM. Oncological aspects of immediate breast reconstruction following mastectomy for malignancy. Arch Surg (Chicago, IL: 1960). 1989;124(7):819–23; discussion 823-814.
43. Slavin SA, Love SM, Goldwyn RM. Recurrent breast cancer following immediate reconstruction with myocutaneous flaps. Plastic Reconstr Surg. 1994;93(6):1191–204; discussion 1205-1197.
44. Evans GR, Schusterman MA, Kroll SS, et al. Reconstruction and the radiated breast: is there a role for implants? Plastic Reconstr Surg. 1995;96(5):1111–5; discussion 1116–1118.
45. Schuster RH, Kuske RR, Young VL, Fineberg B. Breast reconstruction in women treated with radiation therapy for breast cancer: cosmesis, complications, and tumor control. Plastic Reconstruct Surg. 1992;90(3):445–52; discussion 453–444.
46. Victor SJ, Brown DM, Horwitz EM, et al. Treatment outcome with radiation therapy after breast augmentation or reconstruction in patients with primary breast carcinoma. Cancer. 1998;82(7):1303–9.
47. Nguyen TT, Hoskin TL, Habermann EB, Cheville AL, Boughey JC. Breast cancer-related lymphedema risk is related to multidisciplinary treatment and not surgery alone: results from a large cohort study. Ann Surg Oncol. 2017;24(10):2972–80.
48. Pezner RD, Patterson MP, Hill LR, et al. Arm lymphedema in patients treated conservatively for breast cancer: relationship to patient age and axillary node dissection technique. Int J Radiation Oncol Biol Physics. 1986;12(12):2079–83.
49. Bertelli G, Venturini M, Forno G, Macchiavello F, Dini D. Conservative treatment of postmastectomy lymphedema: a controlled, randomized trial. Ann Oncol. 1991;2(8):575–8.
50. Rockson SG. Precipitating factors in lymphedema: myths and realities. Cancer. 1998;83(12 Suppl American):2814–6.
51. Booth CM, Clemons M, Dranitsaris G, et al. Chemotherapy-induced nausea and vomiting in breast cancer patients: a prospective observational study. J Support Oncol. 2007;5(8):374–80.
52. National Cancer Institute NIH. Side effects of cancer treatment. 2018.
53. Burstein HJ. The distinctive nature of HER2-positive breast cancers. N Engl J Med. 2005;353(16):1652–4.
54. Lee MC, Gray J, Han HS, Plosker S. Fertility and reproductive considerations in premenopausal patients with breast cancer. Cancer Control. 2010;17(3):162–72.
55. Abusief ME, Missmer SA, Ginsburg ES, Weeks JC, Partridge AH. The effects of paclitaxel, dose density, and trastuzumab on treatment-related amenorrhea in premenopausal women with breast cancer. Cancer. 2010;116(4):791–8.
56. Barnabei A, Strigari L, Marchetti P, et al. Predicting ovarian activity in women affected by early breast cancer: a meta-analysis-based nomogram. Oncologist. 2015;20(10):1111–8.
57. Su HC, Haunschild C, Chung K, et al. Prechemotherapy anti-mullerian hormone, age, and body size predict timing of return of ovarian function in young breast cancer patients. Cancer. 2014;120(23):3691–8.

58. Oktay K, Sonmezer M. Chemotherapy and amenorrhea: risks and treatment options. Curr Opin Obstetr Gynecol. 2008;20(4):408–15.
59. Zavos A, Valachis A. Risk of chemotherapy-induced amenorrhea in patients with breast cancer: a systematic review and meta-analysis. Acta oncologica. (Stockholm, Sweden). 2016;55(6):664–70.
60. Petrek JA, Naughton MJ, Case LD, et al. Incidence, time course, and determinants of menstrual bleeding after breast cancer treatment: a prospective study. J Clin Oncol. 2006;24(7):1045–51.
61. Ruddy KJ, Gelber SI, Tamimi RM, et al. Prospective study of fertility concerns and preservation strategies in young women with breast cancer. J Clin Oncol. 2014;32(11):1151–6.
62. Loren AW, Mangu PB, Beck LN, et al. Fertility preservation for patients with cancer: American Society of Clinical Oncology clinical practice guideline update. J Clin Oncol. 2013;31(19):2500–10.
63. Quinn GP, Vadaparampil ST, Gwede CK, et al. Discussion of fertility preservation with newly diagnosed patients: oncologists' views. J Cancer Survivorship. 2007;1(2):146–55.
64. Quinn GP, Vadaparampil ST, Lee JH, et al. Physician referral for fertility preservation in oncology patients: a national study of practice behaviors. J Clin Oncol. 2009;27(35):5952–7.
65. Waimey KE, Smith BM, Confino R, Jeruss JS, Pavone ME. Understanding fertility in young female cancer patients. J Women's Health (2002). 2015;24(10):812–8.
66. BreastCancer.org. Fertility issues. 2018. https://www.breastcancer.org/treatment/side_effects/fertility_issues
67. Ganz PA, Coscarelli A, Fred C, Kahn B, Polinsky ML, Petersen L. Breast cancer survivors: psychosocial concerns and quality of life. Breast Cancer Res Treatment. 1996;38(2):183–99.
68. Adler NE, Page AEK. Cancer care for the whole patient: meeting psychosocial health needs. The National Academies Collection: reports funded by National Institutes of Health. Washington, DC: National Academies Press (US) National Academy of Sciences; 2008.
69. Andersen BL, DeRubeis RJ, Berman BS, et al. Screening, assessment, and care of anxiety and depressive symptoms in adults with cancer: an American Society of Clinical Oncology guideline adaptation. J Clin Oncol. 2014;32(15):1605–19.
70. Hegel MT, Moore CP, Collins ED, et al. Distress, psychiatric syndromes, and impairment of function in women with newly diagnosed breast cancer. Cancer. 2006;107(12):2924–31.
71. Wu X, Wang J, Cofie R, Kaminga AC, Liu A. Prevalence of posttraumatic stress disorder among breast cancer patients: a meta-analysis. Iranian J Public Health. 2016;45(12):1533–44.
72. Gonzalez-Angulo AM, Timms KM, Liu S, et al. Incidence and outcome of BRCA mutations in unselected patients with triple receptor-negative breast cancer. Clin Cancer Res. 2011;17(5):1082–9.
73. Davies C, Godwin J, Gray R, et al. Relevance of breast cancer hormone receptors and other factors to the efficacy of adjuvant tamoxifen: patient-level meta-analysis of randomised trials. Lancet (London, England). 2011;378(9793):771–84.
74. Nichols HB, Berrington de Gonzalez A, Lacey JV Jr, Rosenberg PS, Anderson WF. Declining incidence of contralateral breast cancer in the United States from 1975 to 2006. J Clin Oncol. 2011;29(12):1564–9.
75. Sledge GW Jr, Hu P, Falkson G, Tormey D, Abeloff M. Comparison of chemotherapy with chemohormonal therapy as first-line therapy for metastatic, hormone-sensitive breast cancer: an Eastern Cooperative Oncology Group study. J Clin Oncol. 2000;18(2):262–6.
76. Mauri D, Pavlidis N, Polyzos NP, Ioannidis JP. Survival with aromatase inhibitors and inactivators versus standard hormonal therapy in advanced breast cancer: meta-analysis. J Nat Cancer Inst. 2006;98(18):1285–91.
77. Turner NC, Ro J, André F, et al. Palbociclib in hormone-receptor–positive advanced breast cancer. N Engl J Med. 2015;373(3):209–19.

Care of the Breast Cancer Survivor

20

Sarah Merriam and Deborah DiNardo

Learning Objectives

1. Apply current practice guidelines for the care of breast cancer survivors in the primary care setting.
2. List the goals and components of a survivorship care plan.
3. Employ appropriate screening strategies for surveillance for breast cancer recurrence.
4. Assess and manage the physical and psychological sequelae of breast cancer treatment including vasomotor symptoms, sexual dysfunction, depression, anxiety, PTSD, and bone health.
5. Evaluate and treat common sexual problems in breast cancer survivors, incorporating appropriate physical exam skills and evidence-based communication techniques.
6. Counsel breast cancer survivors regarding strategies for overall health promotion, including weight, physical activity, nutrition, alcohol intake, and smoking cessation which in turn may reduce future breast cancer risk.

Rachel is a 48-year-old perimenopausal woman with a past medical history of mild depression in remission. She was diagnosed with breast cancer last week, after feeling a left breast lump and being referred for a diagnostic mammogram and biopsy.

Excluding skin cancers, breast cancer is the most commonly diagnosed malignancy among US women, representing 15% of all new cancer cases in the USA. It accounts for nearly one in three cancers in women and is the second leading cause of cancer death among women. The lifetime risk for diagnosis of female breast cancer is 12%, or one in eight women, and approximately 266,120 new cases of breast cancer were expected among US women in 2018 [1]. Because of early detection and advances in treatment, long-term survival is common, with 89.7% of all women diagnosed with breast cancer surviving 5 years. Survival over the same time frame for women with localized breast cancer (stage 1) is even higher at 98.9%. Accordingly, the number of women living with breast cancer in the USA is large and ever-growing, estimated at around 3.4 million in 2015 [1].

A cancer survivor is defined as "any person with a history of cancer, from the time of diagnosis through the remainder of their life" [2]. Importantly, survivorship is a distinct phase of cancer care which involves the surveillance for and the assessment and management of mental, physical, spiritual, and social aspects of cancer diagnosis and treatment [3]. Unfortunately, major gaps in the care provided to survivors have been described.

In 2006, the Institute of Medicine (IOM) report entitled "From Cancer Patient to Cancer Survivor: Lost in Transition" underscored the quality gaps which exist in cancer survivorship care, including inadequate support for physical and emotional difficulties associated with cancer and its treatment, and poor communication and coordination between oncologists and primary care providers [3]. Breast cancer survivors also describe a feeling of uncertainty as they transition from the intensive and active phase of breast cancer treatment to primary care follow-up [4]. Primary care providers themselves report feeling ill-equipped to provide optimal care for breast cancer survivors, in part due to insuf-

S. Merriam · D. DiNardo (✉)
VA Pittsburgh Healthcare System, Department of Medicine, Pittsburgh, PA, USA

University of Pittsburgh School of Medicine, Pittsburgh, PA, USA
e-mail: sarah.merriam@va.gov; deborah.dinardo@va.gov

S. A. Tilstra et al. (eds.), *Sex- and Gender-Based Women's Health*, https://doi.org/10.1007/978-3-030-50695-7_20

ficient knowledge of the consequences of cancer treatment [5]. Recognizing the importance of survivorship care, multiple organizaions, including the IOM, American Society of Clinical Oncology (ASCO), American Cancer Society (ACS), and the Commission on Cancer, have highlighted the importance of addressing the needs of breast cancer survivors following active treatment. Survivorship care plans (SCPs) have been recommended as one way to improve survivorship care [3, 6–8].

The goal of a SCP is to decrease fragmentation of survivorship care and to assign responsibility for managing different aspects of survivorship care to various providers in the healthcare team. The role of the SCP has become increasingly important due to increasing numbers of breast cancer survivors and longer durations of treatment with endocrine-based therapies. The logistical challenges that result from caring for this population are quickly outpacing the ability of oncologists to provide all follow-up care needed. Thus, the role of the primary care provider in providing posttreatment follow-up, timely and appropriate surveillance, and management of late and long-term effects of therapy is critical. A 2015 joint guideline from ASCO and ACS recommends that SCPs should discuss the following elements [9]:

- Surveillance for breast cancer recurrence.
- Screening for second primary cancers.
- Assessment and management of both physical and psychosocial long-term and late effects of breast cancer and treatment.
- Health promotion.
- Care coordination and practice implications.

Despite patient and provider receptivity toward SCPs, implementation has been limited, with fewer than half of cancer programs using SCPs and less than one-third of primary care providers routinely receiving SCPs as patients complete active treatment [10]. Barriers to SCP implementation are well documented. A major challenge is the shortage of staffing and resources [11]. Although calls to implement SCPs have been made by multiple medical societies, there is no agreed-upon standardized model. Ideally, a SCP would be provided by the patient's oncology team to the patient, which can then be shared with the PCPs and other providers throughout life.

Evidence regarding the efficacy of SCPs in improving patient outcomes (quality of life, functional status), patient satisfaction, or continuity and coordination of care is mixed. Interventions focusing solely upon the delivery of a SCP have failed to impact the aforementioned outcomes [12–14]. However, an intervention which utilized a SCP in conjunction with a single coaching encounter utilizing motivational interviewing techniques to engage breast cancer survivors appeared to have a positive impact on self-reported health, physical function, emotional function, and depressive symptom burden over a 3-month follow-up [15]. Cancer survivors themselves endorse high levels of patient satisfaction with SCPs and report using the materials provided to make health behavior choices and to improve communication with providers [16, 17]. Additional research, to provide evidence about the optimal way to deliver survivorship care to the large and growing population of women with breast cancer, is needed. Meanwhile, given the large number of survivors, the unique role of PCPs in building a long-term relationship, the recommendations of the IOM, and the cited data regarding patient satisfaction with SCPs, we endorse SCPs as a valuable tool to assist PCPs in taking care of cancer survivors.

One year later, Rachel, now 49 years old, presents for her first visit following completion of combined chemotherapy and radiation for stage II, hormone receptor-positive invasive ductal carcinoma. She underwent breast-conserving surgery with axillary lymph node dissection, chemotherapy (anthracycline and taxane containing), and whole breast radiation. Her tumor was estrogen and progesterone receptor positive, HER2/neu negative. She has just started taking tamoxifen. She feels well and has no physical complaints. She brings her SCP with her to the visit.

The aim of surveillance after curative treatment for breast cancer is the early detection of local or regional recurrences and of second primary cancers. Because breast cancer is a heterogeneous disease, the incidence of recurrence is influenced by numerous factors, including age, tumor grade, stage at diagnosis, nodal involvement, hormone receptor status, and treatment of the primary tumor.

In general, the risk for breast cancer recurrence peaks around 4% approximately 2 years after the primary tumor in women with stage I–III invasive breast cancer [18]. However, patients remain at risk for recurrence for as long as they live. Breast cancer survivors are also at increased risk for new primary breast cancers and for local tumor recurrences. The risk of a contralateral breast cancer has been estimated to be between 0.5% and 1.0% per year [19], though this may be an overestimate given these studies were performed during an era of less effective systemic treatments and prior to the use of extended hormonal therapy treatments.

Surveillance for breast cancer recurrence includes three components: the history and physical exam, screening for local recurrence or a new primary breast cancer, and laboratory tests and additional imaging. Before considering each of these aspects of screening individually, it is important to make clear that the decision to perform surveillance should consider the patient's functional status and personal preferences.

The History and Physical Exam

The frequency of follow-up for breast cancer survivors should be determined in conjunction with the patient's oncologist and consider the patient's age, her diagnosis, and her treatment protocol. In general, the patient should have a detailed history and physical exam every 3–6 months for the first 3 years after primary therapy, every 6–12 months for the next 2 years, and annually thereafter (Table 20.1) [9]. The surveillance physical exam should include a clinical breast exam and regular gynecologic follow-up [20]. Postmenopausal women on selective estrogen receptor modulator (SERM) therapies, like tamoxifen, are at increased risk for endometrial hyperplasia and endometrial cancer. Therefore, guidelines recommend that patients taking SERMs be counseled to report any vaginal spotting or bleeding to their provider. Of note, in the absence of abnormal uterine bleeding, screening with pelvic exam, endometrial biopsy, or transvaginal ultrasound is not routinely recommended, even in patients taking SERMS (see chapter on gynecologic cancer).

Follow-up visits should include a detailed cancer-related review of systems [9]. The signs and symptoms of local or regional cancer recurrence and of metastatic disease should be reviewed (e.g., new lumps in the underarm or neck, changes in the contour/shape/size of the breast, swelling of the breast or arm, bone pain, persistent headaches, chest or abdominal pain). The patient should be instructed to contact her provider if any of these symptoms occur between follow-up visits.

Primary care physicians should also continually review and update the patient's cancer family history, with a goal of identifying women who are at increased risk for a second primary breast cancer and/or genetic syndromes [9]. The presence of a genetic mutation increases the risk of future breast, ovarian, or other malignancies and dictates an accelerated cancer screening and prevention program for affected individuals. (See Chap. 17 on Primary Prevention of Breast Cancer.) A referral to a genetic counselor for consideration of testing for gene mutations should be made in breast cancer survivors with any of the following characteristics [21]:

- Age <50 years at the time of diagnosis *OR* age <60 years at the time of diagnosis of triple-negative breast cancer.
- A personal history of bilateral breast cancer.
- A personal history of ovarian cancer at any age.
- A history of ovarian cancer in any first-degree or second-degree relative.
- A first-degree relative with breast cancer diagnosed <50 years.
- Two or more first-degree or second-degree relatives diagnosed with breast cancer at any age.
- A history of breast cancer in a male relative.
- Having at least one grandparent of Ashkenazi Jewish heritage.

Table 20.1 Frequency of clinical follow-up, including cancer-related history and physical exam, for breast cancer survivors after curative therapy

Years after primary curative therapy	History and exam frequency by oncologist or primary care clinician
1–3	Every 3–6 months
4–5	Every 6–12 months
>5	Annually

Surveillance

Mammography is recommended annually for all breast cancer survivors to screen for local recurrence or a new primary breast cancer. For women who have received a unilateral mastectomy, mammography should be performed on the intact breast; the reconstructed breast does not require imaging [9]. For women who have received lumpectomies, mammography should be performed on both breasts. More frequent follow-up may be warranted if an abnormality is found.

There is no evidence to suggest that screening MRI improves outcomes in asymptomatic patients with a history of breast cancer. Of significant import, the use of breast MRI for screening is restricted to women who meet the high-risk criteria, defined as women with a lifetime risk of a second primary breast cancer greater than 20%, as would be the case for a woman with a BRCA1/BRCA2 mutation or a very strong family history of breast cancer [9, 20, 22]. (See Chap. 18 on Breast Cancer Screening.) Additionally, there is a significant increased risk of false-positive findings on breast MRI, which may lead to unnecessary additional imaging and unnecessary breast biopsies.

Laboratory Tests and Additional Imaging

Primary care providers should NOT offer routine lab tests, tumor markers, or imaging studies (e.g., bone scan, chest X-ray, PET scan, MRI scan) for the detection of disease recurrence as a part of routine screening of breast cancer survivors who have completed therapy for early-stage disease [9]. None of these have been demonstrated to improve survival or quality of life in asymptomatic women when compared to standard clinical follow-up.

Rachel comes back to clinic 1 year later and wants to discuss management of her hot flashes. She notes that over the past year, her hot flashes have become more frequent and severe, and she now finds them disabling. She is waking multiple times per night with drenching sweats, having to change her sheets and her clothes. She also reports some sexual problems with her husband. Vaginal dryness has caused sex to become uncomfortable and her libido is decreased.

Vasomotor Symptoms

Breast cancer survivors may experience vasomotor symptoms as a result of therapy-induced menopause (premature cessation of ovarian function from chemotherapy or as a side effect of hormonal therapies), surgical menopause from oophorectomy, or natural menopause. Breast cancer patients with therapy-induced menopause experience more frequent and more severe hot flashes than do women undergoing natural menopause. For example, between 50% and 70% of young women treated with tamoxifen will experience severe hot flashes [23]. Though vasomotor symptoms are not life-threatening, they can greatly impact quality of life and can result in early discontinuation of breast cancer treatment [24]. Hot flashes are thought to result from thermoregulatory dysfunction at the level of the hypothalamus precipitated by estrogen withdrawal, caused by menopause or by medications such as aromatase inhibitors (AIs) or SERMs. While the pathophysiology and management of vasomotor symptoms in this population are similar to those described in the general population (see Chap. 8 on Menopause), some factors specific to breast cancer survivors warrant further discussion.

Though hormone replacement therapy is the most effective treatment for control of menopausal symptoms, its use is relatively contraindicated in patients with breast cancer [9]. Selective serotonin reuptake inhibitors (SSRIs), serotonin and norepinephrine reuptake inhibitors (SNRIs), and anticonvulsants (e.g., gabapentin) are three classes of drugs which have been found to be safe and efficacious in treating vasomotor symptoms in breast cancer survivors in placebo-controlled, double-blinded, randomized clinical trials [9, 25].

Nonhormonal Treatments for Vasomotor Symptoms

SSRIs/SNRIs

The SNRIs venlafaxine (75 mg daily) and desvenlafaxine (100 mg daily) have been shown to reduce hot flash frequency and severity by 50–67% when compared to placebo and are generally well-tolerated [25]. The SSRIs citalopram (10 mg daily) and escitalopram (10 and 20 mg daily) have also been shown to reduce hot flash burden by 50–55% compared to 20–30% with placebo and are similarly well-tolerated [25]. It is important to note that the SSRI paroxetine is a potent inhibitor of the cytochrome P450 2D6 (CYP2D6) enzyme pathway, which may reduce the conversion of tamoxifen to active metabolites. Though the clinical importance of this interaction remains controversial, paroxetine is not recommended for use in women taking tamoxifen [9]. Fluoxetine, duloxetine, and bupropion also inhibit CYP2D6, but to a lesser degree, and are thus avoided by many experts. Sertraline, citalopram, escitalopram, and venlafaxine are thought to be the safest choices among the SSRI/SNRI class for women on tamoxifen.

Anticonvulsants

Gabapentin at a dose of 900 mg/day in three divided doses has been demonstrated to decrease hot flashes by 35–50% compared to placebo [25]. Gabapentin may also be used as a single nighttime dose for nocturnal hot flashes. In one randomized crossover trial, gabapentin was as effective as venlafaxine in reducing hot flashes, but venlafaxine was preferred by patients [25]. Pregabalin (75 mg or 150 mg twice daily) has also been demonstrated to reduce hot flashes to a similar degree as gabapentin, though the side effect burden (e.g., dizziness, lower extremity edema, weight gain) and increased cost compared to gabapentin makes this regimen less attractive [25].

Clonidine

Though the antihypertensive agent clonidine has been demonstrated in older trials to decrease hot flashes more than placebo, the efficacy of this medication is less than the aforementioned classes. This, along with its significant side effect profile, limits clonidine's utility.

Complementary and Alternative Therapies

Complementary and alternative medications including black cohosh, isoflavones, other phytoestrogens, evening primrose oil, flaxseed, ginseng, and dong quai have been found to be minimally effective in treating hot flashes [9]. Several recent studies have examined the effect of acupuncture on the reduction of menopausal symptoms in patients with breast cancer [26–28]. Overall, data indicate that acupuncture has a small but positive effect in reducing the frequency and severity of hot flashes and burden of menopausal symptoms. Other non-pharmacological interventions including cognitive behavioral therapy, yoga, paced breathing, and hypnosis have been purported to have a beneficial effect on hot flashes, though high-quality evidence supporting their effectiveness is currently lacking [29].

Sexual Dysfunction and Vulvovaginal Symptoms

Sexual dysfunction is defined as "a heterogeneous group of disorders that are typically characterized by a clinically significant disturbance in a person's ability to respond sexually or experience sexual pleasure" [30]; See Chap. 9 on Female Sexual Function and Dysfunction. Sexual concerns are common among breast cancer survivors.

Between one- and two-thirds of breast cancer survivors experience sexual concerns, including decreased libido, arousal and/or lubrication concerns, orgasmic concerns, and dyspareunia [9].

Epidemiology and Risk Factors

The etiology of sexual complaints in survivors, similar to non-survivors, is often multifactorial and may include biological, interpersonal, and psychological facets. Hormonal alterations, as a result of chemotherapy or hormonal therapy, can lead to vaginal atrophy, dryness, and pain. Over time, these changes may lead to dyspareunia and subsequent low libido and arousal difficulties. Breast cancer survivors may also have a negative perception of body image because of treatment (e.g., the loss of part or all of a breast, postoperative scarring or lymphedema, therapy-induced early menopause and hair loss, and others). Accordingly, these body image issues can significantly impact sexual function as related to poorer self-esteem and mental health. Anxiety, distress, or depression as a result of a diagnosis of breast cancer or fear of recurrence can also impact survivors' sexual function. Further, problems with sexual intimacy may be impacted by relationship discord, lack of communication, or other relationship challenges.

Diagnosis

Unfortunately, primary care providers report feeling both uncomfortable and inadequately prepared to discuss sexual function with female cancer survivors [31]. The 5 As is an evidence-based framework for communicating about health behaviors that has been adapted to guide communication about sexual dysfunction in female cancer survivors [32]. This counseling model underscores five core components of communication about sexual health (Fig. 20.1). Sexual difficulties may be reported as a temporary condition or may become a more serious disorder.

The physical exam remains an essential component of evaluation of sexual dysfunction. In addition to looking for signs of contributing general medical conditions, the gynecologic exam is important to determine the etiology of any pain complaints. Specifically, the primary care provider should look for signs of vulvovaginal atrophy, vaginismus (a painful spasmodic contraction of the vaginal walls in response to pressure), postoperative or postradiation changes (e.g., vaginal stenosis or atrophy), evidence of primary gynecologic disease (e.g., endometriosis or vaginitis), or evidence of organ prolapse. (See Chap. 9 on Female Sexual Function and Dysfunction for further information.)

Management

Treatment of sexual dysfunction is dictated by the type of sexual dysfunction and by the suspected underlying cause(s). (Please refer to Chap. 9 on Female Sexual Function and Dysfunction for a detailed review of the management of sexual dysfunction.) Just like in non-survivors, often treatment will be multimodal, including psychoeducational support, pharmacotherapy, sexual or marital counseling, and physical therapy [9]. Patient education is an essential component of any treatment plan, including a discussion of normal sexual function and treatment options.

Nonhormonal treatments remain the mainstay of pharmacotherapy for vaginal dryness in breast cancer survivors. Combining as-needed use of water-based lubricants with consistent (3–5×/week) use of a vaginal moisturizer may provide more benefit than either agent alone [9]. Due to concerns regarding the possibility of systemic absorption, topical estrogens should be reserved for patients who are not responsive to nonhormonal treatments [9]. Low-dose estradiol 10 mcg vaginal tablets or the low-dose 2 mg (7.5 mcg/24 hrs) estradiol vaginal ring is preferred to estrogen creams, which have more variable absorption. Although low-dose vaginal estrogens do not result in sustained serum estrogen levels exceeding the menopausal range, the decision to utilize these therapies should be made in coordination with the patient's oncologist with a discussion of the risks

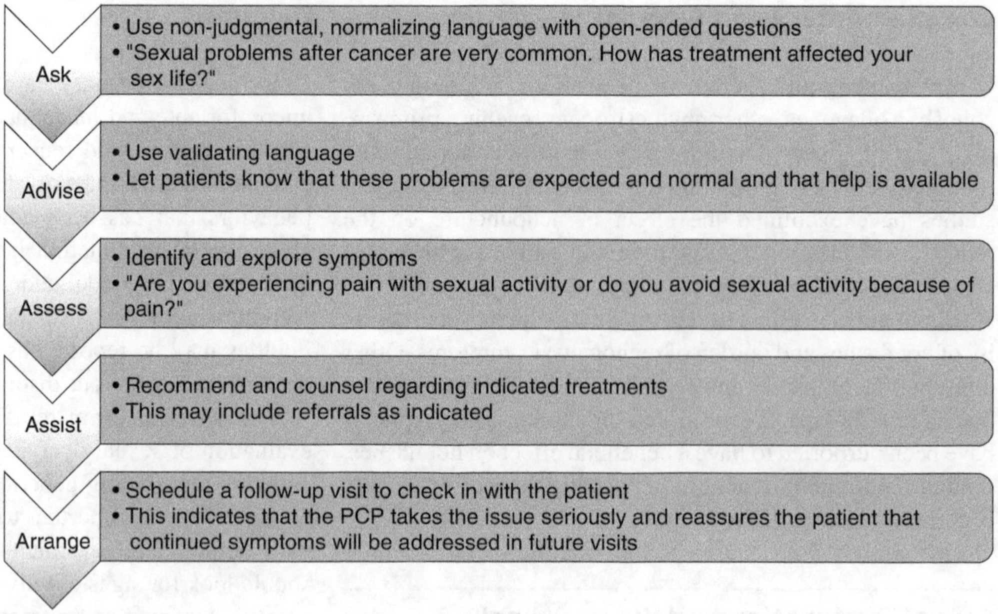

Fig. 20.1 The 5 As framework for evaluating sexual dysfunction in female cancer survivors [32]

and benefits. Regardless of the type of treatment pursued, patients should be counseled that improvement in dryness might require 6–12 weeks of therapy.

Referral to pelvic floor physical therapy may be of additional benefit to breast cancer survivors with sexual dysfunction for relaxation techniques and to improve pelvic muscle floor strength, tone, and vaginal elasticity [9]. Patients with vaginal fibrosis or stenosis as a result of pelvic radiation may benefit from vaginal dilators, foreplay, the use of erotica, and/or dilation with lubrication prior to insertion. Many cancer centers have clinicians specializing in sexual health for cancer patients or may provide referrals for patients who experience sexual difficulties during or after cancer treatment.

Finally, it is essential to attend to psychological and interpersonal factors affecting sexual function in cancer survivors. Referral to a sexual counselor, marital counselor, or psychotherapist should be offered to all patients to address underlying body image, anxiety, stress, and mood changes, all of which can affect sexual function [9]. Specialized clinics and clinicians who are skilled in addressing sexual issues for cancer survivors are available in some medical centers.

While exploring the impact of her sexual dysfunction and hot flashes on her quality of life, Rachel becomes tearful. On further questioning, she relates that she's unsure where to go with her life now that she has "beat cancer." She constantly worries she will have a recurrence, is hopeless about the future, and feels guilty that she is not doing "more with her life."

Distress, Depression, and Anxiety

Epidemiology and Risk Factors

Breast cancer survivors are at risk for a range of mental health problems including distress, depression, anxiety, and post-traumatic stress disorder (PTSD). Distress in this context is defined as "a multifactorial unpleasant experience of a psychological, social, and/or spiritual nature," while depression and anxiety are defined as they are in the general population [9]. According to a 2013 systematic review of observational studies, the median prevalence of depression and anxiety in the breast cancer survivor population ranged from 10% to 22% (with broad range of estimates across studies) depending on the measurement scale being used [33]. Importantly, these problems can occur at any time across the survivorship continuum, not only during the time surrounding diagnosis and treatment but also at any time during the phase of survivorship following treatment completion.

While many of the predisposing factors for depression and anxiety in this population are similar to those described in the general population (see Chap. 33 on Depressive and Anxiety Disorders), some factors specific to cancer survivors warrant further discussion. First, fear of recurrence (FOR) can be a significant contributor and has been documented at higher levels in those whose cancer diagnosis is more recent, in those receiving chemotherapy, and in those experiencing more symptoms [34]. The risk of depression in breast cancer survivors is increased and has been associated with younger age at the time of cancer diagnosis, lower socioeconomic status, and prior history of psychiatric disease [35]. PTSD, which can develop after experiencing a frightening or life-threatening situation, is also common in cancer survivors and can persist or worsen over time. Estimates suggest that between 20% and over 80% of breast cancer patients experience symptoms of PTSD.

Diagnosis

The primary care provider, whose contact with survivors spans the continuum from diagnosis through treatment and beyond, is ideally positioned to play a key role in the identification and appropriate management of distress, depression, and anxiety in breast cancer survivors. Per the American Cancer Society/American Society of Clinical Oncology (ACS/ASCO) Breast Cancer Survivorship Guidelines, primary care providers should screen for the presence of psychological distress in all survivors while probing more deeply in those who are at higher risk based on the factors discussed above [9]. The 2014 ASCO anxiety and depression guideline adaptation recommends screening at the time of cancer diagnosis and "at appropriate intervals, and as clinically indicated, especially with changes in disease or treatment status (i.e., post-treatment, recurrence, progression) and transition to palliative and end-of-life care" [36].

Use of the National Comprehensive Cancer Network (NCCN) *Distress Thermometer and Problem List for Patients* is recommended for the initial screening and monitoring of distress. Scores on this scale range from 0 (no distress) to 10 (extreme distress); in completing the screen, patients are asked to circle the number that best describes how much distress they have been experiencing in the last week. A score of 4 or higher indicates the presence of clinically significant distress [37]. There is also a checklist to question which activities and situations cause the most distress for patients. The tool is freely accessible and downloadable for use in patient care, but cannot be used in publications. Please refer to the NCCN.org website for more info and free download [38].

For depression and anxiety, screening can be performed using validated screening tools available for use in the general population, such as the Patient Health Questionairre-9 (PHQ-9) for depression and the Generalized Anxiety Disorder-7 (GAD-7) for anxiety [39, 40].

For depression, ASCO recommends, as outlined in an algorithm specific to adults with cancer, starting with two specific questions from the PHQ-9 to assess for the classic symptoms of anhedonia and low mood. Providers should administer the remaining seven questions to those with a positive screen, with the expectation that 25–30% of patients will require this step [36]. Importantly, a cutoff score of ≥8 for the PHQ-9 is recommended (as opposed to the more traditional ≥9 cutoff) as this is the threshold for at least moderate depression based on a study of this tool's diagnostic accuracy in cancer outpatients [41]. For anxiety, the traditional cutoff score of ≥10 on the GAD-7 is used to identify at least moderate symptomatology, as in the general population [41]. Despite the usefulness of screening tools, providers should have a high index of suspicion and employ expert interviewing skills to detect depression of anxiety that the patient may not have disclosed on the questionnaires. (Please refer to Chap. 33 on Depressive and Anxiety Disorders for a more detailed discussion of the general principles of screening for depression and anxiety.)

Management

When screening is positive, further assessment and/or management is indicated. Treatment should be individualized, considering severity of symptoms and functional impact of those symptoms as well as patient preferences. The 2014 ASCO anxiety and depression guideline adaptation includes care maps for adults with cancer and depression or anxiety, respectively [41]. Pharmacological, psychological, and psychosocial therapies are the mainstays of treatment just as they are in patients without a cancer history. Primary care providers should become familiar with the resources available within their individual practice settings, including awareness of any psycho-oncology or mental health resources geared toward cancer survivors. Pharmacologic treatments are essentially the same as for the general population. As discussed in the section on vasomotor symptoms, the use of the certain SSRIs, especially paroxetine, should be avoided in women taking tamoxifen due to the potential for interaction leading to reduced tamoxifen active metabolites [9]. Care should also be taken in women with sexual dysfunction when prescribing SSRIs which have frequent sexual side effects including low libido, lack of arousal, or delayed orgasm.

Rachel comes back in follow-up a few months later. She is now engaged with an individual therapist and reports that both her mood and hot flashes are much improved having started treatment with venlafaxine for combined benefit. She is doing well, with no other complaints today, and would like to discuss recommendations for overall health promotion and cancer prevention.

Health Promotion

Health promotion is critical to the well-being of breast cancer survivors, most of whom will experience long-term survival [42]. Pursuit of a healthy lifestyle can not only reduce the risk of cancer recurrence and second cancers but also have a positive impact on cancer-related symptoms and on overall mortality [43–50]. The ACS/ASCO Breast Cancer Survivorship Guidelines make recommendations regarding weight, physical activity, nutrition (including recommendations regarding alcohol consumption), and smoking cessation for breast cancer survivors (Table 20.2) [9]. These recommendations provide a framework that primary care providers can use for counseling and to answer important questions breast cancer survivors may have about healthy behaviors and their potential impact on health and disease prevention. Each category is discussed briefly below.

Weight

Counseling regarding maintenance of a healthy weight is particularly important for breast cancer survivors. Many survivors, like the rest of the population, are overweight or obese. Obesity is an established risk factor for breast cancer recurrence, second cancer recurrence, and a multitude of other medical comorbidities [51]. Additionally, weight loss has been associated with improvements in symptoms and in quality of life in cancer survivors. Primary care providers should, therefore, counsel breast cancer survivors to achieve or maintain a healthy weight [52].

Physical Activity

A minority of cancer survivors meet the ACS guidelines for physical activity. High-quality data suggests that physical activity improves quality of life and physical functioning, and observational data supports a connection between physical activity and reduced breast cancer-specific and all-cause mortality [53, 54]. For these reasons, primary care providers should communicate physical activity guidelines with all survivors, as outlined in Table 20.2.

Nutrition and Alcohol

Breast cancer survivors should be advised to consume a diet rich in vegetables, fruits, whole grains, and legumes due to the association of good nutrition with reduced all-cause mortality [55–57]. Importantly, achievement of weight loss as a result of dietary change may be required in order for breast cancer survivors to experience benefits in terms of breast cancer recurrence and prognosis [58, 59]. Regarding alcohol consumption, the ACS recommends that breast cancer survivors should limit intake to no more than one drink per day [9]. Other organizations site recent data that alcohol consumption of any amount increases cancer risk; therefore, some survivors may choose to limit intake even more or abstain from all alcoholic beverages [60].

Smoking Cessation

Observational data suggests that, in addition to the other well-established health consequences associated with smoking, increased breast cancer-specific and overall mortality are associated with smoking at the time of breast cancer diagnosis [61]. As such, primary care providers should work to motivate and encourage smoking cessation and provide support with pharmacotherapy and/or multimodal tobacco cessation programs according to local availability and patient preference.

Table 20.2 ACS/ASCO health promotion guideline for breast cancer survivors, adapted from ACS/ASCO Breast Cancer Survivorship Guidelines [9]

Lifestyle category	Counseling recommendations
Weight and obesity	Achieve and maintain a healthy weight If overweight or obese, limit consumption of high-calorie foods and beverages and increase physical activity to promote and maintain weight loss
Physical activity	Engage in regular physical activity consistent with the ACS guideline and specifically: Avoid inactivity and return to normal daily activities as soon as possible following diagnosis Aim for at least 150 min of moderate or 75 min of vigorous aerobic exercise per week Include strength training exercises at least 2 days per week; emphasize strength training for women treated with adjuvant chemotherapy or hormone therapy
Nutrition	Achieve a dietary pattern that is high in vegetables, fruits, whole grains, and legumes; low in saturated fats; and limited in alcohol consumption
Smoking	Avoid smoking If smoking, refer to cessation counseling and resources

During her next visit, Rachel states that her oncologist has stopped the tamoxifen and started anastrozole because she is now definitively postmenopausal and did not tolerate raloxifene. She asks for advice regarding guidelines for bone health assessment and management in survivors who are receiving aromatase inhibitor therapy.

Bone Health

Epidemiology and Risk Factors

Breast cancer survivors often possess additional risk factors for bone loss beyond the well-established risk factors for women in general: age, personal fracture history, family history of fracture or osteoporosis, and lifestyle factors such as smoking, alcohol intake, insufficient exercise, etc. (please refer to Chap. 25 on Osteoporosis for a detailed discussion of osteoporosis risk factors in the general population). Potential specific risk factors for breast cancer survivors include the following treatments: chemotherapy (and consequent risk for chemotherapy-induced premature menopause), drugs that suppress gonadal function, oophorectomy causing premature menopause, glucocorticoids, and/or antiestrogen therapies such as aromatase inhibitors [62]. Existing reports estimate that up to 80% of breast cancer survivors experience some degree of bone loss [63, 64]. Furthermore, according to a recent review, aromatase inhibitor therapy leads to a two- to fourfold increase in bone loss compared to expected postmenopausal bone loss [65]. Breast cancer survivors receiving aromatase inhibitors are thus at increased risk for fracture and experience increased morbidity and mortality [66–70]. As aromatase inhibitor therapy and other therapies which cause bone loss continue to proliferate (see Chap. 19 on Breast Cancer Diagnosis and Management), a further increase in fracture risk for breast cancer survivors must be anticipated.

Diagnosis

Current guidelines recommend that all postmenopausal breast cancer survivors being treated with aromatase inhibitors be referred for a baseline DXA scan, regardless of age, for assessment of bone mineral density [9]. Additionally, all women (regardless of menopausal status) who have received treatments that can suppress ovarian function should undergo assessment with DXA. DXA scans should be repeated every 2 years, with consideration of shortening the interval to 1 year if major risk factors change such as use of glucocorticoids or continued aromatase inhibitor use [9].

Management

Once bone mineral density has been assessed with DXA, primary care providers should consider the results in the context of other risk factors for bone loss to direct treatment. While many risk factors for bone loss exist in this population, it remains unclear how best to account for them in the context of treatment decisions. The World Health Organization Fracture Risk Assessment Tool (FRAX, http://www.sheffield.ac.uk/FRAX) [71] is a widely used tool for fracture risk assessment in the general population, but its value for use in the breast cancer survivor population has been questioned. The FRAX tool has not been validated to assess fracture risk in breast cancer survivors and may underestimate risk in this population, at least in part because the "secondary osteoporosis" option in the tool does not adequately account for aromatase inhibitor-associated bone loss [65].

Several guidelines make recommendations regarding the management of bone loss in breast cancer survivors. A joint position statement from several interdisciplinary cancer and bone societies was released in 2017, to update an evidence-based algorithm for both fracture risk assessment and the treatment of bone loss in this high-risk population; see Table 20.3 [65]. Notably, these guidelines highlight the important role that the primary care provider plays in providing counseling about modifiable risk factors for bone loss. Specifically, providers should counsel all survivors about engaging in physical activity including weight-bearing exercise, to avoid tobacco products, to limit alcohol intake, and to ensure adequate calcium and vitamin D supplementation (if dietary intake is inadequate) [9, 65]. The recommendations differ slightly from general bone health advice because survivors may be at increased risk for rapid bone loss.

If a breast cancer survivor meets criteria for treatment with antiresorptive therapy, either based on DXA t-score or based on risk factors as indicated in Table 20.3, treatment with a bisphosphonate or denosumab is recommended. While the 2015 ACS/ASCO guidelines do not recommend one agent over another, more recent consensus guidelines suggest that intravenous zoledronic acid, administered once every 6 months, is first line. This recommendation is made based on available efficacy data in this specific patient population as well as on tolerability. Cost and availability, however, may limit its use. Oral bisphosphonates (which are limited by issues with compliance and by lack of efficacy data for aromatase inhibitor-induced bone loss) and denosumab (which is limited by cost, a paucity of efficacy data, and rebound effect after treatment termination) are alternative treatment options.

Importantly, recent consensus guidelines recommend continuation of antiresorptive therapy for as long as a survivor is receiving aromatase inhibitor therapy (up to 5 years)

Table 20.3 Guidelines for management of bone loss in breast cancer survivors receiving treatments known to accelerate bone loss, according to the joint position statement of the IOF, CABS, ECTS, IEG, ESCEO, IMS, and SIOG, 2017 [65]

Risk category	Recommendation
T-score > −2.0 and no additional risk factors	Exercise Calcium and vitamin D if not present adequately in diet Check BMD and risk factors every 2 years or every 1 year if risk changes
T-score ≤ −2.0 *OR* any two of the following risk factors: Age >65 T-score <1.5 Smoking (current or history of) BMI <20 Family history of hip fracture Personal history of fragility fracture at age ≥50 years Oral glucocorticoid use ≥6 months	Exercise Calcium and vitamin D Bisphosphonate or denosumab therapy Check BMD every 2 years

[65]. Providers should also be aware that some survivors may be receiving intravenous bisphosphonates as a component of adjuvant breast cancer therapy or as a component of management for metastatic bone disease. (See Chap. 19 on Breast Cancer Diagnosis and Management for more information regarding adjuvant use of bisphosphonates in breast cancer treatment.) Finally, while SERMs such as raloxifene are approved for treatment of postmenopausal osteoporosis in the general population, combining SERMs with aromatase inhibitor therapy has been shown to impair the effectiveness of the aromatase inhibitor [72]. As such, SERMs should not be used to treat osteoporosis in survivors who are receiving an aromatase inhibitor [9].

Other Late and Long-Term Complications

Additional late and long-term effects of breast cancer treatment including lymphedema, cardiotoxicity, fatigue, cognitive dysfunction, and neuropathy may occur and should be considered as part of a comprehensive SCP. Evaluation and treatment options are presented in Table 20.4.

Table 20.4 Additional recommendations for breast cancer survivorship care, from the American Cancer Society/American Society of Clinical Oncology [9, 73, 74]

	Description and epidemiology	Management
Lymphedema	Arm, breast, or chest wall swelling as a result of blockage of lymphatic fluid from the arm and/or breast Can range in severity from mild to severe Incidence varies widely, estimated over 40% Risk factors: Lymph node dissection (axillary > sentinel), breast surgery, radiation therapy, obesity	Counsel how to prevent or reduce the risk of lymphedema, including weight loss (if overweight or obese) Refer patients with clinical symptoms or swelling suggestive of lymphedema to a knowledgeable therapist (e.g., a physical or occupational therapist or lymphedema specialist)
Cardiotoxicity	Postmenopausal women are at increased risk of mortality attributed to CVD (risk is increased due to radiation therapy), which manifests ~7 years after diagnosis of breast cancer Patients at elevated risk of left ventricular (LV) dysfunction include patients treated with: Doxorubicin ≥250 mg/m^2 Radiation ≥30 Gy Lower-dose anthracycline with lower-dose radiation (<30Gy) Treatment with lower-dose anthracycline or trastuzumab AND any of the following: Multiple CV risk factors Age ≥ 60 years at cancer treatment Compromised cardiac function (e.g., diminished LV ejection fraction, history of myocardial infarction, moderate to severe valvular heart disease) before or during treatment	Monitor and treat other nontreatment-related CVD risk factors (HTN, DM, dyslipidemia, and lifestyle) aggressively Counsel breast cancer survivors on healthy lifestyle modifications, potential cardiac risk factors, and when to report concerning symptoms Routine screening in asymptomatic patients at low risk for CVD beyond history and physical exam is not warranted Asymptomatic patients at elevated risk of LV dysfunction may undergo imaging 6–12 months following completion of cancer therapy Symptomatic patients should be assessed with echocardiography
Cognitive impairment	Includes symptoms such as difficulty with concentration, executive function, and memory Reported by 75% of patients during treatment and 35% after treatment Cause is multifactorial	Ask patients about cognitive difficulties, and assess for reversible contributing factors Refer patients with signs of cognitive impairment for neurocognitive evaluation Refer patients with cognitive problems for rehabilitation including cognitive therapy or cognitive training Data regarding pharmaceuticals are inconsistent
Fatigue	One of the most prevalent (30–90%) and distressing long-term effects of cancer treatment, which can significantly impact quality of life May last long after treatment ends and can significantly interfere with quality of life	Assess for fatigue and treat any secondary causes Counsel patients to engage in regular physical activity and refer for cognitive behavioral therapy if no identifiable cause of fatigue is determined
Musculoskeletal health	Difficulties with ipsilateral upper extremity (e.g., rotator cuff injury, adhesive capsulitis, and axillary web syndrome) are common after surgery and can impact quality of life and function Up to 50% of women receiving aromatase inhibitor therapy report arthralgias and myalgias, which can be severe enough that 20% discontinue treatment and are often nonresponsive to NSAID therapy	Assess for musculoskeletal symptoms Treat musculoskeletal pain and aromatase inhibitor-associated pain as indicated, considering physical therapy and acupuncture

Table 20.4 (continued)

	Description and epidemiology	Management
Neuropathy	Neuropathy is common (30–40%) following surgery and after treatment with taxane- or platinum-based chemotherapeutic agents	Comprehensively assess the patient's pain history to determine the most likely underlying cause, with dedicated inquiry regarding presence of the characteristic symptoms of peripheral neuropathy (numbness and tingling in the hands or feet) Offer a combination of physical activity and pharmacologic therapy, as indicated, for patients with neuropathic pain
Infertility	Especially important to consider in breast cancer survivors of childbearing age Risk of infertility varies according to age and treatments received	Premenopausal women who desire pregnancy and have been unable to conceive for ≥6 months should be referred to a fertility specialist Future fertility concerns are ideally addressed prior to treatments

Summary Points

1. Key components of a breast cancer survivorship plan include defining a surveillance plan for recurrence or new primary breast cancers, addressing and managing late and long-term complications of treatment, providing psychosocial support, and counseling regarding lifestyle modifications and strategies for overall health promotion.
2. In addition to annual mammograms, patients should be followed to assess for signs and symptoms of recurrence with a periodic history and physical exam. Routine blood tests, advanced imaging, and tumor markers are NOT recommended for surveillance testing in asymptomatic patients.
3. Breast cancer survivors face many potential late and long-term complications of therapy, including lymphedema, cardiotoxicity, premature menopause, fatigue, cognitive dysfunction, depression, anxiety, neuropathy, vasomotor symptoms, and loss of bone mineral density.
4. Sexual dysfunction is common in breast cancer survivors and is often multifactorial. In conjunction with a gynecological exam, the "5 As" framework can be employed to identify and explore symptoms of female sexual dysfunction and to provide counseling regarding treatment options.
5. Women with breast cancer are likely to have long-term survival and thus it is important for the primary care provider to assess and make recommendations related to healthy behaviors including weight, activity, nutrition, smoking cessation, and alcohol use.

Review Questions

1. Many breast cancer patients become "permanent survivors" and have at least some component of their care transitioned back to primary care. Which of the following accurately defines a breast cancer survivor?
   A. A patient whose cancer has been in remission for 5 years or more is a survivor.
   B. A patient who has been diagnosed with breast cancer is a survivor.
   C. A patient whose cancer is in remission is a survivor if she remains cancer-free.
   D. A patient whose cancer is in remission is a survivor for the rest of her life.

   The correct answer is B. The American Cancer Society defines a cancer survivor as "Any person with a history of cancer, from the time of diagnosis through the remainder of their life." Survivorship is a distinct phase of cancer care, involving the surveillance for and assessment/management of mental, physical, spiritual, and social aspects of cancer diagnosis and treatment [2].
2. A 64-year-old woman with stage I, hormone receptor-negative invasive ductal carcinoma s/p lumpectomy with sentinel node biopsy, XRT, and chemotherapy 1 year ago. Her most recent mammogram was negative 2 months ago and there was no sign of clinical disease at her oncology appointment that same day. She presents to primary care for her first follow-up appointment after curative therapy to transition to cancer survivorship care. She feels well and has no physical complaints. Which of the following best describes your breast cancer surveillance plan for this asymptomatic patient during the first 3 years after primary curative therapy?
   A. A clinic visit to assess for signs and symptoms of recurrence with clinician breast exam every 3–6 months, mammogram every 6 months, and annual CT of the chest, abdomen, and pelvis.
   B. A clinic visit to assess for signs and symptoms of recurrence with clinician breast exam every 3–6 months with annual mammography.
   C. A clinic visit to assess for signs and symptoms of recurrence with clinician breast exam every 3–6 months with annual breast MRI, annual FDG-PET scan, and annual bloodwork for CEA and CA 15–3.

D. An annual clinic visit to assess for signs and symptoms of recurrence with clinician breast exam, annual mammography, and annual CT of the chest, abdomen, and pelvis.

The correct answer is B. In general, the patient should have a detailed history and physical exam every 3–6 months for the first 3 years after primary therapy, every 6–12 months for the next 2 years, and annually thereafter (Table 20.1) [9]. The surveillance physical exam should include a clinical breast exam and regular gynecologic follow-up. Because postmenopausal women on SERM therapies, like tamoxifen, are at increased risk for endometrial hyperplasia and endometrial cancer, guidelines recommend that these patients be counseled to report any vaginal spotting or bleeding. Of note, in the absence of abnormal uterine bleeding, routine pelvic exams (more than the usual recommendation guidelines) and transvaginal ultrasounds are not recommended and may lead to unwarranted biopsies. Follow-up visits should also update any family history of cancer and include a detailed cancer-related review of systems including signs and symptoms of local or regional cancer recurrence (e.g., new lumps in the underarm or neck, changes in the contour/shape/size of the breast, swelling of the breast or arm, bone pain, persistent headaches, chest or abdominal pain) [9].

Mammography is recommended on an annual basis to screen for local recurrence or a new primary breast cancer. Primary care providers should NOT offer routine lab tests, tumor markers, or imaging studies (e.g., bone scan, chest X-ray, PET scan, MRI scan) for the detection of disease recurrence as a part of routine screening of breast cancer survivors [9]. None of these have been demonstrated to improve survival or quality of life in asymptomatic women when compared to standard clinical follow-up.

3. A 40 year-old woman with a history of early stage hormone receptor-positive breast cancer treated with lumpectomy and XRT followed by adjuvant chemotherapy. She is currently in year 3 of tamoxifen therapy. She wants to discuss management of her hot flashes. She notes that her hot flashes have become worse over the last year, and she now finds them disabling. She is waking multiple times per night with drenching sweats, having to change her sheets and her clothes. How would you counsel her regarding her treatment options?
   A. Systemic hormone therapy is a safe and effective treatment for hot flashes in breast cancer survivors.
   B. Paroxetine is an option, especially if she also has symptoms of anxiety or depression.
   C. Pharmacologic treatment may not be needed – vasomotor symptoms in breast cancer survivors tend to be more short-lived and less severe than in postmenopausal women without breast cancer.
   D. Gabapentin at bedtime may be an option, especially if her symptoms are most bothersome at night.

The correct answer is D. Breast cancer patients experience more frequent and more severe hot flashes than do women undergoing natural menopause. Because her hot flashes are disabling, they warrant treatment now [9]. Systemic hormone therapy is contraindicated in this patient with hormone receptor-positive breast cancer. Paroxetine is a potent inhibitor of the cytochrome P450 2D6 enzyme pathway, which may reduce the conversion of tamoxifen to active metabolites and is not recommended for use in women taking tamoxifen. Other SSRI/SNRI treatments such as venlafaxine may be effective. Gabapentin has been demonstrated to decrease hot flashes when compared to placebo and would be an appropriate way to treat the patient's hot flashes at this time [25].

4. A 35-year-old woman with a history of early-stage node-positive breast cancer, who completed lumpectomy with adjuvant chemotherapy and XRT 6 months ago. She is now on tamoxifen. She reports some sexual problems with her husband. Sex has become painful. She also notices a feeling of vaginal dryness most of the time. Prior to her diagnosis and treatment, she was satisfied with her sex life. Which of the following is TRUE regarding treatment of vaginal dryness and pain with intercourse?
   A. Vaginal estrogen preparations are considered first line for treatment of these symptoms in breast cancer survivors.
   B. In patients who report painful intercourse, vaginal lubricants should be applied as needed before intercourse.
   C. Vaginal dryness in breast cancer survivors is often self-limited and thus may not require pharmacotherapy.
   D. Vaginal lubricants should not be used in patients who are already using a vaginal moisturizer.

The correct answer is B. Systemic hormone therapy is contraindicated in this patient with hormone receptor-positive breast cancer. Due to concerns regarding the possibility of systemic absorption, topical estrogens should be reserved for patients who are not responsive to nonhormonal treatments [9]. Combining as-needed use of water-based lubricants prior to intercourse with consistent (3–5×/week) use of a vaginal moisturizer may provide more benefit than either agent alone, to improve vaginal dryness and resultant pain with intercourse.

References

1. National Cancer Institute. SEER Cancer Stat Facts Female Breast Cancer Bethesda; 2018 [cited 2018 May 3]. https://seer.cancer.gov/statfacts/html/breast.html%5D
2. American Cancer Society. Treatment & Surivorship Facts & Figures 2016–2017 Atlanta;2016 [cited 2018 Jan 22]. https://www.cancer.org/content/dam/cancer-org/research/cancer-facts-and-statistics/cancer-treatment-and-survivorship-facts-and-figures/cancer-treatment-and-survivorship-facts-and-figures-2016-7.pdf
3. Institute of Medicine and National Research Council. From cancer patient to cancer survivor: lost in transition. Washington, DC: The National Academies Press; 2006.
4. Institute of Medicine. Implementing cancer survivorship care planning: workshop summary. Washington, DC: The National Academies Press; 2007.
5. Nissen MJ, Beran MS, Lee MW, Mehta SR, Pine DA, Swenson KK. Views of primary care providers on follow-up care of cancer patients. Fam Med. 2007;39(7):477–82.
6. Mayer DK, Shapiro CL, Jacobson P, McCabe MS. Assuring quality cancer survivorship care: We've only just begun. Am Soc Clin Oncol Educ Book. 2015:e583–91.
7. American Cancer Society. National Cancer Survivorship Resource Center systems policy and practice: clinical survivorship care overview. Washington, DC: The George Washington Cancer Institute; 2011.
8. American College of Surgeons. Cancer program standards 2016: ensuring patient-centered care [Internet]. Chicago, IL: American College of Surgeons; 2015.
9. Runowicz CD, Leach CR, Henry NL, Henry KS, Mackey HT, Cowens-Alvarado RL, et al. American Cancer Society/American society of clinical oncology breast cancer survivorship care guideline. J Clin Oncol. 2016;34(6):611–35.
10. Forsythe LP, Parry C, Alfano CM, Kent EE, Leach CR, Haggstrom DA, et al. Use of survivorship care plans in the United States: associations with survivorship care. J Natl Cancer Inst. 2013;105(20):1579–87.
11. Mayer DK, Birken SA, Check DK, Chen RC. Summing it up: an integrative review of studies of cancer survivorship care plans (2006–2013). Cancer. 2015;121(7):978–96.
12. Boekhout AH, Maunsell E, Pond GR, Julian JA, Coyle D, Levine MN, et al. A survivorship care plan for breast cancer survivors: extended results of a randomized clinical trial. J Cancer Surviv. 2015;9(4):683–91.
13. Nicolaije KA, Ezendam NP, Vos MC, Pijnenborg JM, Boll D, Boss EA, et al. Impact of an automatically generated cancer survivorship care plan on patient-reported outcomes in routine clinical practice: longitudinal outcomes of a pragmatic, cluster randomized trial. J Clin Oncol. 2015;33(31):3550–9.
14. Hershman DL, Greenlee H, Awad D, Kalinsky K, Maurer M, Kranwinkel G, et al. Randomized controlled trial of a clinic-based survivorship intervention following adjuvant therapy in breast cancer survivors. Breast Cancer Res Treat. 2013;138(3):795–806.
15. Kvale EA, Huang CS, Meneses KM, Demark-Wahnefried W, Bae S, Azuero CB, et al. Patient-centered support in the survivorship care transition: outcomes from the Patient-Owned Survivorship Care Plan Intervention. Cancer. 2016;122(20):3232–42.
16. Hill-Kayser CE, Vachani CC, Hampshire MK, Di Lullo G, Jacobs LA, Metz JM. Impact of internet-based cancer survivorship care plans on health care and lifestyle behaviors. Cancer. 2013;119(21):3854–60.
17. Palmer SC, Stricker CT, Panzer SL, Arvey SA, Baker KS, Casillas J, et al. Outcomes and satisfaction after delivery of a breast cancer survivorship care plan: results of a multicenter trial. J Oncol Pract. 2015;11(2):e222–9.
18. Geurts YM, Witteveen A, Bretveld R, Poortmans PM, Sonke GS, Strobbe LJA, et al. Patterns and predictors of first and subsequent recurrence in women with early breast cancer. Breast Cancer Res Treat. 2017;165(3):709–20.
19. Simone NL, Dan T, Shih J, Smith SL, Sciuto L, Lita E, et al. Twenty-five year results of the national cancer institute randomized breast conservation trial. Breast Cancer Res Treat. 2012;132(1):197–203.
20. Khatcheressian JL, Hurley P, Bantug E, Esserman LJ, Grunfeld E, Halberg F, et al. Breast cancer follow-up and management after primary treatment: American Society of Clinical Oncology clinical practice guideline update. J Clin Oncol. 2013;31(7):961–5.
21. Moyer VA. Force USPST. Risk assessment, genetic counseling, and genetic testing for BRCA-related cancer in women: U.S. Preventive Services Task Force recommendation statement. Ann Intern Med. 2014;160(4):271–81.
22. Saslow D, Boetes C, Burke W, Harms S, Leach MO, Lehman CD, et al. American Cancer Society guidelines for breast screening with MRI as an adjunct to mammography. CA Cancer J Clin. 2007;57(2):75–89.
23. Francis PA, Regan MM, Fleming GF. Adjuvant ovarian suppression in premenopausal breast cancer. N Engl J Med. 2015;372(17):1673.
24. Barron TI, Connolly R, Bennett K, Feely J, Kennedy MJ. Early discontinuation of tamoxifen: a lesson for oncologists. Cancer. 2007;109(5):832–9.
25. Leon-Ferre RA, Majithia N, Loprinzi CL. Management of hot flashes in women with breast cancer receiving ovarian function suppression. Cancer Treat Rev. 2017;52:82–90.
26. Chiu HY, Shyu YK, Chang PC, Tsai PS. Effects of acupuncture on menopause-related symptoms in breast cancer survivors: a meta-analysis of randomized controlled trials. Cancer Nurs. 2016;39(3):228–37.
27. Chien TJ, Hsu CH, Liu CY, Fang CJ. Effect of acupuncture on hot flush and menopause symptoms in breast cancer- a systematic review and meta-analysis. PLoS One. 2017;12(8):e0180918.
28. Chen YP, Liu T, Peng YY, Wang YP, Chen H, Fan YF, et al. Acupuncture for hot flashes in women with breast cancer: a systematic review. J Cancer Res Ther. 2016;12(2):535–42.
29. Tao WW, Tao XM, Song CL. Effects of non-pharmacological supportive care for hot flushes in breast cancer: a meta-analysis. Support Care Cancer. 2017;25(7):2335–47.
30. American Psychiatric Association. Diagnostic and statistical manual of mental disorders. 5th ed. Washington, DC: American Psychiatric Association; 2013.
31. Bober SL, Recklitis CJ, Campbell EG, Park ER, Kutner JS, Najita JS, et al. Caring for cancer survivors: a survey of primary care physicians. Cancer. 2009;115(18 Suppl):4409–18.
32. Bober SL, Carter J, Falk S. Addressing female sexual function after cancer by internists and primary care providers. J Sex Med. 2013;10(Suppl 1):112–9.
33. Zainal NZ, Nik-Jaafar NR, Baharudin A, Sabki ZA, Ng CG. Prevalence of depression in breast cancer survivors: a systematic review of observational studies. Asian Pac J Cancer Prev. 2013;14(4):2649–56.
34. McGinty HL, Goldenberg JL, Jacobsen PB. Relationship of threat appraisal with coping appraisal to fear of cancer recurrence in breast cancer survivors. Psychooncology. 2012;21(2):203–10.
35. Ewertz M, Jensen AB. Late effects of breast cancer treatment and potentials for rehabilitation. Acta Oncol. 2011;50(2):187–93.
36. Andersen BL, DeRubeis RJ, Berman BS, Gruman J, Champion VL, Massie MJ, et al. Screening, assessment, and care of anxi-

ety and depressive symptoms in adults with cancer: an American Society of Clinical Oncology guideline adaptation. J Clin Oncol. 2014;32(15):1605–19.

37. Patel D, Sharpe L, Thewes B, Bell ML, Clarke S. Using the distress thermometer and hospital anxiety and depression scale to screen for psychosocial morbidity in patients diagnosed with colorectal cancer. J Affect Disord. 2011;131(1–3):412–6.
38. NCCN. https://www.nccn.org/patients/resources/life_with_cancer/pdf/nccn_distress_thermometer.pdf. Accessed 15 Dec 2018.
39. Kroenke K, Spitzer RL, Williams JB. The PHQ-9: validity of a brief depression severity measure. J Gen Intern Med. 2001;16(9):606–13.
40. Spitzer RL, Kroenke K, Williams JB, Lowe B. A brief measure for assessing generalized anxiety disorder: the GAD-7. Arch Intern Med. 2006;166(10):1092–7.
41. Thekkumpurath P, Walker J, Butcher I, Hodges L, Kleiboer A, O'Connor M, et al. Screening for major depression in cancer outpatients: the diagnostic accuracy of the 9-item patient health questionnaire. Cancer. 2011;117(1):218–27.
42. DeSantis CE, Lin CC, Mariotto AB, Siegel RL, Stein KD, Kramer JL, et al. Cancer treatment and survivorship statistics, 2014. CA Cancer J Clin. 2014;64(4):252–71.
43. Chan DS, Vieira AR, Aune D, Bandera EV, Greenwood DC, McTiernan A, et al. Body mass index and survival in women with breast cancer-systematic literature review and meta-analysis of 82 follow-up studies. Ann Oncol. 2014;25(10):1901–14.
44. Protani M, Coory M, Martin JH. Effect of obesity on survival of women with breast cancer: systematic review and meta-analysis. Breast Cancer Res Treat. 2010;123(3):627–35.
45. McTiernan A, Irwin M, Vongruenigen V. Weight, physical activity, diet, and prognosis in breast and gynecologic cancers. J Clin Oncol. 2010;28(26):4074–80.
46. Wei EK, Wolin KY, Colditz GA. Time course of risk factors in cancer etiology and progression. J Clin Oncol. 2010;28(26):4052–7.
47. Patterson RE, Cadmus LA, Emond JA, Pierce JP. Physical activity, diet, adiposity and female breast cancer prognosis: a review of the epidemiologic literature. Maturitas. 2010;66(1):5–15.
48. Kellen E, Vansant G, Christiaens MR, Neven P, Van Limbergen E. Lifestyle changes and breast cancer prognosis: a review. Breast Cancer Res Treat. 2009;114(1):13–22.
49. Barbaric M, Brooks E, Moore L, Cheifetz O. Effects of physical activity on cancer survival: a systematic review. Physiother Can. 2010;62(1):25–34.
50. Lahart IM, Metsios GS, Nevill AM, Carmichael AR. Physical activity, risk of death and recurrence in breast cancer survivors: a systematic review and meta-analysis of epidemiological studies. Acta Oncol. 2015;54(5):635–54.
51. Irwin ML, McTiernan A, Bernstein L, Gilliland FD, Baumgartner R, Baumgartner K, et al. Physical activity levels among breast cancer survivors. Med Sci Sports Exerc. 2004;36(9):1484–91.
52. Demark-Wahnefried W, Rogers LQ, Alfano CM, Thomson CA, Courneya KS, Meyerhardt JA, et al. Practical clinical interventions for diet, physical activity, and weight control in cancer survivors. CA Cancer J Clin. 2015;65(3):167–89.
53. Schmid D, Leitzmann MF. Association between physical activity and mortality among breast cancer and colorectal cancer survivors: a systematic review and meta-analysis. Ann Oncol. 2014;25(7):1293–311.
54. Underwood JM, Townsend JS, Stewart SL, Buchannan N, Ekwueme DU, Hawkins NA, et al. Surveillance of demographic characteristics and health behaviors among adult cancer survivors – Behavioral Risk Factor Surveillance System, United States, 2009. MMWR Surveill Summ. 2012;61(1):1–23.
55. Kroenke CH, Fung TT, Hu FB, Holmes MD. Dietary patterns and survival after breast cancer diagnosis. J Clin Oncol. 2005;23(36):9295–303.
56. Kwan ML, Weltzien E, Kushi LH, Castillo A, Slattery ML, Caan BJ. Dietary patterns and breast cancer recurrence and survival among women with early-stage breast cancer. J Clin Oncol. 2009;27(6):919–26.
57. Vrieling A, Buck K, Seibold P, Heinz J, Obi N, Flesch-Janys D, et al. Dietary patterns and survival in German postmenopausal breast cancer survivors. Br J Cancer. 2013;108(1):188–92.
58. Chlebowski RT, Blackburn GL, Thomson CA, Nixon DW, Shapiro A, Hoy MK, et al. Dietary fat reduction and breast cancer outcome: interim efficacy results from the Women's Intervention Nutrition Study. J Natl Cancer Inst. 2006;98(24):1767–76.
59. Pierce JP, Natarajan L, Caan BJ, Parker BA, Greenberg ER, Flatt SW, et al. Influence of a diet very high in vegetables, fruit, and fiber and low in fat on prognosis following treatment for breast cancer: the Women's Healthy Eating and Living (WHEL) randomized trial. JAMA. 2007;298(3):289–98.
60. Kwan ML, Kushi LH, Weltzien E, Tam EK, Castillo A, Sweeney C, et al. Alcohol consumption and breast cancer recurrence and survival among women with early-stage breast cancer: the life after cancer epidemiology study. J Clin Oncol. 2010;28(29):4410–6.
61. Berube S, Lemieux J, Moore L, Maunsell E, Brisson J. Smoking at time of diagnosis and breast cancer-specific survival: new findings and systematic review with meta-analysis. Breast Cancer Res. 2014;16(2):R42.
62. Gralow JR, Biermann JS, Farooki A, Fornier MN, Gagel RF, Kumar R, et al. NCCN task force report: bone health in cancer care. J Natl Compr Cancer Netw. 2013;11(Suppl 3):S1–50; quiz S1.
63. Kanis JA, McCloskey EV, Powles T, Paterson AH, Ashley S, Spector T. A high incidence of vertebral fracture in women with breast cancer. Br J Cancer. 1999;79(7–8):1179–81.
64. Chen Z, Maricic M, Bassford TL, Pettinger M, Ritenbaugh C, Lopez AM, et al. Fracture risk among breast cancer survivors: results from the Women's Health Initiative Observational Study. Arch Intern Med. 2005;165(5):552–8.
65. Hadji P, Aapro MS, Body JJ, Gnant M, Brandi ML, Reginster JY, et al. Management of Aromatase Inhibitor-Associated Bone Loss (AIBL) in postmenopausal women with hormone sensitive breast cancer: joint position statement of the IOF, CABS, ECTS, IEG, ESCEO IMS, and SIOG. J Bone Oncol. 2017;7:1–12.
66. Coleman RE, Banks LM, Girgis SI, Kilburn LS, Vrdoljak E, Fox J, et al. Skeletal effects of exemestane on bone-mineral density, bone biomarkers, and fracture incidence in postmenopausal women with early breast cancer participating in the Intergroup Exemestane Study (IES): a randomised controlled study. Lancet Oncol. 2007;8(2):119–27.
67. Forbes JF, Cuzick J, Buzdar A, Howell A, Tobias JS, Baum M. Effect of anastrozole and tamoxifen as adjuvant treatment for early-stage breast cancer: 100-month analysis of the ATAC trial. Lancet Oncol. 2008;9(1):45–53.
68. Rabaglio M, Sun Z, Price KN, Castiglione-Gertsch M, Hawle H, Thurlimann B, et al. Bone fractures among postmenopausal patients with endocrine-responsive early breast cancer treated with 5 years of letrozole or tamoxifen in the BIG 1-98 trial. Ann Oncol. 2009;20(9):1489–98.
69. Amir E, Seruga B, Niraula S, Carlsson L, Ocana A. Toxicity of adjuvant endocrine therapy in postmenopausal breast cancer patients: a systematic review and meta-analysis. J Natl Cancer Inst. 2011;103(17):1299–309.
70. Bliuc D, Nguyen ND, Milch VE, Nguyen TV, Eisman JA, Center JR. Mortality risk associated with low-trauma osteoporotic fracture and subsequent fracture in men and women. JAMA. 2009;301(5):513–21.
71. The World Health Organization Fracture Risk Assessment Tool (FRAX, http://www.sheffield.ac.uk/FRAX).

72. Baum M, Budzar AU, Cuzick J, Forbes J, Houghton JH, Klijn JG, et al. Anastrozole alone or in combination with tamoxifen versus tamoxifen alone for adjuvant treatment of postmenopausal women with early breast cancer: first results of the ATAC randomised trial. Lancet. 2002;359(9324):2131–9.
73. Mehta LS, Watson KE, Barac A, Beckie TM, Bittner V, Cruz-Flores S, et al. Cardiovascular disease and breast cancer: where these entities intersect: a scientific statement from the American Heart Association. Circulation. 2018;137(8):e30–66.
74. Armenian SH, Lacchetti C, Barac A, Carver J, Constine LS, Denduluri N, et al. Prevention and monitoring of cardiac dysfunction in survivors of adult cancers: American Society of Clinical Oncology clinical practice guideline. J Clin Oncol. 2017;35(8):893–911.

Part IV

Common Medical Conditions

Cardiovascular Disease in Women Part 1: Sex and Gender Differences in Cardiovascular Conditions and Risk Factors

21

Alexandra M. Goodwin, Agnes Koczo, Sarah A. Jones, Melissa A. McNeil, and Brigid M. Dolan

Learning Objectives

1. Discuss the impact of cardiovascular disease on women including disease burden and costs of care.
2. Identify CVD risk factors unique to female patients, including those related to menstrual and reproductive health history.

Angela is a 65-year-old woman who is presenting to establish care after her previous physician retired. Her best friend recently had a heart attack, prompting her to read about heart disease in women. She was surprised to learn that women die of heart disease more than they die of other causes and wants to learn more.

Introduction

Physicians caring for women patients must consider CVD risk assessment during the course of routine primary care due to the high morbidity and mortality conferred by cardiovascular diseases. CVD affects about 47.8 million women in the United States and is the number one cause of death overall for American women [1]. Though mortality rates for CVD have decreased, overall CVD in women accounts for about 1 in 3.3 deaths; coronary artery disease specifically accounts for 1 in 8.3 deaths [1, 2]. Direct annual medical costs in the United States attributable to CVD in women are approximately $272.5 billion and rising [3].

The scope of the problem is broad and extends outside of the physician's office. Women are more likely than men to die from myocardial infarction (MI) outside of the hospital. More women have died of ischemic heart disease since 1984 in comparison with their male counterparts [4]. While still low, women's recognition that CVD is the predominant cause death for women has doubled since 1997. Significantly, awareness remains lower in African American and Hispanic populations when compared to White women [5]. Importantly, physicians themselves may have falsely low perception of women's cardiovascular risk, impacting downstream treatment choices and management of CVD risk factors [2, 6, 7]. Part of this misperception may lie in the differential presentation of cardiovascular conditions in women. The incidence and clinical presentations of a number of cardiovascular diseases prevalent in women are briefly discussed in the following paragraph.

For many of the cardiovascular diseases noted below, it is important to recognize that disparities exist within groups of women. For example, Black women in the United States have a higher prevalence of ischemic heart disease when compared to Hispanic and White women (7%, 5.9%, 4.6%, respectively) [8]. A combination of factors including social and environmental factors, clinician implicit bias, and health care system factors all have been hypothesized to play a role

A. M. Goodwin (✉)
New York University, Bellevue Hospital Center, Department of General Internal Medicine and Clinical Innovation, New York, NY, USA
e-mail: alexandra.goodwin@nyulangone.org

A. Koczo
University of Pittsburgh Medical Center Montefiore, Department of Internal Medicine, Pittsburgh, PA, USA
e-mail: koczoa@upmc.edu

S. A. Jones · M. A. McNeil
University of Pittsburgh Medical Center, Department of Medicine, Pittsburgh, PA, USA
e-mail: jonessa3@upmc.edu; mcneilma@upmc.edu

B. M. Dolan
Northwestern University Feinberg School of Medicine, Division of General Internal Medicine and Geriatrics, Department of Medicine, Chicago, IL, USA
e-mail: bdolan@nm.org

S. A. Tilstra et al. (eds.), *Sex- and Gender-Based Women's Health*, https://doi.org/10.1007/978-3-030-50695-7_21

in contributing to said health disparities [9]; further work is needed to address these factors and improve cardiovascular health equity.

Ischemic Heart Disease

Cardiovascular disease encompasses a range of disease processes affecting the coronary and peripheral arterial vessels. The most common form of CVD in women is ischemic heart disease, which includes coronary artery disease and coronary vasospasm, among others. Microvascular dysfunction and microvascular ischemia are also more common in women and may lead to delayed diagnosis of cardiac ischemia [10]. "Cardiac syndrome X"—the combination of typical exertional chest pain, normal coronary angiography, and positive response to stress testing—is more common in pre- and postmenopausal women than their age-matched male counterparts. Women, especially young women, may have poorer outcomes after MI [11] and delayed recognition of anginal symptoms.

Heart Failure

Chronic heart failure impacts women and men differently. In comparison to men, women are more likely to develop congestive heart failure symptoms later in life and are also more likely to have heart failure with preserved ejection fraction. The etiology of heart failure in women is less likely to be from ischemic cardiomyopathy than it is in men, with diabetes mellitus and hypertension as predominant comorbid conditions [12].

Takotsubo Cardiomyopathy

Gender differences in cardiovascular disease are not limited to the common, widespread conditions discussed above. Takotsubo cardiomyopathy (TC), while accounting for only 2–3% of cases of all patients presenting with symptoms of acute coronary syndrome (ACS), preferentially impacts women. In the United States, women are almost nine times as likely as men to develop Takotsubo cardiomyopathy. Postmenopausal women with cardiac risk factors such as diabetes, dyslipidemia, and hypertension were more likely than younger women to develop TC. Age alone conferred an almost fourfold increased risk of the development of this disorder in women over 55 in comparison with controls younger than 55 [13, 14]. This gender-specific impact is not fully understood, but it is posited that postmenopausal women have lost some of the protective effects of estrogen against catecholamine effects on the myocardium.

Spontaneous Coronary Artery Dissection (SCAD)

Women are also differentially impacted by spontaneous coronary artery dissection, with estimates in some case series showing that over 90% of those diagnosed are women [15, 16]. In one long-term study of 87 patients diagnosed with SCAD—one of the most robust available retrospective cohort studies—SCAD presented as a life-threatening condition in greater than 50% of cases. Percutaneous coronary intervention (PCI) in these patients is associated with higher rates of complication, and although long-term survival is better than in those with typical ACS, these patients still have high rates of major adverse cardiac events [17].

Non-atherosclerotic coronary artery disease (NACAD) is an important cause of MI in women under 50, accounting for 30% of MI; in this group, SCAD is the most common etiology, accounting for 24% of MI [16]. Although classically thought of as a disease of younger women, multiple studies have shown the highest prevalence of disease to be in the fifth and sixth decades of life. SCAD should be considered in the differential for ACS and MI [18].

Cerebrovascular Disease

As the fourth leading cause of death for US women, cerebrovascular disease bears particular mention [1]. While stroke is more prevalent in men earlier in life, women over 85 have a higher incidence of stroke and are more likely to be institutionalized or have lasting disability after a stroke than their age-matched male counterparts [19]. An important risk factor for ischemic stroke in women is migraine headache as women with migraine headaches—particularly migraines with aura—have greater risk than those without [20].

Women are less likely than men to receive standard diagnostic workup for possible ischemic CVA upon arrival to an Emergency Department [21]. Similar to differences in MI presentation, women may be less likely than men to present with "typical" stroke symptoms such as gait disturbance and/or imbalance, sensory abnormalities, dysarthria, or aphasia, leading to possible delays in treatment [22]. Women are more likely than men to initially come to medical attention with nontraditional symptoms of stroke such as pain, unclassifiable neurologic symptoms, disorientation, or nonspecific symptoms [23]. There is also some evidence to suggest that women with acute stroke will present to the ED later in their course of symptoms [24].

Asymptomatic carotid stenosis—a potential precursor to ischemic stroke—is less common in women than in men, with a prevalence of about 2.2%, although this value increases with age [25]. Cerebral aneurysms, however, have a higher incidence in women with 22.5 per 100,000 people, according to one large study; women 75–84 years of age have the highest incidence [26]. In comparison with men, women with unruptured or asymptomatic cerebral aneurysms are more likely to present with subarachnoid hemorrhage and are more likely to have multiple aneurysms that present later in life [27].

Peripheral Arterial Disease

Peripheral arterial disease (PAD) was classically thought to have a higher prevalence in men, but recent studies using the ankle-brachial index, a highly sensitive and specific test, demonstrates that women may in fact have higher rates of PAD than men (15.6% vs. 13.4%) [28]. PAD disproportionately impacts the elderly where women comprise an increasing sector of the elderly population, so rates of PAD in women are expected to increase [27, 28–30]. PAD confers a two- to fourfold increase in the rates of cardiovascular morbidity and mortality; thus, it is important to identify and treat [31].

Women are more likely than men to have asymptomatic disease—estimated at about 50% of female patients with PAD—which can lead to delayed diagnosis and treatment. Additionally, it is estimated that only 10% of women with PAD have "classic" anginal symptoms. Their symptoms are more likely to be misinterpreted as arthritis or spinal stenosis. Women have similar rates of traditional risk factors for PAD development such as obesity, tobacco use, hypertension, and dyslipidemia. However, women may have comorbid conditions like depression, osteoporosis, and hypothyroidism that are under-recognized as being associated with an elevated risk of developing PAD, as discussed in a 2014 systematic review. For example, women diagnosed with PAD may have a fourfold increase in their odds of having baseline depression in comparison with men. Rates of PAD may also be increased in patients with subclinical hypothyroidism, which is more likely to impact women than men. Women with a history of hypertension during pregnancy had an adjusted OR of 1.6 (95% CI 1.04–2.49) in comparison with women with normotensive pregnancies, which further underscores the need for inclusion of a reproductive and obstetric history in the assessment of cardiovascular risk [28]. Data from the RATIO (Risk of Arterial Thrombosis in Relation to Oral Contraceptives) study showed an increased risk of PAD development in women aged 18–49 years using oral contraceptives in comparison with no contraceptive use (OR 3.8 [95% CI 2.4–5.8]) [32].

Traditional Cardiovascular Risk Factors

As you take her history, you find that Angela has a BMI of 32 and is a former cigarette smoker. She used to exercise regularly but after moving recently, she has been unable to get into a routine.

In this section, we review traditional risk factors and relevant gender differences. The next sections discuss female-specific risk factors. These risk factors are summarized at the end of this chapter.

Age and Family History of CHD

Like men, women have increased risk of CHD and stroke as they become older. Family history of premature CHD—defined as a first-degree male relative under age 50 or a female under age 60—is also an important consideration [33, 34].

Hypertension

Hypertension is a well-established risk factor for cardiovascular disease. There are not well-described sex differences in how hypertension manifests in men and women outside of hypertensive disorders of pregnancy (see Risk Factors Associated with the Reproductive Life Cycle below). However, women are more likely to develop hypertension later in life and have poorer blood pressure control than men [35].

Dyslipidemia

Postmenopausal women are disproportionately impacted by dyslipidemia and are less likely to be prescribed lipid-lowering therapy. This discrepancy may be attributed to provider bias as well as underestimation of women's CVD risk [36]. One cohort study identified several independent variables associated with decreased statin use: increased age, history of smoking, decreased referrals to cardiologists, and increased reports of adverse events [37]. These findings were supported by the USAGE (Understanding Statin Use in America and Gaps in Patient Education) study, which found that in comparison with man, women are more likely to stop taking a statin or switch agents because of muscle symptoms. Importantly, more women in the USAGE study reported that their physician did not explain their CVD risk in relation to their LDL cholesterol levels in comparison with men prescribed statins (36% vs. 24%; $p < 0.0001$). Among current statin users in the USAGE study, women were also less likely to be prescribed adjunctive therapies such as niacin, fibrates, or fish oil [38]. These pervasive discrepancies—from counseling and medication use to adherence—in the provision and use of statins in women are important targets for advocacy for and adequate treatment of female patients with hyperlipidemia.

Diabetes Mellitus and Metabolic Syndrome

Diabetes mellitus (DM) and metabolic syndrome are key risk factors for cardiovascular disease in women. Overall, men suffer more cardiovascular deaths attributable to diabetes than women. However, women with DM have between three and six times the risk of death from CAD than women without DM. Additionally, female diabetics have a higher risk of death attributable to CAD in comparison with men with DM and fatal MI [39]. This difference may be attenuated when controlling for other traditional risk factors such as obesity, smoking status, and hyperlipidemia [40–42]. The presence of DM may also increase risk of the development of heart failure and PAD in affected women. The exact mechanism of the increased risk of CVD found in diabetic women is not fully understood, but may be related to the impact of DM and metabolic disorder on increased central adiposity, endothelial dysfunction, and inflammation [43].

Smoking

A 2011 meta-analysis showed that when adjusted for other CVD risk factors, women who smoked had a 25% increased risk of the development of coronary artery disease compared to men, with the exception of the youngest cohort of women included in the study (age 30–44). This risk increased by 2% yearly [44]. Identifying female smokers for early intervention is a critical strategy to reduce future CVD risk.

Obesity and Sedentary Lifestyle

Overweight and obesity remain important risk factors in the development of CVD for both women and men [45]. Data from the year 2015 to 2016 from the NHANES survey in the United States show that in comparison with Hispanic men and with non-Hispanic Black and non-Hispanic Asian men, women in these cohorts had a higher prevalence of obesity [46]. Analysis of a large, multiethnic cohort of postmenopausal women shows a "dose effect" of obesity on overall mortality and on the development of CHF: women with severe obesity (BMI 40 or greater) had an 88% increased risk of all-cause mortality. Additionally, their risk of developing CHF was five times higher than normal BMI cohorts. This study also suggests a synergistic effect of obesity and traditional cardiac risk factors such as hypertension, smoking, and diabetes mellitus, finding a 15-fold increase in coronary heart disease in severely obese women with multiple risk factors (smoking, hypertension, diabetes mellitus) in comparison with their normal-weight, low-risk female counterparts [47]. Further, the Framingham Heart Study suggests that being obese increased women's coronary artery disease risk by 64% in comparison to 46% in men [43].

Sedentary lifestyle is also an important risk factor to consider in women patients, as sitting for ≥10 hours each day was associated with greater CVD risk than sitting for <5 hours per day [48]. This may be of particular concern as there is evidence to suggest that women are less physically active than men [8] and thus more vulnerable to the impact of the added CVD conferred by inactivity.

Risk Factors Throughout the Reproductive Life Cycle

You ask about Angela's pregnancy history. She is surprised that you ask, as she had her last child at age 32 and she doesn't recall physicians asking her about pregnancy since then. She had preeclampsia with her last pregnancy and had to deliver the baby at 37 weeks gestational age.

When evaluating a patient's cardiovascular risk, a reproductive and pregnancy history is a crucial, though often overlooked, aspect of data gathering. Data show that internists are less likely to obtain a pregnancy history than gynecologists, though they are more likely to order appropriate follow-up testing once that history is obtained [49]. Recent data indicate that both internists and obstetrician/gynecologists miss opportunities to identify pregnancy-related risk factors and pursue appropriate risk stratification testing for patients. There are multiple factors in a woman's pregnancy history that may impact their cardiovascular risk [50]. As with traditional risk factors, disparities in reproductive risk factors exist between groups of women; non-Hispanic Black women have a greater likelihood of preterm delivery, any hypertensive disorder of pregnancy, or small for gestational age birth when compared to non-Black women in the United States [51].

Risk Factors Associated with Pregnancy

Hypertensive Disorders of Pregnancy

A personal history of preeclampsia occurring with any pregnancy has been linked to an increased risk of major adverse cardiac events and the development of hypertension later in life. Women with one lifetime birth with preeclampsia are almost twice as likely to develop a major coronary event later in life than women who did not have preeclampsia (HR 2.1 [95% CI 1.73–2.65]). When preeclampsia is combined with a small-for-gestational-age infant or preterm delivery, the likelihood of a subsequent major coronary event is further increased (HR 3.3 [95% CI 2.37–4.57]) [52]. The time of preeclampsia diagnosis may impact future disease risk as well. One study found that a diagnosis of preeclampsia before 37 weeks is associated with an eightfold increase in the risk of subsequent ischemic heart disease in comparison with women diagnosed after 37 weeks and may increase the risk of stroke later in life twofold [53]. Preeclampsia itself may increase the subsequent risk of diabetes mellitus later in life; one study found a threefold increase in subsequent type 2 diabetes mellitus in mothers with preeclampsia in comparison with mothers without preeclampsia, even when controlling for multiple factors such as preterm delivery and small for gestational age births [54].

Gestational Diabetes

Gestational diabetes mellitus (GDM) is defined as the onset or recognition of impaired glucose tolerance during pregnancy. Although the exact mechanisms for the development of GDM are unknown, it creates a state of chronic inflammation and cytokine release. Most clinicians recognize that the diagnosis of GDM is a risk factor for the subsequent development of DM [55]. Clinicians also must recognize that the presence of GDM is an independent risk factor for future CVD, even if a patient does not develop non-gestational diabetes. This risk is compounded in a woman with a family history of type 2 diabetes and is attenuated when adjusted for weight gain in pregnancy [56, 57].

Preterm Delivery and Small for Gestational Age Births

Even in the absence of preeclampsia, preterm delivery is associated with an increased risk of maternal cardiovascular disease. Ten percent of pregnancies in the United States result in preterm delivery each year. Women who give birth to a preterm infant have a 20–40% increased risk of future CVD events in comparison with women who did not experience a preterm delivery. This risk almost doubles for women who deliver before 32 weeks of gestation. The risk is slightly decreased when pre- and post-pregnancy cardiovascular risk factors such as hypertension, diabetes mellitus, hypercholesterolemia, and weight gain are taken into account, though according to a major cohort study, these risks only account for <25% of the association between preterm first births and the subsequent development of CVD [58, 59].

Small for gestational age births (SGA) have been shown to increase the risk of subsequent cardiovascular events such as congestive heart failure and hypertensive heart disease. SGA delivery is an independent risk factor for CVD mortality even when controlling for factors such as obesity, diabetes, and the presence of preeclampsia [60].

Spontaneous Pregnancy Loss

Eliciting a history of spontaneous pregnancy loss is also an important component of cardiovascular risk assessment in your female patients. History of recurrent miscarriage (in one study, defined as over three spontaneous pregnancy losses) conferred an almost fivefold increased risk of later MI in comparison with no spontaneous pregnancy loss when adjusted for age, hypertension, BMI, use of tobacco and alcohol, amount of physical activity, and presence of metabolic risk factors. The risk of MI increased by about 40% for each miscarriage. Notably, induced abortion does not confer added risk of MI, nor does miscarriage increase risk of CVA. Having a stillbirth was also associated with an approximately 3.5 times increased risk of MI [55].

Weight Gain and Pregnancy

Obesity and overweight are known risk factors for the development of CVD, as discussed above. In one study, women who retain postpartum weight after 1 year were found to have increased body weight after 15 years, which in turn may confer increased cardiovascular risk [61]. Additionally, multiple studies have shown that increased weight gain in pregnancy and retention of weight even 3 months after pregnancy have adverse effects on BMI, blood pressure, and lipid profiles, which may persist for years [62, 63].

Other Risk Factors Related to the Reproductive Cycle

Menarche and Premenstrual Syndrome

Data are mixed on whether early menarche—defined as menarche occurring over two standard deviations earlier than the mean for other girls of the same race and geographic location—increases subsequent risk of CVD. It may increase the risk of having metabolic syndrome earlier in life, which is itself a risk factor for the development of CVD. In one meta-analysis, with early menarche defined as <12, early menarche was associated with increased risk of overall mortality [64].

Combined Oral Contraceptives

The use of combined oral contraceptive pills (COCs) that contain both estrogen and progesterone not only increases the risk of arterial and venous thromboembolism but also may increase the risk of unwanted cardiovascular outcomes, especially in women with preexisting risk factors for CVD such as uncontrolled hypertension, obesity, or active tobacco use [65]. Women over 35 who are active smokers may have up to ten times greater risk of MI than nonsmoking woman who take COCs. Similarly, this group has an increased risk of both hemorrhagic and ischemic stroke. In women with hypertension, the use of combined oral contraceptive pills may increase the risk of MI twofold [66]. For these reasons, the Centers for Disease Control Medical Eligibility Criteria for Contraceptive Use (MEC) and other guidelines discourage the use of COCs for women with these CVD risk factors [67].

Menopause

Estrogen pays a role in lowering lipids, especially LDL, and also improves endothelial function [68]. The decrease in the amount of circulating estrogen after menopause may mitigate some of these protective effects and contribute to the higher rates of heart disease seen in postmenopausal women. Postmenopausal women, those most at risk for CVD, have a high incidence of obesity, about 40% [69]. Even if a woman does not gain weight after menopause, menopause is associated with redistributed body fat, increasing abdominal fat waist circumference, which is linked to cardiometabolic disease [8].

Hormone Therapy

Hormone therapy (HT) in postmenopausal women has long been a controversial topic in women's health. The proposed beneficial effects of estrogen on the vasculature in vitro and in premenopausal women are discordant with the clinical CVD outcomes observed in postmenopausal women on HT. An evolving understanding distinguishes the beneficial effects of endogenous estrogen in the premenopausal endothelium versus that of exogenous estrogen in postmenopausal women. Epidemiologic evidence demonstrated a tenfold increase in CVD in postmenopausal women, compared to about a fivefold increase in age-matched men [70].

Early interest in the cardioprotective effect of estrogen comes from data in animal models, showing estrogen had numerous positive effects on both the cellular and molecular levels [71, 72]. Proposed mechanisms include increasing nitric oxide synthesis and availability, propagating degradation of oxygen free radicals, and altering the expression of enzymes responsible for the creation of free radial species, thereby functioning as an antioxidant [73, 74].

The beneficial estrogen effect in animal models was further supported by early retrospective observational studies [75–77]. Subsequently, two large randomized clinical trials, the Heart and Estrogen/Progestin Replacement Study (HERS) and the Women's Health Initiative (WHI), both failed to show an overall benefit to HT in either primary or secondary prevention of CVD [78, 79]. Amidst concerns of several individual disease outcomes from these large trials including CVD, endometrial cancer, breast cancer, and thromboembolic disease, there was an overall decline in the use of HT in the 2000s.

Closer analysis of subgroups within the WHI found that women in younger age cohorts had more favorable CVD outcomes giving rise to the timing hypothesis. In the timing hypothesis, HT given within 5–10 years of menopause has different effects than when initiated later into menopause. Age-stratified analysis of the WHI demonstrated statistically significant hazard ratio reduction for CHD mortality at 0.76 for women within 10 years of menopause, 1.10 for women within 10–20 years of menopause, and 1.28 for women more than 20 years since menopause [80]. This was further supported by a large meta-analysis looking at 23 HT clinical trials encompassing nearly 40,000 women [81, 82]. More recent studies have sought to look at subclinical end points of estrogen's effect on CVD, including carotid intimal thickness (CIMT), and have noted a decrease in progression of CIMT as compared to age-matched cohorts when HT is given within 6 years of menopause as compared to when given to women >10 years into menopause, further supporting the timing hypothesis [83].

Long-term outcomes using 18 years of cumulative follow-up data from the WHI trials provided reassuring data for providers who are still unsure about recommending HT. It found no difference in all-cause mortality between hormone users (including both the combination of estrogen plus progesterone and the estrogen alone cohort) and nonusers (27.1% vs. 27.6%; hazard ratio [HR], 0.99 [95% CI, 0.94–1.03]). Similarly, no difference in CVD mortality, CHD mortality, or stroke mortality was found with the CVD-specific death rate in the pooled cohort at 8.9% in the hormone therapy group vs. 9.0% in the nonuser group with HR 1.00 [95% CI, 0.92–1.08], CHD mortality with HR 0.97 [95% CI, 0.86–1.09], and stroke mortality with HR 1.06 [95% CI, 0.9–1.25]. On age-stratified analysis, younger women (aged 50–59) did not exhibit significant differences with respect to all-cause mortality in the pooled cohort on cumulative follow-up (HR 0.89 [95% CI 0.79–1.01]) as compared to older women both in the 60–69 age group (HR 0.98 [95% CI 0.91–1.05]) and in the 70–79 age group (HR 1.03 [95% CI, 0.96–1.10], p value for the trend = 0.06) [84].

Current guidelines do not recommend using estrogen for the primary or secondary prevention of CVD. The use of HT at the lowest effective dose remains appropriate to treat early menopausal symptoms in women who do not have contraindications [85, 86] and, reassuringly, does not appear to negatively impact long-term CVD mortality and may be beneficial if started early in menopause [84]. Refer to the menopause chapter for additional recommendations.

Lactation and CVD Risk Reduction in Women

Lactation following pregnancy is thought to reset maladaptive metabolic changes occurring during pregnancy. The relationship between lactation and subclinical and clinical CVD and cardiovascular risk factors such as hypertension and diabetes has been examined in several studies [87]. Less data exist related to the association of lactation on postpartum weight and dyslipidemia.

Cardiovascular Disease

Markers of subclinical and clinical atherosclerosis, including atherosclerosis and carotid intima-media thickness (CIMT), decrease with lactation. One prospective study examined 846 women without heart disease prior to pregnancy and found a graded inverse association between duration of breastfeeding and CIMT for 20 years postpartum [88]. Another study demonstrated that women with no breastfeeding history had increased odds of developing aortic calcifications (OR 3.85 [95% CI 1.47–10.00]) and coronary calcifications (OR 2.78 [95% CI 1.05–7.14]), of which aortic calcifications remained significant even after controlling for BMI and other cardiovascular risk factors [89].

In addition, the Nurses' Health Study found women with a lifetime breastfeeding duration of >23 months were less likely to experience an acute coronary event compared to their counterparts who never breastfed (HR 0.63 [95% CI 0.51–0.77]). This remained significant after controlling for a number of cardiovascular risk factors [90]. Another large, prospective study with nearly 22,000 Norwegian women found that over 15 years of follow-up, women without heart disease prior to pregnancy had an increased risk of cardiovascular mortality if they never breastfed as compared to women with cumulative lifetime lactation more than 24 months (HR 2.86 [95% CI 1.51–5.39]), but the trend of breastfeeding and mortality benefit was not statistically significant in women who breastfed for a total of 7–12 months [91]. The beneficial associations between lifetime lactation duration with clinical cardiovascular disease and mortality lose significance for women over age 65. This suggests that the risks of age and menopause outweigh the benefits from lactation for women in their later adult years.

Hypertension

Several retrospective and prospective studies have found breastfeeding to have a dose-response relationship (longer total duration of breastfeeding confers the lowest risk) with lowering risk for developing hypertension [92, 93]. Of note, this correlation was not true for women over 64 years of age, in which the risk for hypertension due to aging again seems to outweigh any risk reduction that comes from lactation [94, 95]. While gestational hypertension and preeclampsia increase the risk for hypertension in later adult life, no risk factor schema including lactation histories has been validated; it is unknown whether lactation reduces risk for these high-risk groups.

Diabetes

Women with gestational diabetes (GDM) have a tenfold higher risk of developing diabetes in later life [96, 97]. While a dearth of longitudinal studies in this area exists, emerging data suggest that lactation may be protective against the development of diabetes and cardiometabolic disease [69]. Normal pregnancy confers a state of increased insulin resistance in order to divert nutrition to the fetus by impeding the use and storage of glucose in maternal tissues [98]. Lactation counteracts this by redirecting glucose for milk production [99]. One meta-analysis found that breastfeeding duration and diabetes risk was protective with a hazard ratio 0.89 (95% CI 0.82–0.97), though this was no longer significant when controlling for factors including baseline BMI [100]. Another meta-analysis found a significant dose-dependent nonlinear (1–3 months vs. 6–10 months) decrease in diabetes with lactation, including one study with GDM patients, where improved risk attributed to lactation remained significant even after controlling for BMI [101]. Favorable glucose metabolism has been positively associated with lactation, and insulin resistance has been associated with impaired lactogenesis. These associations confound the results such that the relationship could be women with good glucose metabolism breastfeed more easily rather than breastfeeding is protective for improving glucose metabolism [102].

Stroke

Several studies have examined the impact of breastfeeding on future stroke risk. In a prospective cohort study of 300,000 Chinese women, women who breastfed had a decreased risk of stroke, hemorrhagic or ischemic, when compared to women who had never breastfed (HR, 0.83; 0.79–0.87). Each additional 6 months of breastfeeding was associated with further reduced risk [103]. A recent analysis of the Women's Health Initiative (WHI) Observation Study sought to examine

Table 21.1 Summary of observed effects of lifetime lactation on cardiovascular disease and its risk factors

Lifetime duration of breastfeeding					
		<3 months	3–12 months	12–23 months	>23 months
Cardiovascular disease	Calcification aorta		↓		
	Calcification coronary artery		↓		
	Myocardial infarction				↓
	Stroke	↓		↓	
	Mortality		↓	X	↓
Hypertension			↓	↓	↓

↓ Decrease in risk
X No association. Insufficient evidence to observe trend. See text
Cumulative lifetime breastfeeding for at least 3–12 months is recommended

whether breastfeeding has an impact on the risk of developing stroke in later life. It found that of the 80,191 parous women in the study, about 58% (46,699) reported some history of breastfeeding. The study showed that women who reported any breastfeeding as compared to those who had never breastfed had a 23% lower risk of stroke (adjusted HR 0.77; 95% CI 0.70–0.83) even after adjusting for non-modifiable confounders. A subgroup analysis across races noted that the protective effect of breastfeeding on risk of stroke was strongest for Black women (adjusted HR 0.52; 95% CI 0.37–0.71). A further, graded, inverse relationship was also noted between risk of stroke and duration of breastfeeding among both White and Black women. Specifically, the association was stronger with women who reported longer breastfeeding durations and among non-Hispanic White and non-Hispanic Black women (test for trend $P < 0.01$). This study both supports the protective effect of breastfeeding on stroke risk while highlighting disparities in risk for Hispanic and Black women who have lower rates of breastfeeding and increased rates of stroke relative to their White counterparts [104].

Table 21.1 summarizes the protective effects of lactation on ASCVD and hypertension. We propose counseling reproductive age women that 3–12 months of lifetime lactation can protect against ASCVD and hypertension at least until age 65.

Emerging Risk CVD Risk Factors in Women

> *Angela comes back to see you 4 years later. Just after her visit with you, she began exercising regularly and lost 10 pounds. She was then diagnosed with breast cancer and did not come back to see you due to the many visits she needed for surgery, chemotherapy, and radiation. She is now 1-year status-post completion of those therapies and in remission on anastrozole.*

History of Radiation Therapy

A history of previous mantle field radiation therapy or radiation therapy to the chest wall or breasts increases the risk of developing ischemic heart disease in a dose-dependent fashion that is proportional to the mean amount of radiation delivered, with a 7.4% increase in coronary events for each 1 Gy of radiation delivered. This risk remains increased for about 30 years after the radiation is administered [105]. Women who receive left-sided radiation have a higher risk of developing CVD in comparison to women with right-sided breast cancers [106].

Other Cancer Therapy

Radiation is not the only cancer therapy that confers an increased risk of developing CVD. Anthracyclines and HER2 receptor antagonists are both associated with macrovascular and microvascular cardiotoxicity, risks that may be potentiated by co-administration with radiation therapy. A recent longitudinal prospective cohort study demonstrated steady decline in left ventricular ejection fraction (LVEF) with both doxorubicin and trastuzumab, which showed a 3.8% decline and 2.8% decline in LVEF after 3 years, respectively. Those patients who received both agents had an average decline in their EF of 6.6% [107]. A number of factors are considered to confer additional risk for the development of cardiovascular complications from breast cancer therapies: age greater than 60, presence of two or more CVD risk factors, preexisting valvular dysfunction, history of MI, and preexisting mildly depressed EF (55%) [108]. While the use of aromatase inhibitors has not been found to increase risk of subsequent ischemic heart disease, it does increase the risk of subsequent dysrhythmia, pericarditis, and valvular dysfunction (HR 1.29 [1.11–1.50] [109].

Depression

Depression is an emerging risk factor for the development of CAD and is increasingly being recognized as a prognostic factor in recovery from major cardiovascular adverse events such as MI [110]. The presence of depression and anxiety may be a stronger risk factor in women than in men [111], and early treatment is warranted.

Table 21.2 Summary of cardiovascular risk factors in women

Traditional CVD risk factors	Risk factors associated with pregnancy, estrogens, and the reproductive cycle	Emerging risk factors
Obesity [43–47] Hypertension [35] Smoking status [44] Family history [33, 34] Age [33, 34] Sedentary lifestyle [48] Diabetes mellitus (DM) [39] Metabolic syndrome [43] Dyslipidemia [36–38]	Pregnancy associated: Hypertensive disorders of pregnancy [52–54] Small for gestational age births [58–60] Spontaneous pregnancy loss [55] Preterm delivery [58, 59] Weight retention after pregnancy [61–63] Gestational DM [55–57] Lactation (negative risk factor) [87–104] Reproductive cycle: Use of COCs [65–67] Early menopause [68–70] Early menarche [64] Hormone therapy: Extended use 10 years after the menopausal transition [78–83]	Depression [110, 111] Autoimmune disease [43, 112, 113] Inflammatory conditions [112, 113] Atrial fibrillation [114–116] Provider bias [9–11, 38] Cancer therapy: Aromatase inhibitors [109] Anthracyclines [107, 108] HER2 receptor antagonists [107, 108] Radiation therapy to chest [105, 106]

Autoimmune and Inflammatory Diseases

Both men and women with autoimmune and inflammatory disorders have increased CVD mortality. This is thought to stem from antigen response causing damage to tissues and endothelium [112, 113]. Patients with rheumatoid arthritis (RA) have a 50% higher risk of CVA and a two- to threefold increase in MI when compared to those without autoimmune disease. Patients with systemic lupus erythematosus (SLE) also carry increased risk of MI. The prevalence of autoimmune diseases like RA and SLE is higher in women, and thus women bear the higher burden of this increased CVD risk [43].

Presence of Atrial Fibrillation

While atrial fibrillation is more prevalent in men than in women, women have increased morbidity and all-cause mortality from the condition [114, 115]. Of note, women have increased risk of CVA and MI related to their atrial fibrillation in comparison to age-matched men [116]. Table 21.2 provides a summary of cardiovascular risk factors in women.

Summary Points

1. Women in the United States have high rates of cardiovascular disease which may be under-recognized and undertreated.
2. Women and men are both at increased risk for cardiovascular disease from diabetes, smoking, and sedentary lifestyles, but women face unique risks: cardiometabolic complications of pregnancy and greater incidence of autoimmune and inflammatory disease, depression, and cancer treatments that confer additional risk. A thorough pregnancy history is critical to assessing cardiovascular risk for women patients.

Review Questions

1. Jane is a 58-year-old woman who presents for annual PE. She endorses a healthy diet and regular exercise. She is a nonsmoker and has two healthy adult children. Her past medical history is negative for a history of hypertension, diabetes, stroke, or heart attack. However, her running buddy recently had a heart attack and she is worried that she might as well. On exam, her BMI is 24 and her blood pressure is 118/70.

   You assess her cardiovascular disease risk as:
   A. Low risk
   B. Moderate risk
   C. High risk
   D. Not enough data to calculate risk

   The correct answer is D. While Jane appears to be in good health, she notes at least two prior pregnancies and we do not know her pregnancy history. In addition to checking her lipids, in order to fully determine a patient's cardiovascular disease risk, one must ask a patient if she had any history of preterm delivery, small-for-gestational age delivery, and GDM or hypertensive disorders of pregnancy, including preeclampsia [4, 114].
2. Miriam is a 48-year-old woman who presents to establish care. She reports a history of severe preeclampsia during her first pregnancy in her mid-30s. Her labor was otherwise without incident and her baby was born healthy and at term. Her health history is otherwise unremarkable. She had not mentioned this to her prior internist, but heard about an increase in US maternal morbidity on the radio and now is concerned. She asks if her history of preeclampsia confers any risk to her health now.

   You tell her that compared to a woman with otherwise similar CVD risk factors, her history of preeclampsia increases her risk of developing ischemic heart disease in the next 12 years by roughly how much?
   A. No change
   B. Risk is decreased
   C. Twofold increase
   D. Fourfold increase

   The correct answer is C. A preeclampsia history is a significant risk factor for the development of future CVD. In two separate trials, risk was found to be greater than 50%. Riise et al. found a 60% increased risk of subsequent major adverse cardiac event in women with preeclampsia during their first pregnancy when compared with other women without preeclampsia while controlling for other CVD risk factors. Lykke et al. found an 80% increase in risk of ischemic heart disease in women with preeclampsia during their first delivery, which was corroborated by a meta-analysis showing a RR of 1.81 for preeclamptic women in developing ischemic heart disease after 12 years, which overall shows a roughly twofold increase in risk of IHD development of preeclampsia [52, 54].

3. One of your long-term patients presents for a routine follow-up visit. She is 65 years old, Caucasian, and generally feels well. Her past medical history includes rate-controlled non-valvular atrial fibrillation, for which she also takes rivaroxaban. She is of a normal weight. She has hypertension well controlled on medication.

   All else being similar, which of these aspects of her medical history increases her ASCVD risk in comparison to a male patient with similar demographics and health profile?

   A. Her age
   B. Her atrial fibrillation
   C. Her race
   D. Her hypertension

   The correct answer is B. While this patient's age and hypertension both increase her risk of cardiovascular disease, atrial fibrillation in women has been shown to increase all-cause mortality, cardiovascular mortality and events, and risk of stroke to a greater extent than it does in men with similar risks [114–116].

References

1. Health COoWs. Leading causes of death in females, 2014 (current listing). 2017. https://www.cdc.gov/women/lcod/2014/race-ethnicity/index.htm. Accessed 2/1/2018.
2. Benjamin EJ, Blaha MJ, Chiuve SE, Cushman M, Das SR, Deo R, American Heart Association Council on, Epidemiology and Prevention Statistics Committee and Stroke Statistics, Subcommittee, et al. Heart disease and stroke statistics: 2017 update: a report from the American Heart Association. Circulation. 2017;135:e146–603.
3. Heidenreich PA, Trogden JG, Khavjou OA, Butler J, Dracup K, Ezekowitz MD, et al. Forecasting the future of cardiovascular disease in the United States: a policy statement from the American Heart Association. Circulation. 2011;123:933–44. https://doi.org/10.1161/CIR.0b013e31820a55f5.
4. Shaw LJ, Bairey Merz CN, Pepine CJ, et al. Insights from the NHLBI-Sponsored Women's Ischemia Syndrome Evaluation (WISE) study: part I: gender differences in traditional and novel risk factors, symptom evaluation, and gender-optimized diagnostic strategies. J Am Coll Cardiol. 2006;47(3, Supplement):S4–S20.
5. Mosca L, Mochari-Greenberger H, Dolor RJ, Newby LK, Robb KJ. Twelve-year follow-up of American women's awareness of cardiovascular disease risk and barriers to heart health. Circ Cardiovasc Qual Outcomes. 2010;3(2):120–7. https://doi.org/10.1161/CIRCOUTCOMES.109.915538.
6. Mosca L, Linfante AH, Benjamin EJ, et al. National study of physician awareness and adherence to cardiovascular disease prevention guidelines. Circulation. 2005;111(4):499.
7. Gu Q, Burt VL, Paulose-Ram R, Dillon CF. Gender differences in hypertension treatment, drug utilization patterns, and blood pressure control among US adults with hypertension: data from the National Health and Nutrition Examination Survey 1999–2004. Am J Hypertens. 2008;21(7):789–98.
8. McSweeney JC, Rosenfeld AG, Abel WM, et al. Preventing and experiencing ischemic heart disease as a woman: state of the science: a scientific statement from the American Heart Association. Circulation. 2016;133(13):1302–31.
9. Green AR, Carney DR, Pallin DJ, Ngo LH, Raymond KL, Iezzoni LI, Banaji MR. Implicit bias among physicians and its prediction of thrombolysis decisions for black and white patients. J Gen Intern Med. 2007;22(9):1231–8.
10. Reis SE, Holubkov R, Conrad Smith AJ, et al. Coronary microvascular dysfunction is highly prevalent in women with chest pain in the absence of coronary artery disease: results from the NHLBI WISE study. Am Heart J. 2001;141(5):735–41.
11. Ford ES, Capewell S. Coronary heart disease mortality among young adults in the U.S. from 1980 through 2002: concealed leveling of mortality rates. J Am Coll Cardiol. 2007;50(22):2128–32.
12. Aimo A, Vergaro G, Barison A, et al. Sex-related differences in chronic heart failure. Int J Cardiol. 2018;255:145–51.
13. Deshmukh A, Kumar G, Pant S, Rihal C, Murugiah K, Mehta JL. Prevalence of Takotsubo cardiomyopathy in the United States. Am Heart J. 2012;164(1):66–71.e61.
14. Kato K, Lyon AR, Ghadri J-R, Templin C. Takotsubo syndrome: aetiology, presentation and treatment. Heart. 2017;103(18):1461.
15. Saw J, Ricci D, Starovoytov A, Fox R, Buller CE. Spontaneous coronary artery dissection: prevalence of predisposing conditions including fibromuscular dysplasia in a tertiary center cohort. JACC Cardiovasc Interv. 2013;6(1):44–52. https://doi.org/10.1016/j.jcin.2012.08.017. Epub 2012 Dec 19.
16. Saw J, Aymong E, Mancini GB, Sedlak T, Starovoytov A, Ricci D. Nonatherosclerotic coronary disease in young women. Can J Cardiol. 2014;30(7):814–9. https://doi.org/10.1016/j.cjca.2014.01.011.
17. Tweet MS, Hayes SN, Pitta SR, et al. Clinical features, management, and prognosis of spontaneous coronary artery dissection. Circulation. 2012;126(5):579–88. https://doi.org/10.1161/CIRCULATIONAHA.112.105718.
18. Alfonso F, Paulo M, Lennie V, et al. Spontaneous coronary artery dissection: long-term follow-up of a large series of patients prospectively managed with a "conservative" therapeutic strategy. JACC Cardiovasc Interv. 2012;5(10):1062–70.
19. Petrea RE, Beiser AS, Seshadri S, Kelly-Hayes M, Kase CS, Wolf PA. Gender differences in stroke incidence and poststroke disability in the Framingham heart study. Stroke. 2009;40(4):1032.
20. Schurks M, Rist PM, Bigal ME, Buring JE, Lipton RB, Kurth T. Migraine and cardiovascular disease: systematic review and meta-analysis. BMJ. 2009;339:b3914.
21. Smith MA, Lisabeth LD, Brown DL, Morgenstern LB. Gender comparisons of diagnostic evaluation for ischemic stroke patients. Neurology. 2005;65(6):855.
22. Turtzo LC, McCullough LD. Sex differences in stroke. Cerebrovas Dis (Basel, Switzerland). 2008;26(5):462–74.
23. Labiche LA, Chan W, Saldin KR, Morgenstern LB. Sex and acute stroke presentation. Ann Emerg Med. 2002;40(5):453–60.
24. Reeves MJ, Bushnell CD, Howard G, et al. Sex differences in stroke: epidemiology, clinical presentation, medical care, and outcomes. Lancet Neurol. 2008;7(10):915–26. https://doi.org/10.1016/S1474-4422(08)70193-5.

25. de Weerd M, Greving JP, de Jong AWF, Buskens E, Bots ML. Prevalence of asymptomatic carotid artery stenosis according to age and sex. Stroke. 2009;40(4):1105.
26. Asaithambi G, Adil MM, Chaudhry SA, Qureshi AI. Incidences of unruptured intracranial aneurysms and subarachnoid hemorrhage: results of a statewide study. J Vasc Interv Neurol. 2014;7(3):14–7.
27. Ghods AJ, Lopes D, Chen M. Gender differences in cerebral aneurysm location. Front Neurol. 2012;3:78.
28. Barochiner J, Aparicio LS, Waisman GD. Challenges associated with peripheral arterial disease in women. Vasc Health Risk Manag. 2014;10:115–28.
29. Vavra AK, Kibbe MR. Women and peripheral arterial disease. Women's Health (Lond Engl). 2009;5(6):669–83.
30. Simmons A, Steffen K. Peripheral arterial disease in women. Rev Cardiovasc Med. 2011;12(3):123–31.
31. Higgins JP, Higgins JA. Epidemiology of peripheral arterial disease in women. J Epidemiol. 2003;13(1):1–14.
32. Van Den Bosch MA, Kemmeren JM, Tanis BC, Mali WP, Helmerhorst FM, Rosendaal FR, et al. The RATIO study: oral contraceptives and the risk of peripheral arterial disease in young women. J Thromb Haemost. 2003;1(3):439–44.
33. Mozaffarian D, Benjamin EJ, Go AS, et al. Heart disease and stroke statistics—2015 update. Circulation. 2015;131(4):e29.
34. Goff DC Jr, Lloyd-Jones DM, Bennett G, Coady S, D'Agostino RB, Gibbons R, American College of Cardiology/American Heart Association Task Force on Practice Guidelines, et al. 2013 ACC/AHA guideline on the assessment of cardiovascular risk. Circulation. 2014;129(25 Suppl 2):S49–73. https://doi.org/10.1161/01.cir.0000437741.48606.98.
35. Lloyd-Jones DM, Evans JC, Levy D. Hypertension in adults across the age spectrum: current outcomes and control in the community. JAMA. 2005;294(4):466–72.
36. Safford MM, Gamboa CM, Durant RW, et al. Race–sex differences in the management of hyperlipidemia. The REasons for Geographic And Racial Differences in Stroke study. Am J Prev Med. 2015;48(5):520–7. https://doi.org/10.1016/j.amepre.2014.10.025.
37. Zhang H, Plutzky J, Shubina M, Turchin A. Drivers of the sex disparity in statin therapy in patients with coronary artery disease: a cohort study. PLoS One. 2016;11(5):e0155228.
38. Karalis DG, Wild RA, Maki KC, Gaskins R, Jacobson TA, Sponseller CA, Cohen JD. Gender differences in side effects and attitudes regarding statin use in America and gaps in patient education (USAGE) study. J Clin Lipidol. 2016;10(4):833–41. https://doi.org/10.1016/j.jacl.2016.02.016.
39. Huxley R, Barzi F, Woodward M. Excess risk of fatal coronary heart disease associated with diabetes in men and women: meta-analysis of 37 prospective cohort studies. Br Med J. 2006;332(7533):73–8.
40. Juutilainen A, Kortelainen S, Lehto S, Rönnemaa T, Pyörälä K, Laakso M. Gender difference in the impact of type 2 diabetes on coronary heart disease risk. Diabetes Care. 2004;27(12):2898.
41. Yusuf S, Hawken S, Ounpuu S, Dans T, Avezum A, Lanas F, INTERHEART Study Investigators, et al. Effect of potentially modifiable risk factors associated with myocardial infarction in 52 countries (the INTERHEART study): case-control study. Lancet. 2004;364(9438):937–52.
42. Kanaya AM, Grady D, Barrett-Connor E. Explaining the sex difference in coronary heart disease mortality among patients with type 2 diabetes mellitus: a meta-analysis. Arch Intern Med. 2002;162(15):1737–45.
43. Garcia M, Mulvagh SL, Merz CN, Buring JE, Manson JE. Cardiovascular disease in women: clinical perspectives. Circ Res. 2016;118(8):1273–93.
44. Huxley RR, Woodward M. Cigarette smoking as a risk factor for coronary heart disease in women compared with men: a systematic review and meta-analysis of prospective cohort studies. Lancet. 2011;378(9799):1297–305. https://doi.org/10.1016/S0140-6736(11)60781-2.
45. Berrington de Gonzalez A, Hartge P, Cerhan JR, Flint AJ, Hannan L, MacInnis RJ, et al. Body-mass index and mortality among 1.46 million white adults. N Engl J Med. 2010;363:2211–9.
46. Hales CM, Carroll MD, Fryar CD, Ogden CL. Prevalence of obesity among adults and youth: United States, 2015–2016. NCHS data brief, no 288 Hyattsville, MD: National Center for Health Statistics. NCHS Data Brief. 2017;(288):1–8.
47. McTigue KM, Chang YF, Eaton C, Garcia L, Johnson KC, Lewis CE, et al. Severe obesity, heart disease, and death among white, African American, and Hispanic postmenopausal women. Obesity (Silver Spring). 2014;22:801–10.
48. Chomistek AK, Manson JE, Stefanick ML, Lu B, Sands-Lincoln M, Going SB, et al. Relationship of sedentary behavior and physical activity to incident cardiovascular disease: results from the Women's Health Initiative. J Am Coll Cardiol. 2013;61:2346–54.
49. Wilkins-Haug L, Celi A, Thomas A, Frolkis J, Seely EW. Recognition by women's health care providers of long-term cardiovascular disease risk after preeclampsia. Obstet Gynecol. 2015;125(6):1287–92.
50. Rich-Edwards JW, Fraser A, Lawlor DA, Catov JM. Pregnancy characteristics and Women's future cardiovascular health: an underused opportunity to improve Women's health? Epidemiol Rev. 2014;36(1):57–70.
51. Grobman WA, Parker CB, Willinger M, Wing DA, Silver RM, Wapner RJ, Eunice Kennedy Shriver National Institute of Child Health and Human Development Nulliparous Pregnancy Outcomes Study: Monitoring Mothers-to-Be (nuMoM2b) Network*, et al. Racial disparities in adverse pregnancy outcomes and psychosocial stress. Obstet Gynecol. 2018;131(2):328–35.
52. Riise HK, Sulo G, Tell GS, et al. Incident Coronary Heart Disease After Preeclampsia: Role of Reduced Fetal Growth, Preterm Delivery, and Parity. J Am Heart Assoc. 2017;6(3):e004158. Published 2017 Mar 6. https://doi.org/10.1161/JAHA.116.004158.
53. Bellamy L, Casas J-P, Hingorani AD, Williams DJ. Pre-eclampsia and risk of cardiovascular disease and cancer in later life: systematic review and meta-analysis. BMJ. 2007;335:974.
54. Lykke J, Langhoff-Roos J, Funai E, Triche E, Paidas E. Hypertensive pregnancy disorders and subsequent cardiovascular morbidity and type 2 diabetes mellitus in the mother. Hypertension. 2009;53:944–51.
55. Kharazmi E, Dossus L, Rohrmann S, Kaaks R. Pregnancy loss and risk of cardiovascular disease: a prospective population-based cohort study (EPIC-Heidelberg). Heart. 2011;97(1):49–54.
56. Vrachnis N, Augoulea A, Iliodromiti Z, Lambrinoudaki I, Sifakis S, Creatsas G. Previous gestational diabetes mellitus and markers of cardiovascular risk. Int J Endocrinol. 2012;2012:458610.
57. Tobias DK, Stuart JJ, Li S, et al. Association of history of gestational diabetes with long-term cardiovascular disease risk in a large prospective cohort of US women. JAMA Intern Med. 2017;177(12):1735–42.
58. Tanz LJ, Stuart JJ, Williams PL, et al. Preterm delivery and maternal cardiovascular disease in young and middle-aged adult women. Circulation. 2017;135(6):578–89.
59. Bonamy AK, Parikh NI, Cnattingius S, Ludvigsson JF, Ingelsson E. Birth characteristics and subsequent risks of maternal cardiovascular disease: effects of gestational age and fetal growth. Circulation. 2011;124(25):2839–46.
60. Pariente G, Sheiner E, Kessous R, Michael S, Shoham-Vardi I. Association between delivery of a small-for-gestational-age neonate and long-term maternal cardiovascular morbidity. Int J Gynaecol Obstet. 2013;123(1):68–71.

61. Kew S, Ye C, Hanley AJ, Connelly PW, Sermer M, Zinman B, Retnakaran R. Cardiometabolic implications of postpartum weight changes in the first year after delivery. Diabetes Care. 2014;37(7):1998–2006. https://doi.org/10.2337/dc14-0087.
62. Linné Y, Dye L, Barkeling B, Rössner S. Long-term weight development in women: a 15 year follow-up of the effects of pregnancy. Obes Res. 2004;12(7):1166–78.
63. Fraser A, Tilling K, Macdonald-Wallis C, et al. Associations of gestational weight gain with maternal body mass index, waist circumference, and blood pressure measured 16 y after pregnancy: the Avon Longitudinal Study of Parents and Children (ALSPAC). Am J Clin Nutr. 2011;93:1285–92.
64. Charalampopoulos D, McLoughlin A, Elks CE, Ong KK. Age at menarche and risks of all-cause and cardiovascular death: a systematic review and meta-analysis. Am J Epidemiol. 2014;180(1):29–40.
65. Wilkins-Haug L, Celi A, Thomas A, Frolkis J, Seely EW. Health care providers' recognition of cardiovascular risk. Obstet Gynecol. 2015;125(6):1287–92. https://doi.org/10.1097/AOG.0000000000000856.
66. Stampfer MJ, Colditz GA. Estrogen replacement therapy and coronary heart disease: a quantitative assessment of the epidemiologic evidence. Prev Med. 1991;20:47–63.
67. Curtis KM, Tepper NK, Jatlaoui TC, et al. U.S. medical eligibility criteria for contraceptive use, 2016. MMWR Recomm Rep. 2016;65(No. RR-3):1–104.
68. Binder EF, Williams DB, Schechtman KB, Jeffe DB, Kohrt WM. Effects of hormone replacement therapy on serum lipids in elderly women: a randomized, placebo-controlled trial. Ann Intern Med. 2001;134(9_Part_1):754–60.
69. Gunderson EP. Impact of breastfeeding on maternal metabolism: implications for women with gestational diabetes. Curr Diab Rep. 2014;14(2):460. https://doi.org/10.1007/s11892-013-0460-2.
70. Duvall WL. Cardiovascular disease in women. Mt Sinai J Med. 2003;70(5):293–305.
71. Chandrasekar B, Nattel S, Tanguay JF. Coronary artery endothelial protection after local delivery of 17beta-estradiol during balloon angioplasty in a porcine model: a potential new pharmacologic approach to improve endothelial function. J Am Coll Cardiol. 2001;38(5):1570–6.
72. Mori T, Durand J, Chen Y, Thompson JA, Bakir S, Oparil S. Effects of short-term estrogen treatment on the neointimal response to balloon injury of rat carotid artery. Am J Cardiol. 2000;85(10):1276–9.
73. Huang A, Kaley G. Gender-specific regulation of cardiovascular function: estrogen as key player. Microcirculation. 2004;11(1):9–38.
74. Meyer MR, Fredette NC, Howard TA, et al. G protein-coupled estrogen receptor protects from atherosclerosis. Sci Rep. 2014;4:7564.
75. Grodstein F, Manson JE, Colditz GA, Willett WC, Speizer FE, Stampfer MJ. A prospective, observational study of postmenopausal hormone therapy and primary prevention of cardiovascular disease. Ann Intern Med. 2000;133(12):933–41.
76. Wolf PH, Madans JH, Finucane FF, Higgins M, Kleinman JC. Reduction of cardiovascular disease-related mortality among postmenopausal women who use hormones: evidence from a national cohort. Am J Obstet Gynecol. 1991;164(2):489–94.
77. Henderson BE, Paganini-Hill A, Ross RK. Decreased mortality in users of estrogen replacement therapy. Arch Intern Med. 1991;151(1):75–8.
78. Hsia J, Langer RD, Manson JE, et al. Conjugated equine estrogens and coronary heart disease: the Women's Health Initiative. Arch Intern Med. 2006;166(3):357–65.
79. Hulley S, Grady D, Bush T, et al. Randomized trial of estrogen plus progestin for secondary prevention of coronary heart disease in postmenopausal women. Heart and Estrogen/progestin Replacement Study (HERS) research group. JAMA. 1998;280(7):605–13.
80. Rossouw JE, Prentice RL, Manson JE, et al. Postmenopausal hormone therapy and risk of cardiovascular disease by age and years since menopause. JAMA. 2007;297(13):1465–77.
81. Salpeter SR, Walsh JM, Greyber E, Salpeter EE. Brief report: coronary heart disease events associated with hormone therapy in younger and older women. A meta-analysis. J Gen Intern Med. 2006;21(4):363–6.
82. Rossouw JE, Anderson GL, Prentice RL, et al. Risks and benefits of estrogen plus progestin in healthy postmenopausal women: principal results from the Women's Health Initiative randomized controlled trial. JAMA. 2002;288(3):321–33.
83. Hodis HN, Mack WJ, Shoupe D, et al. Methods and baseline cardiovascular data from the Early versus Late Intervention Trial with Estradiol testing the menopausal hormone timing hypothesis. Menopause. 2015;22(4):391–401.
84. Manson JE, Aragaki AK, Rossouw JE, et al. Menopausal hormone therapy and long-term all-cause and cause-specific mortality: the Women's Health Initiative randomized trials. JAMA. 2017;318(10):927–38.
85. Stuenkel CA, Davis SR, Gompel A, et al. Treatment of symptoms of the menopause: an endocrine society clinical practice guideline. J Clin Endocrinol Metab. 2015;100(11):3975–4011.
86. Kaunitz AM, Manson JE. Management of menopausal symptoms. Obstet Gynecol. 2015;126(4):859–76.
87. Perrine CG, Nelson JM, Corbelli J, Scanlon KS. Lactation and maternal cardio-metabolic health. Annu Rev Nutr. 2016;36:627–45.
88. Gunderson EP, Quesenberry CP Jr, Ning X, et al. Lactation duration and midlife atherosclerosis. Obstet Gynecol. 2015;126(2):381–90.
89. Schwarz EB, McClure CK, Tepper PG, et al. Lactation and maternal measures of subclinical cardiovascular disease. Obstet Gynecol. 2010;115(1):41–8.
90. Stuebe AM, Michels KB, Willett WC, Manson JE, Rexrode K, Rich-Edwards JW. Duration of lactation and incidence of myocardial infarction in middle to late adulthood. Am J Obstet Gynecol. 2009;200(2):138.e1–8.
91. Natland Fagerhaug T, Forsmo S, Jacobsen GW, Midthjell K, Andersen LF, Ivar Lund Nilsen T. A prospective population-based cohort study of lactation and cardiovascular disease mortality: the HUNT study. BMC Public Health. 2013;13:1070.
92. Ram KT, Bobby P, Hailpern SM, et al. Duration of lactation is associated with lower prevalence of the metabolic syndrome in midlife – SWAN, the study of women's health across the nation. Am J Obstet Gynecol. 2008;198(3):268.e1–6.
93. Natland ST, Nilsen TI, Midthjell K, Andersen LF, Forsmo S. Lactation and cardiovascular risk factors in mothers in a population-based study: the HUNT-study. Int Breastfeed J. 2012;7(1):8.
94. Lupton SJ, Chiu CL, Lujic S, Hennessy A, Lind JM. Association between parity and breastfeeding with maternal high blood pressure. Am J Obstet Gynecol. 2013;208(6):454.e1–7.
95. Zhang BZ, Zhang HY, Liu HH, Li HJ, Wang JS. Breastfeeding and maternal hypertension and diabetes: a population-based cross-sectional study. Breastfeed Med. 2015;10(3):163–7.
96. Bellamy L, Casas JP, Hingorani AD, Williams D. Type 2 diabetes mellitus after gestational diabetes: a systematic review and meta-analysis. Lancet. 2009;373(9677):1773–9.
97. Feig DS, Zinman B, Wang X, Hux JE. Risk of development of diabetes mellitus after diagnosis of gestational diabetes. CMAJ. 2008;179(3):229–34.
98. Buchanan TA. Glucose metabolism during pregnancy: normal physiology and implications for diabetes mellitus. Isr J Med Sci. 1991;27(8–9):432–41.

99. Butte NF, Hopkinson JM, Mehta N, Moon JK, Smith EO. Adjustments in energy expenditure and substrate utilization during late pregnancy and lactation. Am J Clin Nutr. 1999;69(2):299–307.
100. Aune D, Norat T, Romundstad P, Vatten LJ. Breastfeeding and the maternal risk of type 2 diabetes: a systematic review and dose-response meta-analysis of cohort studies. Nutr Metab Cardiovasc Dis. 2014;24(2):107–15.
101. Jager S, Jacobs S, Kroger J, et al. Breast-feeding and maternal risk of type 2 diabetes: a prospective study and meta-analysis. Diabetologia. 2014;57(7):1355–65.
102. Nommsen-Rivers LA, Glueck C, Huang B, Wang P, Dolan LM. Lactation sufficiency is predicted by fasting plasma glucose at 1 month postpartum. FASEB. 2014;28(131):1.
103. Peters SAE, Yang L, Guo Y, Chen Y, Bian Z, Du J, et al. Breastfeeding and the risk of maternal cardiovascular disease: a prospective study of 300 000 Chinese women. J Am Heart Assoc. 2017;6(6):e006081. https://doi.org/10.1161/JAHA.117.006081.
104. Jacobson LT, Hade EM, Collins TC, Margolis KL, Waring ME, Van Horn LV, et al. Breastfeeding history and risk of stroke among parous postmenopausal women in the Women's Health Initiative. J Am Heart Assoc. 2018;7(17):e008739. https://doi.org/10.1161/JAHA.118.008739.
105. Darby SC, Ewertz M, McGale P, et al. Risk of ischemic heart disease in women after radiotherapy for breast cancer. N Engl J Med. 2013;368(11):987–98. https://doi.org/10.1056/NEJMoa1209825.
106. Henson KE, McGale P, Taylor C, Darby SC. Radiation-related mortality from heart disease and lung cancer more than 20 years after radiotherapy for breast cancer. Br J Cancer. 2013;108(1):179–82. https://doi.org/10.1038/bjc.2012.575.
107. Narayan HK, Finkelman BS, French B, et al. Detailed echocardiographic phenotyping in breast cancer patients: associations with ejection fraction decline, recovery, and heart failure symptoms over 3 years of followup. Circulation. 2017;135(15):1397–412. https://doi.org/10.1161/CIRCULATIONAHA.116.023463.
108. Mehta LS, Watson KE, Barac A, et al. Cardiovascular disease and breast cancer: where these entities intersect: a scientific statement from the American Heart Association. Circulation. 2018;137(8):e30–66. https://doi.org/10.1161/CIR.0000000000000556.
109. Haque R, Shi J, Schottinger JE, et al. Cardiovascular disease after aromatase inhibitor use. JAMA Oncol. 2016;2(12):1590–7.
110. Musselman DL, Evans DL, Nemeroff CB. The relationship of depression to cardiovascular disease: epidemiology, biology, and treatment. Arch Gen Psychiatry. 1998;55:580–92.
111. Nabi H, Hall M, Koskenvuo M, Singh-Manoux A, Oksanen T, Suominen SKM, Vahtera J. Psychological and somatic symptoms of anxiety and risk of coronary heart disease: the health and social support prospective cohort study. Biol Psychiatry. 2010;6:378–85.
112. Gianturco L, Bodini BD, Atzeni F, Colombo C, Stella D, Sarzi-Puttini P, et al. Cardiovascular and autoimmune diseases in females: the role of microvasculature and dysfunctional endothelium. Atherosclerosis. 2015;241:259–63.
113. del Rincón I, Polak JF, O'Leary DH, Battafarano DF, Erikson JM, Restrepo JF, Molina E, Escalante A. Systemic inflammation and cardiovascular risk factors predict rapid progression of atherosclerosis in rheumatoid arthritis. Ann Rheum Dis. 2015;74:1118–23.
114. Magnussen C, Niiranen TJ, Ojeda FM, et al. Sex differences and similarities in atrial fibrillation epidemiology, risk factors, and mortality in community cohorts. Circulation. 2017;136(17):1588.
115. Poli D, Antonucci E. Epidemiology, diagnosis, and management of atrial fibrillation in women. Int J Womens Health. 2015;7:605–14. https://doi.org/10.2147/IJWH.S45925.
116. Emdin C, Wong C, Hsiao A, Altman DG, Peters S, Woodward M, et al. Atrial fibrillation as a risk factor for cardiovascular disease and death in women compared with men: systematic review and meta-analysis of cohort studies. BMJ. 2016;352:h7013.

Cardiovascular Disease in Women Part 2: Prevention, Identification, and Treatment of Cardiovascular Disease

22

Agnes Koczo, Alexandra M. Goodwin, Melissa A. McNeil, and Sarah A. Jones

Learning Objectives

1. Counsel women that atherosclerotic cardiovascular disease (ASCVD) is preventable with lifestyle modification.
2. Identify and treat eligible women with lipid management and aspirin for primary prevention of ASCVD.
3. Assess cardiovascular risk, including appropriate use of coronary artery calcium (CAC) to improve ASCVD risk assessment.
4. Recognize sex and gender disparities in prevention, diagnosis, and treatment of ASCVD among women.

Introduction

Cardiovascular disease (CVD) is the leading cause of death for *both* women and men in the United States [1], killing more women than all forms of cancer combined [2]. In 2013, this was 400,000 deaths or one death per minute with an estimated 44 million women in the United States living with or at risk of heart disease [2]. CVD is also costly; estimated indirect and direct costs totaled over $100 billion (USD) in 2010 for ischemic heart disease (IHD) alone [3]. Strokes and cerebrovascular accidents (CVAs) are also costly and life-altering events with risks for lost independence and permanent disability. Despite programs like the American Heart Association's *Go Red for Women* initiative, both patients and physicians often fail to recognize opportunities for better ASCVD prevention, diagnosis, and management [3]. Primary care providers meet at-risk women decades before they meet a cardiologist or neurologist so the opportunities for prevention belong to us in primary care.

In Chap. 21, Part 1 of Cardiovascular Disease in Women, we discussed the range of cardiovascular conditions and their impact on women, as well as detailed both sex and gender differences in traditional risk factors and female-specific risk factors. In this chapter, Part 2, we discuss how to address these risk factors in prevention and use them to assess risk. Additionally, we review approaches to pharmacologic prevention, diagnosis, and management.

Ann is a 55-year-old woman presenting to establish care in your clinic. Unfortunately, her mother died last year from her second myocardial infarction at the age of 78. Ann helped to care for her mother in the last few years and wants to know how she can reduce her risk of a heart attack. Ann does not smoke. Her BMI is 28, and a busy work schedule keeps her from regular exercise.

Prevention of Atherosclerotic Vascular Disease

Given that 80% of ASCVD is preventable, it is incumbent on primary care to counsel women on risk reduction through lifestyle modification and pharmacologic prevention. Focusing first on risk reduction, the American Heart Association (AHA)/American College of Cardiology (ACC) provides a framework through "Life's Simple 7" [4]. These include the following:

A. Koczo · M. A. McNeil · S. A. Jones (✉)
University of Pittsburgh Medical Center, Department of Internal Medicine, Pittsburgh, PA, USA
e-mail: koczoa@upmc.edu; mcneilma@upmc.edu; jonessa3@upmc.edu

A. M. Goodwin
New York University, Bellevue Hospital Center, Department of General Internal Medicine and Clinical Innovation, New York, NY, USA
e-mail: alexandra.goodwin@nyulangone.org

S. A. Tilstra et al. (eds.), *Sex- and Gender-Based Women's Health*, https://doi.org/10.1007/978-3-030-50695-7_22

1. Not smoking (quit >12 months).
2. Healthy diet pattern.
3. Sufficient physical activity (>150 min/week moderate or >75 min/week vigorous intensity).
4. Normal body weight (BMI <25).
5. Normal total cholesterol (initially <200 with an updated goal <178).
6. Normal blood pressure (<120/80).
7. Normal fasting blood glucose (<100).

A woman can calculate her score using the AHA online tool, MyLifeCheck [5], and track her progress toward these goals [6].

Almost half of US deaths from heart disease, stroke, and type 2 diabetes can be attributed to poor dietary habits such as high sodium intake, high consumption of processed meats and sugar-sweetened beverages, as well as low intake of nuts and seeds or omega-3 fats in seafood, vegetables, and fruits [7]. In 2015–2016, rates of US adult obesity approached 40%, with 44.7% of women aged 40–59 and 43.1% of women aged 60 and over being obese [8]. While there was not a statistically significant difference, these rates are higher than aged-matched men at 40.8% and 38.5%, respectively [8]. In the Framingham Heart Study, obesity increased the risk of CAD in women by 64%, compared to 46% in men [9]. Conversely, in good news, the benefit of even small exchanges of sedentary behaviors can be marked. For instance, exchanging 10 minutes of sedentary time for 10 minutes of light-intensity activity is associated with 9% lower mortality risk [7]. This improvement with a small change is particularly important for women, who, compared to men, are less likely to have healthcare provider encouragement to exercise and have less experience in team activities and group exercise [3].

Blood pressure (BP) guidelines have changed rapidly in the last few years and remain controversial. The initial Life's Simple 7 called for goal blood pressure <120/80 [4]. In 2014, the Eighth Joint National Committee (JNC 8) proposed less restrictive hypertension management goals [10]. For hypertensive adults <60 years of age, regardless of comorbid diabetes or chronic kidney disease, goal BP is <140/90 [10]. For adults over the age of 60, goal BP is <150/90 [10]. In 2017, the AHA/ACC recommended a systolic BP target <130 as their meta-analysis showed less cardiovascular events with this goal [11], and we suggest using this goal whenever possible.

Both JNC 8 and AHA/ACC BP recommendations are the same for women and men. However, disparities in hypertension management exist between women and men. More than 75% of women over age 60 have hypertension, and menopause is a risk factor for hypertension [3]. Yet, hypertension is not diagnosed in women as often as men and is not as well controlled in women when compared to men [12]. Also, hypertension is more difficult to control in women who are obese, an important comorbid risk for ASCVD, when compared to women with a normal BMI [13].

The counseling for behavioral changes as well as the diagnosis and treatment of cardiometabolic disease should continue over the lifetime of her primary care. See Fig. 22.1.

Fig. 22.1 Atherosclerotic cardiovascular disease prevention across the adult lifespan

	20s	30s	40s	Risk factors associated with menopause	50s	60s	70s	80+
Counsel on the benefits of breastfeeding	•	•	•					
Collect an obstetric and gynecologic history to identify complications that increase ASCVD risk (PCOS, GDM, pre-eclampsia, premature menopause)	•	•	•		•	•	•	•
Identify ASCVD risk factors in lifestyle (diet, BMI, activity, tobacco) and counsel on modification	•	•	•	BMI often increases	•	•	•	•
Screen and treat hypertension	•	•	•	Prevalence increases	•	•	•	±
Screen high risk women for diabetes and treat (obese, PCOS, GDM)	•	•	•		•	•	•	±
Screen lipids to calculate 10-year ASCVD risk and treat with statin therapy if indicated			•	HT may change lipid profile	•	•	•	±
Treat with aspirin for primary prevention if indicated					•	±		

Key:
Bullets indicate appropriate steps. Consider steps marked ±.
ASCVD = Atherosclerotic Cardiovascular Disease
BMI = Body Mass Index
GDM = Gestational Diabetes Mellitus
HT = Hormone Therapy
PCOS = Polycystic Ovarian Syndrome

Since you last saw Ann, she has started walking four mornings per week for 30 to 45 minutes and stopped eating an after-work snack, and her BMI improved to 26. She wishes to understand more clearly her risk for a heart attack.

You calculate Ann's risk using the Pooled Cohort Equation. With normal blood pressure, total cholesterol 236, and HDL 45, her 10-year ASCVD risk is 8.1%. She wants to know what more she can do to reduce her risk.

Risk Assessment

In 2013, the American College of Cardiology (ACC) and American Heart Association (AHA) proposed calculating risk based on the ASCVD Pooled Cohort Equations (referred to as the PCE risk estimator in this chapter), which has largely replaced the Framingham risk score (FRS). The PCE estimator uses data derived from the Coronary Artery Risk Development in Young Adults (CARDIA), Framingham, Atherosclerosis Risk in Communities (ARIC), and Cardiovascular Health Study (CHS) databases in the United States and has been validated, including in women [14]. It is available at http://tools.acc.org/ascvd-risk-estimator-plus [15].

The PCE risk estimator also broadened the risk categorization from coronary artery disease (CAD) risk to ASCVD risk, which includes stroke and other vascular diseases. It calculates the 10-year risk of hard CVD-related endpoints such as myocardial infarction (MI), CAD, and nonfatal CVA in patients without known CVD [16].

An alternative risk calculator is the Reynolds risk calculator [17], available at http://www.reynoldsriskscore.org [18]. This calculator generates a 10-year CVD risk score, using the additional variables of a high sensitivity C-reactive protein (hsCRP) and a family history of heart disease. For adults with diabetes, a hemoglobin A1C is included. Recognizing that inflammation is a central component of atherosclerosis pathogenesis, the Reynolds calculator incorporates a hsCRP result. High-sensitivity CRP is an inflammatory biomarker test that is not routinely completed and is controversial as a screening test.

This model was derived from a cohort of more than 24,000 healthy US women over the age of 45, who were followed for 10 years, and was applied to recategorizing women of intermediate risk according to Adult Treatment Panel III, a previous cholesterol management model [19]. The Reynolds risk calculator can be used in conjunction with the PCE risk estimator to add nuance to risk prediction and shared decision-making between patients in this population and their providers, as it was found to reclassify intermediate-risk women into higher- or lower-risk subgroups [20]. When compared with the Framingham risk score (FRS), approximately 14% of women were elevated in risk category using Reynolds, while 2% were de-escalated [21]. To our knowledge, the Reynolds risk score has not been compared to the PCE risk estimator.

Pharmacologic Primary Prevention of ASCVD

Low-dose aspirin and high-intensity statin use are recommended for secondary prevention of ASCVD events in patients with a history of clinical ASCVD such as acute coronary syndrome (ACS), angina, myocardial infarction (MI), stroke, transient ischemic attack (TIA), and atherosclerotic peripheral vascular disease (PVD) in both women and men [22–24]. This discussion focuses on pharmacologic primary prevention of ASCVD in patients with increased risk of ASCVD or subclinical CVD and summarizes significant guideline changes as of late 2018.

Aspirin

In 2016, the United States Preventive Services Task Force (USPSTF) updated their recommendations on the use of aspirin for the primary prevention of cardiovascular disease (CVD) [25]. Previously, USPSTF recommendations for aspirin as primary prevention were stratified by gender. Aspirin use was limited to ischemic stroke prevention for women, and aspirin for primary prophylaxis has previously been shown to be underutilized in women [26, 27]. The current recommendation is based on a 17–22% reduction in nonfatal MI and CVA and no sex differences in outcomes [25]. CVD risk is calculated using the PCE risk estimator.

- For adults aged 50–59 years, daily low-dose aspirin use (typically 81 mg in the United States) is recommended for those with ≥10% CVD risk, without increased risk of bleeding, with a life expectancy ≥10 years, and with a willingness to take aspirin for at least 10 years (grade B recommendation) [25].
- For adults aged 60–69 years, USPSTF recommends shared decision-making with consideration of daily low-dose aspirin use for those with ≥10% CVD risk, without increased risk of bleeding, with a life expectancy ≥10 years, with a willingness to take aspirin for at least 10 years, and with patients who value the possible benefits over the possible harms (grade C recommendation) [25].
- For adults <50 years of age or >70 years of age, USPSTF finds insufficient data to recommend for or against aspirin use in the primary prevention of CVD and colorectal cancer (CRC) [25].

The 2016 recommendation updates include considerations of a life expectancy ≥10 years and a willingness to take aspirin for at least 10 years, reflecting the finding that CRC prevention is a latent effect with benefit after 5–20 years use [25]. Of note, lose-dose aspirin is typically considered 81 mg in the United States although studied "low-dose aspirin" ranges from 75 mg daily to 325 mg every other day. Lose-dose aspirin remains preferred over higher-dose aspirin, such as 325 mg daily, since risks of bleeding are lower [23].

USPSTF's strongest recommendations focus on ASCVD prevention during a patient's sixth decade while onset of ASCVD events is typically one to two decades later for women. The 2016 updated recommendation changes largely reflect that the benefit of ASCVD risk reduction is attenuated by increased bleeding risks, particularly in the setting of improved overall ASCVD risk reduction with increased statin use and decreased tobacco use. We did not identify studies assessing gender-specific implementation of the USPSTF's 2016 recommendations above.

Interestingly, the benefit of aspirin for primary prevention of ASCVD events continues to be questioned. Recently, the ASCEND trial showed a slight benefit of aspirin for primary prevention of ASCVD events in patients with diabetes although bleeding event risks increased [28], the ARRIVE trial showed that aspirin did not prevent ASCVD events in patients with risk factors for ASCVD disease [29], and the ASPREE trial showed that aspirin did not confer a protective effect for ASCVD event prevention among healthy patients aged 70 years or older [30]. Furthermore, a recent meta-analysis found the number needed to treat to prevent ASCVD events as 265 and the number needed to harm from bleeding events as 210 [31]. We anticipate adjustment to the guidelines with this new data. Recent expert review of these studies prompted Dr. Ridker to conclude, "Thus, beyond diet maintenance, exercise, and smoking cessation, the best strategy for the use of aspirin in the primary prevention of cardiovascular disease may simply be to prescribe a statin instead" [32].

Reviewing the data, we endorse the 2016 USPSTF recommendation. We recognize 50–59 year-old women who cross the CVD risk threshold of ≥10% as high risk, although this relatively young age for women would generally be protective in the PCE risk estimator. The elevated risk likely reflects many CVD risk factors. For the 60–69 year-old women and women over the age of 70, we endorse the shared decision-making that favors protecting women from the harms of bleeding risks by reserving aspirin for primary prevention to only those recognized as very high risk in light of the recent ARRIVE, ASCEND, and ASPREE trials. For the same reasons, we recommend stopping aspirin for women in these age ranges who have taken as aspirin for primary prevention but who are lower risk.

Statins and Non-Statin Adjuvant Therapies

Guidelines for the recommended use of statins as primary prevention of ASCVD events have also been rapidly changing in the past few years. In 2013, the AHA/ACC suggested evaluation of ASCVD risk every 4–6 years and use of the PCE risk estimator to identify at-risk patients likely to benefit from statin therapy [22]. In late 2018, the AHA/ACC proposed new Cholesterol Clinical Practice Guidelines with the three most notable changes of (1) defining "risk enhancers" which are similar to risks identified in Chap. 21 and, (2) formalizing the improvement target for low-density lipoprotein-cholesterol (LDL-C) while on statins (i.e., decrease LDL-C by 30–50% for those on moderate intensity therapy and by ≥50% for those on high-intensity therapy), and (3) recommending non-statin therapies such as ezetimibe, bile acid sequestrants, or proprotein convertase subtilisin/kexin type 9 (PCSK9) inhibitors, when LDL-C targets are not met despite maximum statin dosing [24]. A free smartphone app "American Heart Association On-The-Go" is available with updated 2018 algorithms under Chol Update > Chol Primary Prevention.

Statins are the first-line therapy because of their effectiveness and availability. Statins limit cholesterol biosynthesis. Ezetimibe decreases cholesterol absorption from the small intestine. Bile acid sequestrants prevent bile acid reabsorption causing fecal loss of LDL-C. PCSK9 inhibitors are monoclonal antibodies that bind to the hepatic enzyme PCSK9. PCSK9 causes LDL-C receptor degradation on hepatocytes, increasing LDL-C levels, and PCSK9 inhibitors allow for more LDL-C receptors and thus less LCL-C in circulation.

Summarized treatment recommendations based on the 2018 AHA/ACC Cholesterol Clinical Practice Guidelines are as follows:

- For adults ≥21 years of age with LDL-C ≥190, there is no need to use the PCE risk estimator. Initiate high-intensity statin therapy (class I recommendation). If LDL-C persists at ≥100 mg/dL, consider ezetimibe (class IIa recommendation). If, despite treatment with statin and ezetimibe, LDL-C remains ≥100 mg/dL, consider a bile acid sequestrant and/or PCSK9 inhibitor (class IIb recommendation) [24]. Given the expense of PCSK9 inhibitors and limited safety data for long-term use, primary care providers may consider referral to cardiology when considering PCSK9 inhibitor prescriptions in this population.
- For adults aged 40–75 years with diabetes and with LDL-C 70–189, moderate-intensity statins are recommended, with consideration of high-intensity statin in higher-risk patients (i.e., multiple risk factors or aged 50–75 years of age) (class IIa recommendation). If ASCVD PCE risk is ≥20%, ezetimibe can be added to maximally tolerated statin therapy to achieve at least 50% reduction of LDL-C (class IIb recommendation) [24].

- For adults aged 20–39 years with long-standing diabetes or significant micro- or macrovascular complications, statin therapy may be reasonable (class IIb recommendation) [24].
- For adults aged 40–75 years without diabetes and with LDL-C 70–189, the updated 2018 recommendation is to pursue shared decision-making. If patients favor treatment and the PCE risk is estimated at 7.5–20%, the recommendation is to initiate moderate-intensity statin therapy (class IIb and class I recommendations, respectively). For those with uncertain risk, coronary artery calcium (CAC) may improve the understanding of risk (class IIa recommendation). For individuals with 10-year PCE risk ≥20%, the goal is to reduce LDL-C by more than 50% with maximally tolerated statins and addition of non-statin adjuvant therapies as needed (class I recommendation) [24].
- For adults 75 years of age or older, the PCE risk estimator cannot calculate 10-year risk. Therefore, it may be reasonable to initiate moderate-intensity statin therapy or to continue well-tolerated statin therapy in patients with risk factors (class IIb recommendation). With functional decline or limited life expectancy, it may be reasonable to stop statin therapy (class IIb recommendation).
- In general, repeat lipid measurement after 4–12 weeks of statin therapy can guide dosing with an expectation that moderate-intensity statins will decrease LDL-C by 30–50% and high-intensity statins will decrease LDL-C by more than 50%. For high-risk patients who do not achieve LDL-C ≤70 mg/dL on maximal statin therapy, consider adding ezetimibe, bile acid sequestrants, or PCSK9 inhibitors (class I recommendation) [24].

The USPSTF developed a recommendation for initiation of statin therapy in 2016. USPSTF also adapted its guidelines for initiation of lipid screening to starting at age 40 universally rather than following prior sex-stratified initiation for men at age 35 and women at age 45 [1]. Overall, both AHA/ACC and USPSTF recommend statin therapy for primary prevention in those individuals with an ASCVD PCE risk ≥10%, but AHA/ACC recommends higher-intensity statin therapy than USPSTF does. Additionally, AHA/ACC considers a lower threshold to favor statin therapy in shared decision-making at ASCVD PCE risk of 7.5%. Please see Fig. 22.2 for a summary of these differences.

- For adults aged 40–75 years without known CVD, with at least one CVD risk factor, and with a 10-year ASCVD PCE risk >10%, USPSTF recommends low- to moderate-dose statin therapy for primary prevention of ASCVD (grade B recommendation) [1].
- For adults aged 40–75 years without known CVD, with at least one CVD risk factor, and with a 10-year ASCVD PCE risk between 7.5% and 10%, clinicians may choose to offer statin therapy (grade C recommendation) [1].
- For adults >75 years of age without known CVD, USPSTF finds insufficient evidence to recommend for or against statins for primary prevention [1].

Early studies of statins for primary prevention did not show benefit of statin therapy for women but the trials included limited numbers of younger women who experienced fewer ASCVD events. Subsequent meta-analysis of only trials including women demonstrated protective effects of statins for primary prevention of coronary heart disease events (RR = 0.78, CI 0.64–0.96) and CVD events (RR = 0.63, CI 0.49–0.82) [33, 34]. However, in a Spanish cross-sectional study, lower-dose statins were prescribed to women, and dyslipidemia was less controlled [35]. Reduced statin prescribing and use for secondary prevention of ASCVD events in women has been shown in the United States [36, 37]. While statins are safe in women, women report more myalgias, trial more statin medications (>3), and express less satisfaction with communication about statins than men [38, 39]. These are proposed reasons for this sex disparity and provide an actionable remedy with improved healthcare communication.

Additionally, it is worth noting that a woman is unlikely to satisfy the recommendations for statin initiation for primary prevention during her reproductive years unless she has diabetes due to the significant contribution of age to the PCE. Since many women of childbearing age have diabetes and women are having children later in life, it is important to remember that statins are category X and should be avoided in pregnancy. The AHA/ACC 2018 Cholesterol Clinical Practice Guidelines recommend that women of childbearing age on statin therapy should be counseled on reliable contraception and that statins should be stopped 1–2 months before trying to conceive (class I recommendation) [24]. Statins should be discontinued immediately upon discovery of unintended pregnancy (class I recommendation) [24].

In summary, a woman's risk may be underestimated by the PCE risk estimator as it does not include risk enhancers, and we will suggest strategies to stratify her risk more appropriately in the next section. With better identification of at-risk women, primary care can utilize primary prevention pharmacotherapy to reduce her risk of ASCVD events.

You discuss options for ASCVD prevention with Ann and review the pros and cons of statin therapy. Ann prefers continued lifestyle changes to medication "but only if that is what is best for her health." Since she is at intermediate risk, you review her risk factors more completely. You inquire about her pregnancies and learn that she had high blood pressure with both of her pregnancies and was on medication. She exclusively breastfed each of her children for 3 months before returning to work. She went through menopause 5 years ago. Her LDL is 167. Ann wants to know how this matters for her health.

ASCVD Prevention in Asymptomatic Women of Intermediate Risk

As outlined in Chap. 21, women have unique risk factors for ASCVD such as pregnancy complications like preeclampsia and gestational hypertension as well as a higher prevalence of autoimmune disease. Furthermore, both women and men have risk factors not incorporated into the PCE risk estimator such as LDL-C >160 and a family history of premature ASCVD [22]. When discussing overall risk with a patient who has additional risk(s) absent from the PCE risk estimator or who has a calculated risk in the discrepant zone between the AHA/ACC and USPSTF guidelines, further risk stratification and shared decision-making are needed. See Chap. 2 on High-Value Health Care for discussion on shared decision-making.

Asymptomatic ASCVD can be evaluated using modalities such as coronary artery calcium (CAC), carotid intimal wall thickness (CIMT), and arterial-brachial index (ABI). For brevity, we will focus on CIMT and CAC. CIMT is an ultrasound technique evaluating the thickness of the carotid artery intima and media. It has performed well in research studies with well-trained technicians but has been more difficult to operationalize in clinical settings [40]. Increases in CIMT from 0.1 mm to 1 mm have been shown to increase the risk of MI and stroke in both men and women [40]. While increased rates of annual progression may increase the risk of CV events, serial evaluation is currently not recommended [40]. In its 2010 Guidelines on Assessment of Cardiovascular Risk in Asymptomatic Individuals, the American College of Cardiology Foundation (ACCF)/AHA recommends consideration of CIMT for further risk stratification in intermediate-risk individuals but cautions there are practical challenges, such as the availability of a skilled technician and insurance coverage (grade B recommendation) [40].

In the 2018 Cholesterol Clinical Practice Guidelines, the AHA recommends consideration of CAC for those in the "intermediate-risk" population with ASCVD PCE risk ≥7.5% to <20% for whom the risk decision to start a statin was uncertain [24]. For those in the "borderline risk" population with ASCVD PCE risk 5% to <7.5% with risk enhancers, CAC may be considered if the risk decision is uncertain [24]. The AHA cautions against the use of CAC in populations with low prevalence of detectable CAC, namely, women <50 years old or men <40 years old since the CT scan requires exposure to radiation, albeit a low dose [40]. CAC has been shown to be superior for risk stratification compared to FRS, CIMT, hsCRP, and the ACC/AHA ASCVD Pooled Cohort Equation risk estimator [40, 41]. The scoring has performed consistently for women and men [40].

With a negative CAC test (score = 0), the presence of atherosclerotic plaque or significant luminal obstructive disease is highly unlikely, and the risk of a cardiovascular event in the next 2–5 years is 0.1% per year [42]. Adding risk calculation to CAC, a CAC = 0 with FRS of low to intermediate risk demonstrated low mortality risk for 15 years while a CAC = 0 with high FRS risk was associated with low mortality risk for 5 years [43]. However, AHA/ACC cautions that for individuals with diabetes, if a strong family history of premature ASCVD or cigarette use exists, statin therapy should not be withheld or delayed even if the CAC score is 0 [24]. A CAC score of 1–99 is considered intermediate risk although the AHA/ACC recently recommended favoring statin therapy in those over age 55 years [24, 42]. A score of ≥100 is considered high risk for a cardiac event within the next 2–5 years, an annual risk of >2%, and initiation of statin therapy is recommended [24, 42]. Compared to a score of 0, a CAC score of ≥100 conferred a ninefold increased risk of CHD events and sixfold increased risk of CVD events [44].

In the Multi-Ethnic Study of Atherosclerosis (MESA), CAC identified candidates for aspirin and statin primary prophylaxis better than risk calculators. When aspirin was used in individuals with CAC = 0, net harm from bleeding events was observed [44]. Aspirin showed net benefit for individuals with CAC ≥100 with a number needed to treat around 125 for prevention of ASCVD events and number needed to harm of 512 for bleeding events [44]. In those with CAC ≥100, statin use resulted in a reduction of CV events similar to the rates when statins were used for secondary rather than primary prevention [45]. Additionally, the use of CAC may demonstrate cost savings compared to the PCE risk estimator when statins are no longer prescribed for CAC = 0 but are initiated when CAC ≥1 and especially with CAC ≥100 [46].

The ACCF/AHA currently recommends against serial CAC scanning. Although an accelerated rate of CAC progression is associated with increased rates of CV events, serial scanning has not improved outcomes or altered therapy [40]. As the prognostic protection conferred by a CAC score of 0 lasts 2–5 years, repeat risk stratification with CAC could be considered after 5 years if it would change pharmacologic prevention. CAC may become more widespread in the future as the American College of Radiology recommends reporting moderate to severe CAC identified on low-dose lung cancer screening CT, and the Society of Cardiovascular Computed Tomography with the Society of Thoracic Radiology is advocating for CAC to be reported on all non-contrasted CT chest to increase identification of subclinical ASCVD for which interventions could be initiated [41].

Another emerging indicator of subclinical ASCVD disease is breast arterial calcification (BAC), which is variably reported on mammography. BAC was shown to correlate with CAC; particularly, no BAC was found to have 81% negative predictive value for CAC [15]. We recommend further evaluation of CVD risk when a mammography report does make mention of calcifications of the breast arteries.

Using these current tools, we recommend using the Reynolds score and CAC to stratify women of borderline and intermediate risk for whom you are concerned that her ASCVD risk is not accurately captured in the PCE risk estimator (Fig. 22.3). Specifically, we would recommend further risk assessment for women with several risk enhancers (see Chap. 21). For a woman of low risk (<5%), counsel on lifestyle changes and continue to reassess her risk approximately every 5 years. For a woman of high risk (≥20%), she is recommended high-intensity statin therapy. Although the 2018 guidelines increased the risk score threshold in the definition of the intermediate group and decreased the intensity of statin therapy to moderate intensity, this group of high intermediate risk (ASCVD PCE risk of 10–19.9%) is high enough risk for a strong recommendation of moderate-intensity statin therapy. If the woman remains uncertain after discussion, CAC could be considered, consistent with the 2018 Cholesterol Clinical Practice Guidelines [24].

For women of borderline risk and low intermediate risk (ASCVD PCE risk of 5–9.9%), we recommend CAC as a tool to enhance your shared decision-making. CAC has performed better than many risk calculators including the PCE, performs as well in women as in men, has been shown to increase medication adherence and lifestyle change, and is cost-effective [40, 41, 44–49]. Since women are more likely to have issues with statin use, we believe this additional risk assessment can better inform shared decision-making with women.

As outlined in Fig. 22.3, for a woman of borderline risk (ASCVD PCE risk of 5–7.%) who does not have additional risk enhancers, Reynolds risk score could be used to further assess her risk, noting than CRP ≥ 2 mg/L is considered a risk enhancer. If her risk does not increase, she can be managed similarly as a woman of low risk. If it does increase, CAC can be used to stratify her risk. For women of high intermediate risk (ASCVD PCE risk of 7.5–9.9%), we recommend CAC to stratify when no additional risk enhancers exist. If the risk enhancers are present, these increase her risk enough to strengthen the recommendation for moderate-intensity statin therapy. If a patient remains uncertain after discussion, CAC could be considered, consistent with the 2018 Cholesterol Clinical Practice Guidelines [24].

A CAC score of 0 provides strong reassurance of low risk. A CAC score of 1–99 prompts shared decision-making about primary prevention with aspirin and statin therapy. A CAC score of 100 or greater reclassifies as high risk; these women likely benefit from low-dose aspirin and statin therapy (Fig. 22.3). On a practical note, often insurance will cover the hsCRP needed for the Reynolds risk score but may not cover the CAC (estimated cost $100–$400). With addition of CAC to the 2018 Cholesterol Clinical Practice Guidelines, insurance coverage for this test may improve. Therefore, patient preference, the degree of risk uncertainty, cost and availability of CAC, as well as likelihood of changing management are important in considering use of this additional risk assessment tool.

Ann undergoes CT chest, and her CAC score is 110. You recommend high-intensity statin therapy and aspirin given her CAC ≥ 100. Her CAC ≥ 100 reclassifies her as high risk despite her intermediate 10-year ASCVD risk from the PCE risk estimator. She agrees to take these medications to reduce her risk of heart attack and stroke.

Several years later, at age 59, Ann presents to the clinic with increasing difficulty completing her morning walks. She feels that she needs to rest once or twice during the walk. She has not regained any weight. She does not have chest pain or trouble breathing. A sense of fatigue prompts her to rest.

Diagnosis and Treatment of ASCVD in Symptomatic Women

Ischemic Heart Disease

Although most patients with acute myocardial infarction present with chest pain, women are more likely to present with variable features. A symptom prodrome with shortness of breath,

Fig. 22.2 Statins for primary prevention: comparing AHA/ACC and USPSTF recommendations [1, 24]. (Adapted from data in US Preventive Services Task Force et al. [1] and Grundy et al. [24])

	10-year ASCVD Risk for ages 40-75			
	5-7.4%	7.5-9.9%	10-19.9%	≥20%
AHA/ACC: If LDL 70-189,	Borderline Risk: Shared decision-making	Intermediate Risk: Moderate intensity statin if shared decision-making favors statin		High Risk: High intensity statin
USPSTF: If ≥ 1 CVD Risk Factor,		Shared decision-making	Low-moderate intensity statin	

Key:
AHA/ACC = American Heart Association/American College of Cardiology
ASCVD = Atherosclerotic Cardiovascular Disease
CVD = Cardiovascular Disease
USPSTF = United States Preventative Services Task Force

unusual fatigue, discomfort in the jaw/teeth, or discomfort in the arms may develop weeks to months before a major cardiac event [50]. During the acute event, similar symptoms often recur, and over 25% of women never report chest pain or discomfort [51]. Symptoms also are likely to occur at rest or with stress rather than with exertion [5, 17]. When presenting acutely, women are more likely to have acute coronary syndrome (ACS) with atypical symptoms and lack EKG findings [3]. In contrast to obstructive lesions which are candidates for revascularization, women have nonobstructive CAD more often and the resulting vascular dysfunction and myocardial IHD that results is less well understood [3, 52]. This may, in part, explain why women's early and late morbidity and mortality after CV events are worse than that of men [3, 52].

While presentation with acute myocardial ischemia is more likely to occur in the emergency department, the primary care clinician is more likely to encounter women with the symptom prodrome or stable ischemic heart disease (SIHD) of nonobstructive CAD. In women who have non-acute symptoms, the AHA recently published a consensus statement for noninvasive imaging for women based upon four levels of risk [52, 53]:

- A low-risk woman is premenopausal, less than age 60 with atypical angina, and without diabetes mellitus. She can be offered reassurance about her low risk, and imaging may be deferred.
- A low intermediate-risk woman is in her 50s with a functional limitation to her activities of daily living (ADLs) or is 60–69 years old. Exercise treadmill testing (ETT) is appropriate if she has a normal baseline EKG and can be expected to achieve the exercise requirements.
- A high intermediate-risk woman is in her 60s with functional limitation of her ADLs. Similar to a high-risk woman, stress imaging is appropriate.
- A high-risk woman either has peripheral artery disease, has poorly controlled diabetes, or is greater than 70 years old.

Extensive comorbidities elevate a woman's categorization by one level [52, 53].

We endorse additional high-risk features as ASCVD risk ≥20% (by PCE risk estimator) or CAC ≥100. The sensitivity and specificity for detecting obstructive CAD on ETT are decreased for women given a higher likelihood of not achieving maximal exercise requirements and lower baseline QRS voltage, yet the negative predictive value remains high [3, 54]. When stress imaging is planned for high intermediate- to high-risk women, we recommend exercise myocardial perfusion imaging, exercise stress echocardiography, or cardiac MRI, with a preference for exercise stress imaging given the prognostic benefit of evaluating her exercise tolerance [52, 53]. Figure 22.4 illustrates risk-stratified diagnostic recommendations for women presenting with SIHD.

Guideline-directed medical therapy (GDMT) remains the same for women and women [55]. However, women with CAD are less likely to initiate statin therapy and to persist with statin therapy for at least a year. Lacking an evaluation by cardiology, reporting more adverse reactions, being older at event onset, and not smoking were the factors linked to women's discontinuation of statin therapy [36]. Between 2014 and 2015, 47% of women filled a statin prescription upon 30 days after hospital discharge for MI compared to 56% of men [37]. Additionally, in a recent meta-analysis, women are less likely to be referred to cardiac rehabilitation after MI that men (0.68, 95% CI 0.62–0.74) [56].

Although Ann's atypical symptoms and age would have made her a low-risk candidate, suitable for reassurance, her elevated CAC score escalated her risk such that she undergoes exercise myocardial perfusion imaging with abnormalities that prompt left heart catheterization. She has an area with 50% stenosis of her left anterior descending artery (LAD) but no obstructing lesions. Her cardiologist recommends GDMT including secondary prevention with continued low-dose aspirin and high-intensity statin for prevention of an acute ASCVD event. She is thankful that she did not have a heart attack like her mother.

Emerging Diagnostics in IHD

In addition to the risk-stratified diagnostic recommendations identified above, there are several emerging imaging modalities for patients who are at least intermediate risk for ischemic heart disease, particularly if they have indeterminate or inability to exercise precluding exercise treadmill testing. Stress cardiac MRI, positron emission tomography (PET), and coronary CT angiography (CCTA) have emerged as effective diagnostic modalities for ischemic heart disease including for nonobstructive coronary and microvascular disease, both of which disproportionately affect women [57–59]. Research to assess the prognostic (and thus management) value of both the ischemic burden by perfusion modalities and the extent of plaque in CCTA continues to evolve [47]. Decision-making on which imaging modality to select also depends on several factors including type of imaging available at an institution, exposure to ionizing radiation, and expertise in imaging interpretation (Fig. 22.4).

Stroke

For both women and men, control of hypertension is an important modifiable risk factor to reduce the risk of stroke.

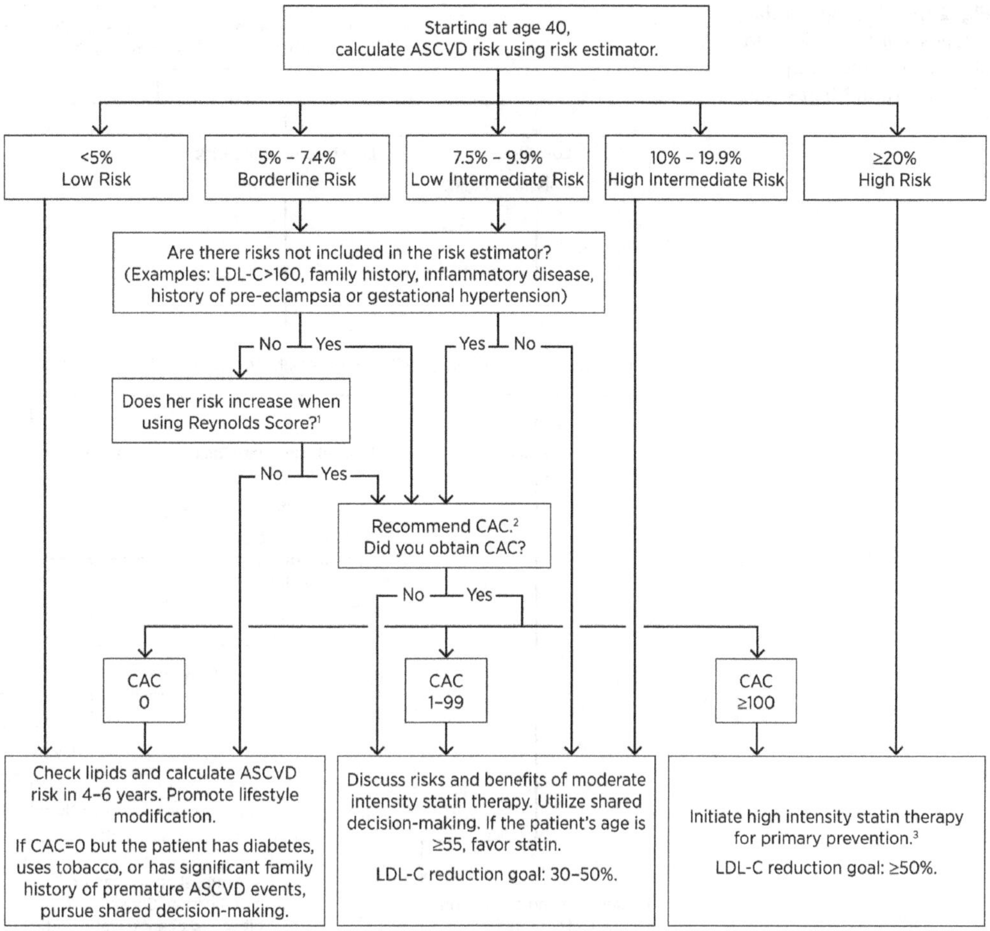

Notes:

1. High sensitivity CRP needed for Reynolds Score.
2. Consider CAC testing based on patient preference, degree of uncertainty in risk assessment, availability, cost, and likelihood of changing next steps.
3. If CAC≥100, add low dose aspirin for primary prevention. If risk solely based on risk estimator and no CAC, consider aspirin for primary prevention as discussed in the text.

Key:

ASCVD = Atherosclerotic Cardiovascular Disease
CAC = Coronary Artery Calcium
CRP = C-Reactive Protein
LDL-C = Low Density Lipoprotein Cholesterol
PCE = Pooled Cohort Equation

Fig. 22.3 Additional ASCVD risk stratification of asymptomatic women for initiation of statin therapy [24]. (Adapted from Grundy et al. [24])

While conditions of blood pressure dysregulation during pregnancy, such as pregnancy-induced hypertension, preeclampsia, and eclampsia, increase the risk of acute stroke during pregnancy, we will focus on the long-term risk conferred by these conditions. Pregnancy-induced hypertension and preeclampsia are associated with two- to tenfold increased risk of hypertension in the 5–30 years after the complicated pregnancy [60]. Similarly, the risk of CVD event in 10 years after pregnancy had an odds ratio of 13 when comparing women with preeclampsia to those with an uncomplicated pregnancy in a 2012 study [61]. Thus, we again emphasize the importance of taking an obstetric history to identify women with an elevated risk for hypertension and stroke.

Women have unique risk factors for stroke including a small increased risk with combined hormonal contraceptive use and an increased risk for migraine with aura. These observations prompted the Centers for Disease Control to recommend against combined hormonal contraceptives in women with a history of migraine with aura [60, 62]. Hormone therapy in menopausal women should not be used for stroke prevention but may be considered for vasomotor symptom management. A recent evaluation of the Women's Health Initiative showed no increase in stroke mortality [60, 63].

Stroke diagnosis and treatment guidelines remain the same for women and men [64]. Of note, women are less likely to undergo carotid endarterectomy (CEA) which is thought to be related to the smaller diameter of women's internal carotid arteries and shorter segments of stenosis as well as less frequent high-grade stenosis [60]. For those that qualify for CEA with symptomatic stenosis, women have

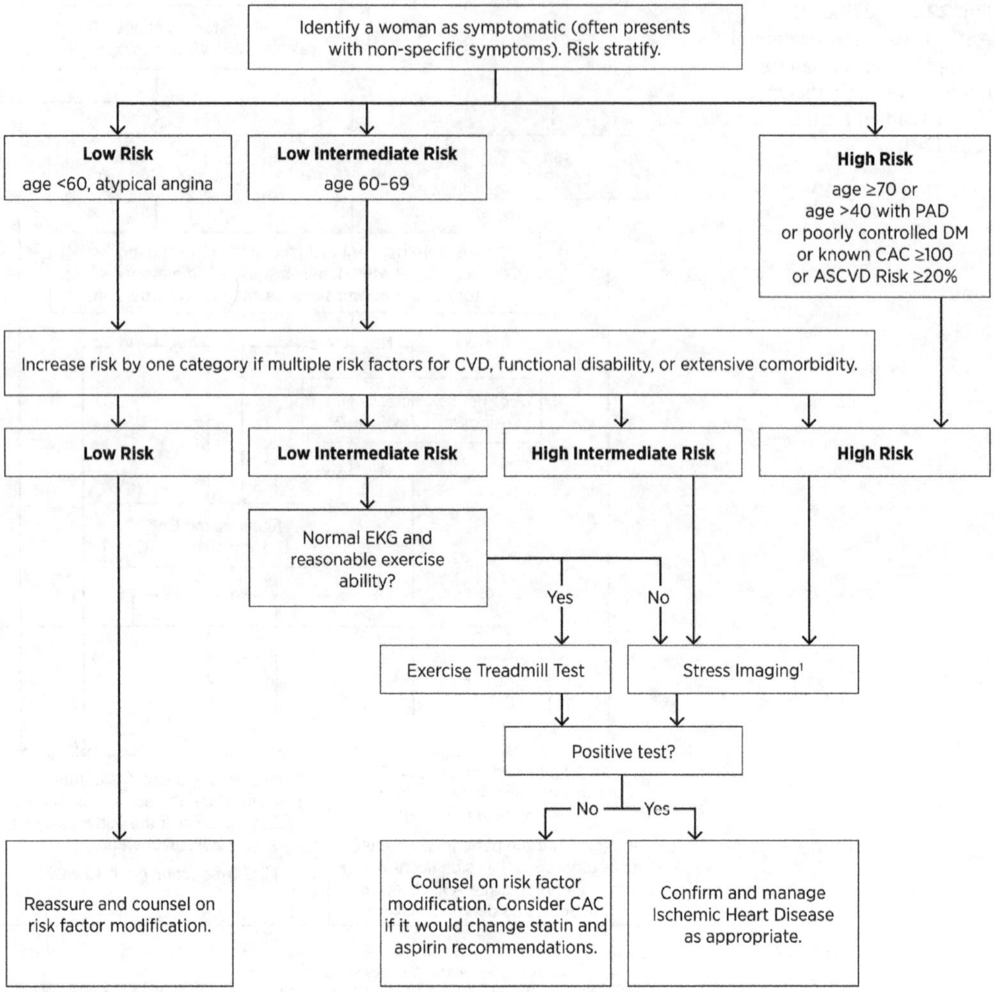

Fig. 22.4 Strategy for the diagnosis of ischemic heart disease in women [52]. (Adapted from Mieres et al. [53])

Notes:
1. Perform exercise stress imaging if patient can exercise.

Key:
ASCVD = Atherosclerotic Cardiovascular Disease
CAC = Coronary Artery Calcium
CVD = Cardiovascular Disease
DM = Diabetes Mellitus
EKG = Electrocardiogram
PAD = Peripheral Artery Disease

been shown to undergo CEA less often and experience a delay in time to surgery compared to men [60].

Addressing Disparities

Throughout these two chapters on cardiovascular disease, the leading cause of death for women in the United States, we highlighted distinguishing features of ASCVD in women. This includes identifying unique risk factors related to pregnancy and menopause as well as risk factors more prevalent in women, like autoimmune disease. It recognizes that our risk assessment tools underestimate risk in women, that we are not optimizing our primary or secondary risk reduction strategies for women, that we are less likely to recognize the presentation of ASCVD in women, and that the pathophysiology of ASCVD is different in women. These disparities are opportunities.

In reading this book, clearly you are interested in excellent primary care for women. We would empower you to remedy these disparities in cardiovascular care for women with the following ideas:

1. Rewrite the illness script.
   CVD is the leading cause of death for women in the United States [1]. Use the rewrite to prioritize risk reduction for women. Also, use the rewrite to hear atypical symptoms in your patient's history and diagnose her disease. Consider that women of color face even greater disparities in cardiovascular care and rewrite the illness script again.
2. Identify that traditional risk assessment may not fit your patient.

Offer additional risk stratification as outlined in this chapter to help identify women with underestimated risk and then to prescribe appropriate pharmacotherapies for primary prevention and to motivate lifestyle changes.

3. Recognize opportunities for patient education.

   Lack of physician encouragement to exercise and inadequate communication about statin medications are two opportunities identified for primary care to engage women for ASCVD risk reduction [3, 39]. Likely there are more. Celebrate *Go Red for Women* month in your clinic each February.

4. Get with the guidelines.

   This campaign is being applied to help us checklist various disease management strategies and can be a quick reminder to review your patient's ASCVD event management and secondary prevention strategies.

5. Recruit and research.

   When trials are recruiting patients to address questions about ASCVD, encourage your eligible female patients to enroll, improving our evidence to guide better outcomes for women. Consider being active in ongoing research or developing new research questions for ASCVD in women.

Summary Points

1. Eighty percent of cardiovascular disease (CVD) is thought to be preventable. The American Heart Association's Life's Simple 7 outlines smoking, diet, BMI, activity, blood pressure, cholesterol, and blood sugar as targets for reducing risk of ASCVD.
2. The USPSTF recommends low-dose aspirin for primary prevention of ASCVD in women who are aged 50–59 years with ≥10% CVD risk, without increased risk of bleeding, with a life expectancy ≥10 years, and with a willingness to take aspirin for at least 10 years. The USPSTF recommends low- to moderate-dose statin therapy for primary prevention of ASCVD in women aged 40–75 years without known CVD but with a 10-year ASCVD PCE risk ≥10% and with at least one CVD risk factor. AHA/ACC recommends high-intensity statin therapy for women aged 40–75 without diabetes and with a 10-year ASCVD PCE risk ≥20% and shared decision-making about moderate-intensity statin when the 10-year ASCVD PCE risk is 7.5–19.9%.
3. Women's risk of ASCVD is underestimated by commonly used risk calculators, and guidelines vary on suggested thresholds to initiate statin therapy. Coronary artery calcium (CAC) is a noninvasive strategy to identify women with subclinical ASCVD or at risk for ASCVD who may benefit from aspirin and statin therapy.
4. When women present with acute coronary syndrome (ACS), they are more likely than men to have nonobstructive ischemic heart disease (IHD) leading to atypical symptoms which can delay diagnosis and treatment of acute myocardial infarction (MI). Women are typically 10 years older than men when presenting with first stroke or MI. Women have worse short- and long-term mortality after these events, and treatment is less likely to follow guidelines.

Review Questions

1. A non-Hispanic Caucasian 50-year-old woman presents to establish care. She is healthy, takes no medications, and has two healthy children delivered in her late 20s without complications. She reports no history of MI in either of her parents. She recently had her HDL measured at 80 and her LDL at 140. In addition to learning more about her risk of cardiovascular events including MI and CHD death, she also wants to know her risk of stroke/death from stroke. Which is most appropriate risk calculator to apply in this setting to use to calculate her 10-year ASCVD risk?

   A. Framingham
   B. Reynolds risk
   C. Pooled cohort equation
   D. Ellington cardiac index

   The correct answer is C. As a general risk calculator for all-comers, the pooled cohort equation risk estimator (which uses data derived from the CARDIA, Framingham, ARIC, CHS databases in the United States) has the highest level of evidence and is the strongest recommendation from the ACC and AHA. The ACC/Framingham risk calculator does not predict risk of CVA or CVA death. The Reynolds risk calculator could be an option for this patient if an hsCRP were available and/or more data points about risk could help with clinical decision-making. Of note, this patient is a candidate for risk assessment using the pooled cohort equation as she has no known ASCVD and has no prior major cardiac events.
2. A 64-year-old African-American woman is establishing care and wants to improve her health and is interested in cholesterol-lowering medications. She has a history of an upper gastrointestinal bleed (UGIB) from overuse of non-steroidal anti-inflammatories (NSAIDs). She smokes ½ pack of cigarettes per day. She has high blood pressure, which is well controlled on two medications. Her BMI is 26. She wants to reduce her risk for heart attack and stroke. She has no symptoms of heart disease. You calculate her ASCVD risk as 14% over the next 10 years using the Pooled Cohort Equation. In addition to lifestyle changes, what pharmacologic strategy do you recommend to reduce her risk, since she does not plan to stop smoking?

A. A moderate-intensity statin and aspirin 325 mg
B. A moderate-intensity statin and aspirin 81 mg
C. No statin but a daily aspirin
D. A moderate-intensity statin but no aspirin

The correct answer is D. According to the USPSTF recommendations for primary prevention of ASCVD, she would not qualify for aspirin 81 mg given that she's in her 60s and has an increased risk of bleeding with her history of UGIB. Both USPSTF and AHA/ACC would recommend at least a moderate-intensity statin given ASCVD PCE risk >10% if shared decision-making favors the statin [22, 24, 25] which we would encourage given she intends to keep smoking.

3. At this visit, she also tells you that her concern for her heart attack and stroke risk is because a good friend recently had a heart attack. Her friend was only a few years older than she is and had similar health issues. She noticed her friend was increasingly tired in the weeks preceding her heart attack but that she never had any chest pain, even when she drove to the emergency department. Her friend had felt tired, weak, and nauseated. She wants to know if this is usual.

   How do you counsel her?

   A. Counsel her that heart disease is the number one cause of death for men but not women.
   B. Counsel her that women often present with symptoms other than typical angina or chest pain with exertion.
   C. Counsel her that her lifestyle changes and medical therapy unfortunately do not substantially reduce her risk.
   D. Counsel her that her friend should have used hormone therapy to reduce her risk of heart attack and stroke.

   The correct answer is B. Women often present with atypical symptoms of CVD. Heart disease is the leading cause of death for both women and men. Eighty percent of cardiovascular disease is thought to be preventable. Hormone therapy is not used for primary prevention of ASCVD disease events because events were shown to be increased.

4. A 64-year-old non-Hispanic Caucasian woman returns for her annual exam. She has a history of hypertension and rheumatoid arthritis (RA). She had two pregnancies without complication and did not breastfeed her children. Her 10-year ASCVD risk using the Pooled Cohort Equation is 7.4%. You decide to send her for coronary artery calcium CT as her history of RA is a risk enhancer so you worry that PCE underestimates her risk.

   What will you do with the results?

   A. If it is 0, indicating no identifiable disease, counsel that she does not need an aspirin and a statin.
   B. If it is 1–99, indicating mild disease, practice shared decision-making about aspirin and statin and repeat CAC-CT in one year.
   C. If it is 100–399, indicating moderate disease, recommend daily aspirin and statin and repeat CAC-CT in one year.
   D. If it is >400, indicating severe disease, recommend aspirin and statin and send her for left heart catheterization.

   The correct answer is A. Her risk of a cardiovascular event in the next 2–5 years is <0.1% with a score of 0. For choice B, shared decision-making is appropriate for CAC score of 1–99, and for choice C, recommendation of aspirin and statin therapy is appropriate as long as she does not have increased risks for bleeding or a contraindication to statin therapy. For both choices B and C, the AHA does not recommend serial CAC-CT as it has not been shown to change outcomes or decision-making [40, 42]. For choice D, primary prophylaxis recommendations are appropriate. However, given that she is asymptomatic, the AHA does not recommend using CAC to guide plans for revascularization [42].

References

1. US Preventive Services Task Force, Bibbins-Domingo K, Grossman DC, Curry SJ, Davidson KW, Epling JW Jr, et al. Statin use for the primary prevention of cardiovascular disease in adults: US preventive services task Force recommendation statement. JAMA. 2016;316(19):1997–2007.
2. Lundberg GP, Dunbar SB, Wenger NK. Guidelines for the reduction of cardiovascular disease in women. J Obstet Gynecol Neonatal Nurs. 2016;45(3):402–12.
3. McSweeney JC, Rosenfeld AG, Abel WM, Braun LT, Burke LE, Daugherty SL, et al. Preventing and experiencing ischemic heart disease as a woman: state of the science: a scientific statement from the American Heart Association. Circulation. 2016; 133(13):1302–31.
4. Benjamin EJ, Blaha MJ, Chiuve SE, Cushman M, Das SR, Deo R, et al. Heart disease and stroke statistics-2017 update: a report from the American Heart Association. Circulation. 2017; 135(10):e146–603.
5. AHA Heart Score Calculator. MyLifeCheck. Available at https://www.heart.org/en/healthy-living/healthy-lifestyle/my-life-check%2D%2Dlifes-simple-7
6. Bairey Merz CN, Shaw LJ, Reis SE, Bittner V, Kelsey SF, Olson M, et al. Insights from the NHLBI-Sponsored Women's Ischemia Syndrome Evaluation (WISE) study: part II: gender differences in presentation, diagnosis, and outcome with regard to gender-based pathophysiology of atherosclerosis and macrovascular and microvascular coronary disease. J Am Coll Cardiol. 2006;47(3 Suppl):S21–9.
7. Benjamin EJ, Virani SS, Callaway CW, Chang AR, Cheng S, Chiuve SE, et al. Heart disease and stroke statistics-2018 update: a report from the American Heart Association. Circulation. 2018;137(12):e67–e492. https://doi.org/10.1161/CIR.0000000000000558.
8. Hales CM, Carroll MD, Fryar CD, Ogden CL. Prevalence of obesity among adults and youth: United States, 2015–2016. NCHS Data Brief. 2017;288:1–8.
9. Garcia M, Mulvagh SL, Merz CN, Buring JE, Manson JE. Cardiovascular disease in women: clinical perspectives. Circ Res. 2016;118(8):1273–93.
10. James PA, Oparil S, Carter BL, Cushman WC, Dennison-Himmelfarb C, Handler J, et al. 2014 evidence-based guideline for the management of high blood pressure in adults: report from the

panel members appointed to the Eighth Joint National Committee (JNC 8). JAMA. 2014;311(5):507–20.

11. Reboussin DM, Allen NB, Griswold ME, Guallar E, Hong Y, Lackland DT, et al. Systematic review for the 2017 ACC/AHA/AAPA/ABC/ACPM/AGS/APhA/ASH/ASPC/NMA/PCNA guideline for the prevention, detection, evaluation, and management of high blood pressure in adults: a report of the American College of Cardiology/American Heart Association Task Force on Clinical Practice Guidelines. J Am Coll Cardiol. 2018;71(19):2176. https://doi.org/10.1016/j.jacc.2017.11.005.
12. Kim JK, Alley D, Seeman T, Karlamangla A, Crimmins E. Recent changes in cardiovascular risk factors among women and men. J Womens Health (Larchmt). 2006;15(6):734–46.
13. Diaconu CC, Paraschiv B. Clinical characteristics of obese patients with hypertension and chronic ischemic heart disease. Rom J Intern Med. 2014;52(4):251–5.
14. ASCVD Risk Estimator Plus. http://tools.acc.org/ascvd-risk-estimator-plus
15. Margolies L, Salvatore M, Hecht HS, Kotkin S, Yip R, Baber U, et al. Digital mammography and screening for coronary artery disease. JACC Cardiovasc Imaging. 2016;9(4):350–60.
16. Action to Control Cardiovascular Risk in Diabetes Study Group, Gerstein HC, Miller ME, Byington RP, Goff DC Jr, Bigger JT, et al. Effects of intensive glucose lowering in type 2 diabetes. N Engl J Med. 2008;358(24):2545–59.
17. Reynolds Risk Calculator. http://www.reynoldsriskscore.org
18. Shaw LJ, Shaw RE, Merz CN, Brindis RG, Klein LW, Nallamothu B, et al. Impact of ethnicity and gender differences on angiographic coronary artery disease prevalence and in-hospital mortality in the American College of Cardiology-National Cardiovascular Data Registry. Circulation. 2008;117(14):1787–801.
19. Ridker PM, Buring JE, Rifai N, Cook NR. Development and validation of improved algorithms for the assessment of global cardiovascular risk in women: the Reynolds Risk Score. JAMA. 2007;297(6):611–9.
20. Ridker PMBJ, Rifai N, Cook NR. Development and validation of improved algorithms for the assessment of global cardiovascular risk in women: the Reynolds Risk Score. JAMA. 2007;297:611–9.
21. Tattersall MC, Gangnon RE, Karmali KN, Keevil JG. Women up, men down: the clinical impact of replacing the Framingham Risk Score with the Reynolds Risk Score in the United States population. PLoS One. 2012;7(9):e44347.
22. Stone NJ, Robinson JG, Lichtenstein AH, Bairey Merz CN, Blum CB, Eckel RH, et al. 2013 ACC/AHA guideline on the treatment of blood cholesterol to reduce atherosclerotic cardiovascular risk in adults: a report of the American College of Cardiology/American Heart Association Task Force on Practice Guidelines. J Am Coll Cardiol. 2014;63(25 Pt B):2889–934.
23. Hennekens CH, Dyken ML, Fuster V. Aspirin as a therapeutic agent in cardiovascular disease: a statement for healthcare professionals from the American Heart Association. Circulation. 1997;96(8):2751–3.
24. Grundy SM, Stone NJ, Bailey AL, Beam C, Birtcher KK, Blumenthal RS, et al. 2018 AHA/ACC/AACVPR/AAPA/ABC/ACPM/ADA/AGS/APhA/ASPC/NLA/PCNA guideline on the management of blood cholesterol: a report of the American College of Cardiology/American Heart Association Task Force on Clinical Practice Guidelines. J Am Coll Cardiol. 2019;73(24):3168–209. https://doi.org/10.1016/j.jacc.2018.11.002.
25. Bibbins-Domingo K, Force USPST. Aspirin use for the primary prevention of cardiovascular disease and colorectal cancer: U.S. Preventive Services Task Force recommendation statement. Ann Intern Med. 2016;164(12):836–45.
26. Rivera CM, Song J, Copeland L, Buirge C, Ory M, McNeal CJ. Underuse of aspirin for primary and secondary prevention of cardiovascular disease events in women. J Womens Health (Larchmt). 2012;21(4):379–87.
27. Force USPST. Aspirin for the prevention of cardiovascular disease: U.S. Preventive Services Task Force recommendation statement. Ann Intern Med. 2009;150(6):396–404.
28. ASCEND Study Collaborative Group, Bowman L, Mafham M, Wallendszus K, Stevens W, Buck G, Barton J, et al. Effects of aspirin for primary prevention in persons with diabetes mellitus. N Engl J Med. 2018;379(16):1529–39. https://doi.org/10.1056/NEJMoa1804988.
29. Gaziano JM, Brotons C, Coppolecchia R, Cricelli C, Darius H, Gorelick PB, et al. Use of aspirin to reduce risk of initial vascular events in patients at moderate risk of cardiovascular disease (ARRIVE): a randomised, double-blind, placebo-controlled trial. Lancet. 2018;392(10152):1036–46.
30. McNeil JJ, Wolfe R, Woods RL, Tonkin AM, Donnan GA, Nelson MR, ASPREE Investigator Group, et al. Effect of aspirin on cardiovascular events and bleeding in the healthy elderly. N Engl J Med. 2018;379(16):1509–18. https://doi.org/10.1056/NEJMoa1805819.
31. Zheng SL, Roddick AJ. Association of aspirin use for primary prevention with cardiovascular events and bleeding events: a systematic review and meta-analysis. JAMA. 2019;321(3):277–87.
32. Ridker PM. Should aspirin be used for primary prevention in the post-statin era? N Engl J Med. 2018;379(16):1572–4.
33. Bukkapatnam RN, Gabler NB, Lewis WR. Statins for primary prevention of cardiovascular mortality in women: a systematic review and meta-analysis. Prev Cardiol. 2010;13(2):84–90.
34. Mora S, Glynn RJ, Hsia J, MacFadyen JG, Genest J, Ridker PM. Statins for the primary prevention of cardiovascular events in women with elevated high-sensitivity C-reactive protein or dyslipidemia: results from the Justification for the Use of Statins in Prevention: An Intervention Trial Evaluating Rosuvastatin (JUPITER) and meta-analysis of women from primary prevention trials. Circulation. 2010;121(9):1069–77.
35. Moreno-Arellano S, Delgado-de-Mendoza J, Santi-Cano MJ. Sex disparity persists in the prevention of cardiovascular disease in women on statin therapy compared to that in men. Nutr Metab Cardiovasc Dis. 2018;28(8):810–5.
36. Zhang H, Plutzky J, Shubina M, Turchin A. Drivers of the sex disparity in statin therapy in patients with coronary artery disease: a cohort study. PLoS One. 2016;11(5):e0155228.
37. Peters SAE, Colantonio LD, Zhao H, Bittner V, Dai Y, Farkouh ME, et al. Sex differences in high-intensity statin use following myocardial infarction in the United States. J Am Coll Cardiol. 2018;71(16):1729–37.
38. Gulati M, Merz CN. New cholesterol guidelines and primary prevention in women. Trends Cardiovasc Med. 2015;25(2):84–94.
39. Karalis DG, Wild RA, Maki KC, Gaskins R, Jacobson TA, Sponseller CA, et al. Gender differences in side effects and attitudes regarding statin use in the Understanding Statin Use in America and Gaps in Patient Education (USAGE) study. J Clin Lipidol. 2016;10(4):833–41.
40. Greenland P, Alpert JS, Beller GA, Benjamin EJ, Budoff MJ, Fayad ZA, et al. 2010 ACCF/AHA guideline for assessment of cardiovascular risk in asymptomatic adults: a report of the American College of Cardiology Foundation/American Heart Association Task Force on Practice Guidelines. J Am Coll Cardiol. 2010;56(25):e50–103.
41. Hecht HS, Cronin P, Blaha MJ, Budoff MJ, Kazerooni EA, Narula J, et al. 2016 SCCT/STR guidelines for coronary artery calcium scoring of noncontrast noncardiac chest CT scans: a report of the Society of Cardiovascular Computed Tomography and Society of Thoracic Radiology. J Cardiovasc Comput Tomogr. 2017;11(1):74–84.
42. Budoff MJ, Achenbach S, Blumenthal RS, Carr JJ, Goldin JG, Greenland P, et al. Assessment of coronary artery disease by cardiac computed tomography: a scientific statement from the American Heart Association Committee on Cardiovascular Imaging and Intervention, Council on Cardiovascular Radiology and Intervention, and Committee on Cardiac Imaging, Council on Clinical Cardiology. Circulation. 2006;114(16):1761–91.

43. Valenti V, Ó Hartaigh B, Heo R, Cho I, Schulman-Marcus J, Gransar H, et al. A 15-year warranty period for asymptomatic individuals without coronary artery calcium: a prospective follow-up of 9,715 individuals. JACC Cardiovasc Imaging. 2015;8(8):900–9.
44. Miedema MD, Duprez DA, Misialek JR, Blaha MJ, Nasir K, Silverman MG, et al. Use of coronary artery calcium testing to guide aspirin utilization for primary prevention: estimates from the multi-ethnic study of atherosclerosis. Circ Cardiovasc Qual Outcomes. 2014;7(3):453–60.
45. Martin SS, Blaha MJ, Blankstein R, Agatston A, Rivera JJ, Virani SS, et al. Dyslipidemia, coronary artery calcium, and incident atherosclerotic cardiovascular disease: implications for statin therapy from the multi-ethnic study of atherosclerosis. Circulation. 2014;129(1):77–86.
46. Roberts ET, Horne A, Martin SS, Blaha MJ, Blankstein R, Budoff MJ, et al. Cost-effectiveness of coronary artery calcium testing for coronary heart and cardiovascular disease risk prediction to guide statin allocation: the Multi-Ethnic Study of Atherosclerosis (MESA). PLoS One. 2015;10(3):e0116377.
47. Kalia NK, Miller LG, Nasir K, Blumenthal RS, Agrawal N, Budoff MJ. Visualizing coronary calcium is associated with improvements in adherence to statin therapy. Atherosclerosis. 2006;185(2):394–9.
48. Kalia NK, Cespedes L, Youssef G, Li D, Budoff MJ. Motivational effects of coronary artery calcium scores on statin adherence and weight loss. Coron Artery Dis. 2015;26(3):225–30.
49. Mamudu HM, Paul TK, Veeranki SP, Budoff M. The effects of coronary artery calcium screening on behavioral modification, risk perception, and medication adherence among asymptomatic adults: a systematic review. Atherosclerosis. 2014;236(2):338–50.
50. McSweeney J, Cleves MA, Fischer EP, Moser DK, Wei J, Pettey C, et al. Predicting coronary heart disease events in women: a longitudinal cohort study. J Cardiovasc Nurs. 2014;29(6):482–92.
51. McSweeney JC, O'Sullivan P, Cleves MA, Lefler LL, Cody M, Moser DK, et al. Racial differences in women's prodromal and acute symptoms of myocardial infarction. Am J Crit Care. 2010;19(1):63–73.
52. Mieres JH, Shaw LJ, Wenger NK. Noninvasive testing in women with suspected ischemic heart disease: ten highlights to guide quality clinical care. Clin Cardiol. 2014;37(9):515–6.
53. Mieres JH, Gulati M, Bairey Merz N, Berman DS, Gerber TC, Hayes SN, et al. Role of noninvasive testing in the clinical evaluation of women with suspected ischemic heart disease: a consensus statement from the American Heart Association. Circulation. 2014;130(4):350–79.
54. Kwok Y, Kim C, Grady D, Segal M, Redberg R. Meta-analysis of exercise testing to detect coronary artery disease in women. Am J Cardiol. 1999;83(5):660–6.
55. Fihn SD, Gardin JM, Abrams J, Berra K, Blankenship JC, Dallas AP, et al. 2012 ACCF/AHA/ACP/AATS/PCNA/SCAI/STS guideline for the diagnosis and management of patients with stable ischemic heart disease: executive summary: a report of the American College of Cardiology Foundation/American Heart Association Task Force on Practice Guidelines, and the American College of Physicians, American Association for Thoracic Surgery, Preventive Cardiovascular Nurses Association, Society for Cardiovascular Angiography and Interventions, and Society of Thoracic Surgeons. J Am Coll Cardiol. 2012;60(24):2564–603.
56. Colella TJ, Gravely S, Marzolini S, Grace SL, Francis JA, Oh P, et al. Sex bias in referral of women to outpatient cardiac rehabilitation? A meta-analysis. Eur J Prev Cardiol. 2015;22(4):423–41.
57. Liu A, Wijesurendra RS, Liu JM, Greiser A, Jerosch-Herold M, Forfar JC, et al. Gadolinium-free cardiac MR stress T1-mapping to distinguish epicardial from microvascular coronary disease. J Am Coll Cardiol. 2018;71(9):957–68.
58. Feher A, Sinusas AJ. Quantitative assessment of coronary microvascular function: dynamic single-photon emission computed tomography, positron emission tomography, ultrasound, computed tomography, and magnetic resonance imaging. Circ Cardiovasc Imaging. 2017;10(8):e006427.
59. Murthy VL, Naya M, Taqueti VR, Foster CR, Gaber M, Hainer J, et al. Effects of sex on coronary microvascular dysfunction and cardiac outcomes. Circulation. 2014;129(24):2518–27.
60. Meschia JF, Bushnell C, Boden-Albala B, Braun LT, Bravata DM, Chaturvedi S, et al. Guidelines for the primary prevention of stroke: a statement for healthcare professionals from the American Heart Association/American Stroke Association. Stroke. 2014;45(12):3754–832.
61. Smith GN, Pudwell J, Walker M, Wen SW. Ten-year, thirty-year, and lifetime cardiovascular disease risk estimates following a pregnancy complicated by preeclampsia. J Obstet Gynaecol Can. 2012;34(9):830–5.
62. Curtis KM, Tepper NK, Jatlaoui TC, Berry-Bibee E, Horton LG, Zapata LB, et al. U.S. medical eligibility criteria for contraceptive use, 2016. MMWR Recomm Rep. 2016;65(3):1–103.
63. Manson JE, Aragaki AK, Rossouw JE, Anderson GL, Prentice RL, LaCroix AZ, et al. Menopausal hormone therapy and long-term all-cause and cause-specific mortality: the Women's Health Initiative randomized trials. JAMA. 2017;318(10):927–38.
64. Powers WJ, Rabinstein AA, Ackerson T, Adeoye OM, Bambakidis NC, Becker K, et al. 2018 Guidelines for the early management of patients with acute ischemic stroke: a guideline for healthcare professionals from the American Heart Association/American Stroke Association. Stroke. 2018;49(3):e46–e110.

Urinary Incontinence

23

Katherine E. Twist and Halle G. Sobel

Learning Objectives

1. Describe the impact of urinary incontinence on daily life.
2. Define the types of urinary incontinence in women.
3. Evaluate a woman with symptoms of urinary incontinence.
4. Manage urinary incontinence.
5. Appropriately seek specialty consultation for urinary incontinence.

Preeti is a 65-year-old female who has type 2 diabetes, obesity, hypertension, and hyperlipidemia. She presents for an annual exam. On reviewing her pre-visit questionnaire, you note in the review of systems that she checked off urinary incontinence and she has gained 10 pounds over the last 5 years.

Background and Epidemiology

Urinary incontinence is a common condition defined as an involuntary loss of urine. It is frequently underdiagnosed but can negatively affect the quality of life in psychological, social, and sexual aspects. Nearly half of all women will experience urinary incontinence at some point during their lifetime, but only 25% of women with the condition will seek treatment [1].

Risk factors include increasing age, obesity, and tobacco use. Conditions unique to women that also increase the risk of urinary incontinence include pregnancy, pelvic floor trauma such as vaginal delivery, menopause, and hysterectomy. Other contributors to incontinence include urinary tract infections (UTIs), functional or cognitive impairment, chronic cough, and constipation [2].

Urinary incontinence is associated with a high societal cost as it is estimated at exceeding $82 billion in the year 2020 [2]. The impaired quality of life can take the form of falls, fractures, sleep disturbances, depression, and UTIs. Older women with lower urinary tract symptoms are about twice as likely to experience falls as those without symptoms [3–5].

Though it can be easily screened for and often managed in a primary care setting, urinary incontinence is frequently underreported and underdiagnosed. Women often do not volunteer symptoms because of embarrassment, lack of understanding about the disease, or misconceptions about treatment, so it is important to ask about urinary leakage [6, 7].

Normal Anatomy and Physiology

The lower urinary tract consists of a urinary bladder and the urethra. Normal urinary function depends on functioning anatomy, muscular supports in the pelvic floor, and neural communications from the central nervous system and peripheral ganglia.

Functional anatomy of the urinary system includes the bladder and urethra. The bladder is composed of a muscular layer called the detrusor muscle. The detrusor in the bladder dome is innervated by both sympathetic beta-adrenergic receptors and parasympathetic muscarinic receptors. When the parasympathetic system is stimulated, muscarinic receptors are activated causing detrusor contraction and bladder emptying. The urethra consists of an internal sphincter which

K. E. Twist (✉)
University of Kentucky, Department of Internal Medicine, Lexington, KY, USA
e-mail: k.twist@uky.edu

H. G. Sobel
Robert Larner MD, College of Medicine at The University of Vermont, Department of General Internal Medicine, Burlington, VT, USA

S. A. Tilstra et al. (eds.), *Sex- and Gender-Based Women's Health*, https://doi.org/10.1007/978-3-030-50695-7_23

is made up of smooth muscle and an external sphincter which is under external/voluntary control.

The bladder and surrounding pelvic structures are held in place by a group of muscles that support the pelvic viscera, including the coccygeus and layers of the levator ani. Collectively, these muscles are referred to as the "pelvic floor."

Complex neural pathways between the central nervous system (CNS) and peripheral ganglia maintain urethral closure and affect detrusor muscle function for the storage and release of urine. Bladder storage is primarily mediated in the spinal cord, whereas micturition is controlled by reflex mechanisms in the brain [8].

Preeti acknowledges urinary leakage before she can make it to the bathroom and also urinary leakage with coughing and sneezing.

Pathophysiology of Urinary Incontinence

Urinary incontinence is classified based on a combination of clinical manifestations and the underlying abnormal mechanism. However, the distinction between the different types is not always clear [2].

Stress Incontinence

Stress incontinence occurs when increased intra-abdominal pressure puts enough force on the urinary bladder that the urethra can no longer resist the flow of urine. It is typically caused by urethral hypermobility, which is often due to impaired pelvic floor support. Risk factors include vaginal delivery, obesity, and conditions that increase intra-abdominal pressure such as chronic constipation, heavy lifting, and high impact exercise [9–14].

Urgency Incontinence

Urgency incontinence is characterized by a sudden desire to pass urine that is difficult to hold. It is caused by detrusor overactivity [15]. While usually idiopathic, it can be associated with systemic neurologic conditions like Parkinson's disease, multiple sclerosis, or pelvic or spinal nerve injury [16].

Mixed Incontinence

Mixed incontinence is a combination of stress and urge symptoms due to detrusor overactivity combined with impaired urethral function. Patients have a combination of symptoms with this condition and may be affected by stress and urgency to varying degrees.

Overflow Incontinence

Overflow incontinence occurs due to incomplete bladder emptying from either impaired detrusor contractility or bladder outlet obstruction. Symptoms can be similar to stress and urge incontinence but may also be associated with incomplete emptying of the bladder. In females, this condition typically occurs with underlying systemic neurologic disease or anatomic abnormalities like urethral obstruction [16].

Functional Incontinence

Patients with functional incontinence have a normal voiding system, but they have a physical or psychological impairment to mobilizing to a toilet, such as patients with limited mobility or dementia.

Preeti's leakage is intermittent and has been present for years after the birth of her two children but notes she has had worsening symptoms over the past 2 years. Not only does it occur with coughing and sneezing, but occasionally, she will note a sudden urge to urinate that seems almost uncontrollable and is associated with leakage. As you proceed with your evaluation, you note she has symptoms of both stress and urgency incontinence.

Differential Diagnosis and Contributing Factors

Though the diagnosis of urinary incontinence specifically refers to involuntary urine loss, there are a number of conditions that can result in similar lower urinary tract symptoms. Urinary tract infections are frequent causes of incontinence and should be ruled out in a primary care setting. (See Chap. 24 on Urinary Tract Infections.) Other conditions that cause inflammation in the lower urinary tract and nearby structures can also result in similar symptoms, such as interstitial cystitis and vaginitis [17]. (See Chap. 12 Vaginitis and Vulvar Problems.)

Urinary frequency and urgency can also be precipitated by systemic diseases including uncontrolled diabetes mellitus as the osmotic effect of glucosuria results in polyuria and polydipsia. Many commonly prescribed medications can cause urinary symptoms by interfering with the bladder or sphincter function, increasing pressure within the bladder, or impairing mobilization. Such classes include diuretics, ACE inhibitors, sedatives-hypnotics, antidepressants, antipsychotics, and antihistamines. The urethral sphincter tone can be reduced with alpha-blocking medications and can result in stress urinary incontinence [18]. The genitourinary syndrome of menopause, previously called vulvovaginal atrophy, can cause urinary frequency, urgency, and urgency incontinence [19]. (See Chap. 8 on Menopause.)

Neurologic impairment in the spinal cord can also result in incontinence and, though rare, should not be missed. Spinal cord trauma as well as a neoplasm or abscess would result in overflow incontinence and usually other neurologic symptoms.

Pelvic Organ Prolapse

Pelvic organs can prolapse or descend into the vagina or beyond its walls. A cystocele is the prolapse of the bladder and can be seen on a speculum exam when using only the posterior blade as anterior descent of the wall on Valsalva maneuver. A rectocele is the prolapse of the rectum, which is seen on a speculum exam when using only the anterior bladder as a posterior descent of the wall on Valsalva. The prevalence of pelvic organ prolapse is highly dependent on age and parity. Obesity, history of hysterectomy, White or Latina groups, and occupations with heavy lifting are also risk factors for symptomatic prolapse. See Chap. 3 on the Sex and Gender Specific History and Examination for details on diagnosing and documenting the severity of pelvic organ prolapse.

Pelvic organ prolapse is associated with a weakened pelvic floor which can increase urethral mobility and thus the risk for incontinence. Prolapse can also potentially restrict urine flow and result in overflow incontinence symptoms as well. Women with pelvic organ prolapse may present with the sensation of something falling out of the vagina or a bulge.

Management of pelvic organ prolapse depends on the presence of symptoms. If prolapse is discovered on exam but is asymptomatic, no specific therapy is necessary. If prolapse is symptomatic (i.e., urinary dysfunction, bowel dysfunction, or the pressure sensation), conservative therapy includes pessaries and pelvic floor muscle exercises, both discussed below. Women who have symptoms of prolapse that persist despite conservative therapy are surgical candidates.

Preeti urinates about every 4 hours during the day and gets up once per night. She denies any dysuria, pelvic pain, pressure, or other vaginal symptoms. She reports her last hemoglobin A1c was 7.5%. Her current medications include metformin, lisinopril-hydrochlorothiazide, simvastatin, and aspirin.

Diagnostic Strategies

History

The first step to evaluating urinary incontinence occurs with a detailed patient history. Many women do not report symptoms or think symptoms are due to normal aging. Thus, a proactive approach to questioning patients, especially women, is imperative [19].

The two most common urinary incontinence types, stress and urgency, can be determined by a brief validated questionnaire which takes little time in an office visit. Additional questions should include a review of voiding habits as well as the amount and type of fluid intake [20].

If a patient has difficulty describing symptoms or the diagnosis is unclear, encourage the patient to keep a voiding diary. The patient should be instructed to record the quantity and timing of fluid intake for 1–3 days. This will assist in determining if there are fluid modifications that can be recommended to the patient.

Exam

The pelvic exam can provide additional information as to the cause and/or contributing factors to the incontinence. In postmenopausal women, it is useful to evaluate for atrophy and consider treatment with local estrogen to improve urethral hypermobility. Pelvic organ prolapse beyond the vagina is associated with a higher risk of urinary retention, and referral to a specialist may be warranted. Pelvic floor integrity can be evaluated during the bimanual pelvic exam by asking a patient to contract her pelvic floor muscles. If the patient has a difficult time isolating these muscles or she can only achieve a poor contraction, she may benefit from a formal pelvic floor therapy program [21, 22].

Laboratory Studies

A urinalysis should be used as an initial diagnostic test to evaluate for a urinary tract infection. Additionally, a urinalysis can detect hematuria, pyuria, and glucosuria which often represent comorbid conditions that may need to be treated separately [23].

Other Diagnostic Strategies

In the authors' experience, the large majority of patients can be managed based on history, exam, and urinalysis without consultation. When diagnosis is still unclear, other diagnostic studies can be used and are often in conjunction with an incontinence specialist. A simple urinary stress test can be done in the office: a woman with a comfortably full bladder strains or coughs while in a standing or lithotomic position. Leakage during this maneuver highly suggests stress incontinence [24].

Other special diagnostic testing like urodynamic studies are often performed by urologists and are not recommended for the uncomplicated disease. They can be used in patients with unclear diagnosis, with suboptimal response to standard treatments, or before undergoing significant and irreversible invasive treatments [23, 25].

A post-void residual (PVR) test should be obtained if symptoms point toward incomplete emptying or exam findings demonstrate a distended bladder. Within 10 minutes of a measured void, the PVR is obtained either by ultrasound or catheterization. While definitions vary, experts typically consider normal residual as either <100 mL left in the bladder when the patient has voided >200 mL or one-third of the total voided volume with lesser voids [23].

Preeti's vital signs are significant for a BMI of 37, blood pressure 137/79, pulse 68. She is neurologically intact. Pelvic exam reveals pale, thin vaginal mucosa, and poor muscle tone with Kegel contraction. A urinalysis is normal. She completes a brief questionnaire in the office, which indicates she has stress-predominant mixed urinary incontinence.

Treatment Strategies

The goal of treatment in patients with urinary incontinence is to achieve or improve continence. General strategies for any type of incontinence include conservative management as a reasonable initial approach and include pelvic floor strengthening as well as behavior and lifestyle modifications. We recommend these therapies because they are low-cost strategies that address the underlying condition and are often without adverse effects.

Pelvic Floor Therapy

Pelvic floor muscle strengthening exercises, including Kegels, are recommended as first-line treatment for stress and mixed urinary incontinence [2]. Pelvic floor muscle training can also offer modest benefit in urgency incontinence.

Strengthening the pelvic floor provides a support system against which the urethra may close. For stress urinary incontinence, muscle strengthening helps compensate for anatomic weakness and defects. For urgency incontinence, it intensifies the pelvic floor muscle contractions to improve continence when the bladder detrusor muscle is contracting.

Kegel exercises are a low-cost, low-risk intervention, but they do require personal engagement from the patient. To perform, the patient consciously contracts the levator ani muscles as if trying to stop the flow of urine. It is recommended to gradually build up to performing three sets of 10 contractions which are held for 10 seconds each. The patient should not interrupt urine stream while doing the exercises. The addition of weighted vaginal cones, biofeedback, or other feedback with a trained physiotherapist can potentially improve cure rates because a patient has greater awareness of muscular activity [26, 27].

For anticipated events that may result in stress incontinence such as coughing or sneezing, patients can perform a Knack maneuver. This maneuver consists of a patient preemptively contracting the pelvic floor and holding the contraction through the episode of increased abdominal pressure [19].

Bladder Training and Scheduled Voiding

Most patients are recommended to perform bladder training and scheduled voiding as it is a simple, low-cost intervention. Bladder training can be offered as first-line therapy for urgency incontinence, and these include timed voiding and urge suppression. Patients should schedule voiding every 2–3 hours or as needed for fluid intake to reduce the risk of incontinence episodes. Urge suppression helps reduce the urge to urinate and improve bladder control. When the urge to urinate occurs, the patient is recommended to become still, sit down and breathe deeply to relax, and then contract the pelvic floor muscles quickly and strongly 5–10 times. Once the urge to urinate goes away, the patient can either walk calmly to the bathroom or wait until the urge returns again.

Dietary and Other Lifestyle Changes

For most patients, dietary changes should be recommended and include avoiding excess fluid intake and reducing caffeine and alcohol [23, 28]. Fluid intake should occur in small amounts of 4–5 ounces per hour for up to 2 liters per day of predominantly water. Modest weight loss (>5% reduction in body weight) should be recommended in obese patients, as this has been shown to reduce the incidence of incontinence episodes [23, 29].

Other General Treatments

Using absorbent products can be beneficial in social situations and is recommended for light urinary incontinence; if contact dermatitis develops, topical zinc oxide can be used as a barrier. Patients should also be evaluated and treated for underlying problems that contribute to increased intra-abdominal pressure, including tobacco abuse/chronic cough and constipation.

Topical estrogen is recommended in patients with the genitourinary syndrome of menopause who have urinary incontinence. The topical estrogen is thought to increase urethral blood flow and potentially collagen deposition to improve urethral coaptation [19, 30]. Systemic estrogens do not have a role in the treatment of urinary incontinence; some studies indicate a worsening of incontinence with systemic estrogen. See Chap. 8 on Menopause for details on topical and systemic estrogen.

Treatments for Stress Incontinence

Medications

There are currently no FDA-approved medications for stress incontinence, and the American College of Physicians recommends against its use [2].

Pessaries

Pessaries are commonly used to treat pelvic organ prolapse but can also help support the bladder neck so the urethrovesicular junction is stabilized [19]. Data are limited regarding the value of pessaries for incontinence, but they may be preferable for patients who only have stress incontinence during specific situations such as exercise [31]. When referring for pessary placement, look for a gynecology or urology colleague that regularly fits pessaries.

Surgery/Invasive Options

For patients with persistent symptoms despite conservative measures, surgical procedures and injection of bulking agents can often improve incontinence symptoms. Selection of appropriate candidates is critical because, while surgery is often efficacious for stress incontinence, its effects may be time-limited in some women, and these procedures put women at risk for postoperative voiding difficulty or urge incontinence [32].

Surgical intervention with mid-urethral slings or other similar procedures can be highly effective but more invasive than other measures. A mid-urethral sling is the most studied anti-incontinent operation and consists of the insertion of a synthetic mesh sling in a 30-minute outpatient procedure and has documented short- and long-term efficacy [33].

Injection of bulking agents can also potentially reduce symptoms of stress incontinence. This is usually an in-office procedure using local anesthesia and a cystoscope and entails injecting bulking material under the urethral mucosal layer to increase outflow resistance. Success rates are lower with bulking agents compared to sling procedures [34].

Treatments for Urgency Incontinence

Medications

For patients in whom bladder training is unsuccessful, medications can be used as second-line therapy for urgency incontinence [35]. There are six FDA-approved anticholinergic medications that block muscarinic receptors in the smooth muscle of the bladder to inhibit detrusor contractions, and these include darifenacin, fesoterodine, oxybutynin, solifenacin, tolterodine, and trospium. The only contraindications to these medications are untreated narrow-angle glaucoma, urinary retention, and gastric retention, although some evidence suggests these medications may aggravate existing cardiac arrhythmias and be associated with dementia. Use caution in starting the medication in older adults because of side effects such as drowsiness, hallucinations, cognitive impairment, and dementia [23].

Dry mouth is the most common side effect due to anticholinergic effects and can affect 20–50% of patients [36]. In addition, constipation, abdominal pain, dyspepsia, fatigue, dry eye, and dry skin can also occur. Due to bothersome side effects, less than 50% of patients continue taking the medication beyond 6 months [37].

Most efficacy data have been limited to short-term industry-supported studies, but all appear to have similar efficacy. The choice of agent relies on the side-effect profile, insurance formulary, or patient cost. Oxybutynin and tolterodine are generic anticholinergics that typically have lower cost. When available, extended-release formulations typically have more favorable side-effect profiles [23].

A newer agent, mirabegron, is a beta-3 agonist that stimulates beta-3 adrenergic receptors through the sympathetic nervous system to promote smooth muscle relaxation of the bladder. It has not been shown to be more effective than anticholinergics, but it does result in less dry mouth and constipation [16], and we recommend its use as second-line therapy when anticholinergics are not tolerated. Recent evidence suggests that mirabegron with anticholinergics may be synergistic in women who have insufficient response with monotherapy alone [38]. Adverse effects associated with mirabegron are less common and can include hypertension, nasopharyngitis, headache, and UTI [19]. As this is a newer agent, potential long-term effects and adverse reactions in patients with other significant comorbidities are less well understood.

Other Options

Other treatment options when lifestyle and medication therapy fail include percutaneous tibial nerve stimulation, botox injection, and sacral neuromodulation. (See below on when to refer.)

Percutaneous tibial nerve stimulation is an office procedure involving electrical stimulation via an acupuncture needle delivered in twelve 30-minute weekly sessions followed by monthly maintenance therapy. It has similar efficacy to anticholinergic medications and low rates of transient local adverse events [39].

OnabotulinumtoxinA can also be injected into the bladder to block the presynaptic release of acetylcholine to decrease muscarinic receptor activation involved in detrusor contraction. This is inserted through a cystoscope with local anesthetic in a provider's office. It is usually as effective as anticholinergic medication and lasts for 6–12 months. Risks of this procedure include urinary retention and urinary tract infections [40].

Sacral neuromodulation is an outpatient surgical procedure involving an implanted electrode placed along the third sacral nerve root to deliver nerve stimulation. A short-term test will determine whether this procedure is successful and tolerable to the patient, and if so, a permanent stimulator can be implanted and last up to 5 years.

Strategies for Mixed Incontinence

The initial management of mixed incontinence should focus on the predominant component, either stress or urgency, and should be conservative in nature [41]. Though there are no randomized controlled trials to evaluate patients with mixed incontinence, combined pelvic floor muscle therapy with bladder training is recommended as a low-cost and low-risk, noninvasive therapy [2, 36, 42].

As second-line therapy, anticholinergic medications can also be useful when managing mixed incontinence; however, this treatment tends to be more useful for urgency symptoms [42]. More invasive procedures and surgeries include urethral bulking, retropubic urethropexies, pubovaginal slings, and mid-urethral slings. These typically have mixed results and are considered if conservative management fails [42]. The overactive bladder aspect may not improve with surgery [41].

Preeti is treated with pelvic floor muscle strengthening by referring to a pelvic physical therapist and a recommendation to void every 2 hours during the day, as well as avoiding excessive fluid intake. Her hydrochlorothiazide is discontinued, and lisinopril was titrated to manage her blood pressure. She denies cough or constipation. She is referred to a dietician to assist in weight management. After completing physical therapy, she reported a 75% decrease in incontinent episodes.

When to Refer and Other Team Members Who Can Help

The vast majority of urinary incontinence can be evaluated and managed in the primary care setting. As mentioned, many women benefit from a referral to a physical therapist if they are having trouble with pelvic floor exercises. A rare urgent evaluation should occur if there are signs of an acute neurosurgical emergency occurring with the urinary incontinence. Cauda equina syndrome, acute trauma, suspected abscess, or other causes of spinal cord compression would necessitate immediate evaluation and management by a specialist.

Urology or urogynecology referral should be considered for patients who have persistent symptoms despite appropriate treatments and who are considering more invasive treatments. Patients who may have a suspected bladder neoplasm or otherwise unexplained hematuria should also be evaluated outside of the primary care domain. Patients with a history of prior radical pelvic surgery or radiation or prior pelvic incontinence surgery are more likely to fail conservative measures and may benefit from earlier specialist referral.

Finally, in cases of significant pelvic organ prolapse or symptomatic prolapse that persists despite a trial of pessaries and pelvic floor therapy, patients should be referred for surgical evaluation. The risk of urinary retention is elevated in severe prolapse, and these patients typically have limited benefit with conservative treatments.

Summary Points

1. Urinary incontinence is common in women, affecting up to half of all women at some point in their lifetime, yet it remains underreported with only a quarter of those affected seeking treatment.
2. The most common types of incontinence are diagnosed primarily by history and are stress, urge, mixed, and overflow.
3. To evaluate urinary incontinence, first collect a detailed history of the amount and circumstances of the episodes. Order a UA, to rule out secondary causes.
4. Pelvic floor muscle exercises are recommended as initial treatment for stress and mixed incontinence. For urgency incontinence, bladder training is first-line therapy followed by medication therapy with anticholinergics or beta-3 agonists.
5. Refer if a spinal cord problem is suspected or if symptoms persist despite appropriate treatments.

Review Questions

1. A 50-year-old woman with a BMI of 41.0 presents to your office with a 3-day history of urinary leakage with coughing and sneezing. She has not noted any blood in

her urine but does have mild dysuria. She has had three vaginal deliveries in the past without complications. She has been on lisinopril for 1 year for hypertension.

What is the first best step in evaluating her urinary leakage?

A. Discontinue the ACE inhibitor and reevaluate
B. Pelvic exam
C. Pelvic floor physical therapy referral
D. Urinalysis

The correct answer is D. The initial evaluation of a patient with new urinary incontinence should include a urinalysis to rule out underlying infection.

2. A 60-year-old overweight female with mixed urge and stress incontinence comes in for a follow-up visit on her symptoms. At your suggestion, she has lost 5 lbs and has participated in pelvic floor physical therapy for 6 months with slight improvement in symptoms, but they are still bothersome. Prior urine studies have been normal. She takes amlodipine, atorvastatin, and vitamin D.

What is the best next step?

A. Order tolterodine
B. Refer for a pessary fitting
C. Refer for urodynamic studies
D. Urinary incontinence pads

The correct answer is A. This patient has already done first-line therapy which included pelvic floor physical therapy, and she has lost weight which was also recommended as part of lifestyle change. It is reasonable to consider pharmacologic therapy as the next step in her treatment plan [35].

3. A 58-year-old menopausal woman comes in for an annual exam. You inquire about urinary incontinence and find that she wears a liner daily for mild urine leakage. She leaks urine daily without trigger as well as when she coughs, sneezes, or laughs. She has a history of osteoporosis and allergic rhinitis for which she takes occasional antihistamines. On exam, you find mildly thin and dry vaginal mucosa and no signs of pelvic organ prolapse. A urinalysis is normal. What is the best next step in managing her symptoms?

A. Order oral estrogen
B. Order oxybutynin
C. Refer to pelvic physical therapy
D. Refer to urology or urogynecology

Correct answer: C. The clinician should recommend pelvic floor physical as this is an effective behavioral therapy for urinary incontinence [2]. Topical estrogen could also be tried in this patient, but oral estrogen is not recommended for vaginal atrophy.

References

1. Minassian VA, Stewart WF, Wood GC. Urinary incontinence in women: variation in prevalence estimates and risk factors. Obstet Gynecol. 2008;111(2 Pt 1):324–31.
2. Qaseem A, Dallas P, Forciea MA, Starkey M, Denberg TD, Shekelle P, Clinical Guidelines Committee of the American College of Physicians. Nonsurgical management of urinary incontinence in women: a clinical practice guideline from the American College of Physicians. Ann Intern Med. 2014;161(6):429–40.
3. Brown JS, McGhan WF, Chokroverty S. Comorbidities associated with overactive bladder. Am J Manag Care. 2000;6(11 Suppl):S574–9.
4. Wagner TH, Hu TW, Bentkover J, LeBlanc K, Stewart W, Corey R, et al. Health-related consequences of overactive bladder. Am J Manag Care. 2002;8(19 Suppl):S598–607.
5. Gibson W, Hunter KF, Camicioli R, Booth J, Skelton DA, Dumoulin C, et al. The association between lower urinary tract symptoms and falls: forming a theoretical model for a research agenda. Neurourol Urodyn. 2018;37(1):501–9.
6. Abrams P, Kelleher CJ, Kerr LA, Rogers RG. Overactive bladder significantly affects quality of life. Am J Manag Care. 2000;6(11 Suppl):S580–90.
7. Ricci JA, Baggish JS, Hunt TL, Stewart WF, Wein A, Herzog AR, Diokno AC. Coping strategies and health care-seeking behavior in a US national sample of adults with symptoms suggestive of overactive bladder. Clin Ther. 2001;23(8):1245–59.
8. Shah AP, Mevcha A, Wilby D, Alatsatianos A, Hardman JC, Jacques S, Wilton JC. Continence and micturition: an anatomical basis. Clin Anat. 2014;27(8):1275–83.
9. Handa VL, Blomquist JL, Knoepp LR, Hoskey KA, McDermott KC, Muñoz A. Pelvic floor disorders 5-10 years after vaginal or cesarean childbirth. Obstet Gynecol. 2011;118(4):777–84.
10. Handa VL, Harvey L, Fox HE, Kjerulff KH. Parity and route of delivery: does cesarean delivery reduce bladder symptoms later in life? Am J Obstet Gynecol. 2004;191(2):463–9.
11. Lawrence JM, Lukacz ES, Liu IL, Nager CW, Luber KM. Pelvic floor disorders, diabetes, and obesity in women: findings from the Kaiser Permanente Continence Associated Risk Epidemiology Study. Diabetes Care. 2007;30(10):2536–41.
12. Lukacz ES, et al. Parity, mode of delivery, and pelvic floor disorders. Obstet Gynecol. 2006;107(6):1253–60.
13. Nygaard IE, Shaw JM. Physical activity and the pelvic floor. Am J Obstet Gynecol. 2016;214(2):164–71.
14. Rortveit G, Daltveit AK, Hannestad YS, Hunskaar S. Vaginal delivery parameters and urinary incontinence: the Norwegian EPINCONT study. Am J Obstet Gynecol. 2003;189(5):1268–74.
15. Abrams P, Andersson KE, Birder L, Brubaker L, Cardozo L, Chapple C, et al.; Members of committees; fourth international consultation on incontinence. Fourth international consultation on incontinence recommendations of the international scientific committee: evaluation and treatment of urinary incontinence, pelvic organ prolapse, and fecal incontinence. Neurourol Urodyn. 2010;29(1):213–40.
16. Lukacz ES, Santiago-Lastra Y, Albo ME, Brubaker L. Urinary incontinence in women: a review. JAMA. 2017;318(16):1592–604.
17. Khandelwal C, Kistler C. Diagnosis of urinary incontinence. Am Fam Physician. 2013;87(8):543–50.
18. Kashyap M, Tu le M, Tannenbaum C. Prevalence of commonly prescribed medications potentially contributing to urinary symptoms

in a cohort of older patients seeking care for incontinence. BMC Geriatr. 2013;13:57.
19. Shih E, Hirsch H, Thacker HL. Medical management of urinary incontinence in women. Cleve Clin J Med. 2017;84(2):151–8.
20. Brown JS, Bradley CS, Subak LL, Richter HE, Kraus SR, et al.; Diagnostic Aspects of Incontinence Study (DAISy) Research Group. The sensitivity and specificity of a simple test to distinguish between urge and stress urinary incontinence. Ann Intern Med. 2006;144(10):716.
21. Dumoulin C, Hay-Smith J, Habée-Séguin GM, Mercier J. Pelvic floor muscle training versus no treatment, or inactive control treatments, for urinary incontinence in women: a short version Cochrane systematic review with meta-analysis. Neurourol Urodyn. 2015;34(4):300–8.
22. Hay-Smith EJ, Herderschee R, Dumoulin C, Herbison GP. Comparisons of approaches to pelvic floor muscle training for urinary incontinence in women. Cochrane Database Syst Rev. 2011;(12):CD009508.
23. Syan R, Brucker BM. Guideline of guidelines: urinary incontinence. BJU Int. 2016;117(1):20–33.
24. Harvey MA, Versi E. Predictive value of clinical evaluation of stress urinary incontinence: a summary of the published literature. Int Urogynecol J Pelvic Floor Dysfunct. 2001;12(1):31–7.
25. Winters JC, Dmochowski RR, Goldman HB, Herndon CD, Kobashi KC, Kraus SR, et al.; American Urological Association; Society of Urodynamics, Female Pelvic Medicine & Urogenital Reconstruction. Urodynamic studies in adults: AUA/SUFU guideline. J Urol. 2012;188(6 Suppl):2464–72.
26. Herbison GP, Dean N. Weighted vaginal cones for urinary incontinence. Cochrane Database Syst Rev. 2013;(7):CD002114.
27. Herderschee R, Hay-Smith EJ, Herbison GP, Roovers JP, Heineman MJ. Feedback or biofeedback to augment pelvic floor muscle training for urinary incontinence in women. Cochrane Database Syst Rev. 2011;(7):CD009252.
28. Imamura M, Williams K, Wells M, McGrother C. Lifestyle interventions for the treatment of urinary incontinence in adults. Cochrane Database Syst Rev. 2015;(12):CD003505.
29. Subak LL, Wing R, West DS, Franklin F, Vittinghoff E, Creasman JM, et al. PRIDE Investigators.Weight loss to treat urinary incontinence in overweight and obese women. N Engl J Med. 2009;360(5):481–90.
30. Weber MA, Kleijn MH, Langendam M, Limpens J, Heineman MJ, Roovers JP. Local oestrogen for pelvic floor disorders: a systematic review. PLoS One. 2015;10(9):e0136265.
31. Lipp A, Shaw C, Glavind K. Mechanical devices for urinary incontinence in women. Cochrane Database Syst Rev. 2011;(7):CD001756.
32. Jonsson Funk M, Siddiqui NY, Kawasaki A, Wu JM. Long-term outcomes after stress urinary incontinence surgery. Obstet Gynecol. 2012;120(1):83.
33. Ford AA, Rogerson L, Cody JD, Ogah J. Mid-urethral sling operations for stress urinary incontinence in women. Cochrane Database Syst Rev. 2015;(7):CD006375.
34. Kirchin V, Page T, Keegan PE, Atiemo K, Cody JD, McClinton S. Urethral injection therapy for urinary incontinence in women. Cochrane Database Syst Rev. 2012;(2):CD003881.
35. Gormley EA, Lightner DJ, Burgio KL, Chai TC, Clemens JQ, Culkin DJ, et al.; American Urological Association; Society of Urodynamics, Female Pelvic Medicine & Urogenital Reconstruction. Diagnosis and treatment of overactive bladder (non-neurogenic) in adults: AUA/SUFU guideline amendment. J Urol. 2012;188(6 Suppl):2455–63.
36. Culbertson S, Davis AM. Nonsurgical Management of Urinary Incontinence in women. JAMA. 2017;317(1):79–80.
37. Brostrom S, Hallas J. Persistence of antimuscarinic drug use. Eur J Clin Pharmacol. 2009;65(3):309–14.
38. Herschorn S, Chapple CR, Abrams P, Arlandis S, Mitcheson D, Lee KS, et al. Efficacy and safety of combinations of mirabegron and solifenacin compared with monotherapy and placebo in patients with overactive bladder (SYNERGY study). BJU Int. 2017;120(4):562–75.
39. Burton C, Sajja A, Latthe PM. Effectiveness of percutaneous posterior tibial nerve stimulation for overactive bladder: a systematic review and meta-analysis. Neurourol Urodyn. 2012;31(8):1206–16.
40. Visco AG, Brubaker L, Richter HE, Nygaard I, et al. Anticholinergic therapy vs. onabotulinumtoxina for urgency urinary incontinence. N Engl J Med. 2012;367(19):1803–13.
41. Bettez M, Tu le M, Carlson K, Corcos J, Gajewski J, Jolivet M, Bailly G. 2012 update: guidelines for adult urinary incontinence collaborative consensus document for the Canadian urological association. Can Urol Assoc J. 2012;6(5):354–63.
42. Myers DL. Female mixed urinary incontinence: a clinical review. JAMA. 2014;311(19):2007–14.

Urinary Tract Infections

24

Jane S. Sillman and Michael P. Carson

Learning Objectives

1. Diagnose and treat cystitis.
2. Diagnose and treat pyelonephritis.
3. Evaluate and treat recurrent urinary tract infections.

Definitions

Complicated urinary tract infection (UTI): an infection occurring in patients with conditions that increase the risk of failing therapy, as outlined in Table 24.1

Cystitis: infection of the bladder

Pyelonephritis: infection of the kidney

Recurrent urinary tract infections: ≥2 infections in 6 months or ≥3 infections in 1 year

Urethritis: inflammation of the urethra.

Table 24.1 Conditions that qualify urinary tract infections as complicated

Pregnancy
Poorly controlled diabetes
Hospital-acquired infection
Acute kidney injury or chronic kidney disease
Suspected or known urinary tract obstruction
Presence of an indwelling urethral catheter, stent, nephrostomy tube, or urinary diversion
Functional or anatomic abnormality of the urinary tract
Renal transplant
Immunocompromise related to other condition or medical therapy

J. S. Sillman (✉)
Brigham and Women's Hospital, Department of Medicine, Boston, MA, USA
e-mail: jsillman@bwh.harvard.edu

M. P. Carson
Hackensack Meridian School of Medicine at Seton Hall, Jersey Shore University Medical Center, Department of Medicine, Neptune, NJ, USA

Epidemiology

Urethritis and cystitis are both common in sexually active women. The incidence of cystitis in a study of 796 young women was 0.5–0.7 per person-year [1] and was 0.07 per person-year in a 2-year study of 1017 postmenopausal women [2]. Pyelonephritis is less common, and at most, only 3% of cystitis cases progress to pyelonephritis [3].

Microbiology

Cystitis and Pyelonephritis

Seventy-five percent to ninety-five percent of uncomplicated cystitis and pyelonephritis in women are due to *Escherichia coli*. Less common causes include other *Enterobacteriaceae* such as *Proteus mirabilis*, *Klebsiella pneumoniae*, and *Staphylococcus saprophyticus*.

Recurrent Urinary Tract Infection

Most are thought to be due to reinfection rather than relapse. Recurrent uncomplicated episodes of cystitis are common in young healthy women and in older women, while recurrent pyelonephritis is not. Women whose first UTI is caused by *E. coli* are more likely to have a second episode within 6 months than those with a first urinary tract infection due to other organisms [4]. A Finnish study of women ages 17 to 82 who had *E. coli* cystitis showed that 44% had a recurrence within 1 year [5].

Clinical Manifestations of UTIs

Urethritis

This is a common cause of dysuria in sexually active women. The presence of a urethral discharge suggests that the patient may have a sexually transmitted infection. Causes include chlamydia, gonorrhea, trichomonas, candidiasis, and herpes

S. A. Tilstra et al. (eds.), *Sex- and Gender-Based Women's Health*, https://doi.org/10.1007/978-3-030-50695-7_24

simplex. Use of irritating substances like contraceptive gel can also cause noninfectious urethritis.

Cystitis

Symptoms of bladder inflammation/infection may include urinary frequency, urgency, and suprapubic pain. Patients may note hematuria, and suprapubic tenderness may be noted on an exam.

Pyelonephritis

Fever is a defining feature of pyelonephritis. Patients may also have chills and malaise, unilateral costovertebral angle tenderness, nausea, and vomiting with or without typical symptoms of dysuria/cystitis.

Urinalysis shows significant pyuria, and an elevated white blood cell count is supportive of the diagnosis, but not required.

Recurrent Urinary Tract Infection

The symptoms are the same as those of a first episode of cystitis. A postmenopausal patient may also have symptoms of vaginal dryness, burning, and dyspareunia due to estrogen deficiency. The physical exam in a postmenopausal patient may reveal atrophy of the external genitalia, loss of normal rugae in the vagina, and foreshortening of the cervix.

Pathophysiology

The basic pathogenesis of all UTIs is thought to be the same: uropathogens from the fecal flora colonize the vaginal introitus, ascend from the urethra to the bladder, and cause cystitis. The pathogens may also ascend from the ureters to the kidneys, resulting in pyelonephritis. Seeding of the kidneys from bacteremia can also cause pyelonephritis.

While UTIs often occur in women without risk factors, certain factors such as sexual behaviors, genetic predisposition, and postmenopausal atrophy increase risk. In young women, risk factors for cystitis include sexual intercourse, new sex partner, spermicide use, and history of urinary tract infections.

In postmenopausal women, estrogen deficiency increases the risk of urinary tract infections. Hypoestrogenic changes include thinning of the vaginal, urethral, and bladder epithelium, making them more vulnerable to infection. The low glycogen content of the thin vaginal epithelium leads to a reduction in lactic acid production by lactobacilli, resulting in an increase in vaginal pH. These changes lead to the overgrowth of nonacidophilic coliforms and the disappearance of lactobacilli, predisposing to infection [6]. In a case-control study of 149 healthy postmenopausal women with a history of recurrent UTI and 53 controls, the following factors were found to be strongly associated with recurrent UTIs: urinary incontinence (OR 5.0), history of UTI before menopause (OR 4.85), and ABO blood group antigen nonsecretor status (OR 2.9) [7].

Risk factors for pyelonephritis are similar to cystitis and include sexual activity, factors that impede urine flow such as pregnancy or mechanical obstruction, genetic predisposition, high microbial load, pathogen virulence characteristics such as adhesion factors, and possibly diabetes mellitus [3].

Inherited factors can also predispose to UTI. For example, being a nonsecretor of ABO blood group antigens (associated with enhanced adherence of uropathogenic *E. coli* compared with secretors [8], having a first UTI before or at age 15, and a mother with a history of UTIs [9] increase UTI risk. In one case-control study of 213 women, the mean distance from the urethra to anus was significantly shorter in recurrent UTI cases than in controls (4.8 versus 5.0 cm, $p = 0.03$) [10].

Alice is a 25-year-old woman who telephones you because of pain on urination.

Differential Diagnosis of Dysuria

Dysuria often represents cystitis or UTI, but not always. Other diagnoses to consider, with differentiating features, are as follows:

- *Urethritis*: Symptoms may include dysuria and frequency in a sexually active woman. The physical exam may reveal a urethral discharge. A urinalysis may show pyuria but no bacteriuria.
- *Vaginitis*: Symptoms include vaginal discharge, odor or itching, or pain on intercourse. The physical exam will reveal a vaginal discharge and the findings associated with candidiasis, trichomonas, or bacterial vaginosis on normal saline wet mount and KOH prep.
- *Subclinical pyelonephritis*: Suspect subclinical pyelonephritis in patients with symptoms of cystitis for more than 5 days. Subclinical pyelonephritis is more common in pregnant women and in patients with recurrent UTIs, diabetes, immunosuppression, renal tract pathology, or previous UTI before age 12.
- *Pyelonephritis*: Symptoms include fever, chills, and flank pain. The physical exam will reveal costovertebral angle tenderness. Urinalysis shows pyuria and bacteriuria.

- *Nephrolithiasis*: Patients typically present with abdominal or flank pain and hematuria without fever.
- *Pelvic inflammatory disease*: Symptoms include abdominal pain, purulent cervical discharge, and cervical motion tenderness in sexually active women.
- *Structural urethral abnormalities*: These, including urethral diverticula or strictures, can cause frequency or urgency and hematuria, with persistent sterile pyuria.
- *Painful bladder syndrome*: It is a diagnosis of exclusion in women with ongoing dysuria, frequency, or urgency with no evidence of an identifiable cause.

Alice reports that she has had pain on urination and urinary frequency for 1 day. She has never had this before. She denies fever, back pain, or vaginal discharge and is sure that she is not pregnant. She has a new boyfriend and has been having intercourse about once a week. They are using a condom and spermicide consistently for contraception.

Alice asks if you need her to come in and submit a urine sample for testing.

Diagnostic Strategies

Cystitis: Outpatient via Phone

If the patient calls with classic symptoms of cystitis, no symptoms to suggest pyelonephritis, is not pregnant, and has no other known risk factors for a complicated UTI, it is reasonable to treat her empirically over the phone without obtaining a urinalysis or urine culture.

Cystitis: In the Office

The office affords the opportunity of a physical exam. Check for suprapubic or costovertebral angle tenderness.

An office urine dipstick can be performed to identify the presence of leukocyte esterase, an enzyme released by white blood cells. A dipstick positive for leukocyte esterase correlates with >10 leukocytes per high-power field. Nitrite positivity indicates the presence of *Enterobacteriaceae* which convert urinary nitrate to nitrite and is sensitive and specific for detecting ≥100,000 colonies/ml on urine culture [11]. Recent ingestion of beets can turn the urine red resulting in a false-positive nitrite result. A dipstick positive for either leukocyte esterase or nitrite has a sensitivity of 75% and a specificity of 82% for making the diagnosis of a UTI [12]. However, all tests should be used only as a complement to the clinical diagnosis as a negative dipstick does not reliably rule out infection in a patient with classic symptoms.

Microscopic urinalysis Urinalysis is often not needed in women with typical symptoms of acute uncomplicated cystitis but can be helpful when a patient's clinical presentation is atypical. In the lab, an unspun voided midstream urine is examined for pyuria and hematuria. Greater than 10 leukocytes per high-power field is consistent with cystitis or pyelonephritis and absence suggests an alternative diagnosis [13]. Hematuria is common in urinary tract infections but not in urethritis or vaginitis. However, hematuria does not indicate that the patient has a complicated infection or requires extended therapy.

Urine culture In women with uncomplicated cystitis, empiric treatment of common organisms is typically adequate, and urine culture is often not necessary. Obtaining a urine culture prior to therapy is recommended if the patient's symptoms are not typical of a urinary tract infection, if symptoms persist or recur within 3 months of treatment, or if there is concern about a resistant organism or complicated infection [14]. Colony counts as low as 100 colonies/mL can be associated with infection. Organisms typically considered to be contaminants may be considered causal when identified as the sole organism on culture and in high counts such as 10^5 colonies/mL in a voided midstream urine.

Suspected pyelonephritis always requires an *office evaluation* to check vital signs, assess for suprapubic and costovertebral angle tenderness, and obtain a *urine dipstick* and/or urinalysis. In pyelonephritis, the urinalysis will typically be positive for leukocyte esterase and nitrites. In a patient with symptoms suggestive of pyelonephritis, the absence of pyuria suggests the need to evaluate for an obstructing lesion, while white cell casts indicate the presence of an upper tract infection [15]. The *urine culture* is the most important confirmatory test. It typically will show >10,000 colonies of a uropathogen/mL. Lower counts may be present if the patient received prior antibiotics, has extreme urine acidification, or has urinary tract obstruction. *Blood cultures* may be helpful in making the diagnosis in ambiguous cases: e.g., a patient who received prior antimicrobial therapy. In this situation, the blood culture may still be positive though the urine culture has become negative. Though blood cultures can be helpful diagnostically, the presence of bacteremia rarely changes the management of acute pyelonephritis.

Recurrent urinary tract infection Obtain a urinalysis and culture to confirm the diagnosis of a recurrent infection. In a postmenopausal patient with symptoms suggestive of vulvovaginal atrophy, it is reasonable to do a pelvic exam, look for evidence of vaginal atrophy, and consider appropriate therapy.

Complicated UTIs Always obtain a urinalysis and urine culture (Table 24.1).

You tell Alice that you think she has a bladder infection and that you would like to treat her with an antibiotic. You ask if she has received any antibiotics recently and if she has any drug allergies.

Treatment Strategies

Cystitis

Duration of Antibiotic Therapy

A systematic review of the treatment of cystitis in adults ≥65 years of age demonstrated that the optimal regimens were the same as those given to younger adults and 3–6 days were as efficacious as 7–14-day courses [16].

First-Line Therapy

First-line therapy includes trimethoprim-sulfamethoxazole (TMP-SMX), nitrofurantoin, or fosfomycin.

TMP-SMX

The recommended dose is one double-strength tablet (160/800 mg) twice a day for 3 days. Randomized trials demonstrate clinical efficacy of 86–100% with a 3–7-day regimen [17]. Empiric treatment with TMP-SMX is not recommended if local resistance is greater than 20% [18, 19]. However, even if local resistance rates are high, if a past urine culture showed a susceptible organism, TMP-SMX can be used. In some locales, trimethoprim 100 mg twice daily for 3 days is used instead of TMP-SMX, with similar efficacy [20].

Nitrofurantoin Monohydrate Macrocrystals

The recommended dose is 100 mg orally twice a day for 5 days. Randomized trials demonstrate clinical efficacy of 90–95% with a 5–7-day regimen [21]. Nitrofurantoin should not be given if pyelonephritis is suspected as it does not achieve adequate renal tissue levels [3]. It should also not be given if the creatinine clearance is <30 mL/minute. Observational studies show that nitrofurantoin is safe in patients with milder renal dysfunction and that it can be used safely in older women [22].

Fosfomycin

If a single-dose regimen is needed, such as in situations where follow-up or adherence may be difficult, fosfomycin is an option, although its efficacy is inferior to TMP-SMX and nitrofurantoin. The recommended dose of fosfomycin is 3 grams single dose. A recent randomized clinical trial comparing nitrofurantoin 100 mg three times a day for 5 days to a single 3 gm dose of oral fosfomycin showed that 5-day nitrofurantoin resulted in a significantly greater likelihood of clinical and microbiologic resolution at 28 days after therapy completion [23]. In a previous evaluation, fosfomycin's efficacy was also considered to be inferior to the other first-line drugs [24]. Fosfomycin should not be given if pyelonephritis is suspected because it does not achieve adequate renal levels [3].

Second-Line Therapy

Second-line therapy is indicated if there is allergy or intolerance to first-line therapy and includes oral beta-lactams. Appropriate beta-lactams include amoxicillin-clavulanate, cefpodoxime, cefdinir, and cefadroxil for a 7-day course.

Ampicillin and amoxicillin should not be used for empiric treatment as they have poor efficacy and high rates of resistance [20].

Non-Recommended Therapies

Fluoroquinolones

Fluoroquinolones should not be used for the treatment of cystitis as widespread use leads to an increase in resistance to fluoroquinolones and other options are available. In addition, the FDA has concluded that the risks of the fluoroquinolones (such as tendonitis, tendon rupture, peripheral neuropathy, and CNS effects) outweigh their benefits for uncomplicated acute cystitis [25].

Ibuprofen

Ibuprofen was studied but found to be inferior to antibiotics for the treatment of uncomplicated cystitis. In this recent noninferiority study, 400 women with symptoms of uncomplicated UTI were randomized to 3 days of either ibuprofen or pivmecillinam, an antibiotic not approved in the United States. The outcome of self-report of feeling cured by day 4 was reported in 38.7% of the patients in the ibuprofen group and 72.6% in the pivmecillinam group. The adjusted risk difference was 35% (27–43%) in favor of pivmecillinam, which crossed the noninferiority margin [26].

Pyelonephritis

Outpatient management is appropriate for patients with mild to moderate illness who can be treated initially with hydration and antibiotics in an outpatient facility and discharged on antibiotics under close supervision. The duration of therapy does not need to be extended if bacteremia is present.

There is no evidence that bacteremia is associated with a worse prognosis.

First-Line Therapy

Fluoroquinolones are the only oral antibiotics recommended for outpatient empiric treatment of acute uncomplicated pyelonephritis and are an appropriate choice if the likelihood of resistance is expected to be <10% [27]. The following suggest a higher resistance level: antibiograms in the community documenting resistance >10%, if the patient recently traveled to an area with known resistance >10%, and if the patient has taken a fluoroquinolone in the last 3–6 months. Without these risk factors, treatment options include ciprofloxacin 500 mg orally twice daily for 7 days, ciprofloxacin 1000 mg extended release once daily for 7 days, or levofloxacin 750 mg orally once daily for 5 days [27]. These can be given with or without an initial intravenous dose of a long-acting parenteral antibiotic. Women who are initially evaluated in an emergency department may receive initial IV ceftriaxone or a 24-hour dose of an aminoglycoside [27].

Second-Line Therapy

Second-line therapy is appropriate when there is an allergy to first-line therapy or anticipated resistance to fluoroquinolones of greater than 10%. Best choices for second-line therapy are as follows:

- Trimethoprim-sulfamethoxazole 160/800 mg (one double-strength tablet) twice daily if the organism is susceptible. The FDA recommends 14-day duration of treatment [3].
- Oral beta-lactam, if the pathogen is susceptible, for 10–14 days [3].
- If either of these drugs are used before susceptibility data is available, an initial intravenous dose of a long-acting parenteral antibiotic such as ceftriaxone 1 gm or an aminoglycoside, gentamicin or tobramycin, 5 mg per kg should be given.

Extended care in the emergency department or observation unit for more extensive fluid therapy and initial intravenous antibiotics is appropriate for patients initially unable or unwilling to swallow an oral antibiotic, too ill to go home immediately, or with clinically significant hypovolemia.

Inpatient care is indicated if the patient has severe illness with high fever, pain, debility, inability to maintain hydration or take oral medications, pregnancy, or concerns about patient compliance. *Recommended initial treatment* for an inpatient is an intravenous antibiotic such as a fluoroquinolone, an aminoglycoside, an extended-spectrum cephalosporin, extended-spectrum penicillin, or a carbapenem [3]. The decision should be based on local resistance data and adjusted according to susceptibility results. Patients who improve and can take oral fluids can be transitioned to oral antibiotics. Fluoroquinolone serum levels and clinical efficacy are the same with oral and intravenous therapy; therefore, if a patient is able to tolerate food or liquids, she may receive oral therapy.

Pyelonephritis During Pregnancy

Pyelonephritis can progress rapidly and be life-threatening to the mother and the fetus [3]. Most pregnant women with pyelonephritis, especially in the third trimester, should be admitted to the hospital and treated with intravenous antibiotics. Ten percent of pregnant women may develop noncardiogenic pulmonary edema related to the lower oncotic pressure of pregnancy and increased risk for capillary leak of water into the interstitium. A healthy fetus depends on a healthy mother, so the consequences of *not* treating an infection should be considered, and when indicated, any antibiotic can be used. While aminoglycosides are typically avoided in the first trimester and fluoroquinolones are generally avoided throughout pregnancy, they should be used when indicated in patients with intolerance, allergy, or a resistant organism. TMP/SMX is used throughout pregnancy in patients who require it for prophylaxis related to acquired immunodeficiency syndrome (AIDS); therefore, the potential concern about a theoretical risk to the fetus should not outweigh the clear clinical benefit. Cephalosporins and broad-spectrum beta-lactams cover the common organisms and are reasonable first-line choices.

Recurrent Infections in Premenopausal Women

The following strategies can be used:

Non-Pharmacologic Strategies

Change of contraceptive method can be considered in premenopausal women who use spermicides, especially with diaphragms. Decreased use or elimination of spermicide should decrease the risk of UTI [28]. See Chap. 4 on Patient-Centered Contraceptive Counseling.

Postcoital voiding and liberal fluid intake to increase the frequency of urination might be helpful in reducing the risk of recurrent UTI; however, there are no controlled studies.

Pharmacologic Strategies

Prophylactic Antibiotics

Strategies include postcoital, self-treatment, and continuous regimens. Antimicrobial prophylaxis is highly effective in reducing the risk of recurrent UTI but may be associated with the development of resistance so it is reserved for selected patients [29]. Postcoital prophylaxis, intermittent self-treatment, and continuous prophylaxis have all been demonstrated to be effective. A *single low postcoital dose* may be more efficient and acceptable than continuous prophylaxis to women whose UTIs seem to be related to sexual intercourse. In the one placebo-controlled trial, postcoital trimethoprim-sulfamethoxazole 40 mg/200 mg was associated with a lower infection rate compared with placebo (0.3 versus 3.6 per patient-year) [30]. Uncontrolled studies show a similar reduction in infection rates with a single low dose of nitrofurantoin, cephalexin, or a fluoroquinolone. Postcoital prophylaxis can also be used during pregnancy. The preferred treatment during pregnancy is cephalexin 250 mg or nitrofurantoin 50 mg [31].

Intermittent Self-Treatment

Three studies have shown that the presence of a UTI can be accurately diagnosed by women 85–95% of the time and that short-course treatment with trimethoprim-sulfamethoxazole or a fluoroquinolone is highly effective [32]. This strategy should be limited to women who have clearly documented recurrent infections and are motivated and compliant with instructions. They should be told to call their clinician if their symptoms do not completely resolve by 48 hours.

Continuous Antibiotic Treatment

Continuous antibiotic treatment significantly reduces recurrences. A meta-analysis from the Cochrane database evaluated 10 trials involving 430 healthy nonpregnant women with 2 or more UTIs in the past 12 months who were treated with continuous or postcoital antibiotics for 6–12 months and noted the following: clinical recurrences were significantly decreased with RR 0.15, (95% CI 0.08–0.28) and NNT 1.85. The RR for side effects which included vaginal and oral candidiasis and gastrointestinal symptoms was 1.58 (95% CI 0.47–5.28). There was no significant difference between continuous daily and postcoital ciprofloxacin. No conclusions could be made regarding the best antibiotic choice or optimal duration of prophylaxis [33].

Regimens for continuous antibiotic treatment include trimethoprim-sulfamethoxazole 40 mg/200 mg once a day, nitrofurantoin 50 mg once a day, cephalexin 125–250 mg once a day, and ciprofloxacin 125 mg once a day. One trial evaluated the efficacy of fosfomycin 3 gm every 10 days for 6 months in 317 nonpregnant women with recurrent UTIs and was associated with a decrease in the number of UTIs from 2.97 to 0.14/patient-year. The time to first recurrence of a UTI was longer in the fosfomycin group (38 versus 6 days), and the drug was well tolerated [34].

When indicated, a 6-month trial of antibiotics given at night should be considered, but some patients might require treatment for 2 or more years [29]. Use of trimethoprim-sulfamethoxazole for as long as 5 years has been reported to be well-tolerated and effective [35]. Patients need to be warned that long-term use of nitrofurantoin has been associated with pulmonary reactions, hepatitis, and neuropathy. For these reasons, we recommend TMP-SMX if continuous antibiotic treatment is initiated, unless there is a sulfa allergy.

Antimicrobial resistance to the agent being used for prophylaxis is an increasing problem.

Recurrent Infections in Postmenopausal Women

Treatment with topical low-dose estrogen is effective in decreasing recurrent UTIs as it normalizes the vaginal, urethral, and bladder epithelium, as well as the vaginal flora. In a randomized placebo-controlled trial of 93 postmenopausal women with history of recurrent UTI, intravaginal estradiol cream (50 mcg estradiol nightly for 2 weeks, then twice weekly for 8 months) significantly reduced the recurrence of UTI from 5.9 episodes per patient-year to 0.5 [36]. The treatment increased vaginal lactobacilli and decreased *E. coli* vaginal colonization. Topical estrogen is more effective than systemic estrogen in decreasing recurrent urinary tract infections and alleviating the symptoms of genitourinary atrophy. A 2008 Cochrane review evaluated estrogens for preventing recurrent UTIs in postmenopausal women [37]. In 4 studies with a total of 2798 women, oral estrogens did not reduce UTI compared to placebo. Treatment with vaginal estrogens did reduce the number of women with UTIs in two studies with reported RR of 0.25 (95% CI 0.13–0.50) and 0.64 (95% CI 0.47–0.86).

Topical estrogen can be given as a cream, tablet, or estrogen-containing ring. Low-dose therapy with a vaginal cream consists of 50 mcg estradiol/0.5 g cream or 0.3 mg conjugated estrogen/0.5 g cream inserted into the vagina daily for 2 weeks, followed by treatment twice a week. Low-dose therapy with an estrogen tablet involves inserting a 10-mcg estradiol tablet into the vagina daily for 2 weeks, followed by the insertion of the tablet twice a week. The estrogen-containing ring releases 7.5 mcg of estradiol daily into the vagina for 90 days. A new ring is inserted every 90 days. It typically requires 6 weeks of treatment with low-dose vaginal estrogen for vaginal, urethral, and bladder atrophy to improve and for patients to begin to note improvement in their symptoms. See Chap. 8 on Menopause, Sect. on Genitourinary Syndrome.

Postmenopausal women who are unable or reluctant to use topical estrogen can use antibiotic prophylaxis as recommended for premenopausal women. Postcoital prophylaxis or self-treatment at the onset of symptoms of a UTI has the advantage of leading to less antibiotic exposure than continuous daily antibiotic use.

Recurrent UTIs: Other Strategies

Cranberry products are not recommended as there are no data showing efficacy. Similarly, more data are needed before recommending probiotics.

You treat Alice with trimethoprim-sulfamethoxazole, one double-strength tablet twice a day for 3 days, and her symptoms resolve completely. She calls to say that she is feeling fine and asks if she needs any follow-up for this episode of cystitis.

Follow-Up

Cystitis

Symptoms should respond to antibiotic treatment within 48 hours. Women with severe dysuria may benefit from a urinary analgesic such as over-the-counter phenazopyridine three times a day as needed for a 2-day course but should be counseled that it can turn tears and urine orange and potentially stain contact lenses. Follow-up urinalysis and/or cultures are not needed if her symptoms resolved.

Patients whose symptoms persist after 48–72 hours of appropriate antibiotics or who have recurrent symptoms within a few weeks of treatment should be evaluated for the possibility of a complicated infection. Urine culture should be obtained or repeated, and while it is pending, empiric treatment should be given with a different antibiotic.

Advise patients to phone right away if symptoms of cystitis recur and teach them the symptoms of pyelonephritis. Consider the interventions above for women with documented recurrent infections.

Pyelonephritis

If the patient shows clinical worsening or the lack of improvement after 1–2 days of antibiotic therapy, she requires a repeat urine culture and imaging to identify if a stone, obstruction, or other anatomical complication is the reason for the lack of improvement. An ultrasound is more sensitive than computerized tomography (CT) for diagnosis of hydronephrosis, is less expensive, and is available at the bedside. A contrast-enhanced CT is more sensitive for the diagnosis of an abscess, gas formation, and inflammation but should be used with caution in patients with renal dysfunction and impairs the detection of stones. An unenhanced CT is preferred for the detection of stones.

Among women treated as outpatients, schedule reassessment to assess response to therapy and the need for broad-spectrum antibiotics or intravenous therapy [3]. If she shows expected clinical improvement with resolution of all symptoms, a follow-up urine culture is not needed.

When to Refer and Other Team Members Who Can Help

- Co-manage pregnant women with their obstetricians. The obstetricians will determine what kind of fetal monitoring is required, if any.
- Urology should be consulted if hydronephrosis is detected.
- Consult urology and interventional radiology for women with an abscess.
- Women with recurrent urinary tract infections who do not respond to treatment may be candidates for referral to a urologist.
- Patients with persistent hematuria after their infection has been eradicated require imaging of their upper and lower urinary tracts and referral to a urologist for a cystoscopy.
- Postmenopausal women on topical low-dose estrogen who develop vaginal bleeding should be referred for an endometrial biopsy.
- Further evaluation of the urinary tract is recommended if any suspicions arise about possible structural or functional abnormalities of the urinary tract. Possible indications for evaluation include a UTI due to *Proteus* species as it is often associated with the presence of stones, or two recurrences of pyelonephritis. Evaluation should start with a renal ultrasound or CT urogram to rule out nephrolithiasis or obstructive uropathy.

Summary Points

1. Women with the classic symptoms of cystitis such as pain on urination, urinary frequency, and urgency can be empirically treated with a short course of antibiotics. First line is 3 days of TMP/sulfa double-strength twice daily.
2. Women with the classic symptoms of pyelonephritis such as fever, chills, and costovertebral angle tenderness must be evaluated with a urinalysis and urine culture and will require treatment with a 7–14 days of an appropriate antibiotic.
3. Young women with recurrent urinary tract infections can self-treat with one dose of postcoital antibiotics. Other options are to self-treat when they diagnose themselves with a UTI or to take a continuous nightly low dose of an appropriate antibiotic.
4. Recurrent urinary tract infections in postmenopausal women are often due to genitourinary atrophy from estrogen deficiency. Treatment with low-dose topical estrogen is often effective.

Review Questions

1. Which factor is the biggest risk for cystitis in young women?
   A. Wearing spandex
   B. Sexual intercourse
   C. Oral contraceptives
   D. Use of an IUD
   The correct answer is B. Of the choices above, sexual intercourse is the biggest risk factor for cystitis in young women. Sexual intercourse expedites the ascension of uropathogens from the fecal flora to the vaginal introitus and then from the urethra to the bladder.
2. Ellen is a 23-year-old woman who calls your office to report urinary frequency, fever, chills, and right flank pain for 2 days. The most appropriate next step is:
   A. To empirically treat her with a 3-day course of TMP/sulfa because she probably has cystitis
   B. To empirically treat her with a 7-day course of ciprofloxacin because she probably has pyelonephritis
   C. To have her come to your office now for evaluation, including a physical exam, urinalysis, and culture, as she probably has pyelonephritis
   D. To have her come to the emergency department for evaluation and possible inpatient admission
   The correct answer is C. The patient's symptoms of fever, chills, and unilateral flank pain are consistent with acute pyelonephritis. When pyelonephritis is suspected, the patient needs to be seen for evaluation of her vital signs, general status, and abdominal and flank exam, and a urinalysis and culture need to be obtained.
3. Louise is a 30-year-old woman who is sexually active and has had four episodes of cystitis in the past year. She uses an oral contraceptive pill. She asks if something can be done to prevent these recurrent episodes. The next best step is:
   A. To tell her to void immediately after each episode of sexual intercourse
   B. To recommend that she take one low dose of an appropriate antibiotic immediately after each episode of intercourse
   C. To start her on daily cranberry juice
   D. To change her contraceptive method to an IUD
   The correct answer is B. To take one low dose of an appropriate antibiotic immediately after each episode of intercourse. Postcoital antibiotic treatment is very effective in reducing the frequency of recurrent UTIs in young women. Voiding after intercourse is also likely to help, but with four episodes in a year, she is a good candidate for a prophylactic antibiotic strategy.
4. Marie is a 58-year-old woman who has had five episodes of cystitis in the past year. She asks if anything can be done to prevent these recurrent episodes. She became menopausal at age 51 and has had a hysterectomy for fibroids. She notes vaginal dryness and her pelvic exam reveals vaginal atrophy. The next best step is:
   A. To prescribe that she use a vaginal moisturizer every night
   B. To suggest that she use a vaginal lubricant before sexual intercourse
   C. To recommend a trial of low-dose vaginal estrogen
   D. To recommend a trial of systemic estrogen
   The correct answer is C. To recommend a trial of low-dose vaginal estrogen. Low-dose vaginal estrogen is highly effective in reducing the frequency of recurrent UTIs in postmenopausal women.

References

1. Hooton TM, Scholes D, Hughes JP, Winter C, Roberts PL, Stapleton AE, et al. A prospective study of risk factors for symptomatic urinary tract infection in young women. N Engl J Med. 1996;335:468–74.
2. Jackson SL, Boyko EJ, Scholes D, Abraham L, Gupta K, Fihn SD. Predictors of urinary tract infection after menopause: a prospective study. Am J Med. 2004;117(12):903–11.
3. Johnson JR, Russo TA. Acute pyelonephritis in adults. N Engl J Med. 2018;378:48–59.
4. Foxman B, Gillespie B, Koopman J, Zhang L, Palin K, Tallman P, et al. Risk factors for second urinary tract infection among college women. Am J Epidemiol. 2000;151:1194–205.
5. Ikaheimo R, Siitonen A, Heiskanen T, Karkkainen U, Kuosmanen P, Lipponen P, et al. Recurrence of urinary tract infection in a primary care setting: analysis of a 1-year follow-up of 179 women. Clin Infect Dis. 1996;22:91–9.
6. Pandit L, Ouslander JG. Postmenopausal vaginal atrophy and atrophic vaginitis. Am J Med Sci. 1997;314:228–31.
7. Raz R, Gennesin Y, Wasser J, Stoler Z, Rosenfeld S, Rottensterich E, et al. Recurrent urinary tract infections in postmenopausal women. Clin Infect Dis. 2000;30(1):152–6.
8. Kinane DF, Blackwell CC, Brettle RP, Weir DM, Winstanley FP, Elton RA. ABO blood group, secretor state, and susceptibility to recurrent urinary tract infection in women. Br Med J (Clin Res Ed). 1982;285:7–9.
9. Scholes D, Hooton TM, Roberts PL, Stapleton AE, Gupta K, Stamm WE. Risk factors for recurrent urinary tract infection in young women. J Infect Dis. 2000;182(4):1177–82.
10. Hooton TM, Stapleton AE, Roberts PL, Winter C, Scholes D, Bavendam T, et al. Perineal anatomy and urine-voiding characteristics of young women with and without recurrent urinary tract infections. Clin Infect Dis. 1999;29(6):1600–1.
11. Pappas PG. Laboratory in the diagnosis and management of urinary tract infections. Med Clin North Am. 1991;75:313–25.
12. Bent S, Nallamothu BK, Simel DL, Fihn SD, Saint S. Does this woman have an acute uncomplicated urinary tract infection? JAMA. 2002;287:2701–10.
13. Wilson ML, Gaido L. Laboratory diagnosis of urinary tract infections in adult patients. Clin Infect Dis. 2004;38:1150–8.
14. Fihn SD. Clinical practice. Acute uncomplicated urinary tract infection in women. N Engl J Med. 2003;349:259–66.
15. Stamm WE. Measurement of pyuria and its relation to bacteriuria. Am J Med. 1983;75:53–8.

16. Lutters M, Vogt-Ferrier NB. Antibiotic duration for treating uncomplicated, symptomatic lower urinary tract infections in elderly women. Cochrane Database Syst Rev. 2008;(3):CD001535.
17. Kavatha D, Giamarellou H, Alexiou Z, Vlachogiannis N, Pentea S, Gozadinos T, et al. Cefpodoxime-proxetil versus trimethoprim-sulfamethoxazole for short-term therapy of uncomplicated acute cystitis in women. Antimicrob Agents Chemother. 2003;47:897–900.
18. Gupta K. Emerging antibiotic resistance in urinary tract pathogens. Infect Dis Clin N Am. 2003;17:243–59.
19. Metlay JP, Strom BL, Asch DA. Prior antimicrobial drug exposure: a risk factor for trimethoprim-sulfamethoxazole-resistant urinary tract infections. J Antimicrob Chemother. 2003;51:963–70.
20. Warren JW, Abrutyn E, Hebel JR, Johnson JR, Schaeffer AJ, Stamm WE. Guidelines for antimicrobial treatment of uncomplicated acute bacterial cystitis and acute pyelonephritis in women. Infectious Diseases Society of America (IDSA). Clin Infect Dis. 1999;29:745–58.
21. Huttner A, Verhaegh EM, Harbarth S, Muller AE, Theuretzbacher U, Mouton JW. Nitrofurantoin revisited: a systematic review and meta-analysis of controlled trials. J Antimicrob Chemother. 2015;70:2456–64.
22. Singh N, Gandhi S, McArthur E, Moist L, Jain AK, Liu AR, et al. Kidney function and the use of nitrofurantoin to treat urinary tract infections in older women. CMAJ. 2015;187(9):648–56.
23. Huttner A, Kowalczyk A, Turjeman A, Babich T, Brossier C, Eliakim-Raz N, et al. Effect of 5-day nitrofurantoin vs single-dose fosfomycin on clinical resolution of uncomplicated lower urinary tract infection in women. A randomized clinical trial. JAMA. 2018;319(17):1781–9.
24. Fosfomycin for urinary tract infections. Med Lett Drugs Ther. 1997;39:66–8.
25. FDA Drug Safety Communication: FDA advises restricting fluoroquinolone antibiotic use for certain uncomplicated infections; warns about disabling side effects that can occur together. http://www.fda.gov/Drugs/DrugSafety/ucm500143.htm.
26. Ingvild I, Bollestad M, Grude N, Baerheim A, Damsgaard E, Neumark T, et al. Ibuprofen versus pivmecillinam for uncomplicated urinary tract infection in women – a double-blind, randomized non-inferiority trial. PLoS Med. 2018;15(5):e1002569.
27. Gupta K, Hooton TM, Naber KG, Wullt B, Colgan R, Miller LG, et al. International clinical practice guidelines for the treatment of acute uncomplicated cystitis and pyelonephritis in women: a 2010 update by the Infectious Diseases Society of America and the European Society for Microbiology and Infectious Diseases. Clin Infect Dis. 2011;52:e103–20.
28. Hooton TM. Clinical practice. Uncomplicated urinary tract infection. N Engl J Med. 2012;366:1028–37.
29. Nicolle LE, Ronald AR. Recurrent urinary tract infection in adult women: diagnosis and treatment. Infect Dis Clin N Am. 1987;1:793–806.
30. Stapleton A, Latham RH, Johnson C, Stamm WE. Postcoital antimicrobial prophylaxis for recurrent urinary tract infection: a randomized, double-blind, placebo-controlled trial. JAMA. 1990;264(6):703–6.
31. Pfau A, Sacks TG. Effective prophylaxis for recurrent urinary tract infections during pregnancy. Clin Infect Dis. 1992;14(4):810–4.
32. Gupta K, Hooton TM, Roberts PL, Stamm WE. Patient-initiated treatment of uncomplicated recurrent urinary tract infections in young women. Ann Intern Med. 2001;135(1):9–16.
33. Albert X, Huertas I, Pereiro II, Sanfelix J, Gosalbes V, Perrota C. Antibiotics for preventing recurrent urinary tract infection in non-pregnant women. Cochrane Database Syst Rev. 2004;(3):CD001209.
34. Rudenko N, Dorofeyev A. Prevention of recurrent lower urinary tract infections by long-term administration of fosfomycin trometamol. Double blind, randomized, parallel group, placebo controlled study. Arzneimittelforschung. 2005;55:420–7.
35. Nicolle L, Harding G, Thomson M, Kennedy J, Urias B, Ronald A. Efficacy of five years of continuous low-dose trimethoprim-sulfamethoxazole prophylaxis for urinary tract infection. J Infect Dis. 1988;157:1239–42.
36. Raz R, Stamm WE. A controlled trial of intravaginal estriol in postmenopausal women with recurrent urinary tract infections. N Engl J Med. 1993;329:753–6.
37. Perrotta C, Aznar M, Mejia R, Albert X, Ng CW. Oestrogens for preventing recurrent urinary tract infection in postmenopausal women. Cochrane Database Syst Rev. 2008;(2):CD005131.

Bone Health and Osteoporosis

25

Jordana Friedman, Aletia Farmer, and Jacqueline Carey Fister

Learning Objectives

1. Describe the public health impact of osteoporosis with regard to cost, mortality, and quality of life.
2. Screen appropriately for osteoporosis based on age and risk.
3. Diagnose primary and secondary osteoporosis.
4. Utilize a risk assessment tool to calculate fracture risk.
5. Recommend non-pharmacologic measures for fracture prevention.
6. Identify candidates for pharmacologic treatment and appropriately recommend pharmacologic treatment for patients at risk for fracture.

Marianne is a 64-year-old Caucasian woman who comes in for her annual exam. She has a history of hypertension and hyperthyroidism status-post radioactive iodine therapy. She takes hydrochlorothiazide and an over-the-counter multivitamin. Her social history is notable for a 30-pack-year smoking history and a sedentary lifestyle due to caring for her chronically ill husband. On exam, she is 5 feet 9 inches tall and weighs 134 lbs. She asks you if she should have a bone density scan for osteoporosis screening.

Osteoporosis: Epidemiology and Public Health Impact

Osteoporosis is a skeletal disorder characterized by a decrease in bone strength predisposing to an increased risk of fracture. Because of the large number of older adults impacted by osteoporosis and the morbidity and mortality associated with fragility fracture, osteoporosis has both a significant clinical impact and a large socioeconomic impact. According to data from the National Health and Nutrition Examination Survey (NHANES), 10.2 million older Americans were estimated to have osteoporosis in 2010, and 43.4 million additional older Americans were estimated to have low bone mass [1]. There are approximately two million osteoporotic fractures annually in the United States, and 70% of those fractures occur in women [1, 2]. The annual cost associated with osteoporotic fractures exceeds the combined cost of caring for breast cancer, myocardial infarction, and stroke in women 55 years or older [3]. It is estimated that the costs of osteoporotic fractures will exceed 25.3 billion (United States dollars) by 2025 [2, 4]. There is also substantial morbidity and mortality associated with fragility fractures. While mortality can reach 20–24% in the first year after a hip fracture [5], associated morbidity rates are higher and include fracture-related pain, deformity, reduced mobility, and loss of function and independence. Up to 40% of those experiencing hip fracture are unable to walk independently, and up to 33% are totally dependent or living in a nursing home in the year following the fracture [6–8]. Up to 10–20% of community-dwelling patients will require long-term nursing home care after a hip fracture [9].

Physiology of Bone Formation and Remodeling

Bone strength is based on both bone density and bone quality. Bone density is the measurement of bone quantity. Bone quality is determined by factors that influence how well bone

J. Friedman
Northwestern University, Feinberg School of Medicine, Department of Internal Medicine, Chicago, IL, USA
e-mail: jordana.friedman@nm.org

A. Farmer (✉) · J. C. Fister
University of Kentucky, Department of Internal Medicine/Women's Health, Lexington, KY, USA

S. A. Tilstra et al. (eds.), *Sex- and Gender-Based Women's Health*, https://doi.org/10.1007/978-3-030-50695-7_25

can resist fractures including microarchitecture, microscopic damage, quality of bone material, size of mineral crystals, and the rate of bone turnover [10].

Normal Bone Remodeling

In the normal bone remodeling process, bone continues to regenerate through remodeling even after the bone skeleton has reached maturity and linear growth is complete. Remodeling refers to the process by which older bone is removed and replaced by new bone and has three phases: resorption, reversal, and formation. The remodeling cycle starts with resorption, which is the removal of old bone by osteoclasts. When resorption is complete, there is a reversal phase in which a glycoprotein rich substance is deposited on the bone surface to which osteoblasts can adhere. In the formation phase, these adherent osteoblasts produce a new bone structure that subsequently begins to mineralize. The remodeling process has a role in maintaining bone health by repairing microscopic damage and minimizing the effects of aging on bone (Fig. 25.1).

Estrogens and androgens play a role in regulating bone remodeling. Estrogen inhibits bone resorption through cell signaling factors including cytokines and growth factors, which induce osteoclast apoptosis and inhibit osteoclast activity. Testosterone increases cytokines and growth factors that stimulate osteoblast proliferation, inhibit osteoclast activity, and induce osteoclast apoptosis. In women, estrogen is the primary sex steroid involved in the regulation of bone. In premenopausal women, the primary source of estrogens is the ovaries. In postmenopausal women, the primary source of estrogens is adrenal androgens that are peripherally converted to estrogens by aromatase.

Impact of Age and Hormonal Fluctuations

Given the impact of estrogen on bone remodeling, age-related bone loss in women begins in the fifth decade at an average rate of 0.5–1% per year as women begin to approach perimenopause [12, 13]. Menopausal related bone loss begins in the menopause transition 3–5 years before the last menstrual period (LMP) and continues for 3–5 years after the LMP. During menopause, bone loss accelerates as estrogen levels significantly decrease. The loss of estrogen leads to increased osteoclast activity and increased bone resorption [12, 13]. During this time, the average rate of bone loss is 1–2% per year, which can lead to a 10–20% loss over 10 years [12, 13]. Age-related osteoporosis after the sixth decade affects both men and women. During this time, resorption exceeds formation resulting in net bone loss.

Marianne's mother fractured her hip at age 62. She is very concerned today regarding her own risk of fracture and how to prevent fracture.

Identification of Osteoporosis: Risk Factors and Indications for Screening

Osteoporosis can be defined as low bone mass with changes in skeletal microarchitecture that lead to fragility fractures. This definition incorporates pathophysiology and clinical manifestations, providing the rationale for identification and treatment of affected individuals. In practice, osteoporosis is often defined by bone mass alone [14, 15] because bone mass is easily measurable and correlates with fracture risk.

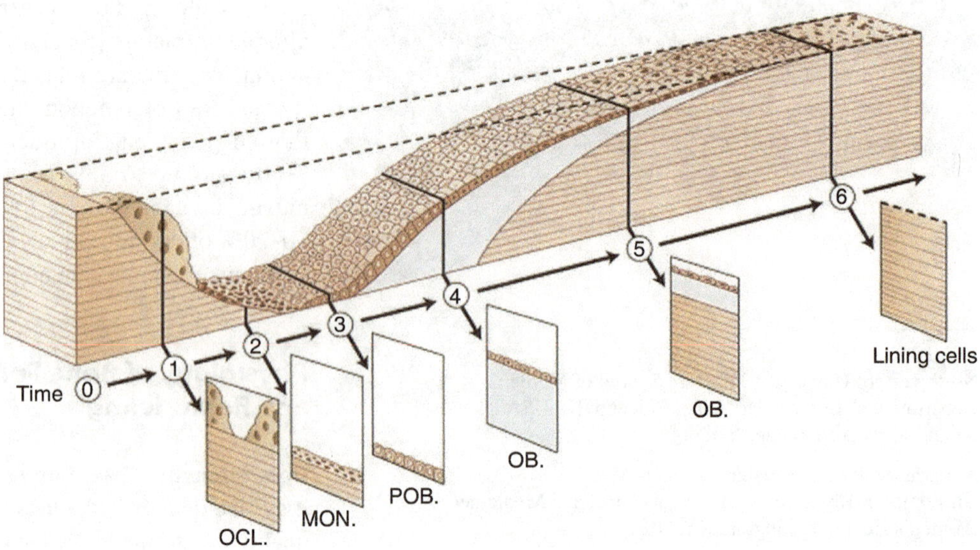

Fig. 25.1 Three-dimensional reconstruction of the remodeling sequence in human trabecular bone. (1). Early bone resorption with osteoclasts (OCL); (2). late bone resorption with mononuclear cells (MON); (3). reversal phase with preosteoblasts (POB); (4). early matrix formation by osteoblasts (OB); (5). late bone formation with mineralization; (6). completed remodeling cycle with reversion to lining cells (Reprinted from Eriksen [11], by permission of Oxford University)

However, clinicians caring for women must remember the more complex definition to minimize overidentification and overtreatment and focus on the goal of preventing fractures and their sequelae.

As noted above, osteoporosis is a common condition with significant clinical impact when it leads to fractures. Because low bone mass is identified with a simple imaging test—the DXA (dual-energy X-ray absorption)—and because effective, low cost therapies with minimal adverse effects exist to mitigate fracture risk, osteoporosis is well suited for population-based screening [16]. As with all screening strategies, it is useful to target individuals who are at risk so that interventions are appropriately applied.

To screen for osteoporosis, clinicians first perform a risk factor assessment. This is often done as part of an annual prevention visit. The most important risk factor for fracture is age, followed by previous fracture; other important factors are glucocorticoid use, parental history of fracture, low body weight, and active tobacco or alcohol use [17]. Since fragility fractures often occur in conjunction with falls, osteoporotic risk assessment includes history-taking on previous falls, neurologic conditions, and gait assessment. During the physical exam, an accurate height measurement should be completed and compared to previous measurements, particularly in older women.

FRAX is a widely accepted risk assessment tool that incorporates multiple clinical risk factors with or without bone density results to help predict fracture risk [18]. The FRAX algorithm estimates the 10-year probability of hip fracture as well as the 10-year probability of a major osteoporotic fracture; this composite includes the hip, spine, shoulder, and wrist. The validated clinical risk factors used in the FRAX algorithm are predictive of osteoporotic fracture independent of bone mineral density (BMD) and include age, body mass index (BMI), previous fracture, a parent with hip fracture, current smoking, glucocorticoids, rheumatoid arthritis, secondary osteoporosis (see below), and consumption of three or more alcoholic units per day.

There are limitations to FRAX. The FRAX algorithm can underestimate fracture risk by only evaluating the risk at the hip and at the major fracture sites that comprise half of all fragility fractures. The algorithm also does not consider the number of fragility fractures and does not directly capture fall risk. In addition, the conditions associated with secondary osteoporosis are not well defined. Finally, the FRAX tool was originally created as a cost-effectiveness model; some analyses suggest that its utility for predicting which patients will fracture may be limited [19].

The United States Preventive Service Task Force (USPSTF) guidelines recommend screening for osteoporosis with BMD measurement for all women 65 years and older [16]. The USPSTF also recommends BMD measurement in younger postmenopausal women who have elevated risk of osteoporosis, as identified by a clinical assessment or a tool such as FRAX. The primary screening tool for BMD measurement is the dual-energy x-ray absorption (DXA) test. DXA is an ionizing radiation test that uses photon beams of two different energies ("dual energy"). A computerized system, specific to the manufacturer, calculates the difference in energies, yielding a density measurement. Because DXA results are specific to the machine and the manufacturer, the T-scores are generally comparable only over time on the same machine, and are not standard across institutions.

Central BMD, that is, DXA at hip and spine, is the standard screening test [16, 20], because most studies of osteoporotic therapies enrolled women based on central BMD measurement. Peripheral measurement, such as at the wrist, is needed only in unusual circumstances when there are structural abnormalities at the standard central sites. The spinal BMD may be difficult to interpret in older adults with significant spinal osteophyte formation; in these cases, the hip BMD is frequently adequate. Ultrasound of the heel cannot reliably identify appropriate candidates for osteoporotic therapies [21] and is therefore not recommended.

Many medical conditions and medications are associated with bone loss because they alter the balance between bone resorption and formation. Secondary osteoporosis describes situations in which bone loss can be attributed to identifiable factors other than aging and menopause. Up to 30% of postmenopausal women with osteoporosis have such an underlying cause [22].

Interpretation of BMD Tests and Diagnosis of Osteoporosis

Osteoporosis can be diagnosed either clinically or based on bone mineral density criteria. A clinical diagnosis of osteoporosis is based on the presence of a fragility fracture. A patient experiences a fragility fracture when the bone fractures with less force than would be expected to result in a fracture; fragility fractures may occur either spontaneously or from minimal trauma, such as the force from a fall from a standing height or less. In the absence of other metabolic diseases, a fragility fracture is diagnostic of osteoporosis, independent of BMD [14]. Traumatic fractures, on the other hand, are not a risk factor for osteoporosis.

The World Health Organization (WHO) has established definitions for osteoporosis and osteopenia based on central DXA measurements. The WHO definitions are based on T-scores in postmenopausal women. The T-score represents the number of standard deviations from the mean of a standardized healthy young adult population. Osteoporosis is defined as a T-score ≤ -2.5. Osteopenia is defined as a T-score between -1.0 and -2.5 [15].

In some patients, the results of a DXA scan will indicate that the patient may have a secondary cause for low bone density. Whereas T-scores compare a patient's BMD to a healthy, young population (that is, the mean density in 25–35 year olds), the Z-score compares a patient's BMD to age- and sex-matched controls. The Z-score thus represents the number of standard deviations from the mean for age- and sex-matched subjects. For example, a patient with a Z-score of −2.0 has a BMD two standard deviations below the average of others who are in her same age group [23]. A Z-score of ≤−2.0 is "below the expected range for age," and this should prompt a work-up for conditions or medications which are leading to this profound degree of low bone mass [14].

Evaluation of Underlying Causes of Osteoporosis

A careful history and physical examination often yield important findings when evaluating a patient for secondary causes of osteoporosis. Patients who consistently drink more than 2 units of alcohol daily are at increased risk of fracture. A patient with lifelong irregular menses and GI distress may have celiac disease leading to malabsorption. Symptoms of bone pain and abdominal discomfort may suggest hypercalcemia and undiagnosed hyperparathyroidism.

Based on one's history and exam, laboratory evaluation can exclude or diagnose secondary causes of osteoporosis such as renal disease, hyperthyroidism, hyperparathyroidism, Cushing's syndrome, celiac disease or other forms of malabsorption, or idiopathic hypercalciuria (Table 25.1). For patients with osteoporosis (based on T-score at or lower than −2.5 or history of fragility fracture), the basic laboratory evaluation includes comprehensive chemistry panel, 25-hydroxyvitamin D, and on occasion serum thyrotropin (TSH). If the clinical scenario suggests secondary osteoporosis or if the Z-score is less than −2, the laboratory evaluation should be expanded, with consideration of parathyroid hormone and 24-hour urine calcium and urine creatinine.

Table 25.1 Laboratory evaluation for secondary osteoporosis

Suspected condition	Suggested evaluation
Vitamin D deficiency	Serum 25-OH vitamin D level
Primary hyperparathyroidism	Serum calcium, serum 25-OH vitamin D level and parathyroid hormone level
Hyperthyroidism	Serum TSH and free T4
Hypercalciuria	24-hour urine calcium and creatinine
Multiple myeloma	Serum and urine protein electrophoresis and serum free light chains
Cushing's syndrome	24-hour urinary cortisol or late-evening salivary cortisol
Celiac disease	Serum anti-tissue transglutaminase antibodies (anti-TTG), anti-endomysial antibodies, and total IgA

Additional laboratory testing, guided by history or examination, may include celiac antibodies, serum and protein electrophoresis, measurement of urinary or salivary cortisol, and other specialized tests to evaluate suspected conditions [14].

Screening Interval

There is limited data to help determine optimal rescreening intervals between BMD testing. The National Osteoporosis Foundation (NOF) advises rescreening every 2 years for most individuals but notes that in some patients who have bone density in the normal or "upper limit of low" range, it is reasonable to lengthen intervals [4]. This recommendation is guided in part by the Study of Osteoporotic Fractures (SOF) which prospectively followed women 67 years and older with no history of hip or clinical vertebral fracture and no prior treatment for osteoporosis. SOF sought to determine the estimated interval during which osteoporosis developed in 10% of the participants prior to fracture. The data showed that the key determinants of screening intervals are baseline T-score and age:

- In study participants with normal BMD or mild osteopenia (T-score between −1.01 and −1.49), osteoporosis developed in less than 10% of women during a rescreening interval of approximately 15 years.
- In women with moderate osteopenia (T-score between −1.50 and −1.99), the screening interval was found to be approximately 5 years.
- For women with advanced osteopenia (T-score between −2.00 and −2.49), the screening interval was 1 year.

The authors suggest using these data to guide interval for rescreening, particularly for patients with mild-to-moderate osteopenia where screening intervals can be lengthened from the commonly used 2-year interval. The study did not take into account risks and benefits of screening or cost-effectiveness [24].

Since the estimated time to the development of osteoporosis decreases with increasing age, one may consider shortening screening intervals for older patients with moderate osteopenia. Although screening intervals were found to be appropriate even after controlling for major risk factors, clinicians may choose to shorten the screening intervals for patients with risk factors not included in the analysis including decreased activity, decreased mobility, or weight loss, particularly if these factors have significantly changed since the original normal BMD was obtained. Patients who are taking steroids or aromatase inhibitors may benefit from more frequent screening or other prevention strategies given the accelerated bone loss experienced by these patients.

Marianne's history of smoking, parental history of hip fracture, and low body weight put her at risk for osteoporosis, and screening is indicated although she is not quite 65 years old. Marianne's bone density scan shows a T-score at the femoral neck of −2.2 (moderately low BMD). Her FRAX score shows a 10-year risk for any major fracture of 19% and hip fracture risk of 3.2%. You discuss the next steps.

Non-Pharmacologic Strategies for Fracture Prevention

A "bone healthy" lifestyle includes adequate intake of calcium and vitamin D, lifelong participation in regular weight-bearing and resistance exercise, the avoidance of tobacco and excessive use of alcohol, and elimination of potential risk factors for falling. Unfortunately, there is variable evidence demonstrating the positive impact of these interventions, as noted below.

Exercise

Regular weight-bearing exercise (for example, walking at least 30 minutes at least three times per week) is recommended for osteoporosis prevention and fracture reduction among women with osteoporosis. Additionally, non-weight-bearing exercise (such as progressive resistance strength training) or a combination of weight-bearing and strength training exercises may be helpful to improve BMD and prevent falls. Studies of early postmenopausal women have shown that strength training leads to small yet significant changes in BMD [25], and evidence suggests a relatively small but possibly important effect of exercise on bone density in postmenopausal women [25]. Exercise should be considered as a preferred intervention for osteoporosis in clinical practice [25] because of these effects and other health benefits unrelated to bone health.

Calcium and Vitamin D

Many societies recommend that women aged 51 and older consume 1200 mg of calcium per day [26]. However, large meta-analyses note that increasing calcium intake either by dietary sources or supplements has minimal effect on bone density within the first year and does not lead to clinically meaningful reductions in fractures [27]. Additionally, based on potential adverse effects associated with calcium supplements including small but significant increased risk of cardiovascular events [28], nephrolithiasis, and constipation, for those who wish to increase calcium intake, dietary calcium is recommended preferentially over calcium supplements.

Vitamin D supplementation is similarly controversial. The USPSTF recommends against daily vitamin D and calcium supplementation for the primary prevention of fractures in noninstitutionalized postmenopausal women [29] given the lack of data for clinical efficacy. Despite these data, many societies including the NOF, AACE, and AGE continue to recommend that adults aged 65 or older consume 800–1000 IU of vitamin D daily for the prevention of falls and fractures [14].

Fall Prevention

Older or frail patients are vulnerable to falls, particularly if recently hospitalized, with musculoskeletal or neurologic disorders including prior stroke, receiving multiple medications that decrease mental alertness, or cognitively impaired. Patients can be referred to physical therapy for gait training when balance or strength is impaired. It is imperative to minimize the use of medications that impair balance. Appropriate correction of visual impairment and walking aids should be encouraged. Home assessments should be performed to reduce the risk of falls [30].

Smoking and Alcohol

Given the impact of tobacco and alcohol use on bone remodeling, addressing these habits during a clinical encounter focused on bone health is appropriate. Patients who consume alcohol in excess of 2 units/day can be counseled that this use increases risk of fragility fracture. Any tobacco use can be discouraged.

Osteoporosis Treatment

Once a diagnosis of osteoporosis is made, either clinically or using BMD measurements, pharmacologic treatment should be offered. Additionally, guidelines recommend pharmacologic treatment for postmenopausal women with have low bone mass (T-score between −1.0 and −2.5 at the femoral neck or lumbar spine) and significantly elevated FRAX risk, defined as a 10-year probability of a hip fracture ≥3% and/or a 10-year probability of major osteoporotic fracture ≥20% [4].

The FDA has approved both antiresorptive and anabolic medications for the treatment of osteoporosis. Unless contraindications exist, oral bisphosphonates are considered first-line treatment for osteoporosis based on their efficacy and

Table 25.2 Osteoporosis treatments

Class	Drug name	Dose	Reduces hip fracture rate?	Number needed to treat to prevent fracture: vertebral (v) and hip (h)	Contraindications (see text for more discussion)
Bisphosphonate	Alendronate (*Fosamax*)	70 mg orally weekly	Yes	15 (v) 9 (h)	GFR <35, GI disorders[a], neurologic or cognitive impairment that impact swallowing function
	Risedronate (*Actonel*)	150 mg orally monthly	Yes		
	Ibandronate (*Boniva*)	150 mg orally monthly	**No**		
	Zoledronic acid (*Reclast*)	5 mg IV once per year	Yes	14 (v) 9 (h)	CKD with GFR <35
Monoclonal antibody	Denosumab (*Prolia*)	60 mg SQ every 6 months	Yes	21 (v) 200 (h)	None
Selective estrogen receptor modulator	Raloxifene (*Evista*)	60 mg orally daily	**No**	16–46 (v) [a]NNT decreases as risk increases	Prior DVT or PE
Anabolic PTH analog	Teriparitide (*Forteo*)	20 mcg SQ daily (limited to 2 years total)	**No**	11 (v) 33 (nonvertebral fracture)	Hyperparathyroidism
	Abaloparatide (*Tymlos*)	3120 mcg SQ daily (limited to 2 years total)	**No**	Limited data exist	None
Antisclerostin antibody	Romosozumab (*Evenity*)	210 mg SQ once monthly (limited to 12 doses)	Yes	18–77 (v) [35] 83 to NS (h) [36]	Uncorrected hypocalcemia

[a]GI (gastrointestinal) disorders: active peptic ulcer disease, uncontrolled reflux, esophageal dysmotility, dysphagia
GFR is glomerular filtration rate, *CKD* is chronic kidney disease, *DVT* is deep venous thrombosis, *PE* is pulmonary embolism, *PTH* is parathyroid hormone, *NS* is non-significant, *IV* is intravenous, *SQ* is subcutaneous

relatively long-term safety data [31–34]. Intravenous bisphosphonates, other antiresorptive agents, and anabolic agents are often reserved for patients who have contraindications to oral bisphosphonates, patients who fracture while on oral bisphosphonates, patients with multiple fractures, or those with very low T-scores (≤−3.0) who are at highest risk of fracture [14]. The authors note that the field of osteoporosis treatment continues to change as new therapies emerge (Table 25.2).

Bisphosphonates

Bisphosphonates prevent bone resorption by binding to hydroxyapatite in bone and inhibiting osteoclast function [32]. Bisphosphonates have high binding affinities for bone and are associated with antiresorptive effects and antifracture protection for years, even after discontinuation [37]. The Fracture Intervention Trial (FIT) was a landmark study of alendronate that demonstrated that alendronate decreases the risk of both vertebral and nonvertebral fractures [31, 32]. In postmenopausal women with low bone density, alendronate decreased the risk of radiographic hip fracture by 44%, and in the subgroup with osteoporosis, alendronate reduced the risk of all clinical fractures by 36% and hip fractures by 56%. Since this trial, studies have shown that alendronate, risedronate, and zoledronic acid decrease both vertebral and nonvertebral fractures. For example, in the VERT trial of postmenopausal women with at least one vertebral fracture, risedronate was shown to decrease the incidence of vertebral fractures by 41–49% and nonvertebral fractures by 36% over 3 years [38, 39]. On the other hand, ibandronate reduced the risk of vertebral fracture, but hip fracture risk reduction was not demonstrated in clinical trials; the use of other available bisphosphonates is preferred.

Alendronate is approved in daily and weekly doses for the prevention and treatment of osteoporosis. Risedronate can be prescribed in daily, weekly, or monthly formulations for the prevention or treatment of osteoporosis.

Gastrointestinal (GI) adverse effects of oral bisphosphonates such as reflux esophagitis can limit tolerance of the medications. Oral bisphosphonates are thought to cause upper GI symptoms due to local effects of the medication on the gastric and esophageal mucosa. The incidence of GI adverse effects is low [40] and can be reduced with proper administration: patients should be counseled to take oral bisphosphonates first thing in the morning with an empty stomach, ingest with 8 ounces of water, and remain upright for 30 minutes afterward. Some patients may have difficulty with one oral agent but be able to tolerate others, so it is reasonable to try switching from alendronate to risedronate if needed. Oral bisphosphonates should be avoided in patients with impaired swallowing, those with esophageal disorders, or those who are unable to follow the dosing instructions. Bisphosphonates are poorly absorbed if taken with food.

Zoledronic acid is administered by yearly IV infusion for the treatment of osteoporosis [33]. When compared with placebo, treatment with zoledronic acid reduces the risk of vertebral fracture by 70%, reduces the risk of hip fracture by 41%, and reduces the risk of nonvertebral fractures by 25% over 3 years in patients with osteoporosis. Yearly infusion of zoledronic acid may be considered for patients who have difficulty with medication adherence, impaired swallowing, or gastrointestinal effects with oral bisphosphonates. Post-infusion symptoms can include fever, flu-like symptoms, myalgias, arthralgias, and headaches. The symptoms occur most commonly occur after the first infusion and typically resolve within 3 days.

Other adverse effects associated with both oral and intravenous bisphosphonates are uncommon but include hypocalcemia, impairment of renal function, musculoskeletal pain, eye inflammation, osteonecrosis of the jaw, and atypical femur fractures. Hypocalcemia is usually transient and is more common with intravenous bisphosphonates. All bisphosphonates can affect renal function and are contraindicated in patients with GFR below 30–35 ml/min.

Osteonecrosis of the jaw (ONJ) and atypical femur fractures are rare but serious adverse effects in patients treated with oral and intravenous bisphosphonates. ONJ is defined as the exposure of maxillofacial bone that remains unhealed over 8 weeks in a patient with bisphosphonate exposure and without radiation exposure [33]. Patients with poor oral hygiene, glucocorticoid therapy, and chemotherapy are at higher risk of developing ONJ. ONJ is mostly seen with IV bisphosphonates especially when used in higher doses in cancer patients for hypercalcemia of malignancy [41]. It is estimated that the risk of ONJ in patients on chronic oral bisphosphonates is between 1 in 1000 and 1 in 263,000 patient-years. It is still unclear whether the risk of ONJ increases with increased duration of exposure to bisphosphonates. Some providers discontinue bisphosphonates prior to invasive dental procedures, but there is limited evidence that discontinuing bisphosphonates prior to invasive dental procedures will reduce the risk of ONJ [33, 42].

Atypical femur fractures are transverse or short oblique fractures located in the subtrochanteric region into the femoral shaft that occur spontaneously or with minimal trauma [43]. The evidence on the incidence and risk factors for atypical femur fractures is inconsistent, but the risk appears to correlate with the duration of bisphosphonate therapy. However, the risk is low even with bisphosphonate use beyond 5 years. In one study, the risk increased from 1.78 atypical femur fractures per 100,000 patient-years in patients treated for 2 years to 113.1 atypical femur fractures per 100,000 patient-years in patients treated for 8–10 years [43]. Evidence supporting the use of bisphosphonates to reduce fracture risk shows that benefits outweigh the risk of atypical fractures: for every subtrochanteric fracture associated with bisphosphonate use, 100 hip fractures were prevented [44]. Clinical decision support tools have been developed to help discuss the benefit and side effect profiles of bisphosphonates with patients, such as the tool provided at https://www.healthdecision.org/tool#/tool/osteoporosis [45].

Because of the safety concerns with long-term use of bisphosphonates, the FDA recommends drug holidays for appropriate patients to reduce potential cumulative adverse effects of bisphosphonates. The Fracture Intervention Trial Long-Term Extension (FLEX) compared 10 years versus 5 years of alendronate therapy and found no significant difference in cumulative risk for nonvertebral fractures at 10 years of follow-up but a lower risk for radiographic vertebral fractures in patients treated for 10 years (2.4% vs. 5.3%) [46]; however, patients at high risk for fracture were excluded from this trial. The subset of patients with T-scores ≤ -2.5 had increased risk for all fractures when bisphosphonates were discontinued at 5 years versus 10 years. In patients treated with zoledronic acid for 3 years, treating with an additional 3 years lowered the risk of radiographic vertebral fractures by 52% compared with 3 years of treatment followed by 3 years of placebo [47]. There was no difference in the rates of other fractures. The decision to initiate a drug holiday should be individualized based on each patient's fracture risk. Patients should be considered for bisphosphonate holiday after 5 years of bisphosphonates. Patients at high risk of vertebral fractures, low T-scores (≤ -2.5), or ongoing or new risk factors for bone loss might benefit from continuing bisphosphonates for up to 10 years.

Denosumab

Denosumab is biologic agent approved for the treatment of osteoporosis in postmenopausal women at high risk of fracture and is given as a twice-yearly subcutaneous injection. Denosumab is a human monoclonal antibody that prevents the receptor activation of nuclear factor-kappa B ligand (RANKL) which is essential in the formation, activation, and survival of osteoclasts [48]. Inhibition of the RANK receptor prevents osteoclast maturation, activation, and survival, thereby decreasing resorption of cortical and trabecular bone [48]. The FREEDOM Trial showed that denosumab given twice yearly for 3 years was associated with a reduction in the risk of vertebral, nonvertebral, and hip fractures in women with osteoporosis [34]. Denosumab reduced the incidence of vertebral fractures by 68%, nonvertebral fractures by 20%, and hip fractures by 40% [34]. Adverse effects with denosumab include cellulitis, rash, hypocalcemia, and rare cases of ONJ and atypical femur fractures. There is a rapid decline in bone density and increased risk of vertebral fracture with discontinuation of denosumab [34, 49]. Thus, if denosumab is discontinued, alternative therapy (such as bisphosphonate) is recommended to maintain BMD and prevent fractures.

Selective Estrogen Receptor Modulator

Raloxifene is a selective estrogen receptor modulator (SERM) that binds to the estrogen receptor and acts as an estrogen agonist on bone. This leads to decreased bone turnover, decreased bone loss, increased bone mineral density (BMD), and decreased risk of vertebral fractures [50]. The MORE trial showed that treatment with raloxifene over 3 years reduced the risk of new vertebral fractures by 55% in women without prevalent baseline fractures. Raloxifene did not reduce hip or nonvertebral fractures and is therefore not considered first-line treatment. Raloxifene increases risk of thromboembolic events threefold and is contraindicated in patients with a history of the thromboembolic disease [50]. Other adverse effects include leg cramps and worsening vasomotor symptoms such as hot flashes and night sweats that can limit use in postmenopausal women. Raloxifene is also contraindicated in lactating women and women who are or may become pregnant [50]. As a result of its efficacy and contraindications, raloxifene's role in the treatment of osteoporosis is limited to those who cannot tolerate other therapies or have other indications for its use (See Chap. 17 on The Primary Prevention of Breast Cancer).

Estrogen Therapy

Estrogen inhibits bone resorption and has been shown to lower the risk of both vertebral and nonvertebral fractures in postmenopausal women [51]. However, estrogens are FDA-approved for prevention but not treatment of osteoporosis given current evidence favoring only early, short-term use of hormone therapy in peri- and postmenopausal women. During the time patients are on estrogen for menopausal symptoms or in patients who are on estrogen therapy for premature ovarian failure, estrogen therapy prevents the rapid bone loss that is associated with loss of estrogen. Once estrogen therapy is discontinued, however, bone loss occurs rapidly; thus, providers should consider starting alternative treatment to maintain BMD.

Anabolic Therapy

Two classes of anabolic therapy are currently FDA-approved for the treatment of osteoporosis: PTH analogs and anti-sclerostin antibodies. Candidates for anabolic therapy include patients with severe osteoporosis at high risk for fracture, patients who fail bisphosphonates, or patients who have contraindications to bisphosphonates.

PTH Analogs

Two PTH analogs are approved for osteoporosis therapy. Teriparatide is a recombinant human parathyroid hormone, and abaloparatide is a synthetic analog of parathyroid hormone-related protein (PTHrP). Both teriparatide and abaloparatide stimulate bone remodeling and, when given as once-daily injections, increase bone formation more than bone resorption [52]. Teriparatide reduces the risk of vertebral fractures by 65% and nonvertebral fractures by 53% with no reduction in hip fractures in postmenopausal women with prior vertebral fracture after an average of 18 months of treatment. Abaloparatide showed similar improvement in bone density and reduction in fracture rates, but the use of teriparatide is preferred due to limited experience and long-term safety data with abaloparatide [53].

When teriparatide is discontinued, significant loss of BMD occurs; thus, an antiresorptive agent (i.e., a bisphosphonate) may be prescribed to preserve the gains in BMD [54]. Treatment with teriparatide is recommended for a maximum of 2 years due to a theoretical risk of osteosarcoma, which was demonstrated in rodent models [52]. The relationship between osteosarcoma and teriparatide in humans is unclear; only three cases of osteosarcoma have been reported out of more than one million patients treated with teriparatide [55].

Potential adverse effects of teriparatide include nausea, headache, orthostatic hypotension, leg cramps, hypercalcemia, hypercalciuria, and gout [52]. Teriparatide should not be used in patients with Paget's disease, hyperparathyroidism, bone metastasis or history of bone malignancies, or a history of nephrolithiasis. In addition to adverse effects, barriers to the use of teriparatide include the need for daily subcutaneous injections and cost.

Anti-Sclerostin Antibodies

Romosozumab is a monoclonal antibody that binds to sclerostin and inhibits its activity. Sclerostin is a glycoprotein produced by osteocytes that inhibits osteoblast activity and bone formation, thus inhibiting sclerostin will enhance osteoblast function [56]. Romosozumab has been shown to stimulate bone formation, decrease bone resorption, and increase BMD. In addition, there is trial evidence of a fracture benefit. In one trial, the romosozumab group reduced absolute vertebral fracture rate by 1.3% (0.5% vs. 1.8% after 12 months of placebo) [35]. In another, romosozumab decreased the incidence of vertebral and nonvertebral fractures compared with alendronate [36]. Patients treated with 12 months of romosozumab followed by 12 months of alendronate had a 48% lower risk of new vertebral fractures and 19% lower risk of nonvertebral fractures compared with women treated with 24 months of alendronate. Adverse reactions with romosozumab include ONJ, atypical femoral fractures, and an increase in cardiovascular events (2.5% in the group treated with romosozumab versus 1.9% in the group treated only with alendronate). In 2019, the FDA granted approval to romosozumab after initial concern with cardiovascular events in patients treated with romosozumab during clinical trials though it remains in limited clinical use at the time of publication.

Marianne agrees to start alendronate 70 mg, once a week for osteoporosis. You counsel her on properly taking the medication and adverse effects and recommend repeating her BMD test in 2 years.

Treatment Monitoring

Treatment monitoring recommendations vary. While several organizations recommend repeat BMD testing 1–2 years after the initiation of therapy [4, 14, 20], the USPSTF recommends a minimum of 2 years between DXA scans to reliably measure changes in BMD [16], and the American College of Physicians (ACP) practice guidelines recommend against monitoring BMD during the initial 5 years of treatment. The ACP recommendations are based on data demonstrating a decrease in fractures with bisphosphonates, raloxifene, and teriparatide treatment regardless of changes in BMD [42]. The authors of this chapter recommend screening no earlier than 2 years after initiating therapy and then extending the interval when BMD is stable or improving. A decline in BMD while on treatment should prompt an investigation into the causes of bone loss including medication nonadherence or underlying conditions that could be contributing, such as celiac disease or other malabsorptive disorders. BMD monitoring should occur at the same facility and on the same machine, when possible, for valid comparison between tests. More frequent screening may be considered in patients at risk for rapid bone loss, including patients taking high-dose steroids or aromatase inhibitors.

Specialized Testing and Referral to a Bone Health Specialist

Markers of Bone Turnover

The use of biochemical markers of bone turnover has been proposed as a tool for evaluating patients with osteoporosis and guiding decisions on screening and treatment. There are several assays that measure biochemical markers of bone turnover. The tests measure products released from osteoclasts and osteoblasts during bone remodeling. Studies show that bone biomarkers can be predictive of the rate of bone loss and may be predictive of fracture risk [57–59]. Markers of bone formation include bone-specific alkaline phosphatase (BSAP), N-terminal propeptide of type I procollagen (PINP), and less so osteocalcin. Markers of resorption include N-telopeptide cross-link (NTX) and C-terminal telopeptide cross-link (CTX). The use of biochemical markers of bone turnover in individual patients has so far been limited by biologic variability and differences in assays [60, 61]. Biochemical markers of bone turnover may have a future role in fracture risk prediction and monitoring medication compliance and efficacy [62].

Referrals

Referral to a bone health specialist should be considered in situations where the clinical presentation and data are inconsistent, for example, when a patient presents with a fragility fracture with normal BMD. Referral should also be considered in patients with complex management needs including patients with osteoporosis who have chronic conditions complicating management (e.g., chronic kidney disease) and patients with recurrent fractures or bone loss while on therapy when secondary causes have been excluded. Generally, bone biopsy is not recommended but may be indicated for a small subset of patients to distinguish between osteoporosis and other bone diseases such as renal osteodystrophy or osteomalacia.

Summary Points

1. Osteoporosis affects about ten million Americans; hip fracture significantly impacts disability (about 40% lose the ability to walk) and mortality (up to 20% within a year of fracture).
2. Screening for osteoporosis with a DXA scan is recommended for all women aged 65 and older; follow-up scans are indicated 2–10 years after the first screening depending on fracture risk and initial results. Women younger than 65 years should be screened when significant risk factors are present, such as current smoking, parental hip fracture, personal history of nontraumatic fracture, prednisone use, or malabsorption.
3. Osteoporosis is diagnosed clinically after a fragility fracture occurs or when the DXA T-score lies at or below −2.5. Low bone mass or osteopenia is defined as a T-score between −1 and −2.5. Most women have primary osteoporosis, occurring after menopause and more common

with increasing age. Secondary osteoporosis occurs due to endocrine, GI, hematologic, or nutritional conditions that affect bone mass.

4. FRAX is an online risk assessment tool to predict the 10-year risk of hip and other major osteoporotic fractures. The inputs in FRAX are race/ethnicity, sex, BMI, smoking status, alcohol or prednisone use, rheumatoid arthritis or other secondary osteoporosis conditions, and personal or family history of fracture.
5. A healthy lifestyle supports bone health, although evidence is insufficient to show these measures prevent osteoporotic fractures: exercise, dietary calcium and vitamin D, and avoidance of tobacco or excessive alcohol.
6. Osteoporosis is generally treated with bisphosphonates, such as once-weekly oral alendronate. Bisphosphonates may also be considered in patients with 10-year hip risk of 3% or greater or 10-year osteoporotic fracture risk of 20% or greater, according to FRAX.
7. If bisphosphonates are contraindicated, not tolerated, or if BMD declines on therapy, newer or anabolic agents may be tried, often in consultation with a specialist.

Review Questions

1. Tammy is a 78-year-old White woman without medical history but with significant alcohol use. She is 5′2″ and 50 kg. She suffered a hip fracture at home slipping on the stairs. She was hospitalized and required surgical intervention and physical therapy. Which of the following best represents her prognosis?
   A. After rehabilitation therapy, she has a 30% likelihood of requiring long-term nursing facility care.
   B. Changing lifestyle (walking most days of the week and avoiding alcohol and tobacco) and adding a calcium/vitamin D supplement daily will halt further loss of bone mass.
   C. Prescribing daily alendronate for a year will increase her bone mass by 50%.
   D. Using FRAX, her 10-year risk of major osteoporotic fracture is 27%.

   The correct answer is D. This woman has significant osteoporotic fracture risk based on her age and alcohol use. Her previous fracture does not qualify for osteoporosis, since it was traumatic, and a DXA would further clarify risk. Among women with osteoporosis, alendronate can improve fracture risk by 40–50%, but the BMD only improves <10% [31]. Lifestyle changes have not been shown to significantly improve age-related BMD decline. Hip fracture significantly contributes to mortality and morbidity, but community-dwelling adults have only about a 10% chance of requiring long-term care after a fracture.
2. Which of the following scenarios best prompts an order for a screening DXA scan for osteoporosis?
   A. A 63-year-old with a history of 5 pack-years of smoking and sedentary lifestyle
   B. A 66-year-old with a DXA last year showing a T-score of −2.0
   C. A 69-year-old with no risk factors but no previous DXA scans
   D. A 72-year-old started on alendronate last year for a high-risk FRAX score
   E. A 75-year-old with treated hyperthyroidism and normal DXA 5 years ago

   The correct answer is C. The USPSTF recommends DXA for osteoporosis screening in women aged 65 or older, with a screening interval of at least 2 years, longer intervals for normal low-risk patients [16]. DXA may be ordered earlier if with significant risk factors such as parental hip fracture, prednisone use, or current smoking. Once started on therapy, DXA scans may be ordered for treatment surveillance, but no more frequent than every 2 years [42].
3. Patriece is a 68-year-old whose mom had a hip fracture when she was in her 80s. Her past medical history is significant only for hypertension and a history of bladder surgery. On DXA, her T-score is −2.2. The best next step is:
   A. After confirming no contraindications such as active ulcers or chronic kidney disease, prescribe a weekly bisphosphonate such as alendronate or risedronate.
   B. Calculate her risk of a 10-year osteoporotic fracture using FRAX.
   C. Complete her social history and ask a review of systems questions for conditions that cause secondary osteoporosis such as malabsorption.
   D. Order a complete chemistry profile, complete blood count, 25-hydroxy vitamin D, and urinary N-telopeptide.

   The correct answer is C. Once a low BMD is found, the first step is to assess for risk factors for osteoporosis and behaviors that contribute to risk in order to understand what part of the bone loss is modifiable (by treating celiac disease, for example) and to use in FRAX calculators to predict future risk. Part of this assessment includes laboratory evaluation, including chemistry, blood counts, and vitamin D, but would not include markers of bone turnover such as N-telopeptide, as the clinical utility of these tests has not yet been defined. FRAX can be used but only after completing the clinical assessment. Alendronate is not indicated at this BMD level without a FRAX predicting high risk [42].
4. Lana has been on alendronate therapy for 5 years for low bone mass. She has tolerated it well. Repeat DXA shows

a T-score of −2.6. Five years ago, the score was −2.4. Which of the following is the best next step?

A. Continue alendronate for another 5 years and recheck DXA then.

B. Re-evaluate for secondary osteoporosis, adequate vitamin D and calcium intake, and adherence to therapy.

C. Refer to an osteoporosis specialist to discuss bisphosphonate failure.

D. Switch to risedronate and recheck DXA in 2 years.

The correct answer is B. If the BMD continues to decline on bisphosphonate therapy, the first step is to check for adherence and adequate dietary calcium and vitamin D. It is also useful to query the patient for any symptoms or signs of a newly acquired secondary osteoporosis condition. Alendronate is generally an effective therapy when taken as prescribed on an empty stomach [32]. If the patient has bone loss or a fracture on bisphosphonate therapy, it is appropriate to consider other agents such as teriparatide, usually in consultation with a specialist. Switching to a different bisphosphonate is useful only when there are adverse effects of one agent; another may not have the same adverse effects.

References

1. Wright NC, Looker AC, Saag KG, Curtis JR, Delzell ES, Randall S, et al. The recent prevalence of osteoporosis and low bone mass in the United States based on bone mineral density at the femoral neck or lumbar spine. J Bone Miner Res. 2014;29:2520–6.
2. Burge R, Dawson-Hughes B, Solomon DH, Wong JB, King A, Tosteson A. Incidence and economic burden of osteoporosis related fractures in the United States, 2005-2025. J Bone Miner Res. 2007;22(3):465–75.
3. Singer A, Exuzides A, Spangler L, O'Malley C, Colby C, Johnston K, et al. Burden of illness for osteoporotic fractures compared with other serious diseases among postmenopausal women in the United States Singer AJ, et al. Mayo Clin Proc. 2015;90:53–62.
4. Cosman F, de Beur SJ, LeBoff MS, et al. Clinician's guide to prevention and treatment of osteoporosis. Osteoporosis Int. 2014;25:2359.
5. Cooper C, Atkinson EJ, Jacobsen SJ, et al. Population-based study of survival after osteoporotic fractures. Am J Epidemiol. 1993;137:1001.
6. Magaziner J, Simonsick EM, Kashner TM, et al. Predictors of functional recovery one year following hospital discharge for hip fracture: a prospective study. J Gereontol. 1995;45:M101.
7. Liebson CL, Tosteson AN, Gabriel SE, et al. Mortality, disability, and nursing home use for persons with and without hip fracture: a population-based study. J Am Geriatr Soc. 2002;50:16.
8. Riggs BL, Melton LJ 3rd. The worldwide problem of osteoporosis: insights afforded by epidemiology. Bone. 1995;17(5 Suppl):505S–11S.
9. Cree M, Soskolne CL, Belsck E, et al. Mortality and institutionalization following hip fracture. J Am Geriatr Soc. 2010;48:283.
10. Licata A. Bone density vs bone quality: what is a clinician to do? Cleve Clin J Med. 2009;76(6):331–6.
11. Eriksen EF. Normal and pathological remodeling of human trabecular bone: three dimensional reconstruction of the remodeling sequence in normals and in metabolic bone disease. Endocr Rev. 1986;7(4):379–408.
12. Greenspan SL, Maitland LA, Myers ER, Krasnow MB, Kido TH. Femoral bone loss progresses with age: a longitudinal study in women over age 65. J Bone Miner Res. 1994;9:1959–65.
13. Finkelstein JS, Brockwell SE, Mehta V, Greendale GA, Sowers MR, Ettinger B, et al. Bone mineral density changes during the menopause transition in a multiethnic cohort of women. J Clin Endocrinol Metab. 2008;93:861–8.
14. Camacho PM, Patek SM, Binkley N, Clarke BL, Harris ST, Hurley DL, et al. American Association of Clinical Endocrinologists and American College of Endocrinology clinical practice guidelines for the diagnosis and treatment of postmenopausal osteoporosis. Endocr Pract. 2016;22(4):1–42.
15. World Health Organization. Who scientific group on the assessment of osteoporosis at primary health care level. Geneva: World Health Organization. 2004. Accessed online 7.23.2019: https://www.who.int/chp/topics/Osteoporosis.pdf.
16. U.S. Preventative Services Task Force. Screening for osteoporosis: U.S. preventive service task force recommendation statement. Ann Intern Med. 2011;154:356–64. US Preventive Services Task Force. Screening for osteoporosis to prevent fractures. US preventive services task force recommendation statement. JAMA. 2018;319(24):2521–31.
17. Cummings SR, Nevitt MC, Browner WS, Stone K, Fox KM, Ensrud KE, et al. Risk factors for fracture in white women. Study of osteoporotic fractures research group. N Engl J Med. 1995;332(12):767.
18. Marques A, Ferreira RJ, Santos E, Loza E, Carmona L, da Silva JA. The accuracy of osteoporotic fracture risk prediction tools: a systematic review and meta-analysis. Ann Rheum Dis. 2015;74(11):1958–67.
19. Crandall CJ, Larson J, LaCroix A, Cauley JA, LeBoff MS, Li W, et al. Predicting fracture risk in younger postmenopausal women: comparison of the Garvan and FRAX risk calculators in the Women's Health Initiative Study. J Gen Intern Med. 2019;34(2):235–42. https://doi.org/10.1007/s11606-018-4696-z.
20. International Society of Clinical Densitometry Official Positions. https://www.iscd.org/official-positions/. Accessed August 10, 2019.
21. Nayak S, Olkin I, Liu H, Grabe M, Gould MK, Allen IE, et al. Meta-analysis: accuracy of quantitative ultrasound for identifying patients with osteoporosis. Ann Intern Med. 2006;144(11):832.
22. Tannenbaum C, Clark J, Scwartzman K, et al. Yield of laboratory testing to identify secondary contributors to osteoporosis in otherwise healthy women. J Clin Endocrinol Metab. 2002;87:4431.
23. Kanis JA, Oden A, Johansson H, Borgeström F, Ström O, McCloskey E. FRAX and its applications to clinical practice. Bone. 2000;44:734–43.
24. Gourlay M, Fine JP, Preisser JS, May RC, Chenxi L, Li-Yung L, et al.; for the Study if Osteoporosis Fractures Research Group. Bone-density testing interval and transition to osteoporosis in older women. N Engl J Med. 2012;366:225–33.
25. Howe TE, Shea B, Dawson LJ, Downie F, Murray A, Ross C, et al. Exercise for preventing and treating osteoporosis in postmenopausal women. Cochrane Database Syst Rev. 2011;(7):CD000333.
26. Tai V, Leung W, Grey A, Reid I, Bolland M. Calcium intake and bone mineral density: systematic reviewand meta-analysis. BMJ. 2015;351:h4183.
27. Bolland MJ, Leung W, Tai V, Bastin S, Gamble G, Grey A, Reid I. Calcium intake and risk of fracture: systematic review. BMJ. 2015;351:h4580.
28. Bolland MJ, Avenell A, Baron JA, et al. Effect of calcium supplements on risk of myocardial infarction and cardiovascular events: meta-analysis. BMJ. 2010;341:c3691.
29. Moyer VA, USPST Force. Vitamin D and calcium supplementation to prevent fractures in adults: U.S. preventive services task force recommendation statement. Ann Intern Med. 2013;158(9):691–6.

30. El-Khoury F, Cassou B, Charles MA, Dargent-molina P. The effect of fall prevention exercise programmes on fall induced injuries in community dwelling older adults: systematic review and meta-analysis of randomised controlled trials. BMJ. 2013;347:f6234.
31. Black DM, Cummings SR, Karpf DB, Cauley JA, Thompson DE, Nevitt MC, et al. Randomized trial of effect of alderonate on risk of fracture in women with exisiting vertebral fratures. Lancet. 1996;348(9041):1535–41.
32. Cummings SR, Black DM, Thompson DE, Applegate WB, Barrett-Connor E, Musliner TA, et al. Effect of alendronate on risk of fracture in women with low bone density but without vertebral fractures: results from the fracture intervention trial. JAMA. 1998;280:2077–82.
33. Black DM, Delmas PD, Eastell R, Reid IR, Boonen S, Cauley JA, et al. Once-yearly zoledronic acid for treatment of postmenopausal osteoporosis. N Engl J Med. 2007;356:1809–22.
34. Cummings SR, San Martin J, McClung MR, Siris ES, Eastell R, Reid IR, et al.; for the FREEDOM Trial. Desosumab for the prevention of fracture in postmenopausal women with osteoporosis. N Engl J Med. 2009;367:1714–23.
35. Cosman F, Crittenden DB, Adachi JD, et al. Romosozumab treatment in postmenopausal women with osteoporosis. N Engl J Med. 2016;376(16):1532.
36. Saag KG, Peterson J, Brandi ML, Karaplis AC, Lorentzon M, Thomas T, et al. Romosozumab or alendronate for fracture prevention in women with osteoporosis. N Engl J Med. 2017;377:1417–27.
37. McClung M, Harris ST, Miller PD, Bauer DC, Davison KS, Dian L, et al. Bisphosphonate therapy for osteoporosis: benefits, risks, and drug holiday. Am J Med. 2013;126:13–20.
38. Harris ST, Watts NB, Genant HK, et al. Effects of risedronate treatment on vertebral and nonvertebral fractures in women with postmenopausal osteoporosis: a randomized controlled trial. Veretebral Efficacy with Risedronate Therapy (VERT) Study group. JAMA. 1999;282:1344–52.
39. Reginster J, Minne HW, Sorensen OH, et al. Randomized trial of the effects of risedronate on vertebral fractures in women with established postmenopausal osteoporosis. Vertebral Efficacy with Risedronate Therapy (VERT) study Group. Osteoporos Int. 2000;11:83–91.
40. Tucci JR, Tonino RP, Emkey RD, et al. Effect of three years of oral alendronate treatment in postmenopausal women with osteoporosis. Am J Med. 1996;101:488.
41. Lee SH, Chang SS, Lee M, Chan RC, Lee CC. Risk of osteonecrosis in the patients taking bisphosphonates for prevention of osteoporosis: a systematic review and meta-analysis. Osteoporos Int. 2014;25(3):1131–9.
42. Qaseem Amir, Forciea MA, McLean RM, Denberg TD; for the clinical Committee of the American College of Physicians. Treatment of low bone density or osteoporosis to prevent fractures in men and women: a clinical practice guideline update from the American College of Physicians. Ann Intern Med. 2017;166:818–39.
43. Dell RM, Adams AL, Greene DF, Funahashi TT, Silverman SL, Eisemon EO, et al. Incidence of atypical nontraumatic diaphyseal fractures of the femur. J Bone Miner Res. 2012;27(12):2544–50.
44. Want Z, Bhattacharya T. Trends in incidence of subtrochanteric fragility fractures and bisphosphonate use among the US elderly 1996-2007. J Bone Miner Res. 2011;26:553–60.
45. HealthDecision. https://www.healthdecision.org/tool#/tool/osteoporosis. Accessed 7.23.2019.
46. Black DM, Schwartz AV, Ensrud KE, et al. Effects of continuing or stopping alendronate after 5 years of treatment: the fracture intervention trial long-term extension (FLEX): a randomized trial. JAMA. 2006;296:2927–38.
47. Black DM, Reid IR, Boonen S, et al. The effect of 3 years versus 6 years of zoledronic acid treatment of osteoporosis: a randomized extension to the HORIZON Pivotal Fracture Trial (PFT). J Bone Miner Res. 2012;27:243–54.
48. Anastasilakis AD, Toulis KA, Anastasilakis CD, Makras P. Long-term treatment of osteoporosis: safety and efficacy appraisal of denosumab. Ther Clin Risk Manag. 2012;8:295–306.
49. Miller PD, Bolognese MA, Lewiecki EM, McClung MR, Ding B, Austin M, et al.; Amg Bone Loss Study Group. Effect of denosumab on bone density and turnover in postmenopausal women with low bone mass after long-term continued, discontinued, and restarting of therapy: a randomized blinded phase 2 clinical trial. Bone. 2008;43(2):222–9.
50. Ettinger B, Black DM, Mitlak BH, Knickerbocker RK, Nickelsen T, Genant HK, et al. Reduction of vertebral fracture risk in postmenopausal women with osteoporosis treated with raloxifene: results from a 3-year randomized clinical trial. Multiple Outcomes of Raloxifene Evaluation (MORE) Investigators. JAMA. 1999;282(7):637–45.
51. Rossouw JE, Anderson GL, Prentice RL, et al. Risks and benefits of estrogen plus progestin in healthy postmenopausal women: principal results from the Women's Health Initiative randomized controlled trial. JAMA. 2002;288:321.
52. Neer RM, Arnaud CD, Zanchetta JR, Prince R, Gaich G, Reginster JY, et al. Effect of parathyroid hormone (1-34) on fractures and bone mineral density in postmenopausal women with osteoporosis. N Engl J Med. 2001;244:1434–41.
53. Miller PD, Hattersley G, Riis BJ, et al. Effect of abaloparatide vs placebo on new vertebral fractures in postmenopausal women with osteoporosis: a randomized clinical trial. JAMA. 2016;316:722.
54. Black DM, Bilezikian JP, Ensrud KE, et al. One year of alendronate after one year of parathyroid hormone (1-84) for osteoporosis. N Engl J Med. 2005;353:555.
55. Cipriani C, Irani D, Bilezikian JP. Safety of osteoanabolic therapy: a decade of experience. J Bone Miner Res. 2012;27:2419.
56. Langdahl B, Libanati C, Crittenden DB, Bolognese MA, Brown JP, Daizadeh NS, et al. Superior gains in bone mineral density and estimated strength at the hip for romosozumab compared with teriparatide in women with postmenopausal osteoporosis transitioning from bisphosphonate therapy: results of the phase 3 open-label structure study. Arthritis Rheumatol. 2016;68(10).
57. Chestnut CH III, Bell NH, Clark GS, et al. Hormone replacement therapy in postmenopausal women: urinary N-telopeptide of type I collagen monitors therapeutic effects and predicts response of bone mineral density. Am J Med. 1997;102:29.
58. Ivaska KK, Lenora J, Gerdhem P, et al. Serial assessment of serum bone metabolism markers identifies women with the highest rate of bone loss and osteoporosis risk. J Clin Endocrinol Metab. 2008;93:2622.
59. Garnero P, Hausherr E, Chapuy MC, et al. Markers of bone resorption predict hip fracture in elderly women: the EPIDOS Prospective Study. J Bone Miner Res. 1996;11:1531.
60. Hlaing TT, Compston JE. Biochemical markers of bone turnover – uses and limitations. Ann Clin Biochem. 2014;51:189.
61. Bell KJ, Hayen A, Irwig L, et al. The potential value of monitoring bone turnover markers among women on alendronate. J Bone Miner Res. 2012;27:195.
62. Vasikaran S, Eastell R, Bruyere O, et al. Markers of bone turnover for the prediction of fracture risk and monitoring of osteoporosis treatment: a need for international reference standards. Osteoporosis Int. 2011;22:391.

Part V

Chronic Pain Disorders

General Approach to Chronic Pain

26

Andrea E. Carter and Melissa A. McNeil

Learning Objectives

1. Review the definition and epidemiology of chronic pain.
2. Assess the biological and psychosocial reasons for gender differences in chronic pain.
3. Describe the evaluation of a patient with chronic pain.
4. Formulate an approach to chronic pain involving collaborative care models and non-pharmacologic therapy.
5. Identify classes of non-opioid medications to use as first-line pharmacotherapy therapy for chronic pain.
6. Determine when to initiate or continue opioids for chronic pain, and assess risk and address harms of opioid use.
7. Discuss the importance of the patient-provider relationship in the treatment of chronic pain.

Kim is a 42-year-old female patient with a history of depression who is presenting to your office to establish care and wants to discuss her total body pain. This pain started at least 10 years ago and has waxed and waned but has been worse in the past year since she started having more stress at work. This pain was diagnosed by her prior primary care provider as fibromyalgia. She is very frustrated by her pain and wants to know how common it is for someone to suffer from chronic pain.

A. E. Carter (✉) · M. A. McNeil
University of Pittsburgh School of Medicine, Division of General Internal Medicine, Pittsburgh, PA, USA
e-mail: carterae@upmc.edu

Definition and Epidemiology of Chronic Pain

Chronic pain has been defined as "an unpleasant sensory and emotional experience associated with actual or potential damage" that persists for longer than 3–6 months [1]. Chronic pain has a significant impact on patients' health and quality of life. Patients with chronic pain have higher rates of depression and anxiety disorders, are more likely to have significant activity limitations, and have more unfavorable perceptions of their health [2]. The cost of chronic pain to society is substantial, accounting for 20% of outpatient visits [3], 12% of all prescriptions [4], and up to $600 billion in annual expenses from healthcare costs and lost productivity [5].

Chronic pain is common, affecting more than 100 million adults in the United States [6, 7]. Data derived from the 2002 National Health and Nutrition Examination Survey (NHANES) showed that chronic pain prevalence estimates were 10% for back pain, 7% for pain in the legs and feet, 4% for pain in the arms and hands, 4% for headache, and 1% for abdominal pain. Women had higher odds than men for headache and abdominal pain [8]. Specific common etiologies of chronic pain in women, including fibromyalgia, chronic pelvic pain, headaches, irritable bowel syndrome, and interstitial cystitis are discussed in detail in separate chapters in this book.

The perception of pain in individual patients is complex. Given this, the approach to evaluating and treating chronic pain must be comprehensive and individualized.

Classification of Chronic Pain

Chronic pain can be classified in many ways, but unfortunately, no single classification system can adequately categorize all types of chronic pain. Often chronic pain is classified based on perceived location (e.g., low back pain, abdominal pain). However, some diagnoses such as fibromyalgia cause widespread pain so categorization based on location alone is not adequate. Chronic pain can also be classified based on the suspected etiology of pain (e.g., postsurgical pain, osteo-

S. A. Tilstra et al. (eds.), *Sex- and Gender-Based Women's Health*, https://doi.org/10.1007/978-3-030-50695-7_26

arthritis), but many types of chronic pain are idiopathic. To address the need for an improved classification system for chronic pain, the International Association for the Study of Pain has suggested a classification system for the upcoming 11th version of the International Classification of Diseases. Their classification system incorporates both perceived location and suspected etiology of pain and includes seven categories: (1) chronic primary pain (e.g. fibromyalgia, irritable bowel syndrome), (2) chronic cancer pain, (3) chronic post-traumatic and postsurgical pain, (4) chronic neuropathic pain, (5) chronic headache and orofacial pain, (6) chronic visceral pain, and (7) chronic musculoskeletal pain [9]. It is important to note that patients often experience more than one type of chronic pain.

Another way to classify chronic pain is to categorize into nociceptive versus neuropathic pain. This classification system is useful in guiding treatment options. Nociceptive pain is caused by damaged tissue and is often due to mechanical or compressive etiologies, musculoskeletal conditions, or inflammation. Patients often describe nociceptive pain as dull or aching. Alternatively, neuropathic pain is caused by damage to the nervous system. Neuropathic pain can be central or peripheral and causes include diabetes mellitus, post-herpetic neuralgia, and spinal stenosis. Patients often describe neuropathic pain as burning, tingling, or electrical [10].

Kim goes on to tell you that she feels her husband does not understand her pain. She wonders if men and women experience pain differently.

Pathophysiology of Chronic Pain

The processing and interpretation of pain is a complex process. During acute pain, tissue injury results in the stimulation of sensory nerve cells called nociceptors. As seen in Fig. 26.1, nociceptors produce a signal at the site of the injury that travels along pain fibers that enter the spinal cord at the dorsal root ganglia and terminate in the dorsal horn. Second-order neurons travel up the contralateral spinothalamic tract and terminate in the thalamus. Third-order neurons travel from the thalamus to the anterior cingulate (C), frontal insular (F), and somatosensory cortex (SS) where pain is perceived. See Fig. 26.1.

Usually, the nociceptive sensory system returns to a normal state once healing is complete after an episode of acute pain. However, chronic pain develops when pain persists long past the expected time of healing due a maladaptive response of this system. When persistent or repeated stimuli are applied to damaged tissues, the threshold for activating nociceptors is lowered, which is called sensitization.

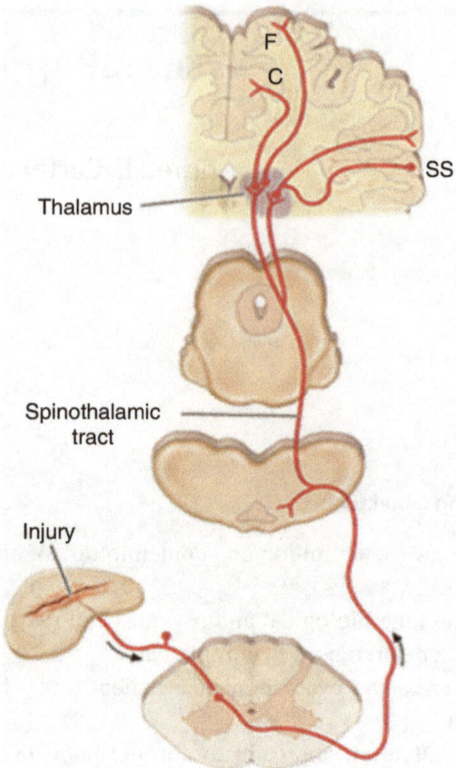

Fig. 26.1 The pain processing pathway. (Reprinted from Rathmell and Fields [11], with permission from McGraw-Hill Education)

Sensitization is an important process contributing to chronic pain [11].

In addition, the experience of chronic pain is very dependent on the patient's individual circumstances. It is important to consider the patient's psychologic, behavioral, emotional, social, economic, and cognitive factors as well as the prior history of pain, coping mechanisms, and support system. All of these factors interact to moderate the patient's experience of chronic pain.

Gender Differences in Chronic Pain

There are significant gender differences in chronic pain. Chronic pain is more common in women than men [6, 7]. In addition, evidence suggests that women experience more severe clinical pain than men [12–14]. The underlying reasons for these gender differences are an area of active research, and the mechanisms have not been fully elucidated.

There are several biological mechanisms that may account for the gender differences. First, the sex hormones have a complex effect on pain sensitivity, and in particular, testosterone may have a modulatory effect on pain [15]. In addition, there are gender differences in the cortical processing of pain [16, 17]. There may also be gender differences in the activation of the opioid receptor system [18].

There are also several psychosocial mechanisms that may account for the gender differences. In particular, there may be gender differences in self-efficacy related to pain and in pain catastrophizing, which is a pain response involving rumination, magnification, and helplessness [19]. Also, sociocultural beliefs may be important as pain expression is generally more socially acceptable among women, which could lead to biased reporting of pain. In addition, women who have experienced childhood abuse [20] or intimate partner violence [21] are more likely to experience chronic pain.

You discuss with Kim that there are indeed significant gender differences in chronic pain. You would like to obtain more information from Kim about her pain.

Clinical History

A thorough history is imperative in the evaluation of a patient with chronic pain. The history should include all the typical components of a medical history with particular attention to details of the characteristics of the pain symptoms, impact of pain on function, and psychosocial factors that could be contributing to chronic pain.

Open-ended questions should be used to determine the nature of the pain. The features of pain in the history of present illness can be recalled using the mnemonic OLD CARTS (Onset, Location/radiation, Duration, Characteristics, Aggravating factors, Relieving factors, Timing, and Severity). Example questions are presented in Table 26.1

In addition to this standard history of present illness, it is critical to understand the impact of the pain on function and psychosocial factors that could be contributing to the pain.

Table 26.1 OLD CARTS mnemonic: History-taking tool to elicit characteristics of pain

Pain features in the history of present illness	Example question(s)
Onset	When did the pain start? Was there an inciting event?
Location	Where is the pain located? Does it radiate anywhere?
Duration	How long has the pain lasted? Are there discrete episodes or is the pain continuous?
Characteristics	What does the pain feel like? Is this pain similar to prior events?
Aggravating factors	What makes the pain worse?
Relieving factors	What makes the pain better?
Timing	How often does the pain occur? Is it temporally related to anything?
Severity	On a scale of 0 to 10, how severe is the pain? Is the pain getting better or worse?

The features of a psychosocial assessment can be recalled using the mnemonic ACT-UP (Activity, Coping, Think, Upset, People's responses) [22]. Example questions are presented in Table 26.2. It is also important to screen for intimate partner violence and sexual abuse, as women experiencing abuse are more likely to experience headaches, back pain, abdominal pain, and pelvic pain [21].

There are several validated multidimensional scales that can be used to evaluate chronic pain. These scales are especially useful to track pain over time and to judge if the pain is improving with treatment. The Brief Pain Inventory is a short, validated questionnaire that measures pain severity and interference with daily activities [23]. The McGill Pain Questionnaire measures pain quality and intensity [24]. These scales can easily be found online and incorporated into a clinic visit for a patient with chronic pain.

Physical Exam

A complete physical examination should be performed in patients with chronic pain. The examination should include a detailed evaluation of the symptomatic areas. It is also important to assess mood during the physical exam. Relevant components of the physical exam for specific types of chronic pain syndromes are described in other chapters.

Diagnostic Workup

Pain is a subjective experience of the patient, and there is no diagnostic test that can confirm the presence of pain. The goal of the diagnostic workup in patients with chronic pain is to identify treatable primary medical conditions causing secondary pain, such as inflammatory bowel disease causing chronic abdominal pain. It is essential to consider "red flag" symptoms in every patient that may reflect pain related to

Table 26.2 ACT-UP mnemonic: History-taking tool to elicit psychosocial aspects of pain [22]

Psychosocial assessment	Example question(s)
Activity	How is your pain affecting the activities in your life such as sleeping, eating, exercising, working, and having fun?
Coping	How are you coping with your pain? Do you have any strategies that help you to manage your pain?
Think	Do you think your pain will get better or worse in the future?
Upset	Does your pain upset your mood? Have you been feeling depressed or anxious?
People's responses	How do other people around you respond when you have pain? Is your pain affecting your relationships?

malignancy, organ dysfunction, infection, or another emergent condition. For example, ask about fever in patients with chronic back to evaluate for osteomyelitis.

Keep in mind that many causes of chronic pain are idiopathic and will not have laboratory or imaging abnormalities. The ordering of tests in chronic pain should be judicious and targeted, and there are times when no tests are indicated. Unfortunately, unnecessary tests are often ordered in chronic pain syndromes. For example, about 12% of outpatients with migraine headaches undergo magnetic resonance imaging of the brain despite clear guidelines from the American College of Radiology recommending against neuroimaging in patients with uncomplicated headache [25].

Suggested diagnostic workup for specific types of chronic pain syndromes is described in other chapters.

Kim's pain is widespread but is usually worst in her neck and shoulders. The pain is predominantly throughout her muscles, but she occasionally has joint pain as well. Most days, she would rate her pain as a 6 out of 10. The pain is worse when she feels stressed out, and she has been having increasing stress at work. She feels that her pain affects her relationship with her husband and also makes her abstain from social activities. She experienced childhood sexual abuse but currently feels safe in her relationship. Although she has a history of depression, she currently feels that her mood is good. When her pain is well controlled, she can walk for exercise, and she would like to get back to doing that. You agree that Kim most likely has fibromyalgia. Kim asks you if there is anything you can do to help her with her pain that doesn't involve taking a pill.

Non-pharmacologic Therapies for Chronic Pain

There are many non-pharmacologic treatments for chronic pain, including exercise, physical therapy, behavioral therapy, complementary or alternative medicine (such as chiropractor therapy and acupuncture), interventional techniques (such as steroid injections and nerve blocks), and surgical approaches. Given the complex nature of chronic pain, the most successful treatments are often multifaceted. Collaborative care interventions in primary care, including provider education, care managers, patient workshops, development of individualized functional goals, and symptom monitoring via telephone visits, have been shown to improve patient outcomes such as pain intensity and pain-related disability [26, 27].

After discussing some non-pharmacologic treatment options for Kim, she wants to pursue cognitive behavioral therapy. She is also interested in trying a medication for her chronic pain and is wondering what types of medications are available.

Non-opioid Pharmacologic Therapies for Chronic Pain

Pharmacologic therapies are often used to treat chronic pain. The major classes of medications used are non-opioid analgesics, opioids, antidepressants, anticonvulsants, and topical agents. Using a combination of medications is often more effective than a single medication.

Non-opioid Analgesics

Non-opioid analgesics include acetaminophen and nonsteroidal anti-inflammatory (NSAID) medications. When prescribing these medications, it is useful to tailor the prescription to the patient's complaints. For patients with constant pain, advise taking the analgesic at set intervals throughout the day. For patients who experience situational pain, advise taking the analgesic prior to the activity that causes pain (such as exercise).

Acetaminophen is available over the counter and is very commonly prescribed for many types of chronic pain. The mechanism of acetaminophen is not well established. The efficacy of acetaminophen is uncertain and has been shown to have very small or no benefit in the treatment of knee osteoarthritis and low back pain [28]. Acetaminophen overdose can lead to irreversible, devastating acute liver failure. Patients can approach toxic levels of acetaminophen ingestion unintentionally and should be counseled extensively about use. The Food and Drug Administration (FDA) lists the maximum safe dose as 4 grams per day, although in 2012, the FDA suggested but did not mandate decreasing the maximum daily dose to 3 grams. Clinically, most providers follow the 3 grams maximum recommendation, and it is thought that the maximum dose should not exceed 2 grams per day in patients with chronic liver disease or heavy alcohol use.

Many types of NSAID medications are also available over the counter and commonly prescribed for many types of chronic pain. NSAIDs act to decrease inflammation by inhibiting the enzyme cyclooxygenase (COX). COX catalyzes the formation of prostaglandin, which is a key messenger molecule in the process of inflammation. NSAIDs are more effective than placebo in treating low back pain [29]. NSAIDs can have adverse gastrointestinal side effects including dyspepsia and gastric ulceration and should be avoided in patients with history of ulcers. For patients with risk factors for gastroduodenal toxicity (older than 60 years of age, concurrent aspirin or glucocorticoid use, dyspepsia, or reflux symptoms), use a COX-2 selective NSAID (e.g., celecoxib) and consider prescribing a concurrent proton-pump inhibitor. NSAIDs can also cause nephrotoxicity due to renal vasoconstriction and should be avoided in patients with chronic renal insufficiency. In addition, the use of both nonselective NSAIDs and COX-2 selective NSAIDs has been associated with an increased risk of adverse cardiovascular events including myocardial infarction, heart failure, and stroke [30]. This risk varies depending on if the patient has baseline cardiovascular disease and on the specific NSAID chosen.

Antidepressants

Antidepressants have analgesic effects related to their effects on the serotonin, norepinephrine, and opioid receptor systems. Antidepressants have been shown to be efficacious in the treatment of neuropathic pain, fibromyalgia, low back pain, and headaches [31–33]. Although they do not have an approved indication for pain, tricyclic antidepressants (TCAs) such as amitriptyline and nortriptyline have long been used to treat chronic pain. TCAs are generally prescribed at lower doses than those used in depression. Adverse effects include sedation, anticholinergic effects (such as dry mouth, constipation, and mental clouding), and cardiac effects (such as prolonged interventricular conduction and prolonged QT interval). Serotonin-norepinephrine reuptake inhibitors (SNRIs), such as duloxetine and venlafaxine, are also frequently used in the treatment of chronic pain. The most frequent adverse effects are nausea, dry mouth, insomnia, constipation, and fatigue. Patients should be counseled that although they may experience side effects immediately, antidepressants may take several weeks to obtain full benefit in the treatment of pain.

Anticonvulsants

Three anticonvulsant medications (gabapentin, pregabalin, and carbamazepine) are approved by the FDA for the treatment of neuropathic pain. Gabapentin and pregabalin bind to voltage-gated calcium channels and inhibit neurotransmitter release. These medications can cause dose-dependent sedation; thus, it is important to start at a low dose and titrate up if needed. Like the antidepressants, the anticonvulsants take several weeks to obtain full benefit. It is important to note that there are rising concerns for gabapentin misuse, abuse, and diversion [34].

Topical Agents

Topical agents are frequently used for chronic pain. They are advantageous in that they avoid systemic side effects and can be delivered directly at the site of pain. Frequently prescribed topical agents include capsaicin, salicylate, lidocaine, and topical NSAIDs.

> *After discussing the medication options with Kim, you decide to prescribe duloxetine in addition to the cognitive behavioral therapy. Kim returns to see you 6 weeks later. She says her pain is markedly improved overall, and she is now back to walking her dog daily. However, her pain is not completely gone. Kim says that about 5 years ago, she was prescribed oxycodone for her chronic pain, and she asks you if you can write her a new prescription for oxycodone.*

Opioids for Chronic Pain

The use of opioids to treat chronic pain has increased despite the lack of convincing evidence that they are effective. About 20% of patients presenting to physician offices with chronic pain receive an opioid prescription [35]; however, a systematic review examining the effectiveness of long-term opioid therapy for chronic pain found no controlled studies that evaluated long-term outcomes related to pain, function, or quality of life [36]. Additionally, the widespread use of prescription opioids has led to a sharp increase in diversion and improper use and ultimately a national epidemic of opioid use disorder and overdose-related deaths—between 2000 and 2014, there was a 200% increase in the deaths from an opioid overdose [37]. To help address this, there is an imperative need for providers to safely prescribe opioids for chronic pain only in patients in whom the benefits outweigh the risks.

In 2016, the Centers for Disease Control and Prevention (CDC) released a guideline for prescribing opioids for chronic pain with the goal of improving communication between providers and patients and reducing the risks associated with long-term opioid therapy [38]. The guidelines recommend preferentially using non-pharmacologic and non-opioid pharmacologic therapy for chronic pain instead of opioids. If opioids are used, they should be combined with these other treatments. Before initiating opioids for chronic pain, providers should explain risks of therapy, discuss side effects, and set realistic treatment goals with patients. Women who have certain psychiatric disorders (depression, bipolar, schizophrenia, attention deficit disorder, or obsessive-compulsive disorder), a personal or family history of drug or alcohol misuse, or a history of preadolescent sexual abuse are more likely to develop opioid misuse [39]. If initiating opioid therapy, always use short-acting opioids at the lowest effective dose, and use an "as needed" dosing regimen as opposed to a fixed dosing schedule such as "every 6 hours." For women with children, it is important to advise storing opioids in a locked medicine cabinet. Patients should be reevaluated within 1–4 weeks of initiating opioid therapy and then at least every 3 months subsequently. If the benefits of pain control are not outweighing the harms of opioid therapy, opioids should be tapered or discontinued. Providers should use caution when prescribing more than 50 morphine milligram equivalents (MME) of opioid daily, and doses higher than 90 MME daily should be avoided as these doses significantly increase the risk of an opioid overdose. To reduce the risk of death from an opioid overdose, consider prescribing naloxone to patients receiving more than 50 MME daily, to patients who are prescribed any other sedating medications such as benzodiazepines, and to patients who have a history of substance use disorder or drug overdose. Providers should also check state prescription drug monitoring programs (PDMP) to identify controlled medications prescribed by other providers and check urine drug testing to identify undisclosed substance use. Patients found to have aberrant behaviors including lost or stolen medications, documented use of multiple physicians, and requests for multiple early refills should be screened for opioid use disorder (see Chap. 32 on Opioid Use Disorder for more information).

Medical Marijuana

The use of medical marijuana is growing in momentum; at the time of this writing, it is legalized in the majority of the United States and in many countries. The indications for medical marijuana use are debated, but its use in cancer patients and in debilitating illnesses are the most widely accepted. The use of medical marijuana in chronic pain for those without a life-limiting or debilitating illness is a subject of investigation by physicians and is desired by many patients. There is data suggesting that Medicare patients filled fewer opioid prescriptions in states with medical cannabis laws [40] and that the legalization of marijuana has been linked to fewer opioid-related deaths [41]. However, the long-term medical and psychosocial implications of medical marijuana use for chronic pain patients are unknown. Traditionally known as the "gateway drug," recent data suggests that medical marijuana use may increase the risk of subsequently developing opioid use disorder [42]. More research is needed to understand the risks and benefits of medical marijuana use in chronic pain disorders.

Depending on the state, providers can become licensed to provide certification exams for patients to enable them to purchase cannabis products from a dispensary. Providers themselves do not prescribe these products. It is important to counsel patients that medical cannabis should not be used in women who are pregnant or lactating, and caution is indicated in patients under 24 years old. It is illegal to drive under the influence of marijuana. The increasing legalization of recreational marijuana use means that patients will be able to legally obtain marijuana without the input of their providers in many instances. A full discussion of marijuana use is beyond the scope of this chapter. The editors recommend that providers become familiar with the uses and effects of medical marijuana. A comprehensive resource guide distributed by the Canadian Government is available online "Information for Health Care Professionals: Cannabis (marihuana, marijuana) and the cannabinoids" at https://www.canada.ca/en/health-canada/services/drugs-medication/cannabis/information-medical-practitioners/information-health-care-professionals-cannabis-cannabinoids.html [43].

You congratulate Kim for reaching her goal of being able to walk her dog due to the improvement in her pain with the duloxetine and cognitive behavioral therapy. You discuss that unfortunately, complete pain relief may not be a realistic expectation and that you are worried about her risk of developing harm from opioids given her risk factors for developing opioid misuse (her age, history of depression, and childhood sexual abuse). After discussing the risks and benefits of opioid therapy, Kim decides against treatment with opioids. You talk about other possible treatments for her fibromyalgia, and Kim decides to try acupuncture.

Importance of Patient-Provider Relationship in Chronic Pain Management

The patient-provider relationship is key in successful treatment of chronic pain. The patient-provider relationship can help promote patient resilience in chronic pain, especially when the provider provides psychologic support and promotes health literacy related to chronic pain and its treatment [44].

It is also important to note that providers often feel an emotional toll when caring for patients with chronic pain [45]. Setting realistic expectations with patients with chronic pain is critical. Being completely pain-free is usually not a realistic goal—a reduction in pain by 30% is considered clinically meaningful [46]. It is often helpful to focus on functional goals, such as returning to work or participating in recreational activities, rather than numeric pain score goals. Frequent visits can be helpful in monitoring pain symptoms, assessing progress toward functional goals, and coordinating multiple treatment approaches.

Summary Points

1. Chronic pain persists for longer than 3 months and is extremely common, affecting more than 50 million adults in the United States. Chronic pain is more common in women than in men, especially headaches, abdominal pain, and widespread pain.
2. The perception of pain depends on many biological and psychosocial factors that are different in women and men, including differences in cortical processing of pain, the endogenous opioid system, catastrophizing, and self-efficacy.
3. Chronic pain should be evaluated with a thorough clinical history including tools to measure pain intensity and impact of pain on function, a thorough physical exam, and additional testing only when indicated.
4. Outcomes in chronic pain are improved by using multifaceted approaches including non-pharmacologic therapies such as physical therapy, behavioral therapy, complementary or alternative medicine, interventional techniques, and surgical approaches.
5. Many classes of medication can be used to treat chronic pain including non-opioid analgesics, topical agents, antispasmodics, opioids, TCAs, SNRIs, and anticonvulsants.
6. The benefits and risks of opioid therapy for chronic pain should be considered carefully in each patient. If opioid therapy is appropriate, methods to reduce the risk of harm should be used including checking urine drug screens and prescription drug monitoring programs, prescribing naloxone when indicated, and tapering or discontinuing opioids when needed.
7. The patient-provider relationship is key in treating chronic pain. It is important to set realistic expectations, focus on functional goals, and arrange for frequent follow-up visits.

Review Questions

1. A 45-year-old female patient presents to your office with widespread musculoskeletal pain involving her ankles, knees, hips, lower back, shoulders, and arms. She has previously been diagnosed with fibromyalgia. Her pain is worse over the past several weeks. On exam, she is afebrile, and vital signs are within the normal range. She has several tender trigger points and has decreased range of motion due to pain. She has no active arthritis on exam.

   What is the next appropriate step in management?

   A. Ask about psychosocial stressors.
   B. Initiate a trial of oxycodone.
   C. Order a serum antinuclear antibody test.
   D. Refer to a rheumatologist.

   The correct answer is A. It is important to assess the biopsychosocial factors that may be contributing to chronic pain. Prior to obtaining a full comprehensive history, it would not be appropriate to initiate opioid therapy, order additional testing, or refer to a specialist.

2. A 65-year-old female patient presents to your office with worsening lower back pain to discuss getting an early refill and increase in the dose of her oxycodone. She has had back pain due to facet joint arthropathy for the past 10 years and is currently taking oxycodone 10 mg every 6 hours as needed for pain. You prescribed a 4-week supply of oxycodone 3 weeks ago, but she has run out of her medications early. On exam, she is afebrile, and vital signs are within the normal range. She has some tenderness to deep palpation of the lumbar vertebrae with otherwise normal back and lower extremity neurologic exam.

   What is the next appropriate step in management?

   A. Prescribe an increased dose of oxycodone.
   B. Order MRI of the lower back.
   C. Screen for signs of opioid use disorder.
   D. Refer to a pain specialist.

   The correct answer is C. It is important to screen for signs of opioid use disorder in patients requesting early refills or increase in the dose of opioid medications. If patients are not displaying signs or symptoms of opioid misuse, it may be appropriate to consider dose escalation, additional diagnostic testing, or referral to a specialist. It is important to discuss anticipatory guidance with all patients on opioids so that they have an action plan should their chronic pain increase between visits. Most of these patients will be tempted to increase the dose of their opioids independently without consultation from a provider which can be dangerous and lead to overdose and the lack of trust and stigmatization from the healthcare system.

3. A 35-year-old female patient presents to your office for the evaluation of chronic abdominal pain. She has crampy abdominal pain most days of the week, and it is associated with constipation. A colonoscopy was performed a year ago which was normal, and she has no family history of gastrointestinal diseases. On exam, she is afebrile, and vital signs are within the normal range. She has mild diffuse tenderness throughout her abdomen without rebound tenderness or guarding.

In addition to starting a trial of lubiprostone, what is the next appropriate step in management?

A. Refer to a gastroenterologist.
B. Recommend dietary manipulation and exercise.
C. Prescribe oxycodone.
D. Order repeat colonoscopy.

The correct answer is B. In patients with chronic pain syndromes, non-pharmacologic treatment strategies are often effective. As this patient is not displaying any concerns for opioid use disorder, it would be appropriate to try non-pharmacologic treatment such as dietary manipulation and exercise prior to prescribing opioids, ordering additional testing, or referring to a specialist [26, 27].

References

1. Merskey H, Bogduk N, International Association for the Study of Pain. Task Force on Taxonomy. Classification of chronic pain: descriptions of chronic pain syndromes and definitions of pain terms. 2nd ed. Seattle: IASP Press; 1994. xvi, 222 pp
2. Gureje O, Von Korff M, Simon GE, Gater R. Persistent pain and well-being: a World Health Organization study in primary care. JAMA. 1998;280(2):147–51.
3. Schappert SM. National Ambulatory Medical Care Survey: 1989 summary. Vital Health Stat. 1992;13:110):1–80.
4. Turk DC. Clinical effectiveness and cost-effectiveness of treatments for patients with chronic pain. Clin J Pain. 2002;18(6):355–65.
5. Institute of Medicine (US) Committee on Advancing Pain Research, Care, and Education. Relieving pain in America: a blueprint for transforming prevention, care, education, and research. The National Academies Collection: reports funded by National Institutes of Health. Washington, DC: National Academies Press; 2011.
6. Tsang A, Von Korff M, Lee S, Alonso J, Karam E, Angermeyer MC, et al. Common chronic pain conditions in developed and developing countries: gender and age differences and comorbidity with depression-anxiety disorders. J Pain. 2008;9(10):883–91.
7. Nahin RL. Estimates of pain prevalence and severity in adults: United States, 2012. J Pain. 2015;16(8):769–80.
8. Hardt J, Jacobsen C, Goldberg J, Nickel R, Buchwald D. Prevalence of chronic pain in a representative sample in the United States. Pain Med. 2008;9(7):803–12.
9. Treede RD, Rief W, Barke A, Aziz Q, Bennett MI, Benoliel R, et al. A classification of chronic pain for ICD-11. Pain. 2015;156(6):1003–7.
10. Reeves AG. Disorders of the nervous system: a primer. 3rd ed. West Lebanon: Imperial Company Printers; 1995. xi, 240 pp.
11. Rathmell JP, Fields HL. Chapter 18. Pain: pathophysiology and management. In: Kasper DL, Fauci A, Hauser S, Longo D, Jameson J, Loscalzo J, editors. Harrison's principles of internal medicine, vol. 1. 19th ed. New York: McGraw Hill Education; 2015. (various pagings).
12. Barnabe C, Bessette L, Flanagan C, Leclercq S, Steiman A, Kalache F, et al. Sex differences in pain scores and localization in inflammatory arthritis: a systematic review and metaanalysis. J Rheumatol. 2012;39(6):1221–30.
13. Fillingim RB, Doleys DM, Edwards RR, Lowery D. Clinical characteristics of chronic back pain as a function of gender and oral opioid use. Spine (Phila Pa 1976). 2003;28(2):143–50.
14. Keefe FJ, Lefebvre JC, Egert JR, Affleck G, Sullivan MJ, Caldwell DS. The relationship of gender to pain, pain behavior, and disability in osteoarthritis patients: the role of catastrophizing. Pain. 2000;87(3):325–34.
15. Craft RM. Modulation of pain by estrogens. Pain. 2007;132(Suppl 1):S3–12.
16. Berman SM, Naliboff BD, Suyenobu B, Labus JS, Stains J, Bueller JA, et al. Sex differences in regional brain response to aversive pelvic visceral stimuli. Am J Physiol Regul Integr Comp Physiol. 2006;291(2):R268–76.
17. Derbyshire SW, Nichols TE, Firestone L, Townsend DW, Jones AK. Gender differences in patterns of cerebral activation during equal experience of painful laser stimulation. J Pain. 2002;3(5):401–11.
18. Zubieta JK, Smith YR, Bueller JA, Xu Y, Kilbourn MR, Jewett DM, et al. Mu-opioid receptor-mediated antinociceptive responses differ in men and women. J Neurosci. 2002;22(12):5100–7.
19. Racine M, Tousignant-Laflamme Y, Kloda LA, Dion D, Dupuis G, Choiniere M. A systematic literature review of 10 years of research on sex/gender and experimental pain perception – part 1: are there really differences between women and men? Pain. 2012;153(3):602–18.
20. Walsh CA, Jamieson E, Macmillan H, Boyle M. Child abuse and chronic pain in a community survey of women. J Interpers Violence. 2007;22(12):1536–54.
21. Campbell J, Jones AS, Dienemann J, Kub J, Schollenberger J, O'Campo P, et al. Intimate partner violence and physical health consequences. Arch Intern Med. 2002;162(10):1157–63.
22. Fishman S, Ballantyne J, Rathmell JP, Bonica JJ. Bonica's management of pain. 4th ed. Baltimore: Lippincott, Williams & Wilkins; 2010. xxxiii, 1661 pp.
23. Keller S, Bann CM, Dodd SL, Schein J, Mendoza TR, Cleeland CS. Validity of the brief pain inventory for use in documenting the outcomes of patients with noncancer pain. Clin J Pain. 2004;20(5):309–18.
24. Dworkin RH, Turk DC, Revicki DA, Harding G, Coyne KS, Peirce-Sandner S, et al. Development and initial validation of an expanded and revised version of the Short-form McGill Pain Questionnaire (SF-MPQ-2). Pain. 2009;144(1–2):35–42.
25. Callaghan BC, Kerber KA, Pace RJ, Skolarus LE, Burke JF. Headaches and neuroimaging: high utilization and costs despite guidelines. JAMA Intern Med. 2014;174(5):819–21.
26. Dobscha SK, Corson K, Perrin NA, Hanson GC, Leibowitz RQ, Doak MN, et al. Collaborative care for chronic pain in primary care: a cluster randomized trial. JAMA. 2009;301(12): 1242–52.
27. Kroenke K, Krebs EE, Wu J, Yu Z, Chumbler NR, Bair MJ. Telecare collaborative management of chronic pain in primary care: a randomized clinical trial. JAMA. 2014;312(3):240–8.
28. Machado GC, Maher CG, Ferreira PH, Pinheiro MB, Lin CW, Day RO, et al. Efficacy and safety of paracetamol for spinal pain and osteoarthritis: systematic review and meta-analysis of randomised placebo controlled trials. BMJ. 2015;350:h1225.
29. Roelofs PD, Deyo RA, Koes BW, Scholten RJ, van Tulder MW. Nonsteroidal anti-inflammatory drugs for low back pain: an updated Cochrane review. Spine (Phila Pa 1976). 2008;33(16):1766–74.
30. Coxib and traditional NSAID Trialists' (CNT) Collaboration, Bhala N, Emberson J, Merhi A, Abramson S, et al. Vascular and upper gastrointestinal effects of non-steroidal anti-inflammatory drugs: meta-analyses of individual participant data from randomised trials. Lancet. 2013;382(9894):769–79.
31. Moore RA, Derry S, Aldington D, Cole P, Wiffen PJ. Amitriptyline for neuropathic pain and fibromyalgia in adults. Cochrane Database Syst Rev. 2012;12:CD008242.
32. Jackson JL, Shimeall W, Sessums L, Dezee KJ, Becher D, Diemer M, et al. Tricyclic antidepressants and headaches: systematic review and meta-analysis. BMJ. 2010;341:c5222.

33. Chou R, Deyo R, Friedly J, Skelly A, Weimer M, Fu R, et al. Systemic pharmacologic therapies for low back pain: a systematic review for an American College of Physicians clinical practice guideline. Ann Intern Med. 2017;166(7):480–92.
34. Smith RV, Havens JR, Walsh SL. Gabapentin misuse, abuse and diversion: a systematic review. Addiction. 2016;111(7):1160–74.
35. Daubresse M, Chang HY, Yu Y, Viswanathan S, Shah ND, Stafford RS, et al. Ambulatory diagnosis and treatment of nonmalignant pain in the United States, 2000–2010. Med Care. 2013;51(10):870–8.
36. Chou R, Turner JA, Devine EB, Hansen RN, Sullivan SD, Blazina I, et al. The effectiveness and risks of long-term opioid therapy for chronic pain: a systematic review for a National Institutes of Health Pathways to Prevention Workshop. Ann Intern Med. 2015;162(4):276–86.
37. Dart RC, Surratt HL, Cicero TJ, Parrino MW, Severtson SG, Bucher-Bartelson B, et al. Trends in opioid analgesic abuse and mortality in the United States. N Engl J Med. 2015;372(3):241–8.
38. Dowell D, Haegerich TM, Chou RCDC. Guideline for prescribing opioids for chronic pain--United States, 2016. JAMA. 2016;315(15):1624–45.
39. Webster LR, Webster RM. Predicting aberrant behaviors in opioid-treated patients: preliminary validation of the Opioid Risk Tool. Pain Med. 2005;6(6):432–42.
40. Bradford AC, Bradford WD, Abraham A, Bagwell Adams G. Association between US state medical cannabis laws and opioid prescribing in the Medicare Part D population. JAMA Intern Med. 2018;178(5):667–72. https://doi.org/10.1001/jamainternmed.2018.0266.29610897.
41. Bachhuber MA, Saloner B, Cunningham CO, Barry CL. Medical cannabis laws and opioid analgesic overdose mortality in the United States, 1999–2010. JAMA Intern Med. 2014;174(10):1668–73. https://doi.org/10.1001/jamainternmed.2014.4005.25154332.
42. Olfson M, Wall MM, Liu SM, Blanco C. Cannabis use and risk of prescription opioid use disorder in the United States. Am J Psychiatry. 2018;175(1):47–53. https://doi.org/10.1176/appi.ajp.2017.17040413. Epub 2017 Sep 26. 28946762.
43. Information for health care professionals: cannabis (marihuana, marijuana) and the cannabinoids. Accessed 9 Dec 2018 at https://www.canada.ca/en/health-canada/services/drugs-medication/cannabis/information-medical-practitioners/information-health-care-professionals-cannabis-cannabinoids.html.
44. Nafradi L, Kostova Z, Nakamoto K, Schulz PJ. The doctor-patient relationship and patient resilience in chronic pain: a qualitative approach to patients' perspectives. Chronic Illn. 2018;14:256–70.
45. Matthias MS, Parpart AL, Nyland KA, Huffman MA, Stubbs DL, Sargent C, et al. The patient-provider relationship in chronic pain care: providers' perspectives. Pain Med. 2010;11(11):1688–97.
46. Ostelo RW, Deyo RA, Stratford P, Waddell G, Croft P, Von Korff M, et al. Interpreting change scores for pain and functional status in low back pain: towards international consensus regarding minimal important change. Spine (Phila Pa 1976). 2008;33(1):90–4.

Irritable Bowel Syndrome

27

Rachel Vanderberg, Amy D. Lu, and Jana G. Hashash

Learning Objectives

1. Review the epidemiology and pathophysiology of irritable bowel syndrome (IBS).
2. Diagnose IBS using the Rome IV criteria.
3. Utilize targeted diagnostic testing in patients presenting with symptoms consistent with IBS.
4. Manage IBS utilizing evidence-based nonpharmacological and pharmacological therapies in a stepwise approach.
5. Design an appropriate interdisciplinary management plan or care team for patients with IBS.

Sloane is a 32-year-old gender-nonconforming natal female (uses they/them/their pronouns) who presents to establish care. They report a 5-year history of intermittent abdominal pain and diarrhea. Five years ago, they had a bout of traveler's diarrhea while on a trip to Mexico. After the initial resolution of symptoms, they began experiencing episodic diarrhea and abdominal cramping.

Epidemiology

Irritable bowel syndrome (IBS) is a symptom-based condition defined by abdominal pain with altered bowel habits in the absence of demonstrable organic disease. The prevalence is between 10% and 15% in North America and is equally distributed between subtypes: constipation predominant (IBS-C), diarrhea predominant (IBS-D), mixed type (IBS-M), and un-subtyped [1]. Women are 1.5–2 times more likely to be affected than males, and the prevalence of IBS decreases with age [2]. IBS is commonly encountered in the primary care setting and accounts for 25–50% of all referrals to gastroenterology. The burden of disease accounts for 3.1 million ambulatory care visits and up to 5.9 million dollars in prescriptions annually [3, 4].

Pathophysiology

The pathophysiology of IBS remains elusive. Traditionally, IBS has been theorized as being a gastrointestinal tract (GI) manifestation of primary brain dysfunction. However, newer epidemiologic studies have noted that GI symptoms may precede mood symptoms, which suggests a dual directionality of gut-brain axis dysfunction. Serotonin (5-HT) is an important and ubiquitous neurotransmitter in the central as well as enteric nervous systems, playing an integral role in GI motility and communication with the brain. Studies have found reduced postprandial 5-HT release in patients with IBS-C compared with those patients with postinfectious IBS and healthy individuals [5]. However, others have shown that alterations in 5-HT metabolism in patients with IBS did not have associations with GI or mood symptoms [6].

Acute enteric infections often precede the onset of IBS, especially IBS-D, and may serve as a trigger for immune activation that is mechanistically different from that of non-infectious IBS. A prospective controlled cohort study of 19,000 individuals exposed to drinking water contaminated with known GI pathogens such as *Norovirus*, *Giardia*, and

R. Vanderberg (✉)
Division of General Internal Medicine, University of Pittsburgh, Pittsburgh, PA, USA
e-mail: vanderbergrh@upmc.edu

A. D. Lu
San Francisco VA Medical Center, University of San Francisco Medical Center, San Francisco, CA, USA

J. G. Hashash
Department of Internal Medicine, Division of Gastroenterology, Hepatology, and Nutrition, University of Pittsburgh, Pittsburgh, PA, USA

American University of Beirut, Beirut, Lebanon

S. A. Tilstra et al. (eds.), *Sex- and Gender-Based Women's Health*, https://doi.org/10.1007/978-3-030-50695-7_27

Campylobacter jejuni showed increased risk of developing IBS-D symptoms in those with preexisting anxiety mediated by T-cell immune activation [7]. Separately, studies have shown increased concentration of cytokines in colonic mucosa as well as peripheral blood of patients with IBS-D [8]. This increased concentration of proinflammatory cytokines was also associated with mood disorders such as anxiety and depression [9].

Many patients with IBS also report diet triggers that initiate or exacerbate their symptoms. Though these are not usually reproducible when rechallenged in a double-blinded manner, certain foods seem to be implicated in the alteration of the gut microbiome and generation of IBS symptoms. Fermentable oligosaccharides, disaccharides, monosaccharides, and polyols (FODMAPs) have been reported to exacerbate symptoms in a subgroup of patients due to proposed fermentation and osmotic effects [10]. In fact, follow-up studies have shown increased small bowel distension and increased water content on MRI when FODMAPs are administered to healthy individuals [11].

Sloane describes experiencing watery bowel movements up to three times a day on at least 3 out of 7 days of the week. They do have occasional normal stools. The diarrhea is accompanied by crampy diffuse abdominal pain that is improved with defecation. They believe intake of certain foods may correlate to timing of their symptoms and have been trialing elimination of dairy products and gluten with limited improvement. Their symptoms have been getting slightly worse over the past year.

Clinical Manifestations and Diagnostic Criteria

Clinical manifestations of IBS encompass a wide range of symptoms including abdominal cramping, bloating, and changes in bowel habits from loose/frequent stools to constipation. Symptoms often change over time and can mimic other disorders. Therefore, diagnosis is usually based on a combination of characteristic symptoms over time and the exclusion of organic diseases. The current diagnostic standard, the Rome IV criteria, describes IBS as recurrent abdominal pain associated with two or more of the following characteristics: abdominal pain related to defecation, abdominal pain associated with changes from baseline stool frequency, and/or abdominal pain associated with a change from baseline stool appearance or form. These criteria should be fulfilled at least 1 day a week for at least 3 months with symptom onset of more than 6 months prior to diagnosis [12].

Classification of a patient's predominant bowel complaint plays an important role in determining further diagnostic testing as well as treatment. As described previously, IBS is classified into four subtypes: IBS-D, IBS-C, IBS-M, or un-subtyped IBS based on stool consistency as assessed by the Bristol Stool Form Scale (BSFS), a validated tool that categorizes stool appearance from a score of 1 (hard and lumpy) to 7 (entirely liquid). This tool can easily be accessed for free on the internet.

It is important to note that the Rome IV updated subtype criteria is explicitly based on *predominant* bowel habits on days with abnormal bowel movements, and not an average of all days. For example, a patient who experiences >25% of abnormal bowel movements consistent with BSFS 6 or 7 can be considered to have IBS-D, while another patient who experiences 25% of abnormal bowel movements consistent with BSFS 1 or 2 has IBS-C. Moreover, another subset of patients may have alternating constipation and diarrheal symptoms (IBS-M) or symptoms that do not fit into any of the other three categories (IBS-un-subtyped). Many IBS-M patients may report extended periods of constipation followed by multiple watery bowel movements only later to be diagnosed with IBS-C with progressive stool accumulation then resulting in eventual bowel purging. A stool diary in these cases can be particularly helpful to elucidate patterns within the chaotic bowel habits these patients may experience [13].

Sloane denies any nocturnal stools, weight loss, rectal bleeding, or family history of gastrointestinal issues. They state they were previously diagnosed with IBS-D. They are wondering if any additional testing should be done at this point.

Differential Diagnosis and Diagnostic Strategies

For patients who present to primary care with symptoms of abdominal pain, constipation, and/or diarrhea, a detailed history and physical exam play a key role in the diagnostic process; oftentimes, no further testing is needed to confidently make a diagnosis of IBS. The differential diagnosis and subsequent diagnostic strategies for IBS are largely dictated by the predominant symptom subtype; however, it is important to keep in mind that conditions can sometimes fall into more than one category. The presence of any alarm features in a patient's medical history including symptom onset after age

50, severe and progressive symptoms, unexplained weight loss, vomiting, nocturnal diarrhea, rectal bleeding, unexplained iron deficiency anemia, or family history of colon cancer, celiac disease, or inflammatory bowel disease indicate the need to exclude organic disease. For patients who fit the Rome IV criteria for IBS without any alarm features, guidelines recommend no further diagnostic workup as it is low yield and unlikely to uncover a new diagnosis [14–16]. However, even in the absence of alarm features, a limited evaluation may still be appropriate to exclude the presence of illnesses that may cause similar symptoms.

Diarrhea-Predominant Symptoms

Table 27.1 outlines the major categories to consider when evaluating a patient with IBS-D [17, 18]. Categorizing diarrhea as inflammatory, malabsorptive/fatty, or watery is a useful framework to navigate the lengthy differential diagnosis for chronic diarrhea and guide additional workup. The first step is to assess for features of inflammatory diarrhea, which include constitutional symptoms, fever, weight loss, and bloody diarrhea. Inflammatory bowel disease, invasive infections, and malignancy all fit into this category. Inflammatory

Table 27.1 Differential diagnosis of IBS-D [17, 18]

Differential diagnoses	Distinguishing features from IBS-D
1. Inflammatory diarrhea – characterized by constitutional symptoms (fever, weight loss) and bloody diarrhea	
Inflammatory bowel disease (IBD)	Family history of IBD Progressive symptoms Extraintestinal manifestations Nutritional deficiencies (iron, vitamin B12, folate, zinc, vitamin D) Elevated inflammatory markers (CRP, ESR) Elevated fecal calprotectin and lactoferrin
Invasive Infections (i.e., *Campylobacter*, *Salmonella*, *Shigella*, enterohemorrhagic *E. coli*)	Historical risk factors: immunocompromised state, travel, animal contact, contaminated food or water ingestion
Malignancy	Older age (but young age does not exclude!) Family history of cancer or familial cancer syndrome
2. Malabsorptive diarrhea – characterized by foul-smelling, fatty, floating, pale, large volume stools; weight loss, + fecal fat, and nutritional deficiencies (iron, vitamin B12, folate, zinc, vitamin D)	
Celiac disease	Dermatitis herpetiformis Responsive to gluten avoidance
Diet-induced	Diet history: symptoms exacerbated by consumption of lactose, high-fructose corn syrup, sugar alcohol additives – sorbitol, mannitol, and xylitol – which are frequently found in sugar-free products such as gum, candy, or soda
Chronic pancreatitis	Historical risk factors: alcohol use, history of recurrent acute pancreatitis
Bile acid malabsorption	Postcholecystectomy Responsive to bile acid sequestrants Difficult to test for outside of research settings; consider empiric treatment
Small bowel bacterial overgrowth (SIBO)	Historical risk factors: anatomic or functional abnormalities including strictures, surgically altered anatomy, motility disorders (DM, scleroderma), systemic disorders (immunocompromised state, chronic pancreatitis, cirrhosis, ESRD)
3. Watery diarrhea – characterized by frequent liquid stools, nocturnal stools, systemic symptoms depending on etiology	
Infectious (i.e., *C. difficile*, *Giardia*, enterotoxigenic *E. coli*, *Cryptosporidium*, *Listeria*, viral)	Historical risk factors: antibiotic use, daycare centers, immunocompromised state/HIV, extremes of age
Drug-induced	Common culprit medications: laxatives, proton pump inhibitors, antibiotics, nonsteroidal anti-inflammatory drugs (NSAIDs), antineoplastic agents, immunosuppression agents, metformin
Metabolic Hyperthyroidism Adrenal insufficiency Neuroendocrine tumors (VIPoma, carcinoid syndrome)	Systemic symptoms related to the metabolic abnormality (i.e., flushing, palpitations, weight loss)
Microscopic colitis	Middle-aged to older patients Can present with large stool volumes (up to 2 L/day) and nocturnal diarrhea May be associated with medication use (i.e., NSAIDs, SSRIs, PPIs)

bowel disease (IBD) may initially present with subtle symptoms such as IBS-D with more than a third of IBD patients also fulfilling Rome criteria for IBS [19]. However, patients with IBD usually experience symptom progression over time underscoring the importance of follow-up and reassessment. Fecal calprotectin is a noninvasive marker of intestinal inflammation that can be used to monitor disease activity in patients with IBD and help differentiate IBD from IBS-D. A complete blood count (CBC) and iron studies can be used to look for subacute blood loss from the GI tract commonly seen in IBD. Serum C-reactive protein (CRP) and erythrocyte sedimentation rate (ESR) should also be considered to evaluate for underlying inflammation; these markers are nonspecific but can indicate underlying inflammation that needs further attention. The probability of active IBD is <1% with fecal calprotectin levels <40 ug/g or with a CRP level <0.5 mg/L [20]. Patients with an invasive infection may have an exposure or travel history. To evaluate for infection, stool studies for bacterial culture, parasites, *Clostridium difficile*, leukocytes, and fecal lactoferrin should be sent. Patients with a strong family history of colon or rectal cancers or cancer syndromes who present with bloody diarrhea/stools should be evaluated early for malignancy regardless of age or accompanying symptoms.

Celiac disease, pancreatic insufficiency, diet-induced bile acid malabsorption, and small bowel bacterial overgrowth (SIBO) are the main causes of malabsorptive diarrhea. Malabsorptive diarrhea can present with foul-smelling "floating" or "greasy" stools, weight loss, and vitamin deficiencies. Checking a fecal fat can help identify malabsorptive diarrhea due to chronic pancreatitis. Celiac disease shares a significant overlap with IBS-D. A recent meta-analysis of 36 studies with 15,256 individuals found an increased likelihood of biopsy-proven celiac disease in patients with IBS with a pooled odds ratio of near 4.5 compared to non-IBS controls [21]. Given its prevalence, serum testing for tissue transglutaminase (tTG) antibodies and total IgA levels for celiac disease should be considered in all IBS-D patients. Total IgA deficiency may affect the validity of antibody testing as tTG antibodies are IgA antibodies. There may also be an overlap between IBS-D and bile acid diarrhea as a systematic review and meta-analysis found positive SeHCAT (23-seleno-25-homotaurocholic acid) testing, which measures radiolabeled bile acid retention, to be present in up to 25% of individuals with IBS-D [22]. Additional testing for lactose intolerance, pancreatic insufficiency, small bacterial overgrowth, tumor syndromes, and bile acid diarrhea is usually carried out after consultation with a gastroenterologist.

Patients presenting with frequent, watery diarrhea should be evaluated for noninvasive infectious causes, microscopic colitis, thyroid disease, endocrinopathies, metabolically active tumors, and medication side effects. A TSH and free T4 level can be checked to evaluate for thyroid disease; if adrenal insufficiency is entertained, the patient can undergo a cosyntropin (ACTH) stimulation test. Stool studies for bacterial culture, parasites, *C. difficile*, leukocytes, and fecal lactoferrin can be helpful if there is clinical suspicion for infectious diarrhea. Microscopic colitis might be considered in older patients with nocturnal stools and comorbid autoimmune disease [23]. Testing for metabolically active tumors such as a VIPoma or carcinoid tumor is most often done under the direction of a specialist. As always, a full medication reconciliation is key to determining any GI medication side effects.

In general, if there is any concern for an underlying IBD, microscopic colitis, or gastrointestinal malignancy, an immediate referral to a gastroenterologist for an endoscopy and/or colonoscopy should be placed as these diseases are most readily diagnosed under direct visualization and biopsy.

Constipation-Predominant Symptoms

The differential diagnosis for patients suffering from IBS-C differs from those who have primary diarrhea symptoms, but the diagnostic strategy is similar. Table 27.2 provides a

Table 27.2 Differential diagnosis of IBS-C [24, 25]

Differential diagnoses	Distinguishing features from IBS-C
1. Primary constipation (also known as chronic idiopathic constipation or functional constipation) – abdominal pain is NOT a prominent complaint	
Normal transit constipation	Regular bowel movements, but subjective complaints of hard stools, difficult evacuation
Slow transit constipation	Defecation may be dramatically infrequent (≤1 bowel movement (BM)/week) May be associated with a pelvic floor injury – childbirth, pelvic surgery
Rectal evacuation disorder Dyssynergic defecation Structural abnormality Functional defecation disorders	Straining even with soft stools, digital manipulation to pass BM
2. Secondary constipation	
Metabolic Hypothyroidism Diabetes mellitus Electrolyte imbalances	Associated signs/symptoms of hypothyroidism, diabetes mellitus Review basic screening lab work: TSH, BMP, Ca
Drug-induced	Common culprit medications: opioids, antihypertensives, antidepressants, antihistamines, and anticholinergics
Neurologic disorders Neuropathy Parkinson's disease Spinal cord injury Multiple sclerosis	Associated neurologic symptoms
Malignancy	Family history Weight loss Bloody stools Change in stool caliber related to structuring

framework of differential diagnoses and distinguishing features to consider in the evaluation of a patient with suspected IBS-C [24, 25]. Again, taking a detailed history assessing for any alarm features as well as performing an appropriate physical exam will help guide whether any additional workup is necessary.

Constipation may be a result of primary, or chronic idiopathic constipation, or secondary to metabolic, drug-induced, neurologic, or malignant etiologies. If a rectal evacuation disorder is suspected such as dyssynergic defecation, we suggest referral to a gastroenterologist for more specialized diagnostic testing. Checking a TSH, free T4, and electrolytes is reasonable to ensure there is not a secondary metabolic condition contributing to constipation. A full medication reconciliation should be performed looking for offending medications as constipation is a common, but often overlooked, side effect of many medications, including many over-the-counter preparations.

While colonic malignancy remains a common concern, meta-analyses of several cross-sectional studies and limited prospective studies have found no increased colon cancer risk in patients with typical IBS-C symptoms when compared to healthy controls [26]. Nevertheless, all patients should be up-to-date with age-appropriate colorectal cancer screening.

You order bloodwork and a stool sample given Sloane's report of slightly worsening diarrhea. CBC, CRP, thyroid testing, and fecal parasite testing all return within normal limits. You call Sloane on the phone to update them about the results. Sloane is relieved to hear that their tests were normal. They would like to avoid taking a medication if possible and asks what you would recommend.

Treatment Strategies

General Considerations

IBS patients frequently report dissatisfaction with their healthcare, particularly in relation to a delay in diagnosis, inadequate education, being perceived by physicians as problematic patients, and a lack of validation of their symptoms or suffering. A positive patient-physician relationship improves both IBS symptoms as well as patient satisfaction [27–29]. Establishing a firm, prompt diagnosis of IBS and educating the patient regarding etiology, diagnosis, and prognosis is an important first step in establishing a working relationship [30–33]. Providers should be aware of patients' potentially prior negative interactions with the healthcare system, validate their symptoms, and display active listening skills and empathy [28, 29]. It is important to set realistic patient expectations and treatment goals, specifically that IBS is not curable, but rather a chronic condition that can be well managed through individualized lifestyle modifications and, at times, medication. Patients should be made aware that although IBS may have a negative impact on their quality of life, this illness is not life-threatening and will not transform into a malignant condition. Continued reassurance provides positive reframing for patients to help patients cope with their symptoms.

There are several nonpharmacological and pharmacological therapies available for IBS. Treatment recommendations should be based on IBS subtype, comorbid conditions, patient preference, and provider expertise/comfort. Given the heterogeneity of IBS, it is important to tailor therapy recommendations to each individual patient through shared decision-making.

Nonpharmacological Interventions

Diet and Exercise

In patients with IBS, true food allergies are rare; however, many patients, regardless of subtype, have food sensitivities or intolerances and benefit from dietary modification. Some patients may independently identify food intolerances. Patients should be asked about dietary triggers and any dietary modifications they have already instituted. For others, maintaining a food/symptom diary can help identify intolerances. Traditional dietary advice includes increasing dietary fiber, taking probiotics, as well as limiting caffeine, alcohol, spicy foods, fatty foods, carbonated drinks, chewing gum, and artificial sweeteners. Fiber can provide relief of diarrhea but is most effective at treating constipation. Soluble (psyllium) fiber should be recommended as insoluble (bran) fiber may exacerbate bloating and gas [34]. A meta-analysis suggests probiotics are beneficial in the treatment of IBS; however, study heterogeneity makes it difficult to give a specific recommendation regarding preparations, species, or strains [35]. Although traditional dietary advice does provide symptom improvement, specialized diets, such as a diet low in FODMAPs, appear to be more effective at reducing gastrointestinal symptoms [36].

Systematic reviews and meta-analyses demonstrate a low-FODMAP diet is effective in reducing gastrointestinal symptoms in most patients with IBS [36, 37]. FODMAPs exacerbate IBS symptoms as they are poorly absorbed by the gastrointestinal tract leading to increased luminal water content, increased fermentation by gut bacteria, and excess gas production. Examples of foods high in FODMAPs can be seen in Table 27.3. A low-FODMAP diet should be initiated with the help of an experienced dietician. Initially, patients are instructed to eliminate all foods high in FODMAPs.

Table 27.3 Examples of high-FODMAP foods versus low-FODMAP foods [35–42]

	High-FODMAP foods	Low-FODMAP foods
Fruits	Avocados, apples, apricots, dates, cherries, figs, mango, pears, peaches, plums, watermelon	Bananas, blueberries, cantaloupe, grapefruit, grapes, kiwi, lemon, lime, mandarin, oranges, passion fruit, pineapple, tangerine
Vegetables	Artichokes, asparagus, beets, broccoli, cabbage, cauliflower, mushrooms, okra, onions, peas	Bell peppers, carrots, corn, cucumbers, eggplant, lettuce, leafy greens, potatoes, pumpkin, tomatoes, zucchini
Grains	Wheat/rye/barley-based breads, cereal, pasta, crackers, cookies	Gluten-free or spelt products, oats, quinoas
Protein	Cashews, legumes, baked beans, kidney beans, lentils	Almonds, eggs, tofu, plain cooked meats, and seafood
Dairy	Cow's milk, soft cheese, margarine	Lactose-free products, hard cheeses
Sweeteners	Honey, high-fructose corn syrup, sorbitol	Maple syrup, table sugar (sucrose), dark chocolate

Symptom improvement is generally seen around 3–4 weeks, although individual response times may be variable. After 4–6 weeks, the patient can reintroduce one high-FODMAP subgroup at a time while monitoring symptoms. Most patients will be able to tolerate some high-FODMAP subgroups and can follow a modified low-FODMAP diet based on individual tolerances. The rechallenge phase and relaxation of dietary restrictions are important as there are concerns about the long-term impact of a low-FODMAP diet on the gut microbiome, nutritional adequacy, and patient compliance [38, 39].

Several randomized double-blind placebo-controlled trials implicate wheat in exacerbating IBS symptoms. Most patients with IBS, even without evidence of celiac disease, experience improvement in gastrointestinal symptoms while on a gluten-free diet [40]. Wheat contains both gluten and high levels of fructans raising the possibility that the improvement achieved on a gluten-free diet may be due to the elimination of high-FODMAP foods rather than the elimination of gluten itself [41]. There is currently stronger evidence to support the efficacy of a low-FODMAP diet; however, a gluten-free diet is also a reasonable recommendation and may be easier for some patients to follow given the availability of products and the clear packaging of gluten-free foods [40, 42]. Moreover, patients should be instructed to avoid gas-producing foods, and in some, avoidance of lactose-rich foods may be needed.

In addition to dietary modifications, exercise is another component of lifestyle modification for patients with IBS. There is limited data that low- to moderate-intensity exercise can be beneficial for IBS symptoms [43–45].

Psychological and Alternative/Complementary Therapies

Underlying gut-brain axis dysfunction can respond to psychological and alternative/complementary therapies. Cognitive behavioral therapy (CBT), hypnotherapy, interpersonal therapy, multicomponent therapy, and dynamic psychotherapy all appear to be effective treatments for IBS [34, 46]. The strongest evidence exists for CBT, and a meta-analysis demonstrated a number needed to treat (NNT) of three [34, 46]. CBT is a highly structured psychotherapy that focuses on identifying and correcting maladaptive information processes and behavioral response patterns. Despite positive treatment outcomes with CBT, access to a psychologist may be difficult or limited for many patients. Thus, researchers are currently investigating the efficacy of psychological care delivered through minimal-contact methods utilizing technology (internet, phones, smartphone apps) and self-help strategies [47].

Two systematic reviews found that CBT-based minimal-contact treatment strategies significantly reduce IBS symptoms as compared to usual care, waitlists, online discussion forums, and symptom monitoring [48, 49]. It is unclear, however, how CBT-based minimal-contact treatment strategies compare to traditional CBT. Data remain limited with regard to relaxation therapy, stress management, and mindfulness training [34, 46]. Chinese herbs and other homeopathic regimens are frequently advertised as treatment for IBS; however, they have not been rigorously studied and cannot yet be recommended as effective treatments for IBS. In several randomized controlled trials, acupuncture compared to sham acupuncture did not improve IBS symptoms [50–52].

In summary, we first recommend nonpharmacological interventions including dietary modification, particularly a low-FODMAP diet, exercise, and, if appropriate, psychological therapy, as first-line treatment to all patients with IBS (Table 27.4). Most patients will achieve satisfactory and adequate relief of symptoms with the nonpharmacological interventions provided.

Sloane decides to try a low-FODMAP diet and start exercising regularly. They return to your office in 3 months and state that these interventions have not helped with symptoms. Sloane is ready to try a medication as they are tired of dealing with frequent diarrhea. At this appointment, Sloane also discloses that they have been struggling with mood symptoms over the past 6 months. They report low energy, difficulty concentrating at work, and difficulty falling asleep.

Table 27.4 Stepwise approach to treatment of IBS [13, 16, 34, 46]

<table>
<tr><td colspan="5">Nonpharmacological Interventions
• Establish a trusting patient-physician relationship
• Set realistic patient expectations and treatment goals
• Dietary Modification(Low FODMAP Diet)
• Exercise
• Psychological (Cognitive Behavioral Therapy)</td></tr>
<tr><td colspan="5">Pharmacological Management</td></tr>
<tr><td></td><td>IBS-C</td><td>IBS-D</td><td></td><td>Pain</td></tr>
<tr><td>Medications that improve stool frequency/ consistency</td><td>Polyethylene Glycol
17gm daily - TID</td><td>Loperamide
Initial: 4 mg, followed by 2 mg after each loose stool; Maintenance 4 to 8 mg/day single dose or divided doses; max 16 mg/day</td><td rowspan="3">+</td><td rowspan="3">• Hyoscyamine 0.125-0.25 mg q4 hrs PRN; max: 1.5 mg/day
• Dicyclomine 20 mg QID x 7 days; then ↑ to 40 mg QID
• Peppermint Oil 187-225 mgTID
<u>TCAs</u>
• Amitriptyline 10-25 mg QPM; may ↑ up to 75 mg
• Nortriptyline 10 mg daily
<u>SSRIs</u>
• Citalopram 40 mg daily
• Fluoxetine 20 mg daily
• Paroxetine 40 mg daily</td></tr>
<tr><td rowspan="2">FDA approved medications that improve global IBS symptoms</td><td>Lubiprostone*
8 mcg BID
Linaclotide*
290 mcg daily</td><td>Rifaximine*
550 mg TID × 14 days; may be retreated 2 times with the same dosing regimen</td></tr>
<tr><td></td><td>Eluxadoline*
75-100mg BID</td></tr>
</table>

*FDA approved for females 18 years or older; Pharmacological management: green = first-line; yellow = second-line; purple = third-line

Pharmacological Interventions

Pharmacological management should be based on the subtype of IBS and the presence of other prominent symptoms such as pain, gas, and bloating, as well as comorbid conditions.

IBS-C

Along with nonpharmacological therapies, we recommend a trial of polyethylene glycol as first-line treatment for IBS-C given its availability and excellent safety profile. Polyethylene glycol 3350, an osmotic laxative, is frequently used to treat constipation. Two small randomized controlled trials in IBS-C patients found that polyethylene glycol improved stool consistency and the number of spontaneous bowel movements per week as compared to placebo; however, these studies failed to show improvement in abdominal discomfort and pain symptoms in the polyethylene glycol arm, and the sample sizes were not clearly adequate [53, 54]. Polyethylene glycol is readily available over the counter, can be easily titrated based on the patient's symptoms, and is generally well-tolerated. There is minimal systemic absorption, and the most frequent side effects associated with its use include abdominal discomfort, bloating, nausea, and diarrhea. The role of polyethylene glycol in the treatment of IBS-C has been questioned by some; however, there is a paucity of evidence that recommends against its use [55]. Other laxatives, especially bowel stimulants, should be avoided as these will likely exacerbate abdominal pain and have a higher risk of leading to dependence.

We recommend intestinal secretagogues as second-line treatment for patients with IBS-C who have failed lifestyle interventions and polyethylene glycol. Intestinal secretagogues, lubiprostone and linaclotide, are FDA approved for the treatment of IBS-C. Both lubiprostone and linaclotide stimulate receptors in the intestinal mucosa that lead to an influx of water into the gut lumen promoting transit. Several randomized clinical trials demonstrate that both drugs significantly improve IBS symptoms compared to placebo with an NNT of 12.5 and 6, respectively [34]. Many of the primary end points of the clinical trials reflect partial improvement in overall IBS symptoms rather than complete resolution of symptoms, so it is important to counsel patients that these medications will not "cure" IBS, but rather mitigate the symptoms. In addition, it is essential to counsel patients about potential side effects related to the use of these secretagogues including nausea and diarrhea. Approximately twice as many patients taking lubiprostone report nausea when compared to placebo [56, 57]. Diarrhea is common with both lubiprostone and linaclotide with a number needed to harm (NNH) of 10 and 6, respectively [34]. Apart from the abovementioned side effects, lubiprostone and linaclotide are generally well-tolerated and have a favorable safety profile; the occurrence of serious adverse events are rare [56–59].

IBS-D

Along with nonpharmacological therapies, we recommend a trial of loperamide as first-line treatment for IBS-D. A trial of ondansetron and a trial of bile acid sequestrants are also reasonable alternatives for symptom control in patients with IBS-D. Medications such as ondansetron (a selective 5-HT3 receptor antagonist), loperamide (a gut-directed opioid-receptor agonist), and bile acid sequestrants are frequently recommended for IBS-D given their antidiarrheal properties, availability, and tolerability; however, the evidence base supporting their use in IBS-D is weak. One randomized controlled trial demonstrated that ondansetron as compared to placebo improves stool frequency and consistency, but does not improve pain scores [60]. Two small randomized controlled trials (n = 20 and n = 90) and one prospective trial examining loperamide compared to placebo found improvement in stool frequency and consistency with mixed effects on pain scores [61–63]. The data is not overwhelming, but loperamide is a reasonable first-line option. Bile acid sequestrants may be beneficial in IBS-D as there appears to be an overlap between IBS-D and bile acid malabsorption; however, formal evidence supporting the uses of bile acid sequestrants in the treatment of IBS-D is currently limited [64].

We recommend rifaximin as second-line therapy in patients with IBS-D who fail nonpharmacological therapy and a trial of symptomatic management with loperamide. There are two FDA-approved treatments for IBS-D: rifaximin, a gut-specific minimally absorbed antibiotic, and eluxadoline, a mixed μ-opioid receptor agonist and δ-receptor antagonist. Rifaximin is FDA-approved as a 14-day treatment course. Presumably, rifaximin alters the gut microbiome to decrease the symptoms of IBS. Compared to placebo, rifaximin provides significant relief of global IBS symptoms; however, approximately two-thirds of patients experience a relapse of symptoms after drug discontinuation [65–67]. Retreatment with another course of rifaximin appears to be both safe and effective, and the FDA has approved up to two repeat courses of rifaximin [67].

We reserve eluxadoline as a third-line agent given the safety concerns. Eluxadoline is an opioid receptor agonist; it acts to decrease intestinal motility and the visceral pain response. Compared to placebo, it is also effective at improving global IBS symptoms; however, sphincter of Oddi dysfunction and pancreatitis can rarely occur (0.5% and 0.4%, respectively) with the use of this drug and have resulted in hospitalization in some patients, specifically those with prior cholecystectomy [68, 69]. Eluxadoline is currently contraindicated in patients with prior cholecystectomy, those with other structural biliary or pancreatic disease, and those with heavy alcohol use.

Pain

In addition to considering subtype-specific therapies, there are several medications that target abdominal pain associated with IBS. Selection of an appropriate agent should be made by considering patient comorbidities and individual patient preferences and by engaging the patient in shared decision-making.

Antispasmodics, peppermint oil, and antidepressants including tricyclic antidepressants (TCAs) and selective serotonin reuptake inhibitor (SSRIs) are effective at reducing both pain and overall IBS symptoms compared to placebo A meta-analysis found that antispasmodics, as a class, are effective at improving IBS symptoms when compared to placebo [33]. However, there was significant heterogeneity among the studies regarding individual antispasmodics. Of all the drugs evaluated, hyoscyamine and dicyclomine are the only agents available in the United States. This meta-analysis included three trials evaluating hyoscyamine with an NNT of 3, while only one trial evaluated dicyclomine with an NNT of 4. Unfortunately, antispasmodics as compared to placebo also have a higher rate of adverse events. There were no serious adverse events; however, anticholinergic side effects including dry mouth, dizziness, and blurred vision were frequent with the use of antispasmodics [34].

Peppermint oil is an attractive alternative to antispasmodics for treating the pain associated with IBS as it is effective (NNT = 3) and has minimal side effects. Heartburn is the most common side effect reported; however, sustained released preparations and enteric-coated preparations of peppermint oil may reduce the frequency of heartburn [34, 70, 71]. In patients with comorbid anxiety or depression, the use of either TCAs or SSRIs may improve both IBS symptoms and mood symptoms. A meta-analysis demonstrated that TCAs and SSRIs are effective at reducing abdominal pain and overall IBS symptoms as compared to placebo, but these medications were more likely to produce adverse events, particularly dry mouth and drowsiness with the use of TCAs [34, 46]. Some gastroenterologists suggest preferentially starting TCAs for IBS-D and SSRIs for IBS-C because constipation and diarrhea are respective class side effects; however, this is not supported by the IBS-specific literature [13]. Serotonin norepinephrine reuptake inhibitors (SNRIs) have a place in some chronic pain conditions but have not been thoroughly studied in patients with IBS.

When to Refer

IBS tends to be a chronic illness, and patients should be educated that there will be periods of time with varying control of symptoms. Most patients treated with the nonpharmacological and pharmacological strategies tend to do well and are happy with their symptom control, but for those who fail to improve despite adherence to diet and medications, referral to a specialist should be considered. Specialists may try different treatment options and often conduct a more extensive evaluation including endoscopy, cross-sectional imaging, and/or more comprehensive laboratory blood testing to exclude other organic diagnoses. In tertiary care centers, IBS patients are often seen in conjunction with a dietician and if need be a psychotherapist. Patients who remain refractory to the treatments prescribed by their primary care physician and the gastroenterologist often benefit from referral to a psychiatrist.

Summary Points

1. IBS is a common clinical condition characterized by abdominal pain associated with altered bowel habits. IBS has four clinical subtypes: IBS-D, IBS-C, IBS-M, and IBS un-subtyped or unclassified. The pathophysiology of IBS is likely multifactorial and is an area of ongoing research.
2. In patients presenting with typical IBS symptoms, no alarm features, and a normal physical exam other than abdominal tenderness, Rome IV criteria can be used to diagnose IBS without additional diagnostic testing.
3. The need for additional diagnostic testing should be tailored to the individual patient based on patient characteristics, IBS subtype, and physician discretion. Red flag symptoms should prompt further evaluation for systemic disease.
4. A stepwise approach is recommended for the treatment of IBS. First-line therapies include nonpharmacological therapies and agents aimed at symptom management such as polyethylene glycol 3350 for IBS-C and loperamide for IBS-D. Several other pharmacological agents are available for second-line therapy including linaclotide or lubiprostone for IBS-C and rifaximin for IBS-D. Antispasmodics, antidepressants, and peppermint oil are helpful in mitigating pain associated with IBS. Patients with refractory IBS or those who develop alarm features should be referred to gastroenterology for additional evaluation.
5. Interdisciplinary support including a dietician and mental health provider should be considered in the management of patients with IBS.

You recommend a trial of a tricyclic antidepressant and close follow-up. Sloane reports an improvement in both their mood and gastrointestinal symptoms at their 6-week follow-up appointment. You recommend continuing the medication for the next several months. Sloane asks you, however, if irritable bowel syndrome can be cured by the medication.

Review Questions

1. A 25-year-old female presents to your clinic with complaints of intermittent abdominal pain associated with diarrhea for the past 6 months. She states she has abdominal pain and loose stools multiple times a day about twice a week. She denies any GI bleeding, nocturnal symptoms, weight loss, or family history of inflammatory bowel disease but notes that her symptoms seem to be worse during times of increased stress. On physical exam, she is afebrile, HR: 70 beats/min, BP: 110/65 mmHg. Abdominal exam reveals normoactive bowel sounds, diffuse mild tenderness, no rebound or guarding, and no masses. Which of the following is the next best diagnostic step?
   A. Colonoscopy
   B. Fecal leukocytes
   C. CT abdomen and pelvis
   D. Apply Rome IV criteria
   E. Watchful waiting

   The correct answer is D. This patient displays no "red flag" features that would indicate underlying GI tract or systemic pathology. The Rome IV criteria can be applied to this patient to facilitate a clinical diagnosis without additional diagnostics as she is presenting with complaints consistent with irritable bowel syndrome without alarm features [16]. Early diagnosis helps accelerate a treatment plan and increases patient satisfaction. Should this patient not respond to first-line treatment or her symptoms progress, additional workup should be pursued.

2. A 51-year-old Caucasian female presents to the clinic to establish care. She reports intermittent abdominal pain and bloating associated with diarrhea. The symptoms have been present for several years, and she denies rectal bleeding, weight loss, and nocturnal symptoms. On average, the symptoms occur once a week. She has a copy of prior medical evaluations which reveal normal thyroid function tests, normal IgA levels, negative celiac disease panel, and normal fecal calprotectin level. She has never had a colonoscopy. She uses loperamide as needed, and this adequately controls her symptoms. Which of the following is the next best step?
   A. No further testing is required.
   B. C-reactive protein.
   C. Colonoscopy.
   D. Fecal elastase.
   E. Stool ova and parasite.

   The correct answer is C. All patients with IBS should undergo age-appropriate colorectal cancer screening. In this Caucasian female with no family history of colon cancer, screening for colon cancer should start at 50 years of age [72].

3. A 45-year-old female with depression and constipation-predominant irritable bowel syndrome returns to your clinic for follow-up. She reports exercising regularly and staying hydrated. Her depression is well controlled with sertraline and cognitive behavior therapy. She has previously tried taking polyethylene glycol twice a day to help with her constipation without significant relief. Most recently, she tried linaclotide for 6 weeks, again, without relief of her symptoms. What is the next best step in management?
   A. Referral to gastroenterology
   B. Switch linaclotide to lubiprostone
   C. Start a gluten-free diet
   D. Start senna

   The correct answer is A. Patients who fail nonpharmacological and pharmacological management should be referred to gastroenterology for further evaluation including other possible etiologies of constipation and/or additional management considerations [24, 25].

References

1. Lovell RM, Ford AC. Global prevalence of and risk factors for irritable bowel syndrome: a meta-analysis. Clin Gastroenterol Hepatol. 2012;10(7):712–721.e4.
2. Lovell RM, Ford AC. Effect of gender on prevalence of irritable bowel syndrome in the community: systemic review and meta-analysis. Am J Gastroenterol. 2012;107(7):991–1000.
3. Everhart JE, Ruhl CE. Burden of digestive diseases in the United States, part II: lower gastrointestinal diseases. Gastroenterology. 2009;136(3):741–54.
4. Agarwal N, Spiegel BM. The effect of irritable bowel syndrome on health-related quality of life and health care expenditures. Gastroentol Clin North Am. 2011;40(1):11–9.
5. Dunlop SP, Coleman NS, Blackshaw E, et al. Abnormalities of 5-hydroxytryptamine metabolism in irritable bowel syndrome. Clin Gastroenterol Hepatol. 2005;3:349–57.
6. Thijssen AY, Mujagic Z, Jonkers DM, et al. Alterations in serotonin metabolism in the irritable bowel syndrome. Aliment Pharmacol Ther. 2016;43:272–82.
7. Wouters MM, Van Wanrooy S, Nguyen A, et al. Psychological comorbidity increases the risk of postinfectious IBS partly by enhanced susceptibility to develop infectious gastroenteritis. Gut. 2016;65:1279–88.
8. Liebregts T, Adam B, Bredack C, et al. Immune activation in patients with irritable bowel syndrome. Gastroenterology. 2007;132:913–20.
9. Zhen Y, Chu C, Zhou S, Qi M, Shu R. Imbalance of tumor necrosis factor-α, interleukin-8 and interleukin-10 production evokes barrier dysfunction, severe abdominal symptoms and psychological disorders in patients with irritable bowel syndrome-associated diarrhea. Mol Med Rep. 2015;12:5239–45.
10. Shepherd SJ, Parker FC, Muir JG, Gibson PR. Dietary triggers of abdominal symptoms in patients with irritable bowel syndrome: randomized placebo-controlled evidence. Clin Gastroenterol Hepatol. 2008;6:765–71.
11. Murray K, Wilkinson-Smith V, Hoad C, et al. Differential effects of FODMAPs (fermentable oligo-, di-, mono-saccharides and polyols) on small and large intestinal contents in healthy subjects shown by MRI. Am J Gastroenterol. 2014;109:110–9.
12. Drossman DA, Hasler WL. Rome IV-functional GI disorders: disorders of gut-brain interaction. Gastroenterology. 2016;150:1257–61.
13. Chey WD, Kurlander J, Eswaran S. Irritable bowel syndrome: a clinical review. JAMA. 2015;313(9):949–58.
14. Longstreth GF, Thompson WG, Chey WD, Houghton LA, Mearin F, Spiller RC. Functional bowel disorders. Gastroenterology. 2006;130(5):1480–91.
15. Spiegel BM, Farid M, Esrailian E, Talley J, Chang L. Is irritable bowel syndrome a diagnosis of exclusion? A survey of primary care providers, gastroenterologists, and IBS experts. Am J Gastroenterol. 2010;105:848–58.
16. Ford AC, Lacy BE, Talley NJ. Irritable bowel syndrome. NEJM. 2017;376:2566–78.
17. Juckett G, Trivedi R. Evaluation of chronic diarrhea. Am Fam Physician. 2011;84(10):1119–26.
18. Camilleri M, Sellin JH, Barrett KE. Pathophysiology, evaluation, and management of chronic watery diarrhea. Gastroenterology. 2017;152(3):515–35.
19. Halpin SJ, Ford AC. Prevalence of symptoms meeting criteria for irritable bowel syndrome in inflammatory bowel disease: systematic review and meta-analysis. Am J Gastroenterol. 2012;107(10):1474–82.
20. Menees SB, Powell C, Kurlander J, Goel A, Chey WD. A meta-analysis of the utility of C-reactive protein, erythrocyte sedimentation rate, fecal calprotectin, and fecal lactoferrin to exclude inflammatory bowel disease in adults with IBS. Am J Gastroenterol. 2015;110(3):444–54.
21. Irvine AJ, Chey WD, Ford AC. Screening for celiac disease in irritable bowel syndrome: an updated systematic review and meta-analysis. Am J Gastroenterol. 2017;112:65–76.
22. Slattery SA, Niaz O, Aziz Q, Ford AC, Farmer AD. Systematic review with meta-analysis: the prevalence of bile acid malabsorption in the irritable bowel syndrome with diarrhoea. Aliment Pharmacol Ther. 2015;42:3–11.

23. Macaigne G, Lahmek P, Locher C, et al. Microscopic colitis or functional bowel disease with diarrhea: a French prospective multicenter study. Am J Gastroenterol. 2014;109(9):1461–70.
24. Sbahi H, Cash BD. Chronic constipation: a review of current literature. Curr Gastroenterol Rep. 2015;17:47.
25. Rao SSC, Rattanakovit K, Patcharatrakul T. Diagnosis and management of chronic constipation in adults. Nat Rev Gastroenterol Hepatol. 2016;13:295–305.
26. Canavan C, Card T, West J. The incidence of other gastroenterological disease following diagnosis of irritable bowel syndrome in the UK: a cohort study. PLoS One. 2014;9:e106478.
27. Ringstrom G, Sjovall H, Simrén M, Ung EJ. The importance of a person-centered approach in diagnostic workups of patients with irritable bowel syndrome: a qualitative study. Gastroenterol Nurs. 2013;36(6):443–51.
28. Dhaliwal SK, Hunt RH. Doctor-patient interaction for irritable bowel syndrome in primary care: a systematic perspective. Eur J Gastroenterol Hepatol. 2004;16(11):1161–6.
29. Kaptchuk TJ, Kelley JM, Conboy LA, Davis RB, Kerr CE, Jacobson EE, et al. Components of placebo effect: randomised controlled trial in patients with irritable bowel syndrome. BMJ. 2008;336(7651):999–1003.
30. Ringström G, Störsrud S, Simrén M. A comparison of a short nurse-based and a long multidisciplinary version of structured patient education in irritable bowel syndrome. Eur J Gastroenterol Hepatol. 2012;24(8):950–7.
31. Ringström G, Störsrud S, Posserud I, Lundqvist S, Westman B, Simrén M. Structured patient education is superior to written information in the management of patients with irritable bowel syndrome: a randomized controlled study. Eur J Gastroenterol Hepatol. 2010;22(4):420–8.
32. Ringström G, Störsrud S, Lundqvist S, Westman B, Simrén M. Development of an educational intervention for patients with Irritable Bowel Syndrome (IBS): a pilot study. BMC Gastroenterol. 2009;9:10.
33. Schmulson MJ, Ortiz-Garrido OM, Hinojosa C, Arcila D. A single session of reassurance can acutely improve the self-perception of impairment in patients with IBS. J Psychosom Res. 2006;61(4):461–7.
34. Ford AC, Moayyedi P, Lacy BE, Lembo AJ, Saito YA, Schiller LR, et al. American College of Gastroenterology monograph on the management of irritable bowel syndrome and chronic idiopathic constipation. Am J Gastroenterol. 2014;109(Suppl 1):S2–S26.
35. Zahedi MJ, Behrouz V, Azimi M. Low FODMAPs diet vs. general dietary advice improves clinical response in patients with diarrhea-predominant irritable bowel syndrome: a randomized controlled trial. Gastroenterol Hepatol. Epub 2017;33(6):1192–9.
36. Marsh A, Eslick EM, Eslick GD. Does a diet low in FODMAPs reduce symptoms associated with functional gastrointestinal disorders? A comprehensive systematic review and meta-analysis. Eur J Nutr. 2016;55(3):897–906.
37. Rao SS, Yu S, Fedewa A. Systematic review: dietary fibre and FODMAP-restricted diet in the management of constipation and irritable bowel syndrome. Aliment Pharmacol Ther. 2015;41(12):1256–70.
38. Tuck C, Barrett J. Re-challenging FODMAPs: the low FODMAP diet phase two. J Gastroenterol Hepatol. 2017;32(Suppl 1):11–5.
39. Barrett JS. How to institute the low-FODMAP diet. J Gastroenterol Hepatol. 2017;32(Suppl 1):8–10.
40. De Giorgio R, Volta U, Gibson PR. Sensitivity to wheat, gluten and FODMAPs in IBS: facts or fiction? Gut. 2016;65(1):169–78.
41. Biesiekierski JR, Peters SL, Newnham ED, Rosella O, Muir JG, Gibson PR. No effects of gluten in patients with self-reported non-celiac gluten sensitivity after dietary reduction of fermentable, poorly absorbed, short-chain carbohydrates. Gastroenterology. 2013;145(2):320–8.
42. Shah SL, Lacy BE. Dietary interventions and irritable bowel syndrome: a review of the evidence. Curr Gastroenterol Rep. 2016;18(8):41.
43. Johannesson E, Ringström G, Abrahamsson H, Sadik R. Intervention to increase physical activity in irritable bowel syndrome shows long-term positive effects. World J Gastroenterol. 2015;21(2):600–8.
44. Johannesson E, Simrén M, Strid H, Bajor A, Sadik R. Physical activity improves symptoms in irritable bowel syndrome: a randomized controlled trial. Am J Gastroenterol. 2011;106(5):915–22.
45. Hajizadeh MB, Tartibian B, Mooren FC, FitzGerald LZ, Krüger K, Chehrazi M, et al. Low-to-moderate intensity aerobic exercise training modulates irritable bowel syndrome through antioxidative and inflammatory mechanisms in women: results of a randomized controlled trial. Cytokine. 2017;102:18–25.
46. Ford AC, Lacy BE, Harris LA, Quigley EMM, Moayyedi P. Effect of antidepressants and psychological therapies in irritable bowel syndrome: an updated systematic review and meta-analysis. Am J Gastroenterol. 2019;114:21–39.
47. Radziwon CD, Lackner JM. Cognitive behavioural therapy for IBS: how useful, how often and how does it work? Curr Gastroenterol Rep. 2017;19:49.
48. Pajak R, Lackner J, Kamboj SK. A systematic review of minimal-contact psychological treatments for symptom management in irritable bowel syndrome. J Psychosom Res. 2013;75(2):103–12.
49. Ahl A, Mikocka-Walus A, Gordon A, Andrews JM. Are self-administered or minimal therapist contact psychotherapies an effective treatment for irritable bowel syndrome (IBS): a systematic review. J Psychosom Res. 2013 Aug;75(2):113–20.
50. Liu JP, Yang M, Liu Y, Wei ML, Grimsgaard S. Herbal medicines for treatment of irritable bowel syndrome. Cochrane Database Syst Rev. 2006;(1):Art. No.: CD004116.
51. Peckham EJ, Nelson E, Greenhalgh J, Cooper K, Roberts E, Agrawal A. Homeopathy for treatment of irritable bowel syndrome. Cochrane Database Syst Rev. 2013;(11):Art. No.: CD009710.
52. Manheimer E, Cheng K, Wieland LS, Min LS, Shen X, Berman BM, Lao L. Acupuncture for treatment of irritable bowel syndrome. Cochrane Database Syst Rev. 2012;(5):Art. No.: CD005111.
53. Chapman RW, Stanghellini V, Geraint M, Halphen M. Randomized clinical trial: macrogol/PEG 3350 plus electrolytes for treatment of patients with constipation associated with irritable bowel syndrome. Am J Gastroenterol. 2013;108(9):1508–15.
54. Awad RA, Camacho S. A randomized, double-blind, placebo-controlled trial of polyethylene glycol effects on fasting and postprandial rectal sensitivity and symptoms in hypersensitive constipation-predominant irritable bowel syndrome. Color Dis. 2010;12(11):1131–8.
55. Shearer J, Ford AC. Polyethylene glycol in constipation-predominant irritable bowel syndrome. Am J Gastroenterol. 2014;109(1):135.
56. Drossman DA, Chey WD, Johanson JF, Fass R, Scott C, Panas R, et al. Clinical trial: lubiprostone in patients with constipation-associated irritable bowel syndrome – results of two randomized, placebo-controlled studies. Aliment Pharmacol Ther. 2009;29(3):329–41.
57. Johanson JF, Drossman DA, Panas R, Wahle A, Ueno R. Clinical trial: phase 2 study of lubiprostone for irritable bowel syndrome with constipation. Aliment Pharmacol Ther. 2008;27(8):685–96.
58. Yang Y, Fang J, Guo X, Dai N, Shen X, Yang Y, et al. Linaclotide in irritable bowel syndrome with constipation: a phase 3 randomized trial in China and other regions. J Gastroenterol Hepatol. Epub 2018;33(5):980–9.
59. Atluri DK, Chandar AK, Bharucha AE, Falck-Ytter Y. Effect of linaclotide in irritable bowel syndrome with constipation (IBS-C):

a systematic review and meta-analysis. Neurogastroenterol Motil. 2014;26(4):499–509.
60. Garsed K, Chernova J, Hastings M, Lam C, Marciani L, Singh G, et al. A randomised trial of ondansetron for the treatment of irritable bowel syndrome with diarrhoea. Gut. 2014;63(10):1617–25.
61. Lavö B, Stenstam M, Nielsen AL. Loperamide in treatment of irritable bowel syndrome--a double-blind placebo controlled study. Scand J Gastroenterol Suppl. 1987;130:77–80.
62. Hovdenak N. Loperamide treatment of the irritable bowel syndrome. Scand J Gastroenterol Suppl. 1987;130:81–4.
63. Efskind PS, Bernklev T, Vatn MH. A double-blind placebo-controlled trial with loperamide in irritable bowel syndrome. Scand J Gastroenterol. 1996;31(5):463–8.
64. Camilleri M, Acosta A, Busciglio I, Boldingh A, Dyer RB, Zinsmeister AR, et al. Effect of colesevelam on faecal bile acids and bowel functions in diarrhoea-predominant irritable bowel syndrome. Aliment Pharmacol Ther. 2015;41(5):438–48.
65. Pimentel M, Lembo A, Chey WD, Zakko S, Ringel Y, Yu J, et al. Rifaximin therapy for patients with irritable bowel syndrome without constipation. N Engl J Med. 2011;364:22–32.
66. Li J, Zhu W, Liu W, Wu Y, Wu B. Rifaximin for irritable bowel syndrome: a meta-analysis of randomized placebo-controlled trials. Medicine. 2016;95(4):e2534.
67. Lembo A, Pimentel M, Rao SS, Schoenfeld P, Cash B, Weinstock LB, et al. Repeat treatment with rifaximin is safe and effective in patients with diarrhea-predominant irritable bowel syndrome. Gastroenterology. 2016;151(6):1113–21.
68. Lembo AJ, Lacy BE, Zuckerman MJ, Schey R, Dove LS, Andrae DA, et al. Eluxadoline for irritable bowel syndrome with diarrhea. N Engl J Med. 2016;374(3):242–53.
69. Cash BD, Lacy BE, Schoenfeld PS, Dove LS, Covington PS. Safety of Eluxadoline in patients with irritable bowel syndrome with diarrhea. Am J Gastroenterol. 2017;112(2):365–74.
70. Khanna R, MacDonald JK, Levesque BG. Peppermint oil for the treatment of irritable bowel syndrome: a systematic review and meta-analysis. J Clin Gastroenterol. 2014;48(6):505–12.
71. Cash BD, Epstein MS, Shah SM. A novel delivery system of peppermint oil is an effective therapy for irritable bowel syndrome symptoms. Dig Dis Sci. 2016;61(2):560–71.
72. Rex DK, Boland CR, Dominitz JA, Giardiello FM, Johnson DA, Kaltenbach T, et al. Colorectal cancer screening: recommendations for physicians and patients from the U.S. multi-society task force on colorectal cancer. Am J Gastroenterol. 2017;122(7):1016–30.

28 Headaches

Rachel Brook and Deborah Kwolek

Learning Objectives

1. Diagnose and treat common primary headache disorders, including migraine, tension-type, and cluster headaches.
2. Identify abortive and preventative treatment options for migraine headaches.
3. Discuss the features of a menstrually associated migraine.
4. Describe the association between migraine and stroke risk in patients with and without aura.
5. Identify the risks and benefits of hormonal contraception use in women with migraines with and without aura.
6. Distinguish primary from secondary headache disorders.

Jennifer, a 22-year-old woman, presents with a new complaint of headache. Her mother and maternal aunt have migraines. Her headache is unilateral, lasts for 2–3 days, and has occurred twice per month over the past year. Her headaches are associated with sensitivity to light and sound, and with nausea, but not vomiting. She has tried ibuprofen without relief. The severity of her headaches has caused her to miss at least 1 day of work per month.

Introduction

Headache is one of the most common complaints in both the primary care and emergency room settings worldwide. Per the Global Burden of Disease study, approximately 3 billion people were diagnosed with either a tension-type headache (TTH) or migraine headache in 2016 [1]. Additionally, headaches were deemed the second highest cause of years lived with disability worldwide [2]. Given the absence of objective diagnostic findings on exam or imaging for most headaches, the diagnosis of the type of headache is often based on clinical criteria. Headaches are generally classified as either primary or secondary according to the International Classification of Headache Disorders third edition (ICHD-3) [3]. Primary headaches are defined as those without any underlying causative disorder. Common primary headache disorders include tension-type, cluster, and migraine. Importantly, many patients may have more than one type of headache disorder. Recognizing "red flag" symptoms which require further evaluation and possible imaging and recognizing the characteristics of secondary headaches are essential. Frequent, severe, or persistent headaches can become a chronic syndrome requiring a multimodal treatment strategy. Components of chronic headache can include lifestyle modifications, dietary changes, physical therapy, treatment of underlying mental health disorders, and medications. Due to the complexity and broad range of headache disorders, this chapter will primarily focus on migraine headaches in the primary care practice.

R. Brook (✉)
David Geffen School of Medicine, UCLA, Department of Internal Medicine, Los Angeles, CA, USA
e-mail: rpbrook@mednet.ucla.edu

D. Kwolek
Harvard Medical School, Massachusetts General Hospital, Department of Medicine, Boston, MA, USA

S. A. Tilstra et al. (eds.), *Sex- and Gender-Based Women's Health*, https://doi.org/10.1007/978-3-030-50695-7_28

The Clinical Evaluation and Differential Diagnosis of Headaches

The evaluation of headaches in the primary care setting begins with a thorough headache history. The history of prior headaches, the onset and duration of the current headache, the frequency of headaches, and any recent changes are noted. Focused questions in which the patient "walks you through" a typical headache episode include frequency, pain (location, quality, severity), pattern (where the pain begins, radiates, and time between those changes), associated symptoms (photophobia, phonophobia, nausea/vomiting, aura), and exacerbating or ameliorating factors. Medication history and use of over-the-counter substances are reviewed, including medications that have been tried previously for headache relief. A family history of headache disorders, new or changed medications, recent trauma or infection, and associated neurologic symptoms are noted. A patient's sleep habits, substance use, psychosocial stressors, and mental health screens are reviewed.

Physical examination includes blood pressure measurement, fundoscopic exam for jugular venous pulsations or papilledema, and neurologic examination. Musculoskeletal examination should include palpation of pericranial and cervical muscles to evaluate for myofascial tenderness or allodynia, temporal arteries that could suggest temporal arteritis, and auscultation for carotid bruits.

"Red flags" which require urgent evaluation include markedly elevated blood pressure, papilledema, nuchal rigidity, fever, chills, head trauma, thunderclap (reaches maximum severity within a few minutes of onset), or worst headache of the patient's life. Although migraines often have neurologic symptoms in the form of an aura, symptoms which come on suddenly, last more than 60 minutes, involve hemiplegia, or are associated with a decreased level of consciousness require imaging to exclude stroke. Additional symptoms which require further investigation include headaches that are positional, that get worse with exertion or sex, that occur after head trauma, that are new after the age of 50, that change in pattern, or that never go away.

Primary Headaches

Tension Headaches

Tension-type headache (TTH) is the most common cause of headaches in the United States (65%), and women tend to have a slightly higher prevalence than men. TTH is often associated with forward posture, eye strain, increased stress, fatigue, or lack of sleep. It can be difficult to distinguish between TTH and mild migraine headaches without aura, and TTH and migraine headaches are often present in the same patient [3, 4].

The pathophysiology of TTH is multifactorial. Episodic tension-type headaches likely involve increased activation and/or sensitization of peripheral pain nociceptors. Over time, patients with chronic TTH may additionally develop altered central pain modulatory mechanisms which then contribute to chronic pain symptoms [3].

Clinical presentation and diagnostic criteria Tension-type headache typically presents as a bilateral headache, and is often described by patients as a "band-like pressure" or tightness of mild to moderate intensity, surrounding their entire head lasting minutes to days [3, 5]. TTH does not typically include nausea and vomiting or sensory hypersensitivity, although photophobia or phonophobia may be present. TTH is not aggravated by routine physical activity such as walking or climbing stairs. Physical examination may be unremarkable; however, patients with TTH may have increased tenderness to palpation of the pericranial muscles or associated trigger points. A cephalic muscle group consisting of the frontal, temporal, lateral pterygoid, and masseter muscles and a neck muscle group including the insertions at the mastoid processes, the sternocleidomastoid and trapezius muscles, and the neck insertions of these muscles are often tender or in spasm. The differential diagnosis of TTH includes cluster headaches, migraine headaches, medication overuse headaches, temporomandibular joint disorders (TMJ), sinus disease, eye disease, chronic post-traumatic headache, and disorders of the cervical spine and cervical muscles [3, 6–8].

The International headache Society (IHS) has published classification guidelines for the diagnoses of headaches. The IHS classifies TTH into three major categories, infrequent, frequent and chronic depending upon the frequency of at least 10 episodes of headache over time. *Infrequent episodic tension type headache* occurs less than one day per month on average, *Frequent episodic tension type headache* occurs 1-14 days per month on average for >3 months and *Chronic tension type headache* occurs more than 15 days per month on average for >3 months. *Chronic tension type headache* can last hours to days, or be unremitting, and evolves from *Frequent episodic tension type headache*. TTH are further subclassified by the presence or absence of pericranial tenderness. The diagnostic criteria for *Infrequent episodic tension type headache* is outlined in Box 28.1, and differs from Frequent and Chronic TTH as described above.

Box 28.1 Diagnostic Criteria for *Infrequent Episodic Tension-Type Headaches*: International Classification of Headache Disorders ICHD-3 [3]

A. At least 10 episodes of headache occurring on <1 day/ month on average (<12 days/year) and fulfilling criteria B-D
B. Lasting from 30 minutes to seven days
C. At least two of the following four characteristics:
   1. bilateral location
   2. pressing or tightening (non-pulsating) quality
   3. mild or moderate intensity
   4. not aggravated by routine physical activity such as walking or climbing stairs
D. Both of the following:
   1. no nausea or vomiting.
   2. no more than one of photobia or phonophobia
E. Not better accounted for by another ICHD-3 diagnosis

Treatment of tension-type headaches Despite its prevalence, most patients do not seek medical attention for TTH. In general, episodic TTHs are of mild severity, do not interfere with activities of daily living, and are infrequent in nature [9]. For patients who seek medical attention, there is a paucity of evidence-based studies to guide abortive and preventative therapy. First-line therapy for abortive treatment includes over-the-counter pain medications: aspirin, acetaminophen, nonsteroidal anti-inflammatory agents (NSAIDs), and combination preparations including caffeine. In evaluating the efficacy of each treatment, an assessment is made of the patients' pain 2–4 hours after medication use [10, 11].

A systematic literature review of abortive treatment options for TTH using the International Headache Society (IHS) definitions of effective treatment was conducted and found that a single dose of acetaminophen (also known as paracetamol) 1000 mg, ibuprofen 400 mg, or ketoprofen 25 mg were more effective than placebo in achieving pain-free intervals after 2 hours [10]. In general, a large initial dose is more effective than repeating small doses, and medication is most effective if given at the onset of the headache. Analgesics using caffeine are considered second-line therapy if the before-mentioned medications are not effective. Triptans are not indicated for the abortive treatment of TTH, although triptans are used in patients with concomitant migraine headaches. Providers should be cautious of overly frequent use of analgesic medications for TTH in order to prevent medication overuse headaches. In general, analgesics should not be used daily for prolonged periods of time. Opioids and butalbital should be avoided in the treatment of TTH [11].

For patients with frequent or chronic TTH, adjunctive treatment options are needed to avoid medication overuse headaches. Cognitive behavioral therapy, relaxation techniques, stress reduction, attention to posture, and physical therapy of the neck and shoulder region may be beneficial. Lack of sleep, lack of exercise, poor posture, and tension from prolonged stooping, or computer work are addressed and corrected as necessary. Massage, myofascial release, spinal manipulation, and acupuncture may be beneficial, but efficacy data is limited. Low-dose amitriptyline, a tricyclic antidepressant, is considered the first-line option for the prevention of chronic or frequent episodic TTH [12]. Mirtazapine and venlafaxine have been used in the preventive treatment of TTH with some reported success. Providers should carefully assess patients for response to therapy and side effects with each intervention or medication trial [11].

Cluster Headaches

Cluster headaches are a rare type of headache which belongs to the *Trigeminal autonomic cephalgia* category. In contrast to tension-type headaches, the prevalence of cluster headaches in the general population is less than 1%. Cluster headaches are one of the few primary headache disorders that occur more commonly in men than in women, but this ratio has decreased in recent years. Traditionally, the prevalence in men vs. women was cited as 6:1; however, data in the 1990s found a ratio closer to 2.1:1 [13]. Despite the low prevalence, cluster headaches are important to diagnose because of specific and effective treatment options and because of the high burden of disease impact on quality of life, including increased suicide ideation [14]. The pathogenesis of cluster headaches is not well understood. Recent evidence has shown that abnormal functioning of the hypothalamus; the trigeminal nerve, parasympathetic pathways, and cerebral vasculature all likely contribute to the development of cluster headaches [15].

Clinical presentation Cluster Headache is defined by the International Classification of Headache Disorders (ICHD) as descibed in Box 28.2. The pain intensity in *Cluster headache* is severe, and the location is unilateral, typically focused in the retro-orbital, periorbital, and temporal region. The quality of the pain is often described as stabbing, boring, or ice pick-like in nature, and classically, attacks are associated with ipsilateral conjunctival lacrimation, conjunctival injection, rhinorrhea, or nasal congestion. *Cluster headache* can be associated with an aura similar to those in migraine headaches, and auras associated with *Cluster headache* are more common in women than in men. *Cluster headache* characteristically has both a circadian and seasonal rhythm occurring at the same time of day, most frequently at night, and around the same time of year, most frequently in spring and autumn. As the name suggests, attacks tend to come in clusters, occurring at least every other day, up to eight times daily, for weeks to months at a time [3, 8]. Differential diagnoses for *Cluster headache* includes paroxysmal hemicranias, trigeminal neuralgia, primary stabbing (ice pick) headache, and unilateral neuralgiform headache [3] which fall under the group category of *Trigeminal autonomic cephalgias*. Cluster-like headaches may occur in the presence of intracranial pathology, and therefore, one non-contrast CT or MRI is recommended as part of the evaluation of suspected *Cluster headache* [16].

The ICHD-3 diagnostic criteria for Cluster headache is listed below: Box 28.2

Box 28.2 Diagnostic Criteria for *Cluster Headache*: International Classification of Headache Disorders ICHD-3 [3]

A. At least five attacks fulfilling criteria B-D:
B. Severe or very severe unilateral orbital, supraorbital, and/or temporal pain lasting 15-180 minutes (when untreated)
C. Either or both of the following:
   1. At least one of the following symptoms or signs, ipsilateral to the headache:
      a) conjunctival injection and/or lacrimation
      b) nasal congestion and/or rhinorrhoea
      c) eyelid oedema
      d) forehead and facial sweating
      e) miosis and/or ptosis
   2. A sense of restlessness or agitation
D. Occuring with a frequency between one every other day and eight per day
E. Not better accounted for by another ICHD-3 diagnosis.

Headache Classification Committee of the International Headache Society (IHS). The International Classification of Headache Disorders, 3rd edition. *Cephalalgia* 38(1), pp. 1–211. Copyright © 2018 by International Headache Society. Reprinted by permission of SAGE Publications, Ltd.

Treatment of Cluster headache Treatment goals for patients with cluster headaches include decreasing both the individual attacks and the duration of the cluster headache episode. Abortive treatments for cluster headaches help resolve individual attacks, but do not alter the length of cluster headache episode. Prophylactic therapies help shorten the episode length and should be started as soon as the cluster headache is diagnosed.

First-line abortive treatment of cluster headaches includes 100% oxygen administration or treatment with triptans. Oxygen therapy is generally well tolerated with minimal side effects; recommended delivery is via a non-rebreather mask or nasal cannula at 6–7 liters per minute. Triptans are also used for abortive treatment of cluster headaches. Subcutaneous sumatriptan has the fastest onset of action and is dosed at 6 mg. Intranasal sumatriptan 20 mg or zolmitriptan 5 mg are also effective with a slightly slower onset of action but fewer side effects. Intranasal medications are sprayed in the nostril on the contralateral side to the headache. In resistant cases, steroids and IV lidocaine have been used although efficacy data is limited [13, 17].

Prophylactic treatments for cluster headaches are started together with abortive treatments. The only evidence-based prophylactic treatment for reducing the duration of cluster headache episodes is verapamil 360 mg oral daily; however, care must be taken concerning blood pressure and bradyarrhythmias. Lithium 800 mg daily is considered to be an alternative treatment if patients have contraindications or adverse reactions to verapamil. Lithium use requires the monitoring of drug levels and renal function, and cannot be used in pregnancy. Additional therapies for resistant or severe cases should be comanaged with a neurologist. Topiramate, gabapentin, lamotrigene, melatonin, prostaglandin, testosterone, and surgical or transcranial stimulation treatments have been tried but have limited data for efficacy [13, 17].

Migraine Headaches

Migraine is the most disabling primary headache disorder, ranking as the third-highest cause of disability worldwide in the 2017 Global Burden of Disease Study [2]. Migraines may begin as early as childhood, peak around ages 35–39, and tend to decrease among women after menopause [18]. Migraines are two to three times more common in women than in men [19] and affect approximately 20% of women [1, 20]. Studies have shown a genetic predisposition in up to 50–90% of patients with migraine [20, 21]. Migraines can be episodic or chronic and are divided into two main subtypes: migraine without aura (MWOA) and migraine with aura (MWA). Migraine with aura is defined as transient neurologic symptoms that precede or accompany the onset of headache, last no more than 60 minutes, and occur in 20–35% of patients with migraine. Typical aura symptoms involve bilateral visual changes, but auras also manifest as disturbances in sensation, motor function, cognitive abilities, concentration, or speech and language [20].

Treatment strategies for migraines include abortive medications, preventive treatments, lifestyle and trigger avoidance strategies; most patients will benefit from a combination of several or all categories of treatment. MWA and MWOA respond to the same treatments. The primary difference clinically is the safety of estrogen-containing contraceptives, which are of concern for patients with an aura, as the risk of stroke may be increased. The management of migraines associated with menses (MAM) which are discussed below includes strategies with hormonal manipulations and choice of triptans which add a layer of complexity to treatment planning.

The pathophysiology of migraines The pathophysiology of migraine involves multiple mechanisms including inflammation of the meninges resulting in increased sensitization of meningeal nerve fibers, abnormalities in cortical activity resulting in a hyperexcitable cortical state, and altered brainstem modulation of the ascending nociceptive pathway [21]. The hyperexcitable cortical state may render genetically predisposed individuals susceptible to the development of a cortical spreading depression. A cortical spreading depression is a wave of neuronal and glial depolarization and subsequent hyperpolarization that incites a cascade of downstream events including vasodilation and altered permeability of the meningeal vessels and the release of pro-inflammatory neuropeptides [20, 21]. Neuropeptides, including calcitonin gene-related peptide (CGRP), substance P, and neurokinin A, contribute to the activation of the trigeminal afferents, which then relay these nociceptive signals to the second- and third-order neurons in the thalamus and cortical pain centers, producing pain. Cortical spreading depression has been most clearly correlated with the aura phase of migraine in patients suffering from migraines *with* aura [3]. While the etiology of migraines remains complex, a large body of evidence has refuted the vascular theory of migraine which had attributed migraine headaches to the dilation of cranial vessels [22].

Clinical presentation of migraines Migraine attacks have been described as an evolution of four phases: a premonitory or prodrome phase, an aura (if present), a headache phase, and a postdrome phase', however, not all patients experience all four stages. The premonitory phase can occur hours prior to the onset of aura or headache. The most common symptoms reported in this phase are fatigue, irritability, difficulty concentrating, mood changes, neck pain, nausea, and sensitivity to light or sound. The presence of these symptoms may alert a patient to the development of a migraine prior to the onset of cephalic pain. The second phase is the aura which includes transient, reversible neurologic symptoms immediately preceding or occurring with the headache. The headache itself is the third phase of a migraine attack. Cephalic pain in migraine attacks is typically unilateral, throbbing, of moderate to severe intensity and lasting 4–72 hours in duration [23].

The phenomenon of *cutaneous allodynia* is a sensation of pain, numbness, tingling, burning, or hypersensitivity of cutaneous nerves on the scalp or elsewhere on the trunk or extremities. Cutaneous allodynia is part of the neurologic manifestations which accompany many migraine headaches.

After the resolution of the headache phase, there is the postdrome phase, which can last up to days after a migraine attack, during which symptoms of fatigue, mood changes, weakness, and cognitive delay may be present [23] (Box 28.3).

Box 28.3 Diagnostic Criteria for *Migraine Without Aura*: International Classification of Headache Disorders ICHD-3 [3]

A. At least five attacks fulfilling the criteria B-D
B. Headache attacks lasting 4–72 hours (when untreated or unsuccessfully treated)
C. Headache has at least two of the following four characteristics:
   1. unilateral location
   2. pulsating quality
   3. moderate or severe pain intensity
   4. aggravation by or causing avoidance of routine physical activity (e.g., walking or climbing stairs)
D. During headache, at least one of the following:
   1. nausea and/or vomiting
   2. photophobia and phonophobia
E. Not better accounted for by another ICHD-3 diagnosis

The differential diagnoses for migraine headaches include tension-type headaches, trigeminal autonomic cephalgias including cluster headaches, and secondary headache disorders including sinus headaches, intracranial lesions, central nervous system (CNS) infections, face or head trauma, or cerebrovascular disorders. In contrast to tension-type and cluster headaches, migraine headaches are more often associated with photophobia, phonophobia, sensitivity to smells, nausea/vomiting, worsening with exertion or physical activity, and interference with daily functioning [3]. Migraines are often incorrectly labeled as sinus headaches by patients and physicians due to the periorbital and sometimes maxillary location of pain.

Migraines with Aura

Migraine with aura is diagnosed by the same criteria as *Migraine without aura* (MWOA), but with the additional presence of transient neurologic symptoms (Box 28.4).

Box 28.4 Diagnostic Criteria for *Migraine with Aura*: International Classification of Headache Disorders ICHD-3 [3]

Headache meeting the criteria for Migraine without aura, with the following additions:

A. At least two attacks fulfilling criteria B and C
B. One or more of the following fully reversible aura symptoms:
   1. visual
   2. sensory
   3. speech and/or language
   4. motor
   5. brainstem
   6. retinal
C. At least three of the following six characteristics:
   1. at least one aura symptom spreads gradually over ≥5 minutes
   2. two or more aura symptoms occur in succession.
   3. each individual aura symptom lasts 5–60 minutes.
   4. at least one aura symptom is unilateral (note: aphasia is always regarded as a unilateral symptom, dysarthria may or may not be).
   5. at least one aura symptom is positive (scintillations and pins and needs are positive signs of aura).
   6. the aura is accompanied, or followed within 60 minutes, by headache.
D. *Not better accounted for by another ICHD-3 diagnosis.*

According to the International Classification of Headache Disorders, third edition (ICHD-3) [3], the most common auras in migraine manifest clinically as bilateral visual disturbances including scintillations of light, fortification spectra, or a central scotoma. Fortification spectra are defined as zigzag light bands, and a central scotoma is defined as a gray/black or blind spot in the center of one's vision. The second most common type of aura is sensory disturbance, which manifests as unilateral tingling and/or numbness affecting the body, face, or tongue. The third most frequent type of aura involves speech and/or language and may present as partial or complete aphasia.

Less frequent manifestations of auras include motor, brainstem, or monocular retinal presentations. Auras involving motor weakness are classified as hemiplegic migraine and involve unilateral weakness. Brainstem auras present with at least two of the following symptoms: dysarthria, tinnitus, vertigo, diplopia, ataxia (not caused by sensory or motor deficits), decreased level of consciousness (i.e., a Glasgow Coma Score of <13), and/or hearing loss. Retinal migraines present as repeated episodes of monocular visual disturbances, often with unilateral transient blindness or flashing lights [3]. The first time that patients present with sensory disturbances, brainstem, or hemiplegic auras, imaging should be considered. Repeated episodes of auras with migraines, especially the brainstem and hemiplegic auras, are an indication for migraine prophylaxis [24].

Auras typically last 5–60 minutes in duration and precede or occur at the beginning of the onset of cephalic pain. Some patients have symptoms of aura *without* accompanying headache (within 60 minutes of the start of aura symptoms). Occurences of neurologic symptoms without headache, especially when new in onset, changing, or different from a typical aura, should be carefully evaluated for underlying neurologic pathology or transient ischemic attacks (TIAs) [3].

Jennifer is diagnosed with migraine headache without aura based on the character of her headaches. She is told that migraines often run in families. The natural history and pathophysiology of her condition are discussed. Jennifer inquires about treatment options, especially for nausea, and for the debilitating pain which causes her to miss work. She currently suffers approximately two migraines per month.

Treatment of Migraine by the Primary Care Provider

Migraine treatment depends on the severity and chronicity of headache attacks. All patients benefit from stress reduction, attention to sleeping and eating patterns, and the identification of possible triggers. Those with mild to moderate episodic migraines are often successfully managed with abortive therapy alone. Acetaminophen or nonsteroidal anti-inflammatory treatments (NSAIDs) are taken in anticipation of, or at the beginning of each migraine headache. Patients who do not respond to acetaminophen or NSAIDs alone may be given triptans, either alone or in combination with NSAIDs.

Patients with frequent and/or moderate to severe migraines benefit from the addition of preventive medications and increased attention to lifestyle changes. Amitriptyline in low doses is first-line treatment for prevention and is generally well tolerated [12, 18, 23].

Patients with chronic or severe migraines require a global approach and should be co-managed with a neurologist. Elimination diets, botox therapy, biologics, identification of individualized migraine threshold and triggers, lifestyle changes, abortive therapies, and prevention treatments are combined and used in management. Patients with severe chronic migraines may need psychosocial support, psychologic care, work accommodations, or disability to manage the burden of chronic pain and distress.

Migraine Triggers

Migraine triggers Although there are no randomized controlled trials that support specific lifestyle changes for the prevention of migraine, behavioral modifications and reduction of migraine triggers can be a cornerstone in the successful management of migraine headaches. Migraine triggers have been shown to include increased stress, menstruation, caffeine, odors, sleeping late, missed meals, hormone treatment, smoke, alcohol (especially wine), certain foods, nitrates, exercise, weather, and neck pain. Stress is the most frequently noted trigger [24, 25]. Maintaining regular sleep, consistent caffeine intake (or reducing/eliminating caffeine altogether), consistent meals, regular aerobic exercise routine, and decreasing stress levels should be emphasized to patients to help reduce migraine headache attacks [25, 26]. The use of opioids and combination analgesic combination medications (barbiturate-based and over-the-counter) should be minimized, as they can increase migraine frequency and severity, even when taken only once or twice a week [18]. Patients are encouraged to keep a headache log or symptom diary to help them and their provider identify possible triggers. Triggers, once identified, should be vigorously avoided by the patient to help reduce the frequency and severity of migraine headache attacks.

Migraine threshold theory The concept of a migraine threshold is embraced by migraine experts, is popular in the lay public literature, and is a helpful way to explain migraine management to patients. Similar to the seizure threshold, patients are vulnerable to headaches when one event, or a combination of factors, increases brain stimulation toward the migraine threshold for that individual. An individual's threshold and vulnerability to migraines may be genetically determined, and migraineurs have a lower threshold to develop a headache due to hyperexcitability and hypersensitivity. Preventive medication and treatments would increase the threshold, making migraines less common and less severe. An example would be that for a certain individual, drinking wine and skipping a meal together are enough to cause a migraine. The patient can abstain from wine and eat regularly which will decrease migraine frequency. The addition of a preventive treatment or medication might raise the threshold so that minor disturbances in sleep or an occasional glass of wine will no longer cause a headache, whereas a sleepless night will still trigger a migraine [27].

Adjuvant non-pharmacologic treatments In addition to avoiding known triggers for migraine headaches, the American Academy of Neurology recommends various non-pharmacologic treatment options for the prevention of migraine headaches. Behavioral treatments with the best evidence include acupuncture, aerobic exercise, cognitive behavioral therapies, thermal or electromyographic biofeedback, and relaxation techniques [28]. Physical therapy and acupuncture can be particularly helpful if myofascial pain is associated with a patient's migraines [29]. Insufficient evidence was found for transcutaneous electrical nerve stimulation and acupuncture, although these therapies may still be used for the preventative treatment of migraine headaches [28]. Most importantly, behavioral and pharmacologic therapies need to be combined to achieve success in preventing migraine headaches.

Abortive Treatments for Migraine Headaches

Several abortive agents have been validated as effective in the acute treatment of migraines; the treatment is the same whether the migraine is with or without aura (see Table 28.1). The most commonly used agents include acetaminophen, nonsteroidal anti-inflammatory drugs (NSAIDs), the triptans (agonists of the 5-HT1BD receptor), dopamine-agonist based anti-emetics, and less commonly ergotamine-derivative compounds. The role of newer agents is currently being defined. Ditans, which have a high affinity for 5HT1F receptors, and agents which inhibit Calcitonin gene-related peptide (CGRP) activity are newly approved and have some use as abortive and preventive therapies. The first approved ditan is lasmiditan, an oral agent approved for use in the

Table 28.1 Selected therapies for acute migraine [18, 30–43]

Class	Specific treatments	Reported mean therapeutic effects[b]	Common or serious adverse effects	Comments
Triptans [30]	Almotriptan, eletriptan, frovatriptan, naratriptan, rizatriptan, sumatriptan, zolmitriptan	Pain relief by 2 hr, 16–51%; pain-free by 2 hr, 9–32%; free of headache for 24 hr, 9–27%	Chest or facial muscle tightness, lightheadedness; contraindicated in patients with coronary artery disease	Response to and side-effect profile of different triptans varies in individual patients; nasal or subcutaneous delivery may be more effective than oral delivery in patients with nausea or vomiting
Ergots [31, 32]	DHE nasal spray, DHE injection	Pain relief by 2 hr, 20–40% (for DHE nasal spray; limited evidence)	Nausea, dizziness; contraindicated in patients with peripheral vascular disease or coronary artery disease	Intravenous DHE is commonly used for refractory migraine
Acetaminophen [33]		Pain relief by 2 hr, 19%; pain-free by 2 hr, 9%	Minimal with intermittent use	May be more effective in combination with antiemetic agent
NSAIDs [34]	Aspirin, diclofenac, ibuprofen, ketorolac, naproxen	Pain relief by 2 hr, 17–29%; pain-free by 2 hr, 7–20%	Gastric irritation, excessive bleeding	May be effective individually or have additive benefit when taken with triptan; different oral preparations (effervescent or powder) may have improved efficacy
Combinations [35, 36]	Acetaminophen-aspirin-caffeine, sumatriptan-naproxen	Pain relief by 2 hr, 10–17% (limited evidence); pain-free by 2 hr, 20–30%	Same as with NSAIDs and triptans	Caffeine-containing preparations may have increased potential for overuse; combination therapy is more effective than individual agents in some patients
AntiemeticAgents [30, 33, 37]	Chlorpromazine, metoclopramide, prochlorperazine	Pain relief by 2 hr with oral metoclopramide (plus aspirin or acetaminophen), 23%; pain relief by 1–2 hr with intravenous delivery in the emergency department, 24–67%	Sedation, restlessness (akathisia), dystonic reactions	Phenothiazines plus metoclopramide have benefit for headache as well as nausea; ondansetron is commonly used for nausea, but evidence is lacking
Single-pulse TMS [38]	SpringTMS	Pain-free by 2 hr, 17%	No clinically significant adverse effects	Handheld device for patient-delivered therapy; currently FDA-approved for treatment of acute migraine with aura
CGRP receptor antagonists [39, 40] (under investigation)	Rimegepant, ubrogepant	Pain-free by 2 hr, 14–18%	None reported; safety studies are ongoing	Phase 2 studies have been completed

[a]Shown are therapies that have high-quality supporting evidence or are highly recommended in guidelines from the American Headache Society [37, 41], the Canadian Headache Society [42], and the European Federation of Neurological Societies [43], as well as other Food and Drug Administration (FDA)—approved or emerging therapies. Citations are for primary trial data within guidelines except as noted; trials were of variable quality. All approaches are FDA-approved for the treatment of acute migraine except antiemetics and calcitonin gene-related peptide (CGRP) receptor antagonists. DHE denotes dihydroergotamine, NSAIDs nonsteroidal anti-inflammatory drugs, and TMS transcranial magnetic stimulation

[b]Values are the percentage of patients with pain relief or freedom from pain after a single dose of the treatment minus the percentage with pain relief or freedom from pain after placebo administration. In most cases, therapy was administered when pain was already moderate or severe

treatment of acute migraine. Oral, short acting CGRP medications, such as rimegepant and ubrogepant, can also be used as abortive migraine treatments. Long acting CGRP parenteral agents can be used as preventive migraine treatments, and examples include erenumab, fremanezumab, galcanezumab and eptinezumab. Both classes of agents are mildly effective, and there is little data on pregnancy or long-term safety. The number of pharmacologic interventions available for migraine treatments is rapidly increasing, and readers are advised to check the most current prescribing information when making treatment decisions. The following table summarizing traditional abortive treatments for migraines was published in 2017 in the New England Journal of Medicine, and is reprinted here with permission.

Acetaminophen and NSAIDs For patients with mild migraine headaches, acetaminophen and NSAIDs are considered the first-line therapy given both their efficacy and decreased adverse side effects [33, 44].

Triptans For patients with more severe or refractory migraine attacks, triptans are commonly prescribed as first-line abortive migraine treatments. Triptans are serotonin 1b/1d agonists that are considered to be "specific treatments" for headaches by blocking pain pathways in the brainstem and increasing vasoconstriction [45]. There are triptans with a shorter half-life which provide more immediate relief but may have more side effects. Subcutaneous and intranasal preparations are helpful when rapid onset is needed or when there is significant nausea and vomiting. Triptans with a longer half-life are slower in onset but are better tolerated. Longer-acting triptans are often used in the treatment of migraine associated with menses (MAM) starting 1–3 days before the onset of menses and continuing 3–5 days into the menstrual period.

Studies have shown that many patients treated with triptans are not satisfied with their treatment and experience persistence of headache symptoms despite medication compliance [46]. The reasons for the lack of symptom improvement may include the fact that many patients delay the use of triptans until the pain is moderate to severe in intensity, whereas early treatment with triptans has been shown to be crucial to successful treatment of migraine headache [18, 47]. Migraine treatment often requires a global and multimodal approach to treatment, and expectations regarding pain relief should be managed. In difficult cases, the goal of treatment should be increased daily functioning rather than total relief from pain.

A combination of naproxen with a triptan, given at the beginning of the headache, is an effective choice for many patients [41]. There is evidence that the addition of NSAIDs to triptan use may have a synergistic effect, increasing the efficacy of the triptan and resulting in improved control of headache symptoms (40% vs. 17%). While there is limited evidence, triptans remain contraindicated in patients with coronary artery disease (CAD), hemiplegic migraines, history of ischemic stroke, uncontrolled hypertension, pregnancy, or peripheral vascular disease (PVD).

Triptans, however, are considered safer to use than ergot-derived medications in the conditions listed above [48].

Ergot medications Ergotamine and dihydroergotamine (DHE) are infrequently used in the treatment of acute migraines due to a lack of efficacy, side effects, rebound headaches, and contraindications. While both are vasoconstricting agents and 5HT 1b/1d agonists, DHE has been shown to be more effective then ergotamine, with fewer adverse effects, and is available as a nasal spray [49]. Ergots are effective and can be given for refractory migraines in an emergency department setting, particularly in headaches lasting greater than 72 hours [49]. Such treatment is usually followed by steroid administration to prevent the rapid return of headache.

Ergot medications are contraindicated in patients with CAD, peripheral vascular disease, cerebrovascular/ischemic stroke disease, hypertension, and hepatic or renal impairment and have been associated with clinically significant vasospasms. Ergot medications are not recommended for elderly or pregnant patients [18].

Antiemetics Patients with nausea as a prominent feature are prescribed an antiemetic agent, such as chlorpromazine or metoclopramide which treat nausea, and may also contribute to headache relief. Ondansetron is commonly used in the treatment of acute migraine, but it has not been significantly evaluated [18]. When nausea or vomiting limits the use of oral medications, non-oral preparations are used: intranasal, intramuscular, intravenous, or per rectum. In the *emergency room*, IV or IM antiemetics are used as monotherapy for severe migraines. Diphenhydramine is usually given concomitantly to prevent dystonic reactions. Parenteral dexamethasone (10–25 mg) is given as adjunctive treatment to prevent headache recurrence.

Opioids and butalbital should not be prescribed as treatments for acute migraine, per the American Headache Society, due to a lack of studies showing positive efficacy, potential side effects of treatment, and potential for misuse [28]. The doses of commonly used medications are listed in Table 28.2.

The early administration of abortive medications, before the migraine attack becomes severe, will increase treatment efficacy. Medication can be taken prior to the headache or with the onset of the prodrome. If the patient has an aura, abortive treatments should be given at the onset [41, 64] Patients often delay the use of abortive medications in hopes that the headache will not progress into a migraine attack or in an attempt to conserve their medication supply of triptans: insurance coverage may limit the number of triptan pills that will be covered per month. Frequent triptan use has the potential to cause medication overuse headache and can be safely used only 10 days per month in chronic migraine patients [18]. The limitations on the use of abortive treatments underscore the importance of trigger avoidance and lifestyle changes in the management of headaches and the use of preventive medications for frequent headaches.

Jennifer is prescribed a triptan medication. She is encouraged to identify the premonitory phase characteristics of her migraine attacks so that she can take her triptan medication as an abortive treatment. She is told to take NSAIDs as needed with her triptan to help with her migraine pain. Chlorpromazine is prescribed to help with her nausea. Additionally, she was instructed on the importance of cutting out caffeine and starting stress reduction strategies to help manage her migraine triggers.

Referral to a Neurologist

Referral to a neurologist should be considered when previously diagnosed tension-type, cluster, or migraine headaches do not respond to initial therapies, worsen despite treatment, have features that do not allow for clear classification, or display neurologic deficits which differ from the patient's typical aura or prior presentations.

Table 28.2 Doses of medications used for selected abortive treatment in acute migraine [33, 34, 36, 47, 50–63]

Abortive medications	Recommended dosing
Acetaminophen	1000 mg PO x once [33]
NSAIDs	Ibuprofen 400 mg PO once [50] Aspirin 1000 mg PO once [34] Naproxen 500 mg or 825 mg PO once (the 825 mg dose is most effective as a single agent) [51] Ketorolac 30 or 60 mg IV/IM once [52]
Acetaminophen-aspirin-caffeine	Acetaminophen 250 mg/aspirin 250 mg/caffeine 65 mg, 1–2 tablets PO once [53]
Triptans (fast onset at 2 hours)	Sumatriptan tablet: 25/50/100 mg PO once. Repeat in 2 hours later if treatment ineffective. (100 mg dose most effective, but 50 mg dose better tolerated with fewer side effects). Maximum dose is 200 mg per 24H [47, 54, 55] Sumatriptan nasal spray: 20 mg intranasal in single nostril once on the contralateral side from the headache pain. Repeat in 2 hours if treatment ineffective. Maximum dose is 40 mg intranasal per 24H [47] Sumatriptan subcutaneous injection: 4 mg or 6 mg (6 mg more effective). Repeat in 1 hour if treatment ineffective. Maximum dose is 12 mg per 24H [47]. Nasal powder sumatriptan: 22 mg dose. An 11 mg capsule is placed in each nostril. Repeat in 2 hours if treatment ineffective. Maximum dose is 44 mg per 24H [47] Rizatriptan tablet: 5 or 10 mg PO once (10 mg dose being more effective). Repeat dose after 2 hours if treatment ineffective [54, 56] Zolmitriptan tablet: 1/2.5/5/10 mg PO once. Repeat dose in 2 hours if treatment ineffective. Maximum dose is 10 mg per 24H. 2.5 mg is recommended starting dose as side effects correlate with increased dose [54, 57]
Sumatriptan-naproxen combination	Sumatriptan 85 mg and naproxen 500 mg. Take together in a combination pill once. Repeat in 2 hours if treatment ineffective. May also take components separately [36]
Triptans (slower onset)	Frovatriptan tablet: 2.5 mg PO once. Repeat dose in 2 hours if treatment ineffective. Maximum dose is 7.5 mg PO per 24H [54] Naratriptan: 1 mg or 2.5 mg PO once. Repeat dose in 4 hours if treatment ineffective. Maximum daily dose is 5 mg per 24H For short-term prevention of menstrual migraines: use 2.5 mg of frovatriptan, 1 mg of naratriptan, or 2.5 mg zolmitriptan PO BID. Start 1–3 days prior to the onset of menses/symptoms, and continue for 4–7 days [58]
Ergots	DHE nasal spray: 2 mg intranasal once [59] DHE injection: 1 mg subcutaneous injection or 1 mg intravenous injection [60]
Antiemetic agents	Chlorpromazine: 0.1 mg/kg IV once [61, 62] Metoclopramide: 20 mg IV once [63] Prochlorperazine: 10 mg IV once [63]

NSAIDS nonsteroidal anti-inflammatory agents, *PO* per oral, *IV* intravenous, *IM* intramuscular

Jennifer returns 10 months later with increased migraines after stressful changes in her job and home life. Initially, the triptans plus NSAID combination effectively aborted her migraines. However, as the headaches increased in frequency, she began using the medications more frequently than advised. For the past 4 months, Jennifer has been having headaches and using her abortive medication for more than 15 days per month. She says her insurance will not give her more than 9 tablets of triptan per month, and she needs medication for the remainder of the headache days. Jennifer has a BMI of 32, but no other medical conditions. She asks what can be done to decrease her headache burden.

Preventive Treatments for Migraines

Chronic migraineurs and those with frequent or severe episodic headaches are candidates for preventive medication. Chronic migraine refers to migraine headaches lasting >4 hours per day, occurring >15 days per month for more than 3 months at a time, with at least 8 of those days meeting criteria for migraine [3]. Patients with frequent or severe episodic migraine attacks at least once weekly, or greater than 4 days per month, whose migraines are having a negative impact on their quality of life or work, are candidates for preventative treatments [18]. Migraines with severe neurologic symptoms or hemiplegia are also treated with preventive medication.

Prescription medications used to prevent frequent migraines include tricyclic antidepressants, anticonvulsants, beta-blockers, serotonin-reuptake inhibitors, angiotension receptor blockers (i.e., candesartan), NMDA antagonists, botulinum toxin, and calcitonin gene-related peptide (CGRP) antagonists. Tricyclic antidepressants (i.e., amitriptyline), anticonvulsants (i.e., topiramate), and beta-blockers (metoprolol or propranolol) are the most commonly used agents for prevention [18, 65] (Table 28.3).

Antidepressants Tricyclic antidepressants (TCA) and selective norepinephrine and serotonin reuptake inhibitors (SNRI) are recommended by the American Academy of Neurology guidelines for use in migraine prevention [28]. Amitriptyline is the only evidence-proven TCA for migraine prevention, and side effects are minimal at low doses. With higher doses, sedation, dry mouth, constipation, palpitations, weight gain, orthostatic hypotension, and urinary retention may occur. Avoidance of TCAs should be considered in elderly adults [76]. Venlafaxine, an SNRI, is useful for migraine prophylaxis, attention deficit hyperactivity disorder (ADHD), menopausal hot flashes, and depression.

Beta-blockers, including metoprolol, propranolol, and timolol, have been shown to be effective for migraine prevention. Patients are educated that beneficial effects may not be seen for at least 2 weeks, and medications should be trialed for 3 months before being deemed ineffective [77]. Beta-blockers are used with caution in elderly patients, smokers, and patients with low blood pressure or bradycardia, asthma, erectile dysfunction, or depression.

Anticonvulsants, particularly topiramate and valproate, have been shown to reduce migraine headache frequency [78]. Topiramate doses of 100 mg are typically needed for patients to see a reduction in migraine headache frequency. Side effects of topiramate include fatigue, decreased appetite, weight loss, nausea, diarrhea, stomach pain, and difficulty concentrating. Valproate can cause severe weight gain and should be used with caution.

Angiotensin-converting enzyme (ACE) inhibitors and angiotensin II receptor blockers (ARB) can be effective in migraine prevention. There is some evidence that lisinopril (20 mg/day) and candesartan (16 mg/day) can be effective, but sample sizes were small, and use in general practice is limited [79, 80].

Calcium channel blockers are commonly used for migraine prevention; however, there is minimal data, and patients may develop tolerance. Verapamil is the most commonly used calcium channel blocker based on both its efficacy and minimal side effects, but is not considered a first-line medication for migraine prophylaxis [81]. Flunarizine is used outside of the United States.

When selecting an ideal preventive pharmacologic treatment, a patient's comorbidities, medication side effects, efficacy of medication for the prevention of migraines, specific headache characteristics, and a patient's goal for treatment outcomes are taken into consideration [18, 76]. Beta-blockers may be beneficial for patients with anxiety, palpitations, or hypertension. Amitriptyline may be used with concomitant insomnia, depression, irritable bowel syndrome, chronic pain, or mood disorders. Patients with obesity may consider topiramate. Patients with hypertension might be considered for preventive treatment with calcium channel blockers [76].

Herbal remedies There is data to support the use of select supplements for migraine prevention: riboflavin (200 mg PO BID), co-Q10 (300–500 mg PO daily), magnesium (400 mg PO daily), and melatonin (3–10 mg PO daily) [71]. Riboflavin benefits are seen after 3 months of therapy [82].

Butterbur is effective at doses of 75 mg PO BID, but hepatotoxicity was reported with higher doses [83]. Although patients may consider nonprescription herbal therapies to be non-pharmacologic and safe, there is a small risk of toxicity or drug interactions with use [84] (Table 28.4).

Table 28.3 Selected preventive therapies for migraine[a] [17, 18, 28, 66–75]

Class	Specific treatments	Reported mean therapeutic effects[b]	Common or serious adverse effects	Comments
Tricyclic antidepressant [66]	Amitriptyline, nortriptyline	Data not available	Dry mouth, sedation, weight gain, urinary retention	Low doses are typically used (10–50 mg); may be useful in patients with insomnia
Beta-blockers [67, 68]	Metoprolol, nadolol, propranolol[c], timolol[c]	Headache days, −0.4 (meta-analysis for propranolol)	Hypotension, exercise intolerance, sexual dysfunction	May be useful in patients with hypertension, tachycardia, or anxiety
Anticonvulsant agent [69]	Topiramate[c]	Episodic migraine days, −1.1 to −1.3; chronic migraine days, −1.5 to −3.3	Paresthesias, weight loss, cognitive dysfunction, depression	Also used for weight loss; preparations with various half-lives are available
Anticonvulsant agent [70]	Divalproex sodium[c]	Migraine days, −2.6; migraine attacks, −0.6 to −3.4	Tremor, weight gain, hair loss, fetal neural-tube defects	May be efficacious, but adverse effects limit its use
Candesartan [68]		Headache days, −0.7 to −1.7; migraine days, −0.6 to −1.1	Dizziness	Side effects generally acceptable
Flunarizine [66]		Migraine attacks, −1.2 to −1.8	Sedation, weight gain, depression	Not available in the United States
Nonprescription therapies [71]	Coenzyme Q10, magnesium, melatonin, petasites, riboflavin	Migraine attacks: −1.1 with coenzyme Q10, −0.5 to −0.9 with magnesium, −0.8 with petasites or riboflavin	Diarrhea with magnesium	Side effects are generally acceptable, but current evidence of efficacy is poor
Botulinum toxins [72]	OnabotulinumtoxinA[c]	Chronic migraine headache days, −1.4 to −2.3; migraine days, −1.5 to −2.4	Muscle weakness, headache	Delivered by subcutaneous injection at multiple sites; approved for chronic migraine only
Supraorbital nerve stimulation [73]	Cefaly device[c]	Migraine days, −2.1	Local discomfort, skin irritation	Headband with forehead simulation; applied for 20 min daily
Monoclonal antibodies targeting CGRP or its receptor [74, 75] (under investigation)	Eptinezumab, erenumab, fremanezumab, galcanezumab	Episodic migraine headache days, −1.0 to −1.2; high-frequency episodic migraine days, −2.8; days with chronic migraine headache, −2.5; hr with chronic migraine headache, −30.4	Injection-site reactions; safety studies are ongoing	Multiple phase 3 trials have been completed; administered subcutaneously or intravenously every 1–3 mo; rapid onset of efficacy; rates of response of 75% and in some cases 100% have been reported

[a]Shown are therapies that have high-quality supporting evidence or are highly recommended in guidelines from the American Academy of Neurology and the American Headache Society [17, 28], the Canadian Headache Society [66], and the European Federation of Neurological Societies [67], as well as other FDA-approved or emerging therapies. Citations for the primary clinical-trial data are included in these guidelines except where noted. All studies were of episodic migraine unless otherwise specified. Episodic migraine is defined as less than 15 headache days per month, chronic migraine is defined as 15 days or more headache days per month, with migraine features on at least 8 of those days

[b]Values are the number of migraine attacks or number of days or hours with symptoms, per month with the treatment minus the number with placebo; negative values indicated a benefit with the treatment. The mean monthly effect (typically after 3 months of treatment) is summarized

[c]These therapies have been approved by the FDA as preventative therapies for migraine

Guidelines recommend starting the chosen preventative medication at the lowest dose and increasing until beneficial effects are seen or when side effects are no longer tolerable [28]. It is of paramount importance to counsel patients that while side effects can begin immediately, improvement in headaches is not noted until at least 4–6 weeks after initiation of preventive therapy. Medications should be maintained for 12 weeks before treatment failure is diagnosed [28]. If a patient does not respond to or cannot tolerate a particular medication, then a different class of preventives can be prescribed, but one should also continue to assess for other factors that can impede response to preventives, such as the development of medication overuse headache or lifestyle habits which contribute to migraine.

Preventative therapies can effect a 50% reduction in migraine frequency, particularly amitriptyline, but the

Table 28.4 Medications and doses for the prevention of recurrent migraine [28, 43, 69, 70, 82, 83, 85–89]

Preventative category	Medication and dosing
Tricyclic antidepressants	Amitriptyline 10–50 mg PO QHS [28] Nortriptyline 10–50 mg PO QHS [28]
Beta-blockers	Propanolol 40–80 mg PO BID [85] Metoprolol 50–100 mg PO BID [85] Nadolol 20–240 mg PO daily [85]
Anticonvulsants	Topiramate 25–50 mg PO BID daily [69] Zonisamide (not yet FDA approved) [69] Valproic acid 500–1500 mg PO daily [70, 85]
Calcium channel blockers	Flunarizine 5–10 mg PO daily (not available in the United States) [85] Verapamil 80 mg PO QID [43, 86]
Angiotension II receptor blocker	Candesartan 16 mg PO daily [87]
SNRI	Venlafaxine 37.5 mg150 mg PO daily [28, 85]
Nonprescription therapies	Magnesium 600 mg PO daily [88] Riboflavin 400 mg PO daily [82] Butterbur (petasite) 75 mg PO BID [83]
NSAIDs	Naproxen 550 mg PO BID [89]

SNRI Selective serotonin reuptake inhibitor, *NSAIDs* nonsteroidal anti-inflammatory drugs, *PO* per oral, *BID* two times daily, *QID* four times daily, *QHS* at nighttime

response is variable [28, 85]. Adherence to preventative treatment tends to be low: one study involving almost 9000 patients found an adherence rate between 26% and 29% at 6 months [90]. Finding the lowest effective dose, a medication with a beneficial side-effect profile for each individual patient, and counseling about appropriate expectations for time frame of improvement can help increase adherence to therapy.

Botox and Monoclonal Antibodies

When prophylactic medication is ineffective, patients should be referred to a neurologist for consideration of botox or biologic therapy injections.

Botox Multiple reviews have found that botulinum toxin A (onabotulinum toxin A or BoNT-A) injections have efficacy in the preventive treatment of chronic, but not episodic, migraine headaches. Studies have revealed a significant reduction in headache and migraine days, moderate to severe headache days, cumulative headache hours on headache days, and psychological distress and an increase in patients' functioning, vitality, and overall health-related quality of life with the use of botox [65].

The exact mechanism by which BoNT-A reduces migraine days in chronic migraineurs is not yet fully understood. While it was initially thought that BoNT-A may exert positive effects in primary headache disorders by the relaxation of spasmed muscles in the head and neck region, botox has no beneficial effect on tension-type headaches. BoNT-A may directly inhibit peripheral sensitization, thereby indirectly reducing central sensitization, which is central to chronic migraine. The effectiveness of BoNT-A in chronic migraine, as opposed to negative findings in episodic migraine, may relate to the fact that sensitization phenomena play a more important role in chronic versus episodic migraine [65]. Common side effects of botox may include elevated blood pressure, headache, facial paresis, and neck pain/stiffness [91].

Biologic agents Erenumab, galcanezumab fremanezumab, and eptinezumab are human monoclonal antibodies (mAbs) that inhibit calcitonin gene-related peptide (CGRP) receptor activity, which is involved in the etiology of migraine. Erenumab binds to and inhibits the CGRP receptor, and is given by monthly subcutaneous (SQ) injection. Galcanezumab and fremanzumab bind to and inhibit the CGRP ligand, and are given subcutaneously monthy (galcanezumab) or quarterly (fremanezumab). Eptinezumab binds the CGRP ligand and is given as an IV infusion every 3 months. Monoclonal antibodies seem to act faster than other preventative medications for chronic migraine. Fremanezumab reached a significant difference from placebo after only 3 days for daily headache hours. Migraine headache days were clearly reduced and separated from placebo in week two. MAbs have been shown to reduce migraine frequency, the use of abortive medications, and the effects of migraines on daily activities for a 6-month period [92]. In addition to rapid onset and proven efficacy, titration is not needed. Antibodies may also be an alternative for patients who do not tolerate available medication due to substance-specific adverse events [93]. Low-frequency administration of mAbs compared with current oral medication could improve therapy adherence, a problematic issue in migraine prevention [94]. Doses of subcutaneous medications can be self-administered. Given that there is little to no data at present regarding safety with pregnancy and lactation, or concerning long term effects, caution may be indicated in the use of these medications in young women.

Dietary intervention and elimination diets There is growing evidence in favor of food elimination diets to help with migraine prevention and the elimination of migraine triggers. Dietary intervention and simple measures such as the elimination of caffeine can sometimes render patients headache-free. In other cases, the frequency and severity of headaches are lessened, as is the need for preventive and abortive therapies [94]. Alcohol, chocolate, aged cheeses, caffeine, nuts, nitrites/nitrates, aspartame, and monosodium glutamate have all been associated with migraines; therefore, educating patients about these foods is imperative [25]. There is some evidence that keto diets or vegan diets help a subset of patients.

Elimination diets have the goal of looking for specific triggers which vary from person to person. Elimination diets work by eliminating a long list of potential offenders from the diet and gradually adding each food back one at a time as tolerated. The elimination is best attempted with the support and guidance of professionals: patients with frequent, chronic, or severe migraine attacks may benefit from referral to a neurologist and nutritionist as appropriate [95]. Many resources for patient education are available through the National Headache Foundation https://headaches.org/ [96], the American Migraine Foundation https://americanmigrainefoundation.org/ [97], and the Migraine Research Foundation https://migraineresearchfoundation.org/ [98].

Jennifer is counseled on options for preventive therapy and guidelines for the use of abortive medication. She is instructed that abortive medications should be used for less than 10 days per month. Given her current headache frequency and her desire to lose weight (BMI 32), topiramate is prescribed for preventative therapy.

After 6 months, Jennifer returns for a follow-up. The topiramate initially helped reduce her migraine frequency to only once or twice a month, but she has recently noticed that the most severe headaches consistently occur right before the onset of her menses. She has been taking a triphasic combined oral contraceptive for 3 months and is concerned that migraines can be associated with menses. She is concerned about overusing her triptan and NSAIDs based on your previous counseling and wants to know if she should come off her birth control pill.

Migraines: Hormones, Contraceptives, and Risk of Stroke

Migraines in most women are affected by hormones: the woman's intrinsic hormonal cycles and externally given hormones. Up to two-thirds of women with migraine headaches report worsening of headaches in association with menses [99, 100], and headaches associated with the onset of menses can be more severe and more refractory to treatment than migraines not associated with menses. Important issues in patient care include the diagnosis and treatment of menstrual migraines, the safe use of contraceptives in women with migraines with aura (MWA) and migraines without aura (MWOA), and the risk of stroke in migraineurs both with and without the use of hormonal contraception.

Estrogen-Withdrawal Headaches

Migraines that worsen in response to estrogen withdrawal can occur either at the start of a woman's natural menstrual cycle or with withdrawal from exogenous estrogen products, such as the placebo week, during which the birth control pills lack active hormones [101]. In patients taking combined hormonal contraceptives (COC) containing at least 20–25 mcg of estrogen, the placebo week is physiologically equivalent to the withdrawal of estrogen seen in naturally occurring menses [100, 102]. In the case of exogenous estrogen withdrawal, an estrogen-associated or menstrual migraine would be defined as occurring within 5 days of cessation of exogenous estrogen which had been taken for ≥3 weeks, with the headache lasting no more than 3 days.

Menstrually Associated Migraines (MAM)

Menstrually associated migraines (MAM) MAMs are migraines which specifically occur prior to the beginning of menses. MAMs are not associated with aura, and can be more severe, more difficult to treat, longer in duration, and more strongly associated with functional disability than other migraines [101, 103]. Migraines often increase in frequency and/or severity in the perimenopausal period, possibly due to fluctuating estrogen levels [104]. Migraines tend to improve during pregnancy and after menopause. Some studies have shown an improvement in migraine frequency after natural menopause more so than with surgical menopause, but this is not definitive [105].

MAMs occur within the 2 days prior to menses and 3 days after the onset of menses, in at least 2 out of 3 menses cycles. Patients with MAM can have migraines with or without aura at other times of the menstrual cycle. Less commonly, some women have pure *menstrual migraines*, and only have headaches in association with menses [106].

Treatment strategies for MAMs include both abortive and preventive measures. Abortive treatment options for estrogen-associated migraines are similar to non-estrogen-associated migraines, including the use of triptans and NSAIDs (Tables 28.1, 28.2, 28.3, and 28.4). A strategy used in patients with MAMs is to use a long-acting triptan for short-term prophylaxis. Frovatriptan, naratriptan, or zolmitriptan can be used twice a day starting 1–3 days prior to menses and continued for a total of 5–7 days. Studies have shown that administering frovatriptan 1 day prior to the onset of a patient's typical estrogen-associated migraine at a dose of 2.5 mg daily for 5–6 days increased the headache-free duration for patients [28]. Preventative strategies for MAM should include both pharmacologic and non-pharmacologic interventions, as are used in the management of non-estrogen-associated migraines. Hormonal treatments which stabilize and prevent declines in estrogen levels can also be used to combat MAM in selected patients.

Hormonal treatments in menstrually associated migraines (MAMs). The goal of hormone treatments in MAM is to prevent the withdrawal of estrogen that precipitates MAM [101, 107]. It should be noted that MAM is most often not associated with aura, and thus, hormonal contraceptives can be used without concern for increased stroke risk if women have pure *menstrual migraines*, or have MWOA at other times during the cycle. Women who have migraines with aura at other times of the month are discussed below. To prevent MAM, the placebo days for most combined oral contraceptive (COC) options should be minimized in order to reduce migraine frequency. Interventions that can be beneficial include:

- Use of low-dose (10–20 mg ethinyl estradiol (EE)) combined monophasic contraceptives instead of triphasic formulations
- Add back estrogen during the menstrual phase so that the patient has only 2 days of placebo pills
- Use of continuous low-dose combined monophasic contraceptives with a placebo week every 12 weeks
- Use of a vaginal ring for contraception that is changed every 3 weeks to avoid a hormone-free week

For example, if using a COC as preventative therapy for hormone-associated migraines, continuous use of a monophasic COC and skipping the placebo week will prevent the withdrawal of estrogen, which would ordinarily trigger headaches in women with MAM. Progestin does not control estrogen level fluctuations or reliably suppress ovulation; thus, progestin-only treatment options (including oral, injectable, and intrauterine devices) are not an effective method for preventing MAM [108].

Jennifer is diagnosed with menstrually associated migraines, and does not have an aura. She is instructed to discuss with her gynecologist changing from a triphasic to a continuous low-dose monophasic combined oral contraceptive, with a placebo week every 12 weeks. She has a significant reduction in her migraine frequency at 6 months follow-up after changing her contraceptive to the suggested regimen.

Contraceptives in Women with Migraines With and Without Aura and Risk of Stroke

Rena is a healthy 35-year-old woman who has chronic migraines without aura. Her migraines have been well controlled on daily amitriptyline and botox injections every 3 months. She does not use tobacco products and has no history of vascular disease. She now has a partner and would like to be started on contraception. She read that birth control pills can cause strokes in women with migraines and wants to discuss options.

Migraine with and without aura may be an independent risk factor for stroke (with or without contraception use), and assessing women for the presence of comorbidities that increase ischemic stroke risk must be done prior to starting an estrogen-containing contraceptive or combined oral contraceptive (COC) [109]. Given the efficacy of long-acting reversible contraception and the lack of estrogen in their preparations, the contraceptive of choice for many migraine patients is a copper or levonorgestrel IUD [100, 110, 111]. (See Chap. 4 on Patient-Centered Contraceptive Counseling.) In migraine patients taking anticonvulsants for prophylaxis, including topiramate, primidone, oxcarbazepine, barbiturate, and phenytoin, the metabolism of estrogen can be increased, reducing the efficacy of oral combined hormonal contraception. IUDs or other progesterone-based contraceptives do not have a reduction in efficacy with the addition of anticonvulsants and should be encouraged [111, 112].

Quantifying the Risk of Migraine and Stroke

The data associating migraines with an increased risk of stroke suggests that migraine with aura (MWA) carries a higher risk than migraines without aura (MWOA). Quantifying the risk of using estrogen-containing contraceptives in women with migraine has been problematic: studies have not reliably differentiated between those taking high-dose estrogen preparations (50 or greater micrograms of EE) from those taking the low-dose formulations commonly in use today (35 micrograms or less EE). Overall, the respective odds ratios (OR) of ischemic stroke varies by study population and is reported as OR of 2.89, 95% CI 2.42–3.45 in patients with any type of migraine [3, 113, 114]; OR 1.29, 95% CI 0.81–2.06 in MWOA; and OR 2.51, 95% CI 1.52–4.14 in those who have MWA [113, 114]. For comparison sake, the odds ratio of stroke is approximately 2 in those who smoke cigarettes. The absolute rate of stroke in patients with migraines, however, is very low at 17–19 per 100,000 woman years [113].

Importantly, while the relative risk for ischemic stroke in all patients with migraines who use COCs is reported as increased [115], most studies in the past involved patients taking higher doses of estrogen than are present in the COC preparations used today. A meta-analysis that reviewed studies from 1960 to 1999 demonstrated an increased relative risk of ischemic stroke of 1.6 (95% CI 1.4–1.8), in female patients (without migraines) using COC regimens with higher doses of estrogen (50 micrograms or more of ethinyl estradiol). Subgroup analysis from this same study showed no increased risk of stroke in patients taking progestin-only forms of contraception [116]. Current COCs use lower doses of estrogen, between 10 and 30 micrograms of ethinyl estradiol; therefore, further data is needed to assess the risk of dose with modern COC formulations. Recent studies performed with lower-estrogen-dose COC preparations, including hormonal contraceptive patches, vaginal rings, or COC pills, have shown lower odds ratios than those previously published [116].

Specifically, the 2015 Cochrane Review found that in female patients without stroke, the use of COCs containing 20mcg of ethinyl estrogen was associated with a more moderate increased risk of ischemic stroke (RR 1.6, 95% CI 1.4–1.8) [117]. However, given the potential devastating effects of stroke, prior to starting a patient on combined hormonal contraceptives, one should assess additional risk factors for stroke, which include, but are not limited to, age > 35 years, known ischemic heart disease, dyslipidemia, hypertension, obesity (BMI > 30), and systemic diseases associated with increased stroke incidence, cigarette smoking, a family history of arterial disease at <45 years of age, and diabetes mellitus. Patients with migraines with or without aura who have risk factors for stroke should preferentially be prescribed nonhormonal or progestin-only contraceptives [118].

Contraception in Migraines without Aura

The Centers for Disease Control (CDC) Contraception 2016 Medical Eligibility Criteria state that patients with migraine without aura are eligible for all types of contraception, including copper IUD, levonorgestrel IUD, progestin implants, progestin injections, progestin-only contraception pills, or combined hormonal contraception (with no limitations based on patient age) [110]. In patients with aura, the safety of contraception use is more controversial with the CDC recommending progestin-only contraception options.

Table 28.5 lists recommendations for COC use in patients with migraines without aura based on various societal guidelines. For example, the CDC recommends COC in migraine without aura patients who are <35 and without stroke risk factors. However, for patients >35 years old and with stroke risk factors, their recommendation is to weigh the risks of stroke and to discuss alternative contraceptive options with patients [110]. ACOG similarly permits COC use in patients with migraines without aura but emphasizes that all patients should be individually assessed for stroke risk. All guidelines agree that patients over 35 years of age should be individually assessed for risk. Women found to have risk factors for stroke should generally avoid estrogen-containing contraceptives. The major risk factors include hypertension, obesity (BMI > 30), diabetes, hyperlipidemia, cigarette smokers, history of CAD, and history of DVT/PE, sickle cell disease, and connective tissue disorders [118–120].

Zoe is a 39-year-old woman who presents to your clinic to establish care. She does not use tobacco, has no personal or family history of vascular disease or hypercoagulable disorder, and exercises regularly. Her past medical history is significant for migraines with aura. She has no complaints today and is requesting a refill of her COC pills. The pills were prescribed 5 years ago by her gynecologist, and she is asking if the pills are the safest form of contraception for her

Contraception in Migraines with Aura

Systematic reviews have shown that patients with migraines with aura (MWA), without hormone use, have approximately a twofold increased risk for ischemic stroke [122, 123]. A case-control study analyzing a large healthcare claims database of women aged 15–49 who had suffered a stroke between 2006 and 2012 found a cumulative incidence of stroke to be 11/100,000 females. The respective odds ratios (OR) of ischemic stroke were migraine with aura using combined oral contraceptives COC, OR = 6.1 (95% CI 3.1–12.1); migraine with aura without COC, OR = 2.7 (95% CI 1.9–3.7); migraine without aura using COC, OR = 1.9 (95% CI 1.1–2.9); and migraine without aura and without COC, OR = 2.2 (95% CI 1.9–2.7). The study concluded that compared to the general population, all migraine patients had a slightly increased risk of stroke. The risk of stroke was slightly increased in patients who had migraine with aura and in patients who had migraine without aura but were taking COCs. The risk of stroke was highest among patients who had migraines with aura and who were also taking COCs [123]. For this reason, it has been recommended that COCs should continue to be avoided in patients with MWA.

The Women's Health Study found that aura frequency was associated with stroke risk: aura <1/month had a twofold increase in stroke risk, versus frequency 1/week which had a fourfold increase in stroke incidence. It has been suggested that excellent preventive care with a decreased incidence of

Table 28.5 Summary table of society recommendations for combined hormonal contraceptive use in patients with *Migraine without aura* [110–112, 118, 120, 121]

Patient characteristics	ACOG 2019 [118]	Centers for Disease Control 2016 [110]	International Headache Society 2000 [112]	American Headache Society 2019 [121]	World Health Organization 2018 [111]	European Headache Federation 2017 [120]
<35 years No risk factors for ischemic stroke	No contraindication to COC use[b]	No contraindication for COC use	No contraindication to COC use	No contraindication to COC use	No contraindication to COC use	Can use COC with <35mcg of EE. Benefits and risks of contraception must be considered
≥35 years No risk factors for ischemic stroke	Individually assess risk of stroke	Risks and benefits of COC use should be weighed against stroke risk factors	No contraindication for COC use	Individually assess risk of stroke	Individually assess risk of stroke . Consider non-estrogen-containing options	Can use COC with <35mcg of EE. Benefits and risks of contraception must be considered
Patients with risk factors for stroke[a]	Individually assess risk of stroke	Risks and benefits of COC use should be weighed against stroke risk factors	Individually assess risk of stroke . Consider use of progestin-only methods in patients with uncontrolled risk factors for stroke or who are current smokers	Individually assess risk of stroke . Low-dose formulations of COCs (EE < 50mcg) can be considered	Individually assess risk of stroke Consider non-estrogen-containing options	Suggest nonhormonal or progestin-only methods of contraception

[a]Risk factors for stroke: hypertension, obesity (BMI > 30), diabetes, hyperlipidemia, cigarette smoking, history of coronary artery disease, history of deep venous thrombosis or pulmonary embolism, sickle cell disease, and connective tissue disorders
[b]*COC* combined oral contraceptives, *ACOG* American College of Obstetricians and Gynecologists

migraines with aura could also decrease a patient's risk for ischemic stroke, but no clinical data yet supports that theory [107].

Ultimately, given the evidence that migraines with aura independently increase the risk of stroke, the use of COCs remains controversial in this population. Table 28.6 summarizes society guidelines for the use of COC in patients with migraines with auras. All of the societies discourage the use of estrogen-containing contraceptive preparations in all women who have migraine with aura. The International Headache Society might seem the most permissive; however, their recommendation is that all women be individually assessed for risk of stroke.

The use of estrogen-containing contraception in women with migraines with aura is currently not recommended by the major societies listed in Table 6. More research on the use of low-dose COC (<35 mcg of EE) in women with MWA is needed to define risks of harm and benefit [124]. This topic is controversial, and some experts suggest that in a healthy patient without additional stroke risk factors, low-dose estrogen-containing contraceptive options (i.e., < 20 mcg) could be considered. If the patient's migraines are associated with menses, the benefit from the suppression of ovulation and stabilization of estrogen levels might outweigh any additional risk [125]. Other experts suggest that the use of estrogen-containing oral contraceptives should be based on an individualized assessment of risks and benefits, including the frequency of migraine with aura attacks, the relation of migraines to menses, and the presence of additional risk factors for stroke. Arguments in favor of the safety of COC in MWA include that risk of stroke with combined contraceptive use is lower than the risk of stroke with pregnancy, which increases to 34 strokes per 100,000 deliveries [116], and that there is a paucity of data regarding the risk of stroke in patients with MWA taking COCs with low-dose estrogen content. Until more safety data are available, given that there are effective non-estrogen contraceptive options, estrogen use must be used with caution in women with MWA.

Zoe returns with a severe headache which she describes as "the worst headache of her life." She is in the third trimester of her first pregnancy. She lost her balance, fell, and hit her head on the cement this morning, but was not concerned at the time. Vital signs include HR of 93 and BP of 168/102. She has no fever, papilledema, or rash, but she feels unsteady on her feet. She is sent to the emergency room for urgent evaluation and treatment.

Table 28.6 Summary of society recommendations for combined oral contraceptive use in patients with *Migraine with aura* [110–112, 118, 120, 121]

Patient characteristics	ACOG 2019 [118]	Centers for Disease Control 2016 [110]	International Headache Society 2000 [112]	American Headache Society 2019 [121]	World Health Organization 2018 [111]	European Headache Federation 2017 [120]
Patients less than 35 years of age	Consider progestin-only or nonhormonal forms of contraception in women with focal neurologic signs or symptoms	Use of COC contraindicated. Progestin-only or nonhormonal options approved	Low-dose estrogen-containing contraception may be prescribed in women who have simple visual aura	Individually assess risk of stroke	Use of COC contraindicated. Progestin-only or nonhormonal options approved	Suggest nonhormonal or progestin-only methods of contraception
Patients 35 years of age or older	Consider progestin-only or nonhormonal forms of contraception in women with focal neurologic signs or symptoms	Use of COC contraindicated. Progestin-only or nonhormonal options approved	Low-dose estrogen-containing contraception may be prescribed in women who have simple visual aura	Individually assess risk of stroke	Use of COC contraindicated. Progestin-only or nonhormonal options approved	Suggest nonhormonal or progestin-only methods of contraception
Patients with risk factors for stroke[a]	Consider progestin-only or nonhormonal forms of contraception	Use of COC contraindicated. Progestin-only or nonhormonal options approved	Use of COC contraindicated	Individually assess risk of stroke	Use of COC contraindicated. Progestin-only or nonhormonal options approved	Suggest nonhormonal or progestin-only methods of contraception.

[a]Risk factors for stroke: hypertension, obesity (BMI > 30), diabetes, hyperlipidemia, cigarette smoking, history of coronary artery disease, history of deep venous thrombosis or pulmonary embolism, sickle cell disease, and connective tissue disorders
COC combined oral contraceptives, *ACOG* American College of Obstetricians and Gynecologists

Secondary Headaches

In contrast to primary headaches, secondary headaches are those caused by separate underlying conditions. The most common etiologies listed include trauma, vascular pathology, intracranial abnormalities, and medication overuse headaches.

Medication Overuse Headache Disorder

Medication overuse headache refers to headaches that occur more than 15 days per month, for at least 3 months consecutively, in a person with a preexisting primary headache disorder, in conjunction with overuse of an acute symptomatic headache medication on between 10 and 15 days per month depending on the medication. The headache usually resolves with the withdrawal of the offending agent, although it may take months to see improvement. When acetaminophen or NSAIDS are used >15 days/month, this diagnosis is likely. Combination pain relievers containing acetaminophen/butalbital/caffeine can lead to caffeine withdrawal headaches if used >10 days/month. High caffeine intake can lead to caffeine withdrawal headaches, and this is a common cause of first trimester headaches in newly pregnant women who discontinue coffee consumption. (Box 28.5).

Box 28.5 Secondary Headache Subtypes and Differential Diagnosis: International Classification of Headache Disorders (ICHD-3) [3]

- Headache attributed to trauma or injury to the head and/or neck (e.g. whiplash, traumatic brain injury.)
- Headache attributed to cranial and/or cervical vascular disorder (e.g. AVM, non-traumatic intracerebral hemorrhage, giant cell arteritis, sinus venous thrombosis, cervical artery dissection.)
- Headache attributed to nonvascular intracranial disorder (e.g. neoplasm, idiopathic intracranial hypertension.)
- Headache attributed to a substance or its withdrawal
- Headache attributed to infection (e.g. intracranial infection such as meningitis or encephalitis, or systemic infection)
- Headache attributed to disorder of homeostasis (e.g. high altitude headache, sleep apnea headache, arterial hypertension)
- Headache or facial pain attributed to disorder of the cranium, neck, eyes, ears, nose, sinuses, teeth, mouth, or other facial or cranial structure (e.g. temporomandibular joint disease, acute angle closure glaucoma, acute or chronic rhinosinusitis, cervical strain)

- Headache attributed to psychiatric disorder
- Headache Classification Committee of the International Headache Society (IHS). The International Classification of Headache Disorders, 3rd edition. Cephalalgia 38(1), pp. 1–211. Copyright © 2018 by International Headache Society. Reprinted and revised by permission of SAGE Publications, Ltd.

Evaluation of Secondary Headaches

In the evaluation of headaches, signs and symptoms may suggest that an underlying disorder is responsible for the headache. Assessment is made as to whether imaging, lumbar pucture, blood cultures, blood tests, or urgent treatment is required. "Red flags" for all headaches include age > 45 with no prior history of headaches, headache onset with sexual activity, altered mental status, recent trauma, focal abnormality on neurologic exam, findings associated with increased intracranial pressure (i.e., papilledema, pulsatile tinnitus, pain worsening with supine position), first or worst headache of life, pain reaching maximal intensity within seconds to minutes, or systemic symptoms such as fever, abnormal vital signs, or weight loss [126]. Patients who are immunosuppressed or HIV positive have an increased risk of intracranial infection. Papilledema can be a sign of benign intracranial hypertension which is more common in pregnancy or of increased intracranial pressure from a mass or cerebral venous thrombosis.

When Should Imaging Be Performed?

Most headaches can be diagnosed and treated based on history and clinical exam alone. However, imaging should be considered for patients with any "red flag" signs or symptoms to evaluate for underlying secondary causes. Neuroimaging is 98.6% sensitive for diagnosing intracranial pathology in patients with focal neurologic findings on physical examination, the onset of headaches > age 45, or sudden onset of headache [127]. Imaging with CT or MRI is indicated in the following settings: patients who are unresponsive to adequate headache treatment, concern for meningitis (prior to lumbar puncture), positional headaches, symptoms suggestive of cluster headaches or other trigeminal autonomic cephalgias, and headaches located in the temporal region in older adults (in addition to ESR and biopsy). Patients who are pregnant, are immunocompromised, or have a systemic illness including a hypercoagulable disorder should also be imaged [128]. Patients who lack "red flag" signs or symptoms rarely require imaging: neuroimaging reveals a clinically significant intracranial lesion in only 0.18% of cases without concerning features [86].

When imaging is indicated, MRI of the brain with contrast remains the preferred brain imaging modality as it is more sensitive at detecting edema, vascular lesions, or other intracranial pathology than CT scans. CT imaging is used more frequently in the acute setting, such as the emergency department, as it has higher sensitivity to detect acute blood or bony trauma [129].

Zoe is taken to the emergency room, and an emergent noncontrast CT scan is performed. Blood pressure is controlled with intravenous medication, and the fetus is monitored. The CT shows a subdural hematoma which is evacuated by neurosurgery. The mother and fetus tolerate surgery well and are discharged after several days without complication. One month later, Zoe delivers a healthy baby girl.

Summary Points

1. Tension-type headaches typically present as bilateral headaches that are mild to moderate in intensity and are often described by patients as having a "band-like pressure or tightness." Cluster headaches usually present with severe "stabbing" pain that is unilateral, and typically focused in the retro-orbital and periorbital regions. Cluster Headaches classically have associated ipsilateral lacrimation. Most recurring headaches in the primary care setting are migraine headaches.
2. Lifestyle modifications and abortive therapy with triptans and NSAIDS are first-line treatments in acute migraines. NSAIDs with triptans may have a synergistic component and are often used together. Preventative treatments should be considered with >4 migraines/month. First-line agents include tricyclic antidepressants, anticonvulsants, and beta-blockers. The identification and avoidance of triggers are important in the management of migraines. Multimodal management is needed for patients with frequent, severe, or chronic migraines.
3. Menstrual or estrogen-associated migraines refer to migraine attacks that occur in the absence of or decline of estrogen, after having been previously exposed to higher levels of estrogen. Preventative strategies may include an evaluation of the patient's current method of contraception and consideration of hormone treatment options.
4. Migraines with aura are associated with an increased risk of stroke, but the absolute risk is very low.

5. The use of combined oral contraceptives (COCs) should be carefully considered in patients with migraines, especially migraines with auras. Current guidelines recommend against using COCs in patients with migraines who have risks for stoke and in any patient with migraines with aura.
6. Secondary headache disorders are caused by underlying conditions such as allergic rhinitis, trauma, vascular pathology, and other intracranial abnormalities. Imaging should be considered for patients with "red flag" symptoms, focal neurologic findings, age > 45–50 with new onset headache, or sudden/worst headache of life.

Review Questions

1. A 45-year-old woman presents for worsening headaches. The headaches are pulsating in quality, unilateral, and associated with photophobia. She denies any symptoms of aura. She notices the headaches most commonly around her menses, but the headaches occur at other times, especially when she has increased stress. She had infrequent migraines in the past which were successfully treated with naproxen. Her current migraines occur 1–2 times per month. She does not smoke. In addition to counsel regarding stress, triggers, and musculoskeletal components of head pain, which intervention is the best next step to help her headaches?
   A. Placement of copper IUD
   B. Prescription of long-acting triptans in the perimenstrual period
   C. Initiation of a triphasic combined hormonal contraceptive (COC) pill
   D. Behavioral modifications including help with stress management
   The correct answer is B. The patient has a diagnosis of menstrually associated migraine (or MAM). Treatment options for MAM include both standard abortive and preventative treatments for migraines: triptans and lifestyle modifications, and prevention of the estrogen withdrawal that occurs during menses. Placement of copper IUD will not improve her migraines which are partly related to hormonal changes. She has already attempted interventions to reduce stress, so behavioral modification for stress management is not the correct next step. A monophasic COC is preferred over triphasic COCs in estrogen-associated or pure menstrual migraines, in order to maintain a steady dose of estrogen [106, 107].
2. A 24-year-old woman presents to clinic to establish care. Her past medical history is notable only for migraine headaches without aura, with no recent change in frequency or severity. Her only medication is a combined oral contraceptive, for which she is requesting a refill. Her BMI is 23, and she is normotensive on physical exam. She denies smoking, or any personal or family history of stroke, cardiovascular disease, blood clots, or diabetes. What is her best contraceptive option?
   A. Recommend stopping combined hormonal contraceptive pill due to increased stroke risk in women who take combined hormonal contraceptives.
   B. Refill her combined hormonal contraceptive pill.
   C. Inform her that due to increased stroke risk with migraines, she can only use progestin-only or barrier method contraception options.
   D. Consider continuing her oral contraceptive, but counsel the patient on stroke risk factors and the importance of letting you know if she develops aura with her migraines.
   The correct answer is D. Recent evidence has demonstrated that patients with migraines without auras do not have an increased risk of stroke and can receive combined hormonal contraceptive pills if there are no other contraindications or increased stroke risk. She should be screened for additional stroke risk factors and counseled on the importance of letting her provider know if she develops auras with her migraines which carry an increased risk of stroke [122, 123].
3. A 51-year-old woman with a past medical history of essential hypertension, dyslipidemia, and hypothyroidism presents for her annual well-woman exam. You notice on her intake worksheet that she checked the box for headaches. She states that she has recently noticed intermittent headaches with sexual activity. She describes the headaches as intense, throbbing pain, located in the back of her head, with a rapid onset of minutes after sexual activity. The headaches last for a half-hour and then resolve spontaneously. She becomes nauseous with the headaches and has to lie very still when they occur. The headaches have only occurred three times, so she didn't know if it was necessary to discuss. Physical exam is notable for a blood pressure of 163/92 and BMI of 31. Neurologic exam is unremarkable. What is the next best step in her care?
   A. Monitor her symptoms and pursue further evaluation if her headaches worsen in frequency or quality.
   B. Order neuroimaging to evaluate for underlying intracranial pathology.
   C. Discuss that her uncontrolled hypertension is likely the cause of her headaches.
   D. Refer her for a neurology consult.
   The correct answer is B. The patient has new onset of headaches at >50 years of age, with intense pain, rapid onset, and association with sexual activity (i.e., exertion). She should undergo neuroimaging to rule out an underlying intracranial cause of her headaches, given her "red flag" "symptoms. Her uncontrolled hypertension could

be the cause of her symptoms, but intracranial pathologies, including intracranial bleed, must be excluded. Referring her to neurology is also likely appropriate, but she requires urgent evaluation and imaging given her concerning presentation [126, 127].

References

1. GBD 2016 Headache Collaborators. Global, regional, and national burden of migraine and tension-type headache, 1990–2016: a systematic analysis for the Global Burden of Disease Study 2016. Lancet Neurol. 2017;17(11):954–76.
2. Saylor D, Steiner TJ. The global burden of headache. Semin Neurol. 2018;38(2):182–90.
3. ICHD-3: Headache Classification Committee of the International Headache Society (IHS). The International Classification of Headache Disorders, 3rd edition. Cephalalgia. 2018;38:1.
4. Karli N, Zarifoglu M, Calisir N, Akgoz S. Comparison of pre-headache phases and trigger factors of migraine and episodic tension-type headache: do they share similar clinical pathophysiology? Cephalalgia. 2005;25(6):444.
5. Jensen RH. Tension-type headache – the normal and most prevalent headache. Headache. 2018;58(2):33.
6. Aaseth K, Grande RB, Lundqvist C, Russell MB. Pericranial tenderness in chronic tension-type headache: the Akershus population-based study of chronic headache. J Headache Pain. 2014;15:58. https://doi.org/10.1186/1129-2377-15-58.
7. Fernández-De-Las-Peñas C, Cuadrado ML, Pareja JA. Myofascial trigger points, neck mobility, and forward head posture in episodic tension-type headache. Headache. 2007; https://doi.org/10.1111/j.1526-4610.2006.00632.
8. Morris L, editor. Comprehensive review of headache medicine: Oxford University Press; 2008.
9. Bendtsen L, Jensen R. Tension-type headache: the most common, but also the most neglected, headache disorder. Curr Opin Neurol. 2006;19(3):305–9.
10. Moore RA, Derry S, Wiffen PJ, et al. Evidence for efficacy of acute treatment of episodic tension-type headache: methodological critique of randomised trials for oral treatments. Pain. 2014;155:2220.
11. Bendtsen L, Evers S, Linde M, et al. EFNS guideline on the treatment of tension-type headache - report of an EFNS task force. Eur J Neurol. 2010;17:1318.
12. Holroyd KA, O'Donnell FJ, Stensland M, Lipchik GL, Cordingley GE, Carlson BW. Management of chronic tension-type headache with tricyclic antidepressant medication, stress management therapy, and their combination: a randomized controlled trial. JAMA. 2001;285(17):2208–15.
13. Jürgens TP. Comment: sex-specific differences in cluster headache. Neurology. 2017;88(11):1074 LP–1074. http://n.neurology.org/content/88/11/1074.abstract.
14. Obermann M, Holle D, Naegel S, Burmeister J, Diener HC. Pharmacotherapy options for cluster headache. Expert Opin Pharmacother. 2015;16(8):1177–84. https://doi.org/10.1517/14656566.2015.1040392.
15. May A, Schwedt TJ, Magis D, et al. Cluster headache. Nat Rev Dis Primers. 2018;4:18006.
16. Holle D, Obermann M. The role of neuroimaging in the diagnosis of headache disorders. Ther Adv Neurol Disord. 2013;6(6):369–74. https://doi.org/10.1177/1756285613489765.
17. May A, Leone M, Afra J, Linde M, Sándor PS, Evers S, Goadsby PJ, EFNS Task Force. EFNS guidelines on the treatment of cluster headache and other trigeminal-autonomic cephalalgias. Eur J Neurol. 2006;13(10):1066–77.
18. Charles AM. Migraine: clinical practice. N Engl J Med. 2017;377(6):553–61. https://doi.org/10.1056/NEJMcp1605502.
19. Vetvig KG, MacGregor EA. Sex differences in the epidemiology, clinical features, and pathophysiology of migraine. Lancet Neurol. 2017;16(1):76–87.
20. Charles A, Hansen JM. Migraine aura: new ideas about cause, classification, and clinical significance. Curr Opin Neurol. 2015;28(3):255–60. https://doi.org/10.1097/WCO.0000000000000193.
21. Vecchia D, Pietrobon D. Migraine: a disorder of brain excitatory-inhibitory balance? Trends Neurosci. 2012;35(8):507–20. https://doi.org/10.1016/j.tins.2012.04.007.
22. Magis D, Vigano A, Sava S, D'Elia TS, Schoenen J, Coppola G. Pearls and pitfalls: electrophysiology for primary headaches. Cephalalgia. 2013;33(8):526–39. https://doi.org/10.1177/0333102413477739.
23. Charles A. The evolution of a migraine attack - a review of recent evidence. Headache. 2013;53(2):413–9. https://doi.org/10.1111/head.12026.
24. Pelzer N, Stam AH, Haan J, Ferrari MD, Terwindt GM. Familial and sporadic hemiplegic migraine: diagnosis and treatment. Curr Treat Options Neurol. 2013;15(1):13–27. https://doi.org/10.1007/s11940-012-0208-3.
25. Kelman L. The triggers or precipitants of the acute migraine attack. Cephalalgia. 2007;27(5):394–402.
26. Martin PR. Behavioral management of migraine headache triggers: learning to cope with triggers. Curr Pain Headache Rep. 2010;14(3):221–7. https://doi.org/10.1007/s11916-010-0112-z.
27. Burstein R, Jakubowski M, Rauch SD. The science of migraine. J Vestib Res. 2011;21(6):305–14. https://doi.org/10.3233/VES-2012-0433.
28. Silberstein SD, Holland S, Freitag F, et al. Evidence-based guideline update: pharmacologic treatment for episodic migraine prevention in adults: report of the Quality Standards Subcommittee of the American Academy of neurology and the American Headache Society. Neurology. 2012;78:1337.
29. Mauskop A. Nonmedication, alternative, and complementary treatments for migraine. Continuum (Minneap Minn). 2012;18(4):796–806. https://doi.org/10.1212/01.CON.0000418643.24408.40.
30. Cameron C, Kelly S, Hsieh SC, et al. Triptans in the acute treatment of migraine: a systematic review and network meta-analysis. Headache. 2015;55(Suppl 4):221–35. https://doi.org/10.1111/head.12601.
31. Nagy AJ, Gandhi S, Bhola R, Goadsby PJ. Intravenous dihydroergotamine for inpatientm management of refractory primary headaches. Neurology. 2011;77:1827–32.
32. Eller M, Gelfand AA, Riggins NY, Shiboski S, Schankin C, Goadsby PJ. Exacerbation of headache during dihydroergotamine for chronic migraine does not alter outcome. Neurology. 2016;86:856–9.
33. Derry S, Moore RA. Paracetamol (acetaminophen) with or without an antiemetic for acute migraine headaches in adults. Cochrane Database Syst Rev. 2013:CD008040.
34. Kirthi V, Derry S, Moore RA. Aspirin with or without an antiemetic for acute migraine headaches in adults. Cochrane Database Syst Rev. 2013:CD008041.
35. Goldstein J, Hagen M, Gold M. Results of a multicenter, double-blind, randomized, parallel-group, placebo-controlled, single-dose study comparing the fixed combination of acetaminophen, acetylsalicylic acid, and caffeine with ibuprofen for acute treatment of patients with severe migraine. Cephalalgia. 2014;34:1070–8.

36. Law S, Derry S, Moore RA. Sumatriptan plus naproxen for the treatment of acute migraine attacks in adults. Cochrane Database Syst Rev. 2016;4:CD008541.
37. Orr SL, Friedman BW, Christie S, et al. Management of adults with acute migraine in the emergency department: the American Headache Society evidence assessment of parenteral pharmacotherapies. Headache. 2016;56:911–40.
38. Lipton RB, Dodick DW, Silberstein SD, et al. Single-pulse transcranial magnetic stimulation for acute treatment of migraine with aura: a randomised, double-blind, parallel-group, sham-controlled trial. Lancet Neurol. 2010;9:373–80.
39. Marcus R, Goadsby PJ, Dodick D, Stock D, Manos G, Fischer TZ. BMS-927711 for the acute treatment of migraine: a double-blind, randomized, placebo controlled, dose-ranging trial. Cephalalgia. 2014;34:114–25.
40. Voss T, Lipton RB, Dodick DW, et al. A phase IIb randomized, double-blind, placebo-controlled trial of ubrogepant for he acute treatment ofof migraine. Cephalalgia. 2016;36:887–98.
41. Marmura MJ, Silberstein SD, Schwedt TJ. The acute treatment of migraine in adults: the american headache society evidence assessment of migraine pharmacotherapies. Headache. 2015;55(1):3–20. https://doi.org/10.1111/head.12499.
42. Worthington I, Pringsheim T, Gawel MJ, et al. Canadian Headache Society Guideline: acute drug therapy for migraine headache. Can J Neurol Sci. 2013;40(Suppl 3):S1–S80.
43. Evers S, Afra J, Frese A, et al. EFNS guideline on the drug treatment of migraine — revised report of an EFNS task force. Eur J Neurol. 2009;16:968–81.
44. MacGregor EA. In the clinic. Migraine. Ann Intern Med. 2013;159:ITC5.
45. Silberstein SD, Rosenberg J. Multispecialty consensus on diagnosis and treatment of headache. Neurology. 2000;54:1553.
46. Lipton RB, Buse DC, Serrano D, Holland S, Reed ML. Examination of unmet treatment needs among persons with episodic migraine: results of the American Migraine prevalence and prevention (AMPP) study. Headache. 2013;53(8):1300–11. https://doi.org/10.1111/head.12154.
47. Derry CJ, Derry S, Moore RA. Sumatriptan (all routes of administration) for acute migraine attacks in adults - overview of Cochrane reviews. Cochrane Database Syst Rev. 2014:CD009108.
48. Dara J. The safety of Triptans in the treatment of patients with migraine. Am J Med. 2002;12(2):135–40.
49. Raskin NH. Repetitive intravenous dihydroergotamine as therapy for intractable migraine. Neurology. 1986;36:995.
50. Rabbie R, Derry S, Moore RA. Ibuprofen with or without an antiemetic for acute migraine headaches in adults. Cochrane Database Syst Rev. 2013:CD008039.
51. Law S, Derry S, Moore RA. Naproxen with or without an antiemetic for acute migraine headaches in adults. Cochrane Database Syst Rev. 2013:CD009455.
52. Taggart E, Doran S, Kokotillo A, et al. Ketorolac in the treatment of acute migraine: a systematic review. Headache. 2013;53:277.
53. Lipton RB, Stewart WF, Ryan RE Jr, et al. Efficacy and safety of acetaminophen, aspirin, and caffeine in alleviating migraine headache pain: three double-blind, randomized, placebo-controlled trials. Arch Neurol. 1998;55:210.
54. American Headache Society – Acute Treatment of Migraine.: https://americanheadachesociety.org/wpcontent/uploads/2018/05/How_I_Do_It_Acute_Treatment.pdf.
55. Pfaffenrath V, Cunin G, Sjonell G, Prendergast S. Efficacy and safety of sumatriptan tablets (25 mg, 50 mg, and 100 mg) in the acute treatment of migraine: defining the optimum doses of oral sumatriptan. Headache. 1998;38:184.
56. Teall J, Tuchman M, Cutler N, et al. Rizatriptan (MAXALT) for the acute treatment of migraine and migraine recurrence. A placebo-controlled, outpatient study. Rizatriptan 022 Study Group. Headache. 1998;38:281.
57. Rapoport AM, Ramadan NM, Adelman JU, et al. Optimizing the dose of zolmitriptan (Zomig, 311C90) for the acute treatment of migraine. A multicenter, double-blind, placebo-controlled, dose range-finding study. The 017 Clinical Trial Study Group. Neurology. 1997;49:1210.
58. Mannix LK, Savani N, Landy S, et al. Efficacy and tolerability of naratriptan for short-term prevention of menstrually related migraine: data from two randomized, double-blind, placebo-controlled studies. Headache. 2007;47(7):1037–49.
59. Winner P, Ricalde O, Le Force B, et al. A double-blind study of subcutaneous dihydroergotamine vs subcutaneous sumatriptan in the treatment of acute migraine. Arch Neurol. 1996;53:180.
60. Gallagher RM. Acute treatment of migraine with dihydroergotamine nasal spray. Dihydroergotamine Working Group. Arch Neurol. 1996;53:1285.
61. Bigal ME, Bordini CA, Speciali JG. Intravenous chlorpromazine in the emergency department treatment of migraines: a randomized controlled trial. J Emerg Med. 2002;23:141.
62. BET 1: Metoclopramide or prochlorperazine for headache in acute migraine? Emerg Med J. 2013;30:595.
63. Friedman BW, Irizarry E, Solorzano C, et al. Randomized study of IV prochlorperazine plus diphenhydramine vs IV hydromorphone for migraine. Neurology. 2017;89:2075.
64. Goadsby PJ, Zanchin G, Geraud G, et al. Early vs. non-early intervention in acute migraine - "Act when Mild (AwM)." A double-blind, placebo-controlled trial of almotriptan. Cephalalgia. 2008;28(4):383–91. https://doi.org/10.1111/j.1468-2982.2008.01546.x.
65. Sprenger T, Viana M, Tassorelli C. Current prophylactic medications for migraine and their potential mechanisms of action. Neurotherapeutics. 2018;15(2):313–23. https://doi.org/10.1007/s13311-018-0621-8.
66. Pringsheim T, Davenport W, Mackie G, et al. Canadian Headache Society guideline for migraine prophylaxis. Can J Neurol Sci. 2012;39(Suppl 2):S1–S59.
67. Linde K, Rossnagel K. Propranolol for migraine prophylaxis. Cochrane Database Syst Rev. 2004;2:CD003225.
68. Stovner LJ, Linde M, Gravdahl GB, et al. A comparative study of candesartan versus propranolol for migraine prophylaxis: a randomised, triple-blind, placebo controlled, double cross-over study. Cephalalgia. 2014;34:523–32.
69. Linde M, Mulleners WM, Chronicle EP, McCrory DC. Topiramate for the prophylaxis of episodic migraine in adults. Cochrane Database Syst Rev. 2013;6:CD010610.
70. Linde M, Mulleners WM, Chronicle EP, McCrory DC. Valproate (valproic acid or sodium valproate or a combination of the two) for the prophylaxis of episodic migraine in adults. Cochrane Database Syst Rev. 2013:CD010611.
71. Tepper SJ. Nutraceutical and other modalities for the treatment of headache. Continuum (Minneap Minn). 2015;21(4 Headache):1018–31.
72. Aurora SK, Dodick DW, Turkel CC, et al. OnabotulinumtoxinA for treatment of chronic migraine: results from the double-blind, randomized, placebo-controlled phase of the PREEMPT 1 trial. Cephalalgia. 2010;30:793–803.
73. Schoenen J, Vandersmissen B, Jeangette S, et al. Migraine prevention with a supraorbital transcutaneous stimulator: a randomized controlled trial. Neurology. 2013;80:697–704.
74. Hou M, Xing H, Cai Y, et al. The effect and safety of monoclonal antibodies to calcitonin gene-related peptide and its receptor on migraine: a systematic review and meta-analysis. J Headache Pain. 2017;18:42.
75. Tepper S, Ashina M, Reuter U, et al. Safety and efficacy of erenumab for preventive treatment of chronic migraine: a randomised, double-blind, placebo-controlled phase 2 trial. Lancet Neurol. 2017;16:425–34.

76. Silberstein SD, Goadsby PJ. Migraine: preventive treatment. Cephalalgia. 2002;22:491.
77. Rosen JA. Observations on the efficacy of propranolol for the prophylaxis of migraine. Ann Neurol. 1983;13(1):92.
78. Shamliyan TA, Choi JY, Ramakrishnan R, Miller JB, Wang SY, Taylor FR, Kane RL. Preventive pharmacologic treatments for episodic migraine in adults. J Gen Intern Med. 2013;28(9):1225–37.
79. Schrader H, Stovner LJ, Helde G, Sand T, Bovim G. Prophylactic treatment of migraine with angiotensin converting enzyme inhibitor (lisinopril): randomised, placebo controlled, crossover study. BMJ. 2001;322(7277):19.
80. Tronvik E, Stovner LJ, Helde G, Sand T, Bovim G. Prophylactic treatment of migraine with an angiotensin II receptor blocker: a randomized controlled trial. JAMA. 2003;289(1):65.
81. Tfelt-Hansen P. Prophylactic pharmacotherapy of migraine. Some practical guidelines. Neurol Clin. 1997;15(1):153.
82. Schoenen J, Jacquy J, Lenaerts M. Effectiveness of high-dose riboflavin in migraine prophylaxis. A randomized controlled trial. Neurology. 1998;50:466.
83. Lipton RB, Göbel H, Einhäupl KM, et al. Petasites hybridus root (butterbur) is an effective preventive treatment for migraine. Neurology. 2004;63:2240.
84. Puledda F, Shields K. Non-pharmacological approaches for migraine. Neurotherapeutics. 2018;15(2):336–45. https://doi.org/10.1007/s13311-018-0623-6.
85. Pringsheim T, Ba WJD, Becker WJ. Prophylaxis of migraine headache review. Can Med Assoc. 2010;182(7):E269–76. https://doi.org/10.1503/cmaj.081657.
86. Solomon GD, Steel JG, Spaccavento LJ. Verapamil prophylaxis of migraine. A double-blind, placebo-controlled study. JAMA. 1983;250(18):2500.
87. Tronvik E, Stovner LJ, Helde G, et al. Prophylactic treatment of migraine with an angiotensin II receptor blocker: a randomized controlled trial. JAMA. 2003;289:65.
88. Peikert A, Wilimzig C, Köhne-Volland R. Prophylaxis of migraine with oral magnesium: results from a prospective, multi-center, placebo-controlled and double-blind randomized study. Cephalalgia. 1996;16:257.
89. Holland S, Silberstein SD, Freitag F, et al. Evidence-based guideline update: NSAIDs and other complementary treatments for episodic migraine prevention in adults: report of the Quality Standards Subcommittee of the American Academy of Neurology and the American Headache Society. Neurology. 2012;78:1346.
90. Hepp Z, Dodick DW, Varon SF, Gillard P, Hansen RN, Devine EB. Adherence to oral migraine-preventive medications among patients with chronic migraine. Cephalalgia. 2015;35(6):478–88. https://doi.org/10.1177/0333102414547138.
91. Coté TR, Mohan AK, Polder JA, et al. Botulinum toxin type A injections: adverse events reported to the US Food and Drug Administration in therapeutic and cosmetic cases. J Am Acad Dermatol. 2005;53(3):407–15.
92. Goadsby PJ, Reuter U, Hallström Y, et al. A controlled trial of Erenumab for episodic migraine. N Engl J Med. 2017;377:2123–32.
93. Lipton RB, Bigal ME, Diamond M, et al. Migraine prevalence, disease burden, and the need for preventive therapy. Neurology. 2007;68:343–9. https://doi.org/10.1212/01.wnl.0000252808.97649.21.
94. Raffaelli B, Reuter U. The biology of monoclonal antibodies: focus on calcitonin gene-related peptide for prophylactic migraine therapy. Neurotherapeutics. 2018;15(2):324–35. https://doi.org/10.1007/s13311-018-0622-7.
95. Orr SL. Diet and nutraceutical interventions for headache management: a review of the evidence. Cephalalgia. 2016;36(12):1112–33. https://doi.org/10.1177/0333102415590239.
96. National Headache Foundation. https://headaches.org/.
97. The American Migraine Foundation. https://americanmigrainefoundation.org/.
98. The Migraine Research Foundation. https://migraineresearchfoundation.org/.
99. Martin VT, Behbehani M. Ovarian hormones and migraine headache: understanding mechanisms and pathogenesis - part I. Headache. 2006;46(1):3–23.
100. Faubion SS, Batur P, Calhoun AH. Migraine throughout the female reproductive cycle. Mayo Clin Proc. 2018;93(5):639–45.
101. Brandes JL. The influence of estrogen on migraine: a systematic review. JAMA. 2006;295(15):1824–30.
102. https://americanheadachesociety.org/wp-content/uploads/2018/05/Vincent_Martin_-_Menstrual_Martin-1.pdf.
103. Johannes CB, Linet CB, Stewart WF, Celentano DD, Lipton RB, Szklo M. Relationship of headache to phase of the menstrual cycle among young women: a daily diary study. Neurology. 1995;45(6):1076–82.
104. MacGregor EA. Migraine headache in perimenopausal and menopausal women. Curr Pain Headache Rep. 2009;13(5):399–403.
105. Ripa P, Ornello R, Degan D, et al. Migraine in menopausal women: a systematic review. Int J Women's Health. 2015;7:773–82. https://doi.org/10.2147/IJWH.S70073.
106. Ashkenazi A, Silberstein S. Menstrual migraine: a review of hormonal causes, prophylaxis and treatment. Expert Opin Pharmacother. 2007;8(11):1605–13.
107. Calhoun AH. Menstrual migraine: update on pathophysiology and approach to therapy and management. Curr Treat Options Neurol. 2012;14(1):1–14. https://doi.org/10.1007/s11940-011-0153-6.
108. Somerville BW. The role of progesterone in menstrual migraine. Neurology. 1971;21:853. https://doi.org/10.1109/CCNC.2015.7157960.
109. Tepper NK, Whiteman MK, Zapata LB, Marchbanks PA, Curtis KM. Safety of hormonal contraceptives among women with migraine: a systematic review. Contraception. 2016;94(6):630–40. https://doi.org/10.1016/j.contraception.2016.04.016.
110. Centers for Disease Control and Prevention, Curtis KM, Tepper NK, Jatlaoui TC, et al. U.S. medical eligibility criteria for contraceptive use, 2016. MMWR Recomm Rep. 2016;65(RR-3):1–104. https://doi.org/10.15585/mmwr.rr6503a1.
111. Medical Eligibility Criteria for Contraceptive Use –World Health Organization Department of Reproductive Health and Research (WHO/RHR) and Johns Hopkins Bloomberg School of Public Health/Center for Communication Programs (CCP), Knowledge for Health Project. Family planning: a global handbook for providers (2018 update). Baltimore/Geneva: CCP and WHO; 2018. https://www.who.int/reproductivehealth/publications/fp-global-handbook/en/. Accessed 5/27/2019.
112. Bousser MG, Conard J, Kittner S, de Lignières B, MacGregor EA, Massiou H, Silberstein SD, Tzourio C. International Headache Society Taskforce. Recommendations on the risk of ischaemic stroke associated with use of combined oral contraceptives and hormone replacement therapy in women with migraine. Cephalalgia. 2000;20(3):155–6. https://doi.org/10.1046/j.1468-2982.2000.00035.x.
113. Spector JT, Kahn SR, Jones MR, Jayakumar M, Dalal D, Nazarian S. Migraine headache and ischemic stroke risk: an updated meta-analysis. Am J Med. 2010;123(7):612–24. https://doi.org/10.1016/j.amjmed.2009.12.021.
114. Kurth T, Chabriat H, Bousser MG. Migraine and stroke: a complex association with clinical implications. Lancet Neurol. 2012;11(1):92–100. https://doi.org/10.1016/S1474-4422(11)70266-6.
115. Gillum LA, Mamidipudi SK, Johnston SC. Ischemic stroke risk with oral contraceptives: a meta-analysis. JAMA. 2000;284(1):72–8. https://doi.org/10.1001/jama.284.1.72.

116. Carlton C, Banks M, Sundararajan S. Oral contraceptives and ischemic stroke risk. Stroke. 2018;49(4):e157–9. https://doi.org/10.1161/STROKEAHA.117.020084.
117. Roach REJ, Helmerhorst FM, Lijfering WM, Algra A, Dekkers OM. Combined oral contraceptives: the risk of myocardial infarction and ischemic stroke. Cochrane Database Syst Rev. 2014; https://doi.org/10.1002/14651858.CD011054.
118. ACOG practice bulletin No. 206: use of hormonal contraception in women with coexisting medical conditions. Obstet Gynecol. 2019;133(2):e128–50. https://doi.org/10.1097/AOG.0000000000003072.
119. Meschia JF, Bushnell C, Boden-Albala B, et al. American Heart Association Stroke Council; Council on Cardiovascular and Stroke Nursing; Council on Clinical Cardiology; Council on Functional Genomics and Translational Biology; Council on Hypertension. Guidelines for the primary prevention of stroke: a statement for healthcare professionals from the American heart association/American stroke association. Stroke. 2014;45(12):3754–832. https://doi.org/10.1161/STR.0000000000000046.
120. Sacco S, Merki-Feld GS, Ægidius KL, et al. Hormonal contraceptives and risk of ischemic stroke in women with migraine: a consensus statement from the European Headache Federation (EHF) and the European Society of Contraception and Reproductive Health (ESC) [published correction appears in J Headache Pain. 2018 Sep 10;19(1):81]. J Headache Pain. 2017;18(1):108. Published 2017 Oct 30. https://doi.org/10.1186/s10194-017-0815-1.
121. Hutchinson S. Use of oral contraceptives in women with migraine. Fact Sheets from American Headache Society: https://americanheadachesociety.org/resources/headache-fact-sheets/. Accessed 5/27/2019.
122. Calhoun AH, Batur P. Combined hormonal contraceptives and migraine: an update on the evidence. Cleve Clin J Med. 2017;84(8):631–8. https://doi.org/10.3949/ccjm.84a.16033.
123. Champaloux SW, Tepper NK, Monsour M, et al. Use of combined hormonal contraceptives among women with migraines and risk of ischemic stroke. Am J Obstet Gynecol. 2017;216(5):489.e1–7. https://doi.org/10.1016/j.ajog.2016.12.019.
124. Sheikh HU, Pavlovic J, Loder E, Burch R. Risk of stroke associated with use of estrogen containing contraceptives in women with migraine: a systematic review. Headache. 2018;58(1):5–21. https://doi.org/10.1111/head.13229.
125. Calhoun AH. Hormonal contraceptives and migraine with Aura—is there still a risk? Headache. 2017;57(2):184–93. https://doi.org/10.1111/head.12960.
126. Lynch KM, Brett F. Headaches that kill: a retrospective study of incidence, etiology and clinical features in cases of sudden death. Cephalalgia. 2012;32(13):972–8. https://doi.org/10.1177/0333102412455706.
127. Hale N, Paauw DS. Diagnosis and treatment of headache in the ambulatory care setting a review of classic presentations and new considerations in diagnosis and management. Med Clin North Am. 2014;98(3):505–27. https://doi.org/10.1016/j.mcna.2014.01.006.
128. Douglas AC, Wippold FJ, Broderick DF, et al. ACR appropriateness criteria headache. J Am Coll Radiol. 2014;11(7):657–67. https://doi.org/10.1016/j.jacr.2014.03.024.
129. Edlow JA, Panagos PD, Godwin SA, et al. PAIN MANAGEMENT/CLINICAL POLICY Clinical Policy: critical issues in the evaluation and management of adult patients presenting to the emergency department with acute headache. Oct Ann Emerg Med. 2008;52(4):407–36. https://doi.org/10.1016/j.annemergmed.2008.07.001.

Fibromyalgia

29

Anita Leon-Jhong and Sarah A. Tilstra

Learning Objectives

1. Describe current theories on pathogenesis of fibromyalgia.
2. Diagnose fibromyalgia using clinical criteria.
3. Review appropriate, cost-conscious evaluations for musculoskeletal pain.
4. Describe an approach to patient education and expectation setting for treatment and prognosis.
5. Initiate a patient-centered treatment plan for patients with fibromyalgia.

Niteri is a 33 year-old woman who presents to your office to discuss pain "everywhere" that has been ongoing for the past two years. She also complains of overwhelming fatigue, headaches, insomnia, and frequent diarrhea. She has been to several specialists and has been told that her symptoms are "all in her head" and that she needs psychotherapy. Her pain and fatigue have become so severe that she has had to reduce her work hours and is desperate for your help.

Epidemiology

Fibromyalgia is a chronic pain syndrome that affects an estimated 2–6% of the population [1–3]. It is characterized by widespread musculoskeletal pain and fatigue without the presence of abnormalities on physical exam, laboratory tests, or biopsy. It is frequently comorbid with other functional pain syndromes such as irritable bowel syndrome, interstitial cystitis, and chronic migraines. The disorder shows female predominance of approximately 6:1 and prevalence increases with age [1, 3]. Fibromyalgia can be challenging to diagnose, and patients often suffer a delay of more than two years and an average of 3.7 specialist consults before diagnosis, resulting in further anxiety, stress, and healthcare spending [4]. Patients also experience high rates of disability, with over 25% of patients in one US study reporting inability to work [5]. A Dutch study estimated a societal cost of fibromyalgia of €7813 ($9600 USD) per patient per year related to healthcare expenditures and lost work, more than double the cost attributable to patients with other rheumatic disease [6]. While fibromyalgia was previously under the umbrella of rheumatology, current guidelines recommend that primary care providers manage these patients to allow for timely diagnosis and individualized treatment [7]. Recent research has helped to increase understanding of the pathophysiology of fibromyalgia, dispel myths that have hindered patient care, and provide increased options for treatment.

Pathophysiology

The pathophysiology of fibromyalgia is not well understood, but current research suggests a biopsychosocial model, where environmental and psychosocial triggers compound a genetic predisposition toward heightened pain responses [7]. This genetic basis is supported by observations that family members of patients with fibromyalgia have an eightfold greater risk of having fibromyalgia and other chronic pain syndromes compared with the general population [8].

A. Leon-Jhong (✉)
University of Pittsburgh Medical Center, Division of General Internal Medicine, Pittsburgh, PA, USA
e-mail: lyonsab@upmc.edu

S. A. Tilstra
University of Pittsburgh School of Medicine, Division of General Internal Medicine, Department of Medicine, Pittsburgh, PA, USA

S. A. Tilstra et al. (eds.), *Sex- and Gender-Based Women's Health*, https://doi.org/10.1007/978-3-030-50695-7_29

The brain of a patient with fibromyalgia appears to be primed to detect and magnify even minor discomfort, a state referred to as "central sensitization" [9]. Studies using functional MRI show that fibromyalgia patients demonstrate increased activity in brain regions responsible for pain processing in response to mild pressure or heat stimuli [10, 11]. Fibromyalgia patients also undergo pain "catastrophizing," experiencing minor pain as extreme or unbearable, with observed activation of brain areas responsible for attention, anticipation, and emotion [12]. A "hypervigilance" model has been proposed as a means of explaining patients' increased sensitivity to stimuli [13]. Patients also demonstrate reduced ability to modulate pain, possibly due to a deficit in endogenous pain inhibition systems [14, 15]. Brain connectivity may also play a role, with research demonstrating elevated resting brain activity in regions dedicated to pain processing [16].

Environmental and psychosocial triggers have also been identified as important in fibromyalgia pathogenesis. Infections including Lyme disease, HIV, and hepatitis C have been temporally associated with fibromyalgia development [17]. Adverse childhood events and psychosocial distress have also been associated with subsequent development of chronic widespread pain [18, 19]. Female patients with fibromyalgia are more likely to report history of physical and sexual abuse, as well as drug use, compared with their counterparts with other rheumatic diseases [20]. Patients with fibromyalgia have high rates of depression and insomnia, conditions which themselves have been linked to decreased pain tolerance [21]. While there are many unknowns regarding the pathogenesis of fibromyalgia, it is helpful for both provider and patient to recognize that research supports a biologic basis for disease with environmental influences.

Upon further questioning, Niteri reports that her symptoms started about two years ago and have gradually worsened. She cannot think of any particular injury or illness that triggered them. She has an achy pain in her whole body that gets worse after any exercise, so she has cut down her activity. She always feels tired, even upon waking in the morning, and feels she cannot think straight, like her brain is in a "fog." She frequently gets diarrhea and crampy abdominal pain. She describes feeling sad and anxious because of her medical problems.

Clinical Manifestations

The hallmark of fibromyalgia is widespread, chronic musculoskeletal pain. Patients may use phrases like "I hurt all over" or "everything hurts" when describing their symptoms. Pain waxes and wanes over time and may migrate to different areas of the body. Patients may experience paresthetic sensations and be bothered by light touch or tight-fitting clothing [22]. While pain can sometimes start after a trauma or injury, more commonly there is no clear inciting event. Fibromyalgia pain does not localize to a specific joint or muscle and is not associated with signs of inflammation such as joint swelling, effusion, or erythema.

Chronic fatigue is present in a majority of patients with fibromyalgia [1]. "I'm always tired" and "I feel like I haven't slept" may be clues to the diagnosis. Sleep quality is poor and non-restorative and may contribute to low function and mood [23, 24]. Patients fatigue easily and may have poor tolerance for even low levels of exertion. Cognitive disturbance, often referred to as "fibro fog," is also common, with patients reporting inability to focus and memory impairment. Mood disturbances are prevalent, with up to 75% of patients experiencing symptoms of depression and anxiety in their lifetime [25]. All patients with fibromyalgia should be screened and treated for coexisting mood disorders. However, fibromyalgia is not a primary psychiatric condition, and a substantial subset of patients do *not* meet criteria for a mental health diagnosis, though they may feel frustrated or upset by their symptoms. Sexual dysfunction is present in greater than 90% of women with fibromyalgia and may be associated with a spectrum of depressive symptoms [26].

In addition to the core symptoms of pain, fatigue, non-restorative sleep, cognitive dysfunction, and poor mood, patients with fibromyalgia may have other "functional" or "central sensitivity" syndromes, several of which are listed in Table 29.1 [16, 27]. Patients are often noted to have a "pan-positive" review of systems, as they may report abdominal pain and diarrhea suggestive of irritable bowel syndrome, bladder pain and urinary frequency indicating interstitial cystitis, or sensitivity to lights and sounds in the setting of chronic headaches. Physicians should strongly consider a diagnosis of fibromyalgia in patients with other central sensitivity syndromes who report chronic, widespread pain. In addition, identifying these comorbid condi-

Table 29.1 Conditions frequently comorbid with fibromyalgia

Chronic fatigue syndrome (CFS)
Irritable bowel syndrome (IBS)
Interstitial cystitis (IC)
Chronic tension-type headache
Migraine
Temporomandibular disorder (TMD)
Chronic pelvic pain
Sexual dysfunction
Insomnia
Multiple chemical sensitivity (MCS)

tions as they arise may help to prevent unnecessary testing and guide therapy.

On physical exam, you appreciate increased tenderness to palpation over Niteri's abdomen, posterior neck, shoulders, arms, and hips bilaterally. There is no joint swelling or deformity and no peripheral edema. She has normal thyroid and neurologic exams. She appears mildly anxious, but further screening for depression and anxiety disorders is negative. She wonders what tests you plan to order. She is worried about her brain fogginess and inquires about an MRI. Reviewing her previous workup, you note that extensive laboratory testing, X-rays, abdominal CT scan, and EMGs have been normal.

Evaluation and Diagnosis

Establishing the diagnosis of fibromyalgia can be very challenging, as there are no specific abnormalities on physical exam or laboratory testing that confirm the disorder. Furthermore, as noted previously, patients often have a variety of divergent symptoms which may lead to unnecessary referrals and testing if not identified as part of the fibromyalgia syndrome. Providers should therefore have a high index of suspicion for fibromyalgia in any patient who describes chronic, widespread pain.

The American College of Rheumatology (ACR) has developed diagnostic criteria for fibromyalgia; the most updated version is found in Table 29.2. The criteria are useful for research and may be helpful, though not required, for diagnosis in the clinical setting. The original criteria released in 1990 required the presence of "tender points" – specific areas of soft tissue where pain could be elicited by applying modest pressure [28]. However, tender points were not particularly sensitive or specific and are, therefore, no longer recommended for diagnosis or monitoring [7]. The updated ACR criteria focus instead on patient-reported symptoms.

Table 29.2 American College of Rheumatology Diagnostic Criteria for Fibromyalgia 2016 Revisions to 2010/2011 Guidelines [29]

1. Generalized pain present in at least four of five body regions (four body quadrants and axial skeleton)
2. Symptoms present at a similar level for at least 3 months
3. Widespread Pain Index (WPI) ≥ 7 and Symptom Severity Scale (SSS) ≥ 5 or WPI = 4–6 and SSS ≥ 9
4. "A diagnosis of fibromyalgia is valid irrespective of other diagnoses. A diagnosis of fibromyalgia does not exclude the presence of other clinically important illnesses"

The Widespread Pain Index (WPI) measures pain location: patients should endorse pain in at least 7 of 19 body regions. The Symptom Severity Scale (SSS), scored from 0 to 12, asks patients to consider how often they experience fatigue, waking unrefreshed, and cognitive symptoms [29]. Providers should be aware of the WPI and SSS as they may be helpful when the diagnosis of fibromyalgia is unclear or when the patient desires objective evidence of diagnosis. Most patients who describe symptoms suggestive of fibromyalgia can be readily diagnosed based on clinical presentation alone.

The clinical evaluation for fibromyalgia starts with taking a careful history of the patient's symptoms. Pain should be ongoing for at least 3 months and present in a majority of body quadrants (i.e., right, left, upper, lower) plus the axial skeleton. Localized pain suggests a regional pain syndrome. As previously discussed, patients will often endorse additional symptoms such as fatigue, non-restorative sleep, brain fog, mood changes, and other somatic symptoms. Patients should be asked about family history of fibromyalgia and other medical conditions, like autoimmune disease, which may suggest another diagnosis. The physical exam should focus on identifying any musculoskeletal abnormalities which would suggest alternative causes of pain, for example, joint effusions or warmth suggesting inflammatory arthritis. The exam in fibromyalgia patients is generally normal aside from diffuse tenderness of soft tissues. If fibromyalgia is suggested by history and physical exam, no further laboratory or imaging exams are required to make the diagnosis.

Patients wait an average of 2–3 years to receive a fibromyalgia diagnosis and have often have been told that they are "normal" by prior medical providers despite their severe debility [4]. Diagnosing fibromyalgia helps these patients to avoid unnecessary testing and allows them to focus on treatment. There is some evidence that healthcare use decreases after fibromyalgia diagnosis, though not all studies have demonstrated a clear economic benefit [30, 31].

Differential Diagnosis

When evaluating a patient for suspected fibromyalgia, it is helpful to exclude common conditions such as thyroid disease, anemia, severe vitamin deficiency, and primary psychiatric disorders like depression or anxiety. This can be done by taking a careful history and ordering a basic laboratory evaluation. The 2012 Canadian Guidelines for the Diagnosis and Management of Fibromyalgia Syndrome suggest obtaining a complete blood count (CBC), thyroid-stimulating hormone (TSH), creatinine kinase (CK), erythrocyte sedimentation rate (ESR), and C-reactive protein (CRP) [7]. Caution should be exercised when ordering an ESR, CRP, or CK without a specific diagnosis in mind, as elevated results are nonspecific and could lead to additional unnecessary workup. Similarly, routine testing for antinuclear antibody (ANA) is not recommended as it is positive in approximately 10% of both the general population and those with fibromyalgia [32]. Iron studies and vitamin B12 levels can be considered as these deficiencies can mimic the fatigue of fibromyalgia. Lyme disease can also have nonspecific symptoms and should be considered when history and physical are suggestive.

Rheumatologic disorders can generally be distinguished based on history and physical exam. Rheumatoid arthritis, psoriatic arthritis, Sjogren's syndrome, and systemic lupus erythematosus cause pain which is localized to the joints rather than distributed throughout the soft tissue. Joint inflammation or destruction on exam is suggestive of an inflammatory arthritis. Spondyloarthritis presents with pain and stiffness primarily in the axial skeleton. Polymyalgia rheumatica may mimic fibromyalgia pain but is generally localized to proximal muscle groups and has an elevated ESR. Polymyositis can be distinguished from fibromyalgia by the presence of muscle weakness and elevated CK level. As noted in Table 29.2, the presence of another disease state does not exclude the diagnosis of fibromyalgia. In fact, as many as 10–30% of patients with rheumatologic diseases like rheumatoid arthritis and lupus also have fibromyalgia [33].

Based on her history and exam, you diagnose Niteri with fibromyalgia and tell her she does not need any more testing. You explain that although there is no cure for fibromyalgia, you will work together to improve her quality of life. She is relieved to finally have a diagnosis. You ask her what symptoms are bothering her the most currently. She reports pain and difficulty sleeping, so you prescribe a low dose of pregabalin to take at night. You also recommend that she start an exercise program, advising her to start slowly as her symptoms may flare at first. You ask her to see you again in a month to see how she is feeling.

Management

The treatment of fibromyalgia requires a multimodal approach that includes both pharmacologic and non-pharmacologic strategies [34]. One of the most important components of treatment is patient education. Patients may feel uncertain about the diagnosis or have experienced stigma from healthcare providers who implied their symptoms were exaggerated or purely psychological [35]. It can be helpful to frame fibromyalgia as a common condition, likely based in aberrant pain processing. Physicians should validate patients' symptoms and provide reassurance that the pain is not a result of tissue damage [7]. The 2012 Canadian Guidelines recommend that patients be encouraged to live as normal a life as possible, to remain in the workforce, and to develop self-efficacy in coping with their symptoms [7]. It is also important to frame patient expectations on treatment success. Fibromyalgia is generally a chronic condition that may wax and wane over time, but which will likely affect patients throughout their lifetime. The goal of all treatment strategies is an improvement in function and quality of life, rather than a complete elimination of symptoms.

Non-pharmacologic Therapies

Exercise is a cornerstone of fibromyalgia treatment. Numerous studies have demonstrated that exercise training is effective in improving fibromyalgia symptoms [36, 37]. A Cochrane review found high-quality evidence that supervised aerobic exercise training increases physical function and well-being and may decrease pain. Strength and flexibility training require further study to evaluate their effectiveness [38]. Another Cochrane review found that aquatic exercise training is equivalent to land-based programs and may be more tolerable to some patients [39]. Unfortunately, many patients will have difficulty exercising due to chronic fatigue and easy fatigability. Patients with fibromyalgia tend to perceive higher exertion than fitness-matched controls when completing the same activity [40]. Patients may also experience an increase in pain initially when starting an exercise program and should be encouraged to "start low, go slow." For patients who are having difficulty exercising on their own, it may be helpful to prescribe physical therapy or a structured exercise program to get started [7, 41].

Complementary and alternative therapies are used by an estimated 90% of fibromyalgia patients and have some evidence for their efficacy [42]. The European League Against Rheumatism (EULAR) gives a weak recommendation for meditation, mindfulness, cognitive behavioral therapy (CBT), and acupuncture [41]. A randomized trial of tai chi vs. education and stretching found improved quality of life with tai chi that was sustained at 24 weeks [43]. A meta-analysis of six trials of mindfulness-based stress reduction showed short-term improvements in quality of life [44]. Cognitive behavioral therapy was evaluated in a Cochrane review and found to reduce pain, low mood, and disability, with results sustained at 6 months [45]. Another Cochrane review found that acupuncture is safe and reduces pain and stiffness in fibromyalgia patients, but does not perform better than sham acupuncture and has no sustained effect at 6 months [46]. Therapies which are not recommended by EULAR due to lack of evidence for benefit include biofeedback, hypnotherapy, massage, chiropractic, and homeopathy

Table 29.3 Medications recommended for treatment of fibromyalgia by the European League Against Rheumatism (EULAR) [41]

Medication (drug class)	Recommended dose	Summary of study results	Treatment considerations and common side effects (SE)
Amitriptyline (TCA)	10–25 mg/day at bedtime	NNT 4.1 for 50% pain reduction. Very poor quality evidence available [51]	No additional benefit to doses >25 mg. Useful for insomnia. SE: dry mouth, sedation, dizziness, weight gain
Pregabalin (gabapentinoid)	300–600 mg/day	NNT 7.2 for 30% pain reduction. NNT 11 to feel "much or very much improved" [52]	Useful for insomnia and anxiety. SE: dizziness, sedation, weight gain, edema
Cyclobenzaprine (muscle relaxant)	10 mg/day at bedtime or 10 mg TID	NNT 4.8 to feel "improved." Some sleep benefit. No effect on pain [53]	High rate of side effects (85%) and trial dropout. SE: sedation, dry mouth
Duloxetine (SNRI)	60–120 mg/day in morning	NNT 10 for 30% pain reduction. Improved patients' "global impression." No effect on fatigue, sleep, or QOL [54]	Consider in patients with depression or anxiety. SE: nausea, headache, dry mouth, constipation
Milnacipran (SNRI)	100–200 mg/day in divided doses		
Tramadol (opioid)	37.5 mg QID	25% reduction in pain scores when combined with acetaminophen 325 mg [55]	Weak opioid with potential for abuse and diversion. SE: nausea, dizziness, constipation

Adapted and updated from Macfarlane et al. [41]
NNT number needed to treat, *QOL* quality of life, TCA tricyclic antidepressant, *SNRI* serotonin norepinephrine reuptake inhibitor

[41]. In general, complementary and alternative therapies are well tolerated with minimal side effects, so there is little harm to trying them, though they may not be available to all patients.

Pharmacologic Therapies

Several medications have been studied for the treatment of fibromyalgia and should be considered an adjunct to education and exercise. Medications recommended by EULAR are listed in Table 29.3 along with common doses and side effects. Only pregabalin, duloxetine, and milnacipran have FDA indications for fibromyalgia, but others, including venlafaxine and gabapentin, may be considered for off-label use. EULAR recommends against nonsteroidal anti-inflammatory drugs (NSAIDs), selective serotonin reuptake inhibitors (SSRIs), and monoamine oxidase inhibitors (MAOIs) due to lack of evidence for benefit. Low-dose naltrexone (4.5 mg per day) is an emerging therapy which has shown promise for pain relief and is well-tolerated [47]. Synthetic cannabinoids have also demonstrated benefit and may be a future option [48]. Both the EULAR and Canadian Guidelines strongly recommend against opioids, citing their unclear benefit and high risk for adverse effects including addiction and hyperalgesia. Despite this, more than 30% of patients with a fibromyalgia diagnosis receive opioids [49].

When choosing an initial medication, it may be helpful to ask the patient what symptom is most bothersome (i.e., fatigue, sleep, pain, mood) and choose a medication with added benefit for that symptom. Patients with anxiety or depression should consider a serotonin norepinephrine reuptake inhibitor (SNRI), while those with sleep disturbances should try a tricyclic antidepressant (TCA) or gabapentinoid. In general, all medications have only a modest effect on pain and do not produce sustained results once discontinued. In addition, fibromyalgia patients often experience high rates of side effects. It is prudent, therefore, to start at the lowest dose possible and slowly increase as tolerated. A combination of several low-dose medications may be helpful.

Follow-Up and When to Refer

In general, patients with fibromyalgia should receive care from their primary care provider, as referral to a specialist has not been demonstrated to improve outcomes [50]. Patients with an unclear diagnosis and those who are not improving may benefit from seeing a specialist. A multidisciplinary team that includes physical therapy, nursing, and psychology may be the best option for management, but may not be available to many patients. Recognizing that fibromyalgia is a lifelong condition, providers should maintain a close relationship with their patients through regular appointments. This allows for management of new symptoms, identification and care of comorbidities, and support for patients to live the fullest life possible.

Summary Points

1. Fibromyalgia is understood to be a disorder of central pain processing whose pathogenesis involves both genetic and environmental factors.
2. Diagnosis of fibromyalgia is based on patient history of widespread musculoskeletal pain lasting greater than

3 months which is not explained by another condition. Evaluation of tender points is not required for diagnosis.
3. Diagnostic workup in patients suspected of having fibromyalgia should be limited. Delay in diagnosis of fibromyalgia leads to unnecessary testing and patient distress.
4. Treatment aims to improve function and quality of life; patients should be counseled to anticipate modest reductions in pain, but not to expect full resolution of symptoms.
5. Initial management of fibromyalgia includes patient education, initiation of an exercise regimen, and pharmacologic treatment using TCAs, SNRIs, gabapentinoids, cyclobenzaprine, or tramadol. Opioids are not recommended.

Review Questions

1. A 32-year-old woman with a history of depression presents to your office with chief complaint of "hurting all over." On further questioning, she reports pain and swelling in bilateral knees, hips, and wrists which has been ongoing for at least 4 months. She also feels tired easily. Physical exam reveals moderate effusions at her knees and wrists and is otherwise unremarkable. What is the next most appropriate step in management?
   A. Screen for depression symptoms.
   B. Provide a prescription for duloxetine.
   C. Recommend an exercise regimen.
   D. Test for rheumatoid factor and anti-CCP.

   The correct answer is D. This patient does have several risk factors for fibromyalgia (female sex, history of mood disorder) and has some suggestive symptoms (widespread, chronic pain and fatigue). However, her exam is not consistent with diagnosis of fibromyalgia as she has evidence of joint inflammation. Patients with fibromyalgia have a normal physical exam aside from soft-tissue tenderness and have normal lab findings. Therefore, it is most appropriate to work up other causes of her joint inflammation at this time, including rheumatoid arthritis.

2. A 42-year-old woman presents to your office for a follow-up visit. She reports feeling "constantly achy" for the past 6 months and being tired all the time despite sleeping 9 hours per day. Her depression screen is negative. On physical exam, she has significant pain with applied pressure to bilateral occiput, trapezius, sternocleidomastoid, lateral epicondyle, and greater trochanter. Physical exam is otherwise normal. She had a CBC and TSH checked earlier this year for fatigue which were normal. She looked up her symptoms online and is concerned for lupus and Lyme disease. What is next best step in management?
   A. Diagnose fibromyalgia and recommend no further testing.
   B. Check ANA, rheumatoid factor.
   C. Order cervical spine and elbow X-rays.
   D. Order Lyme serology.

   The correct answer is A. This patient has a classic presentation of fibromyalgia with chronic, widespread myalgias and tender points without evidence of joint or muscle inflammation. Diagnosis is based on history and exam alone and does not require any specific laboratory testing [29]. Additional testing should be reserved for patients with signs and symptoms suggestive of alternative conditions such as inflammatory arthritis, osteoarthritis, or thyroid disease. It is important to establish the diagnosis of fibromyalgia as early as possible to help patients avoid unnecessary testing and to initiate treatment.

3. A 36-year-old woman with irritable bowel syndrome and generalized anxiety disorder presents to your office with debilitating body pain and fatigue for the past year. Based on her history and unremarkable physical exam, you suspect fibromyalgia. You order a CBC, TSH, and B12 level which are within normal limits. What is your initial approach to management?
   A. Refer to a rheumatologist.
   B. Start oxycodone.
   C. Start duloxetine.
   D. Begin an intensive exercise program.

   The correct answer is C. The three medications currently approved by the FDA for treatment of fibromyalgia are duloxetine, milnacipran, and pregabalin. TCAs, gabapentin, and cyclobenzaprine have also been studied as first-line therapy. Opioids are not recommended due to lack of efficacy and risk of side effects and addiction. While exercise is a crucial part of treatment, patients should generally start slowly as pain symptoms may flare with overexertion. Referral to specialist can be considered if a patient does not respond to initial therapy.

4. Edith is a 49-year-old woman who has been suffering from generalized body pain for several years. She has seen several providers and undergone many tests which have been unrevealing. You see her in the office today and suspect fibromyalgia. She is skeptical ("are you saying nothing is wrong with me?") but agrees to start duloxetine. She wants to know how soon she can expect to feel better. How do you counsel her?
   A. "We will continue to work together until we find a treatment that fully relieves your pain."
   B. "Because fibromyalgia is a psychiatric condition, you may benefit from cognitive behavioral therapy."
   C. "I expect you will start to feel much better once you begin an exercise program."

D. "Fibromyalgia is a chronic condition, and we will work to improve your function and quality of life."
E. "Fibromyalgia is difficult to treat because there is nothing physically wrong."

The correct answer is D. It is important to counsel patients on the chronic nature of fibromyalgia and establish realistic goals, including incremental improvements in pain, function, and quality of life. Patients should not expect to be pain-free. Cognitive behavioral therapy (CBT) may help in some circumstances, but fibromyalgia is not a primary psychiatric condition. Exercise is helpful in the long term, but patients may actually experience more pain at first, resulting in difficulty with adherence to exercise regimens.

References

1. Wolfe F, Ross K, Anderson J, Russell IJ, Hebert L. The prevalence and characteristics of fibromyalgia in the general population. Arthritis Rheum. 1995;38(1):19–28.
2. White KP, Speechley M, Harth M, Ostbye T. The London Fibromyalgia Epidemiology Study: the prevalence of fibromyalgia syndrome in London, Ontario. J Rheumatol. 1999;26(7):1570–6.
3. Vincent A, Lahr BD, Wolfe F, Clauw DJ, Whipple MO, Oh TH, et al. Prevalence of fibromyalgia: a population-based study in Olmsted County, Minnesota, utilizing the Rochester Epidemiology Project. Arthritis Care Res. 2013;65(5):786–92.
4. Choy E, Perrot S, Leon T, Kaplan J, Petersel D, Ginovker A, Kramer E. A patient survey of the impact of fibromyalgia and the journey to diagnosis. BMC Health Serv Res. 2010;10(1):102.
5. Wolfe F, Anderson J, Harkness D, Bennett RM, Caro XJ, Goldenberg DL, et al. Work and disability status of persons with fibromyalgia. J Rheumatol. 1997;24(6):1171–8.
6. Boonen A, van den Heuvel R, van Tubergen A, Goossens M, Severens JL, van der Heijde D, van der Linden S. Large differences in cost of illness and wellbeing between patients with fibromyalgia, chronic low back pain, or ankylosing spondylitis. Ann Rheum Dis. 2005;64(3):396–402.
7. Fitzcharles MA, Ste-Marie PA, Goldenberg DL, Pereira JX, Abbey S, Choinière M, et al. 2012 Canadian guidelines for the diagnosis and management of fibromyalgia syndrome: executive summary. Pain Res Manag. 2013;18(3):119–26.
8. Arnold LM, Hudson JI, Hess EV, Ware AE, Fritz DA, Auchenbach MB, et al. Family study of fibromyalgia. Arthritis Rheum. 2004;50(3):944–52.
9. Yunus MB. Central sensitivity syndromes: a new paradigm and group nosology for fibromyalgia and overlapping conditions, and the related issue of disease versus illness. Semin Arthritis Rheum. 2008;37(6):339–52. https://doi.org/10.1016/j.semarthrit.2007.09.003.
10. Gracely RH, Petzke F, Wolf JM, Clauw DJ. Functional magnetic resonance imaging evidence of augmented pain processing in fibromyalgia. Arthritis Rheum. 2002;46(5):1333–43.
11. Cook DB, Lange G, Ciccone DS, Liu WC, Steffener J, Natelson BH. Functional imaging of pain in patients with primary fibromyalgia. J Rheumatol. 2004;31(2):364–78.
12. Gracely RH, Geisser ME, Giesecke T, Grant MA, Petzke F, Williams DA, Clauw DJ. Pain catastrophizing and neural responses to pain among persons with fibromyalgia. Brain. 2004;127(4):835–43.
13. McDermid AJ, Rollman GB, McCain GA. Generalized hypervigilance in fibromyalgia: evidence of perceptual amplification. Pain. 1996;66(2-3):133–44.
14. Lautenbacher S, Rollman GB. Possible deficiencies of pain modulation in fibromyalgia. Clin J Pain. 1997;13(3):189–96.
15. Julien N, Goffaux P, Arsenault P, Marchand S. Widespread pain in fibromyalgia is related to a deficit of endogenous pain inhibition. Pain. 2005;114(1-2):295–302.
16. Napadow V, LaCount L, Park K, As-Sanie S, Clauw DJ, Harris RE. Intrinsic brain connectivity in fibromyalgia is associated with chronic pain intensity. Arthritis Rheum. 2010;62(8):2545–55.
17. Buskila D, Atzeni F, Sarzi-Puttini P. Etiology of fibromyalgia: the possible role of infection and vaccination. Autoimmun Rev. 2008;8(1):41–3.
18. Jones GT, Power C, Macfarlane GJ. Adverse events in childhood and chronic widespread pain in adult life: results from the 1958 British Birth Cohort Study. Pain. 2009;143(1-2):92–6.
19. Gupta A, Silman AJ, Ray D, Morriss R, Dickens C, MacFarlane GJ, et al. The role of psychosocial factors in predicting the onset of chronic widespread pain: results from a prospective population-based study. Rheumatology. 2006;46(4):666–71.
20. Boisset-Pioro MH, Esdaile JM, Fitzcharles MA. Sexual and physical abuse in women with fibromyalgia syndrome. Arthritis Rheum. 1995;38(2):235–41.
21. Chiu YH, Silman AJ, MacFarlane GJ, Ray D, Gupta A, Dickens C, et al. Poor sleep and depression are independently associated with a reduced pain threshold. Results of a population based study. Pain. 2005;115(3):316–21.
22. Clauw DJ. Fibromyalgia: a clinical review. JAMA. 2014;311(15):1547–55. https://doi.org/10.1001/jama.2014.3266.
23. Osorio CD, Gallinaro AL, Lorenzi-Filho G, Lage LV. Sleep quality in patients with fibromyalgia using the Pittsburgh Sleep Quality Index. J Rheumatol. 2006;33(9):1863–5.
24. Hamilton NA, Affleck G, Tennen H, Karlson C, Luxton D, Preacher KJ, Templin JL. Fibromyalgia: the role of sleep in affect and in negative event reactivity and recovery. Health Psychol. 2008;27(4):490.
25. Epstein SA, Kay G, Clauw D, Heaton R, Klein D, Krupp L, et al. Psychiatric disorders in patients with fibromyalgia: a multicenter investigation. Psychosomatics. 1999;40(1):57–63.
26. Orellana C, Casado E, Masip M, Galisteo C, Gratacós J, Larrosa M. Sexual dysfunction in fibromyalgia patients. Clin Exp Rheumatol. 2008;26(4):663.
27. Aaron LA, Burke MM, Buchwald D. Overlapping conditions among patients with chronic fatigue syndrome, fibromyalgia, and temporomandibular disorder. Arch Int Med. 2000;160(2):221–7.
28. Wolfe F, Smythe HA, Yunus MB, Bennett RM, Bombardier C, Goldenberg DL, et al. The American College of Rheumatology 1990 criteria for the classification of fibromyalgia. Arthritis Rheum. 1990;33(2):160–72.
29. Wolfe F, Clauw DJ, Fitzcharles MA, Goldenberg DL, Häuser W, Katz RL, et al. 2016 revisions to the 2010/2011 fibromyalgia diagnostic criteria. Semin Arthritis Rheum. 2016;46(3):319–29. https://doi.org/10.1016/j.semarthrit.2016.08.012.
30. Hughes G, Martinez C, Myon E, Taïeb C, Wessely S. The impact of a diagnosis of fibromyalgia on health care resource use by primary care patients in the UK: an observational study based on clinical practice. Arthritis Rheum. 2006;54(1):177–83.
31. Annemans L, Wessely S, Spaepen E, Caekelbergh K, Caubère JP, Lay KL, Taïeb C. Health economic consequences related to the diagnosis of fibromyalgia syndrome. Arthritis Rheum. 2008;58(3):895–902.
32. Yunus MB, Hussey FX, Aldag JC. Antinuclear antibodies and connective tissue disease features in fibromyalgia syndrome: a controlled study. J Rheumatol. 1993;20(9):1557–60.
33. Phillips K, Clauw DJ. Central pain mechanisms in the rheumatic diseases: future directions. Arthritis Rheum. 2013;65(2):291–302.

34. Häuser W, Bernardy K, Arnold B, Offenbächer M, Schiltenwolf M. Efficacy of multicomponent treatment in fibromyalgia syndrome: a meta-analysis of randomized controlled clinical trials. Arthritis Care Res. 2009;61(2):216–24.
35. Åsbring P, Närvänen AL. Women's experiences of stigma in relation to chronic fatigue syndrome and fibromyalgia. Q Health Res. 2002;12(2):148–60.
36. Gowans SE, Voss S, Richardson M. A randomized, controlled trial of exercise and education for individuals with fibromyalgia. Arthritis Care Res. 1999;12(2):120–8.
37. McCain GA, Bell DA, Mai FM, Halliday PD. A controlled study of the effects of a supervised cardiovascular fitness training program on the manifestations of primary fibromyalgia. Arthritis Rheum. 1988;31(9):1135–41.
38. Busch AJ, Barber KA, Overend TJ, Peloso PM, Schachter CL. Exercise for treating fibromyalgia syndrome. Cochrane Database Syst Rev. 2007;(4):CD003786.
39. Bidonde J, Busch AJ, Webber SC, Schachter CL, Danyliw A, Overend TJ, et al. Aquatic exercise training for fibromyalgia. Cochrane Database Syst Rev. 2014;(10):CD011336. https://doi.org/10.1002/14651858.CD011336.
40. Nielens H, Boisset V, Masquelier E. Fitness and perceived exertion in patients with fibromyalgia syndrome. Clin J Pain. 2000;16(3):209–13.
41. Macfarlane GJ, Kronisch C, Dean LE, Atzeni F, Häuser W, Fluß E, et al. EULAR revised recommendations for the management of fibromyalgia. Ann Rheum Dis. 2017;76(2):318–28.
42. Pioro-Boisset M, Esdaile JM, Fitzcharles MA. Alternative medicine use in fibromyalgia syndrome. Arthritis Care Res. 1996;9(1):13–7.
43. Wang C, Schmid CH, Rones R, Kalish R, Yinh J, Goldenberg DL, et al. A randomized trial of tai chi for fibromyalgia. N Engl J Med. 2010;363(8):743–54.
44. Lauche R, Cramer H, Dobos G, Langhorst J, Schmidt S. A systematic review and meta-analysis of mindfulness-based stress reduction for the fibromyalgia syndrome. J Psychosom Res. 2013;75(6):500–10.
45. Bernardy K, Klose P, Busch AJ, Choy EH, Häuser W. Cognitive behavioural therapies for fibromyalgia syndrome. Cochrane Database Syst Rev. 2012;9 https://doi.org/10.1002/14651858.CD009796.pub2.
46. Deare JC, Zheng Z, Xue CC, Liu JP, Shang J, Scott SW, Littlejohn G. Acupuncture for treating fibromyalgia. Cochrane Libr. 2013:CD007070.
47. Younger J, Noor N, McCue R, Mackey S. Low-dose naltrexone for the treatment of fibromyalgia: findings of a small, randomized, double-blind, placebo-controlled, counterbalanced, crossover trial assessing daily pain levels. Arthritis Rheum. 2013;65(2):529–38.
48. Skrabek RQ, Galimova L, Ethans K, Perry D. Nabilone for the treatment of pain in fibromyalgia. J Pain. 2008;9(2):164–73.
49. Fitzcharles MA, Ste-Marie PA, Gamsa A, Ware MA, Shir Y. Opioid use, misuse, and abuse in patients labeled as fibromyalgia. Am J Med. 2011;124(10):955–60.
50. Garcia-Campayo J, Magdalena J, Magallón R, Fernández-García E, Salas M, Andrés E. A meta-analysis of the efficacy of fibromyalgia treatment according to level of care. Arthritis Res Ther. 2008;10(4):R81.
51. Moore RA, Derry S, Aldington D, Cole P, Wiffen PJ. Amitriptyline for fibromyalgia in adults. Cochrane Database Syst Rev. 2015;(7):Art. No.: CD011824. https://doi.org/10.1002/14651858.CD011824.
52. Derry S, Cording M, Wiffen PJ, Law S, Phillips T, Moore RA. Pregabalin for pain in fibromyalgia in adults. Cochrane Database Syst Rev. 2016;(9):Art. No.: CD011790. https://doi.org/10.1002/14651858.CD011790.pub2.
53. Tofferi JK, Jackson JL, O'Malley PG. Treatment of fibromyalgia with cyclobenzaprine: a meta-analysis. Arthritis Care Res. 2004;51:9–13.
54. Welsch P, Üçeyler N, Klose P, Walitt B, Häuser W. Serotonin and noradrenaline reuptake inhibitors (SNRIs) for fibromyalgia. Cochrane Database Syst Rev. 2018;(2):Art. No.: CD010292. https://doi.org/10.1002/14651858.CD010292.pub2.
55. Bennett RM, Kamin M, Karim R, Rosenthal N. Tramadol and acetaminophen combination tablets in the treatment of fibromyalgia pain: a double-blind, randomized, placebo-controlled study. Am J Med. 2003;114:537–45.

Interstitial Cystitis/Bladder Pain Syndrome

30

Sumana Koduri

Learning Objectives

1. Define interstitial cystitis/bladder pain syndrome (IC/BPS) and describe the typical patient presentation.
2. Discuss the differential diagnosis of a patient with irritative voiding symptoms.
3. List the common comorbidities associated with IC/BPS.
4. Review the initial diagnostic strategy and management of a woman with symptoms consistent with suspected IC/BPS.

Ingrid is a 42-year-old woman who presents with complaints of urinary urgency, frequency, and burning. She has pain unless she empties her bladder and voids about every ½–1 hour in order to relieve her symptoms. She wakes up five to eight times a night to urinate. Her symptoms have progressed over the past 2 years. She has been treated for six UTIs and several yeast infections in that time period. She has been going to an urgent care clinic whenever she is symptomatic.

Background

Interstitial cystitis (IC) or bladder pain syndrome (BPS) is a female predominant, debilitating disorder characterized by pain with bladder filling that is partially relieved by emptying, urinary frequency, and urgency. The American Urological Association defines IC/BPS as "an unpleasant sensation (pain, pressure or discomfort) perceived to be related to the urinary bladder, associated with lower urinary tract symptoms of more than six weeks duration, in the absence of infection or other identifiable causes" [1]. Other common symptoms include nocturia, pain with intercourse, chronic pelvic pain, and occasionally hematuria. The terms IC and BPS are interchangeably used in the literature; therefore, the combined abbreviation IC/BPS will be used in this chapter.

Epidemiology

The prevalence of IC/BPS has increased over the years, which corresponds to less stringent criteria for the diagnosis over time. Roughly 2.7–6.5% of Americans suffer from IC/BPS based on a population-based study of the US Census data in 2011 [2]. The ratio of women to men has consistently been ~9:1 in many studies with no racial predilection noted [3]. Most women are diagnosed in their 30s–40s with a mean of 10 years from symptom onset to diagnosis. One study also showed that only 9.7% of patients meeting criteria for IC/BPS were actually given a diagnosis of IC/BPS, exposing the large potential for underdiagnosis [2].

Physiology and Pathophysiology

The pathophysiology of IC/BPS is not well understood. The condition of interstitial cystitis was initially recognized by Hunner in 1915 who described an ulceration noted in the bladder during distension via cystoscope [4]. Later authors found that glomerulations (petechial hemorrhages) in the bladder

S. Koduri (✉)
Medical College of Wisconsin, Froedtert Memorial Lutheran Hospital, Department of Obstetrics and Gynecology, Milwaukee, WI, USA
e-mail: skoduri@mcw.edu

S. A. Tilstra et al. (eds.), *Sex- and Gender-Based Women's Health*, https://doi.org/10.1007/978-3-030-50695-7_30

wall were more commonly seen than an ulceration when the bladder was distended [4].The etiology for the abnormal findings was thought to be from a defective glycosaminoglycan (GAG) protective layer in the bladder mucosa [5]; this causes a "leaky epithelium" in which toxins or substances in the urine could penetrate the mucosa and induce inflammation and symptoms. Subsequent studies, however, have shown that even asymptomatic women can have glomerulations when the bladder is hydrodistended, which has brought this theory into question [6]. Other mediators recognized in IC/BPS include histamine, a defect in the urinary Tamm-Horsfall protein, the peptide inhibitor antiproliferative factor, and inflammation caused by a urinary tract infection [7, 8].

Chronic pelvic pain conditions are frequently present concomitantly in IC/BPS patients, including endometriosis, irritable bowel syndrome, and vulvodynia. For this reason, it has been theorized that a systemic process, central sensitization, may facilitate the development of IC/BPS [9–11]. According to this theory, other conditions that cause pelvic pain upregulate the dorsal horns in the lower spinal cord, particularly at the T10–T12 levels. The visceral convergence of the neurons in this area allows the nociceptive input from the bladder to be amplified, causing increased bladder pain with even normal distension. Once the process of central sensitization has started, it is very difficult to normalize pain processing, and a state of chronic pain perception is maintained. The propensity for developing a chronic pain condition such as IC/BPS is also seen with a tendency to develop chronic pain elsewhere in the body [10, 12]. Studies show that the periaqueductal gray region in the brain is a threat monitor for pain, and it is theorized that dysfunction in this area of the brain may be implicated in development of multiple comorbid pain conditions [13, 14]. The pathophysiology of IC/BPS is complex, and the understanding of the mechanisms involved is still evolving.

Clinical Manifestations

The hallmark symptoms of IC/BPS are bladder pain, urinary frequency, dysuria, and nocturia [15, 16]. The pain tends to be relieved with voiding and felt mostly in the bladder and suprapubic region, but can be referred to other areas within the pelvis including the lower quadrants of the abdomen, the gynecologic organs, or the vulva. Urinary frequency is more often seen in women <30 years old, while nocturia increases as patients age [7]. Typically, symptoms wax and wane over time, lasting for hours to days or weeks. Ninety percent of women describe diet sensitivity to certain foods that can exacerbate their pain – most commonly caffeine, alcohol, soda, artificial sweeteners, spicy foods, and citrus fruits [17]. Flares tend to last hours to days and can be triggered by menstrual cycles, intercourse, stressful situations, and increased physical activity. During pregnancy symptoms can worsen, improve, or remain the same. Women with IC/BPS are commonly misdiagnosed with urinary tract infections, vaginitis, or sexually transmitted infections for months or years before IC/BPS is considered in the differential. Patients are often frustrated with the lack of effective treatment for their symptoms and are eventually referred to a urologist or urogynecologist for persistently negative urinalyses, negative urine cultures, and the lack of response to antibiotics or antifungal therapy.

The development of IC/BPS may coincide with trauma or instrumentation to the pelvic area [18, 19], which patients may not associate with the start of symptoms, including hysterectomy, hysteroscopy, bladder catheterization, cystoscopy, kidney stones, colonoscopy, pregnancy, and other pelvic or abdominal procedures. IC/BPS may also be associated with a history of adverse childhood experiences and sexual trauma/abuse [20]. Commonly, women with IC/BPS have been treated for other known pelvic pain conditions such as endometriosis, dysmenorrhea, or irritable bowel syndrome. Pelvic floor dysfunction, coccydynia, piriformis syndrome, and anismus share a common pathophysiology with IC/BPS, visceral sensitization, and therefore may be seen concomitantly in these patients [18, 21, 22].

The lag from onset of symptoms to appropriate evaluation and diagnosis of IC/BPS can be as long as 5–10 years [2, 15]. Delays in diagnosis are caused by the insidious onset of symptoms, overlapping symptoms of IC/BPS with other diseases, the natural waxing and waning trajectory of IC/BPS, and the lack of provider familiarity with the diagnostic criteria for IC/BPS. A patient's quality of life can be greatly improved with proper diagnosis and control of the predominant symptoms: pain, frequent urination, and nocturia [23].

Differential Diagnosis

The differential diagnosis of IC/BPS is broad due to the complexity of the anatomy in the abdomen and pelvis and includes recurrent urinary tract infections, chronic urethritis, overactive bladder, genitourinary syndrome of menopause, vulvodynia, endometriosis, irritable bowel syndrome, pelvic floor dysfunction, and neuropathic pain. The history and urinalysis are helpful in differentiating these conditions from IC/ BPS, although many of these conditions can coexist with IC/BPS (see Table 30.1).

Urinary tract infection The symptoms of IC/BPS are very similar to those of a urinary tract infection. An uncomplicated urinary tract infection is often empirically treated, but once the symptoms become recurrent, the diagnosis should be questioned. A negative urinalysis and urine culture can rule out recurrent urinary tract infections.

Urethritis An undiagnosed urethritis caused by *N. gonorrhoeae, C. trachomatis*, or atypical bacteria such as mycoplasma (*M. hominis, M.genitalium*) and ureaplasma (*U.*

Table 30.1 Differential diagnosis of interstitial cystitis/bladder pain syndrome and overlapping clinical features [1, 7, 12, 13, 15, 17, 18, 22, 24–30]

	Pelvic pain	Dysuria	Urinary frequency	Pyuria	Hematuria	Nocturia	Dyspareunia	Pearls
Interstitial cystitis/ bladder pain syndrome	+	+	+	+/–	+/–	+	+	Negative urine culture Pain relived with voiding
Urinary tract infection	+	+	+	+	+/–	+/–	+	Positive urine culture Pain worse with voiding
Chronic urethritis/ cystitis	+	+	+	+	+/–	+/–	+	Infectious, immunosuppressed, radiation induced
Sexual transmitted infection(s)	+	+/–	+/–	+/–	+/–	–	+	GC/CH, trichomoniasis, NGU, myco-/ uroplasma
Irritable bowel syndrome	+	–	+/–	–	–	–	+/–	GI > GU symptoms
Overactive bladder	–	–	+	–	–	+/–	–	Usually painless
Genitourinary syndrome of menopause	+	+	+	+/–	+/–	+	+	Atrophy on exam
Vulvodynia	+	–	–	–	–	–	+	Pain without urinary symptoms
Endometriosis	+	–	–	–	+/–	–	+	Concomitant in 50% of patients Rare bladder/urethral endometrial implants
Pelvic floor dysfunction	+	+/–	+/–	–	–	–	+	Spasm can cause dysuria/frequency
Neuropathic pain	+	–	–	–	–	–	+	Central sensitization Can be induced post-procedure
Genitourinary malignancy	+	+/–	+/–	+/–	+/–	+/–	+/–	Consider malignancy in any patient with hematuria

NGU non-gonococcal urethritis, *GI* gastrointestinal, *GU* genitourinary

urealyticum) may mimic symptoms of IC/BPS. Chlamydia and other STIs can be excluded by polymerase chain reaction (specific for organism) in patients at risk [1].

Nephrolithiasis and malignancy A urinalysis is important in detecting microscopic hematuria and screening for urinary tract pathologies. Hematuria should trigger a workup for nephrolithiasis or malignancy which can both present with pain, dysuria, and frequency. Patients with a cancer history should be asked about prior chemotherapy and radiation, as cystitis can cause similar symptoms. Any patient with unexplained hematuria should be evaluated with cystoscopy and upper urinary tract imaging to help differentiate among benign and malignant etiologies [1].

Overactive bladder In the absence of any obvious urinary tract pathology, overactive bladder (OAB) is the most common diagnosis that can be confused with IC/BPS [15]. Urinary frequency is seen in both conditions as are urgency and nocturia. The differentiating symptoms are (1) pain, which is more common in IC/BPS, and (2) incontinence, which can be seen in OAB but not typically in IC/ BPS. The motivation to void for patients with OAB is the strong urgency to void and fear of an incontinent episode, while patients with IC/BPS void frequently to eliminate bladder pain or discomfort [1, 30]. Urodynamics can be helpful in differentiating the two, as uninhibited detrusor contractions will be observed in overactive bladder [30].

Genitourinary syndrome of menopause Genitourinary syndrome of menopause (GSM) is a syndrome encompassing vaginal dryness, dyspareunia, urinary frequency, urgency, nocturia, and dysuria. Vaginal estrogen therapy is found to be 80–90% effective in treating the symptoms of GSM [28]; therefore, IC/BPS is entertained as a diagnosis in postmenopausal women only if symptoms persist after appropriate treatment of GSM.

Painful pelvic and gastrointestinal conditions Endometriosis, vulvodynia, irritable bowel syndrome, and pelvic floor dysfunction may cause bladder pain through central sensitization [18, 22]. When pelvic or abdominal conditions are identified, treatment is initiated in conjunction with the treatment of IC/BPS. The following features are helpful in distinguishing diagnoses:

- Vulvodynia typically manifests with burning/pain in the vulva that may be associated with tampon insertion or with insertion during intercourse.
- Endometriosis is typically associated with dysmenorrhea, dyspareunia (more with deeper thrusting rather than with insertion), mittelschmerz (ovulation pain), and sensitivity

to hormonal changes during a menstrual cycle. Hormonal treatments aimed at suppressing ovulation are very effective in endometriosis and may help differentiate endometriosis from IC/BPS. Laparoscopy may be helpful to diagnose endometriosis, but its presence does not rule out IC/BPS. Up to 50% of patients with endometriosis also have IC/BPS, and hence these two conditions have been termed the "evil twins" [29].

- Irritable bowel syndrome typically causes crampy abdominal pain associated with either constipation and/or diarrhea, fecal urgency, and, rarely, fecal incontinence.
- Pelvic floor dysfunction caused by triggering myofascial points within the pelvic floor muscles may be a result of sensitization from these visceral pain conditions and is present in up to 85% of patients with IC/BPS [24]. Hypertonic pelvic floor dysfunction should be considered in the differential diagnosis of IC/BPS or as a coexisting condition with IC/BPS that will also need treatment.
- Pudendal neuropathy is commonly seen in patients with IC/BPS and pelvic floor dysfunction; it can be challenging to diagnose and to manage. The pain associated with pudendal neuropathy usually worsens with sitting and is relieved with standing [27].
- Somatoform disorder is commonly seen in IC/BPS and should be explored in the differential diagnosis of IC/BPS. These patients tend to have allodynia upon examination. Catastrophizing tendencies are seen commonly in IC/BPS patients and can be a clue that a somatoform disorder may be at play.
- Psychiatric conditions including depression, anxiety, posttraumatic stress disorder, panic disorder, and intimate partner violence are seen more commonly in women with IC/BPS and may manifest as IC/BPS symptomatology [9, 21].

Further reading on these topics can be found in these chapters: Chap. 10 on Fibroids, Endometriosis, Ovarian Cysts, Chap. 12 on Vaginitis and Vulvar Conditions, Chap. 13 on Sexually Transmitted Infections, Chap. 24 on Urinary Tract Infections, Chap. 27 on Irritable Bowel Syndrome, Chap. 31 on Chronic Pelvic Pain, and Chap. 33 on Depressive and Anxiety Disorders.

Ingrid has a long-standing history of anxiety that is well controlled despite a recent divorce. On exam, she has suprapubic tenderness; pelvic examination shows normal external genitalia and vaginal mucosa and hypertonic pelvic floor muscles, with tenderness of the bladder and pelvic floor muscles. The uterus, cervix, and adnexa are nontender. A urine culture and STI screen are obtained as a test of cure for the last UTI and to screen for sexually transmitted infections.

Diagnostic Strategies

The diagnosis of IC/BPS is challenging and anchors on a careful history and physical. IC/BPS is a clinical diagnosis and largely a diagnosis of exclusion. The evaluation should target conditions that also cause pelvic pain and overlap with the symptomatology of IC/BPS. Occasionally, other diagnostic studies or even empiric treatment of comorbid conditions are needed to help narrow the diagnosis.

History

Elements of the history should include a complete urologic, gynecologic, gastrointestinal, and psychiatric history and review of systems. The patient should be asked about a history of urinary tract infections, kidney stones, and the presence of gross hematuria; a gynecologic history includes questions regarding STIs, pelvic inflammatory disease, dyspareunia, endometriosis, structural conditions, and gynecologic or urologic instrumentation. A history of symptoms of IBS should be noted. Questions about comorbid medical and chronic pain conditions and abdominal/pelvic surgeries should be noted. A mental health history including known diagnoses, history of PTSD, history of sexual abuse or trauma, and a history of catastrophizing tendencies should be obtained. A questionnaire including these elements can be completed by the patient and reviewed with the patient at the time of initial presentation [31].

In review of systems, urinary urgency, frequency, significant nocturia, and dysuria should be noted. Pain with a full bladder that is relieved with emptying is indicative of IC/BPS, whereas a feeling of urgency that, if not relieved, may cause an incontinence episode implies an overactive bladder component. Questions about dietary triggers of pain or urgency/frequency and diuretic use, particularly in the evening hours, are important. A 24–48-hour voiding diary including dietary/liquid input and voiding times with output can be particularly helpful. Elements that can cause a flare of symptoms should be elicited if possible, such as stress, the menstrual cycle, sexual activity, or certain activities.

Physical Examination

The goal of the physical exam is to evaluate for comorbid illness and other primary causes of pain that may refer to the pelvis and/or bladder. It is helpful to start with a general physical exam including evaluation of posture, a musculoskeletal examination evaluating the back, and a neurologic exam. Arthritis of the hip can refer pain to the pelvis and can be evaluated with provocative maneuvers in the standing and supine positions.

Thorough abdominal and pelvic exams are essential. The abdominal examination is performed in the supine position. At this time, the bony parts of the pelvis can be palpated particularly on the pubic bone looking for signs of chronic suprapubic pain from osteitis pubis, pubic symphysis relaxation, or rectus muscle inflammation at its insertion to the pubis. One should check for tenderness and masses in the various quadrants of the abdomen to evaluate for abdominal pathology and/or for suprapubic tenderness that is commonly seen in IC/BPS. Any rigidity, guarding, or rebound tenderness can imply an acute process such as diverticulitis, pelvic inflammatory disease, colitis, or an appendicitis and signals a medical emergency. Distension, bowel sounds, ascites, masses, vascular bruits, and superficial vs deep tenderness should be noted. Superficial tenderness may imply a neuropathic process or a musculoskeletal/fascial process. Deeper palpation may help evaluate the deep visceral structures such as the bowel, bladder, and gynecologic organs. The ilioinguinal and iliohypogastric nerves should be evaluated for sensory deficits including hyperalgesia or allodynia, which is the perception of noxious stimuli with light touch.

The pelvic exam is then performed in the lithotomy position. The external genitalia should be inspected for any vulvar lesions, vestibular erythema, skin changes, perianal lesions, fissures, and fistulae. The urethral meatus should be inspected for any lesions or a caruncle. A urethral caruncle is an inferior erythematous protrusion of the urethral mucosa commonly seen in atrophic menopausal women. The absence of labia minora may also indicate genital atrophy or lichen sclerosus. Hypersensitivity or allodynia of the thoracic and lumbar nerves should be evaluated along the mons area, groin, labia, and perirectally, as well as the thighs and lower extremities. Bulbocavernosus and anal wink reflexes should be elicited as part of the pudendal nerve evaluation. A cotton swab may be used to check for tenderness along the vulvar vestibule assessing for vulvar vestibulitis.

It is helpful to first start with a single digit examination of the vagina. First the perineal body is palpated followed by the levator muscles. The various muscles that can be appreciated with the single digit vaginal examination are the puborectalis, obturator internus, iliococcygeus, coccygeus, and piriformis muscles. These muscles should be evaluated for spasm, which is commonly seen in visceral pelvic pain disorders [32]. The urethra and the bladder are then palpated and evaluated for urethral diverticula, urethral tenderness, trigonal tenderness, and bladder tenderness. The technique to help isolate bladder tenderness is shown in Fig. 30.1.

Using a single digit for examination, the cervix is palpated for tenderness, which can be a sign of cervicitis or pelvic infection. The posterior fornix is then evaluated for any uterosacral nodules that may be seen in endometriosis.

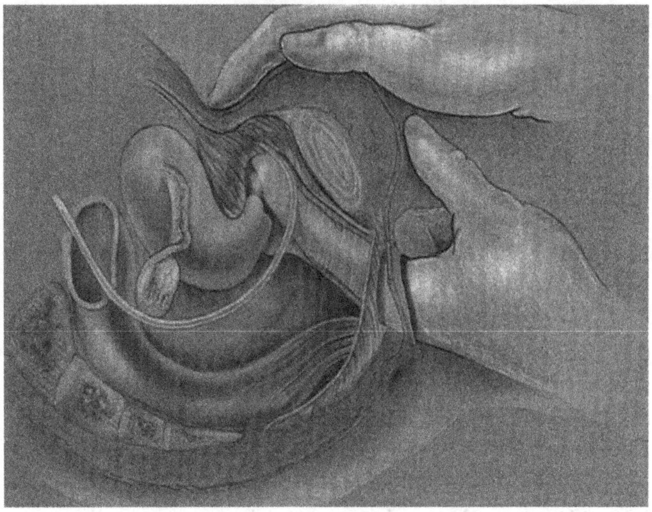

Fig. 30.1 The technique to help isolate bladder tenderness [27]. (Reprinted with permission from Wolters Kluwer, Howard [27])

Uterine tenderness may be present in the setting of pelvic infection, endometritis, or endometriosis. Only after completion of this single digit exam, the traditional bimanual exam with two fingers in the vagina and the second hand on the abdomen is performed (see Chap. 3 on The Female Sex and Gender Specific History and Examination for full details on performing the pelvic exam). Tenderness that is elicited on a bimanual exam, but not the single digit examination, may mistakenly be thought to be pelvic when it is in fact abdominal in origin. The bimanual exam assesses the size, contour, and mobility of the uterus, attempts to palpate any adnexal masses or tenderness, and confirms or better characterizes the tenderness felt on the single digit vaginal examination. A rectal and/or rectovaginal examination is performed last in the lithotomy position to evaluate for any rectal masses or hemorrhoids and to better palpate the adnexa or a retroverted uterus. Any vaginal discharge should be sampled and evaluated with a wet mount, if available, and specimens can be obtained to evaluate for sexually transmitted infections.

Examinations must be performed with gentleness and caution as maneuvers during the pelvic examination may trigger pelvic floor spasm and limit the remainder of the examination. Care should be taken to involve the patient and keep her informed every step of the way, watching for any negative reaction from the patient during the examination. Anxiety or prior negative experiences can trigger a post-traumatic reaction, and the patient may distance herself from the examination. This may limit the information obtained during the evaluation. The presence of any hypertonicity or vaginismus during the examination or at the beginning of the examination should be documented.

Please refer to Chap. 31 on Chronic Pelvic Pain to read more about the gynecologic exam in women with chronic pain.

Testing

Laboratory evaluation is very limited in the diagnosis of IC/BPS, except to rule out an infectious process by urinalysis, urine culture, and/or testing for sexually transmitted infections.

Urinalysis in patients with IC/BPS may be difficult to interpret as up to 40% of patients can have microscopic or gross hematuria [33] which does not necessarily correlate with disease severity or cystoscopic findings [34]. Urinalysis can also be bland or have mild pyuria, though urine cultures should always be sterile [35]. If sterile pyuria persists, other etiologies for urinary symptoms, other than IC/BPS, should be pursued [36, 37]. Urine cytology should be considered if microscopic or gross hematuria is present, as symptoms of IC/BPS can overlap with those of urinary tract malignancy. All other laboratory evaluations should be based on symptomatology, to evaluate for a particular diagnosis rather than to screen for disease. Imaging studies should be conducted with the same intention and specificity, in order to minimize incidental findings. Ultrasound, CT scan, and MRI should be geared toward a specific pathology, keeping in mind the sensitivity and specificity of the test for the condition that is being targeted. Patients should be imaged when there is clinical or physical concern for an abdominal or pelvic mass and in cases of microscopic or gross hematuria.

Focused bladder testing should include a post-void residual to rule out overdistension of the bladder and to obtain a baseline as some treatments can cause retention of urine (e.g., anticholinergic medications). Cystoscopy by a urologist or urogynecologist can be helpful in evaluating for pathology of the urinary tract, particularly during the workup of hematuria, but is not always necessary in the evaluation of IC/BPS. Glomerulations or petechial hemorrhages of the bladder mucosa may be seen in IC/BPS when the bladder is hydrodistended under ~80 cm H_2O pressure for a few minutes and should be documented, but its absence does not rule out IC/BPS [1]. In a patient with bladder pain, the cystoscopy should be done under anesthesia if needed. Urodynamic testing is also considered invasive; it is helpful in ruling out other voiding disorders of the bladder such as overactive bladder and urinary retention, but is not needed to rule out IC/BPS. The classic findings in IC/BPS on urodynamic testing are low bladder capacity and the absence of involuntary detrusor contractions [30].

Based on Ingrid's symptoms and the negative evaluation for other etiologies of her symptoms, she is diagnosed with IC/BPS. She asks about the next step in management.

Treatment Strategies

The goal of treatment for IC/BPS is improvement of symptoms and quality of life. A patient-centered approach is key in management of this syndrome where symptoms can vary from mild to debilitating in the absence of correlating physical findings. The American Urological Association treatment guidelines (Fig. 30.2) have formalized management of IC/BPS into a step-by-step approach [1, 38] to help patients and providers. *Patient education is very important in obtaining patient buy-in.*

All patients should be offered first-line treatment which includes behavioral modification and self-care techniques. Patient education about the disorder can help manage expectations and allow self-assessment of her triggers to manage them appropriately. As approximately 90% of women with IC/BPS report a sensitivity to certain foods, an elimination diet tends to be quite helpful in management [39]. Significant foods to avoid include caffeine, alcohol, soda, artificial sweeteners, and acidic and spicy foods. Acid-reducing products such as baking soda slushes, calcium glycerophosphates, and antacids can be helpful in tolerating certain foods. Stress management should be encouraged due to its association with flares of symptoms. Cognitive behavioral therapy, meditation, and pelvic floor relaxation can be learned.

Symptomatic relief during flares can be obtained from products such as phenazopyridine or methylene blue-containing medications that may be obtained over the counter or as a prescription. These agents act as analgesics for the bladder and can help with the dysuria, urgency, and frequency temporarily, but should not be used long term [1].

The second-line treatments for IC/BPS include physical therapy techniques and medication regimens taken either orally or instilled in the bladder and should be offered in conjunction with first-line treatments. The majority of women with IC/BPS have hypertonic pelvic floor dysfunction and therefore can benefit from manual physical therapy (PT) or pelvic floor physical therapy [18]. PT is geared toward reducing the spasm of the pelvic floor muscles and increasing relaxation and lengthening of the pelvic muscles. PT may be ordered directly by the primary care provider. Strengthening of the pelvic floor muscles through Kegel exercises is strongly discouraged as it can trigger spasm and pain.

Medications that have demonstrated benefit in the treatment of IC/BPS include pentosan polysulfate (PPS), tricyclic antidepressants, cimetidine, and hydroxyzine [1]. Pentosan polysulfate is an oral sulfated polysaccharide that replenishes the defective glycosaminoglycan layer of the bladder mucosa and has shown efficacy in treating the pain and urgency of IC/BPS [40]. PPS can also be instilled intravesi-

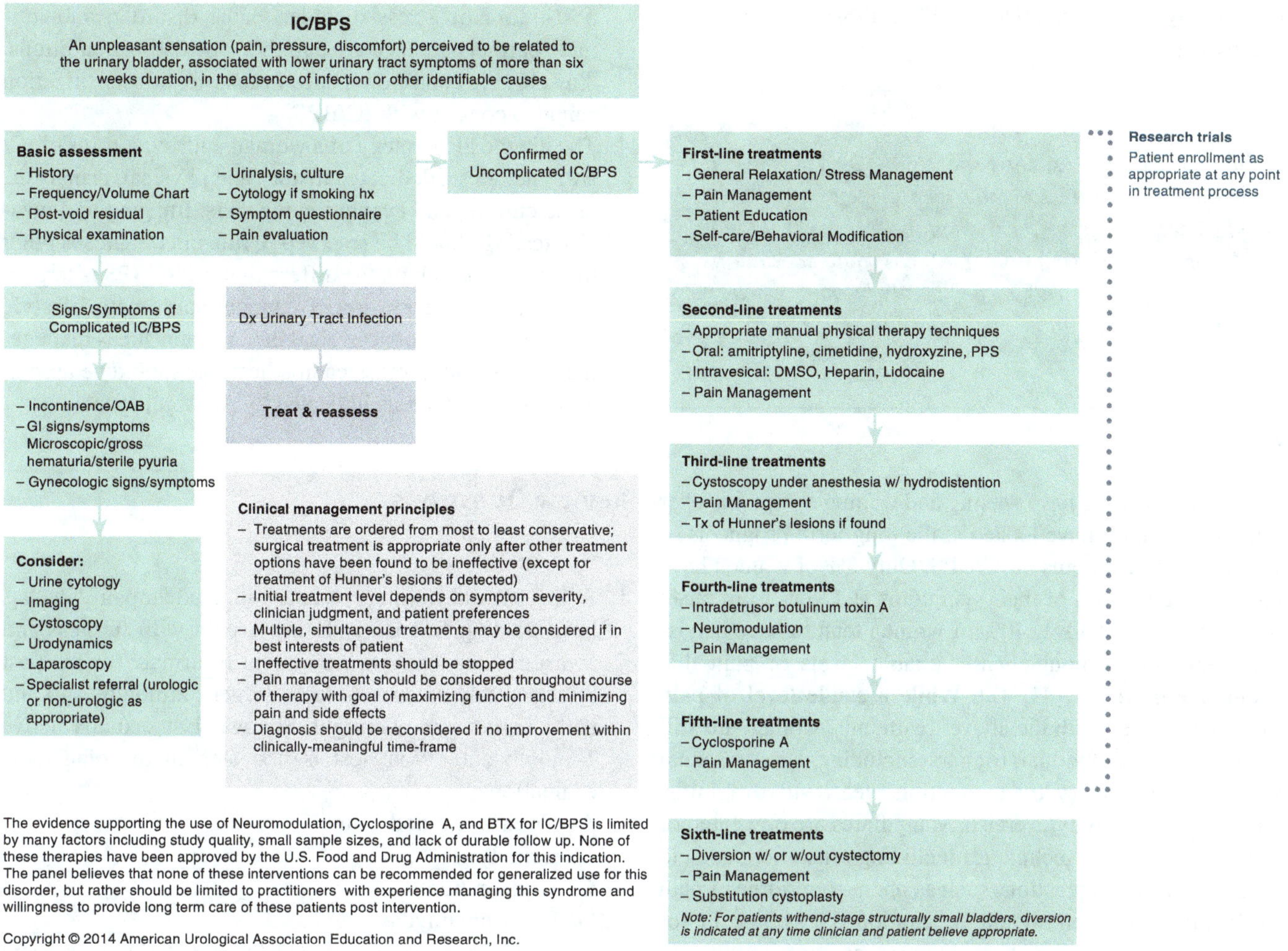

Fig. 30.2 AUA treatment guidelines for bladder pain syndrome algorithm [1, 38]. (Reprinted with permission from the American Urological Association, 2014 AUA Diagnosis and Treatment Interstitial Cystitis/Bladder Pain Syndrome Guidelines, Hanno et al. [38]. © 2015 by American Urological Association Education and Research, Inc)

cally in an attempt to avoid systemic side effects: bleeding, headache, hair loss, nausea, diarrhea, and stomach pain. Tricyclic antidepressants (TCAs) are helpful in treating the chronic pain of IC/BPS, as they are in other chronic pain syndromes. TCAs can improve chronic pain through a neuromodulatory mechanism, and the anticholinergic effects can help with urinary urgency and frequency. TCAs can be quite effective when used long term to decrease frequency of flares, but the CNS side effects of sedation and drowsiness often limit their use. Cimetidine and hydroxyzine are antihistamines and can help episodically or chronically to reduce the frequency of flares [1].

Dimethyl sulfoxide (DMSO), heparin, and lidocaine have been used intravesically to treat IC/BPS by urologists and urogynecologists. Most intravesical treatments are placed in the bladder via a catheter, and the patient is asked to hold the medication in the bladder for at least 30 minutes. Treatments are done at various intervals from weekly to every few months for initial treatment and maintenance therapy.

A referral to a urologist or a urogynecologist should be made if patients are not responding or are responding suboptimally to first-line therapies and/or oral therapies as care beyond these treatments becomes more complex. Invasive therapies such as cystoscopic treatments or neurostimulation can be considered in refractory cases [1]. Intravesical botox injections and cyclosporine A have been used with some success. The specialist and the primary care provider should work together to provide symptom control and pain control. A pain management specialist may also become involved to manage the patient in a multimodal fashion. As a clinical principle, it is best to avoid invasive, non-reversible methods of management until the noninvasive options have been exhausted. Finally, cystectomy is a radical option that has been used as a last resort in patients with intractable pain, although with mixed results [1].

Ingrid decided to start pentosan polysulfate and worked on her stress management techniques. She has had good control of her symptoms for several years. She is now 62-years-old and has noticed that her symptoms are returning, specifically burning when she urinates. Urine cultures have been negative.

Prognosis

IC/BPS is known to have waxing and waning symptoms over time. Few studies have looked at the long-term prognosis of women with symptoms of IC/BPS. Only 8% of women have complete regression of their symptoms at 1 year from onset of symptoms [41]. Over 40% of women tend to have persistent symptoms although with variable levels of pain that occur intermittently [41, 42]. While a stable level of pain may be achieved with the above treatments, women are still vulnerable to individual triggers including stress, sexual activity, diet, urinary tract infection, yeast vulvovaginitis, and strenuous activity/exercise. Many flares are prevented or limited by self-care techniques including relaxation, antacid treatments, and medications such as phenazopyridine or pain medications. Women should be cautioned to come in for evaluation if their "usual" techniques are not working to revisit the diagnosis. A thorough evaluation may need to be reinitiated as these symptoms may be completely independent of the original IC/BPS diagnosis. Treatments may fail to be effective, but also some patients discontinue therapy independently when feeling better, leading to exacerbations of pain and frequency.

Summary Points

1. Interstitial cystitis or bladder pain syndrome (IC/BPS) is a female predominant, debilitating disorder of the bladder characterized by pain with filling that is partially relieved by emptying, urinary frequency, and urgency. Patients often present for evaluation after treatments for UTIs and STIs have failed.
2. The differential diagnosis of IC/BPS is extensive and includes recurrent urinary tract infections, chronic urethritis, overactive bladder, genitourinary syndrome of menopause, vulvodynia, endometriosis, irritable bowel syndrome, pelvic floor dysfunction, and neuropathic pain.
3. Conditions included in the differential diagnosis of IC/BPS can coexist with IC/BPS. Migraine headaches, temporomandibular joint pain, fibromyalgia, depression, post-traumatic stress disorder, panic disorder, and intimate partner violence are common coexisting conditions. Any chronic condition that can cause central sensitization can also coexist with IC/BPS.
4. The diagnostic strategy of a woman with symptoms of IC/BPS includes a dedicated history and physical, urinalysis, urine culture, and evaluation for STIs. Imaging and invasive testing should be reserved to rule out diagnoses other than IC/BPS high on the differential, as IC/BPS is largely a diagnosis of exclusion. Treatment starts with lifestyle changes, pelvic floor physical therapy, and stress management. Oral and intravesical medications should be used in a stepwise fashion as indicated by AUA guidelines.

Review Questions

1. A 42-year-old woman presents with bladder pain. She has been voiding frequently to avoid pain with fullness and awakens four to six times a night to urinate for the past 8 weeks. She underwent knee surgery 2 months ago and had a catheter in overnight. She was last sexually active 1 month ago. What test is first step in the diagnostic evaluation?
   A. Complete blood count.
   B. Urinalysis.
   C. Urine culture.
   D. Urine chlamydia.

   The correct answer is B. In the initial management of a patient with bladder pain and urinary frequency, it is most important to evaluate for a urinary tract infection as a cause of her symptoms. A complete blood count would not aid in the diagnosis of urinary tract infection. A urinalysis should be completed as a first step. If her urinalysis is unremarkable, a urine culture in this patient is not appropriate and thus is not the first step in this evaluation. Urine chlamydia testing would not be the first test given her risk factor of recent catheterization [1].

2. A healthy 65-year-old woman presents with urinary urgency and frequency. She complains of dysuria and has burning in the vulvar area. She had a urinary tract infection 4 months ago, but a recent urinalysis was negative. She is not sexually active. What is a reasonable initial treatment?
   A. Lifestyle changes and avoidance of trigger foods.
   B. Vaginal moisturizers or estrogen therapy.
   C. Antibiotic therapy.
   D. Pentosan polysulfate.

   The correct answer is B. This patient is clearly in her postmenopausal years and is likely to have genitourinary syndrome of menopause (GSM) based on her clinical history and the fact that GSM is much more common than IC/BPS. She does not have a urinary tract infection as urinalysis was negative. GSM is not triggered by certain foods like IC/BPS. Treating GSM might completely resolve her symptoms and should be attempted first with vaginal estrogen or vaginal moisturizers. If her symptoms persist, then one would consider IC/BPS and could treat empirically with pentosan polysulfate after behavioral and lifestyle modifications are made [26].

3. A 42-year-old woman presents with 6-month history of urinary frequency and urgency. She complains of pain in her bladder that is relieved with voiding. She voids frequently to avoid the pain. She has regular menses and finds that her symptoms are worse during her menstrual cycle. Her urinalysis and urine culture are negative. What is a reasonable next treatment after behavioral techniques?
   A. Vaginal estrogen treatment.
   B. Antibiotic suppression.
   C. Cystoscopy with hydrodistension.
   D. Sacral neuromodulation.
   E. Pelvic floor therapy.

   The correct answer is E. This is a typical presentation of a woman with IC/BPS. Based on the AUA treatment algorithm, it is recommended to start with dietary/behavioral techniques for symptom control and then add second-line treatments such as pelvic floor therapy. Answers A and B are not appropriate as the presentation is not consistent with genitourinary syndrome of menopause or recurrent urinary tract infections. Options C and D are reserved for patients that fail conservative therapy [1].

References

1. Hanno PM, Burks DA, Clemens JQ, Dmochowski RR, Erickson D, Fitzgerald MP, et al. AUA guideline for the diagnosis and treatment of interstitial cystitis/bladder pain syndrome. J Urol. 2011;185(6):2162–70.
2. Berry SH, Elliott MN, Suttorp M, Bogart LM, Stoto MA, Eggers P, et al. Prevalence of symptoms of bladder pain syndrome/interstitial cystitis among adult females in the United States. J Urol. 2011;186(2):540–4.
3. Barry MJ, Link CL, McNaughton-Collins MF, McKinlay JB. Overlap of different urological symptom complexes in a racially and ethnically diverse, community-based population of men and women. BJU Int. 2008;101(1):45–51.
4. Peterson A, Hager BH. Interstitial cystitis: report of cases. Cal West Med. 1929;31(4):262–7.
5. Parsons CL, Lilly JD, Stein P. Epithelial dysfunction in nonbacterial cystitis (interstitial cystitis). J Urol. 1991;145(4):732–5.
6. Waxman JA, Sulak PJ, Kuehl TJ. Cystoscopic findings consistent with interstitial cystitis in normal women undergoing tubal ligation. J Urol. 1998;160(5):1663–7.
7. McLennan MT. Interstitial cystitis: epidemiology, pathophysiology, and clinical presentation. Obstet Gynecol Clin N Am. 2014;41(3):385–95.
8. Kuo HC. Potential urine and serum biomarkers for patients with bladder pain syndrome/interstitial cystitis. Int J Urol. 2014;21(Suppl 1):34–41.
9. Chen IC, Lee MH, Lin HH, Wu SL, Chang KM, Lin HY. Somatoform disorder as a predictor of interstitial cystitis/bladder pain syndrome: evidence from a nested case-control study and a retrospective cohort study. Medicine (Baltimore). 2017;96(18):e6304.
10. Clemens JQ. Afferent neurourology: a novel paradigm. Neurourol Urodyn. 2010;29(Suppl 1):S29–31.
11. Lai HH, Gardner V, Ness TJ, Gereau RWT. Segmental hyperalgesia to mechanical stimulus in interstitial cystitis/bladder pain syndrome: evidence of central sensitization. J Urol. 2014;191(5):1294–9.
12. Nickel JC, Tripp DA, Pontari M, Moldwin R, Mayer R, Carr LK, et al. Interstitial cystitis/painful bladder syndrome and associated medical conditions with an emphasis on irritable bowel syndrome, fibromyalgia and chronic fatigue syndrome. J Urol. 2010;184(4):1358–63.
13. Chelimsky G, Heller E, Buffington CA, Rackley R, Zhang D, Chelimsky T. Co-morbidities of interstitial cystitis. Front Neurosci. 2012;6:114. https://doi.org/10.3389/fnins.2012.00114.
14. As-Sanie S, Harris RE, Napadow V, Kim J, Neshewat G, Kairys A, et al. Changes in regional gray matter volume in women with chronic pelvic pain: a voxel-based morphometry study. Pain. 2012;153(5):1006–14.
15. Teichman JM, Parsons CL. Contemporary clinical presentation of interstitial cystitis. Urology. 2007;69(4 Suppl):41–7.
16. Bogart LM, Berry SH, Clemens JQ. Symptoms of interstitial cystitis, painful bladder syndrome and similar diseases in women: a systematic review. J Urol. 2007;177(2):450–6.
17. Shorter B, Lesser M, Moldwin RM, Kushner L. Effect of comestibles on symptoms of interstitial cystitis. J Urol. 2007;178(1):145–52.
18. Peters KM, Carrico DJ, Kalinowski SE, Ibrahim IA, Diokno AC. Prevalence of pelvic floor dysfunction in patients with interstitial cystitis. Urology. 2007;70(1):16–8.
19. Warren JW, Clauw DJ, Wesselmann U, Langenberg PW, Howard FM, Morozov V. Sexuality and reproductive risk factors for interstitial cystitis/painful bladder syndrome in women. Urology. 2011;77(3):570–5.
20. Nickel JC, Tripp DA, Pontari M, Moldwin R, Mayer R, Carr LK, et al. Childhood sexual trauma in women with interstitial cystitis/bladder pain syndrome: a case control study. Can Urol Assoc J. 2011;5(6):410–5.
21. Nickel JC, Tripp DA. International Interstitial Cystitis Study G. Clinical and psychological parameters associated with pain pattern phenotypes in women with interstitial cystitis/bladder pain syndrome. J Urol. 2015;193(1):138–44.
22. Cervigni M, Natale F. Gynecological disorders in bladder pain syndrome/interstitial cystitis patients. Int J Urol. 2014;21(Suppl 1):85–8.
23. El Khoudary SR, Talbott EO, Bromberger JT, Chang CC, Songer TJ, Davis EL. Severity of interstitial cystitis symptoms and quality of life in female patients. J Womens Health (Larchmt). 2009;18(9):1361–8.
24. Butrick CW. Interstitial cystitis and chronic pelvic pain: new insights in neuropathology, diagnosis, and treatment. Clin Obstet Gynecol. 2003;46(4):811–23.
25. Constantine GD, Bruyniks N, Princic N, Huse D, Palmer L, Lenhart G, et al. Incidence of genitourinary conditions in women with a diagnosis of vulvar/vaginal atrophy. Curr Med Res Opin. 2014;30(1):143–8. https://doi.org/10.1185/03007995.2013.850068.
26. Gandhi J, Chen A, Dagur G, Suh Y, Smith N, Cali B, et al. Genitourinary syndrome of menopause: an overview of clinical manifestations, pathophysiology, etiology, evaluation, and management. Am J Obstetr Gynecol. 2016;215(6):704–11.
27. Howard FM. Pelvic pain: diagnosis and management hardcover. 1st ed. Philadelphia: Lippincott, Williams & Wilkins; 2000. xiii, 529 pp.
28. Rahn DD, Carberry C, Sanses TV, Mamik MM, Ward RM, Meriwether KV, et al. Vaginal estrogen for genitourinary syndrome of menopause: a systematic review. Obstet Gynecol. 2014;124(6):1147–56.

29. Tirlapur SA, Kuhrt K, Chaliha C, Ball E, Meads C, Khan KS. The 'evil twin syndrome' in chronic pelvic pain: a systematic review of prevalence studies of bladder pain syndrome and endometriosis. Int J Surg. 2013;11(3):233–7. https://doi.org/10.1016/j.ijsu.2013.02.003.
30. Macdiarmid SA, Sand PK. Diagnosis of interstitial cystitis/ painful bladder syndrome in patients with overactive bladder symptoms. Rev Urol. 2007;9(1):9–16.
31. Bennis S, Hwang S. Office evaluation of pelvic pain. Phys Med Rehabil Clin N Am. 2017;28(3):461–76.
32. Eickmeyer SM. Anatomy and physiology of the pelvic floor. Phys Med Rehabil Clin N Am. 2017;28(3):455–60.
33. Gomes CM, Sanchez-Ortiz RF, Harris C, Wein AJ, Rovner ES. Significance of hematuria in patients with interstitial cystitis: review of radiographic and endoscopic findings. Urology. 2001;57(2):262–5.
34. Stanford EJ, Mattox TF, Parsons JK, McMurphy C. Prevalence of benign microscopic hematuria among women with interstitial cystitis: implications for evaluation of genitourinary malignancy. Urology. 2006;67(5):946–9.
35. Warren JW, Brown V, Jacobs S, Horne L, Langenberg P, Greenberg P. Urinary tract infection and inflammation at onset of interstitial cystitis/painful bladder syndrome. Urology. 2008;71(6):1085–90.
36. Wise GJ, Schlegel PN. Sterile pyuria. N Engl J Med. 2015;372(11):1048–54.
37. Davis R, Jones JS, Barocas DA, Castle EP, Lang EK, Leveillee RJ, et al. Diagnosis, evaluation and follow-up of asymptomatic microhematuria (AMH) in adults: AUA guideline. J Urol. 2012;188(6 Suppl):2473–81.
38. Hanno PM, Erickson D, Moldwin R, Faraday MM, American Urological A. Diagnosis and treatment of interstitial cystitis/ bladder pain syndrome: AUA guideline amendment. J Urol. 2015;193(5):1545–53.
39. Friedlander JI, Shorter B, Moldwin RM. Diet and its role in interstitial cystitis/bladder pain syndrome (IC/BPS) and comorbid conditions. BJU Int. 2012;109(11):1584–91.
40. Mulholland SG, Hanno P, Parsons CL, Sant GR, Staskin DR. Pentosan polysulfate sodium for therapy of interstitial cystitis. A double-blind placebo-controlled clinical study. Urology. 1990;35(6):552–8.
41. Suskind AM, Berry SH, Suttorp MJ, Elliott MN, Clemens JQ. Symptom persistence in a community cohort of women with interstitial cystitis/bladder pain syndrome (IC/BPS): 3-, 6-, 9-, and 12-month follow-up from the RICE cohort. Int Urogynecol J. 2014;25(12):1639–43.
42. Stephens-Shields AJ, Clemens JQ, Jemielita T, Farrar J, Sutcliffe S, Hou X, et al. Symptom variability and early symptom regression in the MAPP study: a prospective study of urological chronic pelvic pain syndrome. J Urol. 2016;196(5):1450–5.

Chronic Pelvic Pain

31

Christina I. Ramirez, Sarah A. Tilstra, and Nicole M. Donnellan

Learning Objectives

1. Define chronic pelvic pain (CPP), including its complex and multifactorial dimensions.
2. Develop a systems-based approach for developing a differential diagnosis of CPP, recognizing that a single diagnosis is often not possible.
3. Describe how to perform a focused history and physical exam in a patient presenting with CPP.
4. Provide examples of initial tests to perform when evaluating a patient with CPP.
5. Discuss treatment options for the multidisciplinary management of CPP.

Sally is a 35-year-old G1P1 woman who presents with pelvic pain. Her menses are regular and last 7–8 days. Her pain started several months after the birth of her daughter 3 years ago. Initially, the pain would only last a couple days at a time and occurred once every few months. Over the last month, the pain has been increasing in intensity and frequency and now is occurring on a daily basis. She is having difficulty concentrating at work due to her pain.

Background

Chronic pelvic pain (CPP) is a prevalent and debilitating condition that impacts women worldwide. It is estimated that CPP affects up to 15% of reproductive age women in the United States [1]. Globally, the prevalence of chronic pelvic pain ranges from 2.1% to 26.6% [2, 3]. CPP is generally defined as noncyclical pain of at least 3–6 months' duration that appears in locations such as the pelvis, anterior abdominal wall, lower back, or buttocks and that is serious enough to cause disability or lead to medical or surgical care [4, 5]. Chronic pelvic pain places a significant burden on the affected individual and on society through economic and healthcare-related costs. In a study by Mathias et al., 15% of women with chronic pelvic pain reported missing paid work. In 1996, this correlated with an estimated cost of $555.3 million dollars due to time lost from work [1]. Women suffering from CPP have significant associated comorbidities and a diminished quality of life. A large study of women with CPP found that 98% met DSM-IV criteria for at least one mental health disorder, 50.5% suffered from a mood disorder, and 38.6% suffered from an anxiety disorder [6]. The large percentage of mental health comorbidities among women with CPP underscores the importance of accurate diagnosis and multidisciplinary care of CPP patients.

There are entire chapters in this book dedicated to a few of the most common causes of chronic pelvic pain including Endometriosis (Chap. 10), Irritable Bowel Syndrome (Chap. 27), Interstitial Cystitis/Bladder Pain Syndrome (Chap. 30), Vulvar Conditions (in Chap. 12), as well as other contributors to pelvic pain such as Depressive and Anxiety Disorders (Chap. 33) and Intimate Partner Violence and Sexual Trauma (Chap. 35). Details of the diagnosis and management of these conditions are outside the scope of this chapter. This chapter will provide a general approach to the patient who presents with pelvic pain and focus on localized causes of CPP such as abdominal wall pain, pelvic floor dysfunction, myofascial pain syndrome, vaginismus, and adhesive disease.

C. I. Ramirez (✉) · N. M. Donnellan
Magee-Womens Hospital of University of Pittsburgh Medical Center, Department of Obstetrics, Gynecology, and Reproductive Sciences, Pittsburgh, PA, USA
e-mail: christina.i.ramirez.mil@mail.mil

S. A. Tilstra
University of Pittsburgh School of Medicine, Division of General Internal Medicine, Department of Medicine, Pittsburgh, PA, USA

S. A. Tilstra et al. (eds.), *Sex- and Gender-Based Women's Health*, https://doi.org/10.1007/978-3-030-50695-7_31

Neuroanatomy of the Pelvis

There are numerous potential etiologies for female chronic pelvic pain, which will be reviewed in further detail within this chapter through a systems-based approach. To best understand the sources and pathophysiology of female chronic pelvic pain, it is imperative to become familiar with the neuroanatomy of visceral and somatic pain pathways within the abdominopelvic region.

The innervation of the pelvis is complex. An intricate relationship exists between the somatic, sympathetic, and parasympathetic nervous systems to allow for appropriate sensation and coordination of dual voluntary and involuntary bodily functions, such as micturition, defecation, and parturition.

The somatic nervous system innervates the skeletal muscles of the pelvis, the abdominal wall, and the skin overlying the external genitalia. The anterior cutaneous branch of the tenth intercostal nerve transmits pain at the level of the umbilicus. The skin overlying the suprapubic region is innervated by cutaneous branches of the iliohypogastric nerve, which is derived from the L1 nerve root [7]. The pelvic floor, which is predominantly made up of the levator ani muscle group (puborectalis, pubococcygeus, and iliococcygeus), is innervated by the S3–S5 nerve roots. The pudendal nerve is the primary sensory and motor nerve of the perineum, which is derived from the S2–S4 nerve roots. Branches of the pudendal nerve provide sensory innervation to the skin of the posterior labia and the clitoris, the urethral and anal sphincters, and the muscles that coordinate orgasm [6–8]. The anterior cutaneous innervation to the labia is supplied by the ilioinguinal nerve (nerve root L1) [8]. Injury to the sacral nerve roots or their branches can result in acute or chronic pain and dysfunction of the innervated tissues. The somatic nervous system most often plays a role in vulvar disease (vulvodynia), vaginismus, myofascial pain syndrome, pelvic floor spasm, and abdominal wall pain.

Visceral pain is unique in that it is poorly localized, can occur without injury (e.g., stretching of the bladder), can be referred to other parts of the body, and is associated with autonomic responses such as nausea, vomiting, and sweating [9]. Visceral pain from the uterus, bladder, and rectum is predominantly transmitted through sympathetic nervous system fibers via the hypogastric plexus [8]. The nerves of the hypogastric plexus return to the spinal cord through the lumbar splanchnics and eventually reach the processing centers in the brain. Conversely, pain signals from the ovary and distal fallopian tubes, which are lateral pelvic structures, and travels through the parasympathetic system through the ovarian plexus to the vagus nerve [8]. Patients with chronic pain can perceive any visceral sensation as pain due to complex dysregulation of pain processing. This may include "central sensitization," where the central nervous system is primed to interpret any pain stimulus in an exaggerated way, and "visceral cross sensitization," where a healthy pelvic organ is influenced by an adjacent diseased organ to perceive pain [6] (Fig. 31.1).

Sally states that her pain is sharp and constant in the lower abdomen. The pain shoots down toward her groin and is aggravated by intercourse. The pain is so intense that she cannot tolerate using tampons. She denies any history of pain with menses (dysmenorrhea), bowel movements (dyschezia), or urination (dysuria).

History

Every woman who presents with chronic pelvic pain will describe her chief complaint and the location and quality of her pain differently. Therefore, a systematic and thorough history is necessary to understand the full scope of the patient's symptoms and concerns. When obtaining the history, it is important to keep the differential diagnoses in mind in order to prevent missing a potential diagnosis. Women may have many different types of pain, and the details of each should be recorded separately. It is important to create

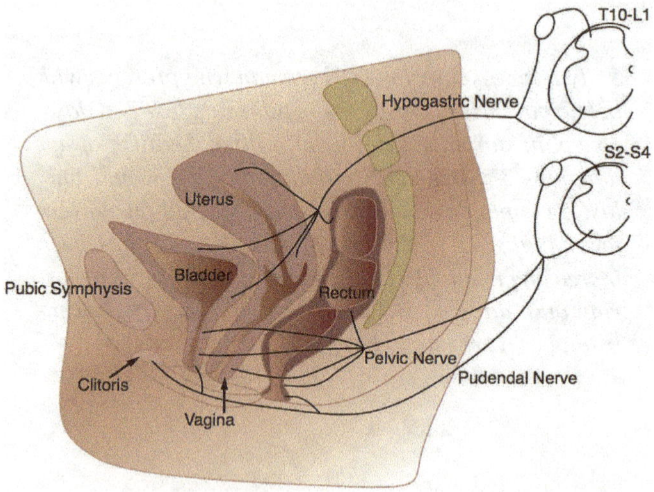

Fig. 31.1 Innervation of the pelvic organs. Sensory axons innervating the vagina reach the spinal cord via pelvic nerves and terminate in sacral spinal cord segments (S2–S4). Axons innervating the uterus travel in the hypogastric nerves and terminate in the thoracolumbar spinal cord segments (T10–L2). The region surrounding the cervix represents a transitional zone and is innervated by fibers that travel in both nerves. Sensory axons from the clitoris and vulva follow the pudendal nerves to sacral spinal cord. Note that sensory information from all pelvic organs may converge onto the same spinal cord neural circuits, DRG (dorsal root ganglia) [10]. (Image reprinted from Jobling et al. [10]: article 17. Special thanks also to Kelly Smith)

a safe, comfortable, and judgment-free space for patients with CPP, as with all patients. The patient should feel that the provider is listening and taking her symptoms seriously. *Whenever possible, history-taking should be performed in the office while the patient is fully clothed.*

A detailed pain history is critical and should include information about the pain characterization: onset, location, duration, timing, what the pain feels like, aggravating and alleviating factors, and prior treatments of each type of pain. Care should be taken to determine the impact of the chronic pain on the patient's quality of life, relationships, and employability. While keeping the differential diagnosis in mind, a complete neurologic, gastrointestinal, urologic, musculoskeletal, gynecologic, and psychiatric review of systems should be obtained. Past medical and surgical history should include any history of chronic pain disorders, psychiatric conditions, and prior abdominal or pelvic surgeries. A detailed obstetric and gynecologic history should include information regarding prior pregnancies and deliveries, menstrual history, sexual history, and any prior diagnoses of endometriosis, fibroids, or sexually transmitted diseases. Pertinent aspects of the patient's social history include occupation, employment disability, support system, screening for history of trauma, and past or present intimate partner violence (see Chap. 35 on Intimate Partner Violence and Sexual Trauma) and drug use (see Chap. 32 on Opioid Use Disorder in Women). Family history should focus on history of chronic pain disorders, substance use, trauma, or psychiatric illnesses.

Physical Exam

The physical exam for a patient with pelvic pain can be a very uncomfortable experience. Prior to beginning the physical exam, it is crucial that the provider create a safe environment for the patient. All components and indications for the different aspects of the physical exam should be explained and verbal consent obtained prior to proceeding with each part of the exam. The patient should also understand that she is in control and that she may pause or stop the exam at any point. Additionally, the patient should be offered a chaperone and/or allowed to have a support person in the room with her if that makes her feel more comfortable with the physical exam.

The focused physical exam should start with a visual assessment of the patient's abdomen while she is lying in the supine position. The abdominal wall should be assessed for any visible masses, areas of asymmetry, skin changes from chronic heat pad usage, and scarring from prior surgical procedures. Next, auscultation for bowel sounds should be performed in all four quadrants. Palpation of the abdomen should proceed from superficial structures down to deep structures. The Carnett's test, in which the examiner palpates each quadrant of the abdomen at rest and then with contraction of the abdominal wall by having the patient raise her head off the bed without using her arms, can be performed to assess for abdominal wall musculoskeletal pain [11]. The Carnett's test is reported to be "positive" if the patient reports reproduction of her pain with palpation of a contracted abdominal wall (as opposed to the relaxed state) and has a diagnostic accuracy of 97% for abdominal wall pain [12]. In contrast, this physical exam finding is positive in less than 10% of patients with a visceral etiology of their chronic pain. When palpating the abdomen at rest, each quadrant should be gently palpated at a superficial and deep level to evaluate for masses, organomegaly, or focal areas of tenderness. Additionally, the patient should be assessed for any signs or symptoms of an acute surgical abdomen: involuntary guarding (tensing of abdominal wall muscles in anticipation of pain with palpation) or rebound tenderness (tenderness when quickly releasing pressure off of the abdominal wall). Patients with evidence of an acute surgical abdomen require immediate evaluation in an emergency room.

The gynecologic exam begins with a visual inspection of the perineum and vulva while the patient is in the dorsal lithotomy position. The external genitalia should be carefully examined for any signs of skin changes, trauma, excoriations, swelling, scarring, pelvic organ prolapse, cystic lesions, and unusual discharge or odor [13]. Next, a Q-tip test should be performed to assess for vulvodynia [14]. This is performed by assessing for reproduction of pain around the introitus when lightly swabbing at the 3 o'clock, 6 o'clock, and 9 o'clock locations. The patient's baseline pain should be assessed on scale from "0" (no pain) to "10" (worst possible pain) and can be used to assess degree of pain improvement following treatment [13].

Assessment of the pelvic floor muscles should also proceed from superficial to deep. The perineal body can be assessed by gently depressing with a single digit just outside the introitus at the 6 o'clock location. The bulbospongiosus muscles can be palpated just deep to the labia majora from 1 o'clock to 5 o'clock on the left and 7 o'clock to 11 o'clock on the right. Next, the deep muscles of the pelvic floor (levator ani, obturator internus, piriformis muscles) should be evaluated. The levator ani muscles can be assessed by placing a single digit within the introitus and gently palpating from 3 to 5 o'clock and 7 to 9 o'clock toward the ischial spines. The obturator internus muscles can be palpated superior to the ischial spines at the 3 o'clock and 9 o'clock positions [13]. The location of any focal areas of muscular tenderness or tight bands should be documented as these may be indicators of pelvic muscle spasm. Muscle testing should also be performed by first palpating the resting tone of the pelvic floor digitally and then asking the patient to maximally contract her pelvic floor muscles (also known as a Kegel). The strength of the muscle contraction should be rated from "0" (no palpable contraction) to "5" (strong muscle contraction) on a modified Oxford scale [15]. The strength of the Kegel can be determined by the degree of squeeze around the examiner's digit as well as the degree of upward lift of the pelvic floor. A weak pelvic floor contraction may be an indication of pelvic floor laxity or uncoordinated pelvic floor muscle movement. The ability to voluntarily relax the pelvic floor is important and can be evaluated by asking the patient to Valsalva or bear down similar to a bowel movement. Pelvic floor relaxation can be determined by degree of relaxation around the examiner's digit as well as visualization of descent of the perineal body. If the patient is unable to do this, pelvic floor dysfunction may be playing a role in the patient's symptoms (Fig. 31.2).

Following assessment of the pelvic floor muscles, a bimanual exam should be performed to assess the uterus, cervix, and adnexa for structural abnormalities. This portion of the exam may be particularly uncomfortable physically or emotionally for women with chronic pelvic pain, and the patient should again be reassured that she can stop or pause the exam at any point. Although a speculum exam is often performed before the bimanual exam in most routine gynecologic assessments, the speculum exam may significantly aggravate chronic pelvic pain symptoms, which can make it more difficult to localize the patient's pain on bimanual exam. Clinical judgment should be used when deciding the order of performing the bimanual and speculum exam.

The bimanual exam is performed by placing one lubricated, gloved digit from the dominant hand vaginally until the

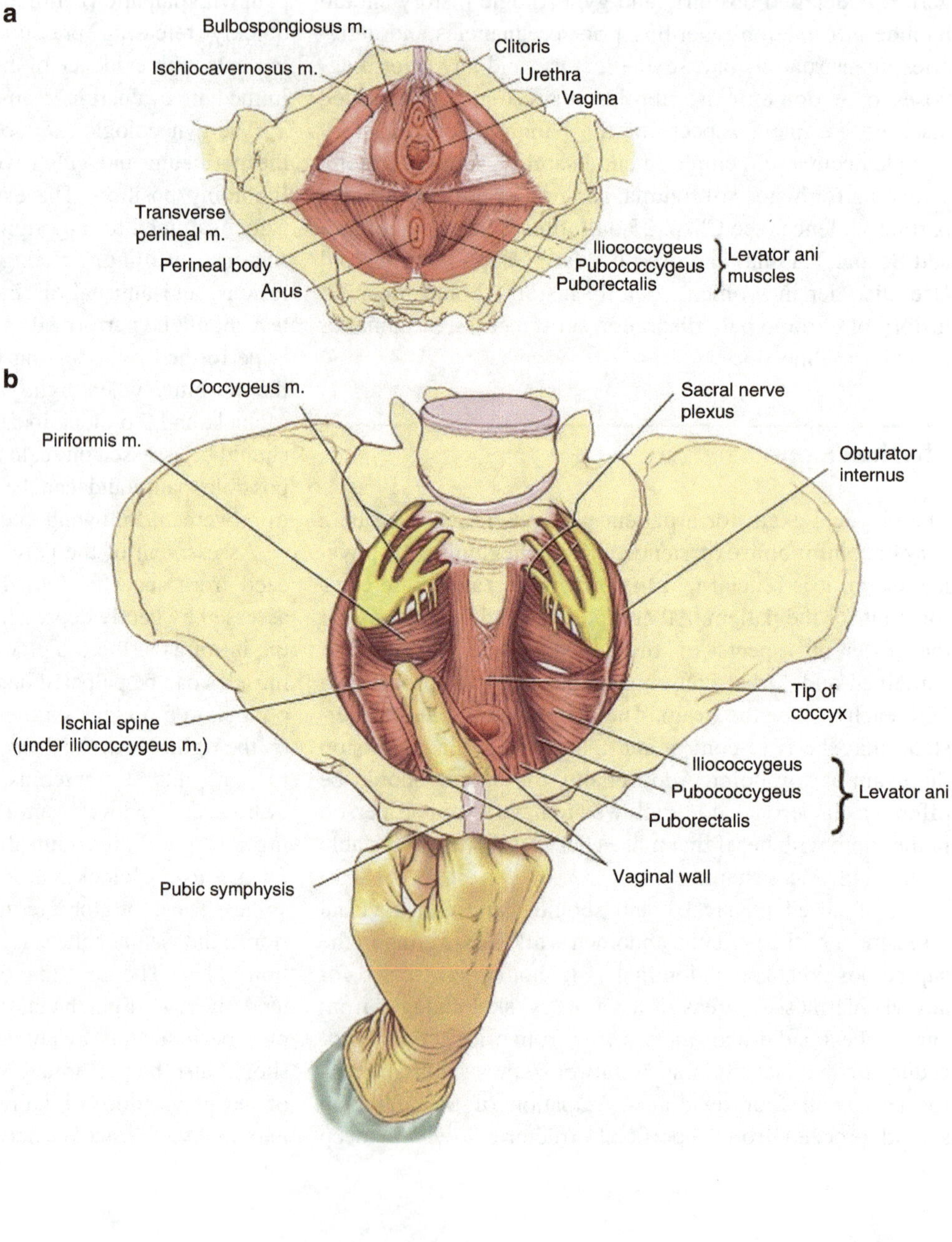

Fig. 31.2 (**a**) Muscles of the pelvic floor. (**b**) Digital palpation of deep pelvic floor muscles. m muscle [16]. (Reprinted from Mayo Clinic Proceedings, Faubion et al. [16], © 2012, with permission from Elsevier)

cervix is palpated. The finger can be lubricated with water or a water-based lubricant. Two vaginal digits may be needed in order to adequately palpate the uterus and cervix; however, this should only be performed if it is tolerated by the patient. Following identification of the cervix, the cervix should be gently pushed laterally or superiorly/inferiorly to assess for cervical motion tenderness. Significant cervical tenderness with minimal palpation may be concerning for acute cervicitis. Next, while placing the nondominant hand on the patient's lower abdomen, the uterine fundus should be palpated while elevating the uterus out of the pelvis with the internal digit(s). The size, shape, mobility, and tenderness of the uterus should be assessed. A uterus that is enlarged and irregularly shaped may indicate adenomyosis or uterine fibroids. Next, the internal digits should be moved to the anterior vaginal fornix at 10 o'clock. With steady pressure, the external hand should sweep the right adnexa into the internal hand from the right anterior superior iliac spine toward the pubic symphysis. An identical assessment should be performed of the left adnexa at the 2 o'clock position within the anterior vaginal fornix. The adnexa should be assessed for size, fullness, mobility, and tenderness. In patients with symptoms concerning for possible endometriosis (dysmenorrhea, deep dyspareunia, infertility), careful palpation retrocervically and along bilateral uterosacral ligaments should be performed to assess for any tenderness or nodularity that may represent deep infiltrating endometriosis.

Next, a vaginal speculum exam should be performed to visually evaluate the cervix and vaginal walls. The cervix should be evaluated for any masses, nodules, erythema, lesions, or purulent discharge. The vaginal walls should be assessed for loss of rugae, which may be consistent with atrophic vaginitis. Additionally, the vaginal vault should be carefully inspected for unusual vaginal discharge. During the speculum exam, cervical swabs for chlamydia, gonorrhea, and trichomoniasis should be obtained routinely, as not all patients with sexually transmitted diseases are symptomatic. Additional samples should be obtained if unusual vaginal discharge is present.

A rectal exam should not be performed routinely for all women presenting with chronic pelvic pain. However, if the patient indicates a history significant for painful or bloody stools or if the bimanual exam is abnormal, then a rectal exam may be warranted to assess for hemorrhoids, rectal lesions, or pelvic masses.

Differential Diagnosis

Providers must keep a broad differential in mind while evaluating for potential etiologies of chronic pelvic pain. A systematic approach enables the primary care provider to more easily organize information. An overview of the common differential diagnoses is outlined in Table 31.1. The following section highlights some of the more common etiologies of chronic pelvic pain, but the authors acknowledge that the differential is very broad and the cause is most often multifactorial.

Table 31.1 Differential diagnosis of conditions contributing to chronic pelvic pain

System	Differential diagnosis of conditions contributing to chronic pelvic pain
Gastrointestinal	Irritable bowel syndrome Constipation Inflammatory bowel disease
Urologic	Painful bladder syndrome/interstitial cystitis Cystitis and urethritis

Musculoskeletal	Abdominal wall pain/myofascial pain syndrome
	Vaginismus
	Pelvic floor muscle spasm
	  Levator ani muscle
	  Piriformis muscle
	  Obturator internus muscle

Gynecologic	Endometriosis Adhesions Vulvovaginitis Vulvodynia Vulvar vestibulitis Vulvovaginal atrophy Leiyomyomas Adenomyosis Pelvic inflammatory disease Adnexal masses
Psychiatric	Depression and anxiety Intimate partner violence and sexual abuse Trauma and post-traumatic stress disorder (PTSD) Drug dependency Somatization

Gastrointestinal Contributors

Gender differences in the gastrointestinal system are well documented. Women exhibit delayed gastrointestinal transit within the stomach and colon when compared to male counterparts [8, 9]. Gastrointestinal disorders including irritable bowel syndrome, chronic constipation, and inflammatory bowel diseases may cause chronic abdominopelvic pain.

Irritable bowel syndrome (IBS) is a functional bowel disorder characterized by chronic abdominal pain related to defecation and frequent changes in baseline stool frequency or appearance [17, 18]. Patients experience visceral pain from alteration in bowels habits, abdominal distention, and cramping. The prevalence is between 10% and 15% in North America and is equally distributed between subtypes: constipation predominant (IBS-C), diarrhea predominant (IBS-D), mixed type (IBS-M), and un-subtyped [19]. Female sex is the best-documented risk factor for IBS;

women are twice as likely to be affected by IBS compared to men [17]. Women often experience exacerbations of IBS-associated abdominal pain during their menses when serum estrogen levels are low, and therefore IBS may be difficult to differentiate from dysmenorrhea (see Chap. 27 on Irritable Bowel Syndrome) [17]. Symptoms change over time and the diagnosis is often made by history and exclusion of other diseases.

Chronic constipation is a characterized by infrequent, painful passage of stools [20]. The global prevalence of constipation is 16% with a greater predisposition among the elderly, women, chronic narcotic users, and individuals who eat low-fiber diets [20]. It is particularly important for clinicians to ask questions regarding regularity and consistency of stools, chronic history of ignoring the urge to defecate, or incomplete evacuation requiring digital assistance [21].

About 3 million Americans carry a diagnosis of ulcerative colitis or Crohn's disease, which together are referred to as inflammatory bowel disease (IBD) [22]. IBD is characterized by potentially severe intestinal inflammation leading to diarrhea, weight loss, nausea, vomiting, and abdominal and pelvic pain. Pain can be acute or chronic, a result of damage to the enteric nervous system from ongoing inflammation or from underlying structural disease, adhesions, or fistulas that are characteristic of Crohn's [23]. Patients can also display extra-intestinal manifestations of IBD such as joint pain, rashes, and ocular disease. IBD can go undiagnosed for years when symptoms are mild and diarrhea is absent and should be considered in all patients presenting with chronic abdominopelvic pain.

Urologic Contributors

Localizing complaints of urinary dysfunction or dysuria on review of systems may indicate a urinary contribution to chronic pelvic pain. Interstitial cystitis or bladder pain syndrome is a common cause of CPP and is diagnosed in patients with pelvic pain for greater than 6 weeks with at least one urinary symptom, such as urgency or frequency (see Chap. 30 on Interstitial Cystitis/Bladder Pain Syndrome). Similar to other chronic pain disorders, bladder pain syndrome is five times more likely to occur in women when compared to men [24]. In patients with more acute urinary discomfort, urinary tract infection (cystitis or urethritis) or urolithiasis may be a more likely diagnosis.

Urinary tract infection is the most common bacterial infection and is more common in women due to the shorter distance between the urethral orifice and the rectum [25]. Patients suffering from acute or recurrent urinary tract infections will often complain of dysuria, hematuria, urinary urgency/frequency, and/or suprapubic pain [25].

Musculoskeletal Contributors

History and physical exam can easily lead to the diagnosis of musculoskeletal or myofascial causes of pain and avoidance of an expensive workup of visceral causes [12]. Chronic abdominal wall pain is typically characterized by focal, superficial tenderness along the abdominal wall [12]. In a study of 2709 patients referred to a gastroenterologist over a 5-year period, 137 patients were diagnosed with chronic abdominal wall pain with 27% experiencing predominantly lower abdominal tenderness [12]. Women were four times more likely than men to present with chronic abdominal wall pain, highlighting the importance of considering the musculoskeletal system in the differential for chronic pelvic pain.

Myofascial pain syndrome is a complex pain disorder where tender bands of hyperirritable skeletal muscle and fascia called "trigger points" cause exquisite local pain and autonomic symptoms. Pain from trigger point presence or manipulation can also cause symptoms at predictable remote sites called "targets" [26]. In women, myofascial pelvic pain is often characterized by dyspareunia, dysuria, and/or dyschezia and may be due to muscle laxity or hypertonicity [27]. Myofascial pain can be triggered by trauma, poor posture, stress on the pelvic floor from obesity and pregnancy, surgery, overuse, underuse, and atrophy [28]. It is estimated that 13.2% of women suffer from pain associated with myofascial pelvic pain [28] with the prevalence as high as 58% in women who suffer from chronic pelvic pain. The most commonly affected pelvic floor muscles include the levator ani, piriformis, and obturator internus [28].

Vaginismus, now known as genito-pelvic pain/penetration disorder, causes chronic pelvic pain with any form of vaginal penetration and can be very distressing for patients and their partners. It includes difficulties with one or more of the following dimensions that are persistent or recurrent: (1) tightening of the pelvic floor muscle when vaginal penetration is attempted; (2) pain, burning, or tension during or when vaginal penetration is attempted; (3) decrease in or no desire for intercourse; and (4) anxiety or fear of pain, pelvic or vulvovaginal, as a result of, during penetration, or in anticipation of penetration [29]. It has long been postulated that vaginismus is caused by spasm of the pelvic floor muscles, occluding the vaginal opening and preventing penetration, but there are few studies documenting differences in pelvic floor tonicity, strength, and presence of spasm between patients diagnosed with vaginismus and those that are not [30]. Risk factors for vaginismus include physical and sexual trauma, relationship issues, pelvic floor dysfunction, anatomical congenital abnormalities, untreated vulvar disease, vaginal atrophy, endometriosis, pelvic infections, and surgical intervention [30].

Gynecologic Contributors

Intra-abdominal adhesions result from direct peritoneal trauma most commonly due to surgery, infections, or inflammation [31]. In normal wound healing, tissue trauma triggers mast cell degranulation and fibrin deposition, which is subsequently degraded within 72 hours [32]. However, adhesions form when fibrinolysis is delayed, resulting in fibroblast infiltration and vascularization [32]. Abdominal or pelvic surgery causes postoperative adhesions in up to 40% of patients [33]. Route of surgery may increase clinical suspicion as studies have demonstrated a higher rate of postoperative adhesions with open surgery when compared to minimally invasive approach (laparoscopic or robotic). Adhesions are an established cause of internal hernias and small bowel obstructions that may result in acute pain [31]. However, the data for chronic pain is not well established. Adhesions may restrict the mobility of affected organs, but it is unclear if adhesions themselves are a direct source of pelvic pain. At least one study demonstrated histologic evidence of nerve fibers in pelvic adhesions in women undergoing gynecologic surgery; however, the prevalence of adhesion innervation was no different between women with and without pelvic pain [34]. Additionally, a cluster analysis in 2018 revealed that the severity of adhesions did correlate with the severity of a patient's pain score [35].

Vulvovaginitis is a group of conditions affecting 15–39% of women and often presents with abnormal vaginal discharge and/or vulvovaginal irritation [36]. The most common causes of vulvovaginitis are bacterial vaginosis, vulvovaginal candidiasis, and trichomoniasis. Bacterial vaginosis results from a shift in the normal vaginal flora resulting in an overgrowth of predominantly anaerobic bacteria and malodorous discharge [36]. Vulvovaginal candidiasis results from a shift in the normal vaginal flora with an overgrowth of yeast species, most commonly *Candida albicans* [36]. Trichomoniasis is caused by a sexually transmitted protozoan *T. vaginalis* and requires treatment of the patient and her partner in order to prevent reinfection (see Chap. 12 on Vaginitis and Vulvar Conditions and Chap. 13 on Sexually Transmitted Infections). Chronic reinfection and irritation of the vaginal mucosa from vaginitis can result in an ongoing pain syndrome.

Vulvodynia is a chronic pain disorder defined as burning vulvar discomfort that occurs in the absence of "relevant visible findings or a specific clinically identifiable neurological disorder" [37]. This condition commonly results in dyspareunia, while in more extreme cases, the patient may be unable to wear certain clothing owing to irritation [38]. Vulvar vestibulitis is a subtype of vulvodynia specifically associated with localized, provoked vulvar pain or discomfort along the vestibule [39]. It is particularly important to exclude and/or treat other potential causes of vulvar pain, such as vulvovaginitis, prior to initiating treatment of vulvodynia.

Further discussion on the remainder of the gynecologic differential for pelvic pain can be found in Chap. 10 on Fibroids, Endometriosis, and Ovarian Cysts; Chap. 8 on Menopause, Atrophic Vaginitis section; Chap. 13 on Sexually Transmitted Infections, PID section; and Chap. 9 on Female Sexual Function and Dysfunction.

Psychiatric Contributors

Women who suffer from chronic pelvic pain are more likely to have a history of major depressive disorder, somatization symptoms, drug use or dependence, and childhood or adult sexual abuse [40]. A survey of 1931 women within a primary care practice found that the prevalence of pelvic pain was two times higher in patients with a history of childhood abuse [41]. Additionally, up to one in three women with pelvic pain will screen positive for post-traumatic stress disorder, which further emphasizes the high risk of psychological comorbidities in women suffering from chronic pelvic pain [42]. Therefore, screening and treatment for psychiatric comorbidities, history of abuse, drug dependency, and post-traumatic stress disorder are crucial during the evaluation and management of women with chronic pelvic pain [43].

Sally is wondering if her pain might be due to endometriosis. She recently heard an advertisement for an endometriosis medication on TV, and the description of the symptoms is similar to what she is experiencing. You explain that while endometriosis is a common cause of pelvic pain, there are many other causes (both gynecologic and non-gynecologic) of pelvic pain. You will need some more information to help determine the etiology of her pain.

Laboratory Testing

There are only a few laboratory tests that should routinely be performed during the assessment of a patient with chronic pelvic pain. All premenopausal women of reproductive age should undergo pregnancy testing for two main reasons: (1) up to 50% of pregnancies in the United States are unintended [44] and (2) a confirmed viable pregnancy will dictate treatment options. Next, a urinalysis or urine dip test should be performed to evaluate for a possible urinary tract infection. Testing for sexually transmitted diseases, specifically for gonorrhea, chlamydia, and trichomoniasis, can either be performed vaginally at the time of the speculum exam or tested with a urine sample. Lastly, if microscopy is available, then a wet mount of the patient's vaginal discharge should be assessed with normal saline and potassium hydroxide to evaluate for yeast, bacterial vaginosis, or an abundance of white blood cells which could signal either acute or chronic abnormal inflammation.

Radiographic Imaging

A transvaginal pelvic ultrasound is the first-line imaging modality during the assessment of chronic pelvic pain [45]. Ultrasound provides a fast, cost-effective, and accurate method of evaluating the reproductive organs and is the imaging modality of choice when assessing pathology of the gynecologic structures [46]. Pelvic ultrasound can also facilitate the diagnosis of uterine leiomyoma, adenomyosis, pelvic inflammatory disease, and adnexal cysts/masses [47]. Ultrasound may have limitations due to variability of operator skill, patient tolerance of the exam, patient obesity, and obscuring bowel gas [47]. If pelvic ultrasound is not feasible or provides limited information, an abdominal/pelvic MRI may be useful in select patients to determine the extent of disease in cases of suspected deep infiltrating endometriosis or a large fibroid uterus [45]. Limitations of MRI include inability to perform in patients with certain metal implants or pacemakers, high cost, and patient tolerance of a small, enclosed space [47]. Abdominal/pelvic computed tomography is commonly used during the evaluation of acute abdominal pain; however, it has limited utility in the evaluation of chronic pelvic pain. Patients with a clinical history concerning for possible gastrointestinal etiology of their pain may benefit the most from additional imaging with CT, as the large and small intestines are not adequately visualized on pelvic ultrasound [45].

Diagnostic Laparoscopy

Diagnostic laparoscopy should not be routinely offered as a first-line assessment for chronic pelvic pain. A detailed history and physical exam with indicated laboratory testing and radiographic imaging will often provide more diagnostic information without exposing the patient to an invasive surgical procedure [48]. Diagnostic laparoscopy is a reasonable next step in patients when the clinical history, physical exam, and noninvasive testing fail to provide a diagnosis. Patients should be counseled that diagnostic laparoscopy fails to find a diagnosis in up to 35% of patients with CPP [48]. Diagnostic laparoscopy may be offered to patients with suspected endometriosis to provide histologic diagnosis and surgical treatment of painful endometriotic implants. Laparoscopy for the evaluation and treatment of adhesive disease will be discussed in further detail below.

Sally's urinalysis and sexually transmitted infection testing are both negative. On exam it is noted that Sally has multiple tender spots along her levator ani, and you are concerned she may be experiencing levator muscle spasm. You recommend that she see a pelvic floor physical therapist for further evaluation and treatment.

Treatment of Chronic Pelvic Pain

Treatment for female chronic pelvic pain can be challenging for both the patient and the provider. As with any other disease, the treatment of chronic pelvic pain should be tailored to the etiological source. The origin of chronic pelvic pain is often complex and multifactorial. A systems-based approach ensures that the provider evaluates the patient in an organized and thorough manner. The optimal treatment of a patient with chronic pelvic pain often requires simultaneous treatments across multiple specialties. For this reason, studies have shown improved patient outcomes with the utilization of an interdisciplinary care team, wherein a team of specialists collaborate in order to achieve a common treatment goal [49]. Many interdisciplinary care teams include a primary care provider, gynecologist, chronic pain specialist, psychologist, and physical therapist [50]. Depending on that patient's specific clinical presentation, the care team may also include a gastroenterologist, urologist, urogynecologist, general surgeon, or psychiatrist. Additionally, it is critical that the provider and patient understand that complete resolution of the pain may not be realistic or a feasible treatment goal [50]. Rather, the goal of chronic pelvic pain management should be overall reduction in pain with associated improvement in quality of life and daily functionality [51]. An exhaustive review of the treatment options for all potential causes of chronic pelvic pain is beyond the scope of this chapter as there are other chapters in this book dedicated to diseases that commonly cause chronic pelvic pain. Please see Chap. 8 on Menopause, Atrophic Vaginitis section; Chap. 10 on Fibroids, Endometriosis, and Ovarian Cysts; Chap. 12 on Vaginitis and Vulvar Conditions; Chap. 13 on Sexually Transmitted Infections, PID section; Chap. 24 on Urinary Tract Infections; Chap. 27 on Irritable Bowel Syndrome; and Chap. 30 on Interstitial Cystitis/Bladder Pain Syndrome.

Musculoskeletal

Patients identified as having abdominal wall myofascial pain based on a positive Carnett's test often require a multimodal approach toward the management of their pain. Patients with evidence of abdominal wall scar tissue from prior trauma or surgery may benefit from manual scar release performed by a trained physical therapist. Additionally, a significant rectus diastasis may occur after pregnancy, which may warrant fitting for an abdominal binder to stabilize and support the abdominal wall muscles. Lifestyle modifications with stretching and exercise are critical as stretching lengthens taut muscles and exercise increases strength and stability. Patients should be screened for repetitive tasks that may be resulting in recurrent microtrauma to abdominal wall muscles. In cases refractory to initial lifestyle modifications, patients may benefit from complementary or alternative medicine treatments with acupuncture, massage, or electrotherapy [26]. Oral and topical nonsteroidal anti-inflammatory drugs are the first-line medical treatment options for chronic myofascial pain [26]. Muscle relaxants such as cyclobenzaprine and tizanidine have been shown to be effective in the treatment of chronic myofascial pain [26]. There is limited data on the utility of topical lidocaine patches, but may be beneficial in patients that demonstrate significant hypersensitivity [26].

Patients with evidence of myofascial pain syndrome of the pelvis and pelvic floor muscle dysfunction often require interdisciplinary management with a pelvic floor physical therapist, urogynecologist, primary care physician, and psychologist. In the acute setting, pharmacologic management of pain with nonsteroidal anti-inflammatory drugs may be helpful, but is unlikely to result in long-lasting pain improvement [52]. Other medications that have been shown to be effective for chronic pelvic pain include tricyclic antidepressants and gabapentin [53]. Muscle relaxants, such as cyclobenzaprine, should be used with caution as they are sedating, nonspecific for the pelvic muscles and may induce urinary retention [14]. Although data is limited to support its use as monotherapy, vaginal diazepam, 5–10 mg BID suppositories, in conjunction with pelvic floor physical therapy has been suggested to benefit patients with contracted or "high-tone" pelvic floor muscle dysfunction [54].

Massage, myofascial release, or directed therapeutic exercise by a trained pelvic floor physical therapist is a critical component of the treatment of pelvic floor dysfunction and pain [55]. Pelvic floor physical therapy is a distinct specialty within physical therapy that requires dedicated training and certification through the Woman's Health Section of the American Physical Therapy Association [14]. The specific therapeutic strategy should be tailored to the patient's symptoms. Hypertonicity may require stretching techniques, vaginal dilators, or manual massage to relax the chronically contracted pelvic muscles [55]. Inadequate muscle control may be treated with biofeedback training, which increases the patient's awareness of her pelvic floor muscles during a state of activation or relaxation [55]. Patients should be counseled that consistent follow-up and adherence with the physical therapy regimen is necessary for adequate treatment. Studies have shown that the pelvic pain improvement with physical therapy is directly correlated with the number of physical therapy visits completed by the patient [56].

In cases refractory to medical and physical therapy, pelvic floor needling or injections may be indicated, an intervention provided by urogynecologists or gynecologists specializing in chronic pelvic pain. Dry needling involves insertion of a needle into the affected myofascial trigger point to produce a local twitch response [26]. A trigger point injection differs such that a local anesthetic (lidocaine, bupivacaine, or ropivacaine) and a steroid (triamcinolone) are administered together at the site of maximum tenderness, often transvaginally into the levator ani muscles [57]. Trigger point injections often provide immediate pain relief and can help to confirm the diagnosis of a pelvic floor spasm [57]. The decision to perform dry needling versus trigger point injections requires clinical judgment as multiple studies and a Cochrane analysis have not shown a difference in effectiveness between the two needling options [58–60].

Like patients with pelvic floor dysfunction, patients suffering with vaginismus (genito-pelvic pain/penetration disorder) should also be treated using a multidisciplinary approach with a pelvic floor physical therapist, urogynecologist, primary care physician, psychologist, and sex therapist. It is important to advise patients to stop engaging in painful sexual activity and seek treatment, as continued painful experiences can increase situational anxiety and result in increased pelvic floor tension and pain [61]. Cognitive behavioral therapy, biofeedback, and mindfulness-based approaches have been shown to be helpful for addressing the pain associated with vaginismus [62–68]. Additional therapies with mixed results include topical lidocaine [69, 70], antidepressants such as tricyclic antidepressants [71], anticonvulsants such as gabapentin [72], or vestibulectomy (excision of the hymenal ring and superficial vulvar mucosa) [72–75], although the latter is reserved for women who have failed multiple less invasive treatments. For refractory cases, pelvic floor injections with botulinum toxin have also been shown to be effective for management of involuntary pelvic floor spasms [76].

Gynecologic

As previously discussed, numerous studies have failed to find a definitive etiologic link between adhesions and chronic pelvic pain. Although there is limited data to guide management options, conservative treatment with non-opioid pain medications, such as nonsteroidal anti-inflammatory drugs or acetaminophen, should be tried first. There is insufficient data to support the use of gabapentin or pregabalin specifically for adhesion-related pain [77]. Adhesive disease is not reliably diagnosed with any imaging modality and can only be confirmed with surgical exploration. Laparoscopy is the least invasive surgical option for the diagnosis and treatment of adhesions. Surgery should be reserved for patients in which other causes of their chronic pain have been ruled out and are at high risk of having adhesions based on a history of prior surgery or inflammatory/infectious processes. For pain relief, short-term success rates for laparoscopic excision of adhesions, or adhesiolysis, are variable between 38% and 87% [78]. However, at least one randomized controlled trial revealed that laparoscopic adhesiolysis resulted in comparable success rates to simple diagnostic laparoscopy [34]. Similarly, complete adhesiolysis does not necessarily correlate with better pain relief when compared to incomplete excision [79]. In contrast, extensive adhesiolysis increases the surgical time and may increase the risk of bleeding, bowel injury, or vascular injury. Patients with chronic pain and suspected intra-abdominal adhesions should be referred to a gynecologic or general surgeon for further evaluation and counseling to determine if laparoscopic evaluation and treatment is indicated. Preoperatively, patients must be counseled that adhesions may or may not be found at time of surgery. Additionally, although adhesiolysis may result in short-term pain improvement, patients must also be aware that recurrence rates may be as high as 26% [78].

Vulvodynia and vulvar vestibulitis are conditions characterized by chronic vulvar pain or discomfort. Initial management steps should include lifestyle modifications with avoidance of vulvar irritants. Such lifestyle modifications include wearing 100% cotton underwear and avoiding synthetic fabrics/tight-fitting pants, using fragrance-free soaps and detergents, using preservative-free emollients for barrier protection, sex counseling, and generally keeping the vulvar area clean and dry [80]. If there is no improvement with initial conservative measures then referral to a gynecologist should be considered for treatment with topical agents: anesthetics, estrogen cream, or compounded tricyclic antidepressants [80]. Additionally, oral tricyclic antidepressants and anticonvulsants have been shown to be effective in improving vulvar pain; however, care should be taken to confirm the patient's current medications to avoid potentially dangerous drug interactions [80]. In patients whose symptoms are refractory to medical management and with pain localization to vestibule, surgical intervention has been shown to be effective [81]. A vulvar vestibulectomy involves excision of the hymenal ring and superficial vulvar mucosa from 3 to 9 o'clock [81]. In addition to lifestyle modification, pharmacologic treatment, and surgical intervention, the patient should also be offered treatment for the psychological effects of vulvodynia. Vulvodynia can be physically and emotionally debilitating to the affected patient, but can also be challenging for her sexual partner and overall sexual health. Therefore, referral to a therapist specializing in sexual disorders is recommended for all women undergoing treatment for vulvodynia [81]. Psychological treatment and support may actually improve pain symptoms, and in fact, at least one study demonstrated that cognitive behavioral therapy resulted in greater long-term reduction in dyspareunia caused by vestibular pain, when compared to vestibulectomy alone [82].

Psychiatric

Psychiatric comorbidities are prevalent in women suffering from chronic pelvic pain. Due to the inherent complexity of chronic pelvic pain, it may be difficult to determine if the psychiatric conditions are precipitating factors, consequences of the chronic pain, or both. When approaching the psychiatric care of patients with chronic pelvic pain, it is crucial that the provider validates that he/she believes in the patient's pain symptoms as patients may become concerned that the provider believes "the pain is just all in her head." Therefore, acknowledgment and treatment of the psychological effects of chronic pelvic pain is just one component of the overall treatment plan. It is appropriate to refer patients with concerns for depression, anxiety, PTSD, and somatization to a behavioral health specialist for long-term management or co-management with their primary care provider. Patients with a history of interpersonal violence, sexual abuse, or drug dependency may need referral to a provider who has expertise in specialized therapy and treatment (see Chap. 33 on Depressive and Anxiety Disorders and Chap. 35 on Intimate Partner Violence and Sexual Trauma). Medications such as tricyclic antidepressants, gabapentin, SSRIs, and SNRIs are commonly used in patients with concomitant pelvic pain and psychiatric comorbidities under the supervision of primary providers comfortable managing these medications or psychiatrists as they harbor properties to treat both neuropathic pain and mood symptoms [83–86].

Following several months of pelvic floor physical therapy, Sally has some improvement in her pelvic pain and is now able to tolerate the use of tampons. She still has significant pain that prevents her from having intercourse, and she confides in you that she has a history of sexual abuse. After confirming that Sally is currently in a safe home situation, you gently recommend that speaking with a therapist may be beneficial. She plans to see a psychiatrist specializing in sexual abuse patients and will continue working with the pelvic floor physical therapist.

Summary Points

1. Chronic pelvic pain is defined as noncyclical pain in the pelvis, anterior abdomen, or lower back lasting for at least 3–6 months' duration.
2. The etiology of chronic pelvic pain is often multifactorial and complicated. In order to avoid misdiagnosis, a systems-based approach should be utilized focusing on gastrointestinal, urologic, neurologic, musculoskeletal, gynecologic, and psychiatric causes which contribute to chronic pelvic pain.
3. The evaluation of chronic pelvic pain includes a comprehensive history detailing the patient's pain symptoms and the effect on her quality of life, personal and family history of chronic pain disorders or psychiatric conditions, surgical history, gynecologic history, sexual history, and pregnancy history. Screening for a history of trauma, past or present intimate partner violence, and substance use is imperative.
4. The physical exam of the CPP patient should include a full abdominal exam, testing for abdominal wall pain, careful visual and Q-tip testing along the vulva, evaluation of the superficial and deep pelvic floor muscles, bimanual exam, and a speculum examination. Particular care should be taken to create a safe, supportive environment during the history and physical exam.
5. Initial testing for the evaluation of chronic pelvic pain should be guided by the patient's symptoms, history, and physical exam. Office laboratory testing, as applicable, should include pregnancy testing, urinalysis, screening for sexually transmitted diseases, and wet mount microscopy of vaginal discharge. Pelvic ultrasound should be considered the first-line imaging modality for chronic pelvic pain. Diagnostic laparoscopy should not routinely be offered for first-line assessment.
6. The treatment for chronic pelvic pain should target the most likely etiological source of the patient's pain, utilizing a patient-centered multidisciplinary team approach which includes a primary care provider, gynecologist, chronic pain specialist, psychologist, and physical therapist. Realistic treatment goals should be established focusing on improvement in quality of life in addition to reduction in pain symptoms.

Review Questions

1. A 30-year-old woman comes to your office reporting pelvic pain and vulvar irritation for the last 10 years that has been worsening over the last several weeks. She researched her symptoms online and took an over-the-counter antifungal for a presumed yeast infection. She is married and denies new sexual partners. She does report a long-standing history of burning pain with intercourse. There are no lesions on her external genitalia and bimanual exam is unremarkable. She reports severe pain from 4 o'clock to 7 o'clock along the posterior fourchette on cotton swab testing. Wet mount with 10% KOH of the vaginal discharge shows no evidence of candidal vaginitis. What is the first-line treatment of vulvodynia?
   A. Nonsteroidal anti-inflammatory drugs
   B. Vulvar care measures: wearing cotton underwear and avoiding vulvar irritants
   C. Vestibulectomy
   D. Topical lidocaine cream
   E. Tricyclic antidepressants

   The correct answer is B. Vulvodynia is a chronic pain disorder that is defined as burning vulvar pain in the absence of relevant visible findings or a specific clinically identifiable neurological disorder. This is a diagnosis of exclusion, and treatable causes of vulvar pain, such as candidal vaginitis, must be ruled out. Other chronic skin conditions, such as lichen sclerosus, lichen planus, and vulvovaginal atrophy, should be first ruled out by careful visual examination of the vulva and perineum. Vulvar lesions may warrant biopsy in order to obtain a tissue diagnosis. Cotton swab testing along the perineum allows for mapping of the location and severity of the patient's vulvodynia symptoms. First-line treatment for suspected vulvodynia includes lifestyle modifications with vulvar care measures that avoid vulvar irritants. Such measures include wearing 100% cotton underwear, avoiding perfumes/dyes in detergents or soaps, avoiding douching, cleaning the vulva with water only, keeping the vulvar area dry throughout the day and applying a preservative-free emollient daily, and rinsing and gently drying the vulva after urination. If lifestyle modifications do not result in improvements, then topical local anesthetics, estrogen cream, or topical tricyclic antidepressants may provide symptomatic relief. Oral tricyclic antidepressants or anticonvulsants may be incorporated as a third-line treatment. Nonsteroidal anti-inflammatory drugs usually provide minimal relief for chronic pain associated with vulvodynia. Surgical resection of the vestibule, or vestibulectomy, should be reserved for patients who have tried and failed medical management options [80, 87].

2. A 45-year-old multiparous woman presents to your office reporting pelvic pain since the birth of her last child 7 years ago. The pain is constant and sharp and radiates to her lower back. Her past medical history is significant for chronic constipation. She has not been sexually active for multiple years due to significant dyspareunia. Pelvic

exam is limited due to discomfort. She has point tenderness along her left and right levator ani muscles. Which of the following is the most appropriate next step in the management of this patient?

A. Recommend strict pelvic rest.
B. Initiation of oral muscle relaxants.
C. Initiation of low-dose long-acting narcotics.
D. Referral to pelvic floor physical therapy.

The correct answer is D. Pelvic floor muscle dysfunction or myofascial pain can often be diagnosed with history and physical exam. Often, the patient will report a history of painful intercourse, painful urination, and/or pain with defecation. Pelvic floor muscle dysfunction may result from either increased muscle tone (muscle spasms) or decreased muscle tone (myofascial laxity). The most commonly affected muscles are the levator ani, obturator, and piriformis muscles which are found deep within the pelvic floor. Patients with pelvic floor dysfunction may require an interdisciplinary team including a pelvic floor physical therapist, urogynecologist, primary care physician, and psychologist. The most important first step in the management of patients with suspected pelvic floor muscle dysfunction is referral of the patient to a certified pelvic floor physical therapist for confirmation of the diagnosis and treatment. Directed therapeutic exercise or myofascial release is recommended over strict pelvic rest, which may actually worsen the pelvic floor dysfunction. Oral muscle relaxants do not specifically target the pelvic floor muscles and are often associated with increased sedation; therefore, their use should be limited. Narcotics in general are unlikely to be effective in treating pelvic floor muscle dysfunction and may worsen the patient's chronic constipation. Patients with pelvic floor muscle spasms, who are refractory to physical therapy, may benefit from pelvic floor injections [27, 28, 55, 56].

3. A 34-year-old multiparous woman presents to your office with progressively worsening lower abdominal and pelvic pain over the past year. She has a medical history significant for fibromyalgia and irritable bowel syndrome. She states that although she experiences the pain daily, her symptoms are worst during her menses and with intercourse. She also reports a history of heavy menstrual bleeding that has been increasing in severity over the past year. On pelvic exam, her uterus is normal size/shape and non-tender. However, she has tenderness in the posterior cul-de-sac and you appreciate tender fullness along the right adnexal region. Her pregnancy test is negative. What imaging study should be ordered first to evaluate her chronic pelvic pain?

A. Transvaginal ultrasound
B. Computed tomography of the abdomen and pelvis
C. Magnetic resonance imaging of the pelvis
D. Abdominal x-ray

The correct answer is A. This patient's symptoms of dysmenorrhea and acute worsening of her chronic pelvic pain with cul-de-sac tenderness and adnexal fullness is concerning for endometriosis. The gold standard for diagnosis of endometriosis is histologic confirmation with tissue biopsy. Radiographic evaluation for pelvic pain should identify structural causes for patient's pain while minimizing unnecessary exposure to ionizing radiation. Transvaginal ultrasound is the optimal initial imaging modality for the evaluation of female pelvic pain because ultrasonography can delineate structural abnormalities within the uterus and adnexae without exposing the patient to radiation. Specifically, ultrasound can distinguish the characteristics of adnexal cysts as simple, complex, hemorrhagic, or endometrioma or exhibits features concerning for malignancy. Additionally, transvaginal ultrasound can be used to detect deep infiltrating endometriosis along the rectovaginal septum. Computed tomography (CT) rarely adds useful additional information to a pelvic ultrasound and exposes the patient to ionizing radiation and significantly increases cost. CT may be useful for further evaluation of patients with an adnexal mass with features concerning for malignancy. Magnetic resonance imaging (MRI) may provide better imaging of deep tissue structures; however, it is significantly more expensive than transvaginal ultrasound and unlikely to be an ideal first imaging study. None of the reproductive organs can be visualized with abdominal x-ray [88–90].

References

1. Mathias SD, Kuppermann M, Liberman RF, Lipschutz RC, Steege JF. Chronic pelvic pain: prevalence, health-related quality of life, and economic correlates. Obstet Gynecol. 1996;87(3):321–7.
2. Latthe P, Latthe M, Say L, Gulmezoglu M, Khan KS. WHO systematic review of prevalence of chronic pelvic pain: a neglected reproductive health morbidity. BMC Public Health. 2006;6:177.
3. Ahangari A. Prevalence of chronic pelvic pain among women: an updated review. Pain Physician. 2014;17:E141–7.
4. Williams RE, Hartmann KE, Steege JF. Documenting the current definitions of chronic pelvic pain: implication for research. Obstet Gynecol. 2004 Apr;103(4):686–91.
5. ACOG practice bulletin No. 51. Chronic pelvic pain. Obstet Gynecol. 2004;103(3):589–605.
6. Origoni M, Leone Roberti Maggiore U, Salvatore S, Candiani M. Neurobiological mechanisms of pelvic pain. Biomed Res Int. 2014;2014:9038484.
7. Brünahl C, Dybowski C, Albrecht R, Riegel B, Höink J, Fisch M, Löwe B. Mental disorders in patients with chronic pelvic pain syndrome (CPPS). J Psychosom Res. 2017;98:19–26.
8. Shoja MM, Sharma A, Mirzayan N, et al. Neuroanatomy of the female abdominopelvic region: a review with application to pelvic pain syndromes. Clin Anatom. 2013;26:66–76.
9. Cervero F, Laird M. Visceral pain. Lancet. 1999;353(9170):2145–8.

10. Jobling P, O'Hara K, Hua S. Female reproductive tract pain: targets, challenges, and outcomes. Front Pharmacol. 2014;5:17. Published online 2014 Feb 13. https://doi.org/10.3389/fphar.2014.00017.
11. Mui J, Allaire C, Williams C, Yong PJ. Abdominal wall pain in women with chronic pelvic pain. J Obstet Gynaecol Can. 2016;38(2):154–9.
12. Costanza CD, Longstreth GF, Liu AL. Chronic abdominal wall pain: clinical features, health care costs, and long-term outcome. Clin Gastroenterol Hepatol. 2004;2(5):395–9.
13. Hartmann D, Sarton J. Chronic pelvic floor dysfunction. Best Pract Res Clin Obstet Gynaecol. 2014;28(7):977–90.
14. Prather H, Dugan S, Fitzgerald C, Hunt D. Review of anatomy, evaluation, and treatment of musculoskeletal pelvic floor pain in women. PM R. 2009;1(4):346–58.
15. Apte G, Nelson P, Brismée JM, Dedrick G, Justiz R, Sizer PS. Chronic female pelvic pain- part 1: clinical pathoanatomy and examination of the pelvic region. Pain Pract. 2011;12(2):88–110.
16. Faubion SS, Shuster LT, Bharucha AE. Recognition and management of nonrelaxing pelvic floor dysfunction. Mayo Clin Proc. 2012;87(2):187–93. https://doi.org/10.1016/j.mayocp.2011.09.004.
17. Meleine M, Matricon J. Gender-related differences in irritable bowel syndrome: potential mechanisms of sex hormones. World J Gastroenterol. 2014;20(22):6725–43.
18. Drossman DA, Hasler WL. Rome IV-functional GI disorders: disorders of gut-brain interaction. Gastroenterology. 2016;150:1257–61.
19. Lovell RM, Ford AC. Global prevalence of and risk factors for irritable bowel syndrome: a meta-analysis. Clin Gastroenterol Hepatol. 2012;10(7):712–721.e4.
20. Forootan M, Bagheri N, Darvishi M. Chronic constipation: a review of literature. Medicine. 2018;97(20):e10631.
21. Wald A. Constipation: advances in diagnosis and treatment. JAMA. 2016;315:185–91.
22. Dahlhamer JM, Zammitti EP, Ward BW, Wheaton AG, Croft JB. Prevalence of inflammatory bowel disease among adults aged≥ 18 years—United States, 2015. MMWR Morb Mortal Wkly Rep. 2016;65:1166–9.
23. Feuerstein JD, Cheifetz AS. Crohn disease: epidemiology, diagnosis, and management. Mayo Clin Proc. 2017;92(7):1088–103.
24. Clemens JQ, Meenan RT, Rosetti MC, Gao SY, Calhoun EA. Prevalence and incidence of interstitial cystitis in a managed care population. J Urol. 2005;173:98–102.
25. Geerlings SE. Clinical presentations and epidemiology of urinary tract infections. Microbiol Spectrum. 2016;4(5):UTI-0002-2012. https://doi.org/10.1128/microbiolspec.UTI-0002-2012.
26. Borg-Stein J, Iaccarino MA. Myofascial pain syndrome treatments. Phys Med Rehabil Clin N Am. 2014;25:357–74.
27. Berghmans B. Physiotherapy for pelvic pain and female sexual dysfunction: an untapped resource. Int Urogynecol J. 2018;29(5): 631–8.
28. Bonder JH, Chi M, Rispoli L. Myofascial pelvic pain and related disorders. Phys Med Rehabil Clin N Am. 2017;28:501–15.
29. American Psychiatric Association. DSM-5 task force. In: Diagnostic and statistical manual of mental disorders: DSM-5. 5th ed. Washington DC: American Psychiatric Association; 2013.
30. Lahaie MA, Boyer SC, Amsel R, Khalife S, Binik YM. Vaginismus: a review of the literature on the classification/diagnosis, etiology and treatment. Womens Health (Long). 2010 Sep;6(5):705–19.
31. Practice Committee of American Society for Reproductive Medicine in collaboration with Society of Reproductive Surgeons. Pathogenesis, consequences, and control of peritoneal adhesions in gynecologic surgery: a committee opinion. Fertil Steril. 2013;99(6):1550–5.
32. Diamond MP, El-Mowafi DM. Pelvic adhesions. Surg Technol Int. 1998;VII:273–83.
33. ten Broek RP, Issa Y, van Santbrink EJ, et al. Burden of adhesions in abdominal and pelvic surgery: systematic review and met-analysis. BMJ. 2013;347:f5588.
34. Kligman I, Drachenberg C, Papadimitriou J, Katz E. Immunohistochemical demonstration of nerve fibers in pelvic adhesions. Obstet Gynecol. 1993;82:566–8.
35. Cheong Y, Saran M, Hounslow JW, Reading IC. Are pelvic adhesions associated with pain, physical, emotional, and functional characteristics of women presenting with chronic pelvic pain? A cluster analysis. BMC Womens Health. 2018;18(1):11.
36. Powell AM, Nyirjesy P. Recurrent vulvovaginitis. Best Pract Res Clin Obstet Gynaecol. 2014;28(7):967–76.
37. Haefner H. Report of the ISSVD terminology and classification of vulvodynia. J Low Genit Tract Dis. 2007;11:48–9.
38. Kliethermes CJ, Shah M, Hoffstetter S, Gavard JA, Steele A. Effect of vestibulectomy for intractable vulvodynia. J Minim Invasive Gynecol. 2016;23(7):1152–7.
39. Tommola P, Unkila-Kallio L, Paavonen J. Long-term well-being after surgical or conservative treatment of severe vulvar vestibulitis. Acta Obstet Gynecol Scand. 2012;91:1086–93.
40. Walker E, Katon W, Harrop-Griffiths, Holm L, Russo J, Hickok LR. Relationship of chronic pelvic pain to psychiatric diagnoses and childhood sexual abuse. Am J Psychiatry. 1988;145(1): 75–80.
41. McCauley J, Kern DE, Kolodner K, et al. Clinical characteristics of women with a history of childhood abuse: unhealed wounds. JAMA. 1997;277(17):1362–8.
42. Meltzer-Brody S, Leserman J, Zolnoun D, Steege J, Green E, Teich A. Trauma and posttraumatic stress disorder in women with chronic pelvic pain. Obstet Gynecol. 2007;109(4):902–8.
43. Meltzer-Brody S, Leserman J. Psychiatric comorbidity in women with chronic pelvic pain. CNS Spectr. 2011;16(2):29–35.
44. Finer LB, Zolna MR. Unintended pregnancy in the United States: incidence and disparities, 2006. Contraception. 2011;84(5):478–85.
45. Juhan V. Chronic pelvic pain: an imaging approach. Diagn Interv Imaging. 2015;96(10):997–1007.
46. Moore J, Copley S, Morris J, Lindsell D, Golding S, Kennedy S. A systematic review of the accuracy of ultrasound in the diagnosis of endometriosis. Ultrasound Obstet Gynecol. 2002;20:630–4.
47. Khatri G, Khan A, Rval G, Chhabra A. Diagnostic evaluation of chronic pelvic pain. Phys Med Rehabil Clin N Am. 2017;28:477–500.
48. Howard FM. The role of laparoscopy as a diagnostic tool in chronic pelvic pain. Baillieres Best Pract Res Clin Obstet Gynaecol. 2000;14(3):467–94.
49. Allaire C, Williams C, Bodmer-Roy S, Ahy S, Arion K, Ambacher K, et al. Chronic pelvic pain in an interdisciplinary setting: 1-year prospective cohort. Am J Obstet Gynecol. 2018;218:114.e1–12.
50. Cheong Y. Chronic pelvic pain: aetiology and therapy. Best Pract Res Clin Obstet Gynaecol. 2006;20(5):695–711.
51. Steege JF, Siedhoff MT. Chronic pelvic pain. Obstet Gynecol. 2014;124(3):616–29.
52. Black CJ, Ford AC. Chronic idiopathic constipation in adults: epidemiology, pathophysiology, diagnosis, and clinical management. Med J Aust. 2018;209(2):86–91.
53. Cheong YC, Smotra G, Williams ACDC. Non-surgical interventions for themanagement of chronic pelvic pain. Cochrane Database of Systematic Reviews 2014;(3). Art. No.: CD008797. https://doi.org/10.1002/14651858.CD008797.pub2.
54. Crisp CC, Vaccaro CM, Estanol MV, Oakley SH, Kleeman SD, Fellner AN, Pauls RN. Intra-vaginal diazepam for high-tone pelvic floor dysfunction: a randomized placebo-controlled trial. Int Urogynecol J. 2013;24(11):1915–23.

55. Nelson P, Apte G, Justiz R III, Brismeé JM, Dedrick G, Sizer PS. Chronic female pelvic pain-part 2: differential diagnosis and management. Pain Pract. 2012;12(2):111–41.
56. Bedaiwy MA, Patterson B, Mahajan S. Prevalence of myofascial chronic pelvic pain and the effectiveness of pelvic floor physical therapy. J Reprod Med. 2013;58(11–12):504–10.
57. Barley J, Han E, Gupta P, Gaines N, Killinger KA, Boura JA, et al. Transvaginal trigger point injections improve pain scores in women with pelvic floor hypertonicity and pelvic pain conditions. Female Pelvic Med Reconstr Surg. 2018;25:392. [Epub ahead of print].
58. Ay S, Evcik D, Tur BS. Comparison of injection methods in myofascial pain syndrome: a randomized controlled trial. Clin Rheumatol. 2010;29(1):19–23.
59. Venancio Rde A, Alencar FG, Zamperini C. Different substances and dry needling injections in patients with myofascial pain and headaches. Cranio. 2008;26(2):96–103.
60. Cummings TM, White AR. Needling therapies in the management of myofascial trigger point pain: a systematic review. Arch Phys Med Rehabil. 2001;82(7):986–92.
61. Fugl-Meyer KS, Bohm-Starke N, Damsted Petersen C, Fugl-Meyer A, Parish S, Giraldi A. Standard operating procedures for female genital sexual pain. J Sex Med. 2013;10(1):83–93.
62. Brotto LA, Bitzer J, Laan E, Leiblum S, Luria M. Women's sexual desire and arousal disorders. J Sex Med. 2010;7(1 Pt 2):586–614.
63. Brotto LA, Basson R. Group mindfulness-based therapy significantly improves sexual desire in women. Behav Res Ther. 2014;57:43–54.
64. Brotto LA, Erskine Y, Carey M, et al. A brief mindfulness-based cognitive behavioral intervention improves sexual functioning versus waitlist control in women treated for gynecologic cancer. Gynecol Oncol. 2012;125(2):320–5.
65. Brotto LA, Basson R, Carlson M, Zhu C. Impact of an integrated mindfulness and cognitive behavioral treatment for provoked vestibulodynia (IMPROVED): a qualitative study. Sex Relatsh Ther. 2013;28(1–2):1–16.
66. Glazer HI, Rodke G, Swencionis C, Hertz R, Young AW. Treatment of vulvar vestibulitis syndrome with electromyographic biofeedback of pelvic floor musculature. J Reprod Med. 1995;40(4):283–90.
67. Bergeron S, Binik YM, Khalife S, et al. A randomized comparison group cognitive-behavioral therapy, surface electromyographic biofeedback, and vestibulectomy in the treatment of dyspareunia resulting from vulvar vestibulitis. Pain. 2001;91(3):297–306.
68. Goldstein AT, Pukall CF, Brown C, Bergeron S, Stein A, Kellogg-Spadt S. Vulvodynia: assessment and treatment. J Sex Med. 2016;13(4):572–90.
69. Danielsson L, Torstensson T, Brodda-Jansen G, Bohm-Starke N. EMG biofeedback versus topical lidocaine gel: a randomized study for the treatment of women with vulvar vestibulitis. Acta Obstet Gynecol Scand. 2006;85(11):1360–7.
70. Goetsch MF, Lim JY, Caughey AB. A practical solution for dyspareunia in breast cancer survivors: a randomized controlled trial. J Clin Oncol. 2015;33(30):3394–400.
71. Reed BD, Haefner HK, Cantor L. Vulvar dysesthesia (vulvodynia). A follow-up study. J Reprod Med. 2003;48(6):409–16.
72. Leo RJ. A systematic review of the utility of anticonvulsant pharmacotherapy in the treatment of vulvodynia pain. J Sex Med. 2013;10(8):2000–8.
73. Goldstein AT, Klingman D, Christopher K, Johnson C, Marinoff SC. Surgical treatment of vulvar vestibulitis syndrome: outcome assessment derived from a postoperative questionnaire. J Sex Med. 2006;3(5):923–31.
74. Bergeron S, Bouchard C, Fortier M, Binik YM, Khalife S. The surgical treatment of vulvar vestibulitis syndrome: a follow up study. J Sex Marital Ther. 1997;23(4):147–52.
75. Kehoe S, Luesley D. Vulvar vestibulitis treated by modified vestibulectomy. Int J Gynaecol Obstet. 1999;64(2):147–52.
76. Ferreira JR, Souza RP. Botulinum toxin for vaginismus treatment. Pharmacology. 2012;89(5–6):256–9.
77. Van den Beukel BA, de Ree R, van Leuven S, Bakkum EA, Strik C, van Goor H, Ten Broek RPG. Surgical treatment of adhesion-related chronic abdominal and pelvic pain after gynaecological and general surgery: a systematic review and meta-analysis. Hum Reprod Update. 2017;23(3):276–88.
78. Vrijland WW, Jeekel J, Van Geldorp HJ, Swank DJ. Abdominal adhesions: intestinal obstruction, pain and infertility. A review. Surg Endosc Ultrasound Intervent Techniques. 2003;17:1017–22.
79. Swank DJ, Van Erp WFM, Repelaer van Driel OJ, et al. A prospective analysis of predictive factors on the results of laparoscopic adhesiolysis in patients with chronic abdominal pain. Surg Laparosc Endosc. 2003;13:88–94.
80. ACOG Committee Opinion No. 673. Persistent vulvar pain. Obstet Gynecol. 2016;128:e78–84.
81. Sadownik LA. Etiology, diagnosis, and clinical management of vulvodynia. Int J Women's Health. 2014;6:437–49.
82. Bergeron S, Khalifé S, Glazer HI, Binik YM. Surgical and behavioral treatments for vestibulodynia: two-and-one-half year follow-up and predictors of outcome. Obstet Gynecol. 2008;111(1):159–66.
83. Moore RA, Derry S, Aldington D, Cole P, Wiffen PJ. Amitriptyline for neuropathic pain and fibromyalgia in adults. Cochrane Database Syst Rev. 2012;12:CD008242.
84. Jackson JL, Shimeall W, Sessums L, Dezee KJ, Becher D, Diemer M, et al. Tricyclic antidepressants and headaches: systematic review and meta-analysis. BMJ. 2010;341:c5222.
85. Chou R, Deyo R, Friedly J, Skelly A, Weimer M, Fu R, et al. Systemic pharmacologic therapies for low back pain: a systematic review for an American College of Physicians Clinical Practice Guideline. Ann Intern Med. 2017;166(7):480–92.
86. Smith RV, Havens JR, Walsh SL. Gabapentin misuse, abuse and diversion: a systematic review. Addiction. 2016;111(7):1160–74.
87. ACOG practice bulletin no 72: vaginitis. (2006, May). Obstet Gynecol. 2006;107:1195–206.
88. Vandermeer FQ, Wong-You-Cheong JJ. Imaging of acute pelvic pain. Clin Obstet Gynecol. 2009;52(1):2–20.
89. ACOG practice bulletin no 114: Management of Endometriosis (July 2010). Obstet Gynecol. 2010;116:223–36.
90. Jeong YY, Outwater EK, Kang HK. Imaging evaluation of ovarian masses. Radiographics. 2000;20:1445–70.

32 Opioid Use Disorder

Alfred Shoukry and Melissa A. McNeil

Learning Objectives

1. Define opioid use disorder.
2. Review the epidemiology of opioid use disorder in women.
3. Identify treatment strategies for opioid use disorder including counseling, abstinence, and medication-assisted treatment.
4. Appropriately prescribe medication-assisted therapy for pregnant women.

Emily is a 32-year-old woman with history of chronic lower back pain who underwent lumbar fusion surgery 3 years ago. She has been on long-standing opioid medications prescribed through your office. In the past year she noticed that she has required higher doses of opioids to manage her pain and has recently started resorting to getting additional pills from friends and family to manage her pain.

Epidemiology

Opioid use in the United States has been rising during the past two decades and has resulted in increasing rates of opioid use disorder. "Opioid use disorder" (OUD) as defined by the DSM V and will be discussed in detail later in this chapter has replaced the prior DSM IV diagnoses of opioid dependence and opioid abuse by accounting for features of both disorders. "Dependence" most often refers to the body's need to use opioids to avoid physical withdrawal symptoms or the need to use more to produce the same effect, also known as "tolerance." "Abuse" refers to the patient's continued use of opioids despite negative social, medical, legal, or occupational problems [1]. Patients with opioid use disorder can misuse opioid prescriptions, use diverted prescription opioid medications, or use illicit opioids such as heroin. It is clear from evaluating changes in opioid use and death from opioids over time that America is facing a major opioid epidemic [2]. In 2015, approximately 91.8 million people in the United States used opioids, 11.5 million people misused them, and 1.9 million people during this period met criteria for opioid use disorder [2]. About 5.1 million people used heroin at some point during their lifetime according to a 2015 estimate. In the United States, opioid-related deaths are increasing with 33,000 deaths related to opioid overdose in 2015 [3]. Most patients who use heroin report previously using prescription drugs for nonmedical uses [4]. Gender has been shown to play a role in opioid use disorder—women tend to initiate illicit drug use at an earlier age, and progress more rapidly to drug dependence than men [5]. Women with serious mental illness or cigarette smoking are more likely to have nonmedical use of prescription opioids [6].

In an effort to gain insight into the factors influencing long-term opioid use, researchers analyzed outcomes of opioid-naive patients treated with opioids; the probability of continued opioid use at 1 year in this group was 5.3%. Factors that increased the risk of continued opioid use in this population included: prescriptions of greater than 90 morphine milligram equivalents, initiation of treatment with tramadol, or treatment with long-acting opioids [7].

Physiology and Pathophysiology

Opioids are natural or synthetic substances that act on the mu, kappa, and delta receptors. They have central and peripheral nervous system effects. Activation of mu receptors in the

A. Shoukry (✉)
UPMC, Department of Internal Medicine, Pittsburgh, PA, USA
e-mail: shoukrya@upmc.edu

M. A. McNeil
University of Pittsburgh Medical Center, Department of Medicine, Pittsburgh, PA, USA

S. A. Tilstra et al. (eds.), *Sex- and Gender-Based Women's Health*, https://doi.org/10.1007/978-3-030-50695-7_32

central nervous system leads to the analgesia, euphoria, and respiratory depression. Opioid receptor activation in the peripheral nervous system can cause constipation and cough suppression. Removal of opioids from mu receptors leads to withdrawal effects including piloerection, joint pain, diaphoresis, mydriasis, diarrhea, and dysphoria [8]. The severity of these withdrawal symptoms is often a barrier that prevents patients who try to stop using opioids.

Natural opioids, including morphine, codeine, and heroin, are drugs extracted directly from the opium poppy plant. Semisynthetic opioids, including oxycodone, hydrocodone, hydromorphone, and oxymorphone, are derived from the opium poppy plant. Synthetic opioids, including methadone, tramadol, and fentanyl, are drugs produced without the poppy plant. Some urine drug assays do not consistently detect semisynthetic and synthetic opioids [9].

Table 32.1 shows the half-lives and duration of effect of some commonly used opioids [10–12]. These properties of opioid medications are important when considering which drug to prescribe, how much to prescribe, and how often to prescribe it. Most opioids are "short-acting" and need to be given several times per day in order to provide adequate pain control for chronic pain. Opioids with a short half-life can have a longer duration of action if there are active metabolites.

Patients receiving opioids chronically may wish to be tapered to off, especially if patients are experiencing adverse effects which include sedation, difficulty with concentration, nausea, mood changes, or constipation. One approach to this would be to taper the opioid dose by 10% per week. In patients who have been on long-term opioids for more than 2 years, the taper can be changed to decreasing the dose by 10% every month [11].

After discussing your concerns with Emily about her using additional pills from her friends and family, she becomes concerned and decides to stop using opioids on her own without a taper. She misses her next scheduled appointment and returns 2 months later. She reports that she experienced nausea, vomiting, diaphoresis, joint pain, and diarrhea after stopping her oxycodone. Due to the severity of her withdrawal symptoms, she started buying opioids illegally.

Table 32.1 Onset, half-life, brand names, and equianalgesic doses of commonly prescribed opioid medications [10, 12, 13]. Onset, half-life, and potency of medication will vary by patient

Drug	Onset	Half-life	Common brand names	Equianalgesic dose
Fentanyl (synthetic)	IM: 7–15 minutes IV: immediate Transdermal patch: 6 hours	IM: 3–4 hours IV: 2–4 hours Transdermal patch: 20–27 hours	Duragesic, Abstral, Fentora, Sublimaze, Subsys	IM: 0.125 Transdermal: variable
Oxymorphone (semisynthetic)	IM: 10–20 minutes PO: Variable	IM: 2–3 hours PO: Variable	Opana (FDA recall of extended-release formulation in 2017)	IM: 1 PO: 10
Hydromorphone (semisynthetic)	IM: 10–20 minutes IV: 5 minutes PO: 15–30 minutes	IM: 2–3 hours PO: Variable	Dilaudid, Exalgo	IM: 1.5 PO: 7.5
Hydrocodone (semisynthetic)	PO: 30–60 minutes	PO: 4 hours	Vicodin, Norco, Lorcet, Lortab, Xodol, Verdrocet (with acetaminophen)	5–10
Oxycodone (semisynthetic)	PO (short-acting formulations): 30–60 minutes	PO (short-acting formulations): 2–3 hours	Percocet, Endocet, Roxicet, Primlev, Xartemis (with acetaminophen) Roxicodone, Oxaydo, Oxycontin, Roxybond, Xtampza	15–30
Oxycodone (semisynthetic)	PO (long acting): 4.5 hours	PO (long acting): 12 hours	Oxycontin	15–30
Codeine (natural)	PO: 10–30 minutes	PO: 3 hours	Tylenol #3, Tylenol #4 (with acetaminophen)	15–30
Morphine (natural)	IM/IV: 5–20 minutes PO: ~ 30 minutes	IM/IV: 2 hours PO: 2–4 hours	MS Contin, Kadian, MorphaBond, Duramorph	IM/IV: 10 PO: 30
Tramadol (synthetic)	PO: <60 minutes	PO: 5–7 hours	Ultram, Zytram, Tridural, Ralivia, Durela	50–100
Methadone (synthetic)	PO: 30–60 minutes	PO: 12–190 hours	Dolophine, Methadose	Variable
Buprenorphine	PO 100 minutes	PO: 24–42 hours	Suboxone, Zubsolv, Bunavail (with naloxone) Subutex (without naloxone)	Variable

Diagnosis

Opioid use disorder (OUD) is formally diagnosed using the *Diagnostic and Statistical Manual of Mental Disorders, Fifth Edition*. This definition now encompasses the previous diagnoses of opioid abuse and opioid dependence from the DSM IV. The DSM V defines opioid use disorder as opioid use that leads to significant impairment and distress as evidenced by two of the following, over a 12-month interval:

1. Patient takes medication in larger quantities than what is recommended, prescribed, or intended.
2. Unable to successfully stop or wean down opiates despite the desire to.
3. Significant efforts are made to secure, use, and recover from opioids.
4. Uncontrollable desire to use opioids, whether or not they are prescribed.
5. Opioid use consistently causes problems in home, school, or work life.
6. Continued use despite social, personal, medical, or psychological problems that result directly from use (social/personal issues = 1, medical/psychological issues = 1).
7. Social or work obligations are compromised due to opioid use.
8. Ongoing use in physically hazardous situations.
9. Physical tolerance to opioids—needing more opioid to produce the same effect or having a diminished effect by consistently using the same dose.
10. Withdrawal—developing physical symptoms of piloerection, joint pain, diaphoresis, mydriasis, diarrhea, and dysphoria after stopping opioids or taking opioids to alleviate these symptoms.

Patients with two to three symptoms present have mild opioid use disorder; four to five symptoms have moderate opioid use disorder; and six or more symptoms have severe opioid use disorder.

Screening

Screening for OUD is an important part of evaluating patients who are prescribed chronic opioids. This can help identify individuals in which the risk of starting or continuing opioids outweighs the benefits of opioid therapy.

Several screening tools exist for identifying patients who are at high risk of misusing opioids and should be administered to patients prior to starting opioid medication to help guide decisions about treatment and follow-up. The Screener and Opioid Assessment for Patients with Pain (SOAPP) is a 14-item patient-reported questionnaire which assess several domains including psychiatric issues, history of substance abuse, problematic medication-related behaviors, family history of substance use, and issues with the provider-patient relationship [14]. The Opioid Risk Tool (ORT) is another patient-reported questionnaire that assesses risk factors for opioid use disorder including personal and family history of substance abuse, age, sexual abuse, and psychological diseases [15]. At the time of publication, both of these tools can be accessed on the Internet for free.

For patients already on opioids, it is important to monitor for aberrant behaviors including lost or stolen medications, documented use of multiple physicians, and requests for early refills. Patients with more aberrant behaviors should prompt further screening for opioid use disorder [15]. The Rapid Opioid Dependence Screen (RODS) is an eight-item tool for screening opioid use disorder in the clinical setting [16]. This tool asks about the pattern of opioid use and its effect on patients' functioning. Patients who screen positive should be asked about the items in the DSM V criteria for the diagnosis of opioid use disorder.

Patients that are not prescribed opioids and are not being evaluated for management of acute or chronic pain can still have opioid use disorder. Frequent visits to the emergency department for pain-related conditions (tooth pain, abdominal pain, trauma), history of mental illness, stress at home, job loss, history of substance use, and family history of substance use should always raise concern for a concomitant substance or opioid use disorder, and patients should be screened appropriately.

History and Physical Exam

When evaluating patients with opioid use disorder, the provider should assess for the type of opioids consumed and the method of consumption. Opioids can be used through intranasal, intravenous, subcutaneous, or intramuscular use or by smoking. Patients using needles should also be asked about needle sharing, disposal, reuse, or other behaviors such as licking needles. The amount of opioid use should also be assessed along with details on the frequency of use and the time of last use. Patients should also be asked about prior attempts at treatment including inpatient rehabilitation, outpatient rehabilitation, or prior medication-assisted treatment (MAT). Other historical elements about medical or legal complications of opioid use should be assessed. Medical complications can include infections such as cellulitis, bacteremia, diskitis, osteomyelitis, epidural abscesses, septic joints, endocarditis, sepsis, HIV, hepatitis B, or hepatitis C. Any surgeries related to orthopedic or valvular infections should be documented. Legal issues can be related to purchasing or distributing opioids or operating vehicles under the influence of substances.

A thorough physical examination should be performed paying particular attention to the potential complications from opioid use. Patients who inject opioids may have track marks on their skin, which are scars or wounds from frequent intravenous injections commonly found on the upper extremities but can be found anywhere there is an accessible vessel. Injection sites should be examined for infection. All joints should be examined for swelling, erythema, warmth, and range of motion. A heart exam can reveal murmurs related to endocarditis. A neurovascular exam should also be done to assess for any neurological deficits which could be related to spine infections, cerebral abscesses, or mycotic aneurysms. The nasal septum should be examined in case of perforation which can occur in patients who use intranasal drugs. Pain should be taken seriously and investigated, especially in the setting of a fever as it can indicate an underlying nidus of infection.

Patients using opioids may be intoxicated or experiencing withdrawal symptoms. Signs of intoxication can include pinpoint pupils, impaired cognition, or drowsiness. Conversely, patients withdrawing from opioids may have lacrimation, rhinorrhea, yawning, hyperactive bowel sounds, piloerection, and tachycardia.

The prescription drug monitoring program should be checked if available to identify any controlled substances that patients are being prescribed.

Laboratory Evaluation

Laboratory evaluation is an important component in the initial evaluation of patients with opioid use disorder. Patients who use opioids intravenously or subcutaneously are at risk for HIV and hepatitis B and C due to sharing needles and drug injection equipment that are contaminated with blood. Active substance use can facilitate disinhibited behaviors such as unsafe sex practices, sex with multiple partners, and sex for drugs placing patients at high risk for STIs [17]. Screening for hepatitis B and C, syphilis, and HIV is indicated. Gonorrhea and chlamydia screening should be offered according to guidelines for high-risk individuals depending on age, sexual exposures, and HIV status [18]. Women should be screened for pregnancy with urine hCG and strongly encouraged to use reliable forms of contraception. A urine drug screen can be helpful to determine if patients are using prescribed medications appropriately and to evaluate for other illicit substances. Having patients return for random drug screens can also provide helpful information about use behaviors. Most labs have different choices for urine drug screens; some of these may not detect semisynthetic opioids (such as oxycodone, hydrocodone, oxymorphone) or synthetic opioids (such as methadone, tramadol, fentanyl). If a urine drug screen returns with unexpected results, a good first step is to discuss the characteristic of the test with the laboratory and discuss the results with the patient, rather than assume use behaviors about the patient.

The history and physical exam should drive any further workup and testing for acute or chronic medical issues at the time of patient presentation. If patients are being considered for medication-assisted treatment (MAT), it is important to evaluate for liver disease, since naltrexone and naloxone are contraindicated in this patient population.

Emily remains motivated to discontinue using illicit opioids, but she feels helpless in her struggle. She has been attending narcotics anonymous meetings but has not been able to discontinue opioids due to intense cravings and the severity of her withdrawal symptoms when she discontinues them. She asks if there are any options available to help her stop using opioids.

Treatment

The approach to treatment for OUD is the same regardless of the severity of OUD. Long-term treatment for opioid use disorder involves a multifaceted approach including addiction counseling and consideration of medication-associated treatment (MAT). Members of a successful treatment team usually include providers from primary care or psychiatry, psychology, peer support groups, social work, and nursing. Factors including the patient's medical comorbidities and preferences can help guide the approach to treatment.

Medically Supervised Withdrawal

Withdrawal symptoms can be severe and a challenging barrier to recovery. Many patients with OUD continue to use opioids only to avoid withdrawal symptoms and not to become intoxicated. Medically supervised withdrawal can help to safely transition patients to abstinence or long-term MAT. Managing patients with opioid use disorder is a complicated task which requires motivational interviewing strategies and a willingness on the patient's part to engage in treatment.

There are two approaches to treating opioid withdrawal: (1) by treating withdrawal with opioid receptor agonists (buprenorphine or methadone) which allows gradual taper of the drug or continuation as part of MAT and (2) by using medications to block the symptoms of opioid withdrawal, allowing the patient to go through withdrawal "cold turkey" from opioids. Alpha-2 agonists (clonidine) help block sympathetic overdrive and decrease sweating, restlessness, anxiety, and rhinorrhea; H_2 blockers such as diphenhydramine or hydroxyzine assist with treating anxiety or restlessness. Loperamide can be used to manage diarrhea, and antiemetics such as ondansetron can be used to manage nausea or vomiting. NSAIDs can help with joint pain, and muscle relaxants such as cyclobenzaprine or baclofen can be helpful with muscle spasms. Opioid agonist therapy is more effective than symptomatic management of withdrawal symptoms and is preferred unless the patient is in an environment such as a prison where opioid agonist therapy is not permitted [19]. Alpha-2 agonists should be avoided in patients with bradycardia or hypotension.

Withdrawal symptoms should be measured serially to assess progress and guide medication therapy. Withdrawal symptoms can be assessed using the structured Clinical Opioid Withdrawal Scale (COWS) [20]. The COWS accounts for resting heart rate, gastrointestinal upset, sweating, tremor, restlessness, yawning, pupil size, anxiety, gooseflesh skin, runny nose, or tearing each on a scale of 1–5. While these withdrawal symptoms can sometimes be severe enough to necessitate inpatient admission for their management, they are not life-threatening. Patients with the following should be considered for admission for medically supervised withdrawal: (1) the patient's home environment is not safe or conducive for patient detoxification; (2) the patient's medical problems need to be monitored during the withdrawal period (e.g., if a patient has chronic renal insufficiency and is having profuse diarrhea from opioid withdrawal, volume status and renal function need to be monitored); (3) there is concern for concomitant drug use with alcohol, benzodiazepines, or barbiturates—acute withdrawal from these substances can be life-threatening; or (4) the patient has severe mental illness or is psychologically unstable.

Medication-supervised withdrawal or tapering patients off opioids is often insufficient for achieving long-term abstinence, and patients forgoing long-term treatment have been found to have higher mortality than ones undergoing MAT due to higher rates of resuming opioid use [21].

Counseling

Current evidence supports the use of MAT for the treatment of opioid use disorder. Addiction counseling can serve as an adjunctive tool or can be used in patients who prefer not to use MAT. Addiction counseling is a loose definition and can take many forms. It can include individual, family, group, cognitive, and behavioral therapies provided by trained physicians, psychologists, counselors, or peer advocates. Patients can enroll in inpatient, intensive outpatient, or outpatient programs depending on their needs. Mutual support groups such as Alcoholics Anonymous and Narcotics Anonymous have played a major role in addiction recovery across America. All of these programs can be used concomitantly with MAT. Methadone and buprenorphine programs typically require patients to participate in some form of addiction counseling.

Some patients may be hesitant to engage in MAT due to stigma previously encountered with other healthcare providers or at mutual support groups which often encourage abstinence-based treatment. This should be explored in a supportive environment and the benefits of medication-assisted treatment should be emphasized.

Medication-Assisted Treatment (MAT)

All patients with OUD can be considered for MAT. The goal of MAT is to allow the patient to be free of physiologic cravings and adverse psychosocial effects of opioids in a controlled environment with a trusted provider. MAT can be started in patients that want to curb cravings that are not currently using opioids and started in patients currently using opioids independently or part of a medically supervised withdrawal program. Long-term treatment of OUD with MAT can consist of opioid antagonist treatment (naltrexone) or opioid agonist treatment (methadone or buprenorphine).

Naltrexone

Naltrexone is a mu-opioid receptor antagonist which helps to lower the rate of opioid use relapse by blocking the euphoric effect of opioids [22]. Since this medication is an antagonist, patients should be abstinent from all opioids for at least 7 days prior to starting. Administering this medication in patients who have used opioids recently can precipitate withdrawal effects. Naltrexone does not have any analgesic effects due to its antagonism of the mu-opioid receptor. When starting naltrexone, a challenge dose of 0.8 mg–1.6 mg IV or IM dose can be given with monitoring over the next 15–30 minutes or a 12.5 mg–25 mg oral dose with monitoring over the next 4 hours. If patients tolerate a test dose without significant withdrawal symptoms as outlined previously, then they can be started on the full oral or intramuscular dose. Naltrexone is available in 50 mg tablets which can block the effect of opioids for 1 day or can be administered in a 380 mg injection which can last for 1 month. Side effects include nausea, abdominal pain, fatigue, or insomnia. Transaminases should be monitored as they can increase while on naltrexone. Women using naltrexone should be counseled on reliable contraception and be screened for pregnancy. In one study, 74% of patients receiving naltrexone had urine samples negative for opioids, compared to 56% of patients receiving counseling and referral to community treatment programs [23]. Naltrexone is typically used as a monthly intramuscular injection.

Buprenorphine

Buprenorphine is a partial mu-opioid receptor agonist which can help to reduce opioid cravings and withdrawal symptoms. It can also help to block euphoric effects if opioids are used in conjunction. Providers can undergo special training to become waivered to prescribe buprenorphine in the outpatient setting. Buprenorphine is most commonly prescribed in an outpatient setting, but increasingly patients are being started on buprenorphine while in the hospital to facilitate MAT when they are admitted for complications from opioid use. The ability to take the medication in outpatient offices makes it more convenient than methadone, which requires daily clinic visits for dosing. This also means that it should be reserved for patients who do not require the frequent follow-up and structure of a methadone clinic.

The most commonly used formulation of buprenorphine is a combination buprenorphine-naloxone film. The naloxone in this formulation is metabolized through first pass metabolism and does not cause withdrawal. If injected, however, the naloxone in this formulation causes withdrawal symptoms. This is used as a deterrent for injecting the medication.

It is optimal to start buprenorphine after patients start to have withdrawal symptoms because starting buprenorphine in patients who are acutely intoxicated can precipitate severe withdrawal symptoms. Because it is a partial agonist, patients being initiated on buprenorphine should attempt to abstain from opioids for about 12–24 hours prior to starting the medication in order for them to develop withdrawal symptoms. If patients are taking longer-acting opioids such as methadone, they may need to wait for longer periods (up to 48–72 hours) before they develop withdrawal symptoms. Patients can typically start with a 4 mg dose of buprenorphine and increase over the course of 1–2 days as needed to curb withdrawal symptoms. Side effects of buprenorphine include fatigue, anxiety, nausea, or constipation. Since buprenorphine is a partial mu-receptor agonist, it does have some mild analgesic effect. In a randomized, double-blind, placebo-controlled efficacy study of buprenorphine for patients with opioid use disorder, the proportion of urine samples that were negative for opioids was 17.8% in patients taking buprenorphine-naloxone compared to 5.8% in patients receiving placebo [24].

Buprenorphine is an effective treatment for opioid use disorder in pregnant women. In this population of patients, buprenorphine monotherapy should be used rather than buprenorphine-naloxone due to limited data regarding naloxone safety during pregnancy. Buprenorphine monotherapy should also be used in patients with cirrhosis due to clearance of naloxone by the liver.

As with naltrexone, if prescribing buprenorphine for women, providers should discuss effective contraception and screen for pregnancy routinely.

Patients interested in buprenorphine therapy can find a provider authorized to prescribe it through the Buprenorphine Treatment Practitioner Locator at the Substance Abuse and Mental Health Services Administration (SAMHSA) website (https://www.samhsa.gov/medication-assisted-treatment/physician-program-data/treatment-physician-locator) [25].

Methadone

Methadone is a full mu-opioid receptor agonist which is restricted to specialized clinics that require daily visits. Given the high degree of monitoring and participation for patients, methadone can be an effective option in patients with severe opioid use disorder and has been associated with a reduced risk of death [26]. It also serves as an effective treatment for special populations including women during pregnancy. Methadone treatment typically has three phases: induction/early stabilization with low doses, late stabilization with increasing doses, and maintenance. Maintenance doses between 80 mg and 100 mg are targeted to minimize cravings while avoiding euphoria and sedation. Side effects include constipation and QT interval prolongation. Methadone has several drug interactions and patient medications must be monitored carefully. Because methadone is most often prescribed by small local clinics, providers may not know that patients are taking methadone, and methadone will not show up on a routine pharmacy dispensing record.

Opioid substitution therapy with methadone or buprenorphine to treat opioid use disorder can help to reduce injection use, needle sharing, and therefore cases of HIV infection [27]. Patients who inject drugs should be considered for pre-exposure prophylaxis (PrEP) to protect against contracting HIV [28]. Patients with history of opioid use disorder should undergo routine urine drug screening regardless of the choice of therapy to ensure that medications they are prescribed are present in their urine, that medications they are not prescribed are absent, and that they are free of other illicit substances. All patients with OUD should also be provided with naloxone in case of relapse or overdose. Naloxone is a short-acting opioid antagonist that can rapidly reverse the effect of opioids in case of overdose. Naloxone can be provided via an intramuscular or intranasal route.

Emily considers methadone or buprenorphine in order to help with withdrawal symptoms and opioid cravings. She opts for buprenorphine because she doesn't feel that she can make it to daily visits for methadone administration. You help her to find a provider waivered to prescribe buprenorphine through the SAMHSA website who is near her home. In addition to MAT, she enrolls in drug and alcohol counseling. She starts to attend Narcotics Anonymous meetings and has been successful in abstaining from opioids. During her follow-up visit, she reports that she would like to become pregnant and would like advice about how to manage her medications.

Opioid Use Disorder During Pregnancy

Early universal screening for opioid use disorder with validated tools is recommended in pregnant women. The 4Ps can serve as a brief screening tool [29].

- **P**arents: One or both parents with a problem with alcohol or drug use?
- **P**artner: Partner with problems with alcohol or drug use?
- **P**ast: Prior difficulties in life due to alcohol or drugs (including prescribed medications)?
- **P**resent: Drug or alcohol use in the past month?

Any questions answered with "yes" should trigger additional questions and potential intervention.

Buprenorphine and methadone are both effective for treating opioid use disorder during pregnancy. Less data are available regarding use of naltrexone in pregnant women.

The American College of Obstetricians and Gynecologists (ACOG) recommends using buprenorphine or methadone for MAT during pregnancy [30]. The use of buprenorphine during pregnancy has the advantage of having lower rates of neonatal withdrawal syndrome compared to methadone [31]. For pregnant women with opioid use disorder who are receiving MAT, abrupt discontinuation is *not recommended* given higher relapse rates than patients who continue MAT [30]. If a pregnant patient wants to wean down her opioid use during pregnancy, she should be closely monitored by her obstetrician and/or maternal fetal medicine physician. Buprenorphine can be started in the outpatient setting. If a pregnant woman is to be started on methadone for MAT, most often she is admitted for methadone induction and titration given the long-acting nature of the drug and risk for respiratory depression. Fetal monitoring is important during this time to avoid adverse outcomes.

Most women that have been on MAT during pregnancy choose to continue MAT postpartum. Buprenorphine and methadone are both excreted in low doses in breast milk, and infants should be observed for sedation. ACOG recommends encouraging women on MAT to breastfeed [30]. Similar to pregnancy, naltrexone should be avoided in breastfeeding women. However, naloxone is a short-acting opioid antagonist which can be used for treatment of opioid overdose and should be given to pregnant or breastfeeding women in case of overdose [30]. All women in the postpartum period should be followed closely as this can be a time associated with additional stress, depression, and relapse, regardless of MAT use.

Summary Points

1. Opioid use disorder is defined by problematic opioid use leading to significant impairment over a 12-month period.
2. Opioid use disorder carries significant morbidity and mortality; women are more likely to start using opioids at a younger age and have a more rapid progression toward overt substance use.
3. Treating opioid use disorder is best done by a multidisciplinary team including primary care, psychology, social work, nursing, and peer support services. Medications including buprenorphine, methadone, and naltrexone can be used to treat opioid use disorder.
4. Buprenorphine and methadone are the preferred medications for treatment of opioid use disorder in pregnant or nursing women.

Review Questions

1. A 27-year-old woman with history of opioid use disorder who has been maintained on buprenorphine-naloxone presents to your office for routine follow-up. She has been doing well with buprenorphine-naloxone and has not used any illicit drugs in the past 3 months. A urine drug screen is positive for buprenorphine and negative for other substances. A urine pregnancy test is positive. Which is the most appropriate option for management of her opioid use disorder?
   A. Taper and discontinue buprenorphine-naloxone.
   B. Start methadone for the duration of pregnancy.
   C. Switch buprenorphine-naloxone to buprenorphine only.
   D. Switch to naltrexone intramuscular shots (Vivitrol).

   The correct answer is C. ACOG recommends against discontinuing MAT in patients who are stable even during pregnancy [30]. Both buprenorphine and methadone are acceptable options in pregnant patients. Since naloxone should be avoided during pregnancy, patients receiving buprenorphine-naloxone should be switched to buprenorphine monotherapy. In this case, since the patient has been stable on buprenorphine-naloxone, it would be reasonable to have her continue the same dose of buprenorphine without naloxone [30].

2. A 23-year-old woman presents for follow-up 1 month after right knee surgery. She was prescribed a 1-month supply of oxycodone 5 mg by mouth every 6 hours as needed for pain. She reports that she had breakthrough pain with this dose and took double the prescribed dose for pain relief. What is the most appropriate next step?
   A. Discuss the need to use opioids only as prescribed and explore strategies for pain control.
   B. Inform the patient that she has opioid use disorder and refer her for drug and alcohol counseling.
   C. Refill the patient's oxycodone early.
   D. Add extended-release oxycodone to help with pain.

The correct answer is A. The next best step in this situation is to discuss the patient's opioid use, the need to adhere to prescribed doses and frequency, and to explore strategies for pain control. There is insufficient evidence in this case to diagnose the patient with OUD [32]. Before giving additional short- or long-acting opioids, other pain control strategies should be explored.

3. A 54-year-old woman with history of heroin use presents for consideration of medication-assisted therapy with buprenorphine-naloxone. She reports injecting heroin 1 hour prior to her appointment. Physical examination reveals normal vital signs. The patient is in no apparent distress. She has pinpoint pupils. Cardiovascular exam reveals regular rate and rhythm without murmurs, rubs or gallops. Her skin is dry. She has no tremor on neurologic exam. Urine drug screen is positive for opioids. Laboratory testing reveals normal liver enzymes. What is the next best option in management?
   A. Start buprenorphine-naloxone now by giving the first dose in your office.
   B. Start buprenorphine-naloxone once she has developed mild-moderate withdrawal.
   C. Start buprenorphine-naloxone only after evaluating for underlying medical illness.
   D. Start buprenorphine-naloxone only after the patient completes inpatient rehab and demonstrates an extended period of abstinence.

   The correct answer is B. The patient in this case has evidence of opioid use disorder and would be a suitable candidate for treatment with buprenorphine-naltrexone. Given her recent heroin use and evidence of intoxication on examination, she is at risk for precipitated withdrawal if she is given buprenorphine now. The best approach would be to have the patient wait until she develops withdrawal symptoms and then have her start buprenorphine-naltrexone. There is no need to screen for other illnesses, require her to complete inpatient rehab, or demonstrate an extended period of abstinence prior to initiating MAT.

References

1. Compton WM, Dawson DA, Goldstein RB, Grant BF. Crosswalk between DSM-IV dependence and DSM-5 substance use disorders for opioids, cannabis, cocaine and alcohol. Drug Alcohol Depend. 2013;132(1-2):387–90. https://doi.org/10.1016/j.drugalcdep.2013.02.036. Epub 2013 May 1.
2. Han B, Compton WM, Blanco C, Crane E, Lee J, Jones CM. Prescription opioid use, misuse, and use disorders in U.S. adults: 2015 National Survey on drug use and health. Ann Intern Med. 2017;167(5):293–301. https://doi.org/10.7326/M17-0865. Epub 2017 Aug 1.
3. Rudd RA, Aleshire N, Zibbell JE, Gladden RM. Increases in drug and opioid-involved overdose deaths - United States, 2010-2015. MMWR Morb Mortal Wkly Rep. 2016;64(50-51):1378–82. https://doi.org/10.15585/mmwr.mm6450a3.
4. Jones CM. Heroin use and heroin use risk behaviors among nonmedical users of prescription opioid pain relievers - United States, 2002-2004 and 2008-2010. Drug Alcohol Depend. 2013;132(1-2):95–100. https://doi.org/10.1016/j.drugalcdep.2013.01.007. Epub 2013 Feb 12.
5. Unger A, Jung E, Winklbaur B, Fischer G. Gender issues in the pharmacotherapy of opioid-addicted women: buprenorphine. J Addict Dis. 2010;29(2):217–30. https://doi.org/10.1080/10550881003684814.
6. Tetrault JM, Desai RA, Becker WC, Fiellin DA, Concato J, Sullivan LE. Gender and non-medical use of prescription opioids: results from a national US survey. Addiction. 2008;103(2):258–68. Epub 2007 Nov 27.
7. Shah A, Hayes CJ, Martin BC. Factors influencing long-term opioid use among opioid naive patients: an examination of initial prescription characteristics and pain etiologies. J Pain. 2017;18(11):1374–83. https://doi.org/10.1016/j.jpain.2017.06.010.
8. White JM. Pleasure into pain: the consequences of long-term opioid use. Addict Behav. 2004;29(7):1311–24.
9. Milone MC. Laboratory testing for prescription opioids. J Med Toxicol. 2012;8(4):408–16.
10. Hemmings HC, Egan TD. Pharmacology and physiology for anesthesia: foundations and clinical application. 2nd ed. Philadelphia: Elsevier, Inc. 994 pgs; 2019.
11. Berna C, Kulich RJ, Rathmell JP. Tapering long-term opioid therapy in chronic noncancer pain: evidence and recommendations for everyday practice. Mayo Clin Proc. 2015;90(6):828–42.
12. DiPiro JT. Pharmacotherapy: a pathophysiologic approach. 8th ed. New York: McGraw-Hill Medical; 2011. xxxii, 2668 p.
13. Opioid Oral Morphine Milligram Equivalent (MME) conversion factors. 2019 1/2/2019]; Available from: https://www.cms.gov/Medicare/Prescription-Drug-Coverage/PrescriptionDrugCovContra/Downloads/Opioid-Morphine-EQ-Conversion-Factors-vFeb-2018.pdf.
14. Butler SF, Budman SH, Fernandez K, Jamison RN. Validation of a screener and opioid assessment measure for patients with chronic pain. Pain. 2004;112(1-2):65–75.
15. Webster LR, Webster RM. Predicting aberrant behaviors in opioid-treated patients: preliminary validation of the Opioid Risk Tool. Pain Med. 2005;6(6):432–42.
16. Wickersham JA, Azar MM, Cannon CM, Altice FL, Springer SA. Validation of a brief measure of opioid dependence: the rapid opioid dependence screen (RODS). J Correct Health Care. 2015;21(1):12–26. https://doi.org/10.1177/1078345814557513.
17. Khan MR, Berger A, Hemberg J, O'Neill A, Dyer TP, Smyrk K. Non-injection and injection drug use and STI/HIV risk in the United States: the degree to which sexual risk behaviors versus sex with an STI-infected partner account for infection transmission among drug users. AIDS Behav. 2013;17(3):1185–94. https://doi.org/10.1007/s10461-012-0276-0.
18. Acheampong AB, Striley CW, Cottler LB. Prescription opioid use, illicit drug use, and sexually transmitted infections among participants from a community engagement program in North Central Florida. J Subst Use. 2017;22(1):90–5.
19. Meader N. A comparison of methadone, buprenorphine and alpha(2) adrenergic agonists for opioid detoxification: a mixed treatment comparison meta-analysis. Drug Alcohol Depend. 2010;108(1-2):110–4.
20. Wesson DR, Ling W. The Clinical Opiate Withdrawal Scale (COWS). J Psychoactive Drugs. 2003;35(2):253–9.
21. Evans E, Li L, Min J, Huang D, Urada D, Liu L, et al. Mortality among individuals accessing pharmacological treatment for opioid

dependence in California, 2006-10. Addiction. 2015;110(6):996–1005. https://doi.org/10.1111/add.12863.
22. Lee JD, McDonald R, Grossman E, McNeely J, Laska E, Rotrosen J, Gourevitch MN. Opioid treatment at release from jail using extended-release naltrexone: a pilot proof-of-concept randomized effectiveness trial. Addiction. 2015;110(6):1008–14. https://doi.org/10.1111/add.12894.
23. Lee JD, Friedmann PD, Kinlock TW, Nunes EV, Boney TY, Hoskinson RA, et al. Extended-release naltrexone to prevent opioid relapse in criminal justice offenders. N Engl J Med. 2016;374(13):1232–42.
24. Fudala PJ, Bridge TP, Herbert S, Williford WO, Chiang CN, et al. Buprenorphine/Naloxone Collaborative Study Group. Office-based treatment of opiate addiction with a sublingual-tablet formulation of buprenorphine and naloxone. N Engl J Med. 2003;349(10):949–58.
25. Buprenorphine Treatment Practitioner Locator at the Substance Abuse and Mental Health Services Administration (SAMHSA) website (https://www.samhsa.gov/medication-assisted-treatment/physician-program-data/treatment-physician-locator). Accessed April 2019.
26. Cousins G, Boland F, Courtney B, Barry J, Lyons S, Fahey T. Risk of mortality on and off methadone substitution treatment in primary care: a national cohort study. Addiction. 2016;111(1):73–82. https://doi.org/10.1111/add.13087.
27. Gowing L, Farrell MF, Bornemann R, Sullivan LE, Ali R. Oral substitution treatment of injecting opioid users for prevention of HIV infection. Cochrane Database Syst Rev. 2011;(8):CD004145. https://doi.org/10.1002/14651858.CD004145.pub4.
28. Centers for Disease Control and Prevention. Update to interim guidance for Preexposure Prophylaxis (PrEP) for the prevention of HIV infection: PrEP for injecting drug users. MMWR Morb Mortal Wkly Rep. 2013;62(23):463–5.
29. Ewing H. A practical guide to intervention in health and social services with pregnant and postpartum addicts and alcoholics: theoretical framework, brief screening tool, key interview questions, and strategies for referral to recovery resources. Martinez: Contra Costa County Department of Health Services; 1990.
30. Committee on Obstetric Practice. Committee opinion No. 711: opioid use and opioid use disorder in pregnancy. Obstet Gynecol. 2017;130(2):e81–94. https://doi.org/10.1097/AOG.0000000000002235.
31. Nanda S, Brant R, Regier M, Yossuck P. Buprenorphine: a new player in neonatal withdrawal syndrome. W V Med J. 2015;111(1):16–21.
32. American Psychiatric Association. and American Psychiatric Association. DSM-5 Task Force. Diagnostic and statistical manual of mental disorders : DSM-5. 5th ed. Washington, D.C: American Psychiatric Association; 2013. xliv, 947 p.

Part VI

Mental Health

Depressive and Anxiety Disorders

33

Rebecca Gitlin and Alexandra E. Mieczkowski

Learning Objectives

1. Describe the prevalence of depressive and anxiety disorders among women in the United States, including gender differences in incidence, prevalence, and presentation.
2. Differentiate among depressive disorders, bipolar disorders, and anxiety disorders.
3. Utilize two validated screening measures, PHQ-9 and GAD-7, to assess depressive and anxiety symptoms in the primary care setting.
4. Formulate patient-centered inquiries to gather information about mood or anxiety symptoms, psychosocial context, and goals for treatment.
5. Conduct a suicide risk assessment to determine the presence or absence of suicidal ideation, intent, and plan.
6. Contrast treatments used for depression and anxiety in the primary care setting with respect to anticipated side effects, efficacy, and safety in pregnancy and lactation.
7. Identify patients who require referral to a psychiatrist and those who would benefit from voluntary or involuntary hospitalization.

Monica is a 27-year-old cisgender woman presenting for a primary care appointment to address problems with her sleep. She appears agitated during the appointment and expresses frustration because she "can't sleep" and is "at [her] wit's end."

Introduction

Depressive and anxiety disorders disproportionately affect women and are a significant cause of morbidity in the United States and across the world. Globally, more than 300 million people are affected by depression [1]. Mental health and substance use disorders are the leading global causes of disability and therefore represent an important public health focus [2]. Per the 2016 National Survey on Drug Use and Health (NSDUH), 18.3% of adults in the United States have at least one mental health disorder, and the prevalence is higher in women (21.7%) than in men (14.5%) [3]. Gender disparity statistics are similar for specific types of mental health issues, such as depressive episodes (8.5% prevalence in women relative to 4.8% prevalence in men) and anxiety (23.4% prevalence in women relative to 14.3% prevalence in men). Bipolar disorders have a similar prevalence in both men and women, estimated to be around 2.8% annually [4]. In contrast, women are less likely than men to be diagnosed with a substance use disorder (5.7% prevalence in women versus 10.1% prevalence in men) [3]. Co-occurring substance use and mental health disorders show a similar prevalence among men (3.6%) and women (3.2%).

The prevalence of depression and anxiety is affected by demographic and socioeconomic factors [3]. Younger adults, ages 18–25, are more likely to be affected by depression when compared with older patients. Individuals of American Indian or Alaska Native descent and those who report two or more races are more likely to be affected by depression than

R. Gitlin (✉)
Los Angeles County Department of Mental Health, Los Angeles, CA, USA
e-mail: rgitlin@dmh.lacounty.gov

A. E. Mieczkowski
UPMC Presbyterian Shadyside and Children's Hospital of Pittsburgh of UPMC, Division of General Internal Medicine, General Academic Pediatrics, Pittsburgh, PA, USA

S. A. Tilstra et al. (eds.), *Sex- and Gender-Based Women's Health*, https://doi.org/10.1007/978-3-030-50695-7_33

individuals from other racial/ethnic groups [3]. Similarly, younger adults in the 18–29- and 30–44-year-old age ranges are more likely to be affected by anxiety disorder than older adults (60+). Sexual minorities, those who identify as gay, lesbian, bisexual, or queer, and gender minorities, those identifying as transgender, non-binary, or genderqueer, are disproportionately affected by depression and anxiety compared with heterosexual and cisgender individuals (see Chap. 36 on the Care of Sexual Minority Women and Chap. 37 on Transgender Care) [5].

Social determinants of health that likely contribute to the disproportionate rates of depression and anxiety among women include the greater likelihood of women to earn less income [6], to be exposed to discrimination based on gender and other social identities [6, 7], and to experience marked interpersonal and family-related stress [8, 9]. Women often serve as caregivers for multiple family members of multiple generations and take on more household tasks and responsibilities than men, even when employed full-time [10]. Women are also at increased risk of anxiety and depression in response to life stressors caused by significant life transitions, including having children, starting a new job, or navigating significant changes in relationships.

Pathophysiology

Understanding the pathophysiology of depression and anxiety helps one to understand the factors that may predispose a patient toward mental health disorders and the mechanisms by which treatments work. While scientific research has provided a basic understanding of neurologic macroscopic and microscopic patterns in depression and anxiety, the biological underpinnings of these disorders continue to be elucidated through animal models, human neuroimaging, and neurocognitive modeling. On a macroscopic level, several structures within the brain are thought to be important in the development of depressive and anxiety disorders. Anxiety disorders arise in part from how perceived threats are processed through signaling from and between the hippocampus, amygdala, and cortex [11]. These areas are responsible for multiple actions, including processing emotion and planning responses and actions [12]. Individuals with anxiety disorders have been shown to have hyperactivity in the amygdala on fMRI, an effect which can be further modulated by appropriate or dysfunctional processing by the prefrontal cortex where thoughts help interpret a perceived threat [12].

Sex and Gender-Based Differences

Research studies aiming to determine the etiology behind the greater prevalence of depressive disorders in women have revealed that structural brain changes are variable between the sexes. For example, depressed women had smaller amygdalae than controls but no change in left inferior cingulate gyri, but depressed men had no change in amygdala volume but a decrease in cingulate gyrus volumes [13]. PET imaging has shown differences in serotonin synthesis between female and male patients with major depressive disorder (MDD) [14]. These differences suggest that different causal mechanisms for MDD may exist in women and men, resulting in similar clinical syndromes, but which may benefit from different treatment strategies.

On the microscopic level, environmental and genetic effects on targets such as the serotonin receptor are important; further understanding of these mechanisms will inform future treatments. Microscopic changes at the level of the neuron synapse are implicated in the development and treatment of a variety of disorders discussed in this chapter. Genetic predisposition and environmental factors such as chronic stress and activation of the hypothalamic-pituitary-adrenal (HPA) axis throughout development may influence a person's tendency toward depression or anxiety by exerting effects on serotonin receptor signaling pathways [15]. The CNS signaling system is further complicated by the presence of multiple different subtypes of signaling receptors.

Serotonin Receptors

Recent research has elucidated that multiple serotonin receptor subtypes exist, and signaling may result in both positive and negative effects on depressive and anxiety symptoms depending on which receptors are targeted [16]. Individuals' signaling pathways involving serotonin and norepinephrine, which affect specific CNS structural areas, are pharmacologic targets and will be discussed later in the chapter [12]. Many medications exert effects on transport within the synapse, preventing the reuptake of serotonin or norepinephrine from the synapse. As more is understood about signaling pathways, attempts are being made to more precisely target desired treatment effects or avoid side effects with medications that target specific receptor subtypes. Some of these agents, which may both exert effects as selective serotonin reuptake inhibitors (SSRIs) and agonist or antagonist effects on 5HT1A, 5HT3, and 5HT4 receptor subtypes, will be discussed [17, 18].

Beyond transporter and receptor signaling, patients' genetics can influence the metabolism of medications (e.g., through the hepatic cytochrome P450 system). Individual alleles may determine which medications are efficacious or may be prone to adverse effects for individual patients. For example, individuals with CYP2C19 alleles that result in decreased, normal, or increased metabolism of medications such as citalopram or escitalopram show differing blood levels on exposure to these medications [19]. Such differential metabolism and exposure may influence treatment response. Testing is currently available that can assess an individual's cytochrome P450 alleles and help predict a response to specific medications; however, this is not routinely available for use in primary care clinical practices at present [16]. As testing becomes less expensive and covered by insurance plans, such testing may help guide medication selection.

Gamma-Aminobutyric Acid (GABA) Receptors

Gender-specific signaling through additional pathways, such as the dopaminergic and gamma-aminobutyric acid (GABA) pathways, and hormone regulation through the HPA axis are important to consider. GABA signaling is a critical neural (typically inhibitory) signaling pathway. GABA receptor subtypes are present throughout the brain, particularly in areas known to be important in anxiety pathways: the amygdala and hippocampus, among others. Consequently, GABA receptors serve as a potential therapeutic target in the treatment of anxiety disorders [20]. The hypothalamic-pituitary-adrenal axis has traditionally been thought to play a role in anxiety symptoms, though it is variably implicated in specific disorders [21]. Glucocorticoid and mineralocorticoid receptors are present within the areas of the brain (e.g., the hippocampus) involved in anxiety, and alterations in signaling are implicated in both macro- and microstructural changes and clinical symptomatology [22].

Sex Hormone Influences in the Brain

Hormonal changes associated with reproductive health (e.g., premenstrual, perinatal/postpartum, or perimenopausal status) may have a significant impact on the emergence of depressive or anxiety symptoms through the signaling pathways mentioned. Estrogen and progesterone interact with multiple systems that may be involved in mood or anxiety symptoms [23]. On the macro scale, both the hippocampus and amygdala have estrogen and progesterone receptors, which have been shown to be associated with neuron survival pathways. Additionally, estrogen and progesterone act on several receptors, including $GABA_A$, N-methyl-D-aspartate (NMDA), serotonin, and dopamine receptors involved in mood and anxiety disorders. Times of hormonal change, such as increasing estrogen levels during puberty and relative decreasing levels in the postpartum period and in menopause, may predispose women to changes in mood and anxiety symptoms through these mechanisms. For women, changes in estrogen and progesterone can also negatively affect sleep, which may in turn influence anxiety and depressive symptoms. Changes occurring, for example, over the phases of a menstrual cycle or for women during the menopausal transition can significantly correlate with sleep changes; however, in the latter situation, this may in part be related to vasomotor symptoms as opposed to direct effects [24]. Prolactin interacts with both the HPA and dopaminergic systems; changes in levels may correlate with the emergence and remission of anxiety symptoms [22].

The Importance of Psychiatric Screening and Intervention in Primary Care

Although women are more likely to seek help for mental health problems compared with men [25], many will not seek help from mental health providers due to inadequate access, cultural beliefs about mental healthcare, and/or internalized stigma. Primary care providers may be the only point of contact between a female patient and the healthcare system; hence, it is crucial for primary care providers to gain competence in the screening, diagnosis, and intervention planning for women presenting with depressive and anxiety disorders encountered in the primary care setting.

Monica states that she has difficulty maintaining focus during the day and has no energy, leading to some recent critical feedback from her employer. She worries that her job is in jeopardy.

Differential Diagnosis

Mental health diagnoses are classified into groups of disorders. Diagnostic criteria for each disorder can be found in the *Diagnostic and Statistical Manual of Mental Disorders, Fifth Edition* (DSM-5), published by the American Psychiatric Association [26]. Depressive and bipolar disorders are considered *mood disorders*, and the diagnostic criteria are represented in distinct classification groups in the DSM-5. Anxiety disorders, which are classified as another distinct group of disorders, have high rates of co-occurrence with mood disorders. When the DSM-5 was published in 2013, several changes were made in how disorders were organized and classified. Table 33.1 provides an example of how bipolar, depressive, anxiety, and trauma-related disorders are classified within the DSM-5. Note that each group of disorders is distinct within the DSM-5, whereas bipolar and depressive disorders were grouped together within the *Diagnostic and Statistical Manual of Mental Disorder, Fourth Edition, Text Revision* (DSM-IV-TR), as were anxiety and trauma-related disorders.

Table 33.1 Classification of disorder types in DSM-IV-TR and DSM-5

Mood disorders *(DSM-IV-TR)*		Anxiety disorders *(DSM-IV-TR)*[a]	
Bipolar and related disorders *(DSM-5)*	Depressive disorders *(DSM-5)*	Anxiety disorders *(DSM-5)*	Trauma- and stressor-related disorders *(DSM-5)*
Bipolar I disorder	Major depressive disorder	Generalized anxiety disorder	Post-traumatic stress disorder
Bipolar II disorder	Persistent depressive disorder (dysthymia)	Panic disorder	Acute stress disorder
Cyclothymic disorder	Premenstrual dysphoric disorder	Agoraphobia	Adjustment disorders[b]
		Specific phobia	
		Social anxiety disorder (social phobia)	

[a]Within the DSM-IV-TR, anxiety disorders also included obsessive-compulsive disorder. The DSM-5 has a discreet obsessive-compulsive and related disorders section

[b]Adjustment disorders were described within a distinct section of disorders within the DSM-IV-TR, separate from anxiety disorders

Table 33.2 Diagnostic criteria for major depressive disorder and persistent depressive disorder (dysthymia)

Major depressive disorder	Both disorders	Persistent depressive disorder (dysthymia)
Presence of five or more total symptoms	Symptoms must include *depressed mood* and/or *anhedonia (loss of interest or pleasure in most activities)*	Presence of three or more total symptoms
Symptoms must be present for *2 weeks* or more		Symptoms must be present for *2 years* or more
Additional symptoms may include: Psychomotor slowing or agitation Recurrent thoughts of death or suicidality	Additional symptoms may include: Too much or too little sleep Significant changes in appetite or weight Fatigue or low energy Difficulties concentrating or making decisions Low self-esteem or feelings of worthlessness	Additional symptoms may include: Feelings of hopelessness
	No history of a manic or hypomanic episode	

Full copyrighted criteria are available from the American Psychiatric Association [26]. All of the criteria are required for the diagnosis of major depressive disorder or persistent depressive disorder. The table text summarizes the diagnostic criteria

Based on initial report, it appears that the patient in our case study may be presenting with symptoms of a depressive and/or anxiety disorder, assuming that medical conditions which might contribute to her symptoms have been excluded.

Depressive Disorders

Table 33.2 outlines the diagnostic criteria for two common depressive disorders: major depressive disorder (MDD) and persistent depressive disorder (dysthymia or PDD). Each of these disorders is primarily characterized by low mood and/or anhedonia (decreased interest or pleasure in activities previously enjoyed) [26]. Note the overlap in symptoms between these two diagnoses. The primary differences between the disorders are in *length of time* and *severity*. Major depressive disorder can be diagnosed in a patient experiencing the requisite symptoms for an episode spanning 2 weeks or more; persistent depressive disorder, on the other hand, can only be diagnosed when symptoms have been present for at least 2 years. Additionally, the symptoms of MDD are more likely to be acute and severe in nature compared with PDD. Patients may describe PDD as a "cloud that's been hanging overhead for years," whereas MDD may be characterized by distinct "low" periods of time or shorter duration. MDD will often go into remission after 6 months to a year. PDD tends to be more chronic and can be difficult to treat.

Gender differences may exist in the way depressive disorders present. Compared with men, women may be likely to report an increased appetite, tearfulness, fatigue, and sleep disturbances [27]. Historically, women have been thought to present with more somatic symptoms of depression as opposed to the "pure" mood symptoms seen in men [27]. However, the research is mixed regarding whether these differences are related to a gendered interpretation of symptoms or biological differences [27]; of note, the American Psychiatric Association has not reported any clear differences between men and women in symptom presentation or treatment response [26].

Premenstrual Dysphoric Disorder

A diagnosis of premenstrual dysphoric disorder (PMDD) may be considered when depressive and anxiety symptoms are present and interfering with daily functioning. PMDD is a severe form of premenstrual syndrome (PMS) that interferes with daily functioning. PMDD is characterized by a marked increase in mood dysregulation or subjective affective distress, during the luteal phase of the menstrual cycle, days 14–28. Symptoms begin 1–2 weeks preceding the start of menstruation and typically subside within a few days after menstruation begins. Common symptoms include changes in sleep and/or appetite, irritability, tension, and difficulty concentrating [26, 28]. Women with PMDD do not appear to have differing levels of hormones relative to women without PMDD; rather, it is hypothesized that individual differences in the $GABA_A$ receptor subunits may confer differing levels of sensitivity toward the natural hormone fluctuations of a woman's menstrual cycle, resulting in symptoms [23, 29].

Anxiety and Panic Disorders

Stress and sleeplessness may suggest the presence of an anxiety disorder. Anxiety and depressive disorders can occur separately, though many patients will meet criteria for both. The most common anxiety disorder is generalized anxiety disorder (GAD), which is characterized by excessive and uncontrollable worries that interfere with daily functioning [26]. GAD may or may not include the presence of panic attacks, which are acute episodes of intense anxiety accompanied by distressing physical symptoms. When panic attacks are the primary manifestation of anxiety (without ongoing excessive worried thoughts), and efforts to decrease the likelihood of these attacks is interfering with daily life, a diagnosis of panic disorder may be appropriate. Anxiety disorders are common in women, and research is ongoing to determine specific underlying mechanisms which can inform therapeutic management. As previously discussed, neuroendocrine signaling can be affected by both estrogen and progesterone, and these hormones' interactions at the level of the $GABA_A$ receptor and with the HPA axis may be responsible in part for differential presentations between women and men [22] (Table 33.3).

When asked for more information about her sleep habits, Monica reveals that when she goes to bed, she "can't turn [her] brain off." Despite her lack of sleep, Monica describes feeling "keyed up" and restless throughout the day, and she is unable to wind down and relax at home.

Table 33.3 Diagnostic criteria for generalized anxiety disorder and panic disorder

Generalized anxiety disorder	Panic disorder
Excessive worried thoughts or subjective feelings of anxiety, which are difficult to control	The presence of multiple unexpected panic attacks, characterized by sudden discomfort or fear
Additional symptoms may include: Feeling restless or "on edge" Difficulty concentrating Muscle tension Irritability Being easily fatigued Disturbed or decreased sleep	Additional symptoms may include: Increased heart rate and/or chest pain Sweating Shaking or trembling Shortness of breath Dizziness or light-headedness Nausea or abdominal discomfort
Symptoms are present for 6 months or longer	At least one of the below is present for 1 month or longer following the panic attack(s): Intense worry about future panic attacks Disruptive behavior changes in an effort to avoid future panic attacks

Full copyrighted criteria are available from the American Psychiatric Association [26]. All of the criteria are required for the diagnosis of generalized anxiety disorder or panic disorder. The table text summarizes the diagnostic criteria

Bipolar Disorder and Post-Traumatic Stress Disorder

Changes in mood or increased anxious distress have a broad range of differential diagnoses to consider, including medical conditions (thyroid disorders, cardiac disease, and respiratory distress), substance use disorders, and two important psychiatric conditions: bipolar disorder and post-traumatic stress disorder. The evaluation and ruling out of medical conditions associated with the common symptoms of depressive and anxiety disorders is beyond the scope of this chapter.

Bipolar Disorder

Patients should be screened for any history of a *manic* or *hypomanic episode*, which would suggest a diagnosis of bipolar disorder. Manic and hypomanic episodes are mood episodes that present with abnormal and marked increases in energy or mood, along with other symptoms associated with heightened arousal (e.g., decreased sleep or appetite, racing thoughts, rapid speech) [26]. Mania may also be manifest as excessive irritability. A patient cannot be diagnosed with a primary depressive disorder if she has ever experienced manic/hypomanic episodes. Many patients with bipolar disorder will experience depressive episodes in addition to manic/hypomanic episodes within the course of the illness.

The differentiation between bipolar disorder and a depressive disorder has important implications for treatment. Some medications that are used to treat depressive symptoms, such as selective serotonin reuptake inhibitors (SSRIs, described below), can potentially induce a manic/hypomanic episode. This is an uncommon occurrence, though women with a family history of bipolar disorder may be at particular risk [30]. Additionally, depressive episodes occurring within the context of bipolar disorder can require more complex medication management, such as mood stabilizers or adjunctive pharmacotherapy as compared to PMDD. Patients reporting symptoms of bipolar disorder should be referred for a psychiatric consultation.

Post-Traumatic Stress Disorder

Patients presenting with mood or anxiety symptoms should also be screened for a history of trauma. Depending on the course and characterization of psychiatric symptoms following a traumatic event, a diagnosis of post-traumatic stress disorder (PTSD) may be most appropriate. PTSD, which is often comorbid with mood and/or anxiety disorders, is a syndrome that occurs when symptoms persist following a traumatic event that interferes with a patient's everyday life [26].

Symptoms of PTSD fall into four clusters:

- Re-experiencing the traumatic event through nightmares, flashbacks, or intrusive memories
- Avoiding reminders of the traumatic event through suppressing memories or avoiding places or people that trigger memories of the trauma
- Hyperarousal as manifested by increased startle response, decreased anger threshold, or engagement in reckless or impulsive behaviors
- Negative changes in mood or affect, including feelings of worthlessness, low mood, and affective numbness

Chronic exposure to stress also places women at risk, but a thorough discussion of this topic is beyond the scope of this chapter.

Monica clarifies that she has never experienced an abnormal elevation in her mood or energy level. She reports that she was sexually assaulted at a party in college. She denies any intrusive thoughts or memories of the event and has not avoided any memories or other reminders of the assault.

Clinical Interviewing

Effective diagnostic interviewing uses a patient-centered approach with open and readily understood language that emphasizes a balanced dynamic in verbal exchange between provider and patient. Patient-centered interviewing maximizes patient satisfaction [31] and is distinct from a more traditional, top-down interview. Patient-centered interviewing incorporates open-ended questioning (e.g., "Which concerns would you like to address today?") along with more focused and reflective inquiries (e.g., "Tell me more about feeling like you can't get anything done these days"). It is helpful to practice using language that the patient can relate to, rather than using clinical jargon. Important information to gather includes the following:

- Time course of symptoms/episodes:
  - "When did you first start to notice (changes in) ________? How long have you been experiencing ________?"
- Diagnostic criteria that may not immediately be reported:
  - "Tell me about your sleep and appetite."
  - "You mentioned having panic attacks. How would you describe them? What are some of the changes that happen during the attacks?"
- Interfering with daily functioning:
  - "It sounds like this has been pretty distressing for you. Has it gotten in the way of your ability to live your life the way you were before?"

Screening Tools for Depression and Anxiety

In addition to clinical inquiry, symptom screening measures are helpful in gathering information about a patient's symptoms. These tools are useful both in the diagnosis of depressive and anxiety disorders and in documenting response to treatment. One of the most commonly used measures to assess depressive symptoms is the Patient Health Questionnaire-9 (PHQ-9). The PHQ-9 is a validated screening tool consisting of nine Likert-scale items corresponding with each of the DSM-5 diagnostic criteria for a major depressive episode [32, 33]. It is publicly available and widely used in primary care settings. Scores range from 0 to 27, with higher scores indicating a greater severity in depressive symptoms. To diagnose a depressive disorder, one of the first two items, anhedonia or depressed mood, must be endorsed by the patient. In the absence of anhedonia or depressed mood, the PHQ-9 can indicate the presence of other important symptoms to address, such as changes in appetite, sleep, energy, or concentration (Fig. 33.1).

Similar to the PHQ-9, the GAD-7 is a seven-item anxiety symptom screening measure whose items represent each of the diagnostic criteria for generalized anxiety disorder [33]. Higher scores signify increased severity of anxiety symptoms.

Utilizing these screening measures represents an important opportunity for preventive care. The PHQ-9 and GAD-7 allow providers to gather invaluable data about acute depressive or anxiety symptoms that patients may not choose to self-report during a clinical interview. Endorsement of key items, especially related to low mood, anhedonia, difficulty controlling worried thoughts, and suicidal ideation, can help providers initiate a dialogue about psychiatric distress and possibilities for early intervention. Open dialogue will help patients gain awareness about mood and anxiety symptoms, decrease stigma toward discussing mental health concerns, and potentially prevent exacerbations of distress and associated impairment in patients.

Fig. 33.1 Patient Health Questionnaire-9 (PHQ-9) [32]. (Developed by Drs. Robert L. Spitzer, Janet B.W. Williams, Kurt Kroenke, and colleagues, with an educational grant from Pfizer, Inc)

PATIENT HEALTH QUESTIONNAIRE-9 (PHQ-9)

Over the last 2 weeks, how often have you been bothered by any of the following problems? *(Use "✓" to indicate your answer)*	**Not at all**	**Several days**	**More than half the days**	**Nearly every day**
1. Little interest or pleasure in doing things	0	1	2	3
2. Feeling down, depressed, or hopeless	0	1	2	3
3. Trouble falling or staying asleep, or sleeping too much	0	1	2	3
4. Feeling tired or having little energy	0	1	2	3
5. Poor appetite or overeating	0	1	2	3
6. Feeling bad about yourself—or that you are a failure or have let yourself or your family down	0	1	2	3
7. Trouble concentrating on things, such as reading the newspaper or watching television	0	1	2	3
8. Moving or speaking so slowly that other people could have noticed? Or the opposite—being so fidgety or restless that you have been moving around a lot more than usual	0	1	2	3
9. Thoughts that you would be better off dead or of hurting yourself in some way	0	1	2	3

FOR OFFICE CODING _0_ + ____ + ____ + ____

=Total Score: ____

If you checked off any problems, how difficult have these problems made it for you to do your work, take care of things at home, or get along with other people?

Not difficult at all	Somewhat difficult	Very difficult	Extremely difficult
☐	☐	☐	☐

Monica reports that she has had previous depressive episodes, but none as lengthy and severe as this one. She notes that her current episode began about 18 months ago. Her PHQ-9 score is consistent with moderate depression and her GAD-7 score is consistent with moderate anxiety.

Biopsychosocial Risk Factors

In the treatment of depressive and anxiety disorders, information should be gathered regarding risk factors and life circumstances: psychosocial stressors (recent and chronic), genetic predispositions, health-related behaviors, and access to resources. Contextual factors can impact diagnosis, prognosis, and treatment. A trained medical social worker or mental health provider typically performs assessments in these domains. A therapeutic multidisciplinary team will provide the best comprehensive care for patients. In the biopsychosocial model of care, providers gather data within biological/genetic/medical, psychological/psychiatric, and social/systemic/political influences on a patient's lived experience and overall functioning.

Substance Use

Health-related behavior such as substance use can influence the onset or course of psychiatric symptoms. Substance use disorders often occur in conjunction with psychiatric disorders and can have a cyclical relationship with one another; a patient may self-medicate a mood or anxiety disorder with various substances, and heavy substance use may result in chemical and behavioral changes leading to a mood or anxiety disorder. Because substance use can be highly stigmatized, assessment should be conducted in an open and nonjudgmental way. Examples include the following:

- "Tell me a bit your alcohol and drug use."
- "How often do you drink?" (This is counter to an inquiry such as "Do you drink? If so, how much?")

A family history of psychiatric illness or substance use should also be assessed. Genetic and environmental factors may predispose a patient to psychiatric illness and/or problematic substance use in adulthood, and thus an understanding of the family history is critical for context. Bipolar disorder and substance use disorders are strongly influenced by genetic factors.

Chronic Pain

The presence of chronic or recurrent pain symptoms may serve as a significant contributor to the development or maintenance of psychiatric symptoms. Mood and anxiety symptoms are common among patients who are living with chronic pain [34]. Patients with comorbid chronic pain, depression, and anxiety may have higher levels of pain intensity and lower quality of life than patients with chronic pain but without co-occurring psychiatric distress. Effective treatment planning for these patients necessitates an integration of interventions addressing pain as well as psychiatric symptoms. Thoughtful treatment planning should incorporate assessing risk for medication misuse or addiction, and the selection of therapies should be determined accordingly in collaboration with patients (see Chap. 26 on General Approach to Chronic Pain and Chap. 32 on Opioid Use Disorder).

Stressors

Providers should ask about any salient stressors or other significant life events that may have impacted the onset or exacerbation of psychiatric symptoms. Research suggests that women may be particularly susceptible to depressive or anxiety symptoms in response to stressful events [35]. Depending on the stressor in question, making changes in a patient's environment or other adjustment behavior may obviate the need for pharmacologic treatment or greatly speed recovery when used in conjunction with pharmacologic or psychotherapeutic interventions. A provider might use inquiries such as:

- "You mentioned that these symptoms started about 18 months ago. What else was happening in your life around that time?"
- "Thinking back, can you identify any event or major change that may have impacted your mood or levels of anxiety?"

Due to sociocultural expectations and constraints, women often face a unique and complex intersection of stressors. These may include workplace stress, unhealthy or unhappy romantic relationships, or perceived expectations to "have it all" within professional and family domains. Women may find themselves in a "sandwich generation," wherein family obligations include simultaneously caring for children as well as aging parents. Social isolation, poverty, immigration-related concerns, and discrimination are other common and highly impactful stressors that many women navigate.

When asked about recent events that may be affecting her life, Monica reports that she was unfairly fired from her job shortly before her current symptoms emerged. She described feeling betrayed by her employer and socially isolated, since much of her interpersonal interaction occurred within the context of employment. Though she has since started another job, she continues to feel down and detached at work.

Traumatic Events in Childhood or Adult Life

As noted earlier in this chapter, the primary precipitating factor contributing to a patient's psychiatric symptoms may be a major traumatic event. Exposure to trauma occurs at high lifetime rates and has a marked impact on an individual's overall functioning. The ACE (Adverse Childhood Experiences) Study, conducted by the CDC and Kaiser Permanente [36], examined the impact of childhood trauma on a variety of health-related outcomes in adulthood. ACE trauma categories include (but are not limited to) physical abuse, sexual abuse, neglect, intimate partner violence, household substance misuse, and incarceration of family members. The study found that 64% of study participants endorsed at least one trauma category during childhood, and one in six participants endorsed exposure to at least four trauma categories. Women were found to be 50% more likely than men to have experienced at least six types of trauma during childhood; this disproportionate exposure to trauma often continues during adulthood, as one in three women experience lifetime intimate partner violence (see Chap. 35 on Intimate Partner Violence and Sexual Trauma) [37]. Trauma exposure has a dose-response relationship, and a history of trauma can negatively impact many areas of functioning. Childhood and adulthood trauma are correlated with multiple poor health outcomes, including increased rates of lung and liver disease, alcoholism, intravenous drug use, depression, chronic pain syndrome, and suicide attempts [36, 38].

Trauma Informed Care

Increasing attention is being given to the cultivation of *trauma-informed primary care*, which highlights the awareness of and responsiveness to the ways in which traumatic experiences can affect a patient's engagement in healthcare and ability to effectively participate in other life domains [39]. Figure 33.2 outlines several key aspects of trauma-informed primary care practices. Despite the high rates at which patients are exposed to trauma and the significant impact it has on functioning, most primary care providers do not routinely screen for histories of abuse [40].

Given the salient influence of trauma exposure on healthcare outcomes, providers should consider whether trauma may be a driving force behind the onset of psychiatric symptoms, even if these symptoms do not indicate the presence of post-traumatic stress disorder. Patients should be asked about current, recent, and childhood traumas. It may be helpful to contextualize the importance of asking about these experiences, highlighting the standardization of such inquiry (e.g., "This is something we ask every patient"). Examples of trauma screening questions include the following:

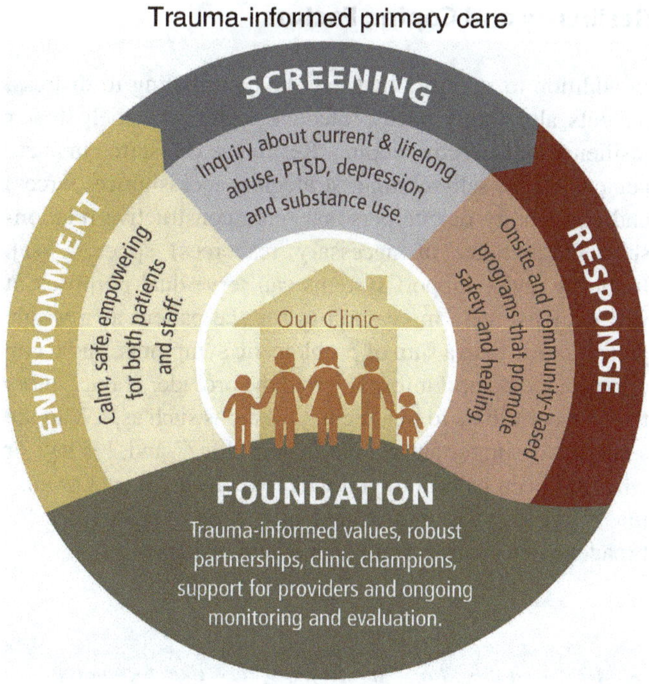

Fig. 33.2 Core elements of the trauma-informed primary care framework [39]. (Reprinted from Women's Health Issues, Machtinger et al. [39], © 2015, with permission from Elsevier)

- "What happens when you and your partner fight? Does your partner ever hit, kick, slap, or push you?"
- "Were you exposed to any violence during childhood?"
- "Have you experienced unwanted sexual attention or sexual contact?"

A patient may not want to discuss past traumatic events or provide many details, and it is important for patients to be able to retain control over their own historical information. Maintaining a trauma-informed approach includes an awareness of the possibility of retraumatizing a patient by pressuring her to disclose more information than is necessary or comfortable. If the patient has a negative reaction to questioning, it may be sufficient to understand that she continues to be impacted by past traumas and allow her to share more information at another time. In the meantime, providers can promote recovery by fostering a safe and responsive clinical environment, including possible referrals for mental health or social services (see Chap. 35 on Intimate Partner Violence and Sexual Trauma).

Resiliency and Coping Factors

In addition to stressors that may be contributing to distress, patients also likely have protective factors that help foster resilience and effective coping. Resilience is fostered in intrapersonal (e.g., self-soothing strategies, accessing resources) and community or interpersonal (e.g., constructive relationships, availability of necessary resources) spheres [41]. Inquiring about support systems can serve dual purposes; it will demonstrate a motivation to see the patient as a whole person rather than a sum of problematic symptoms, and it can also provide helpful information to the provider about factors that can contribute to treatment. Questions such as, "Who are some of the important people in your life?" and, "What, or who, has been helpful to you when you have felt sad or anxious?" are non-assumptive and may open opportunities for broader discussions around coping and resilience.

Monica notes that "it all just feels like too much" sometimes, and she occasionally wonders whether it would easier if she just "weren't here."

Suicide Risk Assessment

Women have significantly higher rates of suicide attempts, though lower rates of dying by suicide, compared with men [26, 42]. Suicide risk assessments are vital within the broader practice of addressing psychiatric distress within any healthcare setting. Conducting a suicide risk assessment can evoke anxiety for many clinicians. Cultivating an understanding of the components of these assessments, along with how to interpret and respond to patients' reports, will help clinicians gain competence and confidence with suicide risk assessment. It is important to remember that *asking about suicide will not make somebody suicidal*, and in fact such inquiry may help mitigate distress associated with suicidal ideation [43]. Generally, the primary components within a comprehensive suicide risk assessment are risk and protective factors, current ideation, plan, means, and intent.

Suicide Risk

The greatest predictor of suicide risk behavior is a history of suicide attempts [44]. Suicide risk assessment should incorporate inquiries about past suicidal ideation (SI) and related behaviors in addition to those occurring in the present. When discussing past risk behaviors, ask about frequency, duration, intensity, outcome, and strategies used to mitigate or stop suicidal or other self-harm behavior.

Protective Factors

Protective factors against suicide are important to include within a risk assessment. These might be treatment-related protective factors, such as displayed hope or motivation to improve symptoms by seeking help. Protective factors are also represented through important roles or relationships (e.g., importance of being a mother, involvement in supportive relationships). Patients experiencing symptoms such as hopelessness may have difficulty identifying these protective factors, which can indicate elevated risk.

Suicidal Ideation

The first step within a present-focused suicide risk assessment is determining the *presence* and *type* of suicidal ideation. *Passive* SI describes a desire to die without a conceived plan. This can manifest as a desire to "disappear" or statements such as, "It wouldn't be so bad if I just didn't wake up one day." *Active* SI refers to a desire to die along with a plan of how a patient might pursue this (e.g., "I think about jumping off a bridge," or, "I've thought about overdosing on my prescription meds"). Inquiring about suicidal ideation is most effective when done in a nonjudgmental and straightforward way. Examples include the following:

- "Sometimes, when people are feeling down, they may have thoughts about dying or about doing something to end their life. Is this something you have experienced?"
- "Have you ever had thoughts of suicide or of doing something to end your life?"

If a patient endorses passive and/or active suicidal ideation, the provider should assess the intensity and frequency of these thoughts. Strategies used to navigate SI can also be assessed. The provider might ask, "What do you do when you have these thoughts of suicide?" Such questions can reveal adaptive coping mechanisms and/or protective factors against self-harm.

Plan and Means to Implement the Plan

The next component of assessing suicide risk is determining the presence of a *plan* and the *means* to implement it. A patient may reveal some of this information while describing any active suicidal ideation, but further probing may be required to elicit additional specific elements to any plan(s) in place. A patient's plan(s) may cover a wide range of access and feasibility; this also needs to be assessed. For example, if a patient states that she imagines ending her life by a self-inflicted gunshot wound, she should be asked whether she owns or has access to a firearm. Described plans may have different levels of specificity. For instance, a patient who reports thinking about jumping off a bridge may or may not have a particular bridge in mind. Patients should also be asked about timelines or dates associated with any plans, in addition to preparatory behaviors she may be engaging in to carry out the plan.

Intent

Finally, *intent* needs to be evaluated by a provider conducting a suicide risk assessment. Determining the level of intent includes (a) asking about whether the patient anticipates implementing any plans she has made to end her life or seriously harm herself and (b) exploring how lethal or harmful a patient believes her plan(s) to be. Here, providers have a key opportunity to identify any ambivalence expressed by a patient. For example, these discussions may include explorations of reasons to live versus reasons to end one's life.

Involuntary Hospitalization

For patients who are exhibiting suicidal ideation or intent, the actions taken by a treatment team are determined by the level of risk. Patients who are deemed to be at imminent risk for suicide or serious self-harm may be voluntarily or involuntarily hospitalized. Regulations pertaining to the implementation and lengths of stay of involuntary hospitalizations vary by state.

Patients may be concerned about what will happen during or after involuntary hospitalization. Generally, involuntary holds will last for several days. These hospitalizations are intended to reduce risk of imminent harm, and they ensure that a patient is evaluated by a psychiatrist and linked to necessary treatment to further mitigate risk. Depending on the acuity and severity of a patient's symptoms, there are several possible outcomes following an involuntary hold. These include an extension of involuntary commitment via a court order, inpatient psychiatric treatment, intensive outpatient programming, and outpatient treatment. Each of these outcomes may involve medication management with a psychiatrist as well as psychotherapy.

Voluntary Hospitalization or Urgent Psychiatric Referral and Safety Planning

Patients who do not warrant involuntary hospitalization may be offered voluntary hospitalization and/or an urgent psychiatry referral. If suicidal ideation is still present with a plan and means, but risk is not imminent, safety planning is an appropriate course of action. Safety plans are completed in collaboration with a patient and are ideally written down for the patient to keep with her. Drafted safety plans may include (a) reaching out for support through calling a crisis hotline or contacting someone in the patient's life, (b) engaging in constructive self-soothing or distracting activities, (c) engaging in ongoing mental health treatment, and/or (d) restricting any access to available means (e.g., keeping a firearm locked in a safe and giving someone else the key, having a friend or family member maintain possession of medications).

Treatment

Monica is told she may be experiencing a depressive disorder with concomitant anxiety. There is no evidence of a prior manic episode, and bipolar disorder has been ruled out as a possible diagnosis. She agrees and asks about available treatments.

Most patients who seek treatment for disorders such as depression and anxiety seek care through their primary care provider [45], and it is therefore essential for providers to understand the range of treatment modalities available to patients. Treatments range from psychotherapy, to medication management, to complementary and alternative treatments. Unfortunately, over a third of patients with major depressive disorder receive no treatment, likely due to the lack of identification of symptoms, further highlighting the need for screening in the primary care setting [46]. A large proportion of patients receives dual treatment with medication management and psychotherapy (44%), while a smaller proportion receives only therapy or medication (13% and 6%, respectively) [46]. Though it is difficult to quantify how many patients use complementary and alternative medicine (CAM) treatments for anxiety and depression specifically, over a third of adults use CAM annually for treatment of issues such as pain, mood, or other symptoms [47].

Lifestyle Behavior Modifications

Mood and anxiety symptoms often present alongside sleep disturbances, changes in diet or weight, and decreases in physical activity. Screening for mood and anxiety symptoms should include assessing these vital lifestyle factors. Psychiatric symptoms and health-related behaviors often show a bidirectional relationship [48]. Making lifestyle changes in sleep, diet, and exercise can be an efficient and effective intervention to implement, with the potential for positive outcomes, which are further maximized by ongoing support, adjunct psychoeducation, or behavioral interventions [49, 50]. Sleep hygiene techniques, including consistent sleep-wake schedules, can be remarkably helpful in reducing the intensity of mood dysregulation or anxiety symptoms [51]. Maintaining a balanced and nutritious diet and engaging in regular physical activity can be particularly valuable aspects of a patient's treatment plan. Physical activity has been shown to improve anxiety and depressive symptoms and may be particularly beneficial for those not interested trying medication or psychotherapy [52, 53]. Modalities such as yoga and mindfulness meditation may also be effective in mitigating depressive or anxious distress [54, 55]. These lifestyle changes are cost-effective and sustainable strategies to integrate into an overall mental health wellness plan.

Medication Management

A variety of pharmacologic treatments are available for the treatment of depressive and anxiety symptoms in the primary care setting, depicted in Table 33.4. Of note, the medical treatment of bipolar disorder includes mood stabilizers and atypical antipsychotics; a thorough discussion of these medications is beyond the scope of this chapter. When a provider and patient have determined that a medication will be used in a patient's treatment plan for depression or anxiety, second-generation antidepressants including SSRIs and SNRIs are considered first line [56]. Choosing which medication to prescribe requires knowledge of the patient's current symptoms, the patient's medical and psychiatric history, the patient's family history, and a working knowledge of medication indications, costs, and potential side effects [57].

Patient's History and Family History

The initial step in determining an appropriate medication for the patient is a careful consideration of the patient's presenting history to ensure that symptoms are consistent with the diagnosis being considered. Prescribed medications should be appropriate for the patient's diagnosis: depression, anxiety, or both. If a primary care provider is unsure about a diagnosis, additional consultation with a psychiatric professional should be obtained prior to considering medication management. Caution should be used with patients who exhibit hypomanic or manic symptoms, which can at times be difficult to differentiate from symptoms of anxiety. As noted throughout this chapter, patients whose symptoms suggest bipolar I or bipolar II disorder will usually require consultation with a psychiatrist. Care should be taken to exclude other diagnoses which may mimic depression or anxiety symptoms, such as thyroid disorders, cardiac disease (e.g., a patient with arrhythmia may present with palpitations), or respiratory diseases such as asthma [58]. Hazardous substance use can also co-occur or mimic these disorders; primary care providers should screen for substance misuse as part of the ongoing evaluation [58, 59].

Evidence is minimal as to whether a patient will respond better to a medication they have used successfully in the past as opposed to another treatment [60]. For patients who are medication naïve, but who may have family members who have been treated with medication for depression, there is face validity to the idea that starting the same or a similar agent may have a higher likelihood of response; however, the literature supporting this is sparse. Some studies have attempted to elucidate whether genetic variations in receptors can predict responses to different medications, but without clear conclusions currently to guide clinical management [60, 61]. Regardless of patient and provider choice, many patients will respond to either a previously used medication or a new medication within the same class, so either may be considered appropriate [57]. If a patient has a bias for or against a medication based on their own, a friend's, or a family member's use and recommendation, a provider should consider this preference through shared decision-making. If a patient has a preconceived prejudice or preference against a medication, in most cases it is unnecessary to push for this medication if other options are available.

Table 33.4 Medications for management of depression and anxiety

Medication class	Indication	Mechanism of action	Class-level side effects/ cautions	Medications within class	Dosage options	Compelling indications	Medication-specific side effects/ cautions
Selective serotonin reuptake inhibitors (SSRI)	Anxiety Depression	Inhibit serotonin reuptake at the synaptic level	GI upset, nausea, vomiting, sexual dysfunction	Citalopram	10 mg 20 mg 40 mg		QTc prolongation especially at high doses and with polypharmacy[a]
				Escitalopram	5 mg 10 mg 20 mg		QTc prolongation especially at high doses and with polypharmacy[a]
				Fluoxetine	10 mg 20 mg 30 mg 40 mg 10 mg/5 ml solution 90 mg (weekly)	OCD Eating Disorders PMDD	Drug interactions: Decreases tamoxifen levels with concomitant use
				Fluvoxamine	25 mg 50 mg 100 mg 150 mg	OCD	Off label for treatment of depression/ anxiety
				Paroxetine	10 mg 20 mg 30 mg 40 mg	OCD PMDD PTSD	Weight gain, daytime somnolence Drug interactions: Decreases tamoxifen levels with concomitant use Contraindicated in pregnancy
				Sertraline	25 mg 50 mg 100 mg 20 mg/1 ml solution	OCD PMDD	
Serotonin partial agonist-reuptake inhibitor (SPARI) and related medications	Depression	Inhibit serotonin reuptake and serotonin receptor modulation	GI upset, nausea, vomiting, low risk for sexual side effects	Vilazodone	10 mg 20 mg 40 mg		
				Vorioxetine	5 mg 10 mg 20 mg		
Serotonin norephinephine reuptake inhibitors (SNRIs)	Anxiety Depression	Inhibit serotonin and norepinephrine reuptake	GI upset, nausea, vomiting, sexual dysfunction	Duloxetine	20 mg 30 mg 40 mg 60 mg	Diabetic nerve pain Fibromyalgia ADHD (possibly)	
				Desvenlafaxine	25 mg 50 mg 100 mg	Major depressive disorder only	
				Levomilnacipran	20 mg 40 mg 80 mg 120 mg	Major depressive disorder only	
				Milnacipran	12.5 mg 25 mg 50 mg 100 mg	Fibromyalgia, depression indication outside of the United States	
				Venlafaxine	37.5 mg 75 mg 150 mg 225 mg	Diabetic Neuropathy Hot flashes ADHD	Safest choice with tamoxifen

(continued)

Table 33.4 (continued)

Medication class	Indication	Mechanism of action	Class-level side effects/ cautions	Medications within class	Dosage options	Compelling indications	Medication-specific side effects/ cautions
Dopamine-norephinephrine reuptake inhibitors	Depression	Prevents dopamine and norepinephrine reuptake at the synaptic level	Lower seizure threshold	Bupropion	75 mg 100 mg 150 mg 200 mg 300 mg 450 mg	Smoking Cessation Low Risk of sexual side effects Off label for weight loss (combination medication)	Do not use in patients with seizure disorder, substance abuse, or eating disorders Decreases tamoxifen levels with concomitant use
Benzodiazepines	Anxiety	GABA agonist	Sedation effects, risk for misuse and addiction	Alprazolam	0.25 mg 0.5 mg 1 mg 2 mg 3 mg 1 mg/ 1 ml solution		Rebound anxiety and potential for misuse, given short half-life
				Clonazepam	0.125 mg 0.25 mg 0.5 mg 1 mg 2 mg	Rapid dissolving available for panic disorder Seizure disorder management	
				Diazepam	2 mg 5 mg 10 mg 5 mg/ 1 ml	Acute seizure treatment Procedural sedation	
				Lorazepam	0.5 mg 1 mg 2 mg 2 mg/ 1 ml solution	Use possible in patients with renal or hepatic impairment	
				Temazepam	7.5 mg 15 mg 22.5 mg 30 mg	Insomnia	
Tetracyclic antidepressants	Depression	Serotonin and norepinephrine reuptake inhibition	Weight gain, sedation	Mirtazapine	7.5 mg 15 mg 30 mg 45 mg		Used in insomnia
Tricyclic antidepressants (TCAs)	Pain, migraines, IBS, no longer used for depression	Serotonin and norepinephrine reuptake inhibition	GI upset, constipation, sedation, overdose may cause fatal cardiac arrythmias	Amitriptyline	10 mg 25 mg 50 mg 75 mg 100 mg 150 mg	Migraine Prophylaxis Irritable bowel syndrome Chronic pain	Dosages above 50 mg are rarely used
				Nortriptyline	10 mg 25 mg 50 mg 75 mg 10 mg / 5 ml solution		Dosages above 50 mg are rarely used

Abbreviations: *NE* norepinephrine, *D* depressive disorders, *A* anxiety disorders

[a]Risk factors for QTc prolongation include female sex, age over 65, high dosages of antidepressant medication, electrolyte disturbances, cardiac or other medical comorbidities, history of QTc prolongation, family history of QTc prolongation, and polypharmacy (see text)

Medication Cost and Generic Drug Availability

Cost is important at both the patient and the health systems level. The American College of Preventive Medicine issued the recommendation to use generic equivalents to expensive brand names when available as part of the Choosing Wisely initiative, estimating the average cost of generic medications to be 80–85% lower than brand name medications [62]. Fortunately, SSRIs, which are first line and have been used for over 20 years, are inexpensive, and generic versions are widely available.

Compelling Indications

Indications and major side effect profiles are highlighted in the following sections and summarized in Table 33.4. Patients may have compelling indications for a given medication, as certain classes may have approvals or be used off label for other diagnoses. Other patients may wish to avoid certain side effects that will guide choice of medication.

Major Classes of Medication

Selective Serotonin Reuptake Inhibitors (SSRIs)

SSRIs have been used in clinical practice for over two decades, and numerous clinical trials have been conducted to guide providers and patients on their efficacy and side effects [63]. SSRIs act at the level of the synapse, inhibiting serotonin reuptake and thereby permitting increased serotonin action. There is significant evidence that SSRIs improve depressive and anxiety symptoms compared to placebo; however, there is no evidence of significant efficacy differences among medications in the class. Side effects and tolerability may differ among medications and therefore are used to guide providers and patients in the choice of initial drug therapy [64, 65]. Individual medications within this class, listed alphabetically, are discussed in detail below.

Citalopram Citalopram is an excellent first line medication for patients with depression, especially when there is significant co-occurring anxiety. It is also effective to treat anxiety alone. Typical doses range between 20 mg and 40 mg, though 10 mg dosage forms are available for slower titration if desired. Citalopram is well tolerated in most patients, is relatively safe in pregnancy, and can be used in patients taking tamoxifen for breast cancer prevention or treatment (see Chap. 17 on The Primary Prevention of Breast Cancer and Chap. 19 on Breast Cancer Diagnosis and Management). When treating anxiety, patients may be offered lorazepam to be used for the first few days to counteract the temporary jitteriness or increased anxiety which may occur at the initiation of citalopram and other SSRIs. As many as 50% of patients may experience unwanted sexual side effects, especially delayed orgasm and lack of libido, when taking citalopram. Adding bupropion to citalopram can help mitigate sexual side effects in many patients.

Citalopram has a greater tendency for QTc prolongation than other SSRIs, and thus an EKG should be performed before the medication is prescribed and after significant increases in dose. Risk factors for QTc prolongation include female sex, age over 65, electrolyte disturbances, a history of any cardiac abnormality, polypharmacy, and higher doses of antidepressants [66]. It is unclear whether patient risk factors such as CYP metabolism place patients at risk or whether this risk is intrinsic to the medication itself, but caution should be used in patients who (1) already have QTc prolongation or (2) are on other QTc prolonging medications [67, 68]. Daily dosages of citalopram of 40 mg or more pose higher risk and should be used with caution.

Escitalopram Escitalopram is the S-enantiomer of citalopram (which is a racemic mix of the L and S enantiomers), and the typical dose range is between 10 mg and 20 mg. It has similar roles in treatment of depression and anxiety and shares the same cautions for QTc prolongation and sexual side effects [69] as citalopram.

Fluoxetine Fluoxetine has stood the test of time as one of the premier first line medications to treat depression and anxiety. Fluoxetine was the first SSRI to be introduced in the United States and among the first in the world when it was developed in the 1970s and approved in 1987 [70]. It has been studied extensively and carries approvals not only for anxiety and depressive disorders, but also for PMDD, obsessive compulsive disorder (OCD), and eating disorders [71]. Fluoxetine may have a stimulating effect and, in some patients, may help promote weight loss. Fluoxetine is relatively safe in pregnancy. Caution should be used in women on tamoxifen treatment, as fluoxetine may decrease tamoxifen levels, although it is safe with raloxifene and aromatase inhibitors (see Chaps. 16, 17, 18, 19, and 20 in the Breast Health and Disease section of this book). Daily dosage forms range from 10 mg to 40 mg, and a weekly 90 mg form is available. The latter may be useful for treatment of PMDD with dosing during the last 1–2 weeks of the menstrual cycle, for women who do not want to take daily medication, or for patients in whom daily dosing is difficult [71, 72].

Fluvoxamine Fluvoxamine is an SSRI which is used in anxiety disorders in the United States, especially OCD, social anxiety disorder, and panic disorder. It has been in use as long as fluoxetine, has been proven safe in children to elderly patients, and has a lower incidence of sexual dysfunction than many other SSRIs [73].

Paroxetine Paroxetine has been studied and approved for a variety of psychiatric conditions: depression and anxiety disorders, PTSD, OCD, and PMDD, with dosage ranges between 10 mg and 60 mg depending on the indication [74]. Paroxetine has lost popularity because of its numerous side effects and teratogenicity. Paroxetine is pregnancy class D due to its association with heart defects and should not be used in patients who are pregnant. It should also be avoided in patients taking tamoxifen, as it can decrease tamoxifen drug levels (citalopram can be considered as an alternative). Paroxetine has been shown to have more sedating effects than other SSRIs [75]. Paroxetine may be associated with significant weight gain, fatigue, daytime somnolence, and severe withdrawal symptoms, more than other SSRIs.

Sertraline Sertraline is a safe and well-tolerated medication. Sertraline is approved for depressive and anxiety disorders in addition to PMDD and OCD. Dosages range from 25 mg to 200 mg daily. It is available in 25 mg, 50 mg, and 100 mg dosages and comes in a solution form [76]. The availability of low-dose tablets and liquid preparations makes sertraline a useful medication with elderly patients. Sertraline is relatively safe in pregnancy and lactation and is not stimulating like fluoxetine. It may cause QTc prolongation, and caution is therefore advised, as with other SSRIs. Nausea can be a limiting side effect, especially at the initiation of treatment, and bedtime dosing can sometimes mitigate this symptom.

Serotonin Partial Agonist-Reuptake Inhibitors (SPARIs) and Related Medications

Serotonin partial agonist-reuptake inhibitors inhibit serotonin reuptake and also have partial agonist activity on serotonin receptors. There is interest in developing classes of medications which provide precise targeting of specific serotonin receptor targets to maximize therapeutic effects and to minimize side effects. At present, these medications are second line to SSRIs and are primarily prescribed by psychiatrists. These medications may be helpful in patients whose symptoms are refractory or those who cannot tolerate SSRIs.

Vilazodone Vilazodone is a selective serotonin reuptake inhibitor and has additional action as a partial agonist of the 5HT1A receptor. It has been approved for depressive disorders [77] and has activity against anxiety. It is available in 10 mg, 20 mg, and 40 mg doses. Therapy is typically started at 10 mg for 7 days and titrated upward as tolerated. Safety and efficacy data suggests that it has similar treatment effects and side effect profiles to SSRIs [78]. Data suggests it is relatively weight neutral and has low risk for sexual side effects [79].

Vortioxetine Vortioxetine is a serotonin receptor antagonist (5-HT3, 5-HT7, and 5-HT1D), partial agonist (5-HT1B) and agonist (5-HT1A), and serotonin transporter inhibitor [80]. It is approved with a dosage range of 5 mg to 20 mg and acts across multiple signaling pathways in the brain to improve symptoms of major depressive disorder and associated anxiety. Like vilazodone, it has a similar side effect profile to SSRIs but may result in less sexual dysfunction than SSRIs.

Serotonin Norepinephrine Reuptake Inhibitors (SNRIs)

SNRIs are first line medications for depression, anxiety, and chronic pain. SNRIs are a class of medications that affect both the serotonin and norepinephrine signaling pathways in the brain and prevent synaptic reuptake of both neurotransmitters, allowing for greater activity [81]. Medications within the class have varying levels of selectivity for the serotonin versus norepinephrine receptors; however, this does not translate into differences in clinical efficacy for depressive and anxiety symptoms. Despite this approval, however, the benefit for anxiety may be offset by the stimulating effect from the norepinephrine reuptake inhibition. SNRIs are used for chronic pain associated with disease processes such as diabetic neuropathy, migraine headaches, and fibromyalgia [82]. SNRIs may also be considered as alternative treatment option for the treatment of ADHD [83, 84].

Duloxetine Duloxetine is approved for depressive, anxiety, and multiple pain disorders including diabetic neuropathy, fibromyalgia, and chronic musculoskeletal pain. Typical doses range from 20 mg to 60 mg daily [85]. Duloxetine seems to have similar efficacy to other SSRI and SNRI family members [86]. Duloxetine may be more effective, but may have more adverse side effects, than vortioxetine [87]. The most common side effects include gastrointestinal symptoms: nausea, vomiting, and diarrhea.

Levomilnacipran and Milnacipran Levomilnacipran is the enantiomer of the racemic milnacipran [88]. The former is approved in the United States for major depressive disorder, while the latter is approved for fibromyalgia [89]. Milnacipran is not approved for MDD in the United States, but it is approved for depression outside of the United States. At lower doses, these medications may be more selective for norepinephrine than other medications within the SNRI class [90].

Venlafaxine and Desvenlafaxine Desvenlafaxine is the enantiomer of the racemic venlafaxine. Both medications are approved to treat depressive and anxiety disorders and have additional uses in ADHD, migraine headache prophylaxis, and for menopausal hot flashes. Venlafaxine shows dose-dependent effects in improving symptoms that may affect mood (such as insomnia) in menopausal women with hot flashes, although hormone replacement is more effective [91]. Venlafaxine may also be a useful prophylactic option in patients with migraines [92]. Venlafaxine may be helpful in patients with ADHD. Venlafaxine should not be used in patients with uncontrolled narrow angle glaucoma. Some research suggests venlafaxine may be associated with the development of hypertension; however, other studies have not shown a clear association [93, 94]. Blood pressure should be monitored, especially in doses above 300 mg/day. Side effects include headache, dizziness, tremor, somnolence, and nausea. High doses of venlafaxine may prolong QTc.

Dopamine-Norephinephrine Reuptake Inhibitors

Bupropion is a medication which is widely used by PCPs for depression and smoking cessation. Bupropion works primarily on the dopamine and NE pathways, preventing reuptake into the synapse and allowing for increased activity of these neurotransmitters [95]. Bupropion can be used first line in patients with depressive symptoms but does not have significant activity against anxiety. Bupropion has several compelling indications in patient care. Bupropion carries an indication for smoking cessation; thus, patients with concomitant tobacco use disorder may derive both mood and tobacco cessation benefits from use [96]. Bupropion does not negatively affect sexual functioning and thus is useful as an add-on to low-dose SSRIs or alone for patients with sexual health concerns. Bupropion can be used (in combination with naltrexone) to assist with weight loss. Bupropion lowers the seizure threshold and is not be used in patients with seizure disorders or in those at risk for development of seizure disorders, including women with eating disorders or substance use disorders [57, 65]. Bupropion reduces the effectiveness of tamoxifen and is general avoided, along with fluoxetine and paroxetine, in this population.

Benzodiazepines

Benzodiazepines, which are GABA agonists, have been used for their anxiolytic properties for decades. Benzodiazepines may be used safely for panic disorder and anxiety in many patients; however, concerns about risk of dependence and adverse effects remain. Generally, it is preferred to give an alternative treatment such as an SSRI as a first line treatment for anxious depression or anxiety. Benzodiazepines may be useful at the initiation of treatment while awaiting the therapeutic effect of SSRIs and to counter temporary increases in anxiety which may occur when SSRIs or other agents are started. The risk for addiction should be assessed prior to prescribing or renewing these medications, and primary care physicians should weigh the risks and benefits associated with their use [97]. Benzodiazepines vary by onset, potency, and half-life, which are important considerations in their clinical use. Availability of additional formulations beyond oral agents, such as sublingual preparations which allow for rapid absorption, may also play into treatment decisions.

The major side effect of benzodiazepines is sedation, and care should be taken in patients who use other sedatives such as alcohol or other prescription sedatives. Collaboration with a geriatric psychiatrist, or at minimum dose adjustment, is strongly encouraged for elderly patients for whom benzodiazepines are being considered. Given the concern about increased risk for falls and other adverse events, other medication options should be discussed [98].

Alprazolam is generally avoided in favor of other benzodiazepines, as it is more addictive and is associated with marked rebound anxiety which limits its use. It is a rapid onset, short-acting medication with high potency, contributing to the addictive potential [99].

These properties may also predispose to its misuse, perhaps more so than other benzodiazepine class members [100]. Patients who have been prescribed alprazolam by another provider may be accustomed to its therapeutic effect with its rapid onset and high potency and may find lorazepam (the first line benzodiazepine) to be less effective by comparison.

Clonazepam Clonazepam is a rapid-onset, intermediate-duration, high-potency benzodiazepine. Because it has a rapid onset, but a longer duration than alprazolam, it may be a better option than alprazolam due to reduced concern about rebound anxiety [99]. Beyond its role in the treatment of anxiety, it is also used in patients with seizure disorders. Clonazepam is available in a rapid dissolving lingual preparation.

Diazepam Diazepam is a fast-acting, long-acting, medium potency benzodiazepine and is used in a variety of clinical situations, including procedural sedation and seizure disorders. It is generally not prescribed for anxiety disorders. It has been used for the acute management of lower back pain; however, the quality of evidence is low, and it may not be superior to placebo for acute or chronic lower back pain [101].

Lorazepam Lorazepam is generally the first line benzodiazepine used for anxiety and panic symptoms [102]. Lorazepam may be useful during times of acute stress, such as bereavement, and for short-term use in severe anxiety or insomnia. It is used as an anxiolytic for airplane travel and as premedication prior to MRIs and other medical procedures. It is a fast-acting, intermediate-duration, high-potency benzodiazepine. Lorazepam, unlike other class members, is metabolized outside of the cytochrome P450 system and thus can more safely be used in patients with renal or hepatic disease [99].

Temazepam Temazepam is an intermediate-onset, intermediate-duration, low-potency benzodiazepine which has traditionally been used for insomnia. While its pharmacology may result in decreased risks of misuse relative to other benzodiazepines, class-specific side effects remain. It currently carries a recommendation from the American Academy of Sleep Medicine for use in insomnia, with acknowledgment of the weak level of evidence to support its use [5].

Miscellaneous Agents

Gabapentin and *pregabalin* have some effectiveness in the treatment of anxiety but are not currently approved for this indication. These medications are discussed in Chap. 26 on General Approach to Chronic Pain.

Mirtazapine (Tetracyclic Antidepressant) Mirtazapine is a second line medication that acts on the serotonin and norepinephrine systems and has been found to be as effective as SSRI treatment. Weight gain and sedation are more common with mirtazapine, and it may be useful in some patients who have insomnia [103].

Tricyclic Antidepressants (TCAs) Tricyclic antidepressants (TCAs) are useful at low doses, alone, or in combination with other medications, for migraine prophylaxis, chronic pain, irritable bowel syndrome, urinary incontinence, and sleep disturbances. TCAs were used to treat depression for decades, but they are no longer used as primary antidepressants due to negative side effects at high doses [104]. TCAs are especially discouraged for use in older adults due to their highly anticholinergic and sedating effects [105]. TCAs prevent serotonin and/or norepinephrine reuptake, and concomitant use with SSRIs may result in increased SSRI levels. TCAs cause QTc prolongation at high doses and have severe cardiac effects when taken as an overdose.

Trazodone Trazodone is a first line treatment for insomnia at low doses but is not typically used as an antidepressant due to the side effects associated with higher doses. It acts through multiple therapeutic mechanisms, including blocking serotonin 2A receptors, histamine receptors, and alpha1 receptors [81].

Additional Considerations

Insufficient Response to One Medication

Some patients may not achieve adequate improvement in their symptoms in response to a single medication, and medication combinations should be considered. Bupropion has been used successfully to augment SSRI effects and to mitigate sexual side effects. Mirtazapine has been studied in combination with venlafaxine for treatment-refractory depression [106]. Antipsychotic medications such as quetiapine or aripiprazole, originally approved for bipolar disorder, may provide additional benefit for patients with difficult to treat symptoms such as insomnia, severe anxiety, and refractory depression [106]. Consultation with a psychiatrist to guide the initiation of bipolar disorder medications and antipsychotics should be sought, although PCPs may become knowledgeable in their use through experience and continuing medical education. A full discussion of combinations of medications is beyond the scope of this chapter.

Patients who have refractory symptoms despite treatment by a PCP, patients with bipolar disorder, or patients with psychotic disorders should be evaluated by a psychiatrist to assist in treatment. Substance misuse, PTSD, and severe psychosocial stressors may also complicate medication management and require the input of mental health professionals and social services.

Hormone Therapy

Given the link to a woman's menstrual cycle, oral contraceptives have been studied and found overall to be an effective option for PMDD [107, 108]. As noted previously, there is clear data that hormone replacement improves hot flashes during the menopausal transition, which may in turn positively affect sleep and mood. (See Chap. 8 on Menopause.)

Insomnia in Depression and Anxiety

Many patients note difficulty with sleep, which coincides with depressive and anxiety symptoms. Symptoms may be adequately addressed through the treatment of the primary disorder; however, additional medication therapy may be needed. Medications useful for insomnia include trazodone, benzodiazepines (short term), zolpidem (5 mg in women), quetiapine, mirtazapine, and low-dose TCAs (if there is another indication such as pain). Caution should be taken with medication interactions, including serotonin syndrome [109].

Serotonin Syndrome

Serotonin syndrome is a set of typically iatrogenic symptoms that can range from mildly uncomfortable to severe and life-threatening. These symptoms occur as a result of excess serotonin in the body. The syndrome is characterized by neurologic (hyperreflexia, clonus), autonomic (tachycardia, diaphoresis, diarrhea), and mental status changes (agitation, delirium). Prevention efforts should include adherence to recommended prescribed doses and avoidance of, or use of caution with, polypharmacy. When introducing a new medication, the lowest dose should be prescribed with an upward titration. In addition, clinicians should have a high index of suspicion for serotonin syndrome when patients develop unexpected symptoms [110]. A full discussion of serotonin syndrome is beyond the scope of this chapter, but a partial list of implicated substances includes SSRIs, SNRIs, MAO inhibitors, triptans, fentanyl, lithium, metoclopramide, St. John's wort, valproate, carbamazepine, cyclobenzaprine, dextromethorphan, amphetamines, levodopa, cocaine, and LSD.

Follow-Up and Treatment Duration

When treating a patient for depression or anxiety, close follow-up within the first weeks of initiating treatment is essential [111]. Follow-up within a week may be useful for patients with severe symptoms; those with milder symptoms may be able to follow up in 4–6 weeks after the initial appointment, with a phone or online check-in to assess response and side effects within the first few weeks. Communication regarding patient expectations of medications is an essential part of the conversation about medication management. It is wise to "start low and go slow" and only start one medication at a time. An exception would be patients with significant anxiety or panic that may benefit from a benzodiazepine to be taken as needed while initiating and adjusting to a new antidepressant.

While some patients may respond to treatment within a couple of weeks, others may require 4–6 weeks, especially for severe depression. If no improvement is seen within 12 weeks of treatment, alternative treatments or additional add-on therapies should be considered [63]. The PHQ-9 and GAD-7 should be serially administered at follow-up appointments to document and monitor response to treatment. Suggested treatment duration is a minimum of 6 months to help prevent the risk of relapse of patients' symptoms [57]. Medications should be tapered slowly, particularly with long-term use, as symptoms may result from abrupt cessation. In some cases of long-term use and recurrent depression, medication discontinuation should not be attempted. The US Preventive Services Task Force and others endorse a collaborative care model in which PCPs work in collaboration with mental health providers to treat patients (discussed below).

Psychotherapy

Psychotherapy is a practice that can be implemented in multiple healthcare settings, using a variety of approaches and techniques. Most commonly, patients are referred to providers within specialty care for psychotherapy treatment. The most commonly known evidence-based psychotherapy treatment is cognitive behavioral therapy (CBT). CBT employs a variety of techniques aiming to help a patient identify and modify maladaptive thoughts and behaviors. This is done within a framework of understanding that thoughts, feelings, and behaviors are bidirectionally interrelated; by changing one component of this triad, the others will alter in turn. Patients being treated with CBT may see significant and constructive changes in how they interpret internal and external stimuli, the kind of "self-talk" they engage in, and become aware of their behavioral responses to stress-inducing situations. CBT can be highly effective in reducing depressive or anxiety symptoms.

Psychotherapeutic approaches such as dialectical behavioral therapy (DBT) for higher-risk or more dysregulated patients, eye movement desensitization and reprocessing (EMDR) for PTSD, interpersonal therapy, mindfulness-based therapy, and others may also be effective for a patient based on individual preferences, cognitive style, or other factors [112, 113]. The detailed discussion of these therapies is beyond the scope of this chapter.

Collaborative Care

Collaborative care models show promise in addressing depressive symptoms within primary care settings [114]. These multidisciplinary and integrated treatment models propose the utilization of multidisciplinary treatment teams consisting of the primary care provider, the patient, a "care manager" (allied mental health professional), and a consulting psychiatrist. Collaborative care is defined as (a) team-driven, (b) population-focused, (c) measurement-guided, and (d) evidence based [115]. Regular follow-up and treatment team meetings facilitate ongoing communication among providers so that treatment can quickly be modified or enhanced to maximize treatment outcomes. Primary care providers and their patients collaboratively formulate a treatment plan to address depressive symptoms, including medication management and/or brief psychotherapy implemented within a primary care setting. The care manager works with the patient and the primary care provider to track symptoms (often using a symptom screening measure such as the PHQ-9), implement brief psychotherapy (solution-focused, cognitive behavioral, or behavioral activation), and maintain close follow-up of treatment progress. Care managers may also ultimately refer patients to specialty care outside the primary care setting. Consulting psychiatrists remain available for recommendations and referrals.

Treatment Planning

Shared Decision-Making

Each patient who seeks care for depression, anxiety, or other psychiatric concerns should have a treatment plan informed by her own preferences and values. Primary care providers are advised to both review options with patients and check in with patients about their thoughts and beliefs. For example, patients may have strong feelings about wanting to avoid medications, while others would prefer medications and do not believe psychotherapy is right for them. The data reviewed in this chapter demonstrates that a variety of treatment modalities may be helpful for depressive and anxiety symptoms. A patient's belief in the efficacy of her treatment plan is also important, highlighting the need to ensure a plan mutually determined by the patient and provider.

Monica begins taking an SSRI and engages in weekly psychotherapy. Six months later, she returns to clinic and reports an improvement in her mood and her sleep. She remarks that she and her long-term partner have been talking about starting a family within the next year.

Preconception Considerations

In women of childbearing age, it is useful to discuss plans for pregnancy during initial treatment planning, including the risks and benefits of medication use in pregnancy. Early discussions regarding plans for medication use and discontinuation may help avert concerns and more urgent discussions in early pregnancy. Patients will benefit from receiving education that depression tends to worsen during pregnancy; thus, medications should be discontinued with care. SSRIs are generally safe in pregnancy, with the exception of paroxetine, but other medications may have a higher level of risk. Proactive planning in regard to medication alternatives during pregnancy is indicated, and patients should be co-managed with obstetricians and psychiatrists during preconception planning, pregnancy, and in the postpartum period.

Psychiatric Management of Mood and Anxiety Disorders During Pregnancy

Please see Chap. 39 on Obstetric Medicine for a discussion regarding medication use and management during pregnancy.

Postpartum Care

The American College of Obstetrics and Gynecology, the American College of Physicians, the American Academy of Pediatrics, and the American Academy of Family Physicians all recommend and support screening and treatment for psychosocial aspects of health affecting mothers to provide the best care for the whole family [116–118]. Providers should screen for symptoms of postpartum depression and mania (in patients with bipolar disorder) in addition to addressing other health concerns in the postpartum period for all women. The Edinburgh Postpartum Depression Scale (EPDS) is a screening tool which has been validated for use in the postpartum setting. The use of psychiatric medications during pregnancy and lactation is covered in Chap. 39 on Obstetric Medicine.

Conclusion

Depressive and anxiety disorders disproportionately affect women and can be treated in the realm of primary care. Primary care providers should be able to recognize risk factors for these disorders and utilize common screening modalities. Primary care providers must carefully consider differential diagnoses, including both psychiatric and medical alternatives. If uncertain, collaboration with a psychiatrist is encouraged. Treatment plans should be individualized, including patients' comorbidities, beliefs, and preferences to arrive at mutually determined plans that may incorporate psychotherapy, medication, lifestyle modifications, or complementary and alternative treatments. After initiation of a treatment plan, patients require close follow-up to ensure improvement in mood or anxiety symptoms.

Summary Points

1. Depressive disorders and anxiety disorders are common and underreported in women seeking care in the primary care setting; annually, 8.5% of women present with depressive disorders and 23.4% present with anxiety disorders. Women may be hesitant to seek out mental healthcare on their own; thus, the assessment and treatment of depressant and anxiety symptoms in primary care is vital.
2. Bipolar disorder and post-traumatic stress disorder are key differential diagnoses to consider for patients presenting with depressive or anxiety symptoms; differentiation between these disorders is critical given that treatment is pharmacologically and behaviorally distinct and usually requires psychiatric consultation.
3. Patient-centered inquiries are important components of a comprehensive clinical interview and diagnostic assess-

ment. These include open-ended questions, reflective statements, clarifying questions, and emotion-seeking approaches. Screening tools such as the PHQ-9 and GAD-7 are helpful adjuncts in the diagnosis and monitoring of depressive and anxiety disorders.

4. Suicide risk assessments are essential to any provider-patient exchange related to emotional or psychiatric distress. These assessments include determining the presence of any ideation (passive and active), intent, and/or plan. Suicide risk is determined through direct and nonjudgmental inquiries.
5. The treatment of depressive and anxiety disorders is individualized based on symptom acuity and severity and patient preference. The choice to prescribe psychotropic medication, recommend behavioral and lifestyle changes, or refer for psychotherapy is made using shared decision-making. Complex or severe symptoms may necessitate a referral to a psychiatrist or psychotherapist.
6. Referral to a psychiatrist is appropriate when patients fail to respond to standard treatment modalities or demonstrate symptoms concerning for complex psychiatric disease including bipolar disorder or psychosis.

Review Questions

1. A 27-year-old woman presents to clinic with acute distress. She declares that she has been "feeling crazy" lately and that her thoughts and emotions feel "out of control." She mentions that her boyfriend called her "bipolar" during their most recent argument and asks whether she might have bipolar disorder. What definitively differentiates a bipolar disorder from a depressive disorder?
   A. Hospitalization or arrest
   B. A manic, hypomanic, or mixed episode
   C. Markedly decreased sleep
   D. Impulsive or destructive behavior

   The correct answer is B. The diagnosis of bipolar disorders requires a least one episode of hypomania or mania for bipolar II and bipolar I disorder, respectively. While hospitalization, arrest, or impulsive behavior may occur in patients with bipolar disorder; these history points are not required for the diagnosis of the bipolar disorder. Markedly decreased sleep may occur in many psychiatric disorders, including depression or anxiety, and is not specific to bipolar disorder; the same is true with impulsive or destructive behavior [26].
2. A 55-year-old woman presents for her routine physical appointment and is asked to complete a Patient Health Questionnaire-9 (PHQ-9) at check-in. The PHQ-9 is:
   A. A validated assessment measure for diet and exercise
   B. A validated screening tool for anxiety symptoms
   C. A validated screening tool for depressive symptoms
   D. A validated assessment measure for substance use

   The correct answer is C. The Patient Health Questionnaire (PHQ) is commonly used in primary care as a screening tool for depression. There are multiple versions which have been adapted for differing patient populations and situations. The PHQ-2 (two-question version) and PHQ-9 have been found to be reasonable screening tools for depression; however, providers should undertake additional discussion with individual patients before making the diagnosis of a depressive disorder [119].
3. A 45-year-old woman is being evaluated for depression. For a person to be diagnosed with major depressive disorder, several symptoms should be present, but at least one of two possible symptoms is required. Which of the following is one of those two required symptoms?
   A. Recurrent thoughts of death, self-harm, or suicide
   B. Marked changes in sleep
   C. Feelings of worthlessness or excessive guilt
   D. Loss of interest or pleasure in previously enjoyed activities or events

   The correct answer is D. The DSM-5 criteria for major depressive disorder require at least one of two symptoms, depressed mood or loss of interest or pleasure, and a total of five of nine symptoms. While thoughts of death, feelings of guilt, changes in sleep, or feelings of worthlessness may be present, they are not required for the diagnosis. Additionally, the diagnosis requires that the episode of symptoms not be attributable to substance use or symptoms of another medical condition. Collaboration within a treatment team as described in the question is important [26].
4. A 34-year-old woman is seen in follow-up in your office for depressive symptoms. She notes that she sometimes feels like it would be better if she weren't "here anymore." What would be the most appropriate patient-centered response to this statement?
   A. Begin following protocol to initiate involuntary hospitalization.
   B. Probe to gather more information about these thoughts.
   C. Do not inquire further, since she did not report an intent to harm herself.
   D. Advise her to increase or change her medication regimen, since it probably is not optimally addressing her depression.

   The correct answer is B. Vague statements such as those made by this patient can have a variety of meanings, and it is important to sensitively gather more information about her symptoms to determine the most appropriate treatment plan. While some patients may have active suicidal intent, not all may, and thus involuntary hospitalization for all patients who make this statement is inappropriate. It is currently unclear if she has intent to harm herself, so failing to inquire further is also inappropriate. While her medication regimen may need to be changed, the next best step is to further discuss the statement she made to gather more specific information about these thoughts, as well as any thoughts or plans of self-harm [120].

References

1. World Health Organization. Depression [homepage on the Internet]. 2017. [cited 2018 Feb 21]. Available from http://www.who.int/mediacentre/factsheets/fs369/en/.
2. World Health Organization. 10 facts on mental health. No date [cited 2018 Feb 21]. Available from: http://www.who.int/features/factfiles/mental_health/mental_health_facts/en/index1.html.
3. Substance Abuse and Mental Health Services Administration. Key substance use and mental health indicators in the United States: results from the 2016 National Survey on drug use and health (HHS Publication No. SMA 17-5044, NSDUH Series H-52). Rockville: Center for Behavioral Health Statistics and Quality, Substance Abuse and Mental Health Services Administration; 2017. Retrieved from https://www.samhsa.gov/data/.
4. Merikangas KR, Akiskal HS, Angst J, et al. Lifetime and 12-month prevalence of bipolar spectrum disorder in the National Comorbidity Survey Replication. Arch Gen Psychiatry. 2007;64(5):543–52.
5. American Psychiatric Association. Mental health disparities: LGBTQ [Internet]. 2017. [updated 2017; cited 2018 Jun 27]. Available from: https://www.psychiatry.org/psychiatrists/cultural-competency/mental-health-disparities.
6. Belle D, Doucet J. Poverty, inequality, and discrimination as sources of depression among U.S. women. Psychol Women Q. 2003;27(2):101–13.
7. Pabayo R, Kawachi I, Gilman S. State-level income inequality and depression among a cohort of American adults. J Epidemiol Community Health. 2014;68(2):110–5.
8. Shih JH, Eberhart NK, Hammen CL, Brennan PA. Differential exposure and reactivity to interpersonal stress predict sex differences in adolescent depression. J Clin Child Adolesc Psychol. 2006;35(1):103–15.
9. Stewart AJ, Salt P. Life stress, life-styles, depression, and illness in adult women. J Pers Soc Psychol. 1981;40(6):1063–9.
10. Hochschild A, Machung A. The second shift. New York: Avon Books; 1989.
11. Avery MC, Krichmar JL. Neuromodulatory systems and their interactions: a review of models, theories, and experiments. Front Neural Circuits. 2017;11:108.
12. Garner M, Möhler H, Stein DJ, Mueggler T, Baldwin DS. Research in anxiety disorders: from the bench to the bedside. Eur Neuropsychopharmacol. 2009;19(6):381–90.
13. Hastings RS, Parsey RV, Quendo MA, Arango V, Mann JJ. Volumetric analysis of prefrontal cortex, amygdala, and hippocampus in major depression. Neuropsychopharmacology. 2004;29(5):952–9. Available from: https://www.nature.com/articles/1300371. Accessed 18 June 2018.
14. Frey BN, Skelin I, Skai Y, Nishikawa M, Diksic M. Gender differences in alpha-[11C]MTrp brain trapping, an index of serotonin synthesis, in medication-free individuals with major depressive disorder: a positron emission tomography study. Psychiatry Res. 2010;183(2):157–66. Available from: https://doi.org/10.1016/j.pscychresns.2010.05.005.
15. Caspi AR, Holmes A, Uher R, Moffitt TE. Genetic sensitivity to the environment: the case of the serotonin transporter gene and its implications for studying complex diseases and traits. Am J Psychiatry. 2010;167(5):509–27. Available from: https://doi.org/10.1176/appi.ajp.2010.09101452.
16. Amidfar M, Colic L, Walter M, Kim YK. Complex role of the serotonin receptors in depression: implications for treatment. In: Kim YK, editor. Understanding Depression. Singapore: Springer; 2018. p. 83–95.
17. Pearce EF, Murphy JA. Vortioxetine for the treatment of depression. Ann Pharmacother. 2014;48(6):758–65. Available from: https://doi.org/10.1177/1060028014528305.
18. Stahl SM. Mechanism of action of the SPARI vilazodone: serotonin 1A partial agonist and reuptake inhibitor. CNS Spectr. 2014;19(2):105–9. Available from: https://doi.org/10.1017/S1092852914000169.
19. Chang M, Tybring G, Dahl M, Lindh J. Impact of cytochrome P450 2C19 polymorphisms on citalopram/escitalopram exposure: a systematic review and meta-analysis. Clin Pharmacokinet. 2014;53(9):801–11. Available from: https://doi.org/10.1007/s40262-014-0162-1.
20. Engin E, Beham RS, Rudolph U. An emerging circuit pharmacology of $GABA_A$ receptors. To be published in Trends in Pharmacol Sci. [Preprint] 2018. Available from: https://linkinghub.elsevier.com/retrieve/pii/S0165-6147(18)30076-2. Accessed 18 June 2018.
21. Jacobson L. Hypothalamic-pituitary-adrenocortical axis: neuropsychiatric aspects. Compr Physiol. 2014;4(2):715–38. Available from: https://doi.org/10.1002/cphy.c130036.
22. McEwen BS, Nasca C, Gray JD. Stress effects on neuronal structure: hippocampus, amygdala, and prefrontal cortex. Neuropsychopharmacology. 2016;41(1):3–23. Available from: https://doi.org/10.1038/npp.2015.171.
23. Barth C, Villringer A, Sacher J. Sex hormones affect neurotransmitters and shape the adult female brain during hormonal transition periods. Front Neurosci. 2015;9(37):1–20. Available from: https://doi.org/10.3389/fnins.2015.00037.
24. Mong JA, Cusmano DM. Sex differences in sleep: impact of biological sex and sex steroids. Philos Trans R Soc Lond Ser B Biol Sci. 2016;371(1688):1–11. Available from: https://doi.org/10.1098/rstb.2015.0110.
25. Susukida R, Mojtabai R, Mendelson T. Sex differences in help seeking for mood and anxiety disorders in the National Comorbidity Survey-Replication. Depress Anxiety. 2015;32(11):853–60.
26. American Psychiatric Association. Diagnostic and statistical manual of mental disorders. 5th ed. Washington, DC: Author; 2013.
27. Romans SE, Tyas J, Cohen MM, Silverstone T. Gender differences in the symptoms of major depressive disorder. J Nerv Ment Dis. 2007;195(11):905–11.
28. Appleton SM. Premenstrual syndrome: evidence-based evaluation and treatment. Clin Obstet Gynecol. 2018;61(1):52–61.
29. Walsh S, Ismaili E, Naheed B, O'Brien S. Diagnosis, pathophysiology and management of premenstrual syndrome. Obstet Gynecol. 2015;17:99–104.
30. Scott J. A re-examination of antidepressant treatment-emergent mania in bipolar disorders: evidence of gender differences. Acta Psychiatr Scand. 2017;135(5):479–88.
31. Lyles JS, Dwamena FC, Lein C, Smith RC. Evidence-based patient-centered interviewing. J Clin Outcomes Manag. 2001;8(7):28–34.
32. Kroenke K, Spitzer RL, Williams JBW. The PHQ-9: validity of a brief depression severity measure. J Gen Intern Med. 2001;16(9):606–13.

33. Kroenke K, Spitzer R, Williams J, Lowe B. The patient health questionnaire somatic, anxiety, and depressive symptom scales: a systematic review. Gen Hosp Psychiatry. 2010;32:345–59.
34. Bair MJ, Wu J, Damush TM, Sutherland JM, Kroenke K. Association of depression and anxiety alone and in combination with chronic musculoskeletal pain in primary care patients. Psychosom Med. 2008;70(8):890–7.
35. Phillips AC, Carroll D, Der G. Negative life events and symptoms of depression and anxiety: social causation and/or stress generation. Anxiety Stress Coping. 2015;28(4):357–71.
36. Centers for Disease Control and Prevention Division of Violence Prevention. Adverse childhood experiences study. c2014 [cited 2018 Feb 18]. Available from https://www.cdc.gov/violenceprevention/acestudy/.
37. Black MC, Basile KC, Breiding MJ, et al. National intimate partner and sexual violence survey: 2010 summary report. Atlanta: Center for Disease Control and Prevention National Center for Injury Prevention and Control; 2011.
38. Kendler KS, Kuhn JW, Prescott CA. Childhood sexual abuse, stressful life events and risk for major depression in women. Psychol Med. 2004;34(8):1475–82.
39. Machtinger EL, Cuca YP, Khanna N, Dawson-Rose C, Kimberg LS. From treatment to healing: the promise of trauma-informed primary care. Womens Health Issues. 2015;25(3):193–7.
40. Weinreb L, Savageau JA, Candim LM, Reed GW, Fletcher KE, Hargraves JL. Screening for childhood trauma in adult primary care patients: a cross-sectional survey. Prim Care Companion J Clin Psychiatr. 2010;12(6):PCC.10m00950. https://doi.org/10.4088/PCC.10m00950blu.
41. Ungar M. Resilience, trauma, context, and culture. Trauma Violence Abuse. 2013;14(3):255–66.
42. Schrijvers D, Bollen J, Sabbe B. The gender paradox in suicidal behavior and its impact on the suicidal process. J Affect Disord. 2011;138(1–2):19–26.
43. Dazzi T, Gribble R, Wessely S, Fear NT. Does asking about suicide and related behaviours induce suicidal ideation? What is the evidence? Psychol Med. 2014;44(16):3361–3.
44. Mann JJ. A current perspective of suicide and attempted suicide. Ann Intern Med. 2002;136(4):302–11.
45. Institute of Medicine (IOM). Crossing the quality chasm: a new health system for the 21st century. Washington, D.C.: National Academy Press; 2001.
46. National Institute of Mental Health (NIMH). Major depression [homepage on the Internet]. c2017 [updated 2017 Nov.; cited 2018 Jan 29]. Available from https://www.nimh.nih.gov/health/statistics/major-depression.shtml#part_155720.
47. National Institute of Health. Complementary and alternative medicine [homepage on the Internet]. c2013 [updated 2013 Mar 29.; cited 2018 Mar 3]. Available from https://report.nih.gov/NIHfactsheets/ViewFactSheet.aspx?csid=85.
48. Lopresti AL, Hood SD, Drummond PD. A review of lifestyle factors that contribute to important pathways associated with major depression: diet, sleep and exercise. J Affect Disord. 2013;148(1):12–27.
49. Casañas R, Catalán R, del Val RL, Real J, Valero S, Casas M. Effectiveness of a psycho-educational group program for major depression in primary care: a randomized controlled trial. BMC Psychiatry. 2012;12:230.
50. Serrano Ripoll MJ, Oliván-Blázquez B, Vicens-Pons E, Roca M, Gili M, et al. Lifestyle change recommendations in major depression: do they work? J Affect Disord. 2015;183(1):221–8.
51. Taylor DJ, Lichstein KL, Weinstock J, Sanford S, Temple JR. A pilot study of cognitive-behavioral therapy of insomnia in people with mild depression. Behav Ther. 2007;38:49–57.
52. Cooney GM, Dwan K, Greig CA, et al. Exercise for depression [Cochrane review]. In: The cochrane library, Issue 9. Oxford: Update Software; 2013.
53. Gartlehner G, Bradley BN, Amick HR, Lohr KN. Comparative benefits and harms of antidepressant, psychological, complementary, and exercise treatments for major depression: an evidence based report for a clinical practice guideline from the American College of Physicians. Ann Intern Med. 2016;165(6):331–41. Available from: https://doi.org/10.7326/L16-0209.
54. De Manincor M, Bensoussan A, Smith CA, et al. Individualized yoga for reducing depression and anxiety, and improving well-being: a randomized controlled trial. Depress Anxiety. 2016;33:816–28.
55. Goran K, Fratini P, Padulo J, Antonio DI, De Giorgio A. Effectiveness of yoga and educational intervention on disability, anxiety, depression, and pain in people with CLBP: a randomized controlled trial. Complement Ther Clin Pract. 2018;31:262–7.
56. Kovich H, Dejong A. Common questions about the pharmacologic management of depression in adults. Am Fam Physician. 2015;92(2):94–110. Available from: https://www.aafp.org/afp/2015/0715/p94.html. Accessed 18 June 2018.
57. Bleakley S. Review of the choice and use of antidepressant drugs. Prog Neurol Psychiatry. 2009;13(1):14–20.
58. Locke AB, Kirst N, Shultz CG. Diagnosis and management of generalized anxiety disorder and panic disorder in adults. Am Fam Physician. 2015;91(9):617–24.
59. Grant BF, Stinson FD, Dawson DA. Prevalence and co-occurrence of substance use disorders and independent mood and anxiety disorders. Arch Gen Psychiatry. 2004;61(8):807–16.
60. Simon GE, Perlis RH. Personalized medicine for depression: can we match patients with treatments? Am J Psychiatry. 2010;167(12):1445–55.
61. Kim H, Lim S-W, Kim S. Monoamine transporter gene polymorphisms and antidepressant response in Koreans with late-life depression. JAMA. 2006;296(13):1609–18.
62. Choosing Wisely: American College of Preventive Medicine. Don't use expensive medications when an equally effective and lower-cost medication is available. Available from: http://www.choosingwisely.org/clinician-lists/american-college-preventive-medicine-name-expensive-medications/. Accessed 1 Feb 2018.
63. Adams S, Miller K, Zylstra R. Pharmacologic Management of Adult Depression. Am Fam Physician. 2008;77(6):785–92.
64. Gale CK, Millichamp J. Clinical evidence handbook: generalized anxiety disorder. Am Fam Physician. 2013;87(2):122–4.
65. Gartlehner G, Hansen RA, Morgan LC, et al. Comparative benefits and harms of second-generation antidepressants for treating major depressive disorder: an updated meta-analysis. Ann Intern Med. 2011;155(11):772–85.
66. Cipriani A, Purgato M, Fukukawa TA, et al. Citalopram versus other anti-depressive agents for depression. Cochrane Database Syst Rev. 2012;7:1–148. Available from: https://doi.org/10.1002/14651858.CD006534.pub2.
67. Kumar Y, Kung S, Shinozaki G. CYP2C19 variation, not citalopram dose nor serum level, is associated with QTc prolongation. J Psychopharmacol. 2014;28(12):1143–8. Available from: https://doi.org/10.1177/0269881114543720.
68. Hutton LMJ, Cave AJ, St-Jean R, Bahn HL. Should we be worried about QTc prolongation using citalopram? A review. J Pharm Pract. 2017;30(3):353–88. Available from: https://doi.org/10.1177/0897190015624862.
69. Sánchez C, Bøgesø KP, Ebert B, Reines EH, Braestrup C. Escitalopram versus citalopram: the surprising role of the R-enantiomer. Psychopharmacology. 2004;174(2):163–76. Available from: https://link.springer.com/article/10.1007%2Fs00213-004-1865-z. Accessed 18 June 2018.

70. Wong DT, Perry KW, Bymaster FP. The discovery of fluoxetine hydrochloride (Prozac). Nat Rev Drug Discov. 2005;4(9):764–74. Available from: https://www.nature.com/articles/nrd1821. Accessed 18 June, 2018.
71. IBM Micromedex (electronic version). Truven Health Analytics. Prozac. Greenwood Village, Colorado, USA. Available from: http://www.micromedexsolutions.com/micromedex2/librarian/CS/F69A39/ND_PR/evidencexpert/ND_P/evidencexpert/DUPLICATIONSHIELDSYNC/105B9C/ND_PG/evidencexpert/ND_B/evidencexpert/ND_AppProduct/evidencexpert/ND_T/evidencexpert/PFActionId/evidencexpert.GoToDashboard?docId=236415&contentSetId=100&title=Fluoxetine+Hydrochloride&servicesTitle=Fluoxetine+Hydrochloride&brandName=PROzac#. Accessed 18 June 2018.
72. Sepede G, Sarchione F, Matarazzo I, Giannantonio MD, Salerno RM. Premenstrual dysphoric disorder without comorbid psychiatric conditions: a systematic review of therapeutic options. Clin Neuropharmacol. 2016;39(5):241–61. Available from: https://doi.org/10.1097/WNF.0000000000000173.
73. IBM Micromedex (electronic version). Truven Health Analytics. Fluvoxamine. Greenwood Village, Colorado, USA. Available from: http://www.micromedexsolutions.com/micromedex2/librarian/CS/593A47/ND_PR/evidencexpert/ND_P/evidencexpert/DUPLICATIONSHIELDSYNC/A857F9/ND_PG/evidencexpert/ND_B/evidencexpert/ND_AppProduct/evidencexpert/ND_T/evidencexpert/PFActionId/evidencexpert.DoIntegratedSearch?SearchTerm=fluvoxamine&UserSearchTerm=fluvoxamine&SearchFilter=filterNone&navitem=searchALL#. Accessed 18 June 2018.
74. IBM Micromedex (electronic version). Truven Health Analytics. Greenwood Village, Paroxetine. Colorado, USA. Available at: http://www.micromedexsolutions.com/micromedex2/librarian/CS/EF0B81/ND_PR/evidencexpert/ND_P/evidencexpert/DUPLICATIONSHIELDSYNC/BD4B77/ND_PG/evidencexpert/ND_B/evidencexpert/ND_AppProduct/evidencexpert/ND_T/evidencexpert/PFActionId/evidencexpert.DoIntegratedSearch?SearchTerm=Paroxetine+Hydrochloride&fromInterSaltBase=true&false=null&false=null&=null#. Accessed 18 June 2018.
75. Marks DM, Park M, Ham B, et al. Paroxetine: safety and tolerability issues. Expert Opin Drug Saf. 2008;7(6):783–94. Available from: https://doi.org/10.1517/14740330802423168.
76. IBM Micromedex (electronic version). Truven Health Analytics. Sertraline. Greenwood Village, Colorado, USA. Available from: http://www.micromedexsolutions.com. Accessed 21 June 2018.
77. IBM Micromedex (electronic version). Truven Health Analytics. Vilazodone. Greenwood Village, Colorado, USA. Available from: http://www.micromedexsolutions.com/micromedex2/librarian/CS/89E138/ND_PR/evidencexpert/ND_P/evidencexpert/DUPLICATIONSHIELDSYNC/E97D84/ND_PG/evidencexpert/ND_B/evidencexpert/ND_AppProduct/evidencexpert/ND_T/evidencexpert/PFActionId/evidencexpert.DoIntegratedSearch?SearchTerm=vilazodone&UserSearchTerm=vilazodone&SearchFilter=filterNone&navitem=searchALL#. Accessed 18 June 2018.
78. Hellerstein DJ, Flaxer J. Vilazodone for the treatment of major depressive disorder: an evidence-based review of its place in therapy. Core Evid. 2015;10:49–62. Available from: https://doi.org/10.2147/CE.S54075.
79. McCormack PL. Vilazodone: a review in major depressive disorder in adults. Drugs. 2015;75(16):1915–23. Available from: https://doi.org/10.1007/s40265-015-0490-y.
80. Sanchez C, Asin KE, Artigas F. Vortioxetine, a novel antidepressant with multimodal activity: review of preclinical and clinical data. Pharmacol Ther. 2015;145:43–57. Available from: https://doi.org/10.1016/j.pharmthera.2014.07.001.
81. Stahl SM. Mechanism of action of trazodone: a multifunctional drug. CNS Spectr. 2009;14(10):536–46.
82. Welsch P, Uceyler N, Klose P, Walitt B, Hauser W. Serontonin and noradrenaline reuptake inhibitors (SNRIs) for fibromyalgia. Cochrane Database Syst Rev. 2018;2:CD 010292.
83. Buoli M, Serati M, Cahn W. Alternative pharmacological strategies for adult ADHD treatment: a systematic review. Exerpt Rev Neurother. 2016;16(2):131–44. Available from: https://doi.org/10.1586/14737175.2016.1135735.
84. Ragguett R, Yim SJ, Ho PT, McIntyre RS. Efficacy of levomilnacipran extended release in treating major depressive disorder. Expert Opin Pharmacother. 2017;18(18):2017–24. Available from: https://doi.org/10.1080/14656566.2017.1410540
85. Ait-Daoud N, Hamby AS, Sharma S, Blevins D. A review of Alprazolam use, misuse and withdrawal. J Addict Med. 2018;12(1):4–10. Available from: https://doi.org/10.1097/ADM.0000000000000350.
86. Li G, Wang D, Ma D. Vortioxetine versus duloxetine in the treatment of patients with major depressive disorder: a meta-analysis of randomized clinical trials. Clin Drug Investig. 2016;36(7):509–17. Available from: https://doi.org/10.1007/s40261-016-0396-9.
87. IBM Micromedex (electronic version) Truven Health Analytics. Duloxetine. Greenwood Village, Colorado, USA. Available from: www.micromedexsolutions.com. Accessed 18 June 2018.
88. Cording M, Derry S, Phillips T, Moore RA, Wiffen PJ. Milnacipran for pain in fibromyalgia in adults. Cochrane Database Syst Rev. 2015;(10):1–41. Available from: https://doi.org/10.1002/14651858.CD008244.pub3.
89. Bernstein CD, Albecht KL, Marcus DA. Milnacipran for fibromyalgia; a useful addition to the treatment armamentarium. Expert Opin Pharmacother. 2013;14(3):905–16. Available from: https://doi.org/10.1517/1456566.2013.779670.
90. Ensrud KE, Guthrie KA, Hohensee C, et al. Effects of estradiol and venlafaxine on insomnia symptoms and sleep quality in women with hot flashes. Sleep. 2015;38(1):97–108. Available from: https://doi.org/10.5665/sleep.4332.
91. Salviz M, Yuce T, Acar H, Karatas A, Aciklain RM. Propranolol and venlafaxine for vestibular migraine prophylaxis: a randomized controlled trial. Laryngoscope. 2016;126(1):169–74. Available from: https://doi.org/10.1002/lary.25445.
92. Ho JM, Gomes T, Straus SE, Austin PC, Mandani M, Jurrlink DM. Adverse cardiac events in older patients receiving venlafaxine: a population based study. J Clin Psychiatry. 2014;75(6):552–8. Available from: https://doi.org/10.4088/JCP.13m08508.
93. Venlafaxine: more dangerous than most "selective" serotonergic antidepressants. Prescrire Int. 2016;25(170):96–9. Available from: https://www.ncbi.nlm.nih.gov/pubmed/27186622. Accessed 18 June 2018.
94. Griffin CE, Kaye AD, Bueno FR, Kaye AD. Benzodiazepine pharmacology and central nervous system-mediated effects. Oschner J. 2013;132(2):214–23. Available at: https://www.ncbi.nlm.nih.gov/pmc/articles/PMC3684331/pdf/i1524-5012-13-2-214.pdf [Accessed 22nd June, 2018].
95. Micromedex 2.0. Truven Health Analytics. Bupropion hydrobromide. Greenwood Village, Colorado, USA. Available at: http://www.micromedexsolutions.com/ (Cited: 2/23/2018).
96. Food and Drug Administration. Highlights of prescribing information: Zyban (bupropion hydrochloride) [homepage from the Internet]. No date [cited 2018 Mar 7]. Available from: https://www.accessdata.fda.gov/drugsatfda_docs/label/2017/020711s045s046s047lbl.pdf#page=37.
97. Benasi G, Guidi J, Offidani E, et al. Benzodiazepines as monotherapy in depressive disorders: a systematic review. Psychother Psychosom. 2018;87(2):65–74.
98. Bilodeau M, Simon T, Beauchamp MH, et al. Duloxetine in adults with ADHD: a randomized-controlled pilot study. J Atten Disord. 2014;18(2):169–75. Available from: https://doi.org/10.1177/1087054712443157.

99. Levin RL, Real LA, Julius R, et al. Safe prescribing of benzodiazepines for anxiety and insomnia. Prescribing guidelines for Pennsylvania. Commonwealth of Pennsylvania. October18, 2016, updated May 15, 2017. Available from: http://www.health.pa.gov/My%20Health/Diseases%20and%20Conditions/M-P/opioids/Documents/PA%20Guidelines%20on%20Benzo%20Prescribing.pdf. Accessed 22 June 2018.
100. Lader M. Benzodiazepine harm: how can it be reduced? Br J Clin Pharmacol. 2012;77(2):295–301. Available from: https://doi.org/10.1111/j.1365-2125.2012.04418.x.
101. Sateia MJ, Buysse DJ, Krystal AD, Neubauer DN, Heald JL. Clinical practice guideline for the pharmacologic treatment of insomnia in adults: an American Academy of Sleep Medicine Clinical Practice Guideline. J Clin Sleep Med. 2017;13(2):307–49. Available from: https://doi.org/10.5664/jcsm.6470.
102. Qaseem A, Wilt TJ, McLean RM, Forciea MA. Noninvasive treatments for acute, subacute and chronic low back pain: a clinical practice guideline from the American College of Physicians. Ann Intern Med. 2017;166(7):514–30. Available from: https://doi.org/10.7327/M16-2367.
103. Holm KJ, Markham A. Mirtazapine: a review of its use in major depression. Drugs. 1999;57(4):607–31.
104. Leucht C, Huhn M, Leucht S. Amitriptyline versus placebo for major depressive disorder. [Cochrane review]. In: The Cochrane Library, Issue 12. Oxford: Update Software; 2012.
105. American Geriatrics Society 2015 Beers Criteria Update Expert Panel. American Geriatrics Society 2015 updated Beers Criteria for potentially inappropriate medication use in older adults. J Am Geriatr Soc. 2015;63(11):2227–46.
106. Preston TC, Shelton RC. Treatment resistant depression: strategies for primary care. Curr Psychiatry Rep. 2013;15:370–7. Available from: https://doi.org/10.1007/s11920-013-0370-7.
107. Hofmeister S, Bodden S. Premenstrual syndrome and premenstrual dysphoric disorder. Am Fam Physician. 2016;94(3):236–40. Available from: https://www.aafp.org/afp/2016/0801/p236.html [Accessed 18th June, 2018].
108. Freeman EW, Halbreih U, Grubb GS, et al. An overview of four studies of a continuous oral contraceptive (levonorgestrel 90 mcg/ethinyl estradiol 20mcg) on premenstrual dysphoric disorder and premenstrual syndrome. Contraception. 2012;85(5):437–45. Available from: https://doi.org/10.1016/j.contraception.2011.09.101.
109. Boyer EW, Shannon M. The Serotonin syndrome. N Engl J Med. 2005;352:1112–20. Available from: https://www.nejm.org/doi/full/10.1056/NEJMra041867. Accessed 22 June 2018.
110. Cipriani A, Koesters M, Furukawa TA, et al. Duloxetine versus other anti-depressive agents for depression. Cochrane Database Syst Rev. 2012:1–96. Available from: https://doi.org/10.1002/14651858.CD006533.pub2.
111. Mitchell J, Trangle M, Degnan B, et al; Institute for Clinical Systems Improvement. Adult depression in primary care. https://www.icsi.org/_asset/fnhdm3/Depr-Interactive0512b.pdf. C2013 [updated 2013 Sep; cited 2018 Feb 23].
112. Goldstone D. Cognitive-behavioural therapy versus psychodynamic psychotherapy for the treatment of depression: a critical review of evidence and current issues. South Afr J Psychol. 2016;47(1):84–96.
113. Hollon SD, Thase ME, Markowitz JC. Treatment and prevention of depression. Psychol Sci Public Interest. 2002;3(2):39–77.
114. Melville JL, Reed SD, Russo J, et al. Improving care for depression in obstetrics and gynecology: a randomized controlled trial. Obstet Gynecol. 2014;123(6):1237–46.
115. American Psychiatric Association, Academy of Psychosomatic Medicine. Dissemination of integrated care within adult primary care settings; the collaborative care model. 2016 Spring.
116. American College of Obstetricians and Gynecologists. Screening for perinatal depression. Committee opinion No. 630. Obstet Gynecol. 2015;125:1268–71.
117. McCarron RM, Vanderlip ER, Rado J. Depression. Ann Intern Med. 2016;165:ITC49–64.
118. Langan RC, Goodbred AJ. Identification and Management of Peripartum Depression. Am Fam Physician. 2016;93(10):852–8.
119. Mitchell AJ, Yadegarfar M, Gill J, Stubbs B. Case finding and screening clinical utility of the Patient Health Questionnaire (PHQ-9 and PHQ-2) for depression in primary care: a diagnostic meta-analysis of 40 studies. BJPsych Open. 2016;2(2):127–38.
120. Norris D, Clark MS. Evaluation and treatment of the suicidal patient. Am Fam Physician. 85(6), March, 2012. 602-605. Hirschfeld RMA and JM Russell. Assessment and treatment of suicidal patients. N Engl J Med. 1997;337:910–5.

Eating Disorders and the Female Athlete Triad

34

Brianna Rossiter and Anna K. Donovan

Learning Objectives

1. Distinguish between the clinical presentations of the three most common eating disorders: anorexia nervosa, bulimia, and binge eating disorder.
2. Identify medical complications of eating disorders that necessitate inpatient evaluation and treatment.
3. Appropriately treat eating disorders with non-pharmacologic and pharmacologic approaches.
4. Describe the female athlete triad and discuss how this syndrome relates to disordered eating.

Gianna is a 33-year-old female who presents to your office as a new patient. She was previously seen in another state and moved here for work in a local law firm. She identifies heartburn and allergies as previous medical conditions. Her only complaint today is poor sleep. Her vital signs on presentation are a heart rate of 62, a blood pressure of 112/74, and a body mass index (BMI) of 16.

Background

Eating disorders (EDs) are classified under the category of "feeding and eating disorders" in the *Diagnostic and Statistical Manual of Mental Disorders* (DSM-5) [1]. These disorders are characterized by a persistent disturbance of eating or behavior regarding eating that results in impaired consumption or absorption of food. Importantly, these eating behaviors must co-exist with a significant impairment of physical health or psychosocial functioning [1]. The most familiar EDs seen by providers—anorexia nervosa (AN), bulimia nervosa (BN), and binge eating disorder (BED)—will be discussed in this chapter. Of note, the DSM-5 no longer uses the umbrella diagnosis of "not otherwise specified" (NOS); instead, EDs not meeting the diagnostic criteria of a particular type are classified as "Other Specified Feeding or Eating Disorder" (OSFED) and "Unspecified Feeding or Eating Disorder" (UFED) [1].

Epidemiology

The prevalence of EDs is challenging to estimate because available data are based on the DSM-4 criteria, which were more restrictive than the current DSM-5 criteria. Additionally, patients with EDs often go to great lengths to conceal their illness, leading to an underestimation of prevalence. Based on the DSM-4 criteria, the US lifetime prevalence estimates of anorexia nervosa, bulimia nervosa, and binge eating disorder are 0.9%, 1.5%, and 3.5%, respectively, among women and 0.3%, 0.5%, and 2.0%, respectively, among men [2]. Both AN and BN are more common in women than in men, with a median age of onset of 18-years-old.

Certain patients are at higher risk for AN and BN than others. For example, a history of dieting is common among individuals who subsequently develop severe EDs. Therefore, activities that emphasize low weight, such as certain sports (dancing, gymnastics, wrestling) and professions (modeling), may place individuals at increased risk of an ED. There is also evidence that genetics play a role in the development of EDs; individuals with a family history of EDs should be considered at higher risk [3, 4]. Additionally, AN and BN are associated with co-existing psychiatric conditions, most

B. Rossiter (✉)
VA Pittsburgh Healthcare System, Pittsburgh, PA, USA

University of Pittsburgh School of Medicine, Department of Medicine, Division of General Internal Medicine, Pittsburgh, PA, USA
e-mail: rossiterbc@upmc.edu

A. K. Donovan
IM Residency Training Program, University of Pittsburgh Medical Center-Presbyterian, Department of Medicine, Division of General Internal Medicine, Pittsburgh, PA, USA

S. A. Tilstra et al. (eds.), *Sex- and Gender-Based Women's Health*, https://doi.org/10.1007/978-3-030-50695-7_34

notably mood disorders and substance use disorders [5]. Bulimia in particular is associated with a history of sexual abuse [5]. Despite the widespread association between AN and higher socioeconomic status, this relationship has not been proven. However, increasing evidence suggests that an association between BN and lower socioeconomic status may exist [6].

Binge eating disorder (BED) is also more common in women than men. Prevalence rates are similar among various demographics irrespective of race, marital status, and employment status. The median age of onset of BED is approximately 23-years-old. Individuals with BED are more likely to have a higher body mass index and obesity when compared to the general population. Similar to AN and BN, over 70% of patients with BED have another co-existing psychiatric disorder [7].

Screening

There are currently no screening recommendations for EDs from major organizations (e.g., USPSTF), and few tools exist for use in the primary care setting [8]. While no major guidelines exist, primary care providers may opt to screen patients considered to be in higher-risk groups epidemiologically; these high-risk individuals include adolescent females, individuals with a family history of EDs, those with rapidly changing or low BMI, those with significant psychiatric illness, and those with high-risk careers like athletes and models [9].

There are currently no recommendations for screening for BED. Patients that should be considered for screening include those with rapid weight gain, high BMI, and underlying mood disorders; however, keep in mind that all patients with BED are not overweight. Screening tools created for use in patients with BED include the BEDS-7 [10], a patient-reported screening tool designed to identify individuals in need of referral to BED specialists. Questions of the BEDS-7 ask about episodes of excessive overeating and the characteristics and emotions that tend to accompany them.

Gianna reports insomnia and poor sleep for the last 10 years that has substantially worsened since moving to the area. She denies any problems falling asleep but awakens at night and cannot fall back to sleep. She reports that she often gets up and does work, or she will go to the kitchen to eat. She often feels guilty in the morning after eating late at night and admits to restricting food the following day.

Pathophysiology

The low population prevalence of EDs makes any prospective study to determine their pathophysiology challenging. A likely pathologic model for EDs is a combination of biologic, psychologic, and environmental factors. For example, anorexia nervosa has been linked to abnormalities in serotonin functioning, with animal models suggesting increased synaptic serotonin release with inhibition of feeding [11]. A number of other neurotransmitters and hormones have also been implicated in the development of AN, including elevated cortisol [12] and decreased oxytocin [13]. Most of the studies to date examining neurochemical changes in AN rely on indirect measures and are therefore challenging to interpret. Regardless of the proposed neurochemical changes, a "multiple-hit hypothesis" in regard to ED pathology is largely accepted [14], with the thought that a certain set of genes expressed under the right sociocultural conditions creates a likely environment for an ED. Similarly to AN, cholecystokinin [15], serotonin [16], and leptin [17] are suggested neurochemicals influencing binge and purge behaviors in BN. Recent data suggests a biologic basis for BED as well. Neuroimaging studies have suggested that individuals with BED have corticostriatal circulatory alterations similar to those seen in substance abuse, suggesting problems with impulse control [18]. Overall, further studies are needed to better understand the pathophysiology of various EDs.

Diagnostic Criteria and Clinical Manifestations

Eating disorders are diagnosed by their clinical features in the DSM-5. When diagnosing EDs, medical comorbidities (most often gastrointestinal disease) and food insecurity must be excluded.

Anorexia Nervosa

Anorexia nervosa is characterized by abnormally low body weight, an intense fear of gaining weight, and a distorted perception of body weight and shape [1]. Patients with AN will put forth significant effort to prevent weight gain even in the setting of a dangerously low BMI. Anorexia can be further categorized as restricting-type or binge eating/purging-type [19]. Restricting-type includes individuals who have not engaged in binge eating or purging behavior, but rather accomplish weight loss through calorie reduction, fasting, and/or excessive exercise. The binge eating/purging subtype encompasses individuals who engage in recurrent episodes of binge eating and purging behavior (described in the bulimia section). The severity of AN is based on BMI, with mild characterized by a BMI between 17 and 18.5 kg/m^2, moderate with a BMI between 16 and 16.99 kg/m^2, severe with a BMI between 15 and 15.99 kg/m^2, and extreme with a BMI under 15 kg/m^2 [1]. The level of severity also reflects the clinical symptoms, the degree of functional disability, and the need for supervision and medical intervention.

Features associated with AN may also include behaviors difficult to observe or assess, including features of extreme preoccupation with food, preference for low-calorie foods, overestimation of calories consumed, and food-related rituals. Food rituals can include behaviors such as cutting food into small pieces prior to eating or eating foods in a particular order. These behaviors can ultimately lead to social withdrawal, excessive exercise, restlessness, dysregulation of emotions, poor sleep, and low libido [20].

Bulimia Nervosa

The DSM-5 criteria for BN include recurrent episodes of binge eating with an accompanying, inappropriate compensatory behavior to prevent weight gain, regardless of a patient's current weight [1, 19]. A binge episode can be challenging to define as it is somewhat subjective based on an individual's determination of a "discrete amount of time" and a "large amount of food" as compared to most people. Regardless, an individual engages in a binge episode when they eat an excessive amount in a small period of time (e.g., 30 minutes to 2 hours). Most importantly, these episodes are defined as a total lack of eating control by the individuals (e.g., they feel that they cannot stop eating). This corresponding lack of control is essential in defining a binge episode. In BN, binge episodes are followed by inappropriate compensatory behaviors including activities such as self-induced vomiting, misuse of laxatives or diuretics, fasting, or excessive exercise. The combination of a binge episode and a compensatory behavior is the cornerstone feature of BN. To diagnose BN, behaviors must occur at least once per week for 3 months [1]. Severity is based on the number of episodes of compensatory behavior per week, with mild having an average of one to three episodes per week while extreme averages more than 14 binge episodes per week [1].

Binge Eating Disorder

Binge eating episodes are also required in the diagnosis of BED [1]. Similar to BN, individuals must feel a lack of control during the episode. In contrast to BN, the defining feature in BED is the significant emotional and/or psychological impairment that follows a binge episode. As noted above, defining an amount of food intake that qualifies as a binge eating episode can be challenging. The DSM-5 attempts to qualify a binge episode under the BED criteria with a binge episode having at least three of the following features: (1) eating well beyond the point of satiety, (2) eating more quickly than one would during a normal meal, (3) eating large amounts of food when one is not particularly hungry, (4) making efforts to cover up the binge or eating alone due to shame or embarrassment, and (5) feeling sad, depressed, or guilty after a binge [1]. Importantly, binge episodes must cause marked mental distress, and, unlike BN, the diagnosis of BED does not include any inappropriate compensatory behaviors. The BED level of severity is based upon the number of binge eating episodes per week: mild, one to three episodes per week; moderate, four to seven per week; severe, eight to 13 per week; and extreme, 14 or more episodes per week [1].

Associated Comorbidities

Psychiatric comorbidity is common among patients with EDs, but can be challenging to distinguish as some are secondary to the ED itself and can resolve with treatment of the ED [2, 21]. Many experts believe that the development of an ED is a way for individuals to exert control over their environment. It is often hard to distinguish if the ED manifests as a pathologic coping mechanism from a primary mood disorder or if the mood disorder is secondary to a primary ED. Ideally, the ED should be treated initially, and, following remission, the patient should be reassessed for any other persistent psychiatric comorbidities. The only exception is the co-existence of a severe substance use disorder, which should be prioritized at the time of initial treatment of the ED to manage withdrawal phenomena [22].

Although the specific rate of comorbid disorders differs between epidemiologic surveys and studies in clinical settings, there is general agreement that patients with AN and BN often suffer from anxiety, mood disorders, obsessive-compulsive disorder, body dysmorphic disorder, and PTSD [23]. The lifetime rates for these comorbidities in patients with EDs exceed the rates in the general population. As an example, the estimated lifetime prevalence of unipolar major depression in the general population is 23% compared to 50% in the ED population [24]. Lifetime rates of substance use disorders are also higher in patients with EDs [22] with alcohol use disorder being most common [25]. Bulimia nervosa is the most common ED associated with prior childhood trauma (e.g., sexual abuse) [26]. Personality disorders associated with EDs have received increasing attention, with the most commonly observed co-occurring personality disorders including histrionic, obsessive-compulsive, avoidant, dependent, and borderline personality types [27]. However, similar to determining prevalence data in EDs, determining the prevalence of personality disorders in individuals with EDs is also challenging. For example, a 2005 meta-analysis found the prevalence of personality disorders to be 0 to 58% among individuals with AN and BN, but documented that these associations are often determined through self-reported instruments that greatly overestimate personality disorder prevalence [28].

Patients with BED are also more likely to have comorbid psychiatric conditions; up to 79% of BED patients have at least one additional psychiatric diagnosis with specific phobia being most common. These prevalence rates are higher than in the general population [29]. Additionally, BED patients are more likely to have co-existing medical diagnoses in addition to psychiatric comorbidities. Specifically, individuals with a history of BED are at increased risk of developing chronic pain, diabetes mellitus, and hypertension [29].

You learn that Gianna lives alone and works as a lawyer in a new law firm. She is a never smoker, rarely drinks, and denies illicit drug use. She swam competitively until college. She has never been pregnant and only briefly used contraceptive pills. She reports that she intermittently would not get her period throughout high school and college and that currently her periods are irregular and very light.

Functional Hypothalamic Amenorrhea

Given that EDs often result in low energy availability from decreased caloric intake and/or excessive energy expenditure, ED patients are at risk of developing functional hypothalamic amenorrhea (FHA). FHA is a cause of secondary amenorrhea that results from abnormalities in pulsatile gonadotropin-releasing hormone (GnRH) secretion, which in turn causes less gonadotropin release (follicle-stimulating hormone and luteinizing hormone). The altered pathways result in complex hormonal changes, most notably, profound hypoestrogenism [30]. Disruption in GnRH drive is postulated to occur from energy deprivation by calorie restriction, excessive exercise, and/or psychological stress, acting to provoke hypothalamic disruption [31]. Importantly, as in every woman with new-onset secondary amenorrhea, other causes such as pregnancy, hypothyroidism, hyperprolactinemia, and polycystic ovary syndrome should first be excluded before diagnosing FHA [30]. Please see Chap. 5 on Menstruation and Secondary Amenorrhea to learn more about secondary amenorrhea.

Given the features of AN, patients with anorexia often have FHA. Importantly, amenorrhea is no longer a criterion for the diagnosis of AN in the DSM-5 [32]; however, it can serve as a surrogate marker for the severity of an eating disorder. Irregular menses or complete loss of menses in a patient who previously menstruated normally should be viewed as a red flag that requires additional history taking regarding food intake, excessive exercise, and restricting or purging behaviors.

The Female Athlete Triad

The female athlete triad is a syndrome often seen in competitive athletes and characterized by functional hypothalamic amenorrhea (FHA) [33]. This syndrome is defined by three components: (a) low energy availability with or without disordered eating, (b) menstrual dysfunction, and (c) low bone density [34, 35]. Patients with the female athlete triad most often have low BMIs and participate in activities where weight and aesthetics are important (dance, gymnastics, figure skating, cross-country, marathon runners). These patients tend to present with oligomenorrhea or amenorrhea in the setting of weight loss or extreme exercise. This causes low energy availability in turn causing dysregulation of gonadotropin-releasing hormone (GnRH) secretion, leading to a state of estrogen deficiency and FHA, much akin to the hormonal dysregulation experienced by patients with anorexia.

All patients with FHA live in an estrogen deficient state and are at increased risk for the consequences of estrogen deficiency, notably low bone density [36, 37]. Low bone density in an athlete can lead to stress fractures, occult fractures, and other musculoskeletal injuries. Evidence of hypothalamic dysfunction manifested clinically as oligomenorrhea, amenorrhea, or a stress fracture should be a red flag and prompt screening for an eating disorder. It is important to note that not every patient with FHA has an eating disorder, and hypothalamic dysfunction is a protective response when the body is in an energy deficient state as the body is unlikely to be able to support a healthy pregnancy.

Treatment of patients with the female athlete triad has several goals: restore normal menses, reverse and treat bone complications, treat underlying psychiatric disorders, and evaluate for any concomitant eating disorders. Most often, decreasing the number of workouts per week and increasing BMI will reinstitute the hypothalamic-pituitary-ovarian axis and normal menses will return. If patients who are overexercising are unwilling to decrease their workouts and do not have a sporting commitment, a provider should assess for the presence of restrictive eating habits and other purging behaviors such as the use of laxatives and vomiting. Psychological evaluation, either with a sports psychologist or therapist, is recommended if the patient has unrealistic performance expectations or places undue training demands on herself.

Combined oral contraceptives can be used to facilitate regular menses, endometrial protection, and pregnancy prevention; however, as per the Endocrine Society Clinical Practice Guidelines, it is not recommended to start oral contraceptive pills for the sole purpose of regaining menses or improving bone mineral density in patients with FHA [30]. Medroxyprogesterone acetate for contraception should be avoided if possible in patients with FHA as it has been associated with low bone mass and osteoporosis in long-term users [38]. Other aspects of bone health in FHA will be discussed later in the chapter.

Gianna is diagnosed with anorexia nervosa and desires treatment. She does not meet inpatient criteria for treatment and you refer her to an intensive outpatient program for patients with eating disorders.

Treatment

Eating disorders can be life-threatening, most often due to medical complications but occasionally secondary to suicide [39]. Unfortunately, complications compound because of patients' frequent refusal of treatment. Similar to patients with substance use disorders, patients must be active and willing participants in treatment to facilitate successful outcomes. Treatment of eating disorders generally involves an interdisciplinary team including, but not limited to, a mental health provider, a dietitian, and a general medical provider. Consultation with a mental health provider with expertise in eating disorders should be considered at the time of diagnosis [19].

Anorexia Treatment Options

Treatment for AN is challenging; standard treatment consists of nutritional rehabilitation and psychotherapy, with only occasional augmentation with pharmacotherapy [40]. Pharmacotherapy is not first-line treatment in AN and is never used alone [18–20]. Psychotherapy is essential, but there is no compelling evidence that one therapeutic modality is clearly superior to others [20, 41]. Options include cognitive behavioral therapy (CBT), group therapy, motivational interviewing, and family therapy. Thus, the choice is based upon availability, patient age, patient preference, and cost.

All patients with AN should be engaged in nutritional rehabilitation for guidance on dietary choices and caloric management. Nutritional rehabilitation is best done at a dedicated ED treatment center with knowledgeable nutritionists. Notably, there is tension between weight restoration and patient anxiety; most patients will be resistant to weight recovery. Caloric requirements in patients with AN are high and vary between 30–40 kcal/kg/day for inpatients and 20 kcal/kg/day for outpatients. These caloric amounts will facilitate weight gain of 1–1.5 kg/week in the inpatient setting and of 0.5 kg/week in the outpatient setting [42].

Adjunctive pharmacotherapy may help reduce symptoms of depression and anxiety in patients who do not respond to psychotherapy and/or treat primary psychiatric disorders [40, 43]. However, distorted thinking about body image and food usually will not respond to pharmacotherapy, nor do drugs delay or prevent subsequent episodes of anorexia nervosa [44]. Patients should be seen often, sometimes weekly, for weight checks, lab monitoring, and assessment of the recovery process [45]. One should consider blinding the patient to weight checks in the office as weight can be a trigger for restrictive behavior, especially in those with a history of AN in remission.

Bulimia Treatment Options

Similar to AN, standard treatment for BN includes nutritional rehabilitation and psychotherapy, with a slightly larger role for pharmacotherapy [40, 46–48]. Notably for patients with BN, management of electrolyte imbalances is essential given purging behaviors. Patients may require high-dose electrolyte replacement from excessive vomiting or laxative use. Patients with BN benefit from nutritional counseling to help disrupt the binging and purging cycle. For patients with bulimia nervosa, CBT is superior to other psychotherapies [46]. Pharmacotherapy alone appears to be less efficacious than psychotherapy alone, but combining the two is the preferred approach [46]. If nutritional rehabilitation and psychotherapy are not available, pharmacotherapy alone is reasonable in the treatment of BN. Selective serotonin reuptake inhibitors (SSRIs) are better tolerated than other medications and recommended over tricyclic antidepressants (TCAs) or monoamine oxidase inhibitors (MAOIs). These medications also help treat a co-existing mood disorder. Bupropion is contraindicated in patients with BN given the risk of seizures secondary to electrolyte disturbances.

Binge Eating Disorder Treatment Options

Management of a patient with BED is twofold: (1) assess for and treat comorbid psychiatric disorders, and (2) treat underlying overweight- and obesity-related comorbidities. Exploring the patient's attitude toward their body weight and shape and their current and future nutritional goals is important. While multiple treatment modalities exist, including psychotherapy, self-help treatment, pharmacotherapy, and behavioral weight loss treatment, psychotherapy is preferred [49]. Studies have indicated that psychotherapy alone is more beneficial than pharmacotherapy alone, with the preferred first-line treatment being cognitive behavioral therapy or interpersonal therapy [50].

Several types of medication have been studied for BED and include SSRIs, antiepileptic drugs (e.g., topiramate), and medications typically indicated for attention deficit hyperactivity disorder (e.g., atomoxetine and lisdexamfetamine) [51]. SSRIs are the preferred medication given their efficacy and tolerability [51]. Additionally, antiepileptics and stimulants have the potential for adverse effects and potential for abuse or dependence. Among antiepileptic drugs, topiramate often reduces hunger and promotes weight loss, resulting in a significant reduction in daily binge episodes and impulsivity. Importantly, topiramate is contraindicated in pregnancy and can lower the efficacy of estrogen and/or progesterone-analog contraceptives. This should be taken into consideration given the prevalence of young women with eating disorders. Drugs that treat attention deficit hyperactivity disorder facilitate function of the dopamine and/or norepinephrine systems, which are involved in eating behavior and subsequent reward that manifests in binge eating [52]. However, these stimulant medications are controlled substances and contraindicated in patients with significant cardiovascular comorbidities.

Gianna presents for her 9-month follow-up visit. She looks tired and withdrawn but does not have any specific complaints. Vital signs at this visit include a heart rate of 52 and blood pressure of 91/76. Patient is orthostatic by HR and BP. BMI is noted to be 15.6. You facilitate immediate admission to an inpatient program for treatment of AN.

Criteria for Hospitalization

Anorexia nervosa is the ED most likely to require inpatient evaluation and stabilization based on potential laboratory and cardiac abnormalities [53]. The goal of hospitalization is to restore nutrition and vital metabolic functions that are compromised by chronic underfeeding. Patients with BN may also require inpatient electrolyte correction given purging behaviors that result in hypokalemia, hypomagnesemia, and hypophosphatemia. The evaluation for inpatient admission for patients with ED starts with the physical examination. Exam findings that suggest severe malnutrition and a need for immediate medical evaluation include low body mass index (<17.5 kg/m^2), a core body temperature <35 °C, a heart rate <60 beats per minute, and/or a systolic blood pressure <90 mmHg. Additional exam findings may include hypoactive bowel sounds, xerosis, brittle hair, hair loss, and lanugo hair growth. Recommended laboratory testing for these patients includes serum electrolytes including calcium, potassium, phosphorus, and magnesium, serum albumin and pre-albumin, liver function tests, thyroid-stimulating hormone, and a pregnancy test in women. Bradycardia should prompt immediate electrocardiogram evaluation to assess for changes related to electrolyte abnormalities and profound malnutrition [54].

If severe exam findings are not present, most medical complications of anorexia nervosa are managed in outpatient or residential care facilities [40]. Other treatment settings that may be available include intensive outpatient (e.g., 2 to 3 hours per weekday) and partial hospitalization (day program that provides 6 to 8 hours of outpatient care per weekday). While there are no evidence-based criteria indicating which patients with anorexia nervosa need hospitalization [53], clinical practice guidelines suggest inpatient hospitalization for adult patients with profound vital sign abnormalities, concern for cardiac dysrhythmia, and/or concern for refeeding syndrome [54]. Profound vital sign abnormalities include a pulse less than 40 beats per minute, a blood pressure <80/60 mmHg, weight <70 percent ideal body weight, or BMI <15 kg/m^2 or signs of marked dehydration. The most concerning cardiac features include an increased PR interval, first-degree heart block, ST wave abnormalities, and a QTc > 499 msec [55].

Refeeding syndrome is a potentially fatal complication of malnutrition that occurs as a result of fluid and electrolyte shifts during aggressive nutritional rehabilitation [56]. The most worrisome electrolyte abnormality in refeeding is hypophosphatemia. AN patients are already phosphate depleted from starvation. Subsequent refeeding causes insulin release resulting in additional cellular uptake of phosphate and worsening hypophosphatemia. This lack of phosphorylated intermediates causes tissue hypoxia and resultant myocardial dysfunction and potential respiratory failure [57]. While it is difficult to determine which ED patients will experience refeeding syndrome, those with lower BMI and starvation in the 5–10 days preceding nutritional support are most at risk [56].

There is currently a lack of evidence regarding the decision for voluntary versus involuntary hospitalization in patients with severe presentations of AN or BN [58, 59]. Assessing the patient's intentional and unintentional risk to self and ability to understand the consequences of their actions and decisions is vital in assessing the need for involuntary inpatient admission.

Early Medical Complications of Eating Disorders

Regardless of the treatment setting, patients with AN and BN exhibit medical complications early in their course. Early complications of anorexia, aside from those already discussed, are broad in clinical scope. Complications range from arrested growth and myocardial atrophy to unplanned pregnancy with neonatal complications to cognitive impairment [60, 61].

Early complications of BN include xerosis, parotid gland swelling, and erosion of dental enamel. Gastrointestinal complications are common with possible loss of gag reflex, ongoing abdominal pain and bloating, Mallory-Weiss syndrome, gastroesophageal reflux disease (GERD), and colonic dysmotility. As noted above, the most common renal and electrolyte complications of BN include dehydration, hypokalemia, hypochloremia, and metabolic alkalosis. Cardiac complications are rare in BN but can include orthostasis resulting in syncope, sinus tachycardia, palpitations, and arrhythmias.

Early medical complications of BED can include insulin resistance, hypertension, hyperlipidemia, and metabolic syndrome [2]. Should patients develop morbid obesity as a result of BED, they are at ongoing risk for resistant hypertension, obstructive sleep apnea, and diabetes.

Gianna presents to your office 5 years after her hospitalization for routine follow-up. She has been doing well and has since married. She is having regular periods and her BMI is 21. She and her husband are interested in getting pregnant.

Sexuality, Fertility, and Pregnancy

A concern for patients with EDs includes future fertility given the suppression of the hypothalamic-pituitary-ovarian axis resulting in hypogonadotropic hypogonadism with amenorrhea (as discussed above). Importantly, reproductive function is restored in approximately 85 percent of women following weight recovery [62], so nutritional support in a treatment protocol is essential. Aside from these hormonal disturbances, eating disorders affect patients' sexuality because of body image issues and low libido. Unexpected pregnancy can occur given irregular menses, as patients may nevertheless ovulate either intermittently or regularly. Pregnancy itself is often a time when eating disorders come to clinical attention given that weight and eating habits are closely monitored at this time. This may be an opportunity for recovery in some, but for other patients, pregnancy is a period of vulnerability for the onset, persistence, or relapse of ED symptoms [63].

Women with eating disorders who consider becoming pregnant should receive preconception counseling about the risks to the patient and child, as well as education about body changes and weight gain during pregnancy. Patients should ideally postpone pregnancy until the disorder and medical complications are stable. The dietary habits of patients with eating disorders must be monitored to ensure proper weight gain and fetal growth, and nutritional guidance should be provided. In addition, patients with ED should be asked about the use of teratogenic medications, including appetite suppressants, diuretics, and excess use of laxatives.

In women with a history of AN and BN, fertility rates appear to be comparable to those in the general population [62]. However, eating disorders appear to be associated with several adverse perinatal outcomes, to both mother and offspring. Maternal AN is associated with slow fetal growth, premature contractions, and infants that are small for gestational age. Maternal BN is associated with premature contractions and low Apgar scores. Alternatively, BED is associated positively with maternal hypertension and large-for-gestational-age infants [64].

Bone Health

Osteoporosis is a common complication of anorexia nervosa. Multiple factors increase risk, including decreased body weight and fat content, elevated cortisol levels, inadequate vitamin D and calcium intake, and amenorrhea and hypoestrogenism. There are both decreased bone formation and increased bone resorption in patients with AN. It places these patients at an increased lifetime risk for fractures. Bone loss may never recover completely even if weight is restored. The degree of osteopenia depends on the age of onset and duration of amenorrhea.

The etiology of bone loss in the patient with anorexia nervosa is multifactorial. In addition to reduced estrogen and progesterone, excess cortisol levels and low levels of insulin growth factor (IGF-1), a correlate for bone formation, are observed. While low estradiol levels contribute to bone loss, the severity of bone loss in women with AN is greater than in those with normal-weight hypothalamic amenorrhea, indicating that, in addition to estradiol deficiency, there are other factors including nutritional deficiencies and hormonal abnormalities that contribute to bone loss [65].

Dual-energy X-ray absorptiometry (DXA) screening is important to assess bone mineral density (BMD). While no guidelines exist for screening, one option is to obtain a baseline DXA measurement with periodic follow-up in females with persistently low weight. Assessment of other risk factors for osteopenia, such as reproductive and family history, smoking, excessive alcohol use, and use of medications affecting bone metabolism, should be assessed [32].

Successful treatments to reverse bone loss in those with anorexia nervosa are lacking. Treatment includes weight normalization and supplemental calcium and vitamin D. Exercise regimens must be individualized; while weight-bearing exercise is generally beneficial to the bone, overexercise in these women can perpetuate weight loss and amenorrhea, thereby leading to bone loss. In addition, women with severe bone loss are at risk for exercise-related stress fractures. Weight gain and restoration of menstrual cycles can independently improve BMD, and they remain the primary goal [66].

The data for use of hormones in FHA specifically secondary to AN is not known, with some studies suggesting modest improvement in bone mineral density and others showing a marginal, if any, effect [67]. In other states of estrogen deficiency, estrogen replacement therapy prevents further bone loss. While oral contraceptives are widely prescribed for this purpose in the clinical setting, the efficacy of combination estrogen-progestin in the treatment of osteopenia of anorexia nervosa lacks sufficient evidence, with multiple studies showing no effect on BMD [68]. There is some data that physiologic transdermal estrogen dosing, which is lower than the dosing of estrogen in contraceptive pills, does improve BMD in adolescent girls and adults with AN [69–71]. Unfortunately, physiologic dosing of estrogen does not protect women from pregnancy. In women with prolonged amenorrhea who do not need pregnancy protection, transdermal physiologic estrogen with cyclic micronized progesterone is a reasonable option to negate the bone loss associated with FHA. Women in need of contraception have two options: (1) insertion of a levonorgestrel IUD combined with transdermal physiologic estrogen or (2) combined oral contraceptive pills. Whether these measures translate into a decrease in fracture risk is unclear and more data are needed.

Prognosis and Relapse

Both anorexia and bulimia are marked by a prolonged course to recovery. In AN, there is an almost 18-fold increase in mortality including a high suicide rate. Recurrent bouts of AN occur in approximately 20 percent of individuals. Mitigating factors include onset of the disorder during adolescence and longer duration of follow-up [40]. The longer-term outcome of BN is only slightly better compared to AN; however, the rate of mortality is low. As a general guideline, it appears that a third of BN patients fully recover, a third experience persistent symptoms without meeting the threshold for a formal diagnosis, and a third transition into a chronic eating disorder [40]. Unlike individuals with AN and BN, who may present to providers with more obvious clinical signs, individuals with BED often go undiagnosed and thus untreated. Without treatment, binge eating disorder is likely to last for many years and to cause a significant impact on weight, health, psychiatric symptoms, and ability to function. In some cases, serious effects of binge eating disorder on health could result in death from suicide or medical complications [1].

Summary Points

1. The three most common eating disorders are anorexia nervosa, bulimia nervosa, and binge eating disorder. Differentiating features include the patient's body weight/BMI at presentation, presence of binge eating, and compensatory behaviors to prevent weight gain.
2. Serious complications of eating disorders include cardiac and hypothalamic-pituitary-ovarian axis dysregulation, electrolyte disturbances, osteoporosis, and gastroparesis. Patients with poor response to outpatient treatment, unstable vital signs, evidence of arrhythmia, weight <70% of ideal body weight, and/or concern for refeeding syndrome should be immediately hospitalized.
3. Patients with eating disorders are best cared for by an interdisciplinary team consisting of a mental health provider, a dietitian, and a primary care provider. Cognitive behavioral therapy and treatment of any underlying mood or substance use disorder is essential for success.
4. Severe energy restriction or expenditure can cause hypothalamic-pituitary-ovarian axis dysfunction, leading to the female athlete triad, a syndrome characterized by (1) low energy availability, (2) menstrual dysfunction, and (3) low bone density.

Review Questions

1. A 19-year-old woman is evaluated during an office visit. She feels the need to diet to achieve a more appropriate body weight and exercises daily. Dietary history suggests that she consumes very little food, but at least twice per week she eats large amounts of high-calorie desserts over the course of 2 hours with compensatory purging behavior by vomiting. Her menses are irregular with 40–60 days between cycles. Physical exam is notable for a BMI of 23 and parotid enlargement.

   Which of the following is the most likely diagnosis?

   A. Anorexia nervosa
   B. Bulimia nervosa
   C. Binge eating disorder
   D. Female athlete triad

   The correct answer is B. Bulimia nervosa is characterized by frequent episodes of binge eating followed by inappropriate compensatory behaviors such as exercise or food restriction due to fear of weight gain. Physical examination may reveal erosion of dental enamel, parotid gland swelling, and Russell sign (scarring or calluses on the dorsum of the hand). Anorexia nervosa is characterized by persistent caloric intake restriction leading to significantly low body weight and a distorted body image. Subtypes include restricting type (no binge eating or purging behaviors) and binge eating/purging type (purging with or without binging). The differentiating factor between bulimia nervosa and the purging subtype of anorexia nervosa is BMI. The diagnostic criteria for anorexia require that the patient be underweight, generally with a BMI less than 18.5. Menstrual irregularities occur in both anorexia nervosa and bulimia nervosa and are present in approximately one half to one third of patients with bulimia. Although amenorrhea previously was a requirement for the diagnosis of anorexia nervosa, it has been removed from the diagnostic criteria in the DSM-5 [1].

2. A 31-year-old female presents to establish care. On review of systems, she acknowledges that she sometimes eats large amounts of food and is unable to stop until she has consumed an entire family-size bag of candy or a bag of potato chips. She says that this eating behavior occurs almost daily when she is stressed. She denies compensatory purging behaviors. She is upset about her weight and would like to lose 15 lbs. Physical exam is normal with the exception of BMI, which is 29. What is the most appropriate treatment option for her condition?
   A. Cognitive behavioral therapy
   B. Family therapy
   C. Orlistat
   D. Atomoxetine

   The correct answer is A. This patient has binge eating disorder (BED). Psychotherapy, particularly cognitive behavioral therapy, is first-line treatment for BED. Reviews have consistently concluded that psychotherapy alone is more beneficial than pharmacotherapy alone in treating binge eating disorder [45]. Medication is also efficacious as a second-line treatment. Additionally, pharmacotherapy may require less time or be less expensive. It is reasonable to use pharmacotherapy as first-line treatment for patients who prefer medication and decline psychotherapy, as well as patients who do not have access to psychotherapy. If pharmacotherapy is selected, the best option is an SSRI. For patients with BED who do not respond to courses of an SSRI, medications such as an anticonvulsant (i.e., topiramate) or a first-line medication for attention deficit hyperactivity disorder (i.e., atomoxetine or lisdexamfetamine) are preferred. However, there have been no head-to-head trials of an SSRI to either topiramate or a stimulant for this indication. Additionally, these medications have greater negative side-effect profiles: topiramate can cause cognitive impairment and somnolence, whereas stimulants can cause anorexia, gastrointestinal distress, headaches, and insomnia and have a potential for abuse. Lastly, anti-obesity medications are not recommended because of lack of efficacy, high remission rates, and adverse effects [72].

3. A 28-year-old woman is evaluated for infertility. She reports having had normal puberty but irregular menses since her teens. She has been unable to become pregnant since marrying 1 year ago despite regular intercourse. During the past year, she has menstruated three times. She was a track athlete in high school and college and still enjoys distance running. On physical examination, blood pressure is 108/72 mm Hg, pulse rate is 52/min, and BMI is 16. There is no evidence of hirsutism or acne. Genital exam is normal. Results of laboratory studies including a prolactin, TSH, LH/FSH, and beta human chorionic gonadotropin are normal. Which of the following is the most appropriate next step in management?
   A. Clomiphene
   B. Pelvic ultrasonography
   C. Referral to a reproductive endocrinologist
   D. Weight gain and decreased exercise

   The correct answer is D. Functional hypothalamic amenorrhea (FHA) is a reversible cause of infertility, which resolves over a period of time after energy availability normalizes or any underlying stress contributing to FHA resolves [73]. Given this patient's low body mass index and irregular menses with normal labs, it is reasonable to recommend weight gain to regain ovulatory function and allow for pregnancy before pursuing alternate diagnoses.

References

1. Association AP. Diagnostic and statistical manual of mental disorders. 5th ed: American Psychiatric Association; 2013.
2. Hudson JI, Hiripi E, Pope HG Jr, Kessler RC. The prevalence and correlates of eating disorders in the National Comorbidity Survey Replication. Biol Psychiatry. 2007;61(3):348–58.
3. Hoek HW. The incidence and prevalence of anorexia nervosa and bulimia nervosa in primary care. Psychol Med. 1991;21(2):455–60.
4. Klump KL, Kaye WH, Strober M. The evolving genetic foundations of eating disorders. Psychiatr Clin North Am. 2001;24(2):215–25.
5. Fairburn CG, Harrison PJ. Eating Dis. Lancet (London, England). 2003;361(9355):407–16.
6. Gard MC, Freeman CP. The dismantling of a myth: a review of eating disorders and socioeconomic status. Int J Eat Disord. 1996;20(1):1–12.
7. Grilo CM, White MA, Masheb RM. DSM-IV psychiatric disorder comorbidity and its correlates in binge eating disorder. Int J Eat Disord. 2009;42(3):228–34.

8. Knapp J, Aerni G, Anderson J. Eating disorders in female athletes: use of screening tools. Curr Sports Med Rep. 2014;13(4):214–8.
9. Swanson SA, Crow SJ, Le Grange D, Swendsen J, Merikangas KR. Prevalence and correlates of eating disorders in adolescents. Results from the national comorbidity survey replication adolescent supplement. Arch Gen Psychiatry. 2011;68(7):714–23.
10. Herman BK, Deal LS, DiBenedetti DB, Nelson L, Fehnel SE, Brown TM. Development of the 7-Item Binge-Eating Disorder Screener (BEDS-7). Prim Care Companion CNS Disord. 2016;18:2.
11. Kaye WH. Anorexia nervosa, obsessional behavior, and serotonin. Psychopharmacol Bull. 1997;33(3):335–44.
12. Kaye WH, Gwirtsman HE, George DT, Ebert MH, Jimerson DC, Tomai TP, et al. Elevated cerebrospinal fluid levels of immunoreactive corticotropin-releasing hormone in anorexia nervosa: relation to state of nutrition, adrenal function, and intensity of depression. J Clin Endocrinol Metab. 1987;64(2):203–8.
13. Demitrack MA, Lesem MD, Listwak SJ, Brandt HA, Jimerson DC, Gold PW. CSF oxytocin in anorexia nervosa and bulimia nervosa: clinical and pathophysiologic considerations. Am J Psychiatr. 1990;147(7):882–6.
14. Klein DA, Walsh BT. Eating disorders: clinical features and pathophysiology. Physiol Behav. 2004;81(2):359–74.
15. Phillipp E, Pirke KM, Kellner MB, Krieg JC. Disturbed cholecystokinin secretion in patients with eating disorders. Life Sci. 1991;48(25):2443–50.
16. Monteleone P, Brambilla F, Bortolotti F, Maj M. Serotonergic dysfunction across the eating disorders: relationship to eating behaviour, purging behaviour, nutritional status and general psychopathology. Psychol Med. 2000;30(5):1099–110.
17. Brewerton TD, Lesem MD, Kennedy A, Garvey WT. Reduced plasma leptin concentrations in bulimia nervosa. Psychoneuroendocrinology. 2000;25(7):649–58.
18. Kessler RM, Hutson PH, Herman BK, Potenza MN. The neurobiological basis of binge-eating disorder. Neurosci Biobehav Rev. 2016;63:223–38.
19. Attia E. In the clinic. Eating Dis. Ann Intern Med. 2012;156(7):ITC4–1.
20. Attia E, Walsh BT. Behavioral management for anorexia nervosa. N Engl J Med. 2009;360(5):500–6.
21. Gregorowski C, Seedat S, Jordaan GP. A clinical approach to the assessment and management of co-morbid eating disorders and substance use disorders. BMC Psychiatry. 2013;13:289.
22. Harrop EN, Marlatt GA. The comorbidity of substance use disorders and eating disorders in women: prevalence, etiology, and treatment. Addict Behav. 2010;35(5):392–8.
23. Kaye WH, Bulik CM, Thornton L, Barbarich N, Masters K. Comorbidity of anxiety disorders with anorexia and bulimia nervosa. Am J Psychiatry. 2004;161(12):2215–21.
24. Fernandez-Aranda F, Pinheiro AP, Tozzi F, Thornton LM, Fichter MM, Halmi KA, et al. Symptom profile of major depressive disorder in women with eating disorders. Aust N Z J Psychiatry. 2007;41(1):24–31.
25. Bulik CM, Klump KL, Thornton L, Kaplan AS, Devlin B, Fichter MM, et al. Alcohol use disorder comorbidity in eating disorders: a multicenter study. J Clin Psychiatry. 2004;65(7):1000–6.
26. Wonderlich SA, Brewerton TD, Jocic Z, Dansky BS, Abbott DW. Relationship of childhood sexual abuse and eating disorders. J Am Acad Child Adolesc Psychiatry. 1997;36(8):1107–15.
27. Tomotake M, Ohmori T. Personality profiles in patients with eating disorders. J Med Investig. 2002;49(3–4):87–96.
28. Cassin SE, von Ranson KM. Personality and eating disorders: a decade in review. Clin Psychol Rev. 2005;25(7):895–916.
29. Kessler RC, Berglund PA, Chiu WT, Deitz AC, Hudson JI, Shahly V, et al. The prevalence and correlates of binge eating disorder in the World Health Organization World Mental Health Surveys. Biol Psychiatry. 2013;73(9):904–14.
30. Gordon CM, Ackerman KE, Berga SL, Kaplan JR, Mastorakos G, Misra M, et al. Functional hypothalamic amenorrhea: an Endocrine Society clinical practice guideline. Biol Psychiatry. 2017;102(5):1413–39.
31. Marcus MD, Loucks TL, Berga SL. Psychological correlates of functional hypothalamic amenorrhea. Fertil Steril. 2001;76(2):310–6.
32. Misra M, Klibanski A. Endocrine consequences of anorexia nervosa. Lancet Diabetes Endocrinol. 2014;2(7):581–92.
33. De Souza MJ, Nattiv A, Joy E, Misra M, Williams NI, Mallinson RJ, et al. 2014 Female athlete triad coalition consensus statement on treatment and return to play of the female athlete triad: 1st international conference held in San Francisco, CA, May 2012, and 2nd international conference held in Indianapolis, IN, May 2013. Clin J Sport Med. 2014;24(2):96–119.
34. Arntfield SL, Slesar K, Dickson J, Charon R. Narrative medicine as a means of training medical students toward residency competencies. Patient Educ Couns. 2013;91(3):280–6.
35. Payne JM, Kirchner JT. Should you suspect the female athlete triad? Patient Educ Couns. 2014;63(4):187–92.
36. Marquez S, Molinero O. Energy availability, menstrual dysfunction and bone health in sports; an overview of the female athlete triad. Nutr Hosp. 2013;28(4):1010–7.
37. Hergenroeder AC, De Souza MJ, Anding RH. The female athlete triad: energy deficiency, physiologic consequences, and treatment. Adolesc Med State Art Rev. 2015;26(1):116–42.
38. Modesto W, Bahamondes MV, Bahamondes L. Prevalence of low bone mass and osteoporosis in long-term users of the injectable contraceptive depot medroxyprogesterone acetate. J Womens Health (Larchmt). 2015;24(8):636–40.
39. Stephen EM, Rose J, Kenney L, Rosselli-Navarra F, Weissman RS. Adolescent risk factors for purging in young women: findings from the national longitudinal study of adolescent health. J Eat Dis. 2014;2:1.
40. American Psychiatric Association. Treatment of patients with eating disorders,third edition. Am J Psychiatry. 2006;163(7 Suppl): 4–54.
41. Hay PJ, Claudino AM, Touyz S, Abd Elbaky G. Individual psychological therapy in the outpatient treatment of adults with anorexia nervosa. Cochrane Database Syst Rev. 2015;(7):Cd003909.
42. Marzola E, Nasser JA, Hashim SA, Shih PA, Kaye WH. Nutritional rehabilitation in anorexia nervosa: review of the literature and implications for treatment. BMC Psychiatry. 2013;13:290.
43. Carlos M. Grilo JEM. The treatment of eating disorders: a clinical handbook Guilford Press: New York. 2011.
44. Bulik CM, Berkman ND, Brownley KA, Sedway JA, Lohr KN. Anorexia nervosa treatment: a systematic review of randomized controlled trials. Int J Eat Disord. 2007;40(4):310–20.
45. Wilson GT, Shafran R. Eating disorders guidelines from NICE. Lancet (London, England). 2005;365(9453):79–81.
46. Bacaltchuk J, Hay P, Trefiglio R. Antidepressants versus psychological treatments and their combination for bulimia nervosa. Cochrane Database Syst Rev. 2001;(4):Cd003385.
47. Shapiro JR, Berkman ND, Brownley KA, Sedway JA, Lohr KN, Bulik CM. Bulimia nervosa treatment: a systematic review of randomized controlled trials. Int J Eat Disord. 2007;40(4):321–36.
48. Bacaltchuk J, Hay P. Antidepressants versus placebo for people with bulimia nervosa. Cochrane Database Syst Rev. 2003;(4):Cd003391.
49. Wilson GT, Grilo CM, Vitousek KM. Psychological treatment of eating disorders. Am Psychol. 2007;62(3):199–216.
50. Vocks S, Tuschen-Caffier B, Pietrowsky R, Rustenbach SJ, Kersting A, Herpertz S. Meta-analysis of the effectiveness of psychological and pharmacological treatments for binge eating disorder. Int J Eat Disord. 2010;43(3):205–17.
51. Reas DL, Grilo CM. Review and meta-analysis of pharmacotherapy for binge-eating disorder. Obesity (Silver Spring, Md). 2008;16(9):2024–38.

52. Wang GJ, Geliebter A, Volkow ND, Telang FW, Logan J, Jayne MC, et al. Enhanced striatal dopamine release during food stimulation in binge eating disorder. Obesity (Silver Spring, Md). 2011;19(8):1601–8.
53. Williams PM, Goodie J, Motsinger CD. Treating eating disorders in primary care. Am Fam Physician. 2008;77(2):187–95.
54. Sachs KV, Harnke B, Mehler PS, Krantz MJ. Cardiovascular complications of anorexia nervosa: a systematic review. Int J Eat Disord. 2016;49(3):238–48.
55. American Psychiatric Association Work Group on Eating Disorders. Practice guideline for the treatment of patients with eating disorders (revision). Am J Psychiatry. 2000;157(1 Suppl):1–39.
56. Mehanna HM, Moledina J, Travis J. Refeeding syndrome: what it is, and how to prevent and treat it. BMJ (Clinical research ed). 2008;336(7659):1495–8.
57. Boateng AA, Sriram K, Meguid MM, Crook M. Refeeding syndrome: treatment considerations based on collective analysis of literature case reports. Nutrition (Burbank, Los Angeles County, Calif). 2010;26(2):156–67.
58. Clausen L, Jones A. A systematic review of the frequency, duration, type and effect of involuntary treatment for people with anorexia nervosa, and an analysis of patient characteristics. J Eat Disord. 2014;2(1):29.
59. Watson TL, Bowers WA, Andersen AE. Involuntary treatment of eating disorders. Am J Psychiatry. 2000;157(11):1806–10.
60. Westmoreland P, Krantz MJ, Mehler PS. Medical complications of anorexia nervosa and bulimia. Am J Med. 2016;129(1):30–7.
61. Mitchell JE, Crow S. Medical complications of anorexia nervosa and bulimia nervosa. Curr Opin Psychiatry. 2006;19(4):438–43.
62. Wolfe BE. Reproductive health in women with eating disorders. J Obstet Gynecol Neonatal Nurs. 2005;34(2):255–63.
63. Astrachan-Fletcher E, Veldhuis C, Lively N, Fowler C, Marcks B. The reciprocal effects of eating disorders and the postpartum period: a review of the literature and recommendations for clinical care. J Womens Health (Larchmt) (2002). 2008;17(2): 227–39.
64. Linna MS, Raevuori A, Haukka J, Suvisaari JM, Suokas JT, Gissler M. Pregnancy, obstetric, and perinatal health outcomes in eating disorders. Am J Obstet Gynecol. 2014;211(4):392.e1–8.
65. Grinspoon S, Miller K, Coyle C, Krempin J, Armstrong C, Pitts S, et al. Severity of osteopenia in estrogen-deficient women with anorexia nervosa and hypothalamic amenorrhea. J Clin Endocrinol Metab. 1999;84(6):2049–55.
66. Misra M, Klibanski A. Anorexia nervosa and bone. J Endocrinol. 2014;221(3):R163–76.
67. Misra M, Klibanski A. Bone health in anorexia nervosa. Curr Opin Endocrinol Diabetes Obe. 2011;18(6):376–82.
68. Golden NH, Lanzkowsky L, Schebendach J, Palestro CJ, Jacobson MS, Shenker IR. The effect of estrogen-progestin treatment on bone mineral density in anorexia nervosa. J Pediatr Adolesc Gynecol. 2002;15(3):135–43.
69. Strokosch GR, Friedman AJ, Wu SC, Kamin M. Effects of an oral contraceptive (norgestimate/ethinyl estradiol) on bone mineral density in adolescent females with anorexia nervosa: a double-blind, placebo-controlled study. J Adolesc Health. 2006;39(6):819–27.
70. Misra M, Katzman D, Miller KK, Mendes N, Snelgrove D, Russell M, et al. Physiologic estrogen replacement increases bone density in adolescent girls with anorexia nervosa. J Bone Miner Res. 2011;26(10):2430–8. https://doi.org/10.1002/jbmr.447.
71. Robinson L, Aldridge V, Clark EM, Misra M, Micali N. Pharmacological treatment options for low bone mineral density and secondary osteoporosis in anorexia nervosa: a systematic review of the literature. J Psychosom Res. 20171;98:87–97. https://doi.org/10.1016/j.jpsychores.2017.05.011. Epub 2017 May 12.
72. Grilo CM, Masheb RM, Salant SL. Cognitive behavioral therapy guided self-help and orlistat for the treatment of binge eating disorder: a randomized, double-blind, placebo-controlled trial. Biol Psychiatry. 2005;57(10):1193–201.
73. Perkins RB, Hall JE, Martin KA. Neuroendocrine abnormalities in hypothalamic amenorrhea: spectrum, stability, and response to neurotransmitter modulation. J Clin Endocrinol Metab. 1999;84(6):1905–11.

Part VII

Selected Populations

Intimate Partner Violence and Sexual Trauma

35

Raquel A. Buranosky and Jennifer S. McCall-Hosenfeld

Learning Objectives

1. Describe the components and dynamics of IPV, including the factors that sustain as well as interrupt the cycle of violence.
2. Identify the clinical signs of IPV and other forms of violence against women (VAW) including sexual violence and human trafficking.
3. Recognize the biopsychosocial, physical, and sexual sequelae of VAW.
4. Using evidence-based strategies perform a patient-centered assessment for IPV.
5. Summarize the primary provider's role in intervention, treatment, and referral for IPV.
6. Develop a strategy for trauma-informed care of people suffering the sequelae of VAW, including PTSD.
7. Outline the key components of safety planning for survivors of IPV.

We recognize that persons of all genders may be victims as well as perpetrators of IPV, sexual violence, and human trafficking. As this chapter was specifically written for a women's health text, and to avoid pronoun confusion, we primarily use the female pronoun to describe victims of VAW. As most perpetrators are male, we also use male pronouns to indicate perpetrators. We encourage healthcare providers to be alert to VAW in all healthcare encounters, with persons of all genders, including gender-fluid and non-conforming individuals.

R. A. Buranosky
University of Pittsburgh Medical Center, Department of Medicine, Pittsburgh, PA, USA

J. S. McCall-Hosenfeld (✉)
The Pennsylvania State University College of Medicine, Department of Medicine, Hershey, PA, USA
e-mail: jmccallhosenfeld@pennstatehealth.psu.edu

Intimate Partner Violence Domains, Prevalence, and Epidemiology

Intimate partner violence (IPV) is a pervasive public health problem that affects the health of a significant proportion of women in the United States and internationally. IPV is defined by the Centers for Disease Control and Prevention (CDC) as physical violence, sexual, stalking, or psychological harm perpetrated by a current or former intimate partner or spouse [1]. There is controversy regarding the distinction of abusive relationships from dysfunctional ones. However, the presence of coercion and control of one partner over another is a key feature in distinguishing the relationships associated with the most severe harm [2].

IPV encompasses many domains, and overlaps between those domains are common. The most recent estimates of IPV prevalence are reported in the National Intimate Partner Violence and Sexual Violence Survey (NISVS) [3–5]. This study described five separate domains of intimate partner violence.

Physical violence are behaviors meant to induce bodily harm, ranging from mild to severe. Examples of these behaviors include slapping and shoving to severe acts such as beating and choking. This form of violence affects approximately 32.4% of US women in their lifetimes, with 3.9% reporting exposure in the past year [3].

Sexual violence includes rape, being made to penetrate someone else, sexual coercion, unwanted sexual contact, and non-contact unwanted sexual experiences. Over 9% of US women report that they have been sexually victimized by an intimate partner in their lifetimes and 0.6% have been sexually victimized in the past year [4].

Stalking is defined by the National Intimate Partner and Sexual Violence Survey (NISVS) as "a pattern of harassing or threatening tactics used by a perpetrator that is both unwanted and causes fear or safety concerns in the victim" [5]. Approximately 15.8% of US women report that they have experienced stalking in their lifetimes, with 4.2% of women reporting stalking victimization in the past year [3]. Women

S. A. Tilstra et al. (eds.), *Sex- and Gender-Based Women's Health*, https://doi.org/10.1007/978-3-030-50695-7_35

reporting stalking note that it is severe enough to cause the victim to be extremely fearful, feeling that she, or someone close to her, is in danger of being harmed or killed [4].

The NISVS defines the experience of physical violence, sexual violence, or stalking collectively as *severe* forms of IPV victimization. These severe forms of abuse from an intimate partner have been experienced by more than one in three US women (35.6%) in their lifetimes [4].

Psychological aggression is defined through behaviors that fall under the following two domains: *expressive aggression* and *coercive control*. Expressive aggression includes behaviors that humiliate the victim often through name-calling and insults. Coercive control is exerted through "behaviors that are intended to monitor and control or threaten an intimate partner" [5]. According to the NISVS, almost half (47.1%) of all US women had experienced psychological aggression in their lifetimes, with 39.3% reporting expressive aggression and 39.7% reporting coercive control [3]. Approximately 14% of US women reported that they had experienced psychological aggression during the past year [4].

Control of reproductive or sexual health was defined by the CDC in 2010 as a form of intimate partner abuse [4]. A man can exert this type of control over his female partner by trying to get her pregnant by either refusing to wear a condom or by not allowing her access to other forms of birth control. Conversely, a female abuser can attempt to control her male partner by becoming pregnant without his consent, such as by falsely stating that she is on birth control when she is not. An additional form of control of reproductive or sexual health is the removal of a condom without a partner's consent, a practice which can transform consensual sexual activity into non-consensual sexual activity (known colloquially as "stealthing") [6].

Risk Factors for IPV

The CDC's social–ecological model is a useful framework for examining risk factors, as well as preventative factors, for being in an abusive relationship. This model considers risk and prevention in the following domains: *individual, relationship, community*, and *societal* [7, 8]. Although there are some identified risk factors for abuse victimization, it is important for providers to be aware that IPV is prevalent in all sectors of the population, and screening should be universally applied, rather than applied only to those who are considered by the provider to be at risk [9].

Of the ***individual*** factors that predispose to both intimate partner violence and sexual violence victimization, one of the most consistent is exposure to violence in youth. Among women who experienced rape, physical violence, or stalking by an intimate partner, 22.4% had their first experiences between 11 and 17 years of age and nearly half (47.1%) had their first experience between ages 18 and 24 [4]. This fact is particularly salient in light of the 2015 Youth Risk Behavior Survey findings showing that among girls in grades 9–12, 11.7% had experienced physical dating violence and 15.6% had experienced sexual dating violence within the past 12 months [10]. Additionally, young people are more likely to experience violence than older individuals. Numerous other individual characteristics are listed by the CDC, including depression, heavy alcohol and drug use, anger and hostility, unemployment, isolation, antisocial or borderline personality traits, and a strong belief in traditional gender roles (e.g., male dominance and aggression in relationships). One of the strongest predictors of perpetration is the individual being a victim themselves of physical or psychological abuse [8].

The association of race and ethnicity with IPV has been questioned. While it is important to remember that IPV is highly prevalent among women of all races and ethnicities, epidemiologic studies have shown some racial and ethnic disparities. Among US women, 56.6% of multiracial, 47.5% of American Indian/Alaska Native, 45.1% of non-Hispanic Black, 37.3% of non-Hispanic White, 34.4% of Hispanic, and 18.3% of Asian or Pacific Islander women reported any lifetime contact of sexual violence, physical violence, or stalking by an intimate partner [3].

Relationship factors that are associated with higher levels of IPV include relationships in which there is a high level of conflict, or instability, such as that caused by divorce or economic uncertainty [8].

Certain ***communities*** may have unique risk factors. For example, rural women are exposed to IPV at levels that are at least as high or higher than non-rural women [11, 12]. Moreover, rural women may be particularly vulnerable to IPV due to limitations in health services, social services, lack of transportation, or long distances to travel for services [12, 13]. Finally, community norms in rural areas may affect women's perceptions of IPV as a health problem and frequency of screening by primary providers [14], making it less likely that women exposed to IPV come to medical attention.

Another ***community*** factor that affects IPV is poverty. Poverty and IPV have a complex relationship, with sequencing of poverty and IPV exposure characterized as a "downward spiral" [15]. Partner violence often follows poverty, as poor women may be financially dependent on an abusive partner. However, IPV likely also contributes to poverty, as abuse can contribute to employment instability [15], which in turn can lead to greater dependence on an abusive partner.

Communities who are marginalized also have high rates of IPV. For example, IPV among sexual minorities should not be dismissed. Bisexual women are 1.8 times more likely to report IPV compared to heterosexual women [16], and IPV prevalence is also higher among lesbian women compared to heterosexual women, although this difference is not statistically significant.

Societal factors known to impact IPV risk including traditional gender norms in which women are expected to be submissive to men, or where men are considered the decision makers, and women are expected to remain at home and out of the workforce [8].

Sexual Violence: Prevalence and Epidemiology

An estimated 19.1% of US women have been raped during their lifetimes, with 36.3% of women reporting other forms of sexual violence (being made to penetrate, sexual coercion, unwanted penetration, unwanted sexual contact (e.g., kissing or fondling).) In addition, 32.1% reported experiencing non-contact unwanted sexual experiences (e.g., being flashed) [3].

Risk factors for sexual violence victimization are similar to those for IPV. Youth is a consistent correlate of rape victimization. Of women experiencing completed rape, 79.6% were less than 25 years of age at the time of the first assault. Of these female victims, 29.9% were between 11 and 17 years of age at time of first rape and 12.3% were at or younger than 10 years of age [17].

As with other forms of IPV, vulnerable populations may be at greater risk for sexual violence victimization perpetrated by an intimate partner. Globally, these factors include being married or cohabitating, consuming alcohol or drugs, involvement in sex work, and poverty. Of note, women's education and economic empowerment reduce vulnerability to intimate partner sexual violence [18].

Campus sexual violence has gained increased media attention recently and deserves special attention. Efforts to describe the frequency of sexual assault on college campuses have been limited by issues with accurate data collection and reporting. However, at least 28% of college campus women report at least one incident of sexual assault, defined as sexualized touching, or attempted or completed penetration [19]. Factors associated with increased risk for sexual assault among college students included sexual minority status, difficulty paying for basic necessities, fraternity or sorority membership, participation in casual sexual encounters, binge drinking, and experiencing sexual assault prior to college [19].

Human Trafficking: Prevalence and Epidemiology

Human trafficking is defined as "the recruitment and movement of individuals—most often by force, coercion, or deception—for the purpose of exploitation" [20]. Among the estimated 2.5 million persons who are subjected to human trafficking, 43% are trafficked for purposes of commercial sexual exploitation and 32% are trafficked for participation in forced labor [21]. Individuals who are trafficked are very often subject to severe forms of physical, sexual, and emotional abuse. Human trafficking disproportionately affects women. Women and girls make up 56% of persons trafficked for the purposes of forced labor, and 98% of the population trafficked for commercial sexual exploitation. Due to the covert nature of human trafficking, epidemiologic data on trafficked individuals is scarce. However, the United States is one of the top 10 destinations for human trafficking internationally [22].

Pathophysiology of IPV

The pathophysiology of IPV is related to control and fear. For a batterer, control is the goal of the abuse, and fear is the tool by which the abuser maintains control. Fear is always present in abusive relationships; thus, identifying fear in the relationship can help to differentiate between relationships that are truly abusive versus those that are dysfunctional [23]. There are two well-established models depicting the dynamics of the abusive intimate partner relationship: the "Cycle of Violence" [24] and the "Power and Control Wheel" [23] (Fig. 35.1).

Cycle of Violence

The "Cycle of Violence" is comprised of three phases as follows: (1) Tension Building, (2) Crisis/Violence, and (3) Honeymoon/Apology. Useful examples of each phase are offered by www.shelterforhelpinemergency [24]. In the *tension building* stage, which usually lasts for weeks to months, stress builds and communication breaks down between partners. Verbal abuse and less severe violence may occur. Victims may sense increasing danger and may try to anticipate the factors that may precipitate more severe violence. During the *crisis/violence* phase, usually lasting for 24–72 hours, violence escalates. Significant injuries, some of which may come to medical attention, are most likely to occur during this phase, and the victim's actions focus on surviving the abuse. The *honeymoon* phase follows the crisis phase. The honeymoon phase may last from days to months and is characterized by the abuser apologizing, asking for forgiveness, promising it will never happen again, and displaying vulnerability.

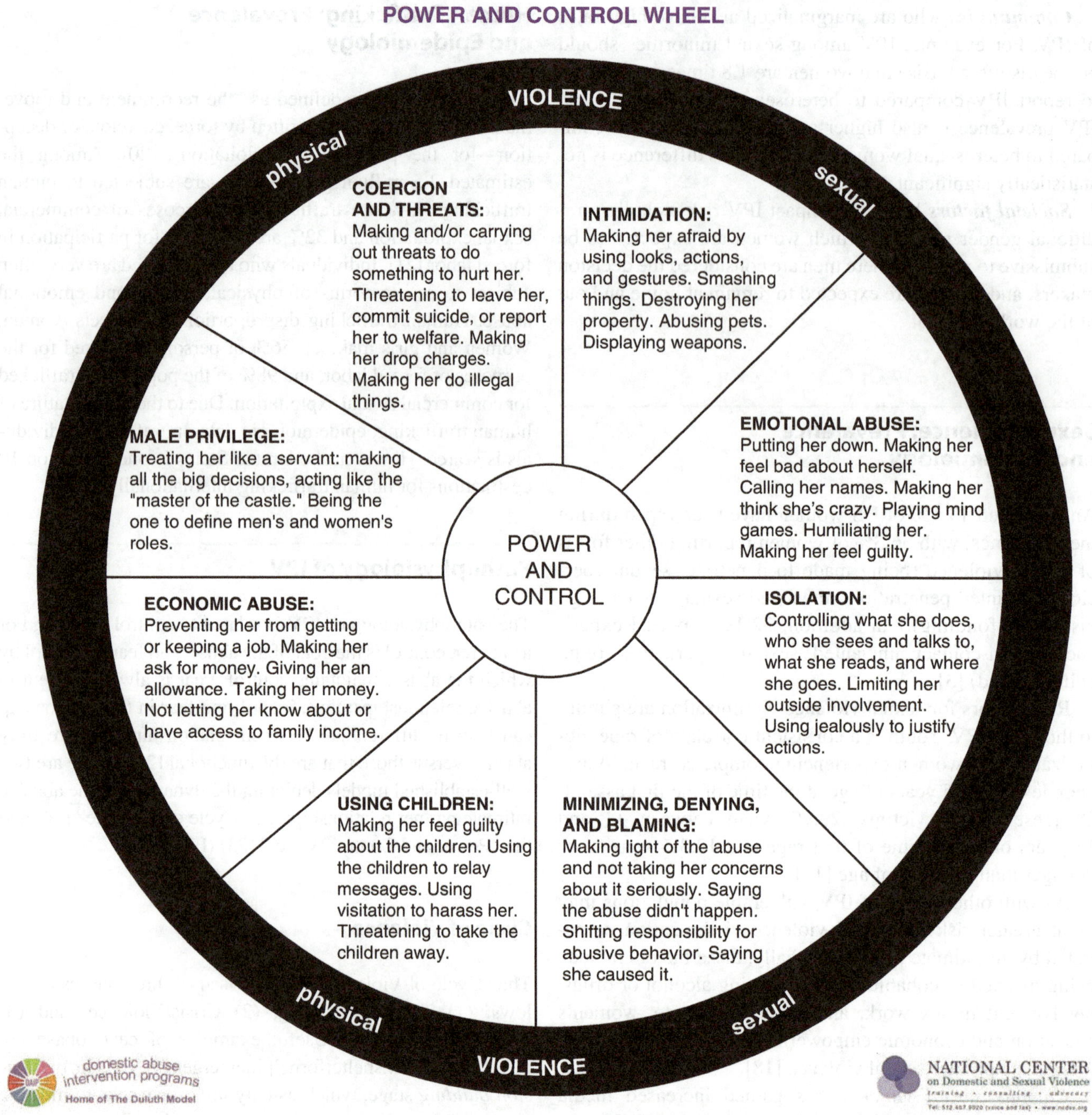

Fig. 35.1 Power and Control Wheel [23, 25]. Produced and distributed by National Center on Domestic and Sexual Violence. www.ncdsv.org, Austin, TX. (Adapted from Domestic Abuse Intervention Project, www.theduluthmodel.org/, 202 East Superior Street, Duluth, MN, 55802. www.theduluthmodel.org)

The cycle of violence model has several important caveats to consider. First, over time the honeymoon period becomes shorter and less frequent and may disappear altogether. Despite this, fear keeps the victim in the cycle. Second, breaking the cycle can have repercussions. When a woman leaves a male perpetrator, there can be up to a fivefold increase in the risk of homicide, which increases to a ninefold increase in risk of homicide when the batterer is extremely controlling during the relationship [26].

Example: Mary's husband comes home to their family seated at the table, trying to be on their best behavior (Tension Building), until a small disagreement arises between the children. The husband throws his plate across the table in anger and it hits the wall behind his wife's head, missing her by inches (Violence). He exclaims, "I work hard all day and all you have to do is keep things in order here." The children run to their rooms. He later apologizes, "You know my job is stressful. I need things to be calm here. If you could do a better job of managing these kids, I wouldn't have to get so angry." The children return to the table, as the tension is reduced (Honeymoon).

Power and Control Wheel

The second model, the Power and Control Wheel, was developed to show types of abuse and the patterns that "are used by a batterer to establish and maintain control over his partner" [23]. As noted previously, violent relationships are sustained by power and control. In the Power and Control Wheel model, fear of physical or sexual violence are the primary agents used to maintain the batterer's control. However, more subtle behaviors such as undermining her self-esteem, preventing her from getting a job, threatening to take away her kids, and isolating her from friends are also used to maintain power and control. All these behaviors are combined in different ways to form patterns of abuse.

Because control is at the core of the batterer's behaviors, occurrences that decrease the batterer's control act as triggers for escalation of violence. Examples of this include a victim gaining financial independence through educational attainment or the batterer sensing a loss of control as his victim is perceived to place the needs of a newborn child over those of the batterer [26].

The Power and Control Wheel is not an "all-inclusive" list of abusive behaviors. Certain populations experience abuse unique to their status. Among sexual minority women, a powerful source of control is the threat of the abuser "outing" the partner, which can bring negative social and economic consequences. Other issues affecting sexual minorities may include legal access to children and the dependence on a tight-knit community in which avoidance of the abuser is not realistic [27]. People with disabilities also experience abusive behaviors unique to their situations, including neglect in daily care, withholding medication or overmedicating, and control of access to healthcare professionals or other services [28].

Clinical Clues

Stress

Providers who are assessing patients for signs of abuse should be alert to assault-related injuries, unusual patterns of injury, and injury that does not match the stated mechanism [29]. In addition to these clinical clues from direct assault, women will often present with issues resulting from stress. Stress leads to impaired immunity, autonomic dysfunction, inflammatory changes, and neurochemical imbalances, which manifest in physical and mental health problems [30]. Conditions such as chronic headaches, chronic abdominal pain, and chronic pelvic pain are common among IPV survivors [31, 32] as are mental health conditions such as anxiety, depression, and post-traumatic stress disorder (PTSD). Signs of acceleration of abuse can either present as exacerbations of these chronic diseases or with acute symptoms such as diarrhea, dizziness, or insomnia [33]. When stress-related complaints are reported, assessing for either ongoing abuse or past abuse is critical.

Adverse Health Conditions

Women who survive IPV are more likely to have poorer physical health status compared to non-abused women. In studies that assess overall physical health with standardized instruments, women with a lifetime history of IPV show substantial decrements in overall health regardless of whether they were exposed to physical, sexual, or psychological abuse. Women with a history of IPV have been shown to have greater frequency of numerous adverse health conditions ranging from cardiovascular disease to diabetes and asthma [34–39].

Mental Health

Depression, anxiety, somatization disorders, and eating disorders are highly prevalent among women who survive IPV [40–43]. A common misconception is that PTSD is a disease more commonly experienced by men; however, women are approximately twice as likely to experience PTSD compared to men, due to a combination of different biological profiles and differing trauma burden [44]. Thus, clinicians should be particularly alert to symptoms of PTSD among survivors of IPV [45]. Although the rate of PTSD among IPV survivors has been difficult to characterize, it is estimated that approximately 64% of women who survive IPV met the criteria for PTSD [46]. Moreover, PTSD in IPV survivors is often comorbid with other mental health disorders such as depression and other anxiety disorders [47, 48].

Adverse Health Behaviors

Adverse health behaviors such as substance abuse, obesity, and noncompliance are elevated in survivors of IPV. In one clinical sample, women who neither smoked nor engaged in problem drinking had a 10% probability of IPV in the preceding 12 months. In contrast, if both smoking and problem drinking were present, the risk of 12-month IPV almost tripled to 27% [49]. The association between IPV and sexual violence and alcohol and other drugs of abuse is complex. Use of drugs or alcohol can create vulnerabilities which predispose women to assault, but also be used as a coping mechanism to address the adverse effects of assault and trauma

[50]. Women with a lifetime history of IPV were also more likely to be identified as obese by a healthcare professional [51] suggesting a relationship between IPV and adverse dietary and exercise patterns. Additionally, women exposed to IPV have been shown to be less likely to attend regular preventive healthcare appointments [35]. One explanation for this may be due to partner interference in healthcare. In one study [52], women who reported IPV were also more than seven times likely to report that their partner had interfered with their healthcare, suggesting that missed clinic appointments or "noncompliance" may be a manifestation of partner control tactics.

Sexual and Reproductive Health

Numerous adverse reproductive health consequences follow IPV. Women who survive IPV are more likely to report dyspareunia [53] and less likely to use their preferred form of contraception [54]. Thus, it is not surprising that these women have increased risk of sexually transmitted infections (STIs), [53] cervical cancer [55], unintended pregnancy [56], and abortion [53]. IPV is associated with reproductive coercion and birth control sabotage, which in turn is associated with unintended pregnancy [57].

Social History Clues

Partner Characteristics

There are partner characteristics and social behaviors that have been linked to an increase in risk of a couple's relationship being or becoming an abusive one. Healthcare providers should be alert to these cues, as their patients often do not identify them as abusive.

A patient may reveal that her partner has a charismatic personality but is living a "double life" in which the abuser is kind in public and cruel in private. Because of this, when abusive behavior does occur, people outside the relationship may find it difficult to believe the woman, causing her to doubt her own intuition. Abusers minimize the impact they have on their partners and may exploit their partners as property or sexual objects. Abusers blame the victim or external factors, such as illicit substance abuse, stress due to jobs or family finances. It is important for the provider to identify these characteristics and to understand the potential that these are signs of an abusive partner [8, 58, 59].

In ***technological abuse***, the batterer controls cell phone and online use. The abuser may restrict access to technology or monitor calls, texts, and emails. An abuser may use GPS to monitor location and track his partner. Cyberbullying, a practice in which abusers use social media to mar personal and professional reputations, is a common and effective means of control [60].

Academic abuse may be identified as behaviors that can reduce the potential for independence through success. Interfering with studying either through guilt ("if you loved me, you wouldn't study so much"), peer pressure (making fun of studying) or through direct interference (frequent texts or calls that deliberately interfere with study schedules) may impact academic performance. An abuser may take all the same classes as his partner as means of monitoring her behaviors and interaction [60]. Some abusers harass their victims at work, making the victim an undesirable employee. Multiple job changes and lack of career advancement can result [60].

Clues to Human Trafficking

Identification of victims of human trafficking in healthcare settings is particularly complicated. Human trafficking is defined by the United Nations as the "recruitment, transportation, transfer, harboring or receipt of persons, by means of threat or…coercion, …abduction, fraud, of deception, of the abuse of power…for the purposes of exploitation" [61]. Many victims of trafficking are forced to be involved in illegal activities such as sex work or drug use, and some are undocumented or using false documents [62]. Thus, trafficked individuals may be less likely to come to medical attention, due to concerns regarding criminal prosecution or legal status. Traffickers are likely to accompany their victims at all times, including to healthcare appointments. Thus, it can be challenging for healthcare providers to determine whether the trafficker is a sex partner, a parent, or an employer [63, 64].

Common red flags for trafficked individuals presenting to healthcare clinics include the following [65]:

1. Chronic untreated medical issues
2. Tattoos indicating tagging or possession
3. Silence, difficulty speaking, or making eye contact
4. Mental health issues
5. Untreated injuries
6. Multiple STIs or abortions
7. Fear or mistrust in the healthcare system
8. Lack of knowledge of local language

Evaluation and Diagnostic Strategy

Trauma-Informed Care

Trauma-informed healthcare service is defined as care which is "influenced by an understanding of the impact of interpersonal violence and victimization on an individual's life and development" [66]. Unfortunately, trauma is pervasive in our society. Healthcare professionals must recognize that all patients, as well as colleagues and co-workers, may be survivors of trauma. Providers practicing trauma-informed care recognize that trauma survivors need support and understanding from those around them. Healthcare providers are also exposed to *vicarious trauma*, which is the emotional trauma that can result from working with trauma victims [27, 67].

The Substance Abuse and Mental Health Services Administration (SAMHSA) offers guidelines to organizations on how to adopt a trauma-informed approach. In this approach, healthcare systems and providers do the following [68].

1. Realize the widespread impact of trauma and understand potential paths for recovery.
2. Recognize the signs and symptoms of trauma in clients, families, staff, and others involved with the system.
3. Respond by fully integrating knowledge about trauma into policies, procedures, and practices.
4. Seek to actively resist re-traumatization.

Thus, providers and healthcare systems are encouraged to adopt universal screening, identification, and response to IPV while considering a trauma-informed approach.

Screening for IPV: Guidelines

Recognizing the adverse health effects associated with IPV, governmental and professional organizations have called for better identification and response to IPV in healthcare settings. These calls date back to 1992, when the American Medical Association (AMA) recommended routine screening for IPV among all women patients [29]. Despite this, routine screening and counseling for IPV was not codified in US policy until 2011, when the Institute of Medicine (IOM) identified IPV screening and intervention as a routine preventive healthcare service for women [69]. Subsequently, these guidelines were adopted as part of comprehensive preventive women's healthcare services under the Affordable Care Act, and in 2013, the United States Preventive Services Task Force (USPSTF) recommended routine screening and follow-up for all women of reproductive age (18–46) for lifetime exposure to IPV [9].

Screening recommendations recognize both ongoing and past violence. Asking patients routinely about IPV increases awareness, decreases isolation, and increases a patient's trust in the healthcare system. Screening, regardless of whether disclosure occurs, can help women who experience abuse. Women who have discussed abuse with a healthcare provider are more likely to plan for their safety and more likely to exit an abusive relationship [70, 71].

To assist providers in implementing screening guidelines, Futures Without Violence, a non-profit organization, created an intervention to outline IPV screening and response in healthcare. The *CUES* intervention includes *Confidentiality, Universal Education, Empowerment, and Support* (www.ipvhealth.org). This approach acknowledges that women do not always disclose IPV to healthcare providers, but that there is value in making the inquiry and offering resources regardless of whether the patient makes a disclosure. *CUES* assists healthcare providers with this process [27].

Case with CUES Intervention

Shu is a 24-year-old undergraduate student who comes in to see you for an urgent visit. She has recurrent diarrhea. A chart review reveals that she has had a comprehensive, but negative work up by her gastroenterologist. She notes that it seems to happen mostly towards the end of the week. She thinks it must be related to fatigue, as she is always more tired by Friday than on Monday.

- *MD: Sometimes symptoms such as diarrhea are signs of stress, good or bad. What is going on in your life over the past couple of months that may be causing stress for you?*
- *Shu: Well, I've been doing a lot of traveling because I spend most weekends with my boyfriend who lives in Cleveland. Also, I am having trouble in choosing a graduate program. My boyfriend really wants me to move to Cleveland, but the program here is better for me. It is causing a lot of tension between us.*
- *MD: Can you see a pattern between the diarrhea and weekends with him?*
- *Shu: Yes! I actually only get this when I am getting ready to see him.*

Confidentiality

The first step is to ensure *Confidentiality*. In this step, the provider ensures that the patient is always seen alone. The provider openly informs the patient that what she discloses will be kept confidential. However, the provider must also note the limits of confidentiality. For example, disclosure of risk of self-harm or harm to others, especially children, is likely to require reporting to authorities. Providers need to be familiar with the mandated reporting requirements within their state and inform patients prior to inquiry of the legal or ethical bounds that inform these discussions. For more information about specifics of mandatory reporting requirements, Futures without Violence offers a compendium of reporting requirements by state https://www.futureswithoutviolence.org/compendium-of-state-statutes-and-policies-on-domestic-violence-and-health-care/ (2013) [72].

- *MD: Before we go any further, I want to let you know that anything you tell me will be kept strictly confidential. This conversation is just between you and me. However, please be aware that there may be limits to this confidentiality. For example, if you give me credible evidence that you are going to harm yourself or another person, I may be required to report this to the authorities. If I must do that, I can make sure that you are in the room and present to hear what is being said. Does that make sense? Do you have any questions before we go forward?*
- *Shu: Yes, that makes sense.*

Universal Education

The next step is *Universal Education*. Providers should start by normalizing the inquiry with a framing statement, so that patients understand why they are being screened and do not feel singled out or stigmatized [73]. Framing statements provide education about violence. For example, the American College of Obstetricians and Gynecologists recommends the following: "We've started talking to all of our patients about safe and healthy relationships because it can have such a large impact on your health" [73].

Futures without Violence recommends having pocket cards on hand and using these to provide universal education about healthy and unhealthy relationships. These cards, available at www.ipv.org, outline the difference between healthy and unhealthy relationships, how unhealthy relationships may affect health, and steps that a victim can take to assess her risks as well as resources she can utilize to improve her safety.

For providers, the pocket cards provide information on beginning a discussion about healthy and safe relationships and exploring how relationships can adversely affect a patient's health. Futures Without Violence suggests giving two cards to each patient, so that the information can be shared with friends and family who may need it [27].

- *MD: I have found that many women in my practice struggle with significant stressors in their relationship. Some of my patients are in relationships that are controlling and even violent. Therefore, I now make sure that I ask all my patients about their relationships, and specifically ask about domestic violence. I like to provide all my patients with information that they can take away which helps them understand healthy relationships. Does this sound like something I can share with you?*
- *Shu: Okay. I understand.*

Empowerment

The goal of *empowerment* is to allow the woman to be the agent of change, giving her the tools to have control over her decisions. This restores control to the patient and reverses one of the cornerstones of IPV, in which the abuser assumes control of her behaviors and decisions. Providers empower women through respectful communication and through affirming their patients' ability to make sound decisions. Keys to empowering patients are the precepts of validation, empathy, respect for autonomy, and education about the health impact of IPV [74, 75].

Validation

To validate the patient's experiences, the healthcare provider should assure the patient that the abusive behavior is a problem that the patient did not create nor is it a problem that they deserve. IPV is sustained when the perpetrator places the blame on the woman, indicating that her behaviors and actions are causal for the abuse suffered. After living under these often-subtle messages, women may internalize this blame, accepting some of the responsibility for the presence of the abuse. By dispelling these myths, the provider empowers the patient [74, 76].

Empathy

Women value an empathetic approach to screening, in which the provider listens attentively, with compassion and kindness. Women often feel ashamed or embarrassed to admit that they are in an abusive relationship to a healthcare provider. Empathy reduces this barrier to disclosure [74–76].

Respect for Autonomy

In offering support, the clinician must respect the patient's decisions, even if the provider does not understand or agree with these decisions. The patient often knows what options will be the safest and most appropriate for her [77]. For example, it may be important for the provider to recognize that in marginalized or vulnerable communities, the patient may prefer counseling that focuses on harm reduction rather than separation from a partner, which may remove her contact with her community [27].

Health Impact

Providers must also assess the impact of the IPV (past or present) on the patient's health [78]. An encounter with a healthcare provider may be the first time that a patient realizes that some of her health issues may be attributable to IPV. Education about the health impact of IPV also helps patients to understand that IPV is appropriately positioned in the healthcare system (in addition to, or instead of the criminal justice system) and that a healthcare provider may be an important ally as both the patient and the provider are working to improve her health.

- *MD: Stress is common during transitions, especially for couples. I'd like to explore this further. I hear that there is tension between you, and I ask all women this question in this situation. Has it gotten to a point now that you feel that your partner is trying to control you in a way that makes you feel afraid of him? Has he done anything to make you feel threatened either physically or emotionally?*
- *Shu: My diarrhea has just been getting worse and worse. He has become very controlling where he won't let me see my friends when he comes to visit. When I cancelled a trip to see him to study for a test, he showed up at my apartment banging on the door and yelling, until my friends threatened to call the police if he didn't leave. I guess I am afraid of him. He hasn't threatened to hurt me but I am just not sure what he is capable of. He is acting so crazy. I am afraid to stay here for graduate school as it will upset him, but I am afraid to live with him by myself in Cleveland.*

Examples of Provider Responses

- *Validate*: I am sorry this is happening to you and want you to know that this abusive behavior is not your fault. No one deserves to be hurt or to feel afraid of his or her partner.
- *Support*: We will work on this together and I want you to know that whatever decisions you make, I will be here to support you. I have information and resources to share with you.
- *Respect*: You have been living with this situation for a while and before I offer my thoughts, what is it that my staff or I can do to help you today with this situation?
- *Health Impact*: All types of stress can contribute to health problems, including diarrhea. Do you think that this is something that is happening to you?

Although the discussion does not require standardized language, if scripted screening questions are preferred, numerous instruments exist which are recommended by the USPSTF as valid and reliable screening tools for domestic violence. These include the following:

1. HARK: Humiliate-Afraid-Rape-Kick HITS [79].
2. HITS: Hurt, Insult, Threaten, Scream [80].
3. OVAT: Ongoing Violence Assessment Tool [81].

Each of these is brief and has a high degree of sensitivity and specificity, making them useful tools for primary care. Additionally, screening can be accomplished via electronic media, and in many cases, this is preferred over face-to-face screening [82].

Support

This final step in CUES is to provide *support*. Key elements of support include referral to specialists and domestic violence advocacy services. Patients should be aware that the National Domestic Violence Hotline [83] (1-800-799-SAFE, www.thehotline.org) is available 24/7, across the United States, and can connect patients with counseling and local services at any time. Healthcare providers should be familiar with their local resources and know how to refer patients if needed.

In addition to referring her to services, the provider should make a follow-up appointment with the patient in the medical office [78]. Women may feel safer coming to a medical appointment versus structured domestic violence services, and in many locations, domestic violence service providers may be able to meet the patient at her medical appointment.

Safety Assessment

A critical aspect of support is exploring the patient's immediate safety, including the pattern and severity of abuse, and the safety of any children, or other household members [78]. If she has disclosed abuse, either the patient may feel safe to leave the office or she may not feel safe going home from the office. Extensive safety planning is outside the purview of most primary care providers; however, it is reasonable to advise women of the tenets of basic safety planning. The basic components of safety planning are listed in Fig. 35.2. Patients should know that if their safety is at immediate risk, they should call 911 or their local emergency response number. Escalation in violence, use of a weapon, and threats of suicide or homicide are all indicators that the patient's immediate safety is threatened. Having an emergency kit available including such items as money, keys, medicines, and legal documentation may be useful to review with patients. Likewise, patients should be directly asked if they are able to safely go home [78].

PATIENT INFORMATION COPY FOR YOUR PATIENT

FROM THE OFFICE OF **DR.** ______________________________

Planning ahead: How to stay safe

If you are being abused, making a safety plan now may help you when you have to act quickly in the future. The following ideas are ways that other women have planned for their safety. Some of these ideas may work for you. You may come up with additional ideas for yourself. You know your own situation better than anyone else, so plan what will work best for you.

- **Hide money** or put it somewhere safe so you can leave quickly.
- **Make copies** of birth certificates, immunization records, Social Security numbers, and other important documents to keep in safe locations away from home such as at work, the homes of trusted family members or friends, or hidden in convenient locations.
- **Hide a spare car key** or bus or subway pass that you can grab quickly.
- **Keep a list** of hotline numbers, or memorize the **1-800-799-SAFE** National Domestic Violence Hotline number.
- **Develop a code** with friends, family, or neighbors to let them know when you need help in an emergency. If you have children, teach them a signal (like a code word) that means they should call the police or go for help. You may want to have a special code for neighbors (like putting on a particular light or opening a certain window) that means you want them to call the police.
- **Plan your exit.** Know which doors, windows, stairwells, elevators, or fire escapes you can use if you have to leave quickly. Practice using them so that they feel familiar to you.
- **Know how to reach the police** and your local women's shelter.
- Every day, **think about where you can go** immediately if you have to leave. Is a neighbor home today? A relative? A friend?
- **Remove weapons** from your home if you can.
- Something to think about: When you cannot get away and your partner becomes violent, **which room is the safest** for you to get to? Is there a room that has a phone and a lock on the door? Can you stay out of rooms with easy weapons, such as the kitchen?
- **Try not to leave without your children.** But if you have to leave your children with the abuser, call the police immediately after you escape.

Adapted from Chang JC. Domestic violence. In: Bieber EJ, Sanfilippo JS, Horowitz IR, editors. Clinical Gynecology. Philadelphia, PA; Elsevier, Inc; 2006:79–89.

For more information

National Domestic Violence Hotline
1-800-799-SAFE
www.thehotline.org

Futures Without Violence
www.futureswithoutviolence.org

National Coalition Against Domestic Violence
www.ncadv.org

CLEVELAND CLINIC JOURNAL OF MEDICINE

This information is provided by your physician and the *Cleveland Clinic Journal of Medicine.* It is not designed to replace a physician's medical assessment and judgment.

For patient information on hundreds of health topics, see the Center for Consumer Health Information web site, www.clevelandclinic.org/health

doi:10.3949/ccjm.81pe.07001 CLEVELAND CLINIC JOURNAL OF MEDICINE VOLUME 81 • NUMBER 7 JULY 2014 447

Fig. 35.2 Planning ahead for safety. (Reprinted with permission from Chang [84])

Part of safety planning is knowing what the risk factors are for severe forms of violence. Risk factors that are associated with femicide [26] include the following:

- Abuser's lack of employment
- Access to a firearm
- Use of illicit drugs
- Recent separation
- Having ever left or asked the partner to leave the relationship
- Living with a non-biologic child of the abuser
- Expression of highly controlling behaviors
- Prior threats with a weapon
- Prior threats to kill his partner

Among these risks, one most important for providers to understand is that separation leads to an increased risk of homicide, especially when the abuser has shown controlling behaviors. For this reason, if the woman is considering leaving her partner, it is important that the physician tell her that she should not confront her partner with this decision. As abusers may retaliate, patients should be advised to leave secretly and notify the abuser later, when all loved ones are in safe places [26]. Trained counselors are best qualified to construct the safest leaving plan for the patient and her family. Thus, establishing and utilizing relationships with domestic violence advocates are critical in helping patients to plan for their safety [85].

- *MD: "Now that you have brought up this fear, do you feel that you would be safe to be at home or do you think that he may do something harmful to you in the next few weeks?"*

1. ***What to do if she discloses IPV and is NOT safe to return home***

There are many options to offer once there is a disclosure. Asking what she has thought of or tried in the past empowers the patient to offer her own solution before listening to the provider's options. A warm referral, which involves contacting an advocate or domestic violence specialist while the patient is in the office with you, ensures that the handoff is made. Many women do not have private access to a phone, so simply offering her the use of the phone in the office can be lifesaving. Many shelters provide not only emergency housing but also offer free legal advocacy, housing, job finding, support groups, and individual counseling. The National Domestic Violence Hotline, 1-800-799-SAFE [83] is available 24/7, has interpreters for most languages, and understands the unique needs of subpopulations such as immigrants, homeless, adolescents, and members of the LGBTQI community.

On-site counseling from a social worker or other trained provider can provide immediate safety planning. When appropriate, hospital admission can be offered to address immediate health issues as well as to protect the patient and to provide for more intensive safety planning by the inpatient social work team or community resource team. In all cases, trained professionals who can help the patient determine the safest course of immediate action, given the individual risks and benefits of her decisions, should conduct detailed safety planning and decision making with the patient. For example, Protection From Abuse orders may reduce harm in some cases; however, at other times, these may only exacerbate the problem without providing the expected protection [85].

Feels "Unsafe" Example

- *Shu: I really don't feel safe to go back to my dorm today and my parents live in Cleveland. I am not sure where he is or what he will do since I haven't spoken to him since this weekend when my friends chased him away. That is probably why the diarrhea has not gone away as it usually does on Mondays!*
- *MD: Since you don't feel safe to return home today, what options, if any, have you thought about as next steps? (Further prompts may depend on her answer). Here are a few things that I can do that have been helpful for my other patients who have had similar problems.*

2. ***What to do if she discloses IPV and IS safe to return home***

There are many reasons women may not wish to leave their partners. They may be economically dependent, they may worry about the safety of children or pets, or they may love their partners [86]. Providers should respect women's decisions about leaving or staying and should not look to IPV disclosure as the primary goal. Leaving is an option, but doing so in the safest way possible is the ultimate goal. Additionally, IPV victims may define "safe" differently than her healthcare providers. Women may prioritize immediate safety, such as "we just got paid and he never hurts me at this time of the month" or "my grandson is visiting for the weekend and he is not abusive when he is around" [87].

Providers should ask the patient if she has thought about what she would do if her situation were to become unsafe on her returning home. Written materials outlining safety planning should be reviewed with the patient. She should only take these home if her abuser will not find them, as this help-seeking behavior may escalate abuse. Basic safety planning can be reviewed (Fig. 35.2). She should be encouraged to trust her fear and to act accordingly. Close follow-up should be planned, with an open invitation for return calls or visits for further discussion or for access to immediate resources such as the phone, staff, or resource materials [88].

Feels "Safe" Example

- *Shu: No, I feel safe to go home. I have good support in my friends, and if I don't make a decision to stay here for school, he should be ok. He is also away for the next few weeks with his family and I have told his parents what he did. They want to talk with him to see if they can help him with our situation.*
- *MD: Well, I can't tell you for sure what may happen in the future with him and your relationship, but I will advise you to always trust your fear. When a partner is concerned that he is losing control, he may increase abuse in an attempt to regain that control. So, if you get to the point of making a separating decision, you will want to do it in a safe way. My office will always be here as a source of support and information, whenever you need it.*

3. ***What to do if she does not disclose abuse***

In many ways, IPV "treatment" in the healthcare setting does not fit the traditional medical model of disease. The goal of screening and intervention for IPV is not to get a disclosure but to build awareness and to provide resources to help patients achieve safety and independence [74, 88]. Women have reported that provider screening and education about IPV is an effective intervention, even if she says "no," as it offers information and a safe place for follow-up if she does need further support [88]. The patient may not be ready to disclose for several reasons including embarrassment, denial, fear of repercussions from her abuser, fear of family separation, and fear of police involvement. Repeat screening has been shown to increase the rate of disclosure [85, 88].

Does Not Disclose Example

- *Shu: I understand what you are saying, and although I understand that my relationship may not be in a good place, I don't feel like I am being controlled and I am not really scared of him.*
- *MD: I'm glad that nothing like this is happening to you. However, IPV is common in women's lives, including my own patients. There are good resources available if this ever happens to you or someone you know. No one deserves to be hurt or afraid of his or her partner. In our practice, we like to provide all our patients with information about where to go in the case of abuse or violence. [Provide a safety card from www.ipvhealth.org, local resources, and/or referral to the National Domestic Violence Hotline.] Because domestic violence is common and we want to get the word out, we encourage all our patients to take two of these cards, in case you discover that a friend or a loved one may need support from domestic violence services.*

4. ***What not to do***

Many providers want to know "what NOT to do" in IPV discussions. Potentially harmful medical interventions include pressuring a patient to leave, contacting legal authorities, or obtaining a restraining order or protection from abuse order (PFA) without the patient's permission, as these might not be the safest options for the individual woman at that time in her life. Further, exposing the patient's help-seeking behaviors to an abusive partner could lead to an escalation of abuse. Providers should refrain from inadvertently showing frustration or anger toward the patient, asking what she did to bring about the abuse or asking why she has not left the partner. These behaviors and questions suggest that the presence and persistence of the abuse is her fault [88–91].

Special Consideration: Forensic Sexual Exam

If the patient reports to you that she has been a victim of sexual assault, she should be offered referral to a facility that offers forensic sexual exam. Forensic sexual assault examiners (Sexual Assault Nurse Examiners, or SANEs and Sexual Assault Forensic Examiners, or SAFEs), are healthcare professionals who are specially trained to guide sexual assault survivors through the healthcare system. They can also help sexual assault providers obtain advocacy and legal services as requested or required by the patient [92]. Moreover, SANEs and SAFEs are specially trained in forensic evidentiary collection as part of post-assault care, especially within 5 days of the rape. Sexual assault evidence kits collected by a trained forensic examiner are more likely to be complete, produce higher quality evidence, and have fewer mistakes that can adversely affect prosecution of a sexual assault case [93, 94]. Medical forensic evidence collected by the sexual assault nurse examiner has been shown to improve rates of successful prosecution of sexual assaults [95]. Rape hotlines can identify which hospitals participate in the SANE program and link patients with legal and medical advocates.

Documentation

Documentation of IPV in the medical record may be particularly worrisome to providers. There are pros and cons to documentation that should be reviewed with the patient [88, 96]. The healthcare record can be a powerful tool in legal cases against abusers. Many providers may not realize the importance of documentation for patients seeking protection and may even be concerned that documentation will increase the probability that they will be involved in litigation. However, good documentation may reduce the likelihood that providers be required to testify in court cases. A factual medical record can help the patient to obtain a Protection from Abuse (PFA) order, help the patient to establish legal safety parameters in child custody cases, and help to make her eligible for special exceptions for healthcare insurance [89].

Providers have appropriate concerns that the information in the medical record could cause the patient harm if found by her abuser. The abuser may have access to the records, request "proxy" status on electronic medical records, or be listed as an emergency contact in the healthcare records. The health insurance policy may be in the abuser's name, in which case the abuser could receive "explanations of benefits" and bills that list billing codes. These potential situations need to be discussed with the patient prior to documentation and billing [97].

Providers' documentation is valuable if it is accurate and factual as it is only admissible in court if it is not considered "hearsay." The "hearsay rule" prohibits out-of-court statements with a few exceptions; one of which is a patient's medical record. Admissible items from the provider as a "medical expert" include the following [88]:

1. *HPI*: Providers should put in quotes what the patient states, including the batterer's name if used. These are called "excited utterances," which are statements made in states of agitation or excitement that are too spontaneous to be prefabricated, and thus are considered credible for use in court.
2. *Physical Exam*: Documentation of injuries should be recorded by photographs, drawings, or detailed descriptions. Optimally, photographs should be taken in close range to show details of the injury as well as from a distance to show the location on her body. The distant photo must include her face to identify that the injury is hers. Knowledge of local protocols and rules for photographic documentation is important. Description of her demeanor is helpful as well and is admissible as part of a medical exam.
3. *Assessment/Plan*: If possible, link the abuse to a medical issue to allow admittance as "medical expert witness." Document the discussion of the abuse and the resources offered to patient as part of the plan. Avoid listing IPV as separate problem in Assessment and Plan to limit the possibility that the patient's insurance is billed as "adult maltreatment/physical abuse" or similar billable labels.

Special Consideration: Caring for Victims of Trafficking

Individuals who are trafficked and present to the healthcare system deserve special consideration. Although a detailed understanding of the care of trafficked individuals is outside the purview of this chapter, there are many principles in caring for victims of trafficking that can reasonably be performed within the healthcare system. For more detail, please refer to the World Health Organization (WHO) Ethical and Safety Recommendations for Interviewing Trafficked Women https://www.unodc.org/documents/human-trafficking/Toolkit-files/08-58296_tool_6-12.pdf [98]. Key points of these guidelines include (but are not limited to) the following (edited for space):

1. Treat all contact with trafficked persons as a potential step toward improving their health
2. Prioritize the safety of trafficked persons, self, and staff by assessing risks
3. Provide respectful, equitable, non-discriminatory care
4. Provide referral information to shelter, legal, counseling, and advocacy services
5. Collaborate care with ancillary services and referral services
6. Ensure privacy and confidentiality in the healthcare encounter
7. Provide information in a way that each patient can understand
8. Obtain voluntary, informed consent from patients
9. Respect the rights, choices, and dignity of each individual
10. Avoid calling authorities, unless the patient has given consent to do so

IPV Course Over Time

Although physical and sexual violence are usually preceded by more subtle controlling behaviors, this trajectory may not be linear, and more severe harm can occur without warning behaviors [88]. IPV exposure is not a state but may change over time. Even when an abusive relationship is terminated, women remain at high risk for victimization by a subsequent partner, as well as the ex-partner [99]. Among women with severe IPV exposure, 39% of women were re-victimized by their index partner within the following year, and 16% were re-victimized by a different partner [100]. However, it is important to recognize that IPV cessation is possible. In one study, approximately half of all women who reported exposure to IPV at baseline did not report IPV exposure during the following year [101]. The properties of IPV may be important in determining whether IPV persists. Women exposed to psychological IPV alone were more likely to remain in an abusive relationship compared to those exposed to both physical and psychological IPV [102]. Thus, investigating for IPV at periodic encounters, providing universal education and resources remain critical throughout women's lives.

Summary Points

1. Intimate partner violence is a pattern of coercive and/or forceful behaviors in which one partner controls another without regard to their health, safety, or human rights. It is sustained by fear and control.
2. Clinical signs of IPV and other forms of violence against women (such as sexual violence, reproductive coercion, and human trafficking) include physical injury, signs of sexual trauma, chronic physical or mental illness, adverse health behaviors, partner's control over access to healthcare, and problems at work or school.
3. Intimate partner violence is multidimensional and includes physical violence, sexual violence, stalking, and psychological aggression. Sequelae that sustain intimate partner violence fall into these subtypes as well and are based on persistent fear of physical harm, of sexual coercion, of being constantly watched, or of harm to professional reputation.
4. A patient-centered evidence-based intervention to approach IPV is the CUES (Confidentiality, Universal Education, Empowerment, and Support) intervention. Assessment of IPV includes normalizing the inquiry through a framing statement, assuring confidentiality, approaching the survivor non-judgmentally and with compassion, validating her experiences, using guideline-informed screening techniques, providing referrals, and providing universal information regardless of the outcome of screening.
5. The primary care provider's role in IPV is to perform universal education and screening. Even without disclosure, screening has been shown to increase a woman's awareness with higher likelihood of future planning for safety and exiting an abusive relationship. Providers should understand that leaving an abusive situation may be associated with an increased risk for violence. Providers should connect patients with trained professionals to assist with safety planning, including social workers, local and national hotlines, and local shelter services.
6. A trauma-informed approach recognizes that trauma is pervasive in our society and acknowledges that trauma survivors can be re-traumatized by well-meaning caregivers and healthcare providers.
7. Safety planning includes ways to stay safe if the patient must currently remain in the relationship and ways to plan to leave safely. Providers can participate in safety planning by providing basic safety tips (having an emergency bag on hand), assessing for recent red flags (escalation of violence, presence of firearms), and giving resources for additional assistance by trained counselors (social work, hotline counselors, in-person shelter counselors, some therapists.).

Shu returns to your clinic 6 months later to fill out a health form prior to graduate school. She reports that she broke up with her boyfriend and is not currently in a relationship. Prior to breaking up, she contacted 1-800-799-SAFE and was referred to a counselor at her local domestic violence shelter. She reports that she worked with the counselor a few times, and eventually made the decision to pursue graduate school in a different city. After breaking up with her partner, her diarrhea improved. She states she feels prepared to enter a new chapter in her life.

Review Questions

1. You have been seeing Sidney in your primary care office for 10 years. Over this time, Sidney has related challenges in her relationship with her partner. You are wondering whether Sidney's partner could be emotionally abusing her. Which of the following questions would be most helpful in distinguishing IPV from a non-abusive (but dysfunctional) relationship.
   A. "Do you feel that you are angry at your partner?"
   B. "Have you ever been afraid of your partner?"
   C. "Are you jealous of your partner?"
   D. "Does your partner use illegal drugs or drink alcohol excessively?"

   The correct answer is B. The pathophysiology of IPV is related to control and fear. Fear is always present in abusive relationships; thus, identifying fear in the relationship can help to differentiate between relationships that are truly abusive versus those that are dysfunctional [23].
2. Which of the following is a form of coercive control?
   A. Suzanne's partner becomes belligerent when she drinks alcohol on the weekends.
   B. Ali's partner insists on reviewing her cell phone use every day when she comes home from work.
   C. Yolanda's ex-partner becomes depressed and refuses to answer the phone or engage in conversation.
   D. Ryan discloses that he and his partner yell at each other daily.

   The correct answer is B. *Coercive control* is a form of psychological aggression in which behaviors are intended to monitor and control or threaten an intimate partner. According to the NISVS, 39.7% of US women reported that they had experienced coercive control during their lifetimes. The other form of psychological aggression is *expressive aggression*, such as name calling, insulting, or humiliating an intimate partner. This has been reported by 39.3% of US women in their lifetimes [3].

3. Lee is new to your practice and makes an urgent appointment to see you. During this appointment, Lee's injuries and demeanor suggest that their partner may have been abusing them. Which of the following is most promising in promoting action-taking for Lee to safely remove themselves from this relationship?
   A. Referral to services.
   B. Counseling the partner.
   C. Reporting the violence to law enforcement.
   D. Advising the patient to leave their partner.

   The correct answer is A. Women have identified increased awareness of options and increased access to support and resources as a possible turning point to promote action taking. Addressing the partner can lead to increase in abuse to the woman, as the disclosure threatens the control that an abuser has in the relationship. Although reporting the violence to law enforcement or counseling her to leave the partner seem like safe options, these may have the negative repercussions of escalating the violence by threatening a partner's control. Homicide rates increase by fivefold when women leave a relationship and any perceived sense of separation has been shown to be a trigger for homicide [88–90].

4. Rochelle is a 45-year-old woman with multiple stress-related symptoms. She answers "yes" when asked if anyone is hurting her physically, emotionally, or sexually at home or making her feel afraid. What do you do next?
   A. Explain that she is unsafe and needs to leave the relationship today with your help.
   B. Ask her why she has not left her partner yet.
   C. Tell her that you are sorry, she does not deserve to be treated that way, and ask her if there is any way that you can help her today.
   D. Call the police to report the partner's behavior to have him arrested.

   The correct answer is C. In the Empowerment component of the CUES (Confidentiality, Universal Education, Empowerment, and Support) intervention developed by Futures Without Violence, providers validate the woman's concerns [27]. Answers (a), (b), and (c), all have possible negative repercussions and should not be discussed until she has been given the opportunity to express her own ideas for solutions. In addition, providers should offer referrals but should never pressure a woman to disclose abuse or to leave the abuser as these actions can exacerbate the abuse.

5. Sarah is a 45-year-old woman with multiple stress-related symptoms. She responds "no" when asked if anyone is hurting her physically, emotionally, or sexually at home or making her feel afraid. What do you do next?
   A. Tell her you are happy that she is not in that situation and normalize the conversation by moving on to asking about other stressors.
   B. Tell her that you are glad this is not happening to her, reinforcing that IPV is common and there are resources available—including your office—should she or her loved ones ever need this support.
   C. Tell her you are happy that she is not in this type of relationship and assure her that there is no reason for you to suspect that she is an abused woman.
   D. Normalize this question by explaining that you are required to ask this question and just need to check the box on the history form and do this for all women.

   The correct answer is B. Women feel that screening and universal education alone are an effective intervention, regardless of disclosure. This model offers a safe place for follow-up if she does need further support. She may not be ready to disclose for reasons including embarrassment, denial, fear of repercussions from her abuser, fear of family separation, and fear of police involvement. However, repeat screening has been shown to increase the rate of disclosure. Although disclosure is not necessary to provide effective intervention, it does help to offer more individualized and appropriate resources for a survivor [85, 88].

References

1. Centers for Disease Control and Prevention. Preventing intimate partner violence, 2019. Available at: https://www.cdc.gov/violenceprevention/pdf/ipv-factsheet508.pdf. Accessed: 29 Feb 2020.
2. Nielsen SK, Hardesty JL, Raffaelli M. Exploring variations within situational couple violence and comparisons with coercive controlling violence and no violence/no control. Violence Against Women. 2016;22(2):206–24.
3. Smith SG, Chen J, Basile KC, et al. The National Intimate Partner and Sexual Violence Survey (NISVS): 2010–2012 state report. Atlanta: Centers for Disease Control and Prevention; 2017.
4. Black MC, Basile KC, Breiding MJ, et al. The National Intimate Partner and Sexual Violence Survey (NISVS): 2010 summary report. Atlanta: National Center for Injury Prevention and Control, Centers for Disease Control and Prevention; 2011.
5. Smith SG, Zhang X, Basile KC, et al. The National Intimate Partner and Sexual Violence Survey: 2015 data brief. Atlanta: National Center for Injury Prevention and Control, Centers for Disease Control and Prevention; 2018.
6. Brodsky A. "Rape adjacent": imagining legal responses to nonconsensual condom removal. Columbia J Gend Law. 2017;32(2):183–210.

7. The Centers for Disease Control and Prevention. The social-ecological model: a framework for prevention. Available at: https://www.cdc.gov/violenceprevention/publichealthissue/social-ecologicalmodel.html. Accessed: 29 Feb 2020.
8. National Center for Injury Prevention and Control, Division of Violence Prevention, Centers for Disease Control and Prevention. Intimate partner violence: risk and protective factors, 2017. Available at: https://www.cdc.gov/violenceprevention/intimatepartnerviolence/riskprotectivefactors.html. Accessed: 13 July 2018.
9. Moyer VA. Screening for intimate partner violence and abuse of elderly and vulnerable adults: U.S. preventive services task force recommendation statement. Ann Intern Med. 2013;158(6):478–86.
10. Kann L, McManus T, Harris WA, et al. Youth risk behavior surveillance – United States, 2015. MMWR Surveill Summ. 2016;65(6):1–174.
11. Breiding MJ, Ziembroski JS, Black MC. Prevalence of rural intimate partner violence in 16 US states, 2005. J Rural Health. 2009;25(3):240–6.
12. Peek-Asa C, Wallis A, Harland K, et al. Rural disparity in domestic violence prevalence and access to resources. J Women's Health. 2011;20(11):1743–9.
13. Averill JB, Padilla AO, Clements PT. Frightened in isolation: unique considerations for research of sexual assault and interpersonal violence in rural areas. J Forensic Nurs. 2007;3(1):42–6.
14. McCall-Hosenfeld JS, Weisman CS, Perry AN, et al. "I just keep my antennae out": how rural primary care physicians respond to intimate partner violence. J Interpers Violence. 2014;29(14):2670–94.
15. Lisa AG, Katya Fels S, Angela MB, et al. When crises collide: how intimate partner violence and poverty intersect to shape women's mental health and coping? Trauma Violence Abuse. 2009;10(4):306–29.
16. Walters ML, Chen J, Breiding MJ. The National Intimate Partner and Sexual Violence Survey: 2010 findings on victimization by sexual orientation. Atlanta: National Center for Injury Prevention and Control, Centers for Disease Control and Prevention; 2013.
17. Breiding MJ, Smith SG, Basile KC, et al. Prevalence and characteristics of sexual violence, stalking, and intimate partner violence victimization – national intimate partner and sexual violence survey, United States, 2011. MMWR Surveill Summ. 2014;63(8):1–18.
18. Jewkes R, Sen P, Garcia-Moreno C. Sexual violence. In: Krug EG, editor. World report on violence and health. Geneva: World Health Organization; 2002.
19. Mellins CA, Walsh K, Sarvet AL, et al. Sexual assault incidents among college undergraduates: prevalence and factors associated with risk. PLoS One. 2017;12(11):e0186471.
20. United Nations. Protocol to prevent, suppress and punish trafficking in persons, especially women and children, supplementing the United Nations Convention against Transnational Organized Crime. Geneva: United Nations; 2000.
21. International Labour Office. A global alliance against forced labour – Global Report on Forced Labour. International Labour Conference 93rd Session 2005. Geneva: International Labour Office; 2005.
22. Hepburn S, Simon RJ. Hidden in plain sight: human trafficking in the United States. Gend Issues. 2010;27(1–2):1–26.
23. Domestic Abuse Intervention Project. FAQs about the wheels, www.theduluthmodel.org/. Available at: https://www.theduluthmodel.org/wheels/faqs-about-the-wheels/. Accessed: 30 July 2018.
24. Cycle of Violence. Available at: http://www.shelterforhelpinemergency.org/cycle-of-violence/#. Accessed: 30 July 2018.
25. Power and Control Wheel. National Center on Domestic and Sexual Violence. Available at: http://www.ncdsv.org/publications_wheel.html. Accessed: 30 July 2019.
26. Campbell JC, Webster D, Koziol-McLain J, et al. Risk factors for femicide in abusive relationships: results from a multisite case control study. Am J Public Health. 2003;93(7):1089–97.
27. www.ipvhealth.org. Accessed: 30 July 2018.
28. Plummer SB, Findley PA. Women with disabilities' experience with physical and sexual abuse: review of the literature and implications for the field. Trauma Violence Abuse. 2012;13(1):15–29.
29. American Medical Association diagnostic and treatment guidelines on domestic violence. Arch Fam Med. 1992;1(1):39–47.
30. Salleh MR. Life event, stress and illness. Malays J Med Sci. 2008;15(4):9–18.
31. Crofford LJ. Violence, stress, and somatic syndromes. Trauma Violence Abuse. 2007;8(3):299–313.
32. Leserman J, Drossman DA. Relationship of abuse history to functional gastrointestinal disorders and symptoms: some possible mediating mechanisms. Trauma Violence Abuse. 2007;8(3):331–43.
33. Plichta SB. Intimate partner violence and physical health consequences: policy and practice implications. J Interpers Violence. 2004;19(11):1296–323.
34. Bonomi AE, Anderson ML, Rivara FP, et al. Health outcomes in women with physical and sexual intimate partner violence exposure. J Women's Health. 2007;16(7):987–97.
35. Breiding MJ, Black MC, Ryan GW. Chronic disease and health risk behaviors associated with intimate partner violence-18 U.S. states/territories, 2005. Ann Epidemiol. 2008;18(7):538–44.
36. Campbell J, Jones AS, Dienemann J, et al. Intimate partner violence and physical health consequences. Arch Intern Med. 2002;162(10):1157–63.
37. Campbell JC, Lewandowski LA. Mental and physical health effects of intimate partner violence on women and children. Psychiatr Clin North Am. 1997;20(2):353–74.
38. Coker AL, Davis KE, Arias I, et al. Physical and mental health effects of intimate partner violence for men and women. Am J Prev Med. 2002;23(4):260–8.
39. Coker AL, Smith PH, Bethea L, et al. Physical health consequences of physical and psychological intimate partner violence. Arch Fam Med. 2000;9(5):451–7.
40. Douge N, Lehman EB, McCall-Hosenfeld JS. Social support and employment status modify the effect of intimate partner violence on depression symptom severity in women: results from the 2006 Behavioral Risk Factor Surveillance System Survey. Womens Health Issues. 2014;24(4):e425–34.
41. McCall-Hosenfeld JS, Winter M, Heeren T, et al. The association of interpersonal trauma with somatic symptom severity in a primary care population with chronic pain: exploring the role of gender and the mental health sequelae of trauma. J Psychosom Res. 2014;77(3):196–204.
42. Schirk DK, Lehman EB, Perry AN, et al. The impact of social support on the risk of eating disorders in women exposed to intimate partner violence. Int J Women's Health. 2015;7:919–31.
43. Pathe M, Mullen PE. The impact of stalkers on their victims. Br J Psychiatry. 1997;170:12–7.
44. Olff M. Sex and gender differences in post-traumatic stress disorder: an update. Eur J Psychotraumatol. 2017;8(sup4):1351204.
45. Duxbury F. Recognising domestic violence in clinical practice using the diagnoses of posttraumatic stress disorder, depression and low self-esteem. Br J Gen Pract. 2006;56(525):294–300.
46. Woods SJ. Intimate partner violence and post-traumatic stress disorder symptoms in women: what we know and need to know. J Interpers Violence. 2005;20(4):394–402.

47. Nixon RDV, Resick PA, Nishith P. An exploration of comorbid depression among female victims of intimate partner violence with posttraumatic stress disorder. J Affect Disord. 2004;82(2):315–20.
48. Lang AJ, Kennedy CM, Stein MB. Anxiety sensitivity and PTSD among female victims of intimate partner violence. Depress Anxiety. 2002;16(2):77–83.
49. Gerber MR, Ganz ML, Lichter E, et al. Adverse health behaviors and the detection of partner violence by clinicians. Arch Intern Med. 2005;165(9):1016–21.
50. Clark CB, Reiland S, Thorne C, et al. Relationship of trauma exposure and substance abuse to self-reported violence among men and women in substance abuse treatment. J Interpers Violence. 2014;29(8):1514–30.
51. Davies R, Lehman E, Perry A, et al. Association of intimate partner violence and health-care provider-identified obesity. Women Health. 2016;56(5):561–75.
52. McCloskey LA, Williams CM, Lichter E, et al. Abused women disclose partner interference with health care: an unrecognized form of battering. J Gen Intern Med. 2007;22(8):1067–72.
53. Letourneau EJ, Holmes M, Chasedunn-Roark J. Gynecologic health consequences to victims of interpersonal violence. Womens Health Issues. 1999;9(2):115–20.
54. Williams CM, Larsen U, McCloskey LA. Intimate partner violence and women's contraceptive use. Violence Against Women. 2008;14(12):1382–96.
55. Coker AL, Sanderson M, Fadden MK, et al. Intimate partner violence and cervical neoplasia. J Women's Health Gend Based Med. 2000;9(9):1015–23.
56. Pallitto CC, Campbell JC, O'Campo P. Is intimate partner violence associated with unintended pregnancy? A review of the literature. Trauma Violence Abuse. 2005;6(3):217–35.
57. Miller E, Decker MR, McCauley HL, et al. Pregnancy coercion, intimate partner violence and unintended pregnancy. Contraception. 2010;81(4):316–22.
58. Hastings JE, Hamberger LK. Personality characteristics of spouse abusers: a controlled comparison. Violence Vict. 1988;3(1):31–48.
59. Signs of Abuse. Women's Center and Shelter of Greater Pittsburgh. Available at: https://www.wcspittsburgh.org/signs-of-abuse. Accessed: 30 July 2018.
60. Types of Abuse. Women's Center and Shelter of Greater Pittsburgh. Available at: https://www.wcspittsburgh.org/types-of-abuse/. Accessed: 30 July 2018.
61. United Nations. Protocol to prevent, suppress, and punish trafficking in persons, especially women and children, supplementing the United Nations Convention against Transnational Organized Crime. New York: United Nations; 2004.
62. Logan TK, Walker R, Hunt G. Understanding human trafficking in the United States. Trauma Violence Abuse. 2009;10(1):3–30.
63. International Organization for Migration. Caring for trafficked persons: guidance for health providers. Geneva: International Organization for Migration; 2009.
64. Safe Horizons. Recognizing human trafficking: guidelines for health care providers. Available at: https://healtrafficking.org/resources/safe-horizons-guidelines-for-healthcare-professionals-recognizing-human-trafficking/. Accessed: 30 July 2018.
65. Toney-Butler TJ, Bhimji SS. Human trafficking. Treasure Island: StatPearls Publishing; 2017.
66. Elliott DE, Bjelajac P, Fallot RD, et al. Trauma-informed or trauma-denied: principles and implementation of trauma-informed services for women. J Community Psychol. 2005;33(4):461–77.
67. Huggard P, Unit G. A systematic review of the measurement of compassion fatigue, vicarious trauma, and secondary traumatic stress in physicians. Australas J Disaster Trauma Stud. 2013;2013:37–44.
68. SAMHSA.GOV. Guiding principles of trauma-informed care. SAMHSA News, 2014. Available at: https://www.samhsa.gov/samhsaNewsLetter/Volume_22_Number_2/trauma_tip/guiding_principles.html. Accessed: 30 July 2018.
69. Institute of Medicine. Clinical preventive services for women: closing the gaps. Washington, DC: National Academies Press; 2011.
70. McCloskey LA, Lichter E, Williams C, et al. Assessing intimate partner violence in health care settings leads to women's receipt of interventions and improved health. Public Health Rep. 2006;121(4):435–44.
71. Gillum TL, Sun CJ, Woods AB. Can a health clinic-based intervention increase safety in abused women? Results from a pilot study. J Women's Health. 2009;18(8):1259–64.
72. Durborow N, Lizdas KC, O'Flaherty A, et al. Compendium of state and U.S. territory statutes and policies on domestic violence and health care. San Francisco: Futures Without Violence; 2013.
73. ACOG Committee Opinion No. 518: Intimate partner violence. Obstet Gynecol. 2012;119(2 Pt 1):412–7.
74. Chang JC. Intimate partner violence: how you can help female survivors. Cleve Clin J Med. 2014;81(7):439–46.
75. Lo Fo Wong S, Wester F, Mol S, Römkens R, Hezemans D, Lagro-Janssen T. Talking matters: abused women's views on disclosure of partner abuse to the family doctor and its role in handling the abuse situation. Patient Educ Couns. 2008;70:386–94.
76. Feder GS, Hutson M, Ramsay J, et al. Women exposed to intimate partner violence: expectations and experiences when they encounter health care professionals: a meta-analysis of qualitative studies. Arch Intern Med. 2006;166(1):22–37.
77. Chang JC, Decker MR, Moracco KE, et al. Asking about intimate partner violence: advice from female survivors to health care providers. Patient Educ Couns. 2005;59(2):141–7.
78. Family Violence Prevention Fund. National consensus guidelines on identifying and responding to domestic violence victimization in health care settings. San Francisco: Family Violence Prevention Fund; 2004.
79. Sohal H, Eldridge S, Feder G. The sensitivity and specificity of four questions (HARK) to identify intimate partner violence: a diagnostic accuracy study in general practice. BMC Fam Pract. 2007;8:49.
80. Sherin KM, Sinacore JM, Li XQ, et al. HITS: a short domestic violence screening tool for use in a family practice setting. Fam Med. 1998;30(7):508–12.
81. Ernst AA, Weiss SJ, Cham E, et al. Detecting ongoing intimate partner violence in the emergency department using a simple 4-question screen: the OVAT. Violence Vict. 2004;19(3):375–84.
82. MacMillan HL, Wathen CN, Jamieson E, et al. Approaches to screening for intimate partner violence in health care settings: a randomized trial. JAMA. 2006;296(5):530–6.
83. National Domestic Violence Hotline, 1-800-799-SAFE. Available at: www.thehotline.org. Accessed: 30 July 2018.
84. Chang JC. Domestic violence. In: Bieber EJ, Sanfilippo JS, Horowitz IR, editors. Clinical gynecology. Philadelphia: Elsevier; 2006. p. 79–89.
85. Chang JC, Cluss PA, Ranieri L, et al. Health care interventions for intimate partner violence: what women want. Womens Health Issues. 2005;15(1):21–30.
86. Anderson DK, Saunders DG. Leaving an abusive partner: an empirical review of predictors, the process of leaving, and psychological well-being. Trauma Violence Abuse. 2003;4(2):163–91.
87. Davidson CA, Buranosky RA, Chang JC. The meaning of "safe": how many women experiencing IPV interpret safety. San Francisco: National Conference on Health and Domestic Violence; 2012.

88. Alpert E. Intimate partner violence, Massachusetts Medical Society Committee on violence intervention and prevention. 6th ed. Waltham: Massachusetts Medical Society; 2015. Available at: http://www.massmed.org/partnerviolence/. Accessed: 30 July 2018.
89. Enos VP. An intervention to improve the documentation of intimate partner violence in medical records. Research report submitted to the US Department of Justice, 2004. Available at: https://www.ncjrs.gov/pdffiles1/nij/grants/207146.pdf. Accessed: 18 Apr 2018.
90. Caralis PV, Musialowski R. Women's experiences with domestic violence and their attitudes and expectations regarding medical care of abuse victims. South Med J. 1997;90(11):1075–80.
91. Hamberger LK, Ambuel B, Marbella A, et al. Physician interaction with battered women: the women's perspective. Arch Fam Med. 1998;7(6):575–82.
92. Ledray LE, Burgess AW, Giardino AP. Medical response to adult sexual assault. St. Louis: STM Learning; 2011.
93. Corum V, Carroll J. Forensic analysts' perspectives: sexual assault kits under the microscope. J Forensic Nurs. 2014;10(1):50–7.
94. Littel K. Sexual assault nurse examiner (SANE) programs: improving the community response to sexual assault victims. Washington, DC: US Department of Justice, Office of Justice Programs, Office for Victims of Crime; 2001.
95. Campbell R, Patterson D, Bybee D, et al. Predicting sexual assault prosecution outcomes: the role of medical forensic evidence collected by sexual assault nurse examiners. Crim Justice Behav. 2009;36(7):712–27.
96. Warshaw C, Ganley AL. Improving the health care response to domestic violence: a resource manual for health care providers, 1996. Available at: http://www.futureswithoutviolence.org. Accessed: 18 Aug 2018.
97. Goldman J, Hudson RM, Hudson Z, Sawires P. Health privacy principles for protecting victims of domestic violence, 2000. Available at: www.futureswithoutviolence.org. Accessed: 14 Aug 2018.
98. Zimmerman C, Watts C. WHO ethical and safety recommendations for interviewing trafficked women. Geneva: World Health Organization; 2003.
99. Johnson H, Hotton T. Losing control, homicide risk in estranged and intact intimate relationships. Homicide Stud. 2003;7(1):58–84.
100. Krause ED, Kaltman S, Goodman LA, et al. Avoidant coping and PTSD symptoms related to domestic violence exposure: a longitudinal study. J Trauma Stress. 2008;21(1):83–90.
101. Parker M, McCall-Hosenfeld JS, Lehmah E. Correlation of actions taken by women in response to intimate partner violence (IPV) and IPV status at 1-year follow-up. Society of General Internal Medicine National Meeting, Denver, CO, 2018.
102. Blasco-Ros C, Sanchez-Lorente S, Martinez M. Recovery from depressive symptoms, state anxiety and post-traumatic stress disorder in women exposed to physical and psychological, but not to psychological intimate partner violence alone: a longitudinal study. BMC Psychiatry. 2010;10:98.

Care of Sexual Minority Women

36

Eloho Ufomata and Carla Spagnoletti

Learning Objectives

1. Describe healthcare disparities and challenges with access to care faced by women who identify as lesbian, gay, or bisexual (LGB).
2. Define the terms "sexual orientation," "sexual behavior," "gender identity," and "gender expression."
3. Elicit information about a patient's sexuality in a sensitive and inclusive manner.
4. Screen and treat sexually transmitted infections in women who have sex with women.
5. Apply guidelines to optimize preventive care in patients who identify as LGB.

Natalie is a 42-year-old woman who presents to establish care. She has a history of depression and obesity. She has not seen a physician in 10 years due to prior unpleasant experiences at providers' offices. Prior to the visit, she called the office staff to inquire about its nondiscrimination policy.

Overview

According to 2016 data from the Gallup poll, about 10 million adults in the United States self-identify as lesbian, gay, bisexual, or transgender (LGBT), of which about 55% are women [1]. This population has steadily been increasing over the years, and the increase in self-identification as LGBT is more noticeable in women than in men. In 2012, 3.5% of women identified as LGBT, while in 2016, 4.4% of women identified as LGBT. This contrasts with 3.4% of men in 2012 vs. 3.7% in 2016 [1]. Of note, definitions of LGB status are varied in studies and may be based on behavioral factors (e.g., women who have sex with women) vs. self-identification (e.g., lesbian). This can make the data in this patient population difficult to interpret. This chapter focuses on sexual minority women, or women who identify as lesbian, bisexual, or gay. There is a separate chapter focusing on the health of transgender individuals (See Chap. 37).

There are health disparities associated with LGB status. Compared to heterosexual adults, LGB adults appear to experience mood disorders at a higher rate and are more likely to have experienced suicidal ideation and self-injurious behaviors [2]. This might be due in part to minority stress, a conceptual framework describing stress related to the experience of being a minority, which could include experienced prejudice, expectations of rejection or discrimination, concealed identity, and internalized negative attitudes such as homophobia [3]. In addition, women who identify as LGB may be at higher risk for breast cancer and cardiovascular disease due to more prevalent risk factors such as obesity and higher rates of tobacco and alcohol use [2]. Individuals who identify as LGB are also at increased risk for discrimination, stigmatization, and violent crimes compared to their heterosexual counterparts. The CDC's National Intimate Partner and Sexual Violence Survey (NISVS): 2010 Findings on Victimization by Sexual Orientation found that lesbian and bisexual women reported intimate partner violence and sexual violence over their lifetimes at rates equal to, or higher than those of, heterosexual women. Bisexual women are most likely to experience intimate partner violence [4].

E. Ufomata (✉)
University of Pittsburgh School of Medicine, Department of Internal Medicine, Pittsburgh, PA, USA
e-mail: ufomataeo@upmc.edu

C. Spagnoletti
University of Pittsburgh, Department of Medicine, Pittsburgh, PA, USA

S. A. Tilstra et al. (eds.), *Sex- and Gender-Based Women's Health*, https://doi.org/10.1007/978-3-030-50695-7_36

Establishing a Welcoming Environment

It is important to note that the majority of Americans have implicit bias which favors heterosexual people over LGB people [5]. A study examining the implicit preferences of healthcare providers found that implicit preferences for heterosexual over lesbian and gay people were common among nurses, physicians, and mental health providers [5]. Lesbians and bisexual women were also significantly more likely than heterosexual women to have unsatisfactory care, as well as to have faced discrimination or disrespect from a healthcare provider [6, 7]. These factors may contribute to a patient's apprehension in establishing care with a new provider and an overall delay in medical care. LGB individuals look for favorable clues when entering healthcare facilities including posted non-discrimination policies, respectful interactions with staff, and gender-neutral bathrooms. They also take note of whether office intake forms are inclusive [8]. Unfortunately, many offices have forms that exclude gender and sexual minority experiences which can discourage disclosure of gender identity, sexual orientation, and sexual behavior. A 2013 survey study piloted a patient intake form in order to validate sexual orientation and gender identity (SOGI) questions [8, 9]. A gender/sexuality diverse group of roughly 400 patients were asked questions about their SOGI and the acceptability of the questions. Most patients believed that the SOGI questions were important, felt that they would answer similar questions in the future, and believed that it was important for their physician to know the information provided [8, 9]. The patients who identified as LGB felt that the questions allowed them to accurately report information about themselves in a comfortable manner [8, 9]. If intake forms are not inclusive, it is critical to obtain a patient's sexual orientation and gender identity during history taking.

Natalie identifies as bisexual and states that she is currently in a monogamous relationship with a woman. She identifies as a woman and prefers to wear clothing from the "men's department."

Terminology

An understanding of the terms used to characterize a person's sexuality and gender is important when eliciting a history from a woman [10].

Sexual orientation is a person's attraction to another person, which could be a physical, romantic, emotional, and/or spiritual attraction. Orientation could be described as lesbian, gay, heterosexual, bisexual, pansexual, polysexual, asexual, among others. A person's sexual orientation should not be assumed based on the perceived sex of the person or the person's partner(s) [11].

Sexual practices are defined by a person's sexual behaviors and guide the clinical assessment of patient risk for sexually transmitted infections (STIs), which drives counseling on risk-reduction strategies, testing protocols, and the identification of anatomical sites from which to collect specimens testing [11]. Sexual orientation and sexual practices can change over time, and do not necessarily "align," although they typically closely correlate.

Gender identity is a person's innate, deeply felt identification as a male person, female person, both male and female, or neither. For patients who identify as cisgender, their gender identity corresponds to that person's assigned sex at birth (i.e., the sex listed on the birth certificate) [11]. For those who identify as transgender, their gender identity is different from their assigned sex at birth (i.e., the sex listed on the birth certificate). For those who identify as gender fluid, their gender identity is not fixed and may be different depending on the context. For those who identify as agender (sometimes referred to as gender neutral), their gender identity does not align with male or female [11]. One question that can be used to determine a patient's gender identity, recommended by the National LGBT Health Education Center is: "Many people are affected by gender issues, so I ask patients if they have any concerns. Is this topic relevant to you?" [12]. Another question is: "It is common to have concerns relating to gender, would you like to discuss your gender identity?" [10].

Gender expression is the way in which a person communicates gender by external means such as clothing, hairstyles, mannerisms, or voice [11]. Many patient's gender expression does not necessarily reflect their gender identity, exemplifying the importance of asking patients, rather than assuming their identity (Table 36.1).

It is imperative that when asking about SOGI, open-ended questions are used and nothing is assumed about the patient, their partners, or their practices.

How to Ask About Sexual Orientation and Gender Identity (SOGI)

Determining a patient's sexual orientation and gender identity (SOGI) is an important component of history taking [10, 13]. When providers do not know a patient's full sexual history, they may not be able to recommend appropriate health services such as vaccinations, screening for cancers, or screening for sexually transmitted infections.

All providers are subject to bias and are influenced by experiences; it is important to be cognizant of how these can affect patient care. Refraining from making assumptions about a patient's sexual orientation and gender identify is critical, as gender does not imply anything about sexuality

Table 36.1 Sexual orientation and gender identity (SOGI) terminology [11]

Term	Definition	Keywords and pearls
Sexual orientation	A person's physical, romantic, emotional, and/or spiritual attraction to another person	Lesbian, gay, heterosexual, bisexual, pansexual, polysexual, asexual, etc. Many terms used and defined by the patient
Sexual practices	A person's sexual behaviors	Ask about partners, the type of sex they engage in, and assess risk for pregnancy and STIs
Gender identity	A person's innate, deeply felt identification as a male person, female person, both male and female, or neither	Cisgender, transgender, gender non-conforming, non-binary, agender, etc. Many terms used and defined by the patient (see Chap. 37)
Gender expression	The way in which a person communicates gender by external means, such as clothing, hairstyles, mannerisms, or voice	May not reflect gender identity

and vice versa. Providers should reflect on phrasing of questions that are commonly used that can imply assumptions, for example "Are you and your boyfriend sexually active?", and form new habits using more inclusive phrasing. This will allow all patient encounters to be approached in a non-judgmental and sensitive way.

The Fenway Institute recommends the following communication techniques when obtaining a patient's SOGI [10]:

1. Set the stage to *normalize* this line of inquiry: "Next, I'd like to ask you some questions about your sexuality. This is routine, confidential and important to your overall health."
2. Use *open, inclusive language* and avoid assuming gender of partners, monogamy, or sexual practices: "Tell me about your sexual partners."
3. Be cognizant of *body language* and other non-verbal cues. Maintain eye contact, be aware of facial expressions or head shaking.
4. *Listen* to how your patients describe themselves, their partners, their practices, and use those same words.

The CDC's "5 Ps" of sexual history is a framework that can be used to learn more about a patient's sexual history [14].

1. PARTNERS: "Are you currently sexually active? Have you ever been sexually active? Are your sex partners men, women, or both?"
2. PRACTICES: "To better understand if you are at risk for STIs, I have a few specific questions. What kind of sexual contact do you have or have you had? Genital (penis in the vagina)? Anal (penis in the anus)? Oral (mouth on penis, vagina, or anus)?"
3. PROTECTION from sexually transmitted infections (STIs): "Do you and your partner(s) use any protection against STIs? If not, why not? If so, what kind? How often do you use protection? In what situations or with whom do you use protection?"
4. PAST HISTORY of STIs: "Have you ever been diagnosed with an STI? What treatment did you receive? Have you ever been tested for HIV or other STIs? Would you like to be tested for STIs?"
5. PREGNANCY planning or prevention: "Do you have concerns about getting pregnant? Are you using any form of birth control (if/when sexually active with men)? Do you want information on birth control?"

Natalie states that she has been with her new partner for a few months. She notes an increase in her vaginal discharge and that it has a "fishy odor." She is diagnosed with bacterial vaginitis utilizing in-office testing. She wonders if her partner could be affected by her diagnosis.

Sexually Transmitted Infections (STIs) in Women Who Have Sex with Women

Women who have sex with women, or WSW, can acquire sexually transmitted infections (STIs). Infected cervicovaginal or anal secretions may be transmitted by digital-vaginal or digital-anal contact and by shared penetrative sex items [15]. It is also important to note a high percentage of WSW have had sex with men in the past; up to one-third in the past 1 year [15]. Women who have sex with women are twice as likely to have bacterial vaginosis (BV) compared to those who are not WSW. Bacterial vaginitis is not considered a sexually transmitted infection per se, but it is thought to be sexually *associated*, which means the risk of BV can increase after sexual encounters. There is a high level of concordance in genital lactobacillus in female sex partners and significant concordant infection rates between female partners (25–50%) [16].

Although less likely than with male-to-female or male-to-male transmission, other STIs, such as chlamydia, gonorrhea, and trichomoniasis, can be transmitted among WSW [16–18]. At least one case study has described the transmission of HIV between females [19]. HPV infection among lesbian women is similar to the general heterosexual population and can be transmitted between female partners (See Chaps. 13 and 14).

Counseling on Safe Sex Practices

Providers should share these simple tips with female patients to help reduce their risk for acquiring STIs [20].

1. Use barrier protection with both male and female partners.
2. Use gloves during digital-genital sex.
3. Use condoms with sex toys.
4. Use latex or plastic barriers (such as dental dams) for oral-genital sex.
5. Properly care for shared penetrative sex toys, by cleaning with hot soapy water between use, but avoid sharing if possible.

Other important preventative measures that should be taken to keep female patients healthy include the following: (1) age-appropriate vaccination against human papilloma virus (HPV) regardless of sexual practices, (2) cervical cancer screening per established guidelines regardless of sexual practices, and (3) STI testing per guidelines. The Center for Disease Control (CDC) recommends chlamydia and gonorrhea screening for all sexually active women yearly until age 25 [15]. They also recommend screening for HIV at least once in a lifetime, regardless of sexual practices [15]. If women are at high risk for HIV, screening at more frequent intervals should occur and concomitant screening for hepatitis C may be considered (See Chaps. 13 and 14).

Natalie presents back a year later at age 43. Her father recently had a heart attack, and she is concerned that this was related to his lifestyle. Because she is obese and inactive, she wants to discuss her overall health and strategies to prevent serious illnesses in the future.

Cardiovascular Disease Risk

There is some data showing that women who are sexual minority, that is lesbian or bisexual, have an increased prevalence of cardiovascular disease. One study found that lesbian and bisexual women are significantly more likely to recall being diagnosed with heart disease compared to heterosexual women [6]. Within this group, bisexual women were younger on average than heterosexual or lesbian women but were still at increased risk compared to heterosexual women, and lesbian women had the highest cardiovascular risk [6]. In addition, a 2016 systematic review found that sexual minority women had higher cardiovascular disease risk compared to men and heterosexual women, which was associated with lifetime tobacco use, alcohol use, illicit drug use, poor mental health, and elevated body mass index [21]. Compared to heterosexual women, lesbian women had higher rates of hypertension and bisexual women had higher rates of hypertension, greater use of blood pressure medication, and were more likely to have diabetes [21]. Unfortunately, there are no specific guidelines for women of sexual minority for the prevention of cardiovascular disease, so routine counseling of lifestyle modification including smoking cessation and weight loss along with aggressive identification of cardiovascular risk factors such as diabetes and hypertension is recommended for these patients (See Chaps. 21 and 22).

Natalie is also interested in cancer screening as a 43-year-old woman. Her last pap test was performed 3 years ago, and she reports that it was normal. She is not sure if she was tested for HPV at that time. In addition, she would like to know more about her risk for breast and ovarian cancer.

Cancer Screening

Cervical Cancer

Data strongly support that human papilloma virus (HPV) infections are common in WSW. A common misconception among patients and some providers is that WSW have a low risk of cervical cancer because they are unlikely to have been exposed to HPV. Transmission can occur between women as it is spread through skin-to-skin contact as well as contact with bodily fluids [16]. HPV has been detected in the genital tract of 13–30% of women who have only had sex with women, which is similar to rates found in the general population [22]. As of 2018, the US Preventive Services Task Force (USPSTF) cervical cancer screening guidelines recommend screening with cervical cytology every 3 years for all persons aged 21–65 who have a cervix, regardless of sexuality or gender identity; alternatively women ages 30–65 can be screened with cervical cytology and HPV co-testing or high-risk HPV testing alone every 5 years (See Chap. 14) [23]. Despite this, WSW are less likely to routinely undergo cervical cancer screening, and lesbians are 87% less likely to have ever received a pap test compared to heterosexual women [24]. Barriers to routine cervical screening include perceived low susceptibility to cervical cancer by these women and their providers, perceived lack of benefits to screening, and an underestimation of the seriousness of cervical cancer [25]. These findings suggest that it is essential for providers to discuss sexual orientation with patients and educate them on their susceptibility to HPV and the benefits of cervical cancer screening. Regarding HPV vaccination, bisexual women were significantly more likely to have HPV vaccination compared to lesbian or heterosexual women, who had similar rates of vaccination [26]. The current recommendation by the CDC is to routinely vaccinate adolescents/young adults starting at age 11 regardless of sexuality [27]. The HPV vaccination series is currently approved through age 26, but the FDA just expanded their recommended coverage of the vaccine series to include all genders aged 9–45 (See Chap. 14) [28].

Breast Cancer

There is no data examining the prevalence of breast cancer as it relates to sexuality; however, the National Academy of Medicine predicts a higher risk of breast cancer in lesbian and bisexual women due to higher prevalence of risk factors such as tobacco use, decreased parity, obesity, and alcohol intake [2]. The screening recommendations are the same for average risk women regardless of sexuality and vary by guideline, beginning at age 40. There is some data suggesting that lesbian and bisexual women are more likely to perceive their risk of breast cancer as lower, to have negative beliefs about breast cancer screening, and that trust or a positive relationship with the provider recommending the test is more likely to affect intentions to follow-through with screening (See Chaps. 17 and 18) [29].

Endometrial and Ovarian Cancer

Screening for endometrial or ovarian cancer is not recommended for asymptomatic women regardless of sexual orientation. There are few data examining the prevalence of endometrial and ovarian cancer in women who identify as lesbian or bisexual; however, the available data is conflicting [30]. Please see Chap. 15 to learn more about the prevention, screening, and management of female cancers.

Summary Points

1. Women who identify as LGB have decreased access to quality healthcare, experience discrimination in medical facilities, and face healthcare disparities. These patients may look for favorable clues that a healthcare environment is welcoming, including non-discrimination policies, inclusive intake forms, and gender-neutral bathrooms.
2. Sexual orientation, sexual practices, gender identity, and gender expression are each unique aspects of a patient's being. Each is important to elicit as part of a patient's history.
3. The 5 Ps (Partners, Practices, Protection from STIs, Past history of STIs, Pregnancy planning or prevention) framework is a good way to acquire a sexual history from patients.
4. Women who have sex with women are at risk for STIs, including bacterial STIs, and HPV. Bacterial vaginosis may be transmitted between female sex partners. STI screening should be performed with attention to sexual practices. Women should receive vaccinations, cervical, and breast cancer screening based on established guidelines, regardless of sexual practices.

Review Questions

1. A 32-year-old woman presents to your office to establish care and for a check-up. She has no symptoms or concerns. As part of her routine history, you gather information about her sexual orientation and gender identity (SOGI) history. You learn that she is attracted to women, she engages in sex with her girlfriend, and they use sex toys during sexual encounters. She has had two male sexual partners in the remote past but is not interested in men romantically or sexually at this time. She identifies as female. On physical exam, you note that she has long hair, is wearing make-up and earrings, and is dressed in a blouse and skirt.

   Which of the following descriptions best summarizes this patient's sexual orientation and gender identity?

   A. She is a cisgender bisexual woman.
   B. She is a transgender bisexual woman.
   C. She is cisgender lesbian woman.
   D. She is a cisgender polysexual woman.
   E. She is a gender-fluid lesbian woman.

   The correct answer is C. Sexual orientation, sexual practices, gender identity, and gender expression are each unique aspects of a patient's sexuality. Each is important to elicit as part of a patient's history. Gathering sexual orientation and gender identity data in a standardized way will allow a better understanding of LGBT health disparities. This will assist the provider in prevention, screening, and detection of conditions that disproportionately affect LGBT people. This patient was assigned female sex at birth, identifies as a female, expresses her gender in a stereotypically feminine manner, is attracted to women, and has had sex with both men and women. Thus, she is a cisgender woman who is lesbian, despite having had sex with men in the past. Sexual orientation is defined as a person's enduring physical, romantic, emotional, and/or spiritual attraction to another person and can be described as lesbian, gay, heterosexual, bisexual, pansexual, polysexual, asexual, and others. A person's sexual orientation should not be assumed based on the perceived sex of that person's partner(s), but rather based on their self-identification, as sexual practices may be fluid. Gender identity is a person's innate, deeply felt identification as a male person, female person, both male and female or neither. Cisgender is the term used when gender identity corresponds to the person's assigned sex at birth (i.e., the sex listed on the birth certificate). Transgender is the term used when gender identity is different from a person's assigned sex at birth (i.e., the sex listed on the birth certificate). Gender fluid is the term used for a person whose gender identity is not fixed and may be different depending on the context. Agender, sometimes referred to as gender neutral, is the term used for a person whose gender identity does not align with male or female [31, 32].

2. A 21-year-old woman presents for a routine annual exam. She last saw her pediatrician at age 17. She is healthy, has no significant past medical history, and has no specific concerns. She has had one lifetime sexual partner who is female, but has not been sexually active for the last 6 months. She recently found out that her former partner has genital herpes. Valerie has never had any lesions. Which of the following should you offer to Valerie as part of routine screening for sexually transmitted infections, per guidelines?
   A. Screening tests for chlamydia and HIV
   B. No screening tests are indicated based on her age and sexual history
   C. Screening test for herpes simplex virus
   D. Screening tests for bacterial vaginosis
   E. Screening test for chlamydia, gonorrhea, and HIV

   The correct answer is E. WSW should not be presumed to be at low or no risk for sexually transmitted infections based on sexual orientation [16]. According to the Centers for Disease Control (CDC), WSW are at risk for acquiring bacterial (chlamydia, gonorrhea, BV), viral (HPV, HSV, and HIV), and protozoal (trichomoniasis) STIs from current and prior partners, both male and female. Report of same-sex-only encounters in women should not deter providers from considering and performing screening for cervical cancer and STIs per current guidelines [15]. There is no utility in screening for HSV based on exposure history in the absence of HSV outbreak [18]. All women should receive cervical cancer screening, regardless of sexual orientation (i.e., women who identify as lesbian, bisexual, or heterosexual), starting at age 21 and continuing through at least age 65. Annual screening of all sexually active women aged <25 years for *C. trachomatis* and *N. gonorrhoeae* is recommended. CDC recommends HIV screening for patients aged 13–64 years at least once as part of routine health care. Although common among WSW, routine screening for BV is not recommended [15].

3. A 51-year-old postmenopausal woman presents to establish care. She is requesting a pap test, and any other screening for gynecologic cancers available. She identifies as a lesbian and has had three female sexual partners in the past year. She was recently tested for STIs, which were negative, and her last pap test was 2 years ago. Her pap result was atypical squamous cells of undetermined significance (ASCUS) with negative HPV testing. She is up-to-date on breast cancer and colon cancer screening per guidelines.

   Which of the following is true regarding gynecologic cancer screening for this patient?
   A. Women who identify as lesbian and bisexual should be screened for cancers more frequently than women who identify as heterosexual.
   B. Women who identify as lesbian or bisexual are less likely to be appropriately screened for cervical cancer compared to heterosexual women.
   C. She should have a repeat pap test and HPV testing done now, since women who identify as lesbian are at higher risk for cervical cancer.
   D. Screening for endometrial cancer is warranted, because she is menopausal.

   The correct answer is B. There is some data that women who identify as lesbian or bisexual are less likely to have appropriate cervical cancer screening, and some of the barriers include perceived low susceptibility to cervical cancer (by women and providers) and perceived lack of benefits to screening and seriousness of cervical cancer [25]. Although weighted prevalence estimates generated using data on 71,112 women from the California Health Interview Survey show that heterosexual women have a significantly lower prevalence of cervical cancer (14%) compared with lesbian women (16.5%) and bisexual women (41.2%), the guidelines are not different based on sexual orientation, and this patient should not be screened more frequently [23]. The American Society for Colposcopy and Cervical Pathology recommends repeating cytology with HPV co-testing at 3 years for a pap test showing ASCUS that is HPV negative. Thus, repeating her pap now would be inappropriate [33]. Routine screening for endometrial cancer in women is not recommended regardless of sexuality [30].

References

1. Gates G. In U.S., more adults identifying as LGBT: Gallup Poll; 2017. Available from: http://news.gallup.com/poll/201731/lgbt-identification-rises.aspx.
2. Institute of Medicine (US) Committee on Lesbian, Gay, Bisexual, and Transgender Health Issues and Research Gaps and Opportunities. The health of lesbian, gay, bisexual, and transgender people: building a foundation for better understanding. Washington, DC: National Academies Press; 2011. Available from: https://www.ncbi.nlm.nih.gov/books/NBK64798/.
3. Meyer IH. Prejudice, social stress, and mental health in lesbian, gay, and bisexual populations: conceptual issues and research evidence. Psychol Bull. 2003;129(5):674–97.
4. Walters ML, Chen J, Breiding MJ. The National Intimate Partner and Sexual Violence Survey (NISVS): 2010 findings on victimization by sexual orientation. Atlanta: National Center for Injury Prevention and Control. Centers for Disease Control and Prevention; 2013. Available from: https://www.cdc.gov/violenceprevention/pdf/nisvs_sofindings.pdf.
5. Sabin JA, Riskind RG, Nosek BA. Health care providers' implicit and explicit attitudes toward lesbian women and gay men. Am J Public Health. 2015;105(9):1831–41.
6. Diamant AL, Wold C. Sexual orientation and variation in physical and mental health status among women. J Womens Health (Larchmt). 2003;12(1):41–9.
7. Dahlhamer JM, Galinsky AM, Joestl SS, Ward BW. Barriers to health care among adults identifying as sexual minorities: a US National Study. Am J Public Health. 2016;106(6):1116–22.
8. Cahill S, Singal R, Grasso C, King D, Mayer K, Baker K, et al. Do ask, do tell: high levels of acceptability by patients of routine collection of sexual orientation and gender identity data in four diverse American community health centers. PLoS One. 2014;9(9):e107104.
9. Bradford JB, Cahill S, Grasso C, Makadon HJ. Policy focus: how to gather data of sexual orientation and gender identity in clinical settings. Boston: The Fenway Institute. Available from: http://thefenwayinstitute.org/documents/Policy_Brief_HowtoGather..._v3_01.09.12.pdf.
10. Makadon H, Mayer K, Potter J, Goldhammer H. Fenway guide to lesbian, gay, bisexual and transgender health. 2nd ed. Boston: The Fenway Institute; 2015.
11. Glossary of LGBT terms for health care teams: National LGBT Health Education Center, a program of the Fenway Institute; 2016.
12. Reisner S. Meeting the needs of transgender people: The National LGBT Education Center, a program of the Fenway Institute; 2012. Available from: http://www.lgbthealtheducation.org/training/online-courses/continuingeducation.
13. Healthy People 2020: Lesbian, gay, bisexual, and transgender health. Office of Disease Prevention and Health Promotion. Available from: https://www.healthypeople.gov/2020/topics-objectives/topic/lesbian-gay-bisexual-and-transgender-health.
14. Centers for Disease Control and Prevention. A guide to taking a sexual history: US Department of Health and Human Services. Available from: https://www.cdc.gov/std/treatment/sexualhistory.pdf.
15. Bolan GA, Workowski KA, Centers for Disease Control. Sexually transmitted diseases treatment guidelines. Special populations – women who have sex with women. MMWR Morb Mortal Wkly Rep. 2015;64:1–37.
16. Gorgos LM, Marrazzo JM. Sexually transmitted infections among women who have sex with women. Clin Infect Dis. 2011;53(Suppl 3):S84–91.
17. Singh D, Fine DN, Marrazzo JM. Chlamydia trachomatis infection among women reporting sexual activity with women screened in Family Planning Clinics in the Pacific Northwest, 1997 to 2005. Am J Public Health. 2011;101(7):1284–90.
18. Xu F, Sternberg MR, Markowitz LE. Women who have sex with women in the United States: prevalence, sexual behavior and prevalence of herpes simplex virus type 2 infection—results from National Health and Nutrition Examination Survey 2001–2006. Sex Transm Dis. 2010;37(7):407–13.
19. Chan SK, Thornton LR, Chronister KJ, Meyer J, Wolverton M, Johnson CK, et al. Likely female-to-female sexual transmission of HIV – Texas, 2012. MMWR Morb Mortal Wkly Rep. 2014;63(10):209–12.
20. NHS UK. Sexual health for lesbian and bisexual women, 2016.
21. Caceres BA, Brody A, Luscombe RE, Primiano JE, Marusca P, Sitts EM, et al. A systematic review of cardiovascular disease in sexual minorities. Am J Public Health. 2017;107(4):e13–21.
22. Marrazzo JM, Koutsky LA, Kiviat NB, Kuypers JM, Stine K. Papanicolaou test screening and prevalence of genital human papillomavirus among women who have sex with women. Am J Public Health. 2001;91(6):947–52.
23. U.S. Preventive Services Task Force. Draft recommendation statement: Cervical cancer: screening; 2017. Available from: https://www.uspreventiveservicestaskforce.org/Page/Document/draft-recommendation-statement/cervical-cancer-screening2.
24. Charlton BM, Corliss HL, Missmer SA, Frazier AL, Rosario M, Kahn JA, et al. Reproductive health screening disparities and sexual orientation in a cohort study of U.S. adolescent and young adult females. J Adolesc Health. 2011;49(5):505–10.
25. Tracy JK, Schluterman NH, Greenberg DR. Understanding cervical cancer screening among lesbians: a national survey. BMC Public Health. 2013;13:442.
26. Polek C, Hardie T. Changing HPV vaccination rates in bisexual and lesbian women. J Am Assoc Nurse Pract. 2017;29(6):333–9.
27. Centers for Disease Control. HPV vaccine recommendations; 2016. Available from: https://www.cdc.gov/vaccines/vpd/hpv/hcp/recommendations.html.
28. US Food and Drug Administration. Gardasil 9. Available from: https://www.fda.gov/biologicsbloodvaccines/approvedproducts/ucm426445.htm. Accessed 30 Nov 2018.
29. Hart SL, Bowen DJ. Sexual orientation and intentions to obtain breast cancer screening. J Womens Health (Larchmt). 2009;18(2):177–85.
30. Quinn GP, Sanchez JA, Sutton SK, Vadaparampil ST, Nguyen GT, Green BL, et al. Cancer and lesbian, gay, bisexual, transgender/transsexual, and queer/questioning (LGBTQ) populations. CA Cancer J Clin. 2015;65(5):384–400.
31. Human Rights Campaign. Sexual orientation and gender identity definitions. Available at: http://www.hrc.org/resources/sexual-orientation-and-gender-identity-terminology-and-definitions. Accessed 11 Jan 2018.
32. The Fenway Institute. Policy focus: why gather data on sexual orientation and gender identity in clinical settings. Available at: http://fenwayhealth.org/documents/the-fenway-institute/policybriefs/Policy_Brief_WhyGather..._v6_01.09.12.pdf. Accessed 11 Jan 2018.
33. Saslow D, Solomon D, Lawson HW, Killackey M, Kulasingam SL, Cain J, et al. American Cancer Society; American Society for Colposcopy and Cervical Pathology; American Society for Clinical Pathology screening guidelines for the prevention and early detection of cervical cancer. Am J Clin Pathol. 2012;137(4):516–42.

Gender Affirming Care

37

Eloho Ufomata and Megan McNamara

Learning Objectives

1. Explain the concepts of sex and gender, gender identity, gender non-conformity, gender dysphoria, and gender affirmation.
2. Describe the importance of using open and inclusive language when eliciting information about a patient's gender identity, transition history, and sexual practices.
3. List strategies for optimizing patient comfort during sensitive parts of the physical exam.
4. Describe the available hormonal treatments, the goals of hormone therapy, as well as associated risks, benefits, and contraindications for gender affirmation.
5. Perform appropriate screening and immunizations for transgender patients according to their natal and surgical anatomy and sexual practices.

Isis is a 45-year-old patient with depression who presents to establish care after a prolonged hiatus from medical care. She tells you that she was assigned male at birth, and although she was named Isiah, she has thought of herself as Isis since childhood and uses the pronouns "she" and "hers." She remembers wanting to wear dresses as a child but her father discouraged her from doing so. She has never felt comfortable as a boy or as a man. She started seeing a therapist on the advice of a friend, changed her legal name, and is dressing in clothing which is more comfortable to her. She is seeking a provider who will be supportive of her and understands how to help.

Gender Identity, Gender Non-Conformity, and Gender Dysphoria

Gender is a concept that encompasses a complex relationship between a person's body or physical sexual characteristics, their identity or a deeply held internal sense of self, and their gender expression or the way they present themselves to the world [1]. Gender is distinct from natal sex, which describes the biological make-up of the individual. People are typically assigned a sex at birth based on the characteristic appearance of their genitalia as male or female, and this is referred to as "natal sex." Sex designation is not always as simple as a male or female binary. Intersex conditions, which may present with ambiguous genitalia at birth, or become evident at puberty, include persons whose chromosomal make-up or anatomy do not fit the usual male XY and female XX binary pattern [1].

Over time, there is physical development into characteristics that are viewed as feminine or masculine which are interpreted within a cultural context as well. Gender identity is an internal sense of self, which could be congruent with the sex assigned at birth or "cisgender," or could be opposite the sex assigned at birth or "transgender" [1]. There are also people who are gender non-conforming, which is an umbrella term for anyone whose gender identity is different from the sex assigned at birth [1]. This illustrates that gender is not necessarily on a binary spectrum, that is, male or female, and people may identify with a non-binary gender identity, meaning they do not identify strictly as a boy or a girl—they could

E. Ufomata (✉)
University of Pittsburgh School of Medicine, Department of Internal Medicine, Pittsburgh, PA, USA
e-mail: ufomataeo@upmc.edu

M. McNamara
Case Western Reserve University School of Medicine, Louis Stokes Cleveland VA Medical Center, Department of Medicine, Cleveland, OH, USA

S. A. Tilstra et al. (eds.), *Sex- and Gender-Based Women's Health*, https://doi.org/10.1007/978-3-030-50695-7_37

identify as both, neither, or as another gender entirely. Some people may not identify with having a gender at all, or as agender. Natal females who consider themselves to be men are referred to as "transgender men." Natal males who consider themselves to be women are referred to as "transgender women." Keep in mind that *patients* determine their own identity, and the best approach is to ask patients about their gender identity and to clarify how they would like to be addressed.

Gender dysphoria is a DSM-V diagnosis which is characterized by a conflict between a person's assigned sex and their gender identity, leading to significant distress and problems with functionality [2]. This diagnosis replaces the former DSM diagnosis of gender identity *disorder* to increase access to care and negate the connotation that gender nonconformity is a pathologic disease. The diagnostic criteria include a duration of at least 6 months and at least two of the following symptoms:

- A significant difference between one's experienced/expressed gender and physical sex characteristics
- A desire to remove one's primary and/or secondary sex characteristics
- A strong desire for the primary and/or secondary physical attributes of the other gender
- A strong desire to be of the opposite gender
- A strong desire to be treated as the opposite gender
- A strong belief that one has the usual feelings and reactions of the opposite gender [2]

The treatment for gender dysphoria includes steps toward gender affirmation, which is a process by which a person can adapt their body to their experienced gender [3, 4]. Treatment options for gender dysphoria include counseling, cross-sex hormones, puberty suppression, and gender affirming surgery [3].

The World Professional Association for Transgender Health (WPATH) and the American Medical Association (AMA) view treatment of gender dysphoria as medically necessary and effective [3, 4]. The current standard of care is an individualized, multidisciplinary approach, according to the patient's desired interventions. Primary care providers, endocrinologists, and surgical subspecialists may provide overall health and wellness support, as well as hormonal and surgical treatments. Mental health professionals may support transition by performing assessment of gender dysphoria, counseling on options for gender identity and expression, management of comorbid mental illness, and assessment of eligibility, preparation, and referral for hormone therapy or surgical treatments [3, 4]. Other professionals in the team-based approach may include speech and language pathologists who can assist with voice coaching, cosmetologists for hair removal and skin care, occupational therapy for adaptation into social circumstances, and social and legal services for legal transitions such as name change [3].

After the second visit to your clinic, Isis speaks to you about how the office staff always calls her "Isaiah" and uses masculine pronouns when referring to her. She is frustrated and feels that your office is not making an effort to treat her respectfully.

Creating a Welcoming Environment

Transgender patients face barriers to accessing optimal healthcare, which leads to disparities in both physical and mental health outcomes. A systematic review of the available literature on primary care for transgender individuals found that there are significant disparities in HIV prevalence compared to cisgender individuals, with significantly higher prevalence in transgender women specifically [5]. In addition, there is increased tobacco use and lower cervical cancer screening [5]. The likely causes of these disparities are multifactorial, with access to care, underinsurance, discrimination, and minority stress playing a role. Data show that transgender individuals who delayed health care due to a fear of discrimination had worse overall health, as well as higher odds of depression, suicidal ideation and suicide attempts in the past year, compared to those who did not delay care [6].

Creating a welcoming environment is an essential first step in establishing open and honest communication with transgender patients. One-third of surveyed transgender individuals in the United States have experienced a negative encounter with a healthcare provider, and 23% avoided seeing a doctor because of concerns about mistreatment [7]. Simple changes such as displaying signs that highlight gender diversity and having brochures that are relevant to LGBTQ individuals can communicate awareness and affirmation [1]. Scheduling personnel or administrative assistants should be trained to use open and inclusive language so that patients have a positive first impression of the clinical environment. Additionally, medical intake forms that query patients about natal sex, gender identity, and sexual orientation, and which use neutral language ("partner" as opposed to "husband"), create an impression of inclusivity even before the face-to-face visit [1]. It is imperative that during the initial encounter, patients should be asked about their preferred name and pronouns, and this information should be used consistently in all verbal and electronic communication among clinical personnel. Transgender and non-binary individuals who experience consistent mis-gendering during a clinical encounter may feel marginalized and refrain from seeking care again.

Obtaining the Medical History

A major goal of the medical history is to understand the patient's gender story and their overall sense of self. Although hormone therapy may improve psychological functioning and quality of life for many transgender individuals [8], it is important to remember that not all patients will choose to transition with medical therapy. Similarly, gender-affirmation surgery may be of interest to only certain individuals [7]; thus, providers should avoid assumptions about a patient's hormonal treatment, prior surgeries, and current anatomy. Use of open-ended questions and non-judgmental language while taking the medical history can facilitate clear and honest communication about these issues.

For patients who are currently using hormonal therapy, it is important to query them about the dose and preparation that is being used, the duration of use, any adverse effects, and goals and expectations of treatment. Patients should be asked about non-prescription or alternative sources of hormone treatment, which may be obtained with little or no clinical oversight [9]. Similarly, providers should inquire about the use of over-the-counter herbal preparations, such as phytoestrogens or dehydroepiandrosterone (DHEA), which are frequently marketed for their hormonal effects [1].

It is important to perform an anatomical inventory on every transgender patient. A thorough understanding of the patient's current anatomy (whether natal or surgical) is essential for providing appropriate preventive care services, such as breast, cervical, and prostate cancer screening. Several options are available for transgender men seeking gender-affirmation surgery, including hysterectomy with salpingoopherectomy, vaginectomy, scrotoplasty, and phalloplasty. Bilateral mastectomy may also be performed. Transgender women may undergo penectomy, orchiectomy, vaginoplasty, vulvoplasty, and breast augmentation [10]. It may also be useful to assess a patient's interest in having gender-affirmation surgery in the future, in order to coordinate referrals and assist with planning [1].

It is important to take a thorough sexual history to accurately assess a patient's risk for sexually transmitted infections, pregnancy, and sexual dysfunction. Prior sections of this text have described techniques for asking sensitive and inclusive questions while taking the sexual history, see Chaps. 3 and 36 for more information. For transgender patients, it is important to frame these questions within the context of current anatomy, as well as the anatomy of their partner(s). The provider should ask patients about the number and gender identity of their partner(s), as well as types of sexual practices and use of barrier protection. Keep in mind that transgender men may be at risk for pregnancy depending on their current anatomy and sexual practices, therefore, assessment of contraceptive use and interest in childbearing is paramount. Simple techniques such as asking the patient's permission, assuring confidentiality, mirroring the patient's language, and using appropriate pronouns to refer to partner(s) (i.e., "they" if appropriate) can facilitate this sensitive conversation.

Performing a Physical Exam

The physical exam should be performed in accordance with the patient's current anatomy. Transgender men who have not undergone hysterectomy require routine pelvic exams for cervical cancer screening according to current recommendations (see Chap. 14) [11]. Additionally, if bilateral mastectomy has not been performed, providers can consider performing a breast exam and screening for breast cancer according to published guidelines for natal women (see Chaps. 17 and 18). Breast examination may be appropriate for transgender women who are taking estrogen, to assess the effects of hormone therapy on breast tissue and development, as well as to assess for galactorrhea. Transgender women who have had gender-affirming surgery retain their prostate, and screening for prostate cancer can be performed according to recommendations for natal males [11].

For some transgender patients, gender-specific aspects of the physical exam can create anxiety. In the absence of clear medical necessity, it is reasonable to defer aspects of the physical exam (i.e., breast, genital, and anal exams) until the patient and provider have developed a strong and trusting relationship [1]. Transgender men, in particular, may experience emotional conflict and distress during gynecologic exams, due to both gender dysphoria as well as physical discomfort related to testosterone-induced vaginal atrophy [12]. Several strategies can be used both before and during the exam to improve the experience for the patient, such as using gender-neutral terms (external pelvic area for vulva, frontal pelvic opening for vagina), having a friend or partner present during the exam, using a small speculum, allowing the patient to self-insert the speculum, and encouraging the patient to communicate any discomfort [13]. These exam strategies are useful if a patient needs a pelvic exam due to a specific complaint such as pain or bleeding or for cervical cancer screening. Chapter 14 discusses the use of a blind sweep HPV test as an alternative for cervical cancer screening in patients who prefer not to have speculum exams.

In contrast, some transgender women find the breast exam to be gender-affirming and are comfortable during this part of the encounter. Nonetheless, it is important for the provider to explain why the exam is being done, to mirror the patient's language, and to provide draping alternatives according to the patient's preference [1].

Isis is interested in beginning affirming hormone therapy. Her goal is to have an appearance which is more feminine, including larger breasts, less facial and body hair, and a more feminine fat distribution. Her physical exam, including her blood pressure, pulse, and body mass index, are entirely normal. The results of her baseline blood work, including lipids, hemoglobin A1c, electrolytes, liver function tests, and prolactin, are within normal limits. Her therapist has confirmed that she meets criteria for gender dysphoria and is supportive of Isis' plans for medical transition. She wonders if you would be willing to start her on hormonal treatment.

Initiation of Hormone Therapy

Guidelines from the World Professional Association for Transgender Health [4] and the Endocrine Society [11] recommend that individuals meet certain criteria before starting on hormone therapy. The WPATH criteria include (1) the presence of persistent, well-documented gender dysphoria; (2) the capacity to make medical decisions and to consent to treatment; (3) of legal adult age; and (4) reasonably well-controlled medical or mental health conditions [4]. The Endocrine Society guidelines are almost identical, although they stipulate that only mental health (and not medical) concerns are well-controlled prior to initiating therapy [11]. To address the first criteria, both guidelines emphasize that providers who prescribe hormone therapy should either be comfortable making the diagnosis of gender dysphoria or consult with a health professional who is skilled in gender dysphoria assessment. Once the diagnosis of gender dysphoria is met, guidelines recommend that the patient be fully informed about the risks and benefits of hormonal treatment, including the impact on medical, mental health, and social outcomes by a knowledgeable provider [11].

For transgender women, the goals of hormone therapy are to reduce natal hormonal levels (testosterone) and replace with hormones of the affirmed gender (estrogen). In the United States, spironolactone is the most commonly used treatment to reduce testosterone levels; gonadotropin-releasing hormone (GnRH) agonists can be used as well, although they are expensive and less convenient to administer. Feminization can be achieved with 17-beta estradiol, also referred to as E2 or Estradiol, which comes in a variety of preparations, including oral, transdermal, and injectable. The starting dose of estradiol should be low and titrated up as patients tolerate. Patient preferences play a role in the route and frequency of administration. Oral dosing is daily. Topical estradiol patches are conveniently changed only one to two times per week but can fall off or cause skin irritation. Parenteral dosing is weekly or biweekly; weekly dosing promotes less variation between peak and trough concentration which may cause less side effects but also requires more frequent injections by the patient. Patients using parenteral estradiol must be educated about safe needle use and disposal to prevent infection and adverse events. The efficacy between all formulations of estradiol is similar. *Ethinyl* estradiol, which is commonly used in combined hormonal contraceptives, should *not* be used for transgender hormone therapy; it is more thrombogenic than 17-beta estradiol, and serum levels cannot be measured for treatment titration [11]. Conjugated Equine Estrogens (CEE), found in Premarin™ products, though used in the past, are also not recommended.

During the first 3–6 months of treatment, patients will likely notice decreased libido and spontaneous erections, body fat redistribution, decreased muscle mass, softening of the skin, decreased testicular size, and breast growth. Over the next 6–12 months, body and facial hair will thin and grow more slowly. It is important to counsel that breast growth is slow and may not fully develop until 2–3 years after initiation of treatment [4]. The effects of hormonal therapy on sperm production and sexual dysfunction are variable, so it is important that patients' interest in child-bearing be assessed prior to initiating treatment [4].

Hormonal therapy with estradiol increases risk for venous thromboembolism (VTE) [14]. Lower doses of estradiol, and the use of transdermal preparations, may be preferable in patients who are at potentially increased risk for VTE [15]. Treatment with estradiol may also be associated with hypertension, increased triglycerides, and impaired glucose tolerance [4]. The effect of estradiol therapy on cardiovascular outcomes is unclear, although guidelines indicate that it is associated with a "moderate risk" for coronary artery disease and cerebrovascular disease [11]. Prior studies that have shown an increased risk for cardiovascular events in transgender women on hormone therapy may have been influenced by the type of estrogen preparation (use of ethinyl estradiol) as well as the subjects' age and associated risk factors, such as smoking [15–17]. In contrast, a more recent retrospective cohort study of mostly non-smoking transfeminine women, investigators noted an increased risk for ischemic stroke as compared to the women in the cisgender matched cohort [14].

Absolute contraindications to feminizing hormone therapy include an estrogen-sensitive active malignancy and end-stage liver disease. In all other instances, it is reasonable to control or reduce medical comorbidities or risk factors as much as possible before starting treatment [4, 11].

Patients on feminizing hormone therapy should have a complete history, physical exam, and laboratory evaluation every 3 months. At each encounter, blood pressure and weight should be monitored, and serum electrolytes, estradiol, and testosterone levels should be measured. The goal of estradiol level is within the range for a reproductive age natal female (100–200 pg/mL) and the testosterone level should be suppressed to less than 50 ng/dL [11]. Estradiol and spironolactone doses can be titrated according to the patient's goals for treatment (i.e., the degree of feminization that she wants to achieve), as well as hormonal levels. After the first year of therapy, and once a stable hormonal regimen is achieved, clinical and laboratory evaluation can occur every 6–12 months. Prolactin levels may increase in patients treated with estradiol; guidelines recommend a baseline measurement and then annual assessment during the transition period [11].

Hormonal Therapy for Transgender Men

The main goals of hormonal therapy for transgender men are (1) to reduce natal hormonal secretion and (2) to replace with hormones consistent with the affirmed gender [11]. For transgender males, testosterone administration is effective in both reducing endogenous estrogen production and achieving testosterone levels within the normal reproductive range for the male gender. Testosterone can be administered as a gel, a patch, or parenterally; oral testosterone is not available in the United States. Like estradiol, patient preferences play a role in the route and frequency of administration. Topical dosing is daily, while parenteral dosing is weekly or biweekly when starting therapy. Weekly parenteral dosing promotes less variation between peak and trough concentration which may cause less side effects but also requires more frequent injections by the patient. Patients using parenteral testosterone must be educated about safe needle use and disposal to prevent infection and adverse events. Topical testosterone delivered in gel form can be absorbed by other people who come into contact with the patient's skin, making it important to keep the dosing site protected from those at risk for adverse effects from masculinizing hormones such as children and females. Testosterone patches can be irritating to the skin and cause a local allergic reaction. Efficacy between all formulations of testosterone is similar.

Testosterone therapy will produce predictable changes in the physical appearance, although the time course of these changes will vary. During the first 6 months of treatment, patients will experience cessation of menses, acne, increased facial and body hair growth, body fat redistribution, clitoral enlargement, and vaginal atrophy. Increased muscle mass, deepening of the voice, and scalp hair loss typically occur during the first year. Some individuals will continue to experience an increase in hair growth and muscle mass for up to 5 years [4].

Testosterone can be associated with adverse effects, including polycythemia, sleep apnea, and excessive weight gain. Additionally, treatment can cause hyperlipidemia, hypertension, impaired glucose tolerance, and severe acne. Absolute contraindications to testosterone include the presence of testosterone-sensitive active malignancy, pregnancy, polycythemia, and unstable coronary artery disease [4]. In all other instances, it is reasonable to control or reduce medical comorbidities or risk factors as much as possible before starting treatment [4, 11].

Patients on masculinizing hormone therapy should have a complete history, physical exam, and laboratory evaluation every 3 months during the first year of treatment. At each encounter, the blood pressure and weight should be monitored, and hemoglobin, hematocrit, and total testosterone levels should be measured at these visits [11]. The desired range of serum testosterone levels is between 400 and 700 ng/dL and the peak should not exceed 1000 ng/dL [11]. The timing of testosterone measurement to assess for adequate levels depends on which type of testosterone is being used. For short-acting parenteral testosterone, levels should be measured mid-way between doses; alternatively, dosing can be based on peak (24-hours after dose) and trough (just before next dose) measurements. For topical testosterone, levels can be measured after consistent daily use of testosterone for 1 week, with the level drawn after 2 hours of dose administration for that day [11]. Testosterone doses can be titrated according to the patient's goals for treatment (i.e., the degree of masculinization that he wants to achieve) as well as hormonal levels. After the first year of therapy, and once a stable hormonal regimen is achieved, clinical and laboratory evaluation can occur every 6–12 months.

Isis starts hormonal treatment with oral estradiol 1 mg twice daily and spironolactone 25 mg twice daily. At her follow-up visit 3 months later, she reports that her mood has dramatically improved, and she has noticed some physical changes, including softening of her skin. She wonders if there is anything else that needs to be "checked" in order to stay healthy. She is sexually active with her primary partner, Kelly, who is a cis female, and engages in oral and penile/vaginal intercourse. She rarely uses condoms, and her last HIV test was 1 year ago.

Screening for Sexually Transmitted Infections

Several studies have shown that there is a high prevalence of HIV among transgender women. According to one systematic review, the pooled prevalence of HIV infection was 19.1% among transgender women worldwide, and the odds for being infected with HIV, as compared to reproductive age adults, was 48.8 [18]. In a US study, 27.7% of transgender women tested positive for HIV infection, and this rate was substantially higher among those who identified as African-American (56.3%) [19]. The CDC recommends screening for HIV and other sexually transmitted infections among transgender individuals according to the patient's sexual practices and anatomy [20]. In patients who engage in frequent unprotected intercourse, particularly anal-receptive intercourse, the risk for syphilis, HIV, gonorrhea, and chlamydia is greatly increased, [21] and screening should be offered every 3–6 months for these infections [22].

Those transgender patients at high risk for acquiring HIV infection may be appropriate candidates for pre-exposure prophylaxis (PrEP) with daily oral tenofovir-emtricitabine to prevent HIV infection. Per the CDC guidelines, patients are "clinically eligible" if they have a documented negative HIV test result, no signs or symptoms of active HIV infection, normal renal function, no co-administration of contraindicated medications, and documentation of hepatitis B status (i.e., either prior infection or vaccination). Providers should counsel these patients about the efficacy of PrEP as well as risk reduction strategies, such as regular condom use and minimization of the number of sexual partners. If a patient is interested in PrEP, a daily fixed dose of tenofovir– emtricitabine (Truvada or Descovy) can be prescribed, with follow-up visits scheduled every 3 months for HIV testing, assessment of renal function, and discussion about adherence and potential side effects [20].

Cancer Screening

In all transgender individuals, screening for breast, cervical, and prostate cancer should be considered within the context of the patient's natal or surgical anatomy.

The recommendations for breast cancer screening among transgender women vary. The Endocrine Society recommends that routine breast cancer screening, including mammography, be performed according to guidelines for natal women [11]. In contrast, recommendations from the University of California San Francisco (UCSF) Transgender Center of Excellence suggest that providers consider the patient's age and duration of hormone therapy when counseling patients about the appropriateness of mammography [21]. Specifically, the UCSF guidelines recommend that screening mammography be performed only in the following situations: (1) the patient is over the age of 50 and (2) the patient has used feminizing hormone therapy for at least 5–10 years [21]. Furthermore, these guidelines recommend mammography biennially (not annually) in patients who meet these criteria and that providers discuss the individual's personal risk factors for breast cancer, as well as the potential for over-diagnosis when considering screening mammography (see Chaps. 17 and 18).

Transgender men who have not undergone mastectomy should be referred for mammography according to guidelines for natal women [11, 21]. The risk for breast cancer among transgender men who have had mastectomy is unclear and may depend on the amount of residual breast tissue that is present after surgery. Some guidelines recommend performing sub- and periareolar breast examinations annually among transgender men who have had a mastectomy [11], whereas other guidelines encourage providers to individualize the discussion about breast cancer risk according to the surgical history and the extent of persistent breast tissue [21].

All guidelines emphasize the importance of cervical cancer screening in transgender men who have not undergone hysterectomy. Screening should occur at intervals as recommended for natal women [11, 21]. Notably, as compared to natal women, transgender men are eight times more likely to have inadequate cytologic sampling during cervical cancer screening, and this is influenced by duration of testosterone therapy [12]. New guidelines, which emphasize the primary role of HPV testing (as compared to cytology), may improve cervical cancer screening among transgender men and also be more acceptable to patients. Self-collection of vaginal HPV samples may be a good option for some patients who are opposed to or unable to tolerate a clinical examination (see Chap. 14) [23, 24].

Transgender women should undergo prostate cancer screening according to guidelines for natal men [11, 21]. The prostate tissue is retained in transgender women who have undergone gender affirming surgery; depending on the type of surgery performed, it may be located anterior to the vaginal wall. In these cases, if digital examination is considered, it should be performed through the neovagina [21].

Preventive Care

Appropriate immunizations are an important part of transgender patients' preventive care, and the immunization schedule from the Centers for Disease Control (CDC) and Advisory Committee on Immunization Practices (ACIP) should be followed based on age, medical comorbidity, or sexual practices. HPV vaccination is covered in Chap. 14.

Bone density testing is recommended for some transgender individuals. According to the Endocrine Society guidelines, it is reasonable to consider screening for osteoporosis among transgender women starting at age 60. Similarly, in transgender men, screening should occur in the setting of treatment non-adherence, cessation of testosterone therapy, or development of additional risk factors for osteoporosis (See Chap. 25) [11].

Summary Points

1. Gender non-conformity is the umbrella term used when a person's gender identity differs from that which was assigned at birth. This can include a person who is transgender. Gender dysphoria is the DSM diagnosis which involves a conflict between a person's physical/assigned gender and the gender with which he/she/they identify.
2. Providers should use open and inclusive language and avoid assumptions when asking transgender patients about their gender identity, history of gender-affirming medical and surgical treatments, and sexual practices. This helps to avoid stigmatization and facilitate trust between provider and patient.
3. Providers should utilize specific strategies such as asking permission and mirroring the patients' language to mitigate the emotional and physical discomfort that some transgender individuals experience during the physical exam.
4. The goals of hormone therapy are to reduce natal hormone levels and to replace with hormones of the affirmed gender, and there are few absolute contraindications to the initiation of hormone therapy. Medical comorbidities and plans for childbearing should be addressed prior to starting hormone therapy.
5. Cancer screening in transgender patients should be individualized according to their natal and surgical anatomy. Screening for sexually transmitted infections and immunizations should be individualized according to natal and surgical anatomy and sexual practices.

Review Questions

1. Jamie is a 45-year-old patient who presents to your office to establish care. Jamie was assigned a female sex at birth but does not identify as either female or male, but rather as both genders. Jamie prefers the pronouns they/them/their/themselves. Jamie dresses in whatever feels comfortable, which typically involves trousers, button down shirts or polos, and has long hair which they typically wear in a ponytail.

   Which of the following best describes Jamie's gender identity?
   A. Non-binary
   B. Gender dysphoric
   C. Transgender
   D. Cisgender
   E. Trans-masculine

   The correct answer is A. The best descriptor of Jamie's gender identity is likely non-binary, which is a term to describe a person whose gender identity falls outside the traditional gender binary [1]. Jamie may be gender fluid, that is, someone who identifies with different genders; or agender, that is, someone who has a neutral gender identity; or non-binary, that is, someone who's gender does not fit into the gender binary [1]. The best way to find out Jamie's exact identity is to ask them. Jamie shows no evidence of gender dysphoria, which is a DSM diagnosis, that involves clinically significant distress due to a conflict between a person's assigned gender and their gender identity [2]. In addition, Jamie is not cisgender, since they do not identify as the assigned female birth sex, or transgender, since they do not identify as male, which is the opposite of their birth sex [1].
2. A 52-year-old transgender female with a medical history significant for obesity, osteoarthritis, and gastroesophageal reflux disease presents for a routine visit. She has been on hormone therapy for 7 years; her regimen includes an estradiol patch, 0.1 mg/24 hours (changed twice weekly) and spironolactone 100 mg twice daily. She has not had gender reassignment surgery. She is currently sexually active with one female partner and engages in oral intercourse but does not use dental dams. Her vital signs and physical exam are entirely normal. Which of the following is the most appropriate next step in her management?
   A. Perform a digital rectal exam for prostate cancer screening
   B. Order a bone density test
   C. Refer for mammography
   D. Perform rectal screening for *Chlamydia*
   E. Order a complete blood count (CBC)

   The correct answer is C. Cross-sex hormone therapy in transgender women may increase the risk for breast cancer. Guidelines from the Endocrine Society recommend that transgender women of average risk for breast cancer receive screening according to recommendations for natal women [11]. The USPSTF currently recommends biennial mammography for natal women aged 50–74 years; thus, it would be appropriate to offer mammography to this patient [11]. The University of California San Francisco Center of Excellence for Transgender Health offers slightly different recommendations and states that appropriate candidates for mammography include transgender women over the age of 50 who have received 5–10 years of feminizing hormone therapy [21]. Per those guidelines, the patient in this case should be offered screening mammography.

   All transgender women, regardless of whether they have had gender-affirming surgery, will have a prostate. According to the Endocrine Society Guidelines, providers should follow recommendations from the USPSTF, which recommends engaging in an informed consent discussion about the benefits and risks of prostate-specific antigen screening with individuals between the ages of 55 and 59. Based on this patient's age, prostate cancer screening would not be currently recommended [11, 25].

Rectal screening for *Chlamydia* is recommended in men who have sex with men and engage in receptive intercourse [10] so rectal screening is not appropriate for this patient.

This patient is at low risk for osteoporosis and has been compliant with her hormone therapy. She should start screening for osteoporosis at the age of 60, which is consistent with the Endocrine Society guidelines for osteoporosis screening in transgender women [11].

An increase in the hemoglobin and hematocrit is commonly seen with administration of testosterone therapy in transgender men but not in transgender women; therefore, routine CBC is not recommended.

3. A 62-year-old transgender female presents to establish care. She has a medical history significant for obesity, hypertension, hyperlipidemia, impaired glucose tolerance, and benign prostatic hypertrophy. She has been using hormonal therapy for 12 years, and her current regimen includes transdermal estradiol (0.1 mg/24 hours, change twice weekly) and spironolactone 100 mg twice daily. She is very satisfied with her hormonal therapy in terms of her emotional well-being as well as her physical appearance. She does not use tobacco, alcohol, or drugs, is not sexually active, and works as a truck driver. On exam, her blood pressure is 146/92 and her pulse is 62. Her physical exam is otherwise normal. On laboratory evaluation, her serum estradiol and testosterone levels are within goal range. Which of the following is the most appropriate next step in her management?
   A. Discontinue estradiol because of the risk for cardiovascular complications
   B. Continue the current hormonal regimen and maximize blood pressure control
   C. Discontinue transdermal estradiol and start oral estradiol to minimize the risk for venous thromboembolism
   D. Increase the dose of transdermal estradiol
   E. Add a GnRH agonist to the hormonal regimen

   The correct answer is B. For many individuals, hormonal therapy may improve the emotional and mental well-being as well as quality of life. Conversely, abrupt discontinuation of hormone therapy can be associated with significant psychological consequences. Thus, hormone therapy should be continued in patients who are medically stable and are doing well on their regimen.

   Cardiovascular risk factors, such as hypertension and hyperlipidemia, are not absolute contraindications to hormonal therapy but should be managed according to published guidelines [11].

   Estradiol increases the risk for venous thromboembolism (VTE), and this should be discussed with the patient prior to initiating hormonal therapy. Transdermal estradiol is theoretically considered to be "safer" than oral estradiol with respect to VTE risk, as it avoids the "first-pass" effect and so is less likely to activate hepatic coagulation factors [14, 15].

   Changes in a patient's hormonal regimen should be guided by their satisfaction with their appearance and well-being, as well as by serum hormone levels. Elevated blood levels of estrogen (exceeding guideline-recommended goal ranges) can increase the risk for VTE, liver dysfunction, and hypertension [4]. This patient is satisfied with her emotional health and physical appearance, and her serum levels are within goal range. Thus, it is not appropriate to increase the dose of transdermal estradiol.

   Several therapies can be used to decrease natal testosterone levels, including spironolactone and GnRH agonists [11]. Spironolactone is often used as first-line therapy due to ease of administration and cost. In this patient, spironolactone has effectively suppressed her testosterone levels to goal range, and thus a GnRH agonist is not indicated.

References

1. Makadon HJ, American College of Physicians. The Fenway guide to lesbian, gay, bisexual, and transgender health. Philadelphia: American College of Physicians; 2008.
2. American Psychiatric Association. Diagnostic and statistical manual of mental disorders: DSM-5. 5th ed. Arlington: American Psychiatric Publishing; 2013.
3. Wylie K, Knudson G, Khan SI, Bonierbale M, Watanyusakul S, Baral S. Serving transgender people: clinical care considerations and service delivery models in transgender health. Lancet. 2016;388(10042):401–11.
4. World Professional Association for Transgender Health. Standards of care for the health of transsexual, transgender, and gender nonconforming people. 7th ed. Minneapolis: World Professional Association for Transgender Health; 2011.
5. Edmiston EK, Donald CA, Sattler AR, Peebles JK, Ehrenfeld JM, Eckstrand KL. Opportunities and gaps in primary care preventative health services for transgender patients: a systemic review. Transgend Health. 2016;1(1):216–30.
6. Seelman KL, Colon-Diaz MJP, LeCroix RH, Xavier-Brier M, Kattari L. Transgender noninclusive healthcare and delaying care because of fear: connections to general health and mental health among transgender adults. Transgend Health. 2017;2(1):17–28.
7. Grant JM, Mottet LA, Tanis J, Harrison J, Herman JL. Transgender aMKIaETARotN, Equality DSWNCfT, and National Gay and Lesbian Task Force. https://www.transequality.org/sites/default/files/docs/resources/NTDS_Report.pdf.
8. White Hughto JM, Reisner SL. A systematic review of the effects of hormone therapy on psychological functioning and quality of life in transgender individuals. Transgend Health. 2016;1(1):21–31.
9. Mepham N, Bouman WP, Arcelus J, Hayter M, Wylie KR. People with gender dysphoria who self-prescribe cross-sex hormones: prevalence, sources, and side effects knowledge. J Sex Med. 2014;11(12):2995–3001.

10. Unger CA. Care of the transgender patient: the role of the gynecologist. Am J Obstet Gynecol. 2014;210(1):16–26.
11. Hembree WC, Cohen-Kettenis PT, Gooren L, Hannema SE, Meyer WJ, Murad MH, et al. Endocrine treatment of gender-dysphoric/gender-incongruent persons: an Endocrine Society Clinical Practice Guideline. J Clin Endocrinol Metab. 2017;102(11):3869–903.
12. Peitzmeier SM, Reisner SL, Harigopal P, Potter J. Female-to-male patients have high prevalence of unsatisfactory Paps compared to non-transgender females: implications for cervical cancer screening. J Gen Intern Med. 2014;29(5):778–84.
13. Potter J, Peitzmeier SM, Bernstein I, Reisner SL, Alizaga NM, Agenor M, et al. Cervical cancer screening for patients on the female-to-male spectrum: a narrative review and guide for clinicians. J Gen Intern Med. 2015;30(12):1857–64.
14. Getahun D, Nash R, Flanders W, et al. Cross-sex hormones and acute cardiovascular events in transgender persons: a cohort study. Ann Intern Med. 2018;169(4):205–13.
15. Streed CG Jr, Harfouch O, Marvel F, Blumenthal RS, Martin SS, et al. Cardiovascular disease among transgender adults receiving hormone therapy: a narrative review. Ann Intern Med. 2017;167(4):256–67.
16. Asscheman H, Giltay EJ, Megens JA, de Ronde WP, van Trotsenburg MA, Gooren LJ. A long-term follow-up study of mortality in transsexuals receiving treatment with cross-sex hormones. Eur J Endocrinol. 2011;164(4):635–42.
17. Weinand JD, Safer JD. Hormone therapy in transgender adults is safe with provider supervision; A review of hormone therapy sequelae for transgender individuals. J Clin Transl Endocrinol. 2015;2(2):55–60.
18. Baral SD, Poteat T, Stromdahl S, Wirtz AL, Guadamuz TE, Beyrer C. Worldwide burden of HIV in transgender women: a systematic review and meta-analysis. Lancet Infect Dis. 2013;13(3):214–22.
19. Herbst JH, Jacobs ED, Finlayson TJ, McKleroy VS, Neumann MS, Crepaz N. Estimating HIV prevalence and risk behaviors of transgender persons in the United States: a systematic review. AIDS Behav. 2008;12(1):1–17.
20. Workowski KA, Bolan GA, Centers for Disease Control and Prevention. Sexually transmitted diseases treatment guidelines. MMWR Recomm Rep. 2015;64(RR-03):1–137.
21. Deutsch MB, Center of Excellence for Transgender Health, Department of Family and Community Medicine, University of California San Francisco. Guidelines for the primary and gender-affirming care of transgender and gender nonbinary people. 2nd ed. San Francisco: University of California, San Francisco; 2016. Available from: www.transhealth.ucsf.edu/.
22. Knight DA, Jarrett D. Preventive health care for men who have sex with men. Am Fam Physician. 2015;91(12):844–51.
23. U.S. Preventive Services Task Force. Draft recommendation statement: Cervical cancer: screening; 2017.
24. Seay J, Ranck A, Weiss R, Salgado C, Fein L, Kobetz E. Understanding transgender men's experiences with and preferences for cervical cancer screening: a rapid assessment survey. LGBT Health. 2017;4(4):304–9.
25. U.S. Preventive Services Task Force. Final update summary: Prostate cancer: screening. U.S. Preventive Services Task Force; 2018.

38 Care of the Female Veteran

Sophia M. Reljanovic and Megan McNamara

Learning Objectives

1. List the key components of a military-focused history.
2. Summarize strategies and available resources for helping female veterans successfully reintegrate from active military service.
3. Describe the rationale for screening and the screening procedures for mental health disorders that are prevalent among female veterans, including post-traumatic stress disorder, military sexual trauma, substance use disorders, mood disorders, and suicidality.
4. List medical conditions that can be influenced by female veterans' military experiences.
5. Identify reproductive health issues specific to women veterans and discuss how the approach to and management of reproductive health may differ in women veterans.

Ava is a 28-year-old female who presents to establish care. She has been experiencing back pain, bilateral knee pain, and insomnia for the last several months. She recently returned from a 2-year deployment to Afghanistan and has had difficulty finding employment. She is currently living with her parents but is not sure how long she will be able to stay with them. Ava frequently feels "on guard" and suspicious, and she worries about the effect that these feelings will have on her relationships.

S. M. Reljanovic (✉)
Case Western Reserve University School of Medicine, Louis Stokes Cleveland VA Medical Center, Department of Women's Health, Cleveland, OH, USA
e-mail: sophia.reljanovic@va.gov

M. McNamara
Case Western Reserve University School of Medicine, Louis Stokes Cleveland VA Medical Center, Department of Medicine, Cleveland, OH, USA

There are approximately 2 million women veterans in the United States, and their numbers are growing rapidly [1]. Women veterans have served in every branch of the military (Army, Navy, Air Force, Marine Corps, Coast Guard, National Guard, and Reserves), and approximately 50% have served in either Gulf War Era I (1990–2001) or Gulf War Era II (2001–present) [2]. There was a striking increase in the number of women on active duty in the armed services during the Gulf War Eras; 20% of the veteran population in the Gulf War Era II (post-September 11, 2001) are women compared to 4% of the veteran population of the pre–Gulf War Era [2]. The care of female veterans extends across their life-span and encompasses all aspects of physical and psychosocial health. Two-thirds of women veterans are aged 35–64, with a peak around 45–54 years old reflecting Gulf War Era veterans [2].

Overview of Health Issues of Women Veterans

Many female veterans receive their care in the civilian setting, so it is essential that all providers are aware of the unique needs of this population [3]. As compared to non-veterans, women who have served in the military are more likely to be obese or overweight, have cardiovascular disease, and report poor health indicators such as tobacco abuse, lack of exercise, and fair or poor overall health [4]. Women veterans who have served in recent conflicts in Iraq and Afghanistan are also prone to developing conditions related to their deployment, including musculoskeletal disorders and mental health issues [3]. Approximately 20–25% of female veterans report military sexual trauma (MST) as a result of unwanted sexual attention or forced sexual encounters [1, 5]. Post-traumatic stress disorder (PTSD) may develop because of exposure to traumatic events, including prior MST [3].

Providers can gain more information about women veterans' experiences by simply inquiring, "Are you currently

S. A. Tilstra et al. (eds.), *Sex- and Gender-Based Women's Health*, https://doi.org/10.1007/978-3-030-50695-7_38

serving or have you ever served in the military?" [3]. Positive responses should be followed up with additional inquiries about when and where the individual served, the type of job she performed, and the effect of military service on her life [1, 3]. Screening for MST and PTSD is imperative, as discussed later in this chapter.

Asking additional questions about the patient's history of musculoskeletal injuries, exposures, and medical or mental health diagnoses during the service period can provide insight into the patient's presenting symptoms. Musculoskeletal pain may be service-related; 60% of Gulf War veterans have been diagnosed with musculoskeletal and connective tissue disorders [3]. Other common conditions associated with Gulf War service include gastrointestinal, neurologic, and respiratory disorders [3].

Chronic pain may impact ability to engage in gainful employment. In 2013, nearly 100,000 women veterans were unemployed, with rates higher among veterans aged 25–34 as compared to their civilian counterparts [2]. Unemployment has been identified as a "root cause" of homelessness among females who have served in the military; additional risk factors include trauma or substance abuse during military service, and post-military medical, mental health, and substance abuse problems [6]. Women who have served in the military are two to four times more likely than their civilian counterparts to be homeless, and the National Coalition for Homeless Veterans reports that the number of homeless women veterans has doubled in recent years [7].

Fortunately, there are many programs to assist veterans, including the Homeless Veterans Reintegration Program, which connects homeless veterans who are reintegrating into civilian life with meaningful employment. Similarly, the HUD-VA Supportive Housing Program can help veterans obtain vouchers for local public housing. Information about these programs can be found at the following website: http://www.nchv.org/images/uploads/HFV%20paper.pdf [8].

Upon further questioning, Ava reports that she served in the Army as a supply truck driver, and that her route was frequently targeted with improvised explosive devices. Although she was never injured, she saw several other trucks explode when they were hit. Since returning home she has had frequent nightmares and feels detached from her family and friends. She has been drinking 3–4 beers every night to help her sleep.

Mental Health

Mental health disorders are common among all veterans. The most prevalent diagnoses include PTSD, depression, anxiety, and substance use disorders.

Post-traumatic Stress Disorder

Although women were not officially deployed in a combat troop role until 2013, many female veterans have held positions that still exposed them to combat [3]. Experiences of combat-related trauma can lead to post-traumatic stress disorder (PTSD). PTSD is a condition that can result after exposure to any traumatic event. It is characterized by re-experiencing the traumatic event through flashbacks or disconcerting and intrusive thoughts [9, 10]. Individuals with PTSD often exhibit avoidance or numbing behaviors in which they will avoid triggers or situations associated with the event or exhibit detachment or estrangement. They frequently also have symptoms of persistently heightened arousal or vigilance [7, 9–11].

It is important to screen all female veterans for PTSD. In a primary care setting, a screening tool such as the Primary Care PTSD screen for DSM-5 (PC-PTSD-5) can be used [7, 12, 13]. The PC-PTSD-5 first screens for a traumatic event experience. If present, the patient answers a series of five questions about experiences over the last month, including (1) nightmares or intrusive thoughts about the event, (2) avoidant behaviors to suppress the event or to avoid triggers that may cause the patient to re-experience the event, (3) hypervigilance, (4) the feeling of being numb or detached from the situation at hand, and (5) guilt related to the event [12]. These questions mirror the diagnostic criteria for PTSD. This tool has a sensitivity of 95% when using a cutoff score of 3 (maximum score = 5), with one point granted for each positive response to a question [12]. A preliminary study evaluating the use of this screening tool among a sample of veterans demonstrated that patients found the questionnaire to be broadly acceptable and easy to understand. Study participants indicated a preference for having this screening completed by their primary care provider rather than by self-report or by another member of the healthcare team such as a nurse or medical assistant [12].

Military Sexual Trauma

Unfortunately, in addition to combat-related trauma, another common cause of trauma among female veterans is military sexual trauma. Military sexual trauma (MST) is defined by the Department of Veterans Affairs as "sexual harassment that is threatening in character or physical assault of a sexual nature that occurred while the victim was in the military, regardless of geographic location of the trauma, gender of the victim, or the relationship to the perpetrator" [3, 14, 15]. Perpetrators are not only limited to other military personnel but may also include civilians, friends, strangers, and intimate partners [5]. As previously noted, national data from VA screening programs for MST demonstrate that about 1 in 4 women and 1 in 100 men reported experiencing MST [15,

16]. There is concern that sexual trauma incidents may be underreported due to concerns about confidentiality, fear of retaliation, and the belief that no action will be taken [7]. Risk factors for MST include: younger age, lower level of education, lower military rank, history of prior abuse, and enlisting to escape an undesirable home environment [3].

All female veterans should be screened for MST because it is common, screening questions are quick and accurate, and effective treatment for MST exists. Screening can be done by asking the following two questions: "When you were in the military, did you ever receive uninvited or unwanted sexual attention (i.e., touching, cornering, pressure for sexual favors, or inappropriate verbal remarks)?" and "When you were in the military, did anyone ever use force or the threat of force to have sex against your will?" If a patient answers "yes" to either one of these questions she should be referred to a mental health provider [1].

For women veterans, MST is one of the most significant risk factors for development of PTSD [16, 17]. Unfortunately, many of the protective factors for PTSD, such as positive social support and a sense of unit cohesion, are lost in instances of sexual trauma that occurs in the military setting [3]. MST is more predictive of PTSD than other types of military trauma, such as combat-related trauma, or civilian sexual trauma [3, 17]. Reports indicate that 40–60% of female survivors of MST will later develop PTSD [18].

In addition to being associated with PTSD, prior MST or other traumatic experiences are also associated with other mental health problems including mood disorders and substance use disorders [7, 17, 19]. Sixty percent of women veterans with a history of MST screen positive for depression and are twice as likely to have alcohol abuse disorder than veterans without MST [20]. Thus, it is important to screen for these comorbid conditions as well. Screening for depression and anxiety can be accomplished with the Patient Health Questionnaire (PHQ-2 or PHQ-9) and the Generalized Anxiety Disorder Scale (GAD-2 or GAD-7), further discussed in Chap. 33. The AUDIT-C screening tool developed by the World Health Organization can be used to assess alcohol abuse. The Department of Veterans Affairs recommends screening all veterans annually for unhealthy alcohol use [21]. The AUDIT-C screening tool is available at the following VA website: https://www.hepatitis.va.gov/provider/tools/audit-c.asp [22].

Treatment

Screening for these conditions can assist in destigmatization and earlier identification which in turn provides opportunity for earlier mental health referral and treatment [13, 23]. Treatment for PTSD, whether due to combat-related trauma or MST, can involve therapy and medication. Trauma-focused cognitive behavioral therapy (CBT) is considered the most effective treatment for PTSD [10, 11]. CBT may involve elements of cognitive processing therapy, prolonged exposure therapy, and eye movement desensitization and reprocessing [10, 11]. Additionally, coping skills training and stress-reduction techniques are often a component of therapy [10, 11].

Results from two recent meta-analyses comparing treatment efficacy of psychotherapy and pharmacotherapy demonstrated that trauma-focused psychotherapies led to greater improvement in PTSD symptoms and longer duration of improvement compared to pharmacotherapy [10, 24, 25]. Also, medications are typically associated with higher risk of adverse reactions and side effects than are psychotherapies [10]. However, in cases where individualized trauma-focused psychotherapies may not be available or may not be an acceptable or agreeable option to patients, medications can certainly be considered as well as non-trauma focused psychotherapy. Furthermore, there is currently insufficient evidence to conclude that pharmacotherapy is superior to non-trauma focused therapy or vice versa [10]. Selective serotonin reuptake inhibitors (SSRIs) are considered first-line medication options to manage PTSD. Sertraline and paroxetine are FDA approved for this indication [10].

Female veterans with a history of MST or a diagnosis of PTSD are eligible for care and treatment at VA medical centers. Early referrals should be made because of the availability of specialized resources. Depending on the VA site, resources can include the following:

- Suicide prevention coordinator
- MST coordinator
- Specialists experienced in treating patients with a history of MST and with expertise in PSTD diagnosis and management

Veterans can also be directed to other PTSD and MST resources:

- VA PSTD website provides information for veterans, family, friends, and providers (https://www.ptsd.va.gov/) [26]
- VA MST website provides information about VA MST resources and has links to helpful articles and fact sheets (https://www.mentalhealth.va.gov/msthome/index.asp) [27]
- Veterans crisis hotline 1-800-273-8255, press #1 [28]

Ava agrees to be referred to a mental health provider and is diagnosed with PTSD. Her symptoms and mood improve significantly with treatment, and she returns to primary care 3 months later to discuss her other medical issues. She has been limiting her activities due to her knee and back pain, and as a result has gained 10 pounds in the last 8 weeks. She is currently taking paroxetine for her PTSD and ibuprofen to manage her pain.

Veterans have a high prevalence of certain medical conditions that can be influenced by prior military service and exposure to hostile military environments. Additionally, a history of trauma and PTSD can frequently have an impact on physical wellbeing. An analysis of VA healthcare utilization among veterans of the War in Iraq and the War in Afghanistan reported that 60% had diagnoses of diseases of the musculoskeletal system and/or connective tissue disorders, 48.7% had diseases of the nervous system, and 37.1% had diseases of the digestive system [3].

Musculoskeletal System

All veterans are at risk for musculoskeletal injuries. Military personnel, regardless of combat experience and gender, chronically expose their bodies to significant physical stress during training, drills, and daily work. Soldiers often have to carry armor, weapons, and supplies for long distances [7, 23], which can lead to acute and overuse injuries. Compared to male veterans, women veterans have higher rates of chronic musculoskeletal pain, physical injuries, and stress fractures [3]. The risk of injury can be compounded by poorly fitting equipment and body armor that is often not designed for the female body type [23].

In addition to musculoskeletal pain resulting from physical injury, there is also high prevalence of functional pain syndromes among veterans. Fibromyalgia prevalence is higher in women with a history of PTSD [3]. One study involving patients with PTSD and fibromyalgia symptoms reported that in two-thirds of the cases, trauma preceded the fibromyalgia symptoms as opposed to 30% of cases in which pain symptoms were followed by trauma or PTSD [29]. This association illustrates that fibromyalgia and PTSD are risk factors for each other and are often comorbid conditions [7]. Keeping this relationship in mind, it is important for providers to remember to screen women with unexplained pain syndromes for psychiatric disorders and history of trauma [3]. Please see Chap. 26 to review the General Approach to Chronic Pain and Chap. 29 to learn more about Fibromyalgia.

Traumatic Brain Injury (TBI)

Traumatic brain injury (TBI) refers to a structural injury or physiological disruption of brain function due to a traumatic external force and is a common injury seen among returning military personnel [30]. Operation Enduring Freedom (2001–2014) and Operation Iraqi Freedom (2003–2011) veterans, in particular, are at risk. Ten to twenty percent of service members report having at least one TBI as a result of their service obligations [7, 13, 31].

There is no diagnostic test for traumatic brain injury [11]. Rather, evaluation involves conducting a thorough history of the inciting incident. History for TBI should include information about the mechanism of injury, course and duration of symptoms, and any treatment or evaluation that was completed at the time of the event [11]. Duration of symptoms including loss of consciousness, altered mental status, and post-traumatic amnesia are used to classify TBI severity [13, 30]. Severity can range from mild to severe with mild symptoms typically improving over a short period of time. However, in some cases, there can be residual symptoms which can include headaches, dizziness, irritability, mood changes such as increased feelings of anxiety or depression, difficulty concentrating, sleep disturbances, and persistent memory problems [11, 13, 30]. Lingering symptoms are related to the degree of brain injury sustained during the initial trauma and may be permanent; the most serious permanent changes can include changes in personality, executive function, or physical health. It is important to note that the symptoms of TBI can overlap with those of PTSD, mood disorders, and substance use disorders [11, 30]. Thus, providers should maintain a high level of suspicion and assess for these conditions which may present simultaneously.

The examination in patients with a history of TBI should include a complete neurologic exam, head and neck exam, and neurocognitive screening [11, 13]. At present, evidence does not support the use of laboratory tests or imaging beyond its potential role in the acute setting immediately following injury, unless symptoms change or worsen, or the patient develops alarm symptoms such as acute vision changes, altered mental status, persistent vomiting, balance issues, or a neurologic deficit [13, 30].

Management of patients with a history of TBI is also based on symptoms [11, 30]. Education about sleep hygiene, referral to neurocognitive therapy, physical therapy, and use of biofeedback and relaxation therapy can often be helpful in addressing symptoms such as sleep disturbances, headaches, irritability, and anxiety [30]. While treatment recommendations often include nonpharmacologic interventions, medications for the complications of TBI can also be of benefit. These may include analgesics for pain (NSAIDs, acetaminophen), treatment of acute or chronic migraine headaches (See Chap. 28), nausea (ondansetron), mood disorders (SSRIs, SNRIs), insomnia (sleep medications), and dizziness (as needed meclizine). A general overarching guideline regarding medication use in persons with a history of TBI includes avoiding medications that lower the seizure threshold or cause confusion or sedation [30]. Lastly, referral to a neurologist or provider that specializes in brain injury can always be considered if the patient has refectory symptoms that are not responding to typical treatment options. Also, referral to a mental health provider can be of benefit, particularly as behavioral health conditions can often present concurrently with post-mild TBI symptoms [30].

Gastrointestinal System

Functional gastrointestinal disorders such as irritable bowel syndrome (IBS) and functional dyspepsia are more common in women veterans compared to civilian women. It is known that stressful events such as experiences during military service can exacerbate functional gastrointestinal disorders. In a study investigating prevalence of IBS and dyspepsia among women veterans, 38% reported IBS and 21% reported dyspepsia [32]. This study also demonstrated a high association between these gastrointestinal disorders and a history of trauma, PTSD, anxiety, and depression [32]. In another study looking specifically at the association between trauma and IBS in women veterans, 56% of women with IBS reported having been forced to have sex against their will versus 42% of women without IBS [33]. Also in the same study, 36% of patients with IBS reported attempted, forced, or unwanted sexual contact versus 21% of patients without IBS [33]. These studies illustrate a clear association between trauma, including MST, and functional gastrointestinal disorders. Please see Chap. 27 to learn more about the diagnosis and management of this disease.

Genitourinary System

Genitourinary concerns are common among women veterans. A review of VA healthcare utilization among War in Iraq and War in Afghanistan veterans reported that 17% had a diagnosis of diseases of the genitourinary system, which often include chronic pelvic pain and menstrual disorders [3]. Again, research shows that there is an association between these conditions and a history of trauma [3]. One study found that among female veterans who reported menstrual disorders, such as premenstrual syndrome, abnormal uterine bleeding, and dysmenorrhea, 71% had experienced MST [3, 34]. This once again illustrates the potential for far-reaching effects of trauma. Women with a history of PTSD and chronic pelvic pain have significantly lower reports of physical functioning and functioning without pain which can in turn impact all aspects of their lives and overall productivity [3]. Please see Chap. 31.

Urinary incontinence is another urogenital concern for which female veterans are at higher risk. Twenty-two percent of women veterans report overactive bladder symptoms which is higher than the prevalence seen in non-veteran women [1]. Women may often need to participate in strenuous activity and heavy lifting as part of their military service and training which can have adverse effects on pelvic support [1]. Not surprisingly, bladder dysfunction has been linked to a history of trauma and mood disorders [1]. Please see Chap. 23 to learn more.

Ava's pain improves with physical therapy and weight loss. She returns to clinic feeling better both mentally and physically. She has stopped drinking alcohol, has been adherent to the paroxetine, and has not used ibuprofen in months. She is in a new relationship with a male partner and is using condoms intermittently but is not interested in getting pregnant. She previously used oral contraceptive pills but discontinued them during deployment, because it was "too hard to remember them." What do you recommend for contraception?

Reproductive Health

Many women veterans experience reproductive health issues, which may be influenced by a variety of factors, including prior military exposure, medical comorbidities, and mental health diagnoses and treatment [1]. In a cross-sectional VA study, common reproductive health diagnoses among women aged 18–44 included menstrual disorders, endometriosis, sexually transmitted infections, urinary disorders, vaginitis, and pregnancy-related conditions, whereas older women veterans experienced menopausal issues and osteoporosis. Women who had a reproductive health diagnosis, as compared to those who did not, were more likely to have a comorbid medical or mental health condition [35].

Family planning and contraceptive counseling are essential for women veterans who want to avoid pregnancy or whose medical or mental health treatments expose them to potentially teratogenic medications. In one study, 37% of reproductive-age women veterans reported an unintended pregnancy, and 11.5% of women at high risk for pregnancy were not using any form of contraception [36]. Contraceptive knowledge among women veterans may be low, and differ according to certain racial and ethnic minority groups [37]. Additionally, women veterans who have been diagnosed with a mental illness or substance use disorder are more likely to be nonadherent to contraception [38].

A variety of contraceptive methods are available to women who receive care at VA centers, including combined hormonal contraceptives (ring, pill, patch), a progestin-only pill, and long-acting reversible contraceptives (LARCs: injection, subdermal implant, intrauterine devices [IUDs]). Providers should consider a patient's medical and mental health comorbidities, as well as the likelihood of adherence, when counseling about various contraceptive methods.

Among 1169 women veterans included in a cross-sectional study, 29% had a medical contraindication to combined hormonal contraceptives, including hypertension, migraine with aura, and smoking over the age of 35 [39]. Similarly, women treated for medical or mental health disorders may be exposed to medications which are associated with adverse pregnancy outcomes. Investigators who conducted a retrospective cohort study found that 12.6% of prescriptions dispensed to female veterans were potentially teratogenic; the most frequent indications for treatment included psychiatric illness, hypertension, and hyperlipidemia. Only 55.7% of women veterans who obtained prescriptions for teratogenic medications received any documented counseling about family planning [40].

LARCs are highly effective forms of contraception which are gaining in popularity among women veterans [36, 41]. IUDs may be an ideal choice among women with medical comorbidities as there are few medical contraindications to use. LARCs' ability to provide long-acting protection without a daily, weekly, or even monthly dosing of medication gives women on active military duty freedom to have efficacious contraception without worrying about how the next dose of medication will be obtained. In particular, LARCs may be preferable for women whose history of PTSD increases their risk for contraceptive non-adherence and whose mental health treatment may increase their risk for adverse fetal outcomes. See more about contraception options and counseling in Chap. 4.

As noted previously, sexually transmitted infections (STIs) are one of the top 5 reproductive health diagnoses among younger women veterans [35]. Compared to their civilian counterparts, women veterans initiate sexual activity at a younger age, have a greater number of both female and male partners, are more likely to report a history of genital warts, and to be seropositive for herpes simplex virus-2 [42]. Providers should consider these factors, as well as the patient's reported sexual practices, when counseling about screening for STIs. Regular condom use is the only way to protect from sexually transmitted infections. Veterans should be screened for STIs according to nationally published guidelines and all women who use condoms inconsistently, regardless of age or partnership, should be counseled about screening for STIs at routine intervals [43].

Summary Points

1. Asking about military service is important in a primary care setting. A military focused history should include a review of the type of military service as well as screening for conditions that are more common among military personnel.
2. Reintegration into civilian life following military service can be challenging for many veterans. VA has many available resources and programs that can be helpful.
3. Certain mental health disorders such as PTSD, MST, substance use disorders, mood disorders, and suicidality are more prevalent among female veterans, and providers should screen for these using validated screening questionnaires.
4. Many medical conditions such as musculoskeletal diagnoses, neurologic disorders, gastrointestinal symptoms, and genitourinary concerns can be impacted by a woman's prior military experience.
5. Female veterans may have unique reproductive health needs. Providers should feel comfortable counseling about a variety of contraceptive methods and STI prevention, recognizing the medical and mental health comorbidities that are more common in women veterans.

Review Questions

1. A 43-year-old female veteran presents for routine primary care. She has a medical history significant for fibromyalgia, irritable bowel syndrome, and is overweight. She was deployed to Afghanistan for 10 months and returned 1 year ago. For the past several months, she has been experiencing discomfort in her lower abdomen which is dull and constant in nature. The discomfort does not worsen with her menses, which have remained normal in flow and duration. She has been sexually abstinent for the last 2 years. The pain has interfered with her ability to work as a teacher.

   On exam, she is afebrile with normal vital signs; cardiovascular, pulmonary, abdominal, and genitourinary exams are normal.

   What is the next best step in her management?

   A. Initiate oral contraceptive pills
   B. Refer to gynecology for diagnostic laparoscopy
   C. Screen for sexually transmitted infections
   D. Refer for pelvic floor physical therapy
   E. Screen for military sexual trauma

   The correct answer is E. This patient's symptoms are consistent with chronic pelvic pain. Although chronic pelvic pain has many causes, it is important to consider an underlying diagnosis of trauma in patients presenting with this syndrome [11, 14]. Mental health disorders are common among female veterans, and approximately 25% have experienced military sexual trauma [14, 15]. Military sexual trauma (MST) is strongly associated with the development of post-traumatic stress disorder (PTSD), which, in turn, has been linked to chronic pelvic pain in some patients. In one study, almost one-third of patients presenting with chronic pelvic pain screened positive for PTSD [3].

While endometriosis is associated with pelvic pain, the discomfort is often cyclical, and associated with other symptoms, such as dyspareunia and dysmenorrhea. Oral contraceptive pills are a reasonable first step in the empiric treatment of endometriosis but are less appropriate here. Diagnostic laparoscopy is recommended for evaluation of endometriosis when the diagnosis is uncertain or medical treatments have not been helpful.

Chronic pelvic pain may be caused by untreated pelvic infections; thus, it is reasonable to consider testing for sexually transmitted infections (STIs). However, this patient has been sexually abstinent for 2 years, and so STIs are less likely. Testing for STIs may be considered in addition to screening for military sexual trauma.

Pelvic physical floor therapy is recommended for patients with chronic pelvic pain attributable to myofascial syndrome or spasm of the pelvic floor muscles.

2. A 32-year-old female veteran presents to your primary care office for follow-up. She has a diagnosis of traumatic brain injury (TBI) following a blast injury during which she lost consciousness for several minutes while deployed to Iraq. Symptoms include chronic headaches, irritability, difficulty sleeping, and trouble concentrating.

   She has been prescribed naproxen as needed for headaches. She currently only gets headaches a couple times a month; severity is described as moderate though she remains functional and symptoms respond well to naproxen. While her headaches have improved, she continues to complain of difficulty staying asleep and increased irritability.

   She is currently employed as a factory worker and feels that these symptoms have started to affect her job performance. She describes a few episodes of angry outbursts with her supervisor and coworkers. Also, she avoids doing tasks that expose her to loud noises, because they make her feel more anxious. Overall, she has been more down and discouraged and feels that no one understands her.

   On exam, she has normal vital signs. Neurologic exam is unremarkable.

   What is the next best step in management?

   A. Start zolpidem
   B. Order a brain MRI
   C. Counsel about sleep hygiene
   D. Refer to mental health for cognitive behavioral therapy
   E. Start a selective serotonin reuptake inhibitor (SSRI)

   The correct answer is D. This patient's symptoms meet DSM 5 criteria for the diagnosis of post-traumatic stress disorder (PTSD) [9]. She had exposure to a traumatic event (blast during deployment) that was potentially life-threatening, she describes symptoms of re-experiencing that event as evidenced by her reaction to loud noises; she exhibits avoidance behaviors and symptoms of hyperarousal. It is important to note that the symptoms of TBI can often overlap with and present in conjunction with symptoms of PTSD. Thus, providers should be vigilant about screening for both diagnoses which have high prevalence among veterans. The most effective treatment for PTSD is cognitive behavioral therapy (CBT). SSRIs, such as sertraline, can be considered as a medication options to manage PTSD [10].

   Options such as counseling about sleep hygiene and zolpidem are sometimes used to manage insomnia in patients with PTSD. However, they are not considered first-line therapy. Neuroimaging is typically not necessary when diagnosing TBI and has no role in diagnosing PTSD. Additionally, this patient is not presenting with any "red flag" headache symptoms such as new onset, thunderclap headache, awakening from sleep with headache, etc., that might warrant a brain MRI.

References

1. Zephyrin LC. Reproductive health management for the care of women veterans. Obstet Gynecol. 2016;127(2):383–92. https://doi.org/10.1097/AOG.0000000000001252.
2. Walker JA, Borbely JM. Women veterans in the labor force. In: Spotlight on statistics. Washington, DC: U.S. Bureau of Labor Statistics; 2014. https://www.bls.gov/spotlight/2014/women-vets/pdf/women-vets.pdf. Accessed June 2018.
3. Levander XA, Overland MK. Care of women veterans. Med Clin North Am. 2015;99(3):651–62. https://doi.org/10.1016/j.mcna.2015.01.013.
4. Lehavot K, Hoerster KD, Nelson KM, Jakupcak M, Simpson TL. Health indicators for military, veteran, and civilian women. Am J Prev Med. 2012;42(5):473–80. https://doi.org/10.1016/j.amepre.2012.01.006.
5. Committee on Health Care for Underserved Women, American College of Obstetricians and Gynecologists. Committee Opinion No. 547: Health care for women in the military and women veterans. Obstet Gynecol. 2012;120(6):1538–42. https://doi.org/10.1097/01.AOG.0000423821.70036.5a.
6. Hamilton AB, Poza I, Washington DL. "Homelessness and trauma go hand-in-hand": pathways to homelessness among women veterans. Womens Health Issues. 2011;21(4 Suppl):S203–9. https://doi.org/10.1016/j.whi.2011.04.005.
7. Johnson BS, Boudiab LD, Freundl M, Anthony M, Gmerek GB, Carter J. Enhancing veteran-centered care: a guide for nurses in non-VA setting. Am J Nurs. 2013;113(7):24–39; quiz 54, 40. https://doi.org/10.1097/01.NAJ.0000431913.50226.83.
8. HUD-VA Supportive Housing Program Information. http://www.nchv.org/images/uploads/HFV%20paper.pdf. Accessed December 2018.
9. American Psychiatric Association. Diagnostic and statistical manual of mental disorders: DSM-5. 5th ed. Arlington: American Psychiatric Publishing; 2013.
10. Department of Veterans Affairs, Department of Defense. VA/DOD clinical practice guideline for the management of post-

traumatic stress disorder and acute stress disorder: Clinician Summary, 2017. https://www.healthquality.va.gov/guidelines/MH/ptsd/VADoDPTSDCPGClinicianSummaryFinal.pdf. Accessed June 2018.
11. Quinlan JD, Guaron MR, Deschere BR, Stephens MB. Care of the returning veteran. Am Fam Physician. 2010;82(1):43–9.
12. Prins A, Bovin MJ, Smolenski DJ, Marx BP, Kimerling R, Jenkins-Guarnieri MA, et al. The primary care PTSD screen for DSM-5 (PC-PTSD-5): development and evaluation within a veteran primary care sample. J Gen Intern Med. 2016;31(10):1206–11. https://doi.org/10.1007/s11606-016-3703-5.
13. Sessums LL, Jackson JL. In the clinic. Care of returning military personnel. Ann Intern Med. 2013;159(1):ITC1–15; quiz ITC16. https://doi.org/10.7326/0003-4819-159-1-201307020-01001.
14. U.S. Department of Veterans Affairs. Military sexual trauma. https://www.mentalhealth.va.gov/mentalhealth/msthome/index.asp. Accessed June 2018.
15. U.S. Department of Veterans Affairs. MST general factsheet, 2015. https://www.mentalhealth.va.gov/docs/mst_general_factsheet.pdf. Accessed June 2018.
16. Kintzle S, Schuyler AC, Ray-Letourneau D, Ozuna SM, Munch C, Xintarianos E, et al. Sexual trauma in the military: exploring PTSD and mental health care utilization in female veterans. Psychol Serv. 2015;12(4):394–401. https://doi.org/10.1037/ser0000054.
17. Goldstein LA, Dinh J, Donalson R, Hebenstreit CL, Maguen S. Impact of military trauma exposures on posttraumatic stress and depression in female veterans. Psychiatry Res. 2017;249:281–5. https://doi.org/10.1016/j.psychres.2017.01.009.
18. Yaeger D, Himmelfarb N, Cammack A, Mintz J. DSM-IV diagnosed posttraumatic stress disorder in women veterans with and without military sexual trauma. J Gen Intern Med. 2006;21(Suppl 3):S65–9.
19. Mankowski J, Everett JE. Women service members, veterans, and their families: what we know now. Nurse Educ Today. 2016;47:23–6.
20. Skinner KM, Kressin N, Frayne S, Tripp TJ, Hankin CS, Miller DR, Sullivan LM. The prevalence of military sexual assault among female veterans' administration outpatients. J Interpers Violence. 2000;15(3):291–310. https://doi.org/10.1177/088626000015003005.
21. Department of Veterans Affairs, Department of Defense. VA/DOD clinical practice guideline for the management of substance use disorder: Clinician Summary, 2015. https://www.healthquality.va.gov/guidelines/MH/sud/VADoDSUDCPGProviderSummaryRevised081017.pdf. Accessed June 2018.
22. The AUDIT-C screening tool. https://www.hepatitis.va.gov/provider/tools/audit-c.asp. Accessed December 2018.
23. Spelman JF, Hunt SC, Seal KH, Burgo-Black AL. Post deployment care for returning combat veterans. J Gen Intern Med. 2012;27(9):1200–9. https://doi.org/10.1007/s11606-012-2061-1.
24. Lee DJ, Schnitzlein CW, Wolf JP, Vythilingam M, Rasmusson AM, Hoge CW. Psychotherapy versus pharmacotherapy for posttraumatic stress disorder: systemic review and meta-analyses to determine first-line treatments. Depress Anxiety. 2016;33(9):792–806. https://doi.org/10.1002/da.22511.
25. Watts BV, Schnurr PP, Mayo L, Young-Xu Y, Weeks WB, Friedman MJ. Meta-analysis of the efficacy of treatments for posttraumatic stress disorder. J Clin Psychiatry. 2013;74(6):e541–50. https://doi.org/10.4088/JCP.12r08225.
26. VA PSTD website. https://www.ptsd.va.gov/. Accessed December 2018.
27. VA MST website resources. https://www.mentalhealth.va.gov/msthome/index.asp. Accessed December 2018.
28. Veterans Crisis Line website. https://www.veteranscrisisline.net/.
29. Häuser W, Galek A, Erbslöh-Möller B, Köllner V, Kühn-Becker H, Langhorst J, et al. Posttraumatic stress disorder in fibromyalgia syndrome: prevalence, temporal relationship between posttraumatic stress and fibromyalgia symptoms, and impact on clinical outcome. Pain. 2013;154(8):1216–23. https://doi.org/10.1016/j.pain.2013.03.034.
30. Department of Veterans Affairs, Department of Defense. VA/DOD clinical practice guideline for the management of concussion-mild traumatic brain injury: Clinician Summary, 2015. https://www.healthquality.va.gov/guidelines/Rehab/mtbi/mTBICPGClinicianSummary50821816.pdf. Accessed June 2018.
31. Terrio H, Brenner LA, Ivins BJ, Cho JM, Helmick K, Schwab K, et al. Traumatic brain injury screening: preliminary findings in a US Army Brigade Combat Team. J Head Trauma Rehabil. 2009;24(1):14–23. https://doi.org/10.1097/HTR.0b013e31819581d8.
32. Savas LS, White DL, Wieman M, Daci K, Fitzgerald S, Laday Smith S, et al. Irritable bowel syndrome and dyspepsia among women veterans: prevalence and association with psychological distress. Aliment Pharmacol Ther. 2009;29(1):115–25. https://doi.org/10.1111/j.1365-2036.2008.03847.x.
33. White DL, Savas LS, Daci K, Elserag R, Graham DP, Fitzgerald SJ, et al. Trauma history and risk of the irritable bowel syndrome in women veterans. Aliment Pharmacol Ther. 2010;32(4):551–61. https://doi.org/10.1111/j.1365-2036.2010.04387.x.
34. Barnard K, Frayne SM, Skinner KM, Sullivan LM. Health status among women with menstrual symptoms. J Womens Health (Larchmt). 2003;12(9):911–9.
35. Katon JG, Hoggatt KJ, Balasubramanian V, Saechao FS, Frayne SM, Mattocks KM, et al. Reproductive health diagnoses of women veterans using department of Veterans Affairs health care. Med Care. 2015;53(4 Suppl 1):S63–7. https://doi.org/10.1097/MLR.0000000000000295.
36. Borrero S, Callegari LS, Zhao X, Mor MK, Sileanu FE, Switzer G, et al. Unintended pregnancy and contraceptive use among women veterans: The ECUUN study. J Gen Intern Med. 2017;32(8):900–8. https://doi.org/10.1007/s11606-017-4049-3.
37. Rosenfeld E, Callegari LS, Sileanu FE, Zhao X, Schwarz EB, Mor MK, Borrero S. Racial and ethnic disparities in contraceptive knowledge among women veterans in the ECUUN study. Contraception. 2017;96(1):54–61. https://doi.org/10.1016/j.contraception.2017.03.008.
38. Callegari LS, Zhao X, Nelson KM, Borrero S. Contraceptive adherence among women Veterans with mental illness and substance use disorder. Contraception. 2015;91(5):386–92. https://doi.org/10.1016/j.contraception.2015.01.013.
39. Judge CP, Zhao X, Sileanu FE, Mor MK, Borrero S. Medical contraindications to estrogen and contraceptive use among women veterans. Am J Obstet Gynecol. 2018;218(2):234.e1–9. https://doi.org/10.1016/j.ajog.2017.10.020.
40. Schwarz EB, Longo LS, Zhao X, Stone RA, Cunningham F, Good CB. Provision of potentially teratogenic medications to female veterans of childbearing age. Med Care. 2010;48(9):834–42. https://doi.org/10.1097/MLR.0b013e3181e57946.
41. Chiles DP, Roberts TA, Klein DA. Initiation and continuation of long-acting reversible contraception in the United States military healthcare system. Am J Obstet Gynecol. 2016;215(3):328.e1–9. https://doi.org/10.1016/j.ajog.2016.03.027.
42. Lehavot K, Katon JG, Williams EC, Nelson KM, Gardella CM, Reiber GE, Simpson TL. Sexual behaviors and sexually transmitted infections in a nationally representative sample of women veterans and nonveterans. J Womens Health (Larchmt). 2014;23(3):246–52. https://doi.org/10.1089/jwh.2013.4327.
43. Centers for Disease Control and Prevention. 2015 sexually transmitted diseases treatment guidelines.

Part VIII

Pregnancy

Obstetric Medicine

39

Lisa B. Bernstein, Michael P. Carson, Meredith O. Cruz, Rachel K. Harrison, Amanda Johnson, Anna Kho, Beth Lewis, and Sarah A. Tilstra

Learning Objectives

- Describe general principles that a provider should follow when caring for pregnant women.
- Explain preconception/interconception interventions that help to minimize risk and contribute to a healthy pregnancy.
- Describe the approach to medication utilization and testing during pregnancy.
- Outline the clinical manifestations, diagnosis, and management of common medical conditions during pregnancy, including hypertension, asthma, venous thromboembolism, diabetes mellitus, thyroid disease, and depression.
- State complications that can occur in the postpartum period and what the primary care provider's main role is in diagnosing and managing each one.

Section 1: Principles of Caring for Pregnant Women

- A healthy fetus depends on a healthy mother. The best approach is to develop a clinical plan as if she were not pregnant; then obtain information to determine how the plan does or does not need to be modified in the setting of pregnancy. Often you will be reassured that the non-pregnant plan is best for the mother and baby. Consider the real benefit to the mother and fetus related to the test or treatment, not just the theoretical or rare risks.
- Refrain from saying "no" when you "don't know." Use evidence-based medicine to answer clinical questions and seek out expert opinion where data is lacking or does not exist.
- Determine if non-pharmacological therapies can be used as first-line treatments; if medications are required, it is important to consider the efficacy and safety profile for pregnant women, which may vary by trimester.
- Do not consider tests, interventions, or medications as "safe" or "unsafe"; consider the clinical setting and then determine which ones may be "reasonable" or "indicated."
- Always consider the consequences and risks of NOT obtaining the test or administering the treatment.

L. B. Bernstein (✉) · A. Kho
Emory University School of Medicine, Department of Medicine, Atlanta, GA, USA
e-mail: lbernst@emory.edu

M. P. Carson
Hackensack Meridian School of Medicine at Seton Hall, Jersey Shore University Medical Center, Department of Medicine, Neptune, NJ, USA

M. O. Cruz
Froedtert and the Medical College of Wisconsin, Department of Obstetrics and Gynecology, Milwaukee, WI, USA

R. K. Harrison
Medical College of Wisconsin, Department of Obstetrics and Gynecology, Milwaukee, WI, USA

A. Johnson
University of Colorado School of Medicine, Department of Obstetrics and Gynecology, Aurora, CO, USA

B. Lewis
Jacobi Medical Center, Department of Obstetrics and Gynecology, Bronx, NY, USA

S. A. Tilstra
University of Pittsburgh School of Medicine, Division of General Internal Medicine, Department of Medicine, Pittsburgh, PA, USA

S. A. Tilstra et al. (eds.), *Sex- and Gender-Based Women's Health*, https://doi.org/10.1007/978-3-030-50695-7_39

Preconception/Interconception Counseling

Aaliyah is a 32-year-old G1P1 female with a history of hypertension, type 2 diabetes, and intermittent asthma who presents to your office for an annual physical exam. She uses condoms for birth control and is interested in having more children. She takes lisinopril 20 mg daily for hypertension and metformin 500 mg twice daily for diabetes, rarely needing her rescue inhaler. She smokes 2 cigarettes per day and drinks 1 glass of wine on the weekends. She had some baby blues after her first pregnancy but did not require any antidepressant medication. Her blood pressure is 124/78 and she is overweight with a body mass index (BMI) of 28 kg/m^2. The remainder of her exam is normal. What is the best way to optimize her health prior to a pregnancy, and how would you counsel her during this preconception time period?

Optimal Timing of Pregnancy Based on Health and Social Factors

In the United States, as many as half of pregnancies are unintended [1]. Primary care providers have the opportunity to educate women in the preconception period to help optimize their health during pregnancy. Every clinic visit for a reproductive age woman is a chance to counsel about issues that may impact a pregnancy including the timing of pregnancy in the setting of chronic health conditions, advanced maternal age, elevated BMI, family history of genetic disorders, sexually transmitted infections (STIs), vaccinations, folic acid supplementation, substance use, caffeine intake, environmental exposures, and intimate partner violence (IPV) [2].

Folic Acid Supplementation

Daily folic acid supplementation of 400 μg (0.4 mg) in pregnant women has been shown to reduce the risk of neural tube defects, cleft lip/palate, genitourinary abnormalities, congenital heart defects, and hydrocephalus in offspring [3–5]. Because the neural tube forms quickly, between 26 and 28 days after conception, folic acid must be started *before* conception. The CDC, National Academy of Medicine, and the USPSTF all recommend that women of childbearing age with an intact uterus, regardless of stated contraception methods, consume 400 μg (0.4 mg) of folic acid daily [6]. Most "prenatal" or "women's" vitamins will contain 400 μg (0.4 mg) or more of folic acid and can be purchased over-the-counter [7].

Reproductive age women with high risk conditions such as intestinal malabsorption, diabetes, liver disease, and those who are taking valproic acid or carbamazepine for seizures should take up to 1000 μg (1 mg) of folic acid for prevention of poor pregnancy outcomes [8, 9]. Women with a history of neural tube defects themselves or a first-degree relative should take 4000 μg (4 mg) of folic acid daily [8, 10, 11]. After the first trimester, when neural tube development is complete, the folic acid dose can be reduced to 0.4 mg daily since high dose folic acid can lead to long-term adverse effects [12]. Women should continue folic acid at 0.4 mg daily after the first trimester through 4–6 weeks postpartum or as long as breastfeeding continues [8].

Advanced Maternal Age

As women age, fertility declines and the risk of pregnancy complications increases. Advanced maternal age is defined as maternal age ≥35 years old and is associated with increased risk of miscarriage, preeclampsia, gestational diabetes, chromosome abnormalities, congenital abnormalities, placenta previa, low birth weight, preterm delivery, small size for gestational age infants, and perinatal mortality [13, 14]. As many women are delaying childbearing until the third and fourth decade, it is important to discuss offsetting the risk of maternal age by optimizing modifiable risk factors.

Body Mass Index (BMI)

Achieving an appropriate BMI prior to pregnancy can improve obstetric outcomes. Women with a BMI ≥ 30 kg/m^2 are more likely to have obese infants, infants with low Apgar scores and congenital anomalies, and higher perinatal mortality. Being thinner is not always better, as women with a low BMI (<18.5 kg/m^2) are at risk for preterm birth and lower birth weight infants compared to women with a normal BMI [15–18]. However, underweight women do have a lower rate of preeclampsia, gestational diabetes, and obstetric interventions [19]. Primary care providers should provide nutritional education and exercise recommendations for women who fall outside the range for a normal BMI.

Family History and Genetic Counseling

Obtaining a family history of inherited disorders and referral to a geneticist for further counseling and testing could be considered for those with a personal or family history of congenital malformations, developmental disability, hemophilia, hemoglobinopathy, cystic fibrosis, polycystic kidney disease, neurofibromatosis, or a similar inheritable condition. Counselors can help determine the need for prenatal testing of the parents or the fetus to inform decisions about family planning, observation of the fetus during pregnancy, and plan for any foreseeable complications upon the child's birth.

Sexually Transmitted Infection (STI) Screening

Depending on the type of infection, treatment may reduce the mother's rate of infertility, pregnancy complications, and congenital infection in the newborn [19]. For example, women with HIV can reduce the rate of maternal-infant HIV transmission if maternal antiretroviral therapy is initiated during the antepartum or intrapartum periods and administered to the infant during the first 6 weeks of life [20].

Women who are contemplating pregnancy should be tested for chlamydia, gonorrhea, hepatitis B and C, human immunodeficiency virus (HIV), syphilis, and trichomonas. It is standard of care to collect these labs at the first prenatal visit [21]; however, if a patient is at high risk for these infections consider testing prior to and throughout pregnancy.

Vaccinations

Women should be vaccinated against vaccine-preventable diseases prior to pregnancy. Live-attenuated vaccines, such as the MMR and varicella vaccines, are contraindicated during pregnancy and must be given in the preconception period [22, 23].

Measles, mumps, rubella (MMR), and varicella: Congenital rubella can be devastating for the fetus and is known to cause deafness, developmental disability, heart defects, and eye problems [24]. Immune status, if unknown, can be determined by checking MMR and varicella titers prior to administration of the vaccine. If the vaccine is needed, pregnancy should be avoided for at least 1 month after each live vaccine dose for MMR and up to 3 months after varicella vaccination [25].

Tetanus, diphtheria, and pertussis (Tdap): All adults over 19 years old who have not previously received the Tdap vaccination should receive one dose, followed by a tetanus and diphtheria (Td) booster every 10 years; Tdap should take the place of one Td shot during adulthood to provide better protection against pertussis as immunity wanes with age [26]. Additionally, pregnant women should receive Tdap vaccination with every pregnancy, preferably during the early part of the 27–36-week gestational range to help protect baby from pertussis during infancy [27, 28].

Influenza: All women regardless of pregnancy status, and who do not have a contraindication, should be vaccinated for influenza. Pregnant women have an exceptionally high rate of morbidity and mortality from influenza, most often from respiratory complications, secondary bacterial infections, and sepsis [29]. Pregnant patients should not receive the live attenuated influenza vaccine since its safety in pregnancy has not been established.

Special populations: For patients at risk for infections with encapsulated organisms, compromised immunity, or high risk occupations, consider immunization against *Haemophilus influenzae*, hepatitis B, meningococcus, and pneumococcus in the preconception period.

Substance Use (Tobacco, Alcohol, Drugs), and Caffeine Intake

It may be very difficult for women who are considering pregnancy or already pregnant to admit to cigarette, alcohol, and substance use. They may fear legal consequences or perceive that they may lose custody of their child at birth. Thus, taking the social history in a confidential and non-judgmental manner is vital.

Cigarette smoking is associated with nearly every obstetric complication including decreased fertility, placental abruption, preterm premature rupture of membranes (PPROM), placenta previa, preterm labor, preterm delivery, low birth weight (LBW), ectopic pregnancy, and stillbirth [30–32]. Smoking reduction, as assessed by maternal nicotine levels, has been associated with greater fetal weight compared to women who continued smoking, and any level of reduction up to 30 weeks gestation can have a beneficial effect on the obstetric risk [33]. At the preconception visit, and at every visit during her pregnancy (if needed), the American College of Obstetricians and Gynecologists (ACOG) and the USPSTF recommend using the Five As intervention to identify smokers and facilitate cessation: *A*sk about her smoking status, *A*dvise her to quit, *A*ssess her readiness to quit, *A*ssist her in quitting, and *A*rrange follow-up visits [34, 35]. Non-pharmacologic methods proven to help pregnant women quit smoking include pamphlets, videos, access to a health educator, and support groups. For some patients, counseling and support by phone (1-800-QUIT-NOW) offers a convenient and flexible way for them to communicate with someone who can encourage desirable health behaviors [36].

When other interventions have been unsuccessful, pharmacotherapy may help patients in their quest to quit smoking. Nicotine replacement therapy (NRT), which includes nicotine lozenges, spray, patches, gum, and an inhaler, may be used as an adjunct to behavioral modification for smoking cessation in the preconception period, even during pregnancy. The benefits of decreasing smoking with NRT are thought to outweigh the risks. NRT and smoking both expose the maternal/fetal unit to nicotine exposure. However, NRT use can decrease exposure to smoke and carcinogens; therefore, while long-term data may not be available, simple logic dictates that NRT use is reasonable during pregnancy. NRT can facilitate cessation in the non-pregnant population, it can reduce the pulmonary effects of smoking on the mother, and was felt to be safe enough for use in a randomized trial. While the trial did not demonstrate that NRT was effective for smoking cessation during pregnancy, it was not found to be more harmful than smoking [37–39].

In pregnancy, there may be a higher rate of left ventricular outflow obstruction in infants exposed to bupropion during the first trimester [40]. As a result, when indicated, it is reasonable to avoid use until after the first trimester. First trimester exposure to varenicline does not appear to be teratogenic, but as the safety in pregnancy has not been established, it is reasonable to recommend discontinuation of the medicine near the time of conception [41].

Alcohol consumption during pregnancy can lead to fetal alcohol spectrum disorder and stillbirth [42], and while women often drink "a glass of wine here-and-there" during pregnancy, there is no known threshold amount of alcohol that is proven safe to consume in pregnancy. A single-item screening tool is a practical way for providers to screen for hazardous alcohol use in women: "How many times in the past year have you had 4 or more drinks in a day?" A response of ≥1 is considered positive [43]. Women who screen positive should be counseled regarding the harm that can occur when alcohol is consumed in pregnancy. Patients that show signs of alcohol use disorder should be provided information regarding appropriate detoxification and treatment services including a list of alcohol rehabilitation resources, and referrals to social work, psychiatry and/or an addiction specialist.

With the legalization of marijuana in some states, both for recreation and medicinal purposes, more women are using marijuana than ever before. Because it is legal, women may not perceive that marijuana is harmful to baby. Babies born to mothers who used marijuana are more likely to have lower birth weights, spend time in the neonatal intensive care unit after birth, be stillborn, and have learning and behavioral issues later in life [44, 45]. ACOG strongly advises against all forms of marijuana use, including medicinal use, during pregnancy [45].

Patients who use other substances such as cocaine, methamphetamines, heroin, and inhalants should be referred immediately to substance use rehab programs, social work, psychiatry, and/or an addiction specialist. Please see Chap. 32 for more information on how to treat opioid use during pregnancy.

Much of the evidence of caffeine's effect on humans is low quality; however, it appears that 200 mg/day or less of caffeine intake is not associated with increased risk of congenital malformations, miscarriage, or growth restriction [46]. Because of this, several organizations, including ACOG and the March of Dimes, recommend limiting caffeine intake to <200 mg/day rather than restricting it entirely [47, 48].

Safety Assessment, Intimate Partner Violence

Intimate partner violence (IPV) affects millions of women regardless of age, economic status, race, religion, sexual orientation, or educational background [49]. As abuse can worsen when a woman is pregnant, it is vital to screen women for IPV and assess for characteristic features of abuse. Injury, bruising, missed appointments, and anxiety/depression can be objective signs that a patient may be a victim of abuse. Please see Chap. 35 to learn more about IPV.

Preexisting Medical Conditions

Women of childbearing age with chronic medical conditions should be advised to seek care for optimization of their medical issues prior to conception. These women should use reliable contraception until their medical issues are controlled to secure the best outcome for them and any future pregnancy. In addition, their medications should be reconciled and adjusted to minimize any potential harm to a developing fetus.

General Approach to the Management of the Pregnant Patient

Physiologic Changes of Pregnancy

The hormonal changes of pregnancy alter maternal physiology as early as 5 weeks gestation and typically resolve by 6 weeks postpartum. Cardiac output increases by three main mechanisms: increase in maternal heart rate, increase in plasma volume, and decrease in systemic vascular resistance. A common finding reflecting this increase in flow is a II/VI systolic pulmonary artery flow murmur at the upper left sternal border. A simple maneuver to document the normal pulmonic arterial flow murmur of pregnancy is that it will become quieter with a deep breath as the chest wall moves away from the pulmonary artery. Diastolic murmurs are not normal and should always be evaluated. The low resistance vascular beds in the uterus and placenta decrease systemic vascular resistance. As plasma volume increases relative to red cell mass, women develop physiologic anemia of pregnancy [50, 51].

Pregnant women often feel dyspneic, even before the uterus restricts diaphragmatic excursion. While the mechanism is not entirely clear, it is likely related to how progesterone affects the respiratory system and acid/base balance. Maternal minute ventilation increases in the first trimester by increasing tidal volume, while maintaining resting maternal respiratory rate. This causes relative hypocapnea, reflecting the normal PCO2 of pregnancy around 30 mmHg. Pulmonary mechanics and spirometry do not change, but the gravid uterus can restrict diaphragmatic excursion later in pregnancy resulting in a decreased residual volume. It is always important to consider all causes of dyspnea in pregnant women before attributing symptoms to benign dyspnea of pregnancy [52].

Gastroesophageal reflux is common due to the progesterone-mediated decrease in lower esophageal sphincter tone. Progesterone also decreases intestinal motility and can lead to severe constipation. Creatinine clearance increases by 50% during pregnancy, which can be associated with worsened proteinuria in women with preexisting renal disease [50, 51].

Prescribing in Pregnancy

Medications are often required for optimal control of a woman's chronic medical issues in order for a successful pregnancy outcome. The US Food and Drug Administration pregnancy safety categories A, B, C, D, and X are no longer used to guide prescribing; instead, providers should consider if a medication is clinically indicated or not, and the implications for the mother and fetus if the medication is used versus withheld [53]. Educate patients that uncontrolled medical issues are often more detrimental to a pregnancy than are the medications used to control them. When treating any medical illness in pregnant women, first consider non-pharmacological interventions and try to limit medications in the first trimester. Most medications cross the placenta; while ample safety data may not be available for all medications, thankfully, few drugs are absolutely contraindicated in pregnancy (Table 39.1) [53, 54].

Table 39.1 Examples of common medications that are relatively or absolutely contraindicated in pregnancy (may not be an exhaustive list of every teratogenic medication) [53–59]

Medication	Risks	Clinical advice
Androgens	Virilization of female fetus	Avoid
Angiotensin converting enzyme (ACE) inhibitors and angiotensin receptor blockers (ARB)	Pulmonary and renal hypoplasia, renal tubular dysgenesis, oligohydramnios, persistent patent ductus arteriosus, intrauterine growth restriction	Avoid
Antiepileptics (carbamazepine, phenobarbital, phenytoin, topiramate, valproic acid)	Neural tube defects, cardiac defects, limb and urinary tract defects, cleft palate	Use when indicated. Monitor maternal levels, coordinate with obstetrician re: fetal monitoring and assessment
Antineoplastics (cyclophosphamide, methotrexate)	Skeletal defects, spontaneous abortion, stillbirth. May be indicated for treatment/exacerbations of autoimmune disorders	Use with caution when indicated
Atenolol	Intrauterine growth restriction, neonatal bradycardia	Avoid as other options are available
Estrogens	Feminization of male fetus	Avoid
Fluconazole	Abnormal facies, cleft palate, congenital heart disease, thin ribs, and long bones	Use with caution when indicated if other treatment options are not available
Isotretinoin and Tazarotene (oral)	Ear, cardiovascular, and skeletal defects; central nervous system dysfunction	Avoid
Lithium	Cardiovascular defects, floppy infant syndrome	Avoid
Methimazole	Retrospective data regarding rare risk of aplasia cutis associated with first trimester use	Drug of choice for Graves' disease during second/third trimesters. Unless intolerant to propylthiouracil, avoid during first trimester
Propylthiouracil (PTU)	Rare risk of maternal drug induced hepatitis	Drug of choice for Graves' disease during first trimester. Unless intolerant to methimazole, avoid during second/third trimesters
Statins	Central nervous system and limb abnormalities	Avoid
Tetracyclines	Permanent discoloration of offspring teeth; maternal hepatic toxicity	Use with caution when indicated if other treatment options are not available
Thalidomide	Limb defects, eye and ear abnormalities, heart defects, neonatal death	Avoid
Warfarin	Nasal and limb hypoplasia, central nervous system abnormalities, spontaneous abortion, fetal hemorrhage	Avoid first trimester. First-line for women with artificial heart valves during second/third trimester. Use with caution

Radiologic Studies

Ionizing Radiation (Computed Tomography, X-Ray)

Exposure to ionizing radiation prior to conception has no measurable impact on future pregnancies [60]. Except for a nuclear medicine thyroid scan, all indicated tests can be obtained during pregnancy [52, 61, 62]. The potential effect on the fetus is dependent on when the ionizing radiation exposure occurred, the dose of radiation, and the status of the fetal cellular repair mechanism at the time of exposure. Overall, exposure below 50 miliGray (mGy)/(5 rads) over the duration of the pregnancy involves no risk of adverse obstetric or fetal outcomes, including implantation failure, major malformations, restricted growth, or developmental delay [61–63]. In order to give providers and patients perspective in simple language on how each test falls well below the upper limit, Table 39.2 lists common imaging studies with the number of maternal studies "permitted" during the entire pregnancy to remain within the safe fetal exposure range [61, 62, 64]. For additional perspective, the table also lists the normal daily background radiation exposure.

Table 39.2 Radiologic studies and the fetal dose of ionizing radiation associated with that study [62]

Radiologic study	Fetal dose of ionizing radiation (mGy)	Number of maternal studies "permitted" during the entire pregnancy to remain within the safe fetal exposure range (equivalent of 50 mGy)
Background radiation exposure/year	0.003	16,667 years
7-hour airline flight (New York USA to London UK)	0.05	1000 7-hour flights
2-hour flight	0.014	3571 2-hour flights
Chest X-ray (2 views)	0.0005–0.01	5000–100,000 studies
CT head	0.001–0.01	5000–50,000 studies
CT chest	0.01–0.66	75–5000 studies
CT pulmonary angiogram	0.01–0.66	75–5000 studies
CT abdomen	1.3–35	1–38 studies
CT pelvis	10–50	1–5 studies
Nuclear medicine		
Ventilation	0.1–0.3	166–500 studies
Perfusion	0.4–0.6	83–125 studies
Mammography	0.001–0.01	5000–50,000 studies
X-ray		
Dental	0.0000001	500 million studies
Abdomen	0.1–3.0	16–500 studies
Chest (2 views)	0.0005–0.01	5000–100,000 studies
Intravenous pyelography	5–10	5–10 studies
Lumbar spine	1.0–10	1–5 studies
Extremity	<0.001	50,000 studies

Adapted with permission from RSNA, Tremblay et al. [62]
CT computed tomography

The clear clinical benefit of any test should not be overshadowed by the potential rare adverse event. Fetal exposure >50–500 mGy poses a slight risk for failure to implant, major malformations, growth restriction, decreased IQ, as well as up to 6% incidence of childhood cancer, depending on the dose. Radiation exposure >500 mGy is associated with >20% incidence of developmental delay and >6% incidence of childhood cancer. Iodinated contrast does cross the placenta, but there are no reports of adverse obstetric or fetal events that have been reported and therefore, when indicated, should be used during pregnancy and lactation without hesitation.

Magnetic Resonance Imaging (MRI)

Magnetic resonance imaging (MRI) testing during pregnancy has not been associated with adverse effects on pregnancy or offspring [65–67]. An expert panel concluded that at ≤1.5 Tesla magnetic field strengths, a clinically indicated MRI should be obtained during any trimester [68]. The risk for women who undergo testing at >1.5 Tesla magnetic field strengths is not clear. Gadolinium crosses the placenta, and a retrospective study found that it may be associated with a "broad range" of rheumatologic, inflammatory, or infiltrative skin disease, and stillbirth [67]. As in non-pregnant women, avoid gadolinium in pregnancy unless it will significantly improve diagnostic performance and serve to modify the care plan [67].

Mammography

A breast ultrasound +/− mammogram is the first indicated test for any breast masses detected during pregnancy, and mammography with appropriate shielding should be reserved for pregnant patients who appear to have a suspicious lesion [69]. Evaluation for suspicious breast masses should not be delayed during pregnancy.

Thyroid Imaging Scans

Thyroid imaging scans using radioiodine isotopes should not be ordered during pregnancy. The fetal thyroid absorbs iodine 400 times more avidly than the adult gland, therefore I-123 and I-131 administered to the mother can result in fetal thyroid ablation or thyroid cancer. In cases were a woman inadvertently received a dose, there is an "all or none" phenomenon where the pregnancy either results in an early loss or continues on without complications [62].

Ultrasonography

Ultrasonography can be used in pregnancy, and there are no long-term harmful effects to the fetus. However, it is recommended that it be used at the lowest acoustic energy necessary that allows adequate diagnostic evaluation and for the shortest time possible [69].

Section 2: Co-management of Medical Issues in Pregnancy

Women with chronic medical conditions, such as diabetes, hypertension, and thyroid disorders, have better obstetric and neonatal outcomes when their condition is well controlled [70–75]. The 35% prevalence of chronic medical conditions present prior to and during pregnancy often leads obstetricians to enlist primary care providers to co-manage pregnant patients [52, 76]. By maintaining an open dialogue and creating a collaborative partnership, the interplay of a patient's medical and obstetric issues will be best addressed. When the provider is not comfortable managing medical issues, she should be referred to a maternal-fetal medicine specialist and/or medical subspecialist to provide proper oversight.

Diabetes

Aaliyah presents a year later for an annual exam. She is planning to become pregnant soon. She is on metformin and lisinopril. Her hemoglobin A1c is 6.8%, blood pressure is 144/78. You change her antihypertensive medication, perform the indicated foot exam, and start a daily prenatal vitamin with 1 mg folic acid.

A few months later, she calls to tell you that she had a positive pregnancy test. How should you change her management for her medical issues now that she is pregnant? What are the risks to her baby if her diabetes or hypertension are uncontrolled?

Epidemiology

Among Americans aged 18–44 years, an estimated 2.6% have diabetes mellitus (DM), 23.7% have pre-diabetes (PreDM), and an additional 1.3% have not yet been diagnosed. Pre-gestational diabetes affects 1–2% of pregnancies in the United States, and 6–15% of women will develop gestational diabetes during their pregnancy [77].

Diabetes can have a major impact on the health of the mother and fetus during pregnancy. There is an increased rate of congenital anomalies which correlate with the maternal HbA1C at the time of conception; there is a 3% rate with an HbA1C ≤ 6.5%, increasing to 3.5% with HbA1C of 7%, 6% with HbA1C of 8%, and nearly 11% with a HbA1C of 10% [78]. Thus, optimizing glucose control before pregnancy is imperative in women with preexisting diabetes, and appropriate contraception should be recommended to women until their disease is well controlled. The American Diabetes Association (ADA) recommends targeting an HbA1C of <6.5% for diabetic women prior to conception to optimize birth outcomes [79].

Patients who are overweight or obese and have a risk factor for the development of gestational diabetes should be screened for pre-diabetes/diabetes prior to conception. Risk factors include previous gestational diabetes, delivering an infant 9 pounds or more, PCOS, metabolic syndrome, hypertension, HbA1C >5.6%, first-degree relative with diabetes, and physical inactivity [80]. There is no standard on how to monitor patients in pregnancy if pre-diabetes is diagnosed. Although screening for gestational diabetes usually is performed at 24–28 weeks of gestation, multiple organizations, including the ADA and ACOG, advocate early screening for women in this high risk category [81].

Pathophysiology and Clinical Manifestations

Multiple placental and maternal hormones including, but not limited to, human placental lactogen, cortisol, and several interleukins are responsible for the relative insulin resistance of pregnancy. This physiologic effect starts early in pregnancy and continues to intensify throughout gestation. During pregnancy, poor glucose control has been associated with miscarriage, fetal growth abnormalities (mostly "large for gestational age"), polyhydramnios, preeclampsia, neonatal hypoglycemia, and respiratory distress syndrome [82]. Pregnant women should monitor home sugars four times per day: fasting and 1 or 2 hours after each meal [83]. The goals are fasting glucose <95 mg/dL, 1-hour postprandial glucose <140 mg/dL or a 2-hour postprandial glucose <120 mg/dL; higher glucose levels have each been associated with poorer fetal outcomes. Additionally, monitoring 2-hour postprandial glucose values has been associated with a lower rate of macrosomia and neonatal hypoglycemia compared to preprandial values [83]. The HbA1c can be used to monitor glycemic control in women with pre-gestational diabetes mellitus, but it is not useful for women with gestational diabetes mellitus.

Treatment

Treatment of diabetes in pregnancy includes tight glucose control without hypoglycemia, keeping up with routine health maintenance, and screening for diabetic complications.

Glucose Control

The mainstay of glucose control is an appropriate diet. Meals should contain a small portion of low glycemic carbohydrates combined with protein to maintain glucose levels and avoid gluconeogenesis. The diet should consist of three larger meals with three snacks spread out throughout the day, including a snack before bed. Long periods of fasting are not recommended, because they may cause gluconeogenesis and elevated blood sugars, but if women are not hungry, it is reasonable to skip snacks. Occasionally, obese women lose weight during pregnancy as they consume an appropriate number of calories prescribed by a clinical nutritionist/provider causing a net negative caloric intake. Pregnant women should be encouraged to engage in 30 minutes of physical activity daily but should not be encouraged to exceed their pre-pregnancy exercise tolerance.

Insulin therapy is the preferred treatment for all pregnant women with diabetes [80] as it does not cross the placenta and provides excellent glucose control. Insulin regimens can vary by patient and their preferences; options include insulin pump therapy with continuous glucose monitoring for women with type 1 diabetes, multiple daily injection dosing using short-acting insulin, or a combination of short- and long-acting insulin. The most well-studied insulins include regular insulin, lispro and aspart (short-acting), NPH (intermediate), and detemir (long-acting). These insulins should be prioritized over other insulin products due to their safety data in pregnancy. Glargine has reassuring data as well, so if the other intermediate/long-acting ones are not available due to intolerance or logistics of the healthcare system, it can be used. Goals for glycemic control are very strict in pregnancy: fasting glucose <95 mg/dL, 1 hour post-prandial glucose <140 mg/dL, and 2-hour post-prandial glucose <120 mg/dL [80]. Patients should be counseled about the signs and symptoms of hypoglycemia and be prescribed glucose tablets or told to carry simple sugar products with them at all times.

Metformin has been used for many years for infertility related to PCOS, and there is reassuring data about its use throughout pregnancy. However, since it freely crosses the placenta, there are concerns that there could be unknown long-term effects on the fetus that have yet to be studied [84, 85]. Metformin is an acceptable alternative for women who refuse insulin. Of women who used metformin as a single agent in early pregnancy, 26–46% were eventually converted to insulin [84, 86]. Glyburide has been used in pregnancy but is inferior to insulin and metformin, with data showing increased risks of macrosomia and hypoglycemia [87]. There is not enough data to determine if other oral or injectable medications for diabetes are safe in pregnancy.

Table 39.3 Health maintenance for pregnant diabetic patients [81]

Pre-conception
Check random urine protein or microalbumin
Refer to ophthalmology to check for diabetic retinopathy
Prescribe prenatal vitamin with folic acid 1 mg/day
Optimize glucose control with target HgbA1c of <6.5%
As soon as pregnancy occurs
Check HbA1c
Continue folic acid 1 mg/day
Check baseline 24-hour urine for protein/creatinine to help monitor for preeclampsia
Refer to ophthalmology to check for diabetic retinopathy
Perform foot exam or refer to podiatry
Monitor finger stick blood glucose at least four times per day
Consider changing oral diabetic regimen to insulin to optimize glucose control
Start aspirin 81 mg daily >12 weeks but <16 weeks gestation

Health Maintenance

Table 39.3 lists the health maintenance for a diabetic patient in anticipation of and during pregnancy. During pregnancy, a 24-hour urine collection for protein is a more sensitive indicator of preeclampsia than the spot urine protein/creatinine ratio. Because cholesterol normally goes up during pregnancy, and cholesterol-lowering medications are avoided in the absence of familial hypertriglyceridemia, there is no need to check lipid levels. A consensus statement suggests that low dose aspirin (81 mg) should be started for prevention of preeclampsia early in pregnancy for all diabetic women, preferably after 12 weeks but before 16 weeks of gestation and be continued until delivery [88]. Diabetic retinopathy may worsen in pregnancy, therefore a dilated retinal exam should be done before or during pregnancy and any diabetic retinopathy should be treated per the standard of care [89].

You suggest Aaliyah continue her prenatal vitamin with 1 mg of folate. You tell her to start measuring her finger stick glucose when she is fasting in the morning and 2 hours after each meal and reinforce the need for good diabetic control during the pregnancy. At about 6 weeks gestation, her finger stick log reveals fasting sugars elevated at about 120 mg/dL with three of her postprandial values elevated to about 140 mg/dL. Although you can increase the metformin, you feel that she is likely to eventually need insulin and start a long-acting insulin before bedtime. At 12 weeks of gestation, you advise her to start aspirin 81 mg daily.

Hypertension

Epidemiology

The incidence of hypertension in the United States ranges from 2.6% to 27.6% in women aged 18–54 years and varies depending on race. Chronic hypertension affects 3–5% of pregnancies, and the risk of preeclampsia in these women is at least 20% [52]. In 2011, the World Health Organization (WHO) estimated that nearly 10% of all maternal deaths in Africa and Asia and 25% of maternal deaths in Latin America were associated with hypertensive disorders of pregnancy [90]. Hypertension in pregnancy is defined as a systolic blood pressure of ≥140 mmHg and/or a diastolic blood pressure of ≥90 mmHg measured on two separate occasions at least 4 hours apart in previously normotensive women [91]. Understanding hypertensive disorders in pregnancy and their complications can prevent unwanted adverse obstetric and fetal outcomes.

Classification

There are four categories of hypertension in pregnancy: (1) chronic hypertension, (2) gestational hypertension, (3) preeclampsia–eclampsia, and (4) preeclampsia–eclampsia superimposed upon chronic hypertension. In general, the risk factors for hypertension in pregnancy are similar to those for preeclampsia [92, 93]. Table 39.4 lists the risk factors for preeclampsia.

Chronic hypertension in pregnancy is defined as hypertension prior to pregnancy, elevated blood pressures before 20 weeks gestation, or hypertension that persists beyond 12 weeks postpartum [91].

Gestational hypertension is defined as hypertension that develops after 20 weeks gestation with no proteinuria or features of preeclampsia. This diagnosis is often assigned retrospectively when elevated blood pressures normalize 3 months postpartum [91].

Preeclampsia is defined as new-onset hypertension, usually after 20 weeks gestation, associated with new proteinuria (≥300 mg protein/24 hours or a spot protein to creatinine ratio ≥0.3 mg/mg or 30 mg/mmol), OR hypertension, with or *without* proteinuria, AND any one of the following examples of end-organ damage: platelet count <100 K/μL; elevated liver enzymes >2x the normal level; new-onset renal insufficiency (creatinine >1.1 mg/dL or a doubling of the creatinine in the absence of other renal disease); pulmonary edema; new-onset cerebral symptoms (e.g., altered mental status, headache, weakness, stroke); or visual disturbances (e.g., photophobia, scotomas, blurry vision, photopsia, temporary blindness, etc.) [91].

Table 39.4 Risk factors for preeclampsia [91, 92, 96]

Pre-gestational (chronic) hypertension
Pre-gestational diabetes
Body mass index of >25 kg/m^2 (overweight) or >30 kg/m^2 (obesity) prior to conception
History of preeclampsia in a previous pregnancy
Chronic kidney disease
Systemic lupus erythematosus
Antiphospholipid antibody
First pregnancy
Multiple gestation pregnancy

Eclampsia is defined as new-onset generalized, tonic-clonic seizures in a patient with preeclampsia. It is one of the manifestations of severe preeclampsia and can occur before, during, or after labor [91].

Preeclampsia–eclampsia superimposed upon chronic hypertension is defined in a pregnant woman with chronic hypertension who has worsening hypertension, new onset proteinuria or features of preeclampsia–eclampsia [91].

Hemolysis, elevated liver enzymes, and low platelet count (HELLP) syndrome shares many features of preeclampsia, but up to 20% of those with HELLP do not have hypertension [94, 95].

Physiology and Pathophysiology

In normal pregnancy, blood pressure decreases by 5–15 mmHg in the first trimester, with a greater decrease in the diastolic blood pressure than the systolic blood pressure. Blood pressure reaches its nadir at approximately 20 weeks, and then gradually comes back to baseline in the third trimester [95, 97, 98]. Any time a previously normotensive pregnant patient has a blood pressure ≥140/90 mmHg after 20 weeks gestation or has a blood pressure reading significantly above their baseline, an evaluation for preeclampsia should be considered [95].

Preeclampsia is a multisystem, progressive process thought to be due to a maladaptive maternal immune response to the invading trophoblast, causing inadequate and shallow placental development. As a result, angiogenic growth factors become altered, the placenta becomes ischemic, and systemic endothelial dysfunction occurs leading to the clinical manifestations that are commonly seen in patients with preeclampsia [99].

Clinical Manifestations

The primary clinical manifestation for the hypertensive disorders in pregnancy is hypertension, which is classified as mild (140–149 mmHg systolic or a 90–99 mmHg diastolic), moderate (150–159 mmHg systolic or 100–109 mmHg diastolic), and severe (≥160 mmHg systolic or ≥110 mmHg diastolic) [100]. Each office visit for these patients, whether it is with an obstetrician or with a primary care provider for medical management of acute or chronic conditions, should include an evaluation for preeclampsia by assessing for signs and symptoms of end-organ damage. A full review of systems should be conducted focusing on visual symptoms, headache, dyspnea, chest pain, abdominal pain, swelling, jaundice, petechiae, and paresthesias; be sure to ask family members for input regarding confusion or disorientation if appropriate. Outpatient blood pressures should be reviewed. The physical exam should focus on manual blood pressure measurement in both arms and uncovering signs of preeclampsia such as visual field defects, pulmonary edema, a cardiac gallop, hepatic tenderness, new onset edema, and abnormal neurologic findings such as altered mental status and clonus. Any pregnant patient with a blood pressure ≥160 mmHg systolic or ≥110 mmHg diastolic should be immediately referred for work-up and management of preeclampsia or hypertension with severe features.

Hypertensive disorders of pregnancy can progress quickly to severe stages and the significant morbidity and mortality associated with them including preterm delivery, intrauterine growth restriction, oligohydramnios, and placental abruption [99]. Preeclampsia can occur before, during, and for up to 2 weeks after pregnancy [101, 102]; thus, women presenting for a postpartum visit with signs of preeclampsia should be thoroughly evaluated and treated.

Women with a history of preeclampsia have a significantly elevated lifetime risk of hypertension, myocardial infarction, congestive heart failure, stroke, peripheral arterial disease, and cardiovascular mortality. Thus, primary providers should be diligent about monitoring for and optimizing cardiovascular risk factors in these women at young ages to help offset their increase in cardiovascular morbidity [99].

Aaliyah is at risk for preeclampsia due to a history of chronic hypertension, gestational diabetes, and an overweight BMI of 28 kg. She reports she had well-controlled hypertension during her first pregnancy and did not develop preeclampsia. At 28 weeks gestation, she has a blood pressure of 148/88 while taking labetalol 400 mg twice daily. She denies headache, visual changes, shortness of breath, chest pain, or decreased urination. You order lab work to evaluate for preeclampsia and instruct her to see her obstetrician for an ultrasound to evaluate fetal growth and amniotic fluid volume, all of which are normal. You discuss warning symptoms for preeclampsia with her, continue her on labetalol 400 mg twice daily and schedule a follow-up visit.

Laboratory Studies

Pregnant patients with chronic hypertension should have baseline laboratory testing early in pregnancy including complete blood count (CBC), comprehensive metabolic profile (CMP), and a 24-hour urine for protein excretion (normal is <300 mg/day during pregnancy) and creatinine clearance. Many patients with chronic hypertension have proteinuria prior to pregnancy, so it is important to quantify the amount of proteinuria in order to follow the trend during pregnancy as worsening proteinuria can suggest progression to preeclampsia. An elevated spot urine protein to creatinine ratio (≥0.3 mg/mg or 30 mg/mmol) above baseline suggests significant proteinuria; repeating a 24-hour urine collection will always be more accurate than a spot urine protein to creatinine ratio due to variability in urine concentration and the sensitivity of testing. Anemia or elevated bilirubin may suggest hemolysis, elevated liver enzymes and low platelets may suggest progression to preeclampsia or possible HELLP syndrome. There should be a low threshold to repeat laboratory testing at any sign or symptom that could indicate the development of preeclampsia.

Treatment

Treatment of hypertensive disorders of pregnancy, depending on their severity, can be done in collaboration with primary care and obstetrics. Target blood pressure *prior to pregnancy* should be per age-appropriate guidelines [103]. Ideally, women of reproductive age with hypertension will already be on a medication not known to be teratogenic in the first trimester of pregnancy.

Once women become pregnant, management changes slightly.

In early pregnancy, there are three approaches one can take in treating *chronic hypertension*, with a goal blood pressure of <160/110 mmHg. The first is to stop pre-pregnancy medication and resume it if the patient's blood pressure rises to ≥160/110 mmHg during pregnancy. The second option is to continue the medication during pregnancy if it has a reasonable safety profile, and the third option is to change the patient's medication to one with a larger body of data regarding its use during pregnancy [52]. Treating to pressures <150/90 mmHg decreases the risk of transient severe hypertension but does not reduce adverse maternal/fetal outcomes [104].

Women with *gestational hypertension* are monitored carefully for signs of end-organ damage as up to half of them can progress to preeclampsia [105]. Because preeclampsia is a progressive disorder of placentation, tight antepartum blood pressure control using non-pregnant goals will not improve obstetric or fetal outcomes in patients with mild–

moderate hypertension defined as pressures <150/100 mmHg [106, 107], and relative hypotension in these patients can be harmful. Should women develop progressive hypertension and concern for preeclampsia during pregnancy, delivery of the placenta is the only definitive treatment and can reverse the course of the disease, although the time to normalization can take days.

Women should work with their primary care providers and obstetricians to determine the most appropriate target blood pressure for them during pregnancy, taking into consideration their baseline blood pressure on and off medications and comorbidities.

Antihypertensive Medications in Pregnancy

Shared decision-making should be used to weigh the potential concrete benefit of any medication against the potential or theoretical effects on the fetus and pregnancy. First-line antihypertensive agents are labetalol, nifedipine, and methyldopa, because they have been well studied and are generally well tolerated. Labetalol is an alpha- and beta-adrenergic blocker and considered first-line treatment with reassuring data regarding its use during pregnancy [100]. It is generally well tolerated, but side effects may include dizziness, fatigue, and rarely hepatocellular injury. Extended-release nifedipine is also well tolerated and reasonable to use [108]. Immediate-release nifedipine could reduce blood pressure quickly and puts women at risk for hypotension. Children whose mothers had taken methyldopa in pregnancy did not show any differences in physical capability, intelligence, sight, or hearing when compared with children whose mothers were untreated, but the side effects of methyldopa (fatigue, drowsiness, drug-induced lupus, and relative lack of potency) make it hard to tolerate [109]. Hydralazine, pindolol, and metoprolol are second-line agents, and third-line medications include clonidine, diltiazem, verapamil, and thiazides.

Antihypertensive medications that are contraindicated in pregnancy include angiotensin converting enzyme (ACE) inhibitors, angiotensin II receptor blockers (ARBs), direct renin inhibitors, and mineralocorticoid receptor antagonists (such as spironolactone and eplerenone). These medicines can cause fetal renal dysplasia, lung hypoplasia, fetal loss, and other adverse outcomes [110–112]. Atenolol, compared to labetalol, was associated with lower birth weight, so is avoided during pregnancy [113].

In summary, primary care providers should be aware of the best medications to use in women of reproductive age, and be proactive about blood pressure monitoring and management for those in early pregnancy. Pregnant patients with known hypertension should be counseled about the signs and symptoms of preeclampsia and encouraged to seek care if concerns arise. All clinic visits should assess for end-organ dysfunction and signs of progression to preeclampsia, and patients should be referred immediately to their obstetrical provider or to emergency services if blood pressure is well above baseline, >160/110 mmHg, labs are abnormal, or symptoms are present.

Thyroid Disease

Hypothyroidism

Epidemiology and Clinical Manifestations

Thyroid disease, most commonly hypothyroidism, affects about 1.5% of the population [114]. It is common for primary providers to help manage hypothyroidism in women who are thinking of getting pregnant or are currently pregnant. Uncontrolled thyroid disease can have major effects on pregnancy as overt maternal hypothyroxinemia (0.3–0.5% of women) has been associated with cognitive effects in offspring, intrauterine growth restriction, preterm labor, and preeclampsia; therefore, the goal is to achieve normal thyroid function prior to and during pregnancy [115, 116]. While some data are conflicting regarding the appropriate management of hypothyroidism in symptomatic vs. asymptomatic women, the potential for adverse outcomes dictates that when a thyroid stimulating hormone (TSH) is obtained during pregnancy and is above the pregnancy-specific norm, treatment to correct it should be initiated.

Subclinical hypothyroidism, the presence of abnormal thyroid function tests without any overt symptoms, is more common (2.0–2.5% of women) and may be associated with increased risk of placental abruption, pregnancy loss, and preterm rupture of membranes [117]. Studies regarding the risk of cognitive effects in offspring are conflicting, and the relationship between subclinical hypothyroidism diagnosed during pregnancy and pregnancy outcomes is unclear. Autoimmune thyroid disease, thyroid disease with high antibody titers, may have a stronger association with adverse pregnancy outcomes than thyroid dysfunction itself. Not all women have antibody positive thyroid disease; euthyroid antibody positive mothers (particularly antithyroid peroxidase or "anti-TPO" antibodies) have an increased risk of spontaneous pregnancy loss and premature delivery, and pregnancy complications increase when the TSH >2.5 mU/L. For anti-TPO negative women, the obstetric risk remains low until the TSH is >5–10 mU/L [58]. Despite these associations, it is not clear that levothyroxine supplementation can modify outcomes in the offspring of these asymptomatic women [118].

Many symptoms common to hypothyroidism are also normally experienced during pregnancy: fatigue, constipation, and weight gain. Therefore, screening for thyroid dysfunction is only indicated for the reasons listed below.

Diagnosis

ACOG does not recommend routine screening for thyroid disease in asymptomatic women. Testing should be reserved for high risk populations: women with appropriate symptoms, history of neck/mantle radiation, a history of thyroid disease or other autoimmune diseases, a strong family history of thyroid disease, and women with a history of miscarriage or infertility [119]. Women with a history of thyroid disease trying to conceive should have their TSH checked in the preconception period to assure appropriate serum thyroxine levels in early pregnancy. One reason to avoid indiscriminately screening during the first trimester is that the first trimester TSH will often be normally decreased (transient hyperthyroidism of pregnancy) because the n-terminal portion of HCG (human chorionic gonadotropin) stimulates the thyroid gland to secrete thyroid hormone, resulting in negative feedback on the pituitary, which responds with decreased TSH output [58]. Thus, inappropriate screening may result in abnormal results that are clinically insignificant. Additionally, prospective maternal screening for hypothyroidism in low-risk women and subsequent treatment did not show any benefit to the offspring [120].

Pregnancy and trimester-specific normal ranges for TSH should be used for diagnosis. When pregnancy-specific TSH ranges are not presented, use 0.4 mU/L less than the upper limit of the normal value for that lab, or 4.0 mU/L as the top normal value. The American Thyroid Association recommends a target TSH of 2.5 mU/L or lower for the first trimester [58]. Total T4 and T3 levels naturally increase during pregnancy to about 1.5 times the upper limit of the non-pregnant normal range. This is caused by an increase of thyroid-binding globulin resulting in increased hormone output by the normal thyroid in order to maintain the same amount of free thyroxine (free T4 and free T3). Free hormone levels are usually physiologically normal in pregnancy; rarely free hormone assays may be falsely lower, especially in the third trimester [121]. Thyroid hormone levels may be assessed using either free T4 and free T3 or by obtaining a Total T4 and T3 Resin Uptake (T3RU) to calculate the Free Thyroxine Index (FTI). FTI = Total T4 (nmol/L) × (%T-Uptake/100).

Treatment

For women with preconception hypothyroidism, it is reasonable to titrate their thyroid hormone replacement dose to target a TSH on the lower end of the normal range as this will allow for the increased thyroxine demand in pregnancy; often <2.5 mU/L is targeted as this is the recommended TSH for the first trimester of pregnancy [58, 122]. The American Thyroid Association suggests that all pregnant women on thyroxine replacement prior to pregnancy increase their levothyroxine dose by 30% as soon as they become pregnant. This can be accomplished by having the patient take two extra tablets of her levothyroxine per week [120] until an adjustment to the daily dose is made by the provider. Women on thyroxine supplementation prior to pregnancy should have their medication adjusted to target a TSH < 2.5 mU/L during the first trimester and <3.0 during the second and third trimesters [58]. TSH levels should be checked with the first positive pregnancy test, every 4 weeks through mid-gestation, and once around 30 weeks if stable. Levels should be checked 4 weeks after each dosing change. Hypothyroxinemia (low free T4, normal TSH) is not considered a pathologic state and should not be treated during pregnancy [58].

Pregnant women incidentally found to have subclinical hypothyroidism or a TSH > 2.5 mU/L should be tested for the presence of anti-TPO antibodies, as they are a marker of adverse pregnancy outcomes and may drive levothyroxine supplementation [58]. Treatment of subclinical hypothyroidism in pregnancy according to the American Thyroid Association guidelines is outlined in Table 39.5.

After delivery, levothyroxine should be adjusted to pre-pregnancy doses and TSH rechecked in 6 weeks. In some women, the dosing may be confounded by postpartum autoimmune thyroiditis, which is more common among TPO-positive women. In women with subclinical hypothyroidism that were started on levothyroxine during pregnancy, medication can be stopped and TSH rechecked 6 weeks after delivery [58].

Hyperthyroidism

Epidemiology

Hyperthyroidism occurs in about 0.2% of the population and is characterized by a suppressed TSH and elevated free T4. Hyperthyroidism complicates 0.1–0.4% of pregnancies, with Graves' disease and transient gestational thyrotoxicosis being the most common causes [123]. Transient gestational

Table 39.5 Treatment of subclinical hypothyroidism in pregnancy [58]

TSH[a]	Anti-TPO[b] antibody status	Management
0.01–2.5 mU/L		No medication
2.6–4.0 mU/L	Negative	No medication
2.6–4.0 mU/L	Positive	May consider treatment with 25–50 μg levothyroxine
4.1–10 mU/L	Negative	May consider treatment with 25–50 μg levothyroxine
4.1–10 mU/L	Positive	Treat with 50 μg levothyroxine

[a]Presumes upper limit of normal range is 4.0 mU/L
[b]TPO = Anti-thyroid peroxidase antibody

hyperthyroidism/thyrotoxicosis is more common than Graves' disease, occurring in 1–3% of pregnancies [58], and is a self-limited phenomenon during the first trimester. The n-terminal portion of HCG is similar in structure to TSH and stimulates the thyroid gland resulting in elevated free T4 levels that will decrease as HCG levels fall during the second trimester [124]. Gestational thyrotoxicosis is more likely to occur in conditions associated with higher HCG levels such as multiple gestation pregnancies, hydatidiform moles, or hyperemesis gravidarum [58]. Other forms of hyperthyroidism, such as toxic multinodular goiter, a hormone secreting adenoma, acute thyroiditis, and medication mismanagement for known hypothyroidism are less common causes during pregnancy but should be considered in the differential.

Clinical Manifestations

Manifestations of hyperthyroidism mimic normal pregnancy and include heat intolerance, palpitations, fatigue, nausea, feelings of anxiety, and mood changes. However, true hyperthyroidism should be suspected in women with a prior history of the disease, a strong family history of thyroid disease, as well as in patients with weight loss, tremor, goiter, or exophthalmos/lid lag on exam. Pregnancy is typically constipating, so an increase in stool frequency (hyperdefecation) also is suggestive of hyperthyroidism. A bruit over the thyroid gland is pathognomonic of Graves' disease. Overt maternal hyperthyroidism has been associated with poor obstetric outcomes such as fetal loss, intrauterine growth restriction, preeclampsia, and preterm labor. Maternal thyroid storm, which can occur in labor or with pregnancy loss, carries a 40% mortality rate [58].

Diagnosis

The TSH in patients with true hyperthyroidism will classically be undetectable, in contrast to transient gestational thyrotoxicosis where the TSH is below the lower limit of normal but still detectable. Free T4 will be elevated and the patient will most likely have clinical signs of hyperthyroidism. A TSH should not be routinely obtained in women with hyperemesis gravidarum as they often have a low but detectable TSH and/or an elevated free T4 that will resolve without medical intervention. When unsure, look for the classic symptoms and findings listed above. Total thyroxine normally increases about 10–20% during pregnancy [125] and is not solely used to diagnose hyperthyroidism.

Nodules should be evaluated with a thyroid ultrasound, and when indicated, fine needle aspirations can and should be obtained during pregnancy. Thyroid radionuclide scans are contraindicated in pregnancy as the fetal thyroid is 400 times more avid for iodine and the fetal gland will be ablated [58].

Treatment

When the diagnosis of hyperthyroidism is confirmed, obtain thyroid-stimulating antibodies/immunoglobulins (TSI) and TPO antibodies as they help distinguish between Graves' disease, Hashitoxicosis, and gestational transient thyrotoxicosis. If thyroid antibodies are negative, a watch-and-wait approach for the first trimester is appropriate if the patient is otherwise stable without suspicion for thyroid storm. Antithyroid medications should not be given for hyperemesis or transient gestational thyrotoxicosis, even when the free T4 is elevated, as hyperemesis should resolve by 14–18 weeks gestation [58].

Graves' disease must be treated with propylthiouracil (PTU) in the first trimester which is then changed to methimazole in the second trimester to avoid the potential for aplasia cutis rarely associated with methimazole [58]. A suppressed TSH can take months to normalize, so monitor levels of free T4 and free T3 or total T4 1–2 weeks after dosing changes, and then at least monthly if the levels have stabilized. In order to minimize fetal exposure to the antithyroid medications, they should be titrated to bring the free T4 into the upper limit of normal range or just above, or until the total T4 is 1.5 times the upper limit of normal. (Example: A woman with Graves' disease has total T4 of 22 μg/dL. Normal range for total T4 at that lab is 5.0–12.0 μg/dL. The clinician will titrate the antithyroid medications to bring the total T4 Level to 18 μg/dL). TSI antibodies cross the placenta and may stimulate the fetal thyroid gland. Therefore, the obstetrician should obtain a fetal thyroid ultrasound around 30 weeks of gestation to assess for a goiter, and newborns should be monitored after birth by pediatricians for symptoms of thyroid dysfunction. In spite of thyroidectomy or radioactive iodine treatment, women with Graves' disease may have persistent TSI antibodies that can cross the placenta and affect the fetal thyroid of any future pregnancies. Therefore, the fetus of subsequent pregnancies requires monitoring and assessment for goiter and postpartum hyperthyroidism [126].

In summary, abnormal thyroid function affects pregnancy outcomes and impacts offspring. Management of hypothyroidism prior to and during pregnancy is often the responsibility of the woman's primary care provider. Hyperthyroidism is very manageable, but primary providers and obstetricians often need to coordinate with specialists for medical management and monitoring of the mother and the fetus.

Asthma

Aaliyah had intermittent asthma prior to pregnancy. What are the risks to her baby if her asthma is uncontrolled? How should you manage her asthma now that she is pregnant?

Epidemiology and Pathophysiology

Asthma is present in up to 8% of pregnant women in the United States [127]. While women with mild and well-controlled asthma can often expect uncomplicated pregnancies, those with uncontrolled moderate or severe asthma are at higher risk for preeclampsia, preterm delivery, and intrauterine growth restriction [128]. Classification of asthma severity in pregnancy is the same as for non-pregnant patients. Based on symptom severity, nocturnal awakenings, and frequency of use of a short-acting beta$_2$-agonist for symptom control, patients are classified as having (1) intermittent, (2) mild persistent, (3) moderate persistent, or (4) severe persistent asthma [129].

During pregnancy, asthma symptoms worsen in one-third of women, improve in one-third and remain unchanged in the remaining one-third [130, 131]. While shortness of breath can be a common complaint in normal pregnancies due to the progesterone-mediated increase in tidal volume, spirometry and airway mechanics do not change [132]. Asthma worsens in pregnancy for the same reasons that asthma can worsen in non-pregnant women: triggers can include exposure to smoking, infection, allergens, changes in environment and weather, exercise, and lack of appropriate medications. Pregnancy rhinitis is an annoying non-pathologic state of chronic nasal congestion that occurs during pregnancy due to changes in the nasal mucosa and can trigger asthma symptoms [133]. Finally, gastroesophageal reflux disease can also worsen during pregnancy and induce asthma symptoms in someone who was previously well controlled.

Classification/Treatment

The classification and treatment of asthma during pregnancy is the same as for non-pregnant patients and appropriate management of asthma in pregnancy can significantly diminish the increased risk of morbidity and mortality for the mother and fetus. The National Asthma Education and Prevention Program Expert Panel recommends four components of effective asthma management: (1) assessment and monitoring, (2) control of risk factors which may worsen symptoms, (3) patient education, and (4) pharmacologic therapy using a stepwise approach. Assessment identifies triggers, symptom frequency, nocturnal awakenings, limitation of activities due to asthma, exacerbations, medication use, and frequency of fetal movement since this can decline with worsening asthma [129]. On the physical exam, note any respiratory distress and auscultate for wheezing or prolonged expiratory phase. Pulmonary function should be evaluated ideally with spirometry at the first visit, though it is fine to rely on peak flow meter readings at subsequent visits if a woman's asthma is fairly well controlled. In fact, the peak flow meter is a tool that can help patients and clinicians differentiate normal symptoms of pregnancy from true airflow obstruction [134].

Patient Education: During each visit, the provider should give anticipatory guidance about warning signs of an impending exacerbation, such as worsening cough, chest tightness, and wheezing, and review proper use of the patient's peak flow meter and metered dose inhalers [134]. Counsel regarding avoidance or treatment of triggers, treat seasonal allergy symptoms, and advise her to rid her home of dust mites. Warn her of the increased risk of symptoms in the setting of a viral upper respiratory illness and discuss having a lower threshold to seek care should her breathing worsen. Smokers should be counseled on cessation as the risks to the fetus from exposure to active or passive cigarette smoke are potentially additive to those from uncontrolled asthma, and maternal smoking increases the risk of childhood asthma in the offspring [135, 136]. Spirometry and lung mechanics are not altered so the standard asthma action plan should be utilized during pregnancy, where the yellow zone is identified by a peak flow value 50–80% of their baseline and the red zone when it is below 50%.

Pharmacologic Therapy: After education, medical therapy is the mainstay of therapy and mirrors that used in non-pregnant patients. Recommendations are based on the stepwise approach based on classification [134]. Patients with mild intermittent asthma have daytime symptoms <2 days/week or <2 nights/month and should use a short-acting β2-agonist (SABA) as needed. Once symptoms occur >3 days/week or >3 nights/month, then the asthma is classified as "persistent" and a low dose inhaled corticosteroid should be added for those with symptoms that are not daily. Once symptoms become present daily or >2 nights/week, then they should be on a long-acting β2-agonist (LABA) plus inhaled steroid OR placed on a medium-potency inhaled steroid. Patient with persistent daily symptoms, nighttime symptoms approaching 7/week, or using SABA multiple times a day should be placed on high dose inhaled corticosteroid plus LABA AND consider addition of other medications or consultation.

For women with more persistent asthma, monthly evaluations of their asthma will allow closer monitoring of symptoms and pulmonary function as well as therapy modifications as needed. As with other medical issues, the better controlled the asthma, the better the outcome for mother and child. Among inhaled corticosteroids, budesonide is preferred, because there is more pregnancy specific data; no data suggest that other inhaled corticosteroids are unsafe in pregnancy, thus a provider also has the option to continue another inhaled corticosteroid that has been effective based on patient preference, price, or insurance coverage [137]. For inhaled long-acting beta$_2$-agonists, salmeterol is preferred but formoterol can also be considered based on patient preference, cost, and response [138]. There are two classes of oral leukotriene modifiers: leukotriene receptor antagonists, such as montelukast and zafirlukast, and 5-lipoxygenase pathway inhibitors, such as zileuton. Montelukast does not appear to be teratogenic and should be used when risk factor modification and inhaled corticosteroids are not adequately controlling symptoms. The adverse consequences related to uncontrolled asthma must be considered when making management decisions; as such, the National Asthma Education and Prevention Program Expert Panel counsels that the benefits of asthma medications used during pregnancy far outweigh their theoretical risks [133, 139–141].

Exacerbations

Asthma exacerbations occur in up to one-third of pregnant asthmatic patients and the likelihood of occurrence correlates with initial classification of a woman's asthma severity [142, 143]. Develop an asthma action plan based on peak flow meter results as it can differentiate dyspnea of pregnancy from asthma exacerbations and give a more reliable indication of severity than her symptoms [134]. If her expiratory flow is in the yellow or red zone, she should use her albuterol rescue inhaler 2–4 puffs every 20 minutes and contact her provider. If in the red zone (Peak Flow <50% baseline), she should call her provider immediately and/or go directly to the nearest emergency department. The goal of therapy is to keep maternal oxygen saturation 95% or higher. Short courses of oral corticosteroids are often used for severe exacerbations, as the risks of maternal hypoxemia and poorly control asthma outweigh the potential risks of oral corticosteroids including pre-term birth and low birth weight [139].

Labor, Delivery, and Postpartum Period

About 10% of patients have an asthma attack during labor. Chronic asthma medications should be continued during labor and delivery. Barring a critically ill mother, cesarean section is reserved for obstetric indications. To prevent maternal adrenal crisis, any woman who received greater than 20 mg of oral corticosteroids daily for more than 3 weeks in the 6 months prior to delivery should be given stress-dose steroids during labor and for 24 hours after delivery. Management of asthma in lactating mothers is the same as for pregnancy.

Venous Thromboembolism

Aaliyah calls you 10 days after her delivery. She tells you that while both of her legs are swollen, the left side is more swollen than the right and she has calf pain. She has no associated chest pain or shortness of breath. You tell her to come to the emergency room for evaluation as you are concerned that she has a deep vein thrombosis. What tests would you run? What tests would you avoid if she was still pregnant? If she has a clot, how would you treat her and for how long?

Epidemiology

Venous thromboembolism (VTE) encompasses deep vein thrombosis (DVT) and pulmonary embolism (PE). In the United States, the rate is 1–2/1000 non-pregnant person-years and 2–4.7/1000 pregnant person-years [144–147]. The risk of VTE is thought to be four to five times higher in pregnancy compared to the same aged non-pregnant women, with the risk being even greater during the postpartum period [148, 149]. In addition to the associated medical costs and necessary treatments associated with VTE, the risks to the mother and infant cannot be understated. Among women who died in pregnancy and postpartum from 2011 to 2013 in the United States, 9.2% of deaths were attributed to thrombotic pulmonary embolism, thus a high level of suspicion is needed [150].

Pathophysiology

VTE risk increases in pregnancy and the postpartum period due to many of the physiologic changes of pregnancy. The majority of thrombogenic factors are increased in pregnancy, including fibrinogen and factors VII and VIII [148], and anticoagulation factors, such as Protein S, decrease in pregnancy [148, 151]. Increased venous stasis, particularly in the lower extremities, results from compression of the venous vasculature and venous return by the growing uterus, and hormonal changes lead to peripheral vasodilation [145]. Compression of the left iliac vein as it passes under the right iliac artery is the reason that 90% of DVTs in pregnancy occur in the left leg, and the risk of VTE after cesarean section is four times that of vaginal delivery.

Medical Conditions Associated with VTE

Those with a prior VTE outside of pregnancy are considered at the highest risk for developing a VTE during pregnancy.

Examples of comorbidities associated with VTE include systemic lupus erythematous, sickle cell anemia, inherited thrombophilias, antiphospholipid syndrome, mechanical heart valve, obesity, tobacco use, hypertension, and cancer [148, 149]. The inherited thrombophilias include Protein C or S deficiency and antithrombin deficiency. Consider a work-up for inherited or acquired thrombophilias in women with a past history of VTE prior to pregnancy to quantify the patient's future VTE risk. Be aware that during pregnancy, Protein C levels increase and Protein S levels are universally low, which will influence the results of the thrombophilia screen if checked after conception [152]. While Factor V Leiden (FVL) and prothrombin gene mutations are more prevalent in patients with VTE, there is no evidence that prophylaxis or full anticoagulation during pregnancy can reduce the rate of recurrent events, and a prospective study showed that FVL is not associated with a higher recurrence risk [153]. Additionally, evidence does not support obtaining homocysteine levels or testing for methylenetetrahydrofolate reductase (MTHFR) gene mutation.

Clinical Manifestations

Bilateral lower extremity edema is common during pregnancy but rapidly progressive unilateral swelling, calf pain or tenderness, calf redness, or warmth warrant an evaluation.

During the third trimester, healthy pregnant women will often complain of shortness of breath due to the expanding uterus and hormonal changes and may have a resting heart rate of 90–100 beats per minute (bpm) due to the increase in cardiac output, but they should not have pleuritic chest pain or shortness of breath that wakes them up at night [154]. These signs, in addition to any change in dyspnea, swelling, or heart rate from baseline are red flags and VTE should always be considered in the evaluation.

Diagnostic Strategy

There are some differences that must be considered from the usual diagnostic work-up of VTE in pregnant women including the sensitivity and safety of testing. The negative predictive value of a d-dimer makes it useful in non-pregnant patients; however, it is frequently elevated during pregnancy, so the false-positive rate limits its utility [148, 155]. Lower extremity duplex ultrasounds are considered safe and are the standard of care for diagnosis of lower extremity DVT [156]. In pregnant patients, if the duplex ultrasound is positive and there is also concern for a concomitant PE, it is reasonable to forgo a CT scan of the chest as this will prevent unnecessary radiation exposure to the fetus as treatment with systemic anticoagulation will be the same for DVT or co-existing DVT and PE.

Based on the patient's presentation and the physician's level of concern for a pulmonary embolism, if chest X-ray has excluded other causes of her symptoms, it is reasonable to proceed to either a ventilation-perfusion (V/Q) scan or a pulmonary computed tomography (CT) angiogram if there is no suggestion of an accompanying DVT [61, 62, 155]. Utilize the tests that are available and with which your radiologists have the most experience. A CT scan may actually be associated with lower fetal doses of radiation than a V/Q scan (Table 39.2) [61, 62, 155]. If the suspicion for DVT/PE is high, and imaging is not immediately available, it is reasonable to initiate anticoagulation.

Acute VTE Management

Utilizing the guidelines from the American Congress of Obstetricians and Gynecologists as well as the American College of Chest Physicians, we have established recommendations for acute VTE treatment as follows [148, 155]:

1. If the patient is hemodynamically unstable, a large blood clot is present, the patient requires surgery, or the patient is nearing delivery, it is necessary for inpatient management of an acute VTE. Some will consider hospitalization for all pregnant women with PE for a short period at diagnosis.
2. Treatment can be initiated with intravenous unfractionated heparin (IV UFH), subcutaneous UFH, or weight-based subcutaneous low molecular weight heparin (LMWH). A Cochrane review found that LMWH was associated with lower rate of recurrent VTE, reduction in the size of thrombi, and lower rates of major hemorrhage but no difference in mortality rates [157].
3. The indications for thrombolytic therapy for life-threatening PE or large occluding DVTs that place an affected limb at risk are the same as for non-pregnant women. Tissue plasminogen activator does not cross the placenta, is the appropriate treatment for these women, and has been used during pregnancy for these indications as well as stroke and myocardial infarction (prior to percutaneous interventions being the standard of care) [158].
4. VTE should be treated at therapeutic doses for 3–6 months after initial diagnosis. If the 3–6-month timeframe ends before delivery, then transition her to a prophylactic dose of LMWH or UFH which will be administered until 6 weeks postpartum [148].

VTE Prophylaxis in Pregnancy

The treatment decisions for VTE prophylaxis throughout pregnancy in women without indications for chronic anticoagulation are complex. Consensus guidelines are based on theoretical risks from retrospective or cohort data, not clinical trials demonstrating efficacy or safety [159, 160]. The known risks of heparin-induced thrombocytopenia and osteoporosis must be considered along with the lack of prospective data demonstrating that aggressive prophylaxis has not been shown to decrease the incidence of recurrent VTE during pregnancy [152, 159, 160] A Cochrane review concluded that "Large scale, high-quality randomised trials of currently used interventions are warranted" [161].

Assessing if the VTE was provoked can help clinicians make treatment decisions. Specifically, assessing if a VTE was provoked by an estrogen-related risk factor such as estrogen-containing contraceptives is a logical step, but there is no data documenting that women with a past VTE related to contraceptive use have a higher in-pregnancy recurrence risk compared to a past VTE related to another cause [152, 159, 160].

American Congress of Obstetricians and Gynecologists Practice Bulletin #138 outlines the approach to women with prior VTE as related to inherited thrombophilias in pregnancy, but a full discussion is beyond the scope of this chapter [152]. The following antepartum treatment scenarios are relatively clear*:*

- Scenario 1: Any indication for lifelong anticoagulation prior to pregnancy:
  - Continue full-dose anticoagulation with LMWH or dose-adjusted UFH
- Scenario 2: "Low risk" thrombophilia (heterozygous factor V Leiden; heterozygous prothrombin gene mutation, protein C or S deficiency) and NO prior VTE:
  - Clinical surveillance
- Scenario 3: "High risk" thrombophilia (antithrombin deficiency; homozygous prothrombin gene mutation or factor V Leiden) and NO prior VTE:
  - Clinical surveillance or prophylactic dose LMWH or UFH
- Scenario 4: VTE prior to pregnancy not on lifelong anticoagulation:
  - Prophylactic dose LMWH or UFH

Prophylactic LMWH doses include enoxaparin 40 mg subcutaneously (SC) once daily, dalteparin 4000 units SC daily, or tinzaparin 4500 units SC daily. Prophylactic UFH doses include 5000–10,000 units SC BID in all trimesters or 5000–7500 units BID in the first trimester, 7500–10,000 units SC BID in the second trimester, and 10,000 units BID in the third trimester [152, 162]. Postpartum, all women treated with any doses of heparin during pregnancy should receive prophylactic dose anticoagulation. Vitamin K antagonists such as warfarin are reserved for women with mechanical heart valves. Warfarin is not recommended for other women who require anticoagulation in pregnancy due to the risks of warfarin embryopathy, miscarriage, and fetal hemorrhage [152].

Labor and Delivery Considerations

Labor and delivery present a unique challenge for anticoagulated women and their providers as the onset of labor is very unpredictable. The duration a woman will be off anticoagulation can be variable; thus, the medical team must strategize around epidural or spinal anesthesia placement and removal. Proactively refer patients for consultation with obstetric anesthesiologists and maternal-fetal medicine specialists to develop a plan. Some obstetricians will change from LMWH to UFH late in the third trimester in anticipation of delivery, as the half-life is 2–4 times longer for LMWH.

After the last heparin injection, the following time should be allowed to pass prior to placement of spinal or epidural anesthesia: Therapeutic LMWH dosing: 24 hours; prophylactic LMWH dosing: 12 hours; intravenous UFH: 4–6 hours [148, 163, 164]. In coordination with anesthesia colleagues, after removal of epidural catheters, low-dose/prophylactic anticoagulation is typically restarted 4–6 hours after a vaginal delivery and 6–12 hours after a cesarean delivery. As the indications are preventative and not to treat an acute clot, should full dose anticoagulation be deemed necessary, waiting 18–24 hours after a cesarean section is preferable [148].

Depression

You remember that Aaliyah had some baby blues after her first pregnancy but did not require any antidepressant medication then or during this pregnancy. She screens positive for postpartum depression at her 8-week follow-up with you.

Introduction

Depression in pregnancy is common. Untreated depression has negative effects on the mother, the developing fetus, and the newborn if the mother's health is not optimized. For patients at high risk of perinatal depression, counseling prior to the development of depressive symptoms is an effective strategy to prevent the onset of depression. For patients who develop perinatal depression, counseling remains an important treatment option while many patients will also benefit from pharmacologic treatment.

Epidemiology

Although it was initially believed that the "glow of pregnancy" was protective against depression, about 12% of women experience depression during pregnancy [165]. Risk factors for depression include a personal or family history of depression or mood disorders, lack of social or financial support, history of trauma and interpersonal violence, having more than three children, if the current pregnancy is unwanted, and if there have been pregnancy complications [166, 167]. ACOG universally recommends screening for depression and mood disorders at least once during pregnancy and more often in high-risk populations [167]. There are several validated screening tools used during the perinatal period; the most universally accepted and most easily administered tool is the Edinburgh Postnatal Depression Scale (EDPS), which is used during pregnancy as well as during the postpartum period. The Edinburgh Scale controls for many of the symptoms that concomitantly occur in pregnancy, such as changing sleep patterns, can be administered in 5 minutes, and has been shown in some studies to have a sensitivity of 100% [168].

Roughly half of the women that suffer from depression during pregnancy remain untreated [169]. Undertreated depression in pregnancy is largely due to stigma, the fear that women will harm their babies with medication, provider discomfort with treatment, and lack of local services. While there are concerns regarding use of psychoactive medications during pregnancy, there is data quantifying the risk and consequences of not taking them. In one study of women with depression controlled with medication who became pregnant, 26% of women who maintained their medication in pregnancy relapsed compared with 68% of those who discontinued their medication [170]. Thus, continuing medications offers many women the best opportunity to maintain their psychological well-being during pregnancy.

Postpartum depression is much more common; about 80% of women suffer from postpartum blues (symptoms <2 weeks) and about 10–16% have postpartum depression (symptoms >2 weeks) [171]. Screening is recommended for all postpartum woman and is most often performed at the 6-week postpartum visit and at pediatrician visits for baby for the first month [168].

Clinical Outcomes

Mothers with depression may have a slight increased risk of poor obstetrical outcomes such as miscarriage, low birth weight, and preterm birth [172, 173]. There are conflicting results about the effect of antenatal depression on neurocognitive development in the offspring, but a growing body of literature has associated perinatal maternal stress, depression, and anxiety disorders with developmental delay [174], behavior problems [175], and cognition [176]. There is evidence that maternal depression is associated with structural differences in newborn gray matter structure based on MRI findings, though the effect size is small [177]. Unquestionably, the worst possible outcome of depression on the fetus is a successful suicide or the consequences of an attempted suicide.

Prevention

For patients at risk of depression, but whose office screening results do not demonstrate active depression, clinicians should discuss measures to prevent perinatal depression. In 2019, the USPSTF recommended offering counseling to women at high risk for perinatal depression even before the onset of depressive symptoms. Counseling, particularly cognitive behavioral therapy or interpersonal therapy, demonstrated reduction in the rate of perinatal depression in high risk groups in several studies. Other strategies for preventing depression, such as education, physical activity, or medications, lacked sufficient data supporting benefits over harms [167].

Treatment: General Principles

There are clear guidelines as outlined in a joint statement by ACOG and the American Psychiatric Society to help with the triage and management of women with new onset or relapsing depression during pregnancy. Non-pharmacologic interventions such as interpersonal therapy and cognitive behavioral therapy should be considered for all women with perinatal depression and has been shown to be effective [178, 179]. Patients who fail therapy show moderate to severe symptoms, have a history of a mood disorder, or have suicidal thoughts should be referred for immediate medical stabilization [180].

In the preconception period, pregnancy should be deferred until the patient's depression has been stable for a period of time, on or off medications. If the patient has been euthymic for at least 6 months on medications and does not have a history of recurrent major depressive disorder, suicide attempt, bipolar disorder, or psychosis, then she may be a candidate to wean her medications prior to conceiving. Otherwise, continuation of medications during pregnancy should be highly encouraged to prevent worsening of depression and its complications [180].

Retrospective data suggests risks associated with antidepressant medications, but prospective data demonstrates that stopping medication can cause significant decompensation in 68% of women [170].

Treatment

The goal of treatment is to use medications that have reputable safety data during pregnancy and that will optimize the patient's mood symptoms. Many women are best treated by medications that have worked for them in the past, assuming that there is an acceptable safety profile for that medication in pregnancy. Changing a stable patient's depression medication is not recommended unless it is highly teratogenic given the risk of recurrent or worsening depressive symptoms. When selecting a medication, it is important to identify the gestational age of the patient as some medications have different effects on the fetus depending on when the medication is started during pregnancy. As with use of any medication in pregnancy, a discussion with the patient about risks and benefits is warranted.

Interpreting the data regarding depression medication use in pregnancy is challenging. Studies are often confounded by healthy controls with the inability to account for the study group's underlying mood disorder, the low absolute number of events of poor outcomes at baseline, and hindsight bias. The relative risk/odds ratios associating medications and potential adverse effects typically range from 1.3 to 1.8, and while statistically significant, they are still subject to the biases and confounding of retrospective studies. Some associations may be pertinent only for women using a particular medication at the time of conception or during a certain trimester, so gestational age of the mother when a medication will be prescribed must be factored into management decisions. The most important factors to consider are the more obvious consequences of withholding an antidepressant medication and the risks that withholding could have on the patient, fetus, and newborn.

Most studies on bupropion (Wellbutrin) in pregnancy are reassuring. Bupropion has not been associated with low birth weight, major congenital malformations, or premature delivery [181]. A few small studies have shown a slight increase in cardiac anomalies, particularly ventricular septal defects [182, 183].

Selective serotonin reuptake inhibitors (SSRIs) have been studied extensively in pregnancy and data continue to be refined. Sertraline is often considered the drug of choice in pregnancy; however, fluoxetine, citalopram, and escitalopram are also commonly used, particularly when a patient has been stable on these medications. Paroxetine should be avoided because of an association with cardiac anomalies [184]; however, if a patient has failed all other antidepressants, continuation of paroxetine can be considered after a risk/benefit conversation with the patient. Neonates who have been exposed to an SSRI, particularly in the third trimester, may have poor neonatal adaption (NAS), often characterized by mild agitation and restlessness, but which can also include gastrointestinal manifestations, respiratory distress, and in very rare cases, seizures [185]. Some patients have weaned or stopped their SSRIs in the third trimester to decrease the risk of their baby developing NAS; there is limited data to support this practice, and third trimester weaning puts the mother at risk of depression relapse during a crucial transition period [186]. Exposure to SSRIs after 20 weeks gestation may be associated with persistent pulmonary hypertension of the newborn (PPHN), which may cause significant newborn morbidity; however, in case-control studies, the absolute rate of this complication was very low at <1% (compared to 0.2% in the general population). Several studies have shown a small risk of postpartum hemorrhage in mothers on SSRIs at the time of delivery [187–189]. Possible associations with SSRIs and neurocognitive outcomes such as ADHD and autism have been reported [190–192]. It is important to note that these studies examining the relationship between neurocognitive outcomes in children of mothers with mental illness are likely confounded by the mother's indication for medications during pregnancy [191, 193], and the magnitude of the effect of medications on outcomes relative to other variables is controversial [192]. More data is needed to tease out this relationship; in the meantime, medications for depression should not be withheld during pregnancy for fear of developing ADHD or autism in offspring.

There is less readily available data about the use of serotonin–norepinephrine reuptake inhibitors (SNRIs) in pregnancy. Most studies have included venlafaxine and duloxetine; there does not appear to be an association with congenital malformations or cardiac defects [194]. SNRIs are associated with a small increased risk of postpartum hemorrhage [189, 195] and poor neonatal adaptation [196]. Venlafaxine has been linked with the development of hypertensive disorders during pregnancy [197, 198]. Women that stay on venlafaxine during pregnancy should be educated about the signs and symptoms of preeclampsia and can consider home blood pressure monitoring should office blood pressure readings start to rise.

Tricyclic antidepressants (TCAs) can also be considered for the treatment of depression in pregnancy. Like SSRIs and SNRIs, TCAs are associated with risk for postpartum hemorrhage [189] and poor neonatal adaptation [199]. Unlike SSRIs, TCAs have been associated with hypertensive disorders of pregnancy including preeclampsia [198, 200]. Nortriptyline has fewer metabolites and may be the preferred tricyclic to use; it is also one of the preferred drugs for breastfeeding women [201] (Table 39.6).

Table 39.6 Antidepressants in pregnancy

Medication class	Specific medications	Reported pregnancy effects	Lactation
SSRI	First-line therapy Sertraline is first choice Citalopram, escitalopram, and fluoxetine also reasonable If not responding to first drug, switch to a different SSRI Avoid paroxetine at time of conception and first trimester	Poor neonatal adaption Postpartum hemorrhage Conflicting data: Autism, ADHD, PPHTN	Sertraline lowest passage to breast milk Citalopram and fluoxetine can produce detectable levels in babies; less preferred but still considered safe Paroxetine is safe
SNRI	Second-line therapy Venlaxafine has more data that duloxetine Can be effective in patients refractory to SSRI	Poor neonatal adaptation Postpartum hemorrhage Hypertension disorders of pregnancy	Low levels detectable in infants. Monitor for drowsiness, adequate weight gain and milestones Do not stop breastfeeding if mother needs these medications and infant is healthy
Dopamine/norepinephrine-reuptake inhibitor	Bupropion	Conflicting data: Low teratogenic risk vs. slight increase in risk of cardiac anomalies	Low levels in breast milk; likely safe
Tricyclic antidepressant	Nortriptyline is first choice Avoid clomipramine	Poor neonatal adaptation Postpartum hemorrhage Hypertension disorders of pregnancy	Crosses breast milk in low levels Nortriptyline preferred agent

ADHD attention deficit hyperactivity disorder, *PPHN* persistent pulmonary hypertension of the newborn, *SNRI* serotonin-norepinephrine reuptake inhibitors, *SSRI* selective serotonin reuptake inhibitors

Section 3: The Postpartum Period

At the time Aaliyah presented to the hospital for delivery, she was on long-acting insulin for control of her diabetes, labetalol for her chronic hypertension, and albuterol as needed for control of her asthma. During labor, she received an insulin drip for optimal control of her glucose. She continued to receive her oral labetalol and had an albuterol inhaler available for use as needed.

Following delivery, Aaliyah's blood pressure increased to a level that was persistently in the range of 150–155 mmHg systolic over 100–105 mmHg diastolic, despite her regular dose of labetalol. She denied any symptoms associated with preeclampsia, such as headache, visual disturbances, or shortness of breath. She had also been started on enoxaparin due to her left lower extremity DVT she suffered 10 days postpartum.

Management issues include

- *Managing the increase in her blood pressure*
- *Managing her diabetic medications in the postpartum period*
- *Postpartum medical therapy for her DVT*
- *Counseling regarding her medications and breastfeeding*

The postpartum period, or puerperium, is the period lasting from delivery of the placenta to 6–12 weeks thereafter. During this time, many changes take place in women, as they return to a non-pregnant physiology. These changes impact management of chronic medical issues and introduce new concerns such as medication safety when breastfeeding.

Breastfeeding

Breastfeeding is considered the gold standard for feeding infants in both developed and developing countries. The American Academy of Pediatrics (AAP) recommends exclusive breastfeeding during the first 6 months of an infant's life, with continued breastfeeding during the first year of life [202].

Physiology of Breastfeeding

During the latter half of pregnancy, the breast has been preparing for lactation by producing small amounts of milk and colostrum, which is a nutrient-rich substance containing minerals, amino acids, and proteins, with low levels of fat and sugar [203]. Both colostrum and breast milk contain high levels of immunologic factors, in particular secretory IgA, which protects the infant against enteric pathogens. Other immunologic factors found in colostrum and milk include complement, macrophages, T- and B-cell lymphocytes, lactoferrin, lactoperioxidase, and lysozymes [203].

Following delivery, progestin levels drop and there is a high-prolactin state, stimulating changes in the breast to produce high quantities of milk. When baby nurses soon after birth, they are only receiving the small quantity of colostrum and milk produced during pregnancy. Around postpartum days 3–5, breast milk production has commenced, the breasts become engorged, and baby becomes the driver of breast milk production. The more often the breasts are stimulated and emptied, the more milk the mother will make. If the nipple is not stimulated by baby (or by pumping) and prolactin and oxytocin are not released by the pituitary, milk remains in the breast, halting further breast milk production.

Benefits of Breastfeeding

Breastfeeding has been shown to decrease the incidence of breast cancer and coronary artery disease and can also help decrease postpartum weight retention. Breastfeeding can have a contraceptive benefit by delaying return of ovulation; however, definitive birth control should be used by women who do not desire pregnancy [203]. Neonatal benefits of breastfeeding include decreased incidence and severity of gastroenteritis, lower respiratory infections, otitis media, bacterial meningitis, urinary tract infections, and necrotizing enterocolitis. It may protect against sudden infant death syndrome (SIDS), type 1 diabetes mellitus, and inflammatory bowel disease, but the evidence does not support that breastfeeding reduces the risk of allergic conditions [204–207].

Complications of Breastfeeding

Half of postpartum women may experience pain from breast engorgement that may persist for 2 weeks in up to 10% of patients [203]. Treatment is supportive with oral analgesics, ice packs, and use of a tight-fitting sports bra or a breast binder. Lactation mastitis, inflammation in the breast most often from blocked milk ducts, occurs in up to 10% of breastfeeding women. It is typically unilateral and can become infected with *Staphylococcus aureus,* coagulase-negative staphylococci, or *Streptococcus viridans* [208]. Mastitis can cause systemic symptoms including high fevers, myalgias, nausea, and weakness. Culture for the causative organism may be obtained from breast milk. Therapy typically resolves the infection within 48 hours, but up to 10% develop a breast abscess. Women should continue breastfeeding, including feeding from the inflamed breast [208].

Contraindications to Breastfeeding

Contraindications to breastfeeding are rare and include active herpes simplex lesions of the breast, active tuberculosis, human immunodeficiency virus (HIV) infection, and active illicit drug use [208]. It is recommended that most women on chemotherapy stop breastfeeding while on treatment but ultimately depends on the regimen and duration of treatment.

Drug Safety in Breastfeeding

Medications are often required postpartum. Primary care providers should have a reference text in the office (electronic or paper—we suggest using the LactMed Database, which is a free online resource maintained by the National Library of Medicine [209], or the reference book *Drugs in Pregnancy and Lactation* edited by Gerald G Briggs and Roger K. Freeman published by Wolters Kluwer) [210] to help guide medication decisions in breastfeeding women and identify obstetric colleagues with whom they can collaborate. While many drugs are secreted into breast milk, the important issue is how much is actually absorbed by the newborn and whether there is evidence of a physiological effect. Typically, maternal medications have no adverse effects on breastfed infants. As an example, warfarin, when indicated, is compatible with breastfeeding but contraindicated in most women during pregnancy.

Dr. Hale's Lactation Risk Category is similar to the FDA's former lactation categories of A, B, C, D, and X. Dr. Hale's categories range from L1 to L5, with L1 being compatible with breastfeeding referenced by controlled studies, L3 being probably compatible without any observed risks, and L5 being hazardous based on observed damage to an infant. Commonly used medications in primary care will be detailed below using Dr. Hale's categories for reference [197].

Pain Medications

Acetaminophen (L1), non-steroidal anti-inflammatory drugs (NSAIDs) (L1), and short-acting opioids such as oxycodone (L3) are considered safe during breastfeeding and are used routinely for postpartum women with no harmful effects reported [203]. In rare cases, opioid medications may result in infant drowsiness.

In 2017, the Food and Drug Administration (FDA) issued a Drug Safety Communication warning that breastfeeding is not recommended while using codeine (L4) and tramadol (L4) due to the risk for infant opioid overdose [211]. In women who are "ultra-rapid metabolizers," normal doses of these medications lead to high maternal serum levels of active metabolites, which are then present in breast milk [212]. Adverse effect reports exist for codeine, and because tramadol has similar metabolism, the recommendation against breastfeeding was made for both medications [212].

Antibiotics

No adverse events have been reported with use of penicillins (L1), cephalosporins (L1), nitrofurantoin (L2), gentamicin (L2), clindamycin (L2), tetracycline (L2), and macrolide (L2) antibiotics [203].

Sulfonamides are considered safe in breastfeeding, and there is experience using them in patients with HIV who require prophylaxis against pneumocystis infections. However, these drugs should be avoided in women who have infants at risk for hyperbilirubinemia, including premature and ill infants, because they displace bilirubin from binding sites on albumin leading to elevated infant bilirubin levels [213].

The concentration of metronidazole (L2) in breast milk is similar to that of the maternal plasma. Discontinuation of breastfeeding for 12–24 hours after single-dose (2 g) therapy may be considered to minimize neonatal exposure to the drug through breast milk, although no adverse effects have been reported [203]. In Utero exposure to doxycycline, (L3) may cause staining of teeth.

Antihypertensive Medications

Labetalol (L2) and propranolol (L2) have low concentrations in breast milk, with no reported adverse effects on the infant, so these are preferred agents for treatment in this category [203]. Other beta-adrenergic blocking agents, such as metoprolol (L3), can be concentrated in breast milk but appear reasonable when indicated.

Angiotensin-converting enzyme inhibitors [enalapril (L2)] and calcium channel blockers [amlodipine (L3)] are secreted into breast milk in low levels but are compatible with breastfeeding.

Thiazide diuretics (L3) are low to undetectable in breast milk and infant serum but may decrease maternal milk production, therefore other antihypertensive agents are preferred if possible [197].

Diabetic Medications

Glyburide (L2) and insulin (L1) are not found in breast milk [214]. Metformin enters breast milk in non-clinically significant amounts [215]. When using oral diabetic medications, monitor infants for signs of hypoglycemia.

Psychiatric Medications

Most psychiatric mediations are present in breast milk at low levels, with non-clinically relevant effects on nursing infants. Testing of serum drug levels in infants is not recommended [216].

SSRIs are found in breast milk at low concentrations, are considered safe for use during breastfeeding, but irritability and one case of transient apnea in an infant whose mother was taking citalopram have been reported [216]. Fluoxetine is (L2 in older children, L3 in neonates), paroxetine (L2–no detectable milk levels), sertraline (L2), and citalopram (L3) may be used when indicated. Long-term studies of exposed infants are lacking.

Tricyclic antidepressants, such as amitriptyline (L2) are considered compatible with breastfeeding, with the exception of doxepin (L5) due to potential respiratory depression [216].

The AAP considers lithium (L4) incompatible with breastfeeding as the breast milk concentration is as high as one-half of the maternal serum concentration, and infant serum levels may be clinically significant leading to lethargy, hypotonia, hypothermia, and cyanosis [203]. Use of other mood stabilizing agents, such as valproic acid (L2) and carbamazepine (L2), is considered compatible with breastfeeding [216]. Studies regarding effects of antipsychotic use in breastfeeding women are limited. Haloperidol (L2) data is limited with some studies showing limited effects and others demonstrating developmental delay later in life [216]. Benzodiazepine (L3) use during breastfeeding is considered moderately safe at low doses [216].

Anticoagulants

UFH (L1), enoxaparin (L2), and warfarin (L2) are safe to take for breastfeeding mothers. Heparin does not cross into breast milk. Warfarin is highly protein-bound, and thus it is found in very low concentrations in breast milk [203].

Postpartum Physiology

Uterus

Within 24 hours after delivery the uterus, when palpated on the abdominal exam, should feel like a hard knot of muscle just below the umbilicus. Lochia rubra is the initial postpartum bloody discharge, followed by 3–10 days of pale mucopurulent lochia serosa, then yellow–white lochia alba. Lochia typically resolves by 6 weeks postpartum which coincides with the uterus returning to its normal size and location within the pelvis [203, 217]. Discharge beyond this, especially in the setting of fevers, chills, or uterine tenderness, should be evaluated by the obstetrical team for retained products of conception.

Ovaries

For women who are not breastfeeding, the average time to return of ovulation is 70–75 days and the majority will resume menstruation within 12 weeks of delivery [217]. In women who are breastfeeding, elevated prolactin levels result in delayed return of ovulation, which occurs on average 6 months after delivery [217]. The exact return of ovulation is influenced by the frequency and duration of breastfeeding and the proportion of supplemental feeds in the infant's feeding regimen.

Coagulation

The hypercoaguable state of pregnancy continues into the postpartum period, with half of all thromboembolic events occurring during this time [203, 217]. The risk for development of VTE is highest in the first week postpartum [218]. D-dimer levels may remain elevated into the postpartum period, limiting their usefulness as a diagnostic test for VTE [217]. Thrombophilia work-ups should ideally be delayed up to 12 weeks postpartum and 6 weeks post-thrombosis [152].

Cardiovascular System

Postpartum blood loss during delivery is balanced by the "autotransfusion" that occurs when the uterus contracts down to the postpartum size. Cardiac output slowly returns to pre-pregnancy levels after delivery, heart rate normalizes within hours after delivery, systolic and diastolic blood pressure slowly increase by about 5% in the first 4 days postpartum [217]. Postpartum leukocytosis is common and the hemoglobin typically drops 1–2 mg/dL after delivery, normalizing by 6 weeks postpartum [217].

Urinary System

The normal pregnancy-related dilation of the renal pelvises and ureters due to hormonal effects of progesterone will return to their pre-pregnancy size by 6 weeks postpartum [203, 217].

Bladder dysfunction may appear in the postpartum period as a result of labor trauma or epidural anesthesia, and urinary retention in the first several hours after delivery is common. Women may also experience incontinence during pregnancy or the postpartum period secondary to the hormonal effects of progesterone on the pelvic floor musculature or trauma to the perineum, which will often resolve by 6 weeks postpartum. However, parity is a risk for stress incontinence that typically presents later in life, affecting 3% of women under 35 and rising to 38% of women >60 [219]. Pelvic floor physical therapy is a great option for young women with postpartum incontinence and will help maintain the strength of the pelvic floor as patients enter menopause.

Nervous/Musculoskeletal System

Transient decreased bone mineralization occurs normally following delivery and resolves by 12–18 months postpartum. Treatments such as calcium supplementation and exercise do not prevent this bone loss [217]. Muscle and joint injuries associated with labor are usually transient, improved with anti-inflammatory medications and physical therapy [203]. Nerve injuries complicate 1% of deliveries such as lumbosacral plexus injury due to compression from the fetal head, or lithotomy positioning in stirrups with hyperflexion of the hips can compress the common fibular nerves. They are more commonly seen in deliveries with a prolonged second stage or pushing in a semi-Fowler position [203]. Symptoms may include sensory deficits, motor deficits, or foot drop and generally resolve by 2 months postpartum [203].

Body Weight

Delivery results in an approximately 10-pound weight loss secondary to delivery of the infant, placenta, amniotic fluid, and blood loss. Women often lose the majority of their weight over the 6 months after delivery, women who gained excessive weight >35 pounds are more likely to have a net weight gain following pregnancy, and the average woman retains about 10 pounds after the pregnancy [217]. Patients should be reassured that aerobic exercise does not adversely affect breast milk production.

Postpartum Care of Medical Complications

Diabetes Mellitus

Patients with a history of type 1 and type 2 diabetes mellitus (DM) can generally be converted back to their pre-pregnancy medication doses or started on half of their pre-delivery dose [10].

Following delivery, most women with gestational diabetes mellitus (GDM) will have normalization of glucose levels. However, up to one-third of these women will demonstrate glucose intolerance with postpartum screening [48]. While the 2-hour oral glucose tolerance test is recommended for women with GDM by ADA and ACOG at 4–12 weeks postpartum because it detects both impaired fasting glucose and impaired glucose tolerance, compliance rates are a dismal 35% [48, 220]. In the United Kingdom, the fasting plasma glucose is recommended due to the convenience factor, and after 12 weeks a HbA1C is recommended. A pilot study found obtaining a HbA1C at the postpartum visit, rather than from the lab, doubled the rate of testing, although additional data is needed to validate this approach [221].

Women with GDM have up to a 70% chance of developing DM later in life [48], though breastfeeding may help reduce the risk of developing future diabetes [222]. Patients who meet criteria for a diagnosis of DM based on postpartum screening should be referred for diabetes education and management. Those who meet criteria for a diagnosis of impaired fasting glucose or impaired glucose tolerance, lifestyle modifications, nutritional therapy, and possible medical therapy to decrease development of DM should be considered [48]. For those with normal results, screening for diabetes should be repeated every 1–3 years [223]. Identifying these patients at risk with a thorough pregnancy history is important as randomized trials demonstrate that lifestyle modification and use of metformin for pre-diabetic women will help prevent the development of overt diabetes [224].

Hypertensive Disorders of Pregnancy

Most preeclampsia-related hypertension normalizes by 6 weeks after delivery, but preeclampsia can present or flare postpartum, so new or recurrent spikes in blood pressure should prompt a clinical assessment. The diagnostic criteria for postpartum preeclampsia are the same. Patients who meet criteria for preeclampsia with severe features in the postpartum period are generally admitted to the hospital for observation, with administration of magnesium sulfate for seizure prophylaxis and initiation of antihypertensive medications as needed.

If hypertension associated with gestational hypertension or preeclampsia does not resolve by 12 weeks postpartum, a diagnosis of chronic hypertension rather than pregnancy-associated hypertension disease should be entertained [225]. Women with pregnancies complicated by gestational hypertension or preeclampsia should return to the office for blood pressure evaluation 7–10 days following delivery or earlier if they develop symptoms of preeclampsia at home [148].

Antihypertensive treatment is recommended in patients who have persistently elevated blood pressures, ≥150 mmHg systolic and/or ≥100 mmHg diastolic [148]. Educate patients regarding signs and symptoms of hypotension as blood pressure returns to pre-pregnancy levels.

More frequent dosing (labetalol three times daily) will prevent spikes in pressure. The rate of blood pressure normalization after delivery is variable, so monitoring and use of holding parameters for antihypertensives will facilitate proper control. It is often prudent to discharge patients with a home blood pressure cuff and the consider the following "Sliding Scale" for women discharged home on antihypertensives related to persistently elevated pressures:

- Check pressure before each dose (three times a day)
- Skip that dose of labetalol if the systolic pressure is <140 mmHg

Preeclampsia and gestational hypertension are major risk factors for development of cardiovascular disease [226, 227]. The Cardiovascular Health After Maternal Placental Syndromes (CHAMPS) study showed a 12-fold increased risk for development of heart disease in women with a prior history of preeclampsia or metabolic syndrome compared to those women without these conditions [228]. This risk is especially increased for women who develop early and severe preeclampsia. Additionally, preeclampsia is a marker for future diabetes, subclinical hypothyroidism, and end-stage renal disease [229–231]. Thus, it is critical that all healthcare providers inquire about a history of hypertensive disorders during pregnancy so that education and lifestyle interventions for these potential conditions become a routine part of our long-term postpartum primary care.

Thyroid Disorders

After delivery, women whose dose of levothyroxine was increased during pregnancy should be placed on the pre-pregnancy dose and have a TSH checked around 4 weeks postpartum.

Graves' disease tends to become less active in the third trimester but may recur in the postpartum period. Flares are treated with antithyroid medications such as methimazole (L3–no evidence of excretion into milk) or propylthiouracil (L2). Radioiodine ablation or surgery may be recommended for non-pregnant women with refractory disease.

Postpartum thyroiditis (PPT) results in transient thyroid dysfunction that develops in the first year after delivery in women who were previously euthyroid and may even occur after pregnancy termination or spontaneous loss. The prevalence ranges from 1% to 17% and women with a history of type 1 diabetes, Graves' disease (treated), and viral hepatitis are at a higher risk for developing PPT [122]. Testing in asymptomatic women found that 10% of women in early second trimester have thyroid peroxidase antibodies and 50% of those women will develop postpartum thyroiditis [232]. However, screening all pregnant women to identify the 5% that may develop a self-limited syndrome is not indicated. PPT usually manifests first as signs and symptoms of hyperthyroidism. The hyperthyroid stage is due to inflammation of the gland with rapid release of pre-formed hormone; thus, initial testing may reveal an elevated free T4 and low TSH. This is followed by a hypothyroid phase with low free T4 and high TSH. PPT is usually a self-limited illness, and most patients will spontaneously return to a euthyroid state. A small subset of patients will progress to permanent hypothyroidism; thus, thyroid function studies must be monitored every 4–6 weeks to assure normalization. Persistent hypothyroidism for more than 1 year following delivery ranges from 2% to 21% [58].

Treatment of PPT is largely supportive, and patients should only be treated if they are symptomatic. Hyperthyroid symptoms may be treated with a β-blocker such as propranolol, which is compatible with breastfeeding [58]. Hypothyroidism should be treated with levothyroxine, with a reasonable starting dose being somewhere between 50 and 100 μg depending on the weight of the patient and degree of symptoms [58]. Subclinical hypothyroidism should be treated according to guidelines, with initiation of thyroid hormone in any patient with a TSH >10 mU/L. There is less clear evidence that treating subclinical hypothyroidism based on a TSH > ~4.5 mU/L (or the upper limit of the reference range) and <10 mU/L provides any clinical benefits, and this decision must be made between the patient and the provider. Keep in mind that less thyroid hormone may be needed when treating women with PPT in the subsequent weeks to months as the thyroid gland heals and PPT resolves. TSH and free T4 should be checked every 4–6 weeks when adjusting medications or monitoring for progression/regression of PPT [122].

Any thyroid dysfunction can affect breast milk production. It is important to maintain a euthyroid state in women who are planning another pregnancy. Women who have had postpartum thyroiditis are at a higher risk for the development of permanent thyroid dysfunction in the future [233].

Venous Thromboembolism

For patients with a history of thromboembolism, timing of anticoagulation therapy in the postpartum period requires balance between the risks of clot formation and bleeding complications. Guidelines state that full-dose anticoagulation with unfractionated or low molecular weight heparin (LMWH) may be restarted 4–6 hours after vaginal delivery or 6–12 hours following cesarean delivery, but one may consider restarting at 18–24 hours in order to avoid postoperative bleeding [148]. For those patients who require anticoagulation at low dose prophylactic doses only during the 6-week postpartum period, LMWH is commonly used, but women who need to continue therapy beyond 6 weeks postpartum may be bridged to warfarin or another oral agent during this time [148].

Postpartum Depression

Postpartum depression, defined as an episode of major depression that occurs within the first 4–6 weeks postpartum, complicates approximately 10–16% of pregnancies [171]. Universal screening for postpartum depression is recommended at the postpartum visit with commonly used screening such as the Edinburgh Postnatal Depression Scale, the Beck Depression Inventory, and the Postpartum Depression Screening Scale [216]. Most pediatrician offices also screen mothers for depression when babies have visits soon after birth. Symptoms of depression in the postpartum period mimic issues that new mothers face including poor sleep, irritability, change in appetite, poor concentration, hopelessness, guilt, fatigue, amotivation, and sadness. Treatment is based on regimens for major depression in non-pregnant women as discussed in the section on peripartum depression, with particular attention to choosing medications that are safe during breastfeeding.

Postpartum psychosis is a rare complication of child birth but considered a medical emergency. Several studies have quoted the incidence between 0.89 and 2.6 per 1000 births across several countries [234]. Mothers present within the first 4 weeks after childbirth, often within a few days, with disorganized thinking and behaviors, hallucinations, paranoia, grandiosity, mood lability, and poor judgment that can affect their health and the health and safety of their child. Risk factors include a history of mood disorder (bipolar, schizophrenia), a family history of a mood disorder, having a history of postpartum psychosis, major obstetrical complications, and stopping mood-stabilizing medications during pregnancy [235]. Evaluation for medical causes of symptoms must be sought as the differential diagnosis includes infection, thyroid disease, toxidromes, alcohol withdrawal, and electrolyte disturbances. Treatment includes immediately psychiatric stabilization, usually in the inpatient setting under the care of a psychiatrist for medication titration or in an intensive outpatient treatment program.

Summary Points

1. A pregnant patient's medical and obstetric issues will be best addressed by maintaining an open dialogue and creating a collaborative partnership with obstetric colleagues and subspecialists.
2. Optimizing a mother's health and well-being prior to and during pregnancy will ensure that her fetus has the best outcome.
3. Rather than considering a medication or test to be "safe" during pregnancy, providers should consider if they are medically indicated or reasonable, and consider the consequences of not pursuing the test or prescribing the medication.
4. Women with hypertension and risk factors for preeclampsia should be educated about and monitored for preeclampsia by their obstetricians and primary providers during pregnancy and in the postpartum period.
5. The management of asthma during pregnancy is the same as for non-pregnant patients.
6. Venous thromboembolism is an important cause of maternal morbidity and mortality. Providers should be familiar with guidelines for prophylaxis in women with a known hypercoaguable state and maintain a high index of suspicion of VTE in any pregnant patient.
7. Tight glycemic control for women with pre-gestational diabetes mellitus can optimize pregnancy outcomes, and women with gestational diabetes require close follow-up to screen for persistent dysglycemia.
8. Thyroid disease is prevalent; therefore, proper preconception, pregnancy, and postpartum management of hypothyroidism, and recognition of hyperthyroidism by

primary care providers can minimize the risk for complications
9. Depression during pregnancy is best managed with a multidisciplinary team and a good understanding that medications can and should be prescribed to optimize outcomes and well-being for the mother and newborn
10. Supporting lactation is important for new mothers. Finding medications safe for breastfeeding babies can be accomplished through a variety of online resources and applications.
11. Primary providers should be monitoring for postpartum complications and for complications associated with diseases diagnosed during pregnancy including pre-eclampsia, postpartum depression and psychosis, VTE, thyroid dysfunction, the development of diabetes, and the progression of hypertension.

Review Questions

Diabetes Questions [78, 236]

A 32-year-old woman with a 6-year history of diabetes is on sitagliptin (Januvia) and metformin to control her blood sugars. She comes to your office because she missed her period. Her last menstrual period was 6 weeks ago. A pregnancy test is positive. Her last HgA1c from a month earlier was 9.5%.

1. If her diabetic control continues to be similar, her risk for a baby with a congenital anomaly will be:
   A. 3% (same as the general population)
   B. 10% (1 per 10)
   C. 25% (1 per 4)
   D. 50% (1 per 2)
   The correct answer is B. As per the chart from the article by Bell, a hemoglobin A1c of 9.5% confers ~10% risk for a major fetal anomaly. This patient should be counseled about the risk to her fetus and the need to better control her blood glucose immediately to decrease her future risk.

2. Which oral medication is commonly used early in pregnancy?
   A. Sitagliptin (Januvia)
   B. Metformin
   C. Glipizide
   D. Acarbose
   The correct answer is B. Because metformin is used for the treatment of women with polycystic ovary syndrome and infertility, it has been commonly used in early pregnancy and there is an abundance of safety data available for its use. However, the standard of care for glucose control during pregnancy is insulin. Given this patient's poorly controlled diabetes, she should immediately be converted to insulin for tighter glycemic control. Sitagliptin (Januvia) is a newer drug, and therefore there is not a much safety data available on this medication in early pregnancy. Glipizide is not well studied in pregnancy and therefore not commonly used. In women who were taking glipizide in pregnancy, there were not shown to be excess anomalies though. Acarbose is not commonly used. There is no literature to support for or against its use; however, because most of its action is in the intestine and it is not well systemically absorbed, it is probably safe to use in pregnancy.

Thyroid Question

1. A 25-year-old G0 female patient was diagnosed with hypothyroidism 4 years ago. She has been taking levothyroxine 75 μg daily for the past 2 years. Her TSH last month was 2.5 mU/L. She calls to tell you that she had a positive pregnancy test. As per American Thyroid Association guidelines, you tell her to:
   A. Discontinue levothyroxine
   B. Continue levothyroxine at the same dose
   C. Increase levothyroxine to 100 μg daily
   D. Increase her to two tablets (150 μg) of levothyroxine daily
   The correct answer is C. As per the ATA, a woman should increase her levothyroxine dosing about 25–30% as soon as she has a confirmed pregnancy; this would be about 100 μg for the patient in this questions. The ATA recommends that this is done empirically even before testing is done. Although women need to increase their levothyroxine dosing in pregnancy, a 200% increase empirically would be too aggressive in a woman who had reasonable control of her hypothyroidism just before pregnancy [58].

Asthma Question

1. A 28-year-old G2P1 with intermittent asthma at baseline in referred to you at 20 weeks gestation complaining of increased cough and wheezing since spring began. She usually only needs her albuterol inhaler once weekly but has been using up to five times per week recently, though not at night. She has no accessory muscle use or wheezing on exam in your office. In addition to educating her on avoiding triggers and giving her a peak flow meter, how would you address her medication regimen at this point?

A. Have her continue using her albuterol rescue inhaler but do not add another medication to minimize risks to the fetus.
B. Start a low-dose inhaled corticosteroid as a chronic controller
C. Start a low-dose inhaled corticosteroid along with a long-acting beta$_2$-agonist as controllers
D. Start a moderate-dose inhaled corticosteroid as a chronic controller
E. Start an oral leukotriene receptor antagonist

The correct answer is B. This patient is now classified as having mild persistent asthma due to her increased symptoms requiring use of her beta$_2$-agonist multiple times per week, though not daily (which would have bumped her up to moderate persistent in severity). Uncontrolled asthma poses significant maternal and fetal risk, so while avoiding triggers might help, at this point, pharmacologic control is warranted. It is reasonable to start with a low-dose inhaled corticosteroid as a chronic controller for mild persistent asthma. In patients with moderate persistent asthma, involving daily symptoms or frequent nocturnal symptoms, there are two options: a moderate dose of inhaled corticosteroid or a combination of a low-dose inhaled corticosteroid and a long-acting beta$_2$-agonist. If this patient were well controlled on a leukotriene receptor antagonist prior to pregnancy, it would be fine to continue it in pregnancy; however, these agents are not first-line to start de-novo in pregnancy [128].

Depression Question

1. A 24-year-old woman is considering pregnancy. She has a significant history of major depression with anxiety since the age of 16. She was hospitalized last year for suicidal ideation. Although she was initially on multiple medications to control her depression, she is currently maintained on sertraline 200 mg daily and finally doing well. What changes should you suggest in her medications before pregnancy?
   A. She should stop her sertraline because SSRIs are associated with major congenital malformations and poor pregnancy outcomes
   B. She should wean her medication to the lowest tolerable dose prior to pregnancy
   C. She should change her sertraline to a less teratogenic medication
   D. She should continue her sertraline as is currently prescribed

   The correct answer is D. SSRIs and sertraline in particular have not been associated with major congenital malformations or poor pregnancy outcomes. They have been associated with poor neonatal adaptation, and in very rare cases, persistent pulmonary hypertension of the newborn. Weaning her dose does not decrease the risk of these outcomes and puts this patient at a high risk of depression relapse during pregnancy, so her dose should be continued at 200 mg as she is doing well. Sertraline is first line for pregnant women and has excellent safety data compared to other antidepressants, so changing her medication is also not indicated. This patient should continue her current medication to optimize her mental health and decrease the risks of depression relapse and its effect on her and her future pregnancy [182].

Anticoagulation Question

1. A 30-year-old woman is considering her first pregnancy. She has a history of bicuspid aortic valve and currently has a mechanical valve in place for which she is on warfarin. She is otherwise healthy. She would like to breastfeed. She is wondering if she should continue the warfarin during the pregnancy and postpartum. When is warfarin appropriate for women in pregnancy and postpartum?
   A. Warfarin is never appropriate for pregnancy or breastfeeding
   B. Warfarin is never appropriate for pregnancy but is compatible with breastfeeding.
   C. Warfarin is appropriate in pregnancy in rare cases but is never appropriate for breastfeeding.
   D. Warfarin is appropriate in pregnancy in rare cases and is compatible with breastfeeding.
   E. Warfarin is recommended in pregnancy and in breastfeeding.

   The correct answer is D. Answers A, B, and C are incorrect as there are scenarios for pregnant women at very high risk of clotting, where remaining on warfarin is appropriate, including this one. Warfarin is considered compatible with breastfeeding. Warfarin is not recommended in pregnancy for most patients who require anticoagulation due to its ability to cross the placenta and the likely increased risks of miscarriage, warfarin embryopathy, and fetal hemorrhage. Warfarin embryopathy includes a constellation of symptoms identified in neonates of mothers on warfarin, particularly those on more than 5 mg/day, including nasal hypoplasia, stippled epiphyses, and limb hypoplasia, as well as long term CNS sequelae. However, warfarin has been shown to be the most efficacious anticoagulant in protecting from acute valve thrombosis, and there have been multiple case reports of patients suffering from thrombosis of their mechanical valves while using unfractionated heparin therapy in pregnancy. Thus, weighing the risks and benefits, most pregnant women with mechanical valves are anticoagulated with warfarin throughout pregnancy [237, 238].

Hypertension Questions

1. A 26-year-old obese female G0P0 with a history of uncontrolled hypertension and diabetes presents for pre-conception counseling. Her diabetes is diet-controlled and her only medication is losartan 50 mg daily. What factors put her at risk for developing preeclampsia?
   A. Age > 20 years old
   B. Nulliparity
   C. History of hypertension
   D. Diabetes
   E. Obesity
   F. C, D, E
   G. B, C, D, and E
   H. All of the above
   The correct answer is G. Hypertension, diabetes, nulliparity, and obesity put the patient at risk for preeclampsia. Other risk factors that are not present in this case include a history of preeclampsia, systemic lupus erythematosus, antiphospholipid antibody, chronic renal disease, and multiple gestation pregnancy [221].
2. A 26-year-old G0P0 obese female with a history of hypertension and diabetes presents for preconception counseling. Her diabetes is diet-controlled and her only medication is losartan 25 mg daily. Her blood pressure in clinic is 129/86 mmHg. What is the next best step in managing her hypertension?
   A. Continue the current dose of losartan
   B. Change losartan to amlodipine
   C. Change losartan to methyldopa
   D. Stop her losartan and monitor her blood pressure closely during pregnancy
   E. Advise the patient to not conceive
   The correct answer is D. Angiotensin II receptor blockers (ARBs) like losartan are contraindicated in pregnancy. These medicines, along with angiotensin converting enzyme (ACE) inhibitors, direct renin inhibitors, and mineralocorticoid receptor antagonists are avoided in pregnancy because they can cause fetal renal dysplasia, lung hypoplasia, fetal loss, and other adverse fetal outcomes. Changing the patient's losartan to methyldopa is an acceptable option, but methyldopa is poorly tolerated due to fatigue, drowsiness, drug induced lupus, and relative lack of potency, so this is probably not the best answer. A better drug would have been labetalol or extended release nifedipine. Because this patient's blood pressure is reasonably controlled on minimal medication, it is acceptable to stop her losartan and monitor her blood pressure clinically, restarting blood pressure medications if needed during pregnancy [110–112].

References

1. Finer LB, Zolna MR. Unintended pregnancy in the United States: incidence and disparities, 2006. Contraception. 2011;84(5):478–85.
2. Bernstein L, Higgins S, Kho A, Umpierrez G, Watkins C Jr. Comprehensive hospital medicine: an evidenced-based approach. In: Williams MV, editor. Medical complications of pregnancy. Philadelphia: Saunders/Elsevier; 2007. p. 837–47.
3. Liu S, Joseph KS, Luo W, Leon JA, Lisonkova S, Van den Hof M, et al. Effect of folic acid food fortification in Canada on congenital heart disease subtypes. Circulation. 2016;134(9):647–55.
4. Ionescu-Ittu R, Marelli AJ, Mackie AS, Pilote L. Prevalence of severe congenital heart disease after folic acid fortification of grain products: time trend analysis in Quebec, Canada. BMJ. 2009;338:b1673.
5. Badovinac RL, Werler MM, Williams PL, Kelsey KT, Hayes C. Folic acid-containing supplement consumption during pregnancy and risk for oral clefts: a meta-analysis. Birth Defects Res A Clin Mol Teratol. 2007;79(1):8–15.
6. Centers for Disease Control and Prevention. Recommendations: women & folic acid; 2019 [cited 2019 7/17/2019]. Available from: https://www.cdc.gov/ncbddd/folicacid/recommendations.html.
7. Czeizel AE, Dudas I. Prevention of the first occurrence of neural-tube defects by periconceptional vitamin supplementation. N Engl J Med. 1992;327(26):1832–5.
8. Wilson RD, Genetics C, Wilson RD, Audibert F, Brock JA, Carroll J, et al. Pre-conception folic acid and multivitamin supplementation for the primary and secondary prevention of neural tube defects and other folic acid-sensitive congenital anomalies. J Obstet Gynaecol Can. 2015;37(6):534–52.
9. MRC Vitamin Study Research Group. Prevention of neural tube defects: results of the Medical Research Council Vitamin Study. Lancet. 1991;338(8760):131–7.
10. ACOG Committee on Practice Bulletins. ACOG Practice Bulletin. Clinical Management Guidelines for Obstetrician-Gynecologists. Number 60, March 2005. Pregestational diabetes mellitus. Obstet Gynecol. 2005;105(3):675–85.
11. Wentzel P, Gareskog M, Eriksson UJ. Folic acid supplementation diminishes diabetes- and glucose-induced dysmorphogenesis in rat embryos in vivo and in vitro. Diabetes. 2005;54(2):546–53.
12. Patel KR, Sobczynska-Malefora A. The adverse effects of an excessive folic acid intake. Eur J Clin Nutr. 2017;71(2):159–63.
13. Salihu HM, Shumpert MN, Slay M, Kirby RS, Alexander GR. Childbearing beyond maternal age 50 and fetal outcomes in the United States. Obstet Gynecol. 2003;102(5 Pt 1):1006–14.
14. Cleary-Goldman J, Malone FD, Vidaver J, Ball RH, Nyberg DA, Comstock CH, et al. Impact of maternal age on obstetric outcome. Obstet Gynecol. 2005;105(5 Pt 1):983–90.
15. Galtier-Dereure F, Boegner C, Bringer J. Obesity and pregnancy: complications and cost. Am J Clin Nutr. 2000;71(5 Suppl):1242S–8S.
16. Stothard KJ, Tennant PW, Bell R, Rankin J. Maternal overweight and obesity and the risk of congenital anomalies: a systematic review and meta-analysis. JAMA. 2009;301(6):636–50.
17. Jeric M, Roje D, Medic N, Strinic T, Mestrovic Z, Vulic M. Maternal pre-pregnancy underweight and fetal growth in relation to institute of medicine recommendations for gestational weight gain. Early Hum Dev. 2013;89(5):277–81.

18. Tabet M, Flick LH, Tuuli MG, Macones GA, Chang JJ. Prepregnancy body mass index in a first uncomplicated pregnancy and outcomes of a second pregnancy. Am J Obstet Gynecol. 2015;213(4):548.e1–7.
19. Sebire NJ, Jolly M, Harris J, Regan L, Robinson S. Is maternal underweight really a risk factor for adverse pregnancy outcome? A population-based study in London. BJOG. 2001;108(1):61–6.
20. Connor EM, Sperling RS, Gelber R, Kiselev P, Scott G, O'Sullivan MJ, et al. Reduction of maternal-infant transmission of human immunodeficiency virus type 1 with zidovudine treatment. Pediatric AIDS Clinical Trials Group Protocol 076 Study Group. N Engl J Med. 1994;331(18):1173–80.
21. American College of Obstetricians. FAQ 133; 2019. Available from: https://www.acog.org/-/media/For-Patients/faq133.pdf?dmc=1&ts=20190717T1903502020.
22. Centers for Disease Control and Prevention. Recommended adult immunization schedule for ages 19 years or older, United States; 2019 [cited 2019 7/17/2019]. Available from: https://www.cdc.gov/vaccines/schedules/hcp/imz/adult.html.
23. Centers for Disease Control and Prevention. General best practice guidelines for immunization: best practices guidance of the Advisory Committee on Immunization Practices (ACIP); 2019 [cited 2019 7/17/2019]. Available from: https://www.cdc.gov/vaccines/hcp/acip-recs/general-recs/contraindications.html.
24. Reef SE, Plotkin S, Cordero JF, Katz M, Cooper L, Schwartz B, et al. Preparing for elimination of congenital Rubella syndrome (CRS): summary of a workshop on CRS elimination in the United States. Clin Infect Dis. 2000;31(1):85–95.
25. McLean HQ, Fiebelkorn AP, Temte JL, Wallace GS, Centers for Disease Control and Prevention. Prevention of measles, rubella, congenital rubella syndrome, and mumps, 2013: summary recommendations of the Advisory Committee on Immunization Practices (ACIP). MMWR Recomm Rep. 2013;62(RR-04):1–34.
26. Kim DK, Riley LE, Harriman KH, Hunter P, Bridges CB. Advisory Committee on Immunization Practices recommended immunization schedule for adults aged 19 years or older – United States, 2017. Am J Transplant. 2017;17(4):1132–5.
27. Centers for Disease Control and Prevention. Updated recommendations for use of tetanus toxoid, reduced diphtheria toxoid, and acellular pertussis vaccine (Tdap) in pregnant women—Advisory Committee on Immunization Practices (ACIP), 2012. MMWR Morb Mortal Wkly Rep. 2013;62(7):131–5.
28. Kim DK, Riley LE, Harriman KH, Hunter P, Bridges CB. Advisory Committee on Immunization Practices recommended immunization schedule for adults aged 19 years or older – United States, 2017. MMWR Morb Mortal Wkly Rep. 2017;66(5): 136–8.
29. Grohskopf LA, Sokolow LZ, Broder KR, Walter EB, Bresee JS, Fry AM, et al. Prevention and control of seasonal influenza with vaccines: recommendations of the Advisory Committee on Immunization Practices – United States, 2017-18 influenza season. MMWR Recomm Rep. 2017;66(2):1–20.
30. Pavlidis N. Lung cancer during pregnancy: an emerging issue. Lung Cancer. 2008;59(3):279–81.
31. Practice Committee of the American Society for Reproductive Medicine. Electronic address asrm@asrm.org, Practice Committee of the American Society for Reproductive Medicine. Smoking and infertility: a committee opinion. Fertil Steril. 2018;110(4): 611–8.
32. Raymond EG, Cnattingius S, Kiely JL. Effects of maternal age, parity, and smoking on the risk of stillbirth. Br J Obstet Gynaecol. 1994;101(4):301–6.
33. Li CQ, Windsor RA, Perkins L, Goldenberg RL, Lowe JB. The impact on infant birth weight and gestational age of cotinine-validated smoking reduction during pregnancy [see comments]. JAMA. 1993;269(12):1519–24.
34. Committee on Underserved Women, Committee on Obstetric Practice. Committee Opinion No. 721: Smoking cessation during pregnancy. Obstet Gynecol. 2017;130(4):e200–e4.
35. Siu AL, Force USPST. Behavioral and pharmacotherapy interventions for tobacco smoking cessation in adults, including pregnant women: U.S. Preventive Services Task Force Recommendation Statement. Ann Intern Med. 2015;163(8):622–34.
36. Vodopivec-Jamsek V, de Jongh T, Gurol-Urganci I, Atun R, Car J. Mobile phone messaging for preventive health care. Cochrane Database Syst Rev. 2012;12:CD007457.
37. Auer C. Health status of children living in a squatter area of Manila, Philippines, with particular emphasis on intestinal parasitoses. Southeast Asian J Trop Med Public Health. 1990;21(2): 289–300.
38. Coleman T, Chamberlain C, Davey MA, Cooper SE, Leonardi-Bee J. Pharmacological interventions for promoting smoking cessation during pregnancy. Cochrane Database Syst Rev. 2015;(12):CD010078.
39. Coleman T, Cooper S, Thornton JG, Grainge MJ, Watts K, Britton J, et al. A randomized trial of nicotine-replacement therapy patches in pregnancy. N Engl J Med. 2012;366(9):808–18.
40. Thyagarajan V, Robin Clifford C, Wurst KE, Ephross SA, Seeger JD. Bupropion therapy in pregnancy and the occurrence of cardiovascular malformations in infants. Pharmacoepidemiol Drug Saf. 2012;21(11):1240–2.
41. Richardson JL, Stephens S, Yates LM, Diav-Citrin O, Arnon J, Beghin D, et al. Pregnancy outcomes after maternal varenicline use; analysis of surveillance data collected by the European Network of Teratology Information Services. Reprod Toxicol. 2017;67:26–34.
42. Kesmodel U, Wisborg K, Olsen SF, Henriksen TB, Secher NJ. Moderate alcohol intake during pregnancy and the risk of stillbirth and death in the first year of life. Am J Epidemiol. 2002;155(4):305–12.
43. Smith PC, Schmidt SM, Allensworth-Davies D, Saitz R. Primary care validation of a single-question alcohol screening test. J Gen Intern Med. 2009;24(7):783–8.
44. Gunn JK, Rosales CB, Center KE, Nunez A, Gibson SJ, Christ C, et al. Prenatal exposure to cannabis and maternal and child health outcomes: a systematic review and meta-analysis. BMJ Open. 2016;6(4):e009986.
45. Committee on Obstetric Practice. Committee Opinion No. 722: Marijuana use during pregnancy and lactation. Obstet Gynecol. 2017;130(4):e205–e9.
46. Brent RL, Christian MS, Diener RM. Evaluation of the reproductive and developmental risks of caffeine. Birth Defects Res B Dev Reprod Toxicol. 2011;92(2):152–87.
47. American College of Obstetricians & Gynecologists. ACOG Committee Opinion No. 462: Moderate caffeine consumption during pregnancy. Obstet Gynecol. 2010;116(2 Pt 1):467–8.
48. ACOG Practice Bulletin No. 190: Gestational diabetes mellitus. Obstet Gynecol. 2018;131(2):e49–64.
49. ACOG Committee Opinion No. 518: Intimate partner violence. Obstet Gynecol. 2012;119(2 Pt 1):412–7.
50. Carson MP, Pagan ER. Effects of pregnancy on common laboratory tests. In: Powrie RO, Greene MF, Camann W, editors. De Swiet's medical disorders in obstetric practice. 5th ed. Hoboken: Wiley-Blackwell; 2010. p. 661–70.
51. Soma-Pillay P, Nelson-Piercy C, Tolppanen H, Mebazaa A. Physiological changes in pregnancy. Cardiovasc J Afr. 2016;27(2):89–94.
52. Carson MP, Ehrenthal D. Medical issues from preconception through delivery: a roadmap for the internist. Med Clin North Am. 2008;92(5):1193–225, xi.
53. Mehta N, Chen K, Powrie RO. Prescribing for the pregnant patient. Cleve Clin J Med. 2014;81(6):367–72.

54. Ciarkowski SL, Stalburg CM. Medication safety in obstetrics and gynecology. Clin Obstet Gynecol. 2010;53(3):482–99.
55. Bullo M, Tschumi S, Bucher BS, Bianchetti MG, Simonetti GD. Pregnancy outcome following exposure to angiotensin-converting enzyme inhibitors or angiotensin receptor antagonists: a systematic review. Hypertension. 2012;60(2):444–50.
56. Myles N, Newall H, Ward H, Large M. Systematic meta-analysis of individual selective serotonin reuptake inhibitor medications and congenital malformations. Aust N Z J Psychiatry. 2013;47(11):1002–12.
57. Holmes LB, Harvey EA, Coull BA, Huntington KB, Khoshbin S, Hayes AM, et al. The teratogenicity of anticonvulsant drugs. N Engl J Med. 2001;344(15):1132–8.
58. Alexander EK, Pearce EN, Brent GA, Brown RS, Chen H, Dosiou C, et al. 2017 Guidelines of the American Thyroid Association for the diagnosis and management of thyroid disease during pregnancy and the postpartum. Thyroid. 2017;27(3):315–89.
59. Mylonas I. Antibiotic chemotherapy during pregnancy and lactation period: aspects for consideration. Arch Gynecol Obstet. 2011;283(1):7–18.
60. Toppenberg KS, Hill DA, Miller DP. Safety of radiographic imaging during pregnancy. Am Fam Physician. 1999;59(7):1813–8, 20.
61. American College of Obstetrics and Gynecology. Committee Opinion No. 723: Guidelines for diagnostic imaging during pregnancy and lactation. Obstet Gynecol. 2017;130(4):e210–e6.
62. Tremblay E, Therasse E, Thomassin-Naggara I, Trop I. Quality initiatives: guidelines for use of medical imaging during pregnancy and lactation. Radiographics. 2012;32(3):897–911.
63. ACOG Committee on Obstetric Practice. ACOG Committee Opinion. Number 299, September 2004 (replaces No. 158, September 1995). Guidelines for diagnostic imaging during pregnancy. Obstet Gynecol. 2004;104(3):647–51.
64. Brent RL. The effect of embryonic and fetal exposure to x-ray, microwaves, and ultrasound: counseling the pregnant and non-pregnant patient about these risks. Semin Oncol. 1989;16(5): 347–68.
65. Strizek B, Jani JC, Mucyo E, De Keyzer F, Pauwels I, Ziane S, et al. Safety of MR imaging at 1.5 T in fetuses: a retrospective case-control study of birth weights and the effects of acoustic noise. Radiology. 2015;275(2):530–7.
66. De Wilde JP, Rivers AW, Price DL. A review of the current use of magnetic resonance imaging in pregnancy and safety implications for the fetus. Prog Biophys Mol Biol. 2005;87(2–3):335–53.
67. Ray JG, Vermeulen MJ, Bharatha A, Montanera WJ, Park AL. Association between MRI exposure during pregnancy and fetal and childhood outcomes. JAMA. 2016;316(9):952–61.
68. Expert Panel on Magnetic Resonance Safety, Kanal E, Barkovich AJ, Bell C, Borgstede JP, Bradley WG Jr, et al. ACR guidance document on MR safe practices: 2013. J Magn Reson Imaging. 2013;37(3):501–30.
69. Reddy UM, Abuhamad A, Saade GR. Fetal imaging. Semin Perinatol. 2013;37(5):289.
70. Kitzmiller JL, Wallerstein R, Correa A, Kwan S. Preconception care for women with diabetes and prevention of major congenital malformations. Birth Defects Res A Clin Mol Teratol. 2010;88(10):791–803.
71. Murphy HR, Roland JM, Skinner TC, Simmons D, Gurnell E, Morrish NJ, et al. Effectiveness of a regional prepregnancy care program in women with type 1 and type 2 diabetes: benefits beyond glycemic control. Diabetes Care. 2010;33(12):2514–20.
72. Ankumah NA, Cantu J, Jauk V, Biggio J, Hauth J, Andrews W, et al. Risk of adverse pregnancy outcomes in women with mild chronic hypertension before 20 weeks of gestation. Obstet Gynecol. 2014;123(5):966–72.
73. Sibai BM. Chronic hypertension in pregnancy. Obstet Gynecol. 2002;100(2):369–77.
74. LaFranchi SH, Haddow JE, Hollowell JG. Is thyroid inadequacy during gestation a risk factor for adverse pregnancy and developmental outcomes? Thyroid. 2005;15(1):60–71.
75. Leung AS, Millar LK, Koonings PP, Montoro M, Mestman JH. Perinatal outcome in hypothyroid pregnancies. Obstet Gynecol. 1993;81(3):349–53.
76. Ehrenthal D, Jurkovitz C, Hoffman M, Weintraub W. More common than we think: chronic medical risks in a representative obstetric population. JGIM. 2007;22(Supplent 1):53.
77. Correa A, Bardenheier B, Elixhauser A, Geiss LS, Gregg E. Trends in prevalence of diabetes among delivery hospitalizations, United States, 1993-2009. Matern Child Health J. 2015;19(3): 635–42.
78. Bell R, Glinianaia SV, Tennant PW, Bilous RW, Rankin J. Periconception hyperglycaemia and nephropathy are associated with risk of congenital anomaly in women with pre-existing diabetes: a population-based cohort study. Diabetologia. 2012; https://doi.org/10.1007/s00125-012-2455-y.
79. American Diabetes Association. 14. Management of diabetes in pregnancy: standards of medical care in diabetes—2019. Diabetes Care. 2019;42(Suppl 1):S165–S72.
80. ACOG Practice Bulletin No. 190 Summary: Gestational diabetes mellitus. Obstet Gynecol. 2018;131(2):406–8.
81. American Diabetes Association. 13. Management of diabetes in pregnancy: standards of medical care in diabetes–2018. Diabetes Care. 2018;41(Suppl 1):S137–S43.
82. Metzger BE, Lowe LP, Dyer AR, Trimble ER, Chaovarindr U, Coustan DR, et al. Hyperglycemia and adverse pregnancy outcomes. N Engl J Med. 2008;358(19):1991–2002.
83. de Veciana M, Major CA, Morgan MA, Asrat T, Toohey JS, Lien JM, et al. Postprandial versus preprandial blood glucose monitoring in women with gestational diabetes mellitus requiring insulin therapy. N Engl J Med. 1995;333(19):1237–41.
84. Rowan JA, Hague WM, Gao W, Battin MR, Moore MP. Metformin versus insulin for the treatment of gestational diabetes. N Engl J Med. 2008;358(19):2003–15.
85. Vanky E, Zahlsen K, Spigset O, Carlsen SM. Placental passage of metformin in women with polycystic ovary syndrome. Fertil Steril. 2005;83(5):1575–8.
86. Spaulonci CP, Bernardes LS, Trindade TC, Zugaib M, Francisco RP. Randomized trial of metformin vs insulin in the management of gestational diabetes. Am J Obstet Gynecol. 2013;209(1):34. e1–7.
87. Balsells M, Garcia-Patterson A, Sola I, Roque M, Gich I, Corcoy R. Glibenclamide, metformin, and insulin for the treatment of gestational diabetes: a systematic review and meta-analysis. BMJ. 2015;350:h102.
88. ACOG Committee Opinion No. 743: Low-dose aspirin use during pregnancy. Obstet Gynecol. 2018;132(1):e44–52.
89. Klein BE, Moss SE, Klein R. Effect of pregnancy on progression of diabetic retinopathy. Diabetes Care. 1990;13(1):34–40.
90. WHO. WHO recommendations for prevention and treatment of pre-eclampsia and eclampsia. WHO guidelines approved by the Guidelines Review Committee. Geneva: WHO; 2011.
91. American College of Obstetricians and Gynecologists, Task Force on Hypertension in Pregnancy. Hypertension in pregnancy. Report of the American College of Obstetricians and Gynecologists' Task Force on Hypertension in Pregnancy. Obstet Gynecol. 2013;122(5):1122–31.
92. Ros HS, Cnattingius S, Lipworth L. Comparison of risk factors for preeclampsia and gestational hypertension in a population-based cohort study. Am J Epidemiol. 1998;147(11):1062–70.
93. Bartsch E, Medcalf KE, Park AL, Ray JG, High Risk of Pre-eclampsia Identification Group. Clinical risk factors for pre-eclampsia determined in early pregnancy: systematic review and meta-analysis of large cohort studies. BMJ. 2016;353:i1753.

94. Reubinoff BE, Schenker JG. HELLP syndrome – a syndrome of hemolysis, elevated liver enzymes and low platelet count – complicating preeclampsia-eclampsia. Int J Gynaecol Obstet. 1991;36(2):95–102.
95. Sibai BM. The HELLP syndrome (hemolysis, elevated liver enzymes, and low platelets): much ado about nothing? Am J Obstet Gynecol. 1990;162(2):311–6.
96. Duckitt K, Harrington D. Risk factors for pre-eclampsia at antenatal booking: systematic review of controlled studies. BMJ. 2005;330(7491):565.
97. Grindheim G, Estensen ME, Langesaeter E, Rosseland LA, Toska K. Changes in blood pressure during healthy pregnancy: a longitudinal cohort study. J Hypertens. 2012;30(2):342–50.
98. Ochsenbein-Kolble N, Roos M, Gasser T, Huch R, Huch A, Zimmermann R. Cross sectional study of automated blood pressure measurements throughout pregnancy. BJOG. 2004;111(4):319–25.
99. ACOG Practice Bulletin No. 202: Gestational hypertension and preeclampsia. Obstet Gynecol. 2019;133(1):e1–e25.
100. American College of Obstetricians & Gynecologists. ACOG Practice Bulletin No. 125: Chronic hypertension in pregnancy. Obstet Gynecol. 2012;119(2 Pt 1):396–407.
101. Yancey LM, Withers E, Bakes K, Abbott J. Postpartum preeclampsia: emergency department presentation and management. J Emerg Med. 2011;40(4):380–4.
102. Matthys LA, Coppage KH, Lambers DS, Barton JR, Sibai BM. Delayed postpartum preeclampsia: an experience of 151 cases. Am J Obstet Gynecol. 2004;190(5):1464–6.
103. Whelton PK, Carey RM, Aronow WS, Casey DE Jr, Collins KJ, Dennison Himmelfarb C, et al. 2017 ACC/AHA/AAPA/ABC/ACPM/AGS/APhA/ASH/ASPC/NMA/PCNA guideline for the prevention, detection, evaluation, and management of high blood pressure in adults: a report of the American College of Cardiology/American Heart Association Task Force on Clinical Practice Guidelines. Hypertension. 2018;71(6):e13–e115.
104. Magee LA, von Dadelszen P, Rey E, Ross S, Asztalos E, Murphy KE, et al. Less-tight versus tight control of hypertension in pregnancy. N Engl J Med. 2015;372(5):407–17.
105. Barton JR, O'Brien JM, Bergauer NK, Jacques DL, Sibai BM. Mild gestational hypertension remote from term: progression and outcome. Am J Obstet Gynecol. 2001;184(5):979–83.
106. Magee LA, von Dadelszen P, Singer J, Lee T, Rey E, Ross S, et al. The CHIPS randomized controlled trial (control of hypertension in pregnancy study): is severe hypertension just an elevated blood pressure? Hypertension. 2016;68(5):1153–9.
107. Abalos E, Duley L, Steyn DW. Antihypertensive drug therapy for mild to moderate hypertension during pregnancy. Cochrane Database Syst Rev. 2014;(2):CD002252.
108. Smith P, Anthony J, Johanson R. Nifedipine in pregnancy. BJOG. 2000;107(3):299–307.
109. Cockburn J, Moar VA, Ounsted M, Redman CW. Final report of study on hypertension during pregnancy: the effects of specific treatment on the growth and development of the children. Lancet. 1982;1(8273):647–9.
110. Cooper WO, Hernandez-Diaz S, Arbogast PG, Dudley JA, Dyer S, Gideon PS, et al. Major congenital malformations after first-trimester exposure to ACE inhibitors. N Engl J Med. 2006;354(23):2443–51.
111. Shotan A, Widerhorn J, Hurst A, Elkayam U. Risks of angiotensin-converting enzyme inhibition during pregnancy: experimental and clinical evidence, potential mechanisms, and recommendations for use. Am J Med. 1994;96(5):451–6.
112. Hunseler C, Paneitz A, Friedrich D, Lindner U, Oberthuer A, Korber F, et al. Angiotensin II receptor blocker induced fetopathy: 7 cases. Klin Padiatr. 2011;223(1):10–4.
113. Xie RH, Guo Y, Krewski D, Mattison D, Walker MC, Nerenberg K, et al. Association between labetalol use for hypertension in pregnancy and adverse infant outcomes. Eur J Obstet Gynecol Reprod Biol. 2014;175:124–8.
114. Vanderpump MP. The epidemiology of thyroid disease. Br Med Bull. 2011;99:39–51.
115. Haddow JE, Palomaki GE, Allan WC, Williams JR, Knight GJ, Gagnon J, et al. Maternal thyroid deficiency during pregnancy and subsequent neuropsychological development of the child. N Engl J Med. 1999;341(8):549–55.
116. Allan WC, Haddow JE, Palomaki GE, Williams JR, Mitchell ML, Hermos RJ, et al. Maternal thyroid deficiency and pregnancy complications: implications for population screening. J Med Screen. 2000;7(3):127–30.
117. Maraka S, Ospina NM, O'Keeffe DT, Espinosa De Ycaza AE, Gionfriddo MR, Erwin PJ, et al. Subclinical hypothyroidism in pregnancy: a systematic review and meta-analysis. Thyroid. 2016;26(4):580–90.
118. Willoughby KA, McAndrews MP, Rovet JF. Effects of maternal hypothyroidism on offspring hippocampus and memory. Thyroid. 2014;24(3):576–84.
119. American College of Obstetricians and Gynecologists. Practice Bulletin No. 148: Thyroid disease in pregnancy. Obstet Gynecol. 2015;125(4):996–1005.
120. Lazarus JH, Bestwick JP, Channon S, Paradice R, Maina A, Rees R, et al. Antenatal thyroid screening and childhood cognitive function. N Engl J Med. 2012;366(6):493–501.
121. Kahric-Janicic N, Soldin SJ, Soldin OP, West T, Gu J, Jonklaas J. Tandem mass spectrometry improves the accuracy of free thyroxine measurements during pregnancy. Thyroid. 2007;17(4):303–11.
122. De Groot L, Abalovich M, Alexander EK, Amino N, Barbour L, Cobin RH, et al. Management of thyroid dysfunction during pregnancy and postpartum: an Endocrine Society clinical practice guideline. J Clin Endocrinol Metab. 2012;97(8):2543–65.
123. Cooper DS, Laurberg P. Hyperthyroidism in pregnancy. Lancet Diabetes Endocrinol. 2013;1(3):238–49.
124. Glinoer D, de Nayer P, Bourdoux P, Lemone M, Robyn C, van Steirteghem A, et al. Regulation of maternal thyroid during pregnancy. J Clin Endocrinol Metab. 1990;71(2):276–87.
125. Soldin OP, Soldin D, Sastoque M. Gestation-specific thyroxine and thyroid stimulating hormone levels in the United States and worldwide. Ther Drug Monit. 2007;29(5):553–9.
126. Peleg D, Cada S, Peleg A, Ben-Ami M. The relationship between maternal serum thyroid-stimulating immunoglobulin and fetal and neonatal thyrotoxicosis. Obstet Gynecol. 2002;99(6):1040–3.
127. Kwon HL, Belanger K, Bracken MB. Asthma prevalence among pregnant and childbearing-aged women in the United States: estimates from national health surveys. Ann Epidemiol. 2003;13(5):317–24.
128. Dombrowski MP, Schatz M. Asthma in pregnancy. Clin Obstet Gynecol. 2010;53(2):301–10.
129. National Heart Lung Blood Institute National Asthma Education Prevention Program Asthma Pregnancy Working Group. NAEPP expert panel report. Managing asthma during pregnancy: recommendations for pharmacologic treatment-2004 update. J Allergy Clin Immunol. 2005;115(1):34–46.
130. Schatz M, Harden K, Forsythe A, Chilingar L, Hoffman C, Sperling W, et al. The course of asthma during pregnancy, post partum, and with successive pregnancies: a prospective analysis. J Allergy Clin Immunol. 1988;81(3):509–17.
131. Gluck JC, Gluck PA. The effect of pregnancy on the course of asthma. Immunol Allergy Clin N Am. 2006;26(1):63–80.
132. Grindheim G, Toska K, Estensen ME, Rosseland LA. Changes in pulmonary function during pregnancy: a longitudinal cohort study. BJOG. 2012;119(1):94–101.

133. Gani F, Braida A, Lombardi C, Del Giudice A, Senna GE, Passalacqua G. Rhinitis in pregnancy. Eur Ann Allergy Clin Immunol. 2003;35(8):306–13.
134. McCarter T. Asthma-The National Surveillance Data and the National Asthma Education and Prevention Program's expert panel report 3. Am Health Drug Benefits. 2008;1(2):35–50.
135. Schatz M, Zeiger RS, Hoffman CP. Intrauterine growth is related to gestational pulmonary function in pregnant asthmatic women. Kaiser-Permanente Asthma and Pregnancy Study Group. Chest. 1990;98(2):389–92.
136. Martinez FD, Wright AL, Taussig LM, Holberg CJ, Halonen M, Morgan WJ. Asthma and wheezing in the first six years of life. The Group Health Medical Associates. N Engl J Med. 1995;332(3):133–8.
137. Yawn B, Knudtson M. Treating asthma and comorbid allergic rhinitis in pregnancy. J Am Board Fam Med. 2007;20(3): 289–98.
138. Cossette B, Beauchesne MF, Forget A, Lemiere C, Larivee P, Rey E, et al. Relative perinatal safety of salmeterol vs formoterol and fluticasone vs budesonide use during pregnancy. Ann Allergy Asthma Immunol. 2014;112(5):459–64.
139. Schatz M, Dombrowski MP, Wise R, Momirova V, Landon M, Mabie W, et al. The relationship of asthma medication use to perinatal outcomes. J Allergy Clin Immunol. 2004;113(6):1040–5.
140. Bracken MB, Triche EW, Belanger K, Saftlas A, Beckett WS, Leaderer BP. Asthma symptoms, severity, and drug therapy: a prospective study of effects on 2205 pregnancies. Obstet Gynecol. 2003;102(4):739–52.
141. Schatz M. The efficacy and safety of asthma medications during pregnancy. Semin Perinatol. 2001;25(3):145–52.
142. Murphy VE, Gibson P, Talbot PI, Clifton VL. Severe asthma exacerbations during pregnancy. Obstet Gynecol. 2005;106(5 Pt 1):1046–54.
143. Schatz M, Dombrowski MP, Wise R, Thom EA, Landon M, Mabie W, et al. Asthma morbidity during pregnancy can be predicted by severity classification. J Allergy Clin Immunol. 2003;112(2):283–8.
144. Beckman MG, Hooper WC, Critchley SE, Ortel TL. Venous thromboembolism: a public health concern. Am J Prev Med. 2010;38(4 Suppl):S495–501.
145. Blondon M, Casini A, Hoppe KK, Boehlen F, Righini M, Smith NL. Risks of venous thromboembolism after cesarean sections: a meta-analysis. Chest. 2016;150(3):572–96.
146. Heit JA, Kobbervig CE, James AH, Petterson TM, Bailey KR, Melton LJ 3rd. Trends in the incidence of venous thromboembolism during pregnancy or postpartum: a 30-year population-based study. Ann Intern Med. 2005;143(10):697–706.
147. Abdul Sultan A, Tata LJ, Grainge MJ, West J. The incidence of first venous thromboembolism in and around pregnancy using linked primary and secondary care data: a population based cohort study from England and comparative meta-analysis. PLoS One. 2013;8(7):e70310.
148. James A, Committee on Practice Bulletins-Obstetrics. Practice Bulletin No. 123: Thromboembolism in pregnancy. Obstet Gynecol. 2011;118(3):718–29.
149. Simpson EL, Lawrenson RA, Nightingale AL, Farmer RD. Venous thromboembolism in pregnancy and the puerperium: incidence and additional risk factors from a London perinatal database. BJOG. 2001;108(1):56–60.
150. Creanga AA, Syverson C, Seed K, Callaghan WM. Pregnancy-related mortality in the United States, 2011-2013. Obstet Gynecol. 2017;130(2):366–73.
151. Oruc S, Saruc M, Koyuncu FM, Ozdemir E. Changes in the plasma activities of protein C and protein S during pregnancy. Aust N Z J Obstet Gynaecol. 2000;40(4):448–50.
152. American College of Obstetricians. ACOG Practice Bulletin No. 138: Inherited thrombophilias in pregnancy. Obstet Gynecol. 2013;122(3):706–17.
153. Clark P, Walker ID, Govan L, Wu O, Greer IA. The GOAL study: a prospective examination of the impact of factor V Leiden and ABO(H) blood groups on haemorrhagic and thrombotic pregnancy outcomes. Br J Haematol. 2008;140(2):236–40.
154. Carson MP, Powrie RO, Rosene-Montella K. The effect of obesity and position on heart rate in pregnancy. J Matern Fetal Neonatal Med. 2002;11(1):40–5.
155. Leung AN, Bull TM, Jaeschke R, Lockwood CJ, Boiselle PM, Hurwitz LM, et al. An official American Thoracic Society/Society of Thoracic Radiology clinical practice guideline: evaluation of suspected pulmonary embolism in pregnancy. Am J Respir Crit Care Med. 2011;184(10):1200–8.
156. Kearon C, Julian JA, Newman TE, Ginsberg JS. Noninvasive diagnosis of deep venous thrombosis. McMaster Diagnostic Imaging Practice Guidelines Initiative. Ann Intern Med. 1998;128(8):663–77.
157. Robertson L, Jones LE. Fixed dose subcutaneous low molecular weight heparins versus adjusted dose unfractionated heparin for the initial treatment of venous thromboembolism. Cochrane Database Syst Rev. 2017;2:CD001100.
158. Leonhardt G, Gaul C, Nietsch HH, Buerke M, Schleussner E. Thrombolytic therapy in pregnancy. J Thromb Thrombolysis. 2006;21(3):271–6.
159. Bates SM, Greer IA, Middeldorp S, Veenstra DL, Prabulos AM, Vandvik PO. VTE, thrombophilia, antithrombotic therapy, and pregnancy: Antithrombotic Therapy and Prevention of Thrombosis, 9th ed: American College of Chest Physicians Evidence-Based Clinical Practice Guidelines. Chest. 2012;141(2 Suppl):e691S–736S.
160. Pabinger I, Grafenhofer H, Kaider A, Kyrle PA, Quehenberger P, Mannhalter C, et al. Risk of pregnancy-associated recurrent venous thromboembolism in women with a history of venous thrombosis. J Thromb Haemost. 2005;3(5):949–54.
161. Bain E, Wilson A, Tooher R, Gates S, Davis LJ, Middleton P. Prophylaxis for venous thromboembolic disease in pregnancy and the early postnatal period. Cochrane Database Syst Rev. 2014;(2):CD001689.
162. American College of Obstetricians and Gynecologists Women's Health Care Physicians. ACOG Practice Bulletin No. 138: Inherited thrombophilias in pregnancy. Obstet Gynecol. 2013;122(3):706–17.
163. Horlocker TT, Wedel DJ, Rowlingson JC, Enneking FK, Kopp SL, Benzon HT, et al. Regional anesthesia in the patient receiving antithrombotic or thrombolytic therapy: American Society of Regional Anesthesia and Pain Medicine Evidence-Based Guidelines (Third Edition). Reg Anesth Pain Med. 2010;35(1):64–101.
164. Leffert L, Butwick A, Carvalho B, Arendt K, Bates SM, Friedman A, et al. The Society for Obstetric Anesthesia and Perinatology consensus statement on the anesthetic management of pregnant and postpartum women receiving thromboprophylaxis or higher dose anticoagulants. Anesth Analg. 2018;126(3):928–44.
165. Bennett HA, Einarson A, Taddio A, Koren G, Einarson TR. Prevalence of depression during pregnancy: systematic review. Obstet Gynecol. 2004;103(4):698–709.
166. Dietz PM, Williams SB, Callaghan WM, Bachman DJ, Whitlock EP, Hornbrook MC. Clinically identified maternal depression before, during, and after pregnancies ending in live births. Am J Psychiatry. 2007;164(10):1515–20.
167. Force USPST, Curry SJ, Krist AH, Owens DK, Barry MJ, Caughey AB, et al. Interventions to prevent perinatal depression: US Preventive Services Task Force Recommendation Statement. JAMA. 2019;321(6):580–7.

168. ACOG Committee Opinion No. 757 Summary: Screening for perinatal depression. Obstet Gynecol. 2018;132(5):1314–6.
169. Ko JY, Farr SL, Dietz PM, Robbins CL. Depression and treatment among U.S. pregnant and nonpregnant women of reproductive age, 2005–2009. J Womens Health (Larchmt). 2012;21(8):830–6.
170. Cohen LS, Altshuler LL, Harlow BL, Nonacs R, Newport DJ, Viguera AC, et al. Relapse of major depression during pregnancy in women who maintain or discontinue antidepressant treatment. JAMA. 2006;295(5):499–507.
171. Gaillard A, Le Strat Y, Mandelbrot L, Keita H, Dubertret C. Predictors of postpartum depression: prospective study of 264 women followed during pregnancy and postpartum. Psychiatry Res. 2014;215(2):341–6.
172. Accortt EE, Cheadle AC, Schetter CD. Prenatal depression and adverse birth outcomes: an updated systematic review. Matern Child Health J. 2015;19(6):1306–37.
173. Grote NK, Bridge JA, Gavin AR, Melville JL, Iyengar S, Katon WJ. A meta-analysis of depression during pregnancy and the risk of preterm birth, low birth weight, and intrauterine growth restriction. Arch Gen Psychiatry. 2010;67(10):1012–24.
174. Deave T, Heron J, Evans J, Emond A. The impact of maternal depression in pregnancy on early child development. BJOG. 2008;115(8):1043–51.
175. Robinson M, Mattes E, Oddy WH, Pennell CE, van Eekelen A, McLean NJ, et al. Prenatal stress and risk of behavioral morbidity from age 2 to 14 years: the influence of the number, type, and timing of stressful life events. Dev Psychopathol. 2011;23(2):507–20.
176. Hay DF, Pawlby S, Waters CS, Sharp D. Antepartum and postpartum exposure to maternal depression: different effects on different adolescent outcomes. J Child Psychol Psychiatry. 2008;49(10):1079–88.
177. Lebel C, Walton M, Letourneau N, Giesbrecht GF, Kaplan BJ, Dewey D. Prepartum and postpartum maternal depressive symptoms are related to children's brain structure in preschool. Biol Psychiatry. 2016;80(11):859–68.
178. Burns A, O'Mahen H, Baxter H, Bennert K, Wiles N, Ramchandani P, et al. A pilot randomised controlled trial of cognitive behavioural therapy for antenatal depression. BMC Psychiatry. 2013;13:33.
179. McGregor M, Coghlan M, Dennis CL. The effect of physician-based cognitive behavioural therapy among pregnant women with depressive symptomatology: a pilot quasi-experimental trial. Early Interv Psychiatry. 2014;8(4):348–57.
180. Yonkers KA, Wisner KL, Stewart DE, Oberlander TF, Dell DL, Stotland N, et al. The management of depression during pregnancy: a report from the American Psychiatric Association and the American College of Obstetricians and Gynecologists. Obstet Gynecol. 2009;114(3):703–13.
181. Chun-Fai-Chan B, Koren G, Fayez I, Kalra S, Voyer-Lavigne S, Boshier A, et al. Pregnancy outcome of women exposed to bupropion during pregnancy: a prospective comparative study. Am J Obstet Gynecol. 2005;192(3):932–6.
182. Alwan S, Reefhuis J, Botto LD, Rasmussen SA, Correa A, Friedman JM, et al. Maternal use of bupropion and risk for congenital heart defects. Am J Obstet Gynecol. 2010;203(1):52.e1–6.
183. Louik C, Kerr S, Mitchell AA. First-trimester exposure to bupropion and risk of cardiac malformations. Pharmacoepidemiol Drug Saf. 2014;23(10):1066–75.
184. Berard A, Iessa N, Chaabane S, Muanda FT, Boukhris T, Zhao JP. The risk of major cardiac malformations associated with paroxetine use during the first trimester of pregnancy: a systematic review and meta-analysis. Br J Clin Pharmacol. 2016;81(4):589–604.
185. Moses-Kolko EL, Bogen D, Perel J, Bregar A, Uhl K, Levin B, et al. Neonatal signs after late in utero exposure to serotonin reuptake inhibitors: literature review and implications for clinical applications. JAMA. 2005;293(19):2372–83.
186. Warburton W, Hertzman C, Oberlander TF. A register study of the impact of stopping third trimester selective serotonin reuptake inhibitor exposure on neonatal health. Acta Psychiatr Scand. 2010;121(6):471–9.
187. Grzeskowiak LE, McBain R, Dekker GA, Clifton VL. Antidepressant use in late gestation and risk of postpartum haemorrhage: a retrospective cohort study. BJOG. 2016;123(12):1929–36.
188. Lindqvist PG, Nasiell J, Gustafsson LL, Nordstrom L. Selective serotonin reuptake inhibitor use during pregnancy increases the risk of postpartum hemorrhage and anemia: a hospital-based cohort study. J Thromb Haemost. 2014;12(12):1986–92.
189. Palmsten K, Hernandez-Diaz S, Huybrechts KF, Williams PL, Michels KB, Achtyes ED, et al. Use of antidepressants near delivery and risk of postpartum hemorrhage: cohort study of low income women in the United States. BMJ. 2013;347:f4877.
190. Clements CC, Castro VM, Blumenthal SR, Rosenfield HR, Murphy SN, Fava M, et al. Prenatal antidepressant exposure is associated with risk for attention-deficit hyperactivity disorder but not autism spectrum disorder in a large health system. Mol Psychiatry. 2015;20(6):727–34.
191. Mezzacappa A, Lasica PA, Gianfagna F, Cazas O, Hardy P, Falissard B, et al. Risk for autism spectrum disorders according to period of prenatal antidepressant exposure: a systematic review and meta-analysis. JAMA Pediatr. 2017;171(6):555–63.
192. Rai D, Lee BK, Dalman C, Golding J, Lewis G, Magnusson C. Parental depression, maternal antidepressant use during pregnancy, and risk of autism spectrum disorders: population based case-control study. BMJ. 2013;346:f2059.
193. Castro VM, Kong SW, Clements CC, Brady R, Kaimal AJ, Doyle AE, et al. Absence of evidence for increase in risk for autism or attention-deficit hyperactivity disorder following antidepressant exposure during pregnancy: a replication study. Transl Psychiatry. 2016;6:e708.
194. Huybrechts KF, Palmsten K, Avorn J, Cohen LS, Holmes LB, Franklin JM, et al. Antidepressant use in pregnancy and the risk of cardiac defects. N Engl J Med. 2014;370(25):2397–407.
195. Hanley GE, Smolina K, Mintzes B, Oberlander TF, Morgan SG. Postpartum hemorrhage and use of serotonin reuptake inhibitor antidepressants in pregnancy. Obstet Gynecol. 2016;127(3):553–61.
196. Grigoriadis S, VonderPorten EH, Mamisashvili L, Eady A, Tomlinson G, Dennis CL, et al. The effect of prenatal antidepressant exposure on neonatal adaptation: a systematic review and meta-analysis. J Clin Psychiatry. 2013;74(4):e309–20.
197. Newport DJ, Hostetter AL, Juul SH, Porterfield SM, Knight BT, Stowe ZN. Prenatal psychostimulant and antidepressant exposure and risk of hypertensive disorders of pregnancy. J Clin Psychiatry. 2016;77(11):1538–45.
198. Palmsten K, Huybrechts KF, Michels KB, Williams PL, Mogun H, Setoguchi S, et al. Antidepressant use and risk for preeclampsia. Epidemiology. 2013;24(5):682–91.
199. Gentile S. Tricyclic antidepressants in pregnancy and puerperium. Expert Opin Drug Saf. 2014;13(2):207–25.
200. Palmsten K, Setoguchi S, Margulis AV, Patrick AR, Hernandez-Diaz S. Elevated risk of preeclampsia in pregnant women with depression: depression or antidepressants? Am J Epidemiol. 2012;175(10):988–97.
201. TOXNET Toxicology Data Network; 2019. Available from: https://toxnet.nlm.nih.gov/.
202. Section on Breastfeeding. Breastfeeding and the use of human milk. Pediatrics. 2012;129(3):e827–41.
203. Cunningham FG, Leveno K, Bloom S, Hauth J, Rouse D, Spong C, editors Chapter 30: The puerperium. In: Williams obstetrics.

23rd ed. New York: McGraw-Hill Professional Publishing; 2010. p. 646–60.

204. Victora CG, Bahl R, Barros AJ, Franca GV, Horton S, Krasevec J, et al. Breastfeeding in the 21st century: epidemiology, mechanisms, and lifelong effect. Lancet. 2016;387(10017):475–90.
205. Koletzko S, Sherman P, Corey M, Griffiths A, Smith C. Role of infant feeding practices in development of Crohn's disease in childhood. BMJ. 1989;298(6688):1617–8.
206. Thompson JMD, Tanabe K, Moon RY, Mitchell EA, McGarvey C, Tappin D, et al. Duration of breastfeeding and risk of SIDS: an individual participant data meta-analysis. Pediatrics. 2017;140(5):e20171324.
207. Yang YW, Tsai CL, Lu CY. Exclusive breastfeeding and incident atopic dermatitis in childhood: a systematic review and meta-analysis of prospective cohort studies. Br J Dermatol. 2009;161(2):373–83.
208. Newton E. Chapter 23: Lactation and breastfeeding. In: Gabbe S, Niebyl J, Simpson J, Landon M, Galan H, Jauniaux E, et al., editors. Obstetrics: normal and problem pregnancies. 6th ed. Philadelphia: Elsevier/Saunders; 2012.
209. National Library of Medicine. Drugs and lactation database (LactMed) [Internet]. Bethesda, MD, 2006. Available from: https://www.ncbi.nlm.nih.gov/books/NBK501922/.
210. Briggs GG, Freeman RK, Yaffe SJ. Drugs in pregnancy and lactation. 11th ed. Philadelphia: Wolters Kluwer; 2017.
211. Committee on Practice Bulletins-Obstetrics. Practice Bulletin No. 177: Obstetric analgesia and anesthesia. Obstet Gynecol. 2017;129(4):e73–89.
212. U.S. Food and Drug Administration. FDA Drug Safety Communication: FDA restricts use of prescription codeine pain and cough medicines and tramadol pain medicines in children; recommends against use in breastfeeding women; 2017. Available from: https://www.fda.gov/drugs/drug-safety-and-availability/fda-drug-safety-communication-fda-restricts-use-prescription-codeine-pain-and-cough-medicines-and.
213. Thyagarajan B, Deshpande SS. Cotrimoxazole and neonatal kernicterus: a review. Drug Chem Toxicol. 2014;37(2):121–9.
214. Feig DS, Briggs GG, Kraemer JM, Ambrose PJ, Moskovitz DN, Nageotte M, et al. Transfer of glyburide and glipizide into breast milk. Diabetes Care. 2005;28(8):1851–5.
215. Briggs GG, Ambrose PJ, Nageotte MP, Padilla G, Wan S. Excretion of metformin into breast milk and the effect on nursing infants. Obstet Gynecol. 2005;105(6):1437–41.
216. ACOG Committee on Practice Bulletins-Obstetrics. ACOG Practice Bulletin: Clinical management guidelines for obstetrician-gynecologists number 92, April 2008 (replaces practice bulletin number 87, November 2007). Use of psychiatric medications during pregnancy and lactation. Obstet Gynecol. 2008;111(4):1001–20.
217. Katz V. Chapter 22: Postpartum care. In: Gabbe S, Niebyl J, Simpson J, Landon M, Galan H, Jauniaux E, et al., editors. Obstetrics: normal and problem pregnancies. 6th ed. Philadelphia: Elsevier/Saunders; 2012.
218. Galambosi PJ, Gissler M, Kaaja RJ, Ulander VM. Incidence and risk factors of venous thromboembolism during postpartum period: a population-based cohort-study. Acta Obstet Gynecol Scand. 2017;96(7):852–61.
219. Anger JT, Saigal CS, Litwin MS, Urologic Diseases of America Project. The prevalence of urinary incontinence among community dwelling adult women: results from the National Health and Nutrition Examination Survey. J Urol. 2006;175(2):601–4.
220. Carson MP, Frank MI, Keely E. Original research: postpartum testing rates among women with a history of gestational diabetes—systematic review. Prim Care Diabetes. 2013;7(3):177–86.
221. Carson MP, Morgan B, Gussman D, Brown M, Rothenberg K, Wisner TA. SUGAR: spotting undiagnosed glucose abnormal results—a new protocol to increase postpartum testing among women with gestational diabetes mellitus. Am J Perinatol. 2015;32(3):299–306.
222. Stuebe AM, Rich-Edwards JW, Willett WC, Manson JE, Michels KB. Duration of lactation and incidence of type 2 diabetes. JAMA. 2005;294(20):2601–10.
223. American Diabetes Association. 2. Classification and diagnosis of diabetes: standards of medical care in diabetes—2018. Diabetes Care. 2018;41(Supplement 1):S13–27.
224. Aroda VR, Christophi CA, Edelstein SL, Zhang P, Herman WH, Barrett-Connor E, et al. The effect of lifestyle intervention and metformin on preventing or delaying diabetes among women with and without gestational diabetes: the diabetes prevention program outcomes study 10-year follow-up. J Clin Endocrinol Metab. 2015;100(4):1646–53.
225. Task Force on Hypertension in Pregnancy. Hypertension in pregnancy. Obstet Gynecol. 2013;122(5):1122–31.
226. Ahmed R, Dunford J, Mehran R, Robson S, Kunadian V. Pre-eclampsia and future cardiovascular risk among women: a review. J Am Coll Cardiol. 2014;63(18):1815–22.
227. Mosca L, Benjamin EJ, Berra K, Bezanson JL, Dolor RJ, Lloyd-Jones DM, et al. Effectiveness-based guidelines for the prevention of cardiovascular disease in women—2011 update: a guideline from the American heart association. Circulation. 2011;123(11):1243–62.
228. Ray JG, Vermeulen MJ, Schull MJ, Redelmeier DA. Cardiovascular health after maternal placental syndromes (CHAMPS): population-based retrospective cohort study. Lancet. 2005;366(9499):1797–803.
229. Feig DS, Shah BR, Lipscombe LL, Wu CF, Ray JG, Lowe J, et al. Preeclampsia as a risk factor for diabetes: a population-based cohort study. PLoS Med. 2013;10(4):e1001425.
230. Levine RJ, Vatten LJ, Horowitz GL, Qian C, Romundstad PR, Yu KF, et al. Pre-eclampsia, soluble fms-like tyrosine kinase 1, and the risk of reduced thyroid function: nested case-control and population based study. BMJ. 2009;339:b4336.
231. Wang IK, Muo CH, Chang YC, Liang CC, Chang CT, Lin SY, et al. Association between hypertensive disorders during pregnancy and end-stage renal disease: a population-based study. CMAJ. 2013;185(3):207–13.
232. Nicholson WK, Robinson KA, Smallridge RC, Ladenson PW, Powe NR. Prevalence of postpartum thyroid dysfunction: a quantitative review. Thyroid. 2006;16(6):573–82.
233. Stagnaro-Green A. Recognizing, understanding, and treating postpartum thyroiditis. Endocrinol Metab Clin N Am. 2000;29(2):417–30, ix.
234. VanderKruik R, Barreix M, Chou D, Allen T, Say L, Cohen LS, et al. The global prevalence of postpartum psychosis: a systematic review. BMC Psychiatry. 2017;17(1):272.
235. Sit D, Rothschild AJ, Wisner KL. A review of postpartum psychosis. J Women's Health (Larchmt). 2006;15(4):352–68.
236. Cassina M, Dona M, Di Gianantonio E, Litta P, Clementi M. First-trimester exposure to metformin and risk of birth defects: a systematic review and meta-analysis. Hum Reprod Update. 2014;20(5):656–69.
237. Chan WS, Anand S, Ginsberg JS. Anticoagulation of pregnant women with mechanical heart valves: a systematic review of the literature. Arch Intern Med. 2000;160(2):191–6.
238. Liu TH, Yan SS, Lee YN. Meigs' syndrome: a case report. Zhonghua Yi Xue Za Zhi (Taipei). 1989;44(5):322–4.

Index

S. A. Tilstra et al. (eds.), *Sex- and Gender-Based Women's Health*, https://doi.org/10.1007/978-3-030-50695-7

H

L

T